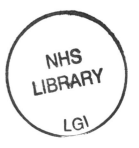

Clinical Pharmacy
and Therapeutics

Commissioning Editor: Ellen Green/Pauline Graham
Development Editor: Janice Urquhart
Project Manager: Elouise Ball
Design Direction: Erik Bigland
Illustration Manager: Merlyn Harvey
Illustrator: David Graham

Clinical Pharmacy and Therapeutics

EDITED BY

Roger Walker BPharm PhD FRPharmS FFPH

Professor of Pharmacy Practice,
Welsh School of Pharmacy, Cardiff University;
Consultant in Pharmaceutical Public Health, National Public Health Service for Wales, Wales, UK

Cate Whittlesea BSc MSc PhD MRPharmS

Senior Lecturer, Pharmacy Practice Department, Pharmacy School of Biomedical and Health Sciences,
King's College London, London, UK

FOURTH EDITION

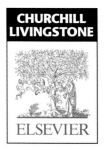

EDINBURGH LONDON NEW YORK OXFORD PHILADELPHIA ST LOUIS SYDNEY TORONTO 2007

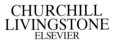

CHURCHILL
LIVINGSTONE
ELSEVIER

An imprint of Elsevier Limited

© Longman Group 1994
© Harcourt Brace and Company Limited 1999
© Harcourt Publishers Limited 2000
© 2003, Elsevier Limited. All rights reserved
© 2007, Elsevier Limited. All rights reserved

First edition 1994
Second edition 1999
Third edition 2003
Fourth edition 2007

ISBN-13: 9780443102851

International Edition ISBN-13: 9780443102868

British Library Cataloguing in Publication Data
A catalogue record for this book is available from the British Library

Library of Congress Cataloging in Publication Data
A catalog record for this book is available from the Library of Congress

Note
Knowledge and best practice in this field are constantly changing. As new
research and experience broaden our knowledge, changes in practice,
treatment and drug therapy may become necessary or appropriate. Readers
are advised to check the most current information provided (i) on procedures
featured or (ii) by the manufacturer of each product to be administered,
to verify the recommended dose or formula, the method and duration
of administration, and contraindications. It is the responsibility of the
practitioner, relying on their own experience and knowledge of the patient,
to make diagnoses, to determine dosages and the best treatment for each
individual patient, and to take all appropriate safety precautions. To the
fullest extent of the law, neither the Publisher nor the Editors assume any
liability for any injury and/or damage to persons or property arising out or
related to any use of the material contained in this book.

The Publisher

ELSEVIER your source for books,
journals and multimedia
in the health sciences
www.elsevierhealth.com

Working together to grow
libraries in developing countries

www.elsevier.com | www.bookaid.org | www.sabre.org

ELSEVIER **BOOK AID** International Sabre Foundation

The
publisher's
policy is to use
**paper manufactured
from sustainable forests**

Printed in China

Preface

In primary and secondary care the use of medicines is the most common intervention in healthcare. Medicines use, however, is not without risk. Drug selection and prescribing is increasingly complex and demanding, and undertaken as part of a multi-disciplinary process that involves pharmacists, doctors, nurses and other members of the healthcare team. All must strive to promote safe, appropriate and cost-effective prescribing that respects patient choice. This book has been written to help the reader understand and address many of these issues. It is unashamedly written from a pharmacy perspective, although we do hope those from other disciplines will also find it of use.

The extension of prescribing rights to pharmacists and other professional groups has meant that former roles and relationships have changed, with groups such as pharmacists needing to acquire additional skills and knowledge. We have tried to provide a foundation for this emerging role with new chapters on the prescribing and clinical pharmacy process.

We have also made considerable effort to update each chapter and ensure the content is relevant to current practice. Selected website addresses have been included to assist those who want to obtain further information. However, knowledge in therapeutics progresses rapidly, changes to dose regimens and licensed indications are frequent and new medicines appear at regular intervals. Yesterday another landmark study was published adding to, or perhaps altering, the evidence base for a specific treatment. Together with the ongoing publication of national guidelines and frameworks, the face of therapeutics is ever changing. It is therefore inevitable that some sections of this book will date more quickly than others.

In practice many licensed drugs are used 'off label' when prescribed for a certain indication or when used in a specific patient group, e.g. children. To omit reference to these agents in the relevant chapter would leave an apparent gap in therapeutic management. As a consequence we have encouraged our authors to refer to relevant drugs and regimens even where 'off label'. There is, however, a downside to this approach. The reader must always use this text critically and with caution. If this is done the book will serve as a valuable learning resource and help the reader understand some of the principles of therapeutics. We hope that, in some small way, this will also assist in achieving positive patient outcomes.

Roger Walker
Cate Whittlesea

Acknowledgements

Undergraduate and postgraduate students were the inspiration for the first edition of this book in 1994. They continue to be the *raison d'etre* and, along with feedback from readers, help sustain our enthusiasm and commitment. To all those who have provided feedback in the past, thank you. For those who would like to comment on this edition, do not hesitate to do so. In this electronic age it is easier than ever and always welcome at walkerR@cardiff.ac.uk or cate.whittlesea@kcl.ac.uk.

We remain indebted to all authors who, through their hard work, patience and tolerance, have contributed to the fourth edition of this book. We are particularly grateful to those for whom this has become a regular commitment and who strive, along with us, to produce an ever better textbook. To our first-time authors, we are very grateful that you agreed to contribute, that you accepted our cryptic editorial comments in good faith and still managed to submit on time. We hope that you will continue to work with us on future editions.

A textbook of this size cannot, of course, be produced without the invaluable help, support and occasional comments of numerous colleagues, particularly those within the National Public Health Service for Wales, the Welsh School of Pharmacy, Cardiff University, and the Department of Pharmacy, King's College London. It would be invidious to name individuals who have helped us, in part for fear of offending anyone we might miss. We do, however, make one exception to this rule. The administrative support from Marilyn Meecham has been invaluable. She co-ordinated the project from the outset and was often called upon to present the polite face of two chastened editors. Thanks Marilyn.

The enormous contribution Clive Edwards made to the first three editions of this book also cannot pass without due acknowledgement. It was with some regret that we embarked on this, the fourth edition, without his involvement at the helm. We did manage to convince him to co-author a chapter but could entice him to do no more. We hope we have maintained the standards Clive set in previous editions.

Finally, and on a personal note, we would like thank our close families for their support and tolerance with our indulgence in editing this text. At times it may have appeared that everything in our lives took second place to 'the book'. We are eternally grateful for their understanding, particularly when we got our priorities in life wrong. Without the unfailing support of Ann and acceptance by Alex, this book would never have materialized.

Roger Walker
Cate Whittlesea

Contributors

Christopher Acomb BSc MPharm MRPharmS MCPP
Pharmacy Department, St James's University Hospital,
Leeds, UK
49. Anaemia

Andrew Alldred BPharm MRPharmS AdvDipClinPharm
Director of Pharmacy, Harrogate District Foundation Trust,
Harrogate, UK
53. Rheumatoid arthritis and osteoarthritis
54. Gout and hyperuricaemia

Rosalyn Anderson BSc MRPharmS DipTher
Senior Pharmacist Medicines Management, NHS Borders,
Melrose, UK
58. Pressure sores and leg ulcers

Sharon D. Andrew BSc MPharm MRPharmS
NHS Liaison Executive, Alcon Laboratories (UK) Ltd, Hemel
Hempstead, UK
55. Glaucoma

C. Heather Ashton DM FRCP
Emeritus Professor of Clinical Psychopharmacology, Royal
Victoria Infirmary, Newcastle upon Tyne, UK
28. Insomnia and anxiety

Catrin Barker BSc MSc PGDipClinPharm
Head of Drug Information, Pharmacy Department, Alder Hey
Children's Hospital, Liverpool, UK
10. Paediatrics

Sasha Beresford BPharm DipPharmPrac
Principal Pharmacist, Clinical Services; Honorary Lecturer.
Northwick Park and St Mark's Hospitals NHS Trust, London, UK
13. Inflammatory bowel disease

Andrew Berrington MRCP MRCPath
Consultant Microbiologist, City Hospitals Sunderland,
Sunderland, UK
35. Respiratory infections

David Branford PhD MRPharmS
Chief Pharmacist, Derbyshire Mental Health Services,
Derby, UK
30. Schizophrenia

David Bryant BSc MSc MRPharmS
Formerly Clinical Pharmacy Team Leader, Leeds Teaching
Hospitals NHS Trust, Leeds, UK; Project Manager, LUTO, UK
53. Rheumatoid arthritis and osteoarthritis

David J. Burn MD FRCP MA MB BS
Consultant Neurologist, Newcastle upon Tyne Hospitals NHS
Trust; Professor of Movement Disorder Neurology, Newcastle
University, Newcastle upon Tyne, UK
32. Parkinson's disease

Brit Cadman BSc DipClinPharm
Principal Pharmacist, Clinical Services, Addenbrooke's NHS
Trust, Cambridge, UK
15. Adverse effects of drugs on the liver

Susan Calvert MRCOG
Consultant Obstetrician and Gynaecologist, Bradford Royal
Infirmary, Bradford, UK
45. Menstrual cycle disorders
46. Menopause and hormone replacement therapy

Laura Cameron BPharm DipPharmPractice MRPharmS
Chemotherapy Preparative Service Manager, St Bartholomew's
Hospital, Barts and The London NHS Trust, London, UK
51. Lymphomas

Toby Capstick BSc MRPharmS ClinDip
Rhueumatology Specialist Pharmacist, Leeds Teaching
Hospitals, St James's University Hospital, Leeds, UK
54. Gout and hyperuricaemia

Neil J. B. Carbarns BSc MB ChB FRCPath
Consultant Medical Microbiologist, Gwent Healthcare NHS
Trust, Department of Clinical Microbiology and Infection
Control, Nevill Hall Hospital, Abergavenny, Wales, UK
36. Urinary tract infections

Mary M. Carr MD BSc FRCP
Consultant Dermatologist, County Durham and Darlington
Foundation NHS Trust, University Hospital of North Durham,
UK
57. Eczema and psoriasis

Jonathan Cooke MPharm PhD MRPharmS
Director of Research and Development, Clinical Director of
Pharmacy and Medicines Management, South Manchester
University Hospitals NHS Trust, Wythenshawe Hospital,
Manchester, UK
8. Pharmacokinetics

Duncan Cripps BPharm PGDipHospPharm
Education and Training Pharmacist, Plymouth Hospitals NHS Trust; Acting Visiting Lecturer, Advanced Programmes in Pharmaceutical Practice and Therapeutics, University of Bath, Bath, UK
25. Asthma
26. Chronic obstructive pulmonary disease

Sarah Cripps BPharm, MSc, MRPharmS
Lead Pharmacist (medicine, cardiac, renal services); Specialist Pharmacist for Gastroenterology, Oxford Radcliffe Hospitals NHS Trust, Oxford, UK
13. Inflammatory bowel disease

J. Graham Davies BPharm MSc PhD MRPharmS
Professor of Clinical Pharmacy and Therapeutics, School of Pharmacy and Biomolecular Sciences, University of Brighton, Brighton UK; Associate Director of Clinical Pharmacy, London, Eastern and South East Specialist Pharmacy Services, UK
1. Clinical pharmacy process

Soraya Dhillon MBE BPharm PhD MRPharmS
Foundation Professor Head, School of Pharmacy, University of Hertfordshire, Hatfield, UK
31. Epilepsy

Sarah J. Dunnett BPharm MRPharmS DipClinPharm
Medical Affairs Manager, Baxter Healthcare, Compton, UK
7. Parenteral nutrition

Jeremy Dwight BSc MD FRCP
Consultant Cardiologist, John Radcliffe Hospital, Oxford, UK
20. Coronary heart disease

Clive Edwards BPharm PhD MRPharmS
Prescribing Adviser, North Tyneside Primary Care Trust, Newcastle upon Tyne, UK
6. Laboratory data

Bridget Featherstone BSc DipClinPharm
Lead Pharmacist for Transplantation and Surgery, Addenbrooke's NHS Trust, Cambridge, UK
15. Adverse effects of drugs on the liver

Martin Fisher MB BS BSc FRCP
Consultant Physician HIV/AIDS, Brighton and Sussex University Hospitals NHS Trust, Brighton, UK
41. HIV infection

Ray Fitzpatrick BSc PhD MRPharmS
Clinical Director of Pharmacy, Royal Wolverhampton Hospitals NHS Trust; Professor of Clinical Pharmacy, Wolverhampton University, Wolverhampton, UK
3. Practical pharmacokinetics

Sharon J. Gardiner MClinPharm
Drug Information Pharmacist, Department of Clinical Pharmacology, Christchurch Hospital, Christchurch, New Zealand
47. Drugs in pregnancy and lactation

Subrata Ghosh MD FRCP FRCP(E)
Professor of Gastroenterology, Imperial College London; Chief of Service, Hammersmith Hospital, London, UK
12. Peptic ulcer disease

Kevin P. Gibbs BPharm DipClinPharm MRPharmS
Principal Pharmacist, Clinical Services, Bristol Royal Infirmary, Bristol, UK
25. Asthma
26. Chronic obstructive pulmonary disease

Richard L. Gower FRCS
Clinical Director for Urological Services, Gwent Healthcare NHS Trust, Royal Gwent Hospital, Newport, Wales, UK
48. Benign prostatic hyperplasia

J. Clive. Graham MB BS MRCP MRCPath
Consultant Medical Microbiologist, Birmingham Children's Hospital, Birmingham, UK
39. Surgical antibiotic prophylaxis

James W. Gray MRCP FRCPath
Consultant Microbiologist, Department of Microbiology, The Birmingham Children's Hospital NHS Trust, Diana, Princess of Wales Children's Hospital, Birmingham, UK
37. Gastrointestinal infections
38. Infective meningitis

Elizabeth Hackett BSc MSc
Principal Pharmacist for Emergency and Metabolic Medicine, Leicester Royal Infirmary, Leicester, UK
44. Diabetes mellitus

Jayne Holden MPharm MRPS
Lead Pharmacist for Haematology, Leeds Teaching Hospitals, Leeds, UK
49. Anaemia

Steve A. Hudson MPharm BPharm FRPharmS
Professor of Pharmaceutical Care, School of Pharmacy, Strathclyde Institute of Biomedical Sciences, Glasgow, UK
21. Congestive heart failure

Graham Jackson MA MB BS FRCP FRCPath MD
Consultant Haematologist, Department of Haematology, Royal Victoria Infirmary, Newcastle upon Tyne, UK
50. Leukaemia

Gail Jones MD MRCP MRCPath
Consultant Haematologist, Royal Victoria Infirmary, Newcastle upon Tyne, UK
50. Leukaemia

Dil Kapur MB ChB FRCA
Consultant in Pain Management, Pain Management Unit, Flinders Medical Centre, Befrod Park, South Australia, Australia
33. Pain

Niall P. Keaney BSc MB PhD FRCP
Honorary Consultant Physician, Sunderland Royal Hospital, Sunderland, UK
27. Drug-induced lung disease

Patrick T. F. Kennedy MB ChB BAO BMedSci MRCP
Specialist Registrar in Hepatology, St Mary's Hospital, London, UK
16. Liver disease

Moira Kinnear Bsc MSc ADCPT MRPharmS
Head of NHS Lothian Pharmacy Education, Research and Development, Western General Hospital, Edinburgh; Lecturer in Clinical Practice, University of Strathclyde, Glasgow, UK
12. Peptic ulcer disease

Heather Leake Date Bsc MSc MRPharmS
Principal Pharmacist HIV/Sexual Health Brighton and Sussex University Hospitals NHS Trust Brighton UK: Honorary Senior Lecturer Scholl of Pharmacy and Biomolecular Sciences University of Brighton, Brighton, UK
41. HIV infection

Anne Lee MPhil MRPharmS
Principal Pharmacist, Scottish Medicines Consortium, NHS Quality Improvement Scotland, Glasgow, UK
4. Drug interactions
5. Adverse drug reactions

Catherine Loughran MPharm MSc
Senior Pharmacist, Haematology and Clinical Governance, Guy's and St Thomas' NHS Foundation Trust, London, UK
51. Lymphomas

John J. McAnaw BSc PhD MRPharmS
Lecturer in Clinical Practice, University of Strathclyde, Glasgow, UK
21. Congestive heart failure

Duncan McRobbie MSc MRPharmS
Principal Clinical Pharmacist, Guy's and St Thomas' Hospital Trust, London, UK
1. Clinical pharmacy process

Pam Magee BSc MSc MRPharmS
Director of Pharmacy, University Hospitals, Coventry and Warwickshire, UK
56. Drug-induced skin disorders

John Marriott PhD BSc MRPharmS
Subject Convenor, Pharmacy and Biology, School of Life and Health Sciences, Aston University, Birmingham, UK
17. Chronic kidney disease and end-stage renal failure
18. Acute renal failure

Kay Marshall BPharm PhD FRPharmS
Senior Lecturer in Pharmacology, School of Pharmacy, University of Bradford, Bradford, UK
45. Menstrual cycle disorders
46. Menopause and hormone replacement therapy

Emma Mason BSc MB ChB MRCP
Lecturer in Palliative Medicine and Pharmacology, Department of Pharmacology and Therapeutics, University of Wales College of Medicine, Cardiff, UK
34. Nausea and vomiting

Lika K. Nehaul LRCPI LRCSI MSc FFPH
Consultant in Communicable Disease Control, National Public Health Service for Wales, Mamhilad House, Pontypool, UK
40. Tuberculosis

Anthony J. Nunn BPharm FRPharmS
Director of Clinical Pharmacy, Pharmacy Department, Alder Hey Children's Hospital, Liverpool, UK
10. Paediatrics
40. Tuberculosis

John O'Grady MD FRCPI
Consultant Hepatologist, Institute of Liver Studies, King's College Hospital, London, UK
16. Liver disease

Mike Page MD FRCP
Consultant Physician, Pontypridd and Rhondda NHS Trust; Honorary Consultant Physician, Cardiff and Vale NHS Trust, Wales, UK
43. Thyroid and parathyroid

Stephen J. Pedler MB ChB FRCPath
Consultant Microbiologist, Royal Victoria Infirmary, Newcastle upon Tyne, UK
42. Fungal infections

Peter Pratt BSc MPhil MRPharmS
Chief Pharmacist, Community Health Sheffield, Pharmacy Services, Michael Carlisle Centre, Sheffield, UK
29. Affective disorders

Philip A. Routledge MD FRCP FRCPE
Professor, Department of General Medicine, Llandough Hospital, Penarth, UK
23. Thrombosis
34. Nausea and vomiting

Paul Rutter MRPharmS
Principal Lecturer, Department of Pharmacy, University of Wolverhampton, Wolverhampton, UK
14. Constipation and diarrhoea

Kordo Saeed MB ChB MSc
Specialist Registrar Microbiology, Southampton General Hospital, Microbiology Department, Southampton, UK

Josemir W. Sander MD MRCP PhD
Professor of Neurology, Queen Square, London, UK
31. Epilepsy

David Scott BSc PhD DipMedEd MRPharmS
Regional Clinical Training Pharmacist, Oxford Radcliffe Hospital, Oxford, UK
20. Coronary heart disease
22. Cardiac arrhythmias

Hamasaraj G. M. Shetty BSc MB BS FRCP(London)
Consultant Physician, University Hospital of Wales, Cardiff, UK
11. Geriatrics
23. Thrombosis

Steve Smith MB ChB FRCP MD
Clinical Director of Renal Services, Birmingham Heartlands Hospital, Birmingham, UK
17. Chronic kidney disease and end-stage renal failure
18. Acute renal failure

June So BSc MRPharmS
Chief Pharmacist, Christie Hospital, Manchester, UK
52. Solid tumours

Ivan H. Stockley BPharm PhD FRPharmS
Consultant Pharmacologist, University of Nottingham Medical School, Nottingham, UK
4. Drug interactions

Barry Strickland-Hodge BSc MSc PhD MRPharmS ACPP AFPMM
Pharmaceutical Adviser, Primary Care, Newham PCT; Senior Pharmacy Lecturer, University of Leeds, Leeds, UK
2. Clinical pharmacy and prescribing

Simon H. L. Thomas BSc MB BS MRCP FRCP FRCP(Edin)
Consultant Physician and Clinical Pharmacologist, Newcastle upon Tyne Hospitals NHS Trust; Reader in Therapeutics, University of Newcastle, Newcastle upon Tyne, UK
5. Adverse drug reactions
19. Hypertension

Stephen Thomas FRCP
Consultant in Diabetes, Guy's and St Thomas' Hospital NHS Foundation Trust, London, UK
44. Diabetes mellitus

Lucy C. Titcomb BSc MRPharmS MCPP
Directorate Pharmacist Ophthalmology, Birmingham and Midland Eye Centre, Stratford upon Avon, UK
55. Glaucoma

Sean Turner BPharm MSc DipClinPharm
Clinical Pharmacist, Princess Margaret Hospital for Children, Perth, Western Australia, Australia
10. Paediatrics

Roger Walker BPharm PhD FRPharmS FFPH
Professor of Pharmacy Practice, Welsh School of Pharmacy, Cardiff University; Consultant in Pharmaceutical Public Health, National Public Health Service for Wales, Wales, UK
24. Dyslipidaemia

Martin P. Ward Platt ChB MD FRCP FRCPCH
Consultant Paediatrician and Senior Lecturer in Child Health, Newcastle Neonatal Service, Royal Victoria Infirmary, Newcastle upon Tyne, UK
9. Neonates

David Webb BPharm MSc MRPharmS
Director, Clinical Pharmacy Specialist Service for London, Eastern and South East, Clinical Pharmacy Support Unit, Pharmacy Department, North West London Hospitals Trust, Harrow, UK
1. Clinical pharmacy process

Ken Woodhouse MD FRCP
Pro Vice Chancellor, External Affairs; Professor of Geriatric Medicine, Cardiff University Academic Centre, Llandough Hospital, Penarth, UK
11. Geriatrics

David J. Woods MPharm
Pharmaceutical Programme Manager, Best Practice Advocacy Centre, Demedin, New Zealand
47. Drugs in pregnancy and lactation

Sheila Woolfrey BSc PhD MRPharmS FCPP DipMPED
Lead Pharmacist Medicine, Wansbeck General Hospital, Northumbria Healthcare NHS Trust, Ashington, Northumbria, UK
33. Pain

Hilary Wynne MA MD FRCP
Consultant Physician, Royal Victoria Infirmary, Newcastle upon Tyne, UK
6. Laboratory data

Contents

GENERAL

Clinical pharmacy process

D. G. Webb   J. G. Davies   D. McRobbie

- Clinical pharmacy comprises a set of functions that promote the safe, effective and economic use of medicines for individual patients.
- The emergence of clinical pharmacy has allowed pharmacists to shift from a product orientated role towards direct engagement with patients and the problems they encounter with medicines.
- The practice of clinical pharmacy is generally an essential component of pharmaceutical care.
- Pharmaceutical care is a co-operative, patient centred system for achieving specific and positive patient outcomes from the responsible provision of medicines. Professionals, other than pharmacists, may lead and/or be key in this process.
- The three key elements of the care process are patient assessment, determining the care plan and evaluating the outcome.
- The ability to consult with patients is a key process in the delivery of pharmaceutical care and requires regular review and development regardless of experience.
- The clinical pharmacy process has been incorporated into a competency framework that can be used to further develop skills and knowledge.

Clinical pharmacy, unlike the discipline of pharmacy, is a comparatively recent and variably implemented form of practice. It encourages pharmacists and support staff to shift their focus from a solely product-oriented role towards more direct engagement with patients and the problems they encounter with medicines. Over the past 20 years there has been an emerging consensus that the practice of clinical pharmacy itself should grow from a collection of patient-related functions to a process in which all actions are undertaken with the intention of achieving explicit outcomes for the patient. In doing so, clinical pharmacy moves to embrace the philosophy of pharmaceutical care (Hepler & Strand 1990).

This chapter provides a practical framework within which a knowledge and understanding of therapeutics and practice can be best utilized. It describes a pragmatic approach to applying both the principles of pharmaceutical care and the specific skills of clinical pharmacy in a manner that does not depend on the setting of the practitioner or patient.

Development of clinical practice in pharmacy

The emergence of clinical pharmacy as a form of practice has been attributed to the poor medicines control systems that existed in hospitals during the early 1960s (Cousins & Luscombe 1995).

Although provoked by similar hospital-centred problems, the nature of the professional response differed between the USA and the UK.

In the USA, the approach was to adopt unit dose dispensing and pursue decentralization of pharmacy services. In the UK the unification of the prescription and the administration record meant this document needed to remain on the hospital ward and required the pharmacist to visit the ward to order medicines. Clinical pharmacy thereby emerged from the presence of pharmacists in these patient areas and their interest in promoting safer medicines use. This was initially termed 'ward pharmacy' but participation in medical ward rounds in the late 1970s signalled the transition to clinical pharmacy.

Medication safety may have been the spur but clinical pharmacy in the 1980s grew because of its ability to promote cost-effective medicines use in hospitals. This role was recognized by the UK government who, in 1988, endorsed the implementation of clinical pharmacy services to secure value for money from medicines. Awareness that support depended, to an extent, on the quantification of actions and cost savings led several groups to develop ways of measuring pharmacists' clinical interventions. Coding systems were necessary to aggregate large amounts of data in a reliable manner and many of these drew upon the eight steps (Table 1.1) of the drug use process (DUP) indicators (Hutchinson et al 1986).

The data collected from these early studies revealed that interventions had very high physician acceptance rates, were made most commonly at the 'select regimen' and 'need for drug' stages of the drug use process, and were influenced by hospital ward type (intensive care and paediatrics having the highest rates), pharmacist grade (rates increasing with grade) and time spent on wards (Barber et al 1997).

Despite the level of activity that intervention monitoring revealed, together with evidence of cost containment and a broadly supportive healthcare system, frustrations began to appear. These, in part, stemmed from a lack of certainty about the fundamental purpose of clinical pharmacy and from tensions between the drive towards specialization in clinical pharmacy and the need to improve services of a more general level in hospitals and other care settings.

Pharmaceutical care

The need to focus on outcomes of medicines use rather than dwelling only on the functions of clinical pharmacy became apparent (Hepler & Strand 1990). The launch of pharmaceutical

Table 1.1 Drug use process (DUP) indicators

DUP stage	Action
Need for a drug	Ensure there is an appropriate indication for each drug and that all medical problems are addressed therapeutically
Select drug	Select and recommend the most appropriate drug based upon the ability to reach therapeutic goals, with consideration of patient variables, formulary status and cost of therapy
Select regimen	Select the most appropriate drug regimen for accomplishing the desired therapeutic goals at the least cost without diminishing effectiveness or causing toxicity
Provide drug	Facilitate the dispensing and supply process so that drugs are accurately prepared, dispensed in ready-to-administer form and delivered to the patient on a timely basis
Drug administration	Ensure that appropriate devices and techniques are used for drug administration
Monitor drug therapy	Monitor drug therapy for effectiveness or adverse effects in order to determine whether to maintain, modify or discontinue
Counsel patient	Counsel and educate the patient or caregiver about the patient's therapy to ensure proper use of medicines
Evaluate effectiveness	Evaluate the effectiveness of the patient's drug therapy by reviewing all the previous steps of the drug use process and taking appropriate steps to ensure that the therapeutic goals are achieved

Table 1.2 Definitions of clinical pharmacy, pharmaceutical care and medicines management

Term	Definition
Clinical pharmacy	Clinical pharmacy comprises a set of functions that promote the safe, effective and economic use of medicines for individual patients. Clinical pharmacy process requires the application of specific knowledge of pharmacology, pharmacokinetics, pharmaceutics and therapeutics to patient care
Pharmaceutical care	Pharmaceutical care is a co-operative, patient-centred system for achieving specific and positive patient outcomes from the responsible provision of medicines. The practice of clinical pharmacy is an essential component in the delivery of pharmaceutical care
Medicines management	Medicines management encompasses the way in which medicines are selected, procured, delivered, prescribed, administered and reviewed to optimize the contribution that medicines make to producing informed and desired outcomes of patient care

care as the 'responsible provision of drug therapy for the purpose of achieving definite outcomes that improve a patient's quality of life' was a landmark in the topography of pharmacy practice. In reality, this was an incremental step forward, rather than revolutionary leap, since the foundations of pharmaceutical care as 'the determination of drug needs for a given individual and the provision not only of the drug required but also the necessary services to assure optimally safe and effective therapy' had been established previously (Brodie et al 1980).

The delivery of pharmaceutical care is dependent on the practice of clinical pharmacy but the key feature of care is that the practitioner takes responsibility for a patient's drug-related needs and is held accountable for that commitment. None of the definitions of pharmaceutical care is limited by reference to a specific professional group. Although pharmacists and pharmacy support staff would expect to, and clearly can, play a central role in pharmaceutical care, it is essentially a co-operative system that embraces the contribution of other professionals and patients (Table 1.2). The avoidance of factionalism has enabled pharmaceutical care to permeate community pharmacy, particularly in Europe, in a way that clinical pharmacy and its bedside connotations did not. It also anticipated healthcare policy in which certain functions, such as the prescribing of medicines, have been extended beyond their traditional professional origins to be undertaken by those trained and identified to be competent to do so.

Medication-related problems

When the outcome of medicines use is not optimal, a classification (Table 1.3) for identifying the underlying medication-related problem (MRP) has been proposed (Hepler & Strand 1990). Some medication-related problems are associated with significant morbidity and mortality. Preventable medication-related hospital admissions in the USA have a prevalence of 4.3%, indicating that gains in public health from improved medicines management would be sizeable (Winterstein et al 2002). In the UK too, preventable medication-related morbidity has been

Table 1.3 Categories of medication-related problems

Untreated indication

Treatment without indication

Improper drug selection

Too little drug

Too much drug

Non-compliance

Adverse drug reaction

Drug interaction

al 1999). The services involved were medicines information, clinical research performed by pharmacists, active pharmacist participation in resuscitation teams and pharmacists undertaking admission medication histories.

In the UK, the focus has been also on prevention and management of MRPs. Recognition that many patients either fail to benefit or experience unwanted effects from their medicines has elicited two types of response from the pharmacy profession. The first has been the re-engineering of pharmaceutical services to introduce schemes for medicines management at an organizational level. These have ranged from specific initiatives to target identified areas of medication risk, such as pharmacist involvement in anticoagulation services, to more general approaches where the intention is to ensure consistency of medicines use, particularly across care interfaces. The second response has been to put in place, and make use of, a raft of postgraduate programmes to meet the developmental needs of pharmacists working in clinical settings.

associated with 4.3% of admissions to a medical unit. In nearly all cases, the underlying MRP was linked to prescribing, monitoring or adherence (Howard et al 2003).

In prospective studies, up to 28% of emergency department visits have been identified as medication related, of which 70% are deemed preventable (Zed 2005). Again, the most frequently cited causes were non-compliance and inappropriate prescribing and monitoring. The cost of drug-related morbidity and mortality in the US ambulatory care (outpatient) population was estimated in 2000 to be $177 billion. Hospital admission accounted for 70% of total costs (Ernst & Grizzle 2001).

The rate for adverse drug events among hospital inpatients in the USA has been quantified as 6.5 per 100 admissions. Overall, 28% of events were judged preventable, rising to 42% of those classified as life threatening or serious (Bates et al 1995). The direct cost of medication errors, defined as preventable events that may cause or lead to inappropriate medicines use or harm, in NHS hospitals has been estimated to lie between £200 and £400 million per year. To this should be added the costs arising from litigation (DH 2004).

The scale of the misadventure that these findings reveal, coupled with current concerns about the costs of drug therapy, creates an opportunity for a renaissance in clinical pharmacy practice, providing that it realigns strongly with patient safety, clinical governance and public health. In practice, community pharmacists may be uniquely placed to help reduce the level of medication-related morbidity in primary care by virtue of their accessibility and existing relationships.

Pharmaceutical consultation

Structured postgraduate education has served to improve the knowledge of clinical pharmacists but fully achieving the goals of pharmaceutical care has proved more challenging. Part of the difficulty has been the requirement to place the patient at the heart of the system, rather than being a relatively passive recipient of drug therapy and associated information. To deliver pharmaceutical care requires more than scientific expertise. It mandates a system that clearly describes the role and responsibilities of the pharmacist and provides the necessary infrastructure to support them in this role and, secondly, a clear process by which the pharmacist can deliver their contribution to patient care.

Pharmaceutical care is predicated on a patient-centred approach to identifying, preventing or resolving MRPs. Central to this aim is the need to establish a therapeutic relationship. This relationship must be a partnership in which the pharmacist takes responsibility for resolving medication-related issues in line with the patient's wishes, expectations and priorities. Table 1.4 summarizes the three key elements of the care process (Cipolle et al 1998).

Benefits of pharmaceutical care

The ability to demonstrate that clinical pharmacy practice improves patient outcomes is of great importance to the pharmaceutical care model. In the USA, for example, pharmacists' participation in physician ward rounds has been shown to reduce adverse drug events by 78% and 66% in general medical (Kucukarslan et al 2003) and intensive care settings (Leape et al 1999), respectively. A study covering 1029 USA hospitals was the first to indicate that both centrally based and patient-specific clinical pharmacy services are associated with reduced mortality rates (Bond et

Table 1.4 Key elements of the care process

Element	Purpose
Assessment	The main goal is to establish a full medication history and highlight actual and potential drug-related problems
Care plan	This should clearly state the goals to optimize care and the responsibilities of both the pharmacist and the patient in attaining the stated goals
Evaluation	This reviews progress against the stated patient outcomes

Medicines-taking behaviour

The need for a care process which ensures that the patient is involved at all stages has become clearer as the extent of non-adherence has been revealed. Significant proportions (between 30% and 50%) of patients with chronic conditions do not take their prescribed medicines as directed. Many factors are thought to influence a patient's decision to adhere to a prescribed regimen. These include the characteristics of the disease and the treatment used to manage it, the patient's beliefs about their illness and their medicines, as well as the quality of the interaction between the patient and healthcare practitioner. Non-adherence can be categorized broadly into two types: intentional and unintentional. Unintentional non-adherence may be associated with physical or sensory barriers to taking medicines, for example, not being able to swallow or unable to read the labels, forgetfulness or poor comprehension. Traditionally, pharmacists have played a key role in helping patients overcome these types of problems, but have been less active in identifying and resolving intentional non-adherence.

Intentional (or deliberate) non-adherence may be due to a number of factors. Recent work in health psychology has shaped our understanding of how patients perceive health and illness and why they often decide not to take their medicines. When people receive information about illness and its treatment, it is processed in accordance with their own belief systems. Often patients' perceptions are not in tune with the medical reality and when this occurs, taking medicines may not make sense to the individual. For example, a patient diagnosed with hypertension may view the condition as one that is caused by stress and, during periods of lower stress, may not take their prescribed medicines (Baumann & Leventhal 1985). Consequently, a patient holding this view of hypertension may be at increased risk of experiencing an adverse outcome such as a stroke.

More recent research has shown that patient beliefs about the necessity of the prescribed medication and concerns about the potential long-term effects have a strong influence on medicines-taking behaviour (Horne 2001). However, a patient's beliefs about the benefits and risks of medicines are rarely explored during consultation, despite evidence of an association between non-adherence and the patient's satisfaction with the consultation process adopted by practitioners (Ley 1988).

Consultation process

There are several comprehensive accounts of functions required to satisfy each stage of the drug use process, but few go on to explore how the pharmacist might create a therapeutic relationship with their patient. The ability of a pharmacist to consult effectively is fundamental to pharmaceutical care and this includes establishing a platform for achieving concordance. Nurturing a relationship with the patient is essential to understanding their medication-related needs.

Descriptions of pharmaceutical consultation have been confined largely to the use of mnemonics such as WWHAM, ENCORE and AS METTHOD (Table 1.5). These approaches provide the pharmacist with a rigid structure to use when questioning patients about their symptoms but, although useful, serve to make the symptom or disease the focus of the consultation rather than the

patient. A common misconception is that healthcare professionals who possess good communication skills are also able to consult effectively with patients; this relationship will not hold if there is a failure to grasp the essential components of consultation technique. Research into patients' perceptions of their illness and treatment has demonstrated that they are more likely to adhere to their medication regimen, and be more satisfied with the consultation, if their views about illness and treatment have been taken into account and the risks and benefits of treatment discussed. The mnemonic approach to consultation does not address adequately the complex interaction that may take place between a patient and a healthcare practitioner.

Undertaking a pharmaceutical consultation can be considered as a series of four interlinked phases, each with a goal and set of competencies (Table 1.6). These phases follow a problem-solving pattern, embrace relevant aspects of adherence research and attempt to involve the patient at each stage in the process. For effective consultation, the practitioner needs also to draw upon a range of communication behaviours (Table 1.7). This approach serves to integrate the agendas of both patient and pharmacist. It provides the vehicle for agreeing the issues to be addressed and the responsibilities accepted by each party in achieving the desired outcomes.

Table 1.5 Mnemonics used in the pharmacy consultation process

WWHAM
Who is it for?
What are the symptoms?
How long has it been going on?
Action taken?
Medicines taken?

AS METTHOD
Age of the patient?
Self or for someone else?
Medicines being taken?
Exactly what do you mean (by the symptom)?
Time and duration of the symptom
Taken any action (medicine or seen the doctor)?
History of any disease?
Other symptoms?
Doing anything to alleviate or worsen the symptom?

ENCORE
Evaluate the symptom, its onset, recurrence and duration
No medication is always an option
Care when dealing with specific patient groups, notably the elderly, the young, nursing mothers, pregnant women, those receiving specific medication such as methotrexate and anticoagulants, and those with particular disease, e.g. renal impairment
Observe the patient for signs of systemic disturbance and ask about presence of fever, loss of weight and any accompanying physiological disturbance
Refer when in doubt
Explain any course of action recommended

Table 1.6   Pharmaceutical consultation process

Element	Goal	Examples of associated competencies
Introduction	Building a therapeutic relationship	Invites patient to discuss medication or health-related issue Discusses structure and purpose of consultation Negotiates shared agenda
Data collection and problem identification	Identifying the patient's medication-related needs	Takes a full medication history Establishes patient's understanding of their illness Establishes patient's understanding of the prescribed treatment Identifies and prioritizes patient's pharmaceutical problems
Actions and solutions	Establishing an acceptable management plan with the patient	Involves patient in designing management plan Tailors information to address patient's perception of illness and treatment Checks patient's understanding Refers appropriately
Closure	Negotiating safety netting strategies with the patient	Provides information to guide action when patient experiences problems with management plan Provides further appointment or contact point

Table 1.7   Consultation behaviours

Active listening

Appropriate use of open and closed questions

Respects patient

Avoids jargon

Demonstrates empathy

Deals sensitively with potentially embarrassing or sensitive issues

Table 1.8   Key postconsultation questions

Do I know more now about the patient?

Was I curious?

Did I really listen?

Did I find out what really mattered to them?

Did I explore their beliefs and expectations?

Did I identify the patient's main medication-related problems?

Did I use their thoughts when I started explaining?

Did I share the treatment options with them?

Did I help my patient to reach a decision?

Did I check that they understood what I said?

Did we agree?

Was I friendly?

The ability to consult with patients is a key process in the delivery of pharmaceutical care and consequently requires regular review and development, regardless of experience. To ensure these core skills are developed, individuals should use trigger questions to prompt reflection on their approach to consulting (Table 1.8).

Clinical pharmacy functions and knowledge

The following practical steps in the delivery of pharmaceutical care are based largely on the drug use process. The 'select regimen' and 'drug administration' indicators have been amalgamated at step 3.

Step 1 Establishing the need for drug therapy

For independent prescribers this step includes establishing a diagnosis and then balancing the risks and benefits of treatment against the risks posed by the disease. Current practice for most pharmacists means that another professional, most frequently a doctor, will have diagnosed the patient's presenting condition and any co-existing disease. The pharmacist's role, therefore, is often one of providing information to the independent prescriber on the expected benefits and risks of drug therapy by evaluating both the evidence base and individual patient factors.

The evidence for one specific mode of therapy may not be conclusive. In this circumstance, the pharmacist will need to call on their understanding of the principles of pharmaceutical science and on clinical experience to provide the best advice possible.

Step 1.1 Relevant patient details

Without background information on the patient's health and social circumstances (Table 1.9) it is difficult to establish the existence of, or potential for, medication-related problems. When this information is lacking a review solely of prescribed medicines

Table 1.9 Relevant patient details

Factor	Implications
Age	The very young and the very old are most at risk of medication-related problems. A patient's age may indicate their likely ability to metabolize and excrete medicines and have implications for step 2 of the drug use process
Gender	This may alter the choice of the therapy for certain indications. It may also prompt consideration of the potential for pregnancy or breast feeding
Ethnic or religious background	Racially determined predispositions to intolerance or ineffectiveness should be considered with certain classes of medicines, e.g. ACE inhibitors in Afro-Caribbean people. Formulations may be problematic for other groups; for example, those based on blood products for Jehovah's Witnesses or porcine-derived products for Jewish patients
Social history	This may impact on ability to manage medicines and influence pharmaceutical care needs; for example, living alone or in a care home or availability of nursing, social or informal carers
Presenting complaint	Symptoms the patient describes and the signs identified by the doctor on examination. Pharmacists should consider whether these might be attributable to the adverse effects of prescribed or purchased medicines
Working diagnosis	This should enable the pharmacist to identify the classes of medicines that would be anticipated on the prescription based on current evidence
Previous medical history	Understanding the patient's other medical conditions and their history helps ensure that management of the current problem does not compromise a prior condition and guides the selection of appropriate therapy by identifying potential contraindications
Laboratory or physical findings	The focus should be on findings that may affect therapy, such as: renal function / liver function / full blood count / blood pressure / cardiac rhythm / Results may convey a need for dosage adjustment or presence of an adverse reaction

will probably be of limited value and risks making a flawed judgement on the appropriateness of therapy for that individual.

Current and co-existing conditions with which the patient presents can be established from various sources. In medical notes, the current diagnosis (Δ) or differential diagnoses (Δ Δ) will be documented, as well as any previous medical history (PMH). Other opportunities to gather information come from discussion with the patient and participation in medical rounds. In primary care, general medical practitioners' computer systems carry information on the patient's diagnosis.

Once the diagnosis and previous medical history are established it is then possible to identify the medicines that would be expected to be prescribed for each indication, based on contemporary evidence. This list of medicines may be compiled from appropriate national or international guidelines, local formularies and knowledge of current practice.

Step 1.2 Medication history

A medication history is the part of a pharmaceutical consultation that identifies and documents allergies or other serious adverse medication events, as well as information about how medicines are taken currently and have been taken in the past. It is the starting point for medication review.

Obtaining accurate and complete medication histories has been shown to have a positive effect on patient care and pharmacists have demonstrated that they can compile such histories

with a high degree of precision and reliability. The benefit to the patient is that prescribing errors of omission or transcription are identified and corrected early, reducing the risk of harm and improving care.

Discrepancies between the history recorded by the medical team and that which the pharmacist elicits fall into two categories: intentional (where the medical team has made a decision to alter the regimen) or unintentional (where a complete record was not obtained). Discrepancies should be clarified with the prescriber or referred to a more senior pharmacist. Table 1.10 lists the key components of a medication history.

Step 2 Selecting the medicine

The issues to be tackled at this stage include clinical and cost-effective selection of a medicine in the context of individual patient care. The list of expected treatments generated at step 1 is now scrutinized for its appropriateness for the patient. This requires three separate types of interaction to be identified: drug–patient, drug–disease and drug–drug. The interactions should be prioritized in terms of likelihood of occurrence and the potential severity of outcome should they occur.

Step 2.1 Identify drug–patient interactions

Many medicines have contraindications or cautions to their use that relate to age groups or gender. Potential drug–patient

Table 1.10   Key components of a medication history

1. Introduce yourself to the patient and explain the purpose of the consultation
2. Identify any allergies or serious adverse reactions and record these on the prescription chart, care notes or patient medication record
3. Ascertain information about prescribed and non-prescribed treatments from: the patient's recall medicines in the patient's possession referral letter (usually from the patient's primary care doctor) copy of prescriptions issued or a repeat prescription list medical notes contact with the appropriate community pharmacist or primary care doctor
4. Ensure the following are recorded: generic name of medicine (unless specific brand is required) dose frequency duration of therapy
5. Ensure items such as inhalers, eye drops, topical medicines, herbal and homeopathic remedies are included, as patients often do not consider these as medicines
6. Ascertain the patient's medication-taking behaviour
7. Consider practical issues such as swallowing difficulties, ability to read labels and written information, container preferences, ordering or supply problems
8. Document the history in an appropriate format
9. Note any discrepancies between this history and that recorded by other healthcare professionals
10. Ascertain if these discrepancies are intentional (from patient, nursing staff, medical staff or medical notes)
11. Non-intentional discrepancies should be communicated to the prescriber
12. Document any other important medication-related information in an appropriate manner; for example, implications of chronic renal failure, dialysis, long-term steroid treatment

interactions should be identified that may arise with any of the medicines that could be used to treat the current and pre-existing conditions. Types of drug–patient interactions may include allergy or previous adverse drug reaction, the impact of abnormal renal or hepatic function or chronic heart failure on the systemic availability of some medicines, and patients' preferences for certain treatment options, formulations or routes of administration.

Step 2.2 Identify drug–disease interactions

A drug–disease interaction may occur when a medicine has the potential to make a pre-existing condition worse. Older people are particularly vulnerable, due to the co-existence of several chronic diseases and exposure to polypharmacy. Prevention of drug–disease interactions requires an understanding of the pharmacodynamic properties of medicines and an appreciation of their contraindications.

Step 2.3 Drug–drug interactions

Medicines may affect the action of other medicines in a number of ways. Those with similar mechanisms of action may show

an enhanced effect if used together whilst those with opposing actions may reduce each other's effectiveness. Metabolism of one medicine can be affected by a second that acts as an inducer or inhibitor of the cytochrome P450 enzyme system.

The practitioner should be able to identify common drug interactions and recognize those medicines with increased risk of potential interaction, such as those with narrow therapeutic indices or involving hepatic P450 metabolic pathways. It is important to assess the clinical significance of drug interactions and consider the options for effective management.

The list of potential, evidence-based treatments should be reviewed for possible drug–patient, drug–disease and drug–drug interactions. The refined list can then be compared with the medicines that have been prescribed for the patient. The practitioner should explore any discrepancies to ensure the patient does not experience a medication-related problem. This may necessitate consultation with medical staff or other healthcare professionals, or referral to a more senior pharmacist.

Step 3 Administering the medicine

Many factors influence the effect that a medicine has at its locus of action. These include the rate and extent of absorption, degree of plasma protein binding and volume of distribution, and the routes of metabolism or excretion. Factors affecting bioavailability may include the extent of absorption of the drug from the gastrointestinal tract in relation to food and other medicines, or the amount adsorped onto intravenous infusion bags and giving sets when used to administer medicines parenterally.

The liver has extensive capacity for drug metabolism, even when damaged. Nevertheless, the degree of hepatic impairment should be assessed from liver function tests and related to potential changes in drug metabolism. This is particularly important for medicines that require activation by the liver (pro-drugs) or those whose main route of elimination is transformation into water-soluble metabolites.

Table 1.11 summarizes the main pharmaceutical considerations for step 3. At this point, the practitioner needs to ensure the following tasks have been completed accurately.

Step 3.1 Calculating the appropriate dose

Where doses of oral medicines require calculation, this is usually a straightforward process based on the weight of the patient. However, medicines to be administered parenterally may require more complex calculations, including knowledge of displacement values (particularly for paediatric doses) and determination of appropriate concentrations in compatible fluids and rates of infusion.

Step 3.2 Selecting an appropriate regimen

Giving medicines via the oral route is the preferred method of administration. Parenteral routes carry significantly more risks, including infection associated with vascular access. This route, however, may be necessary when no oral formulation exists or when the oral access is either impossible or inappropriate because of the patient's condition.

Although simple regimens (once- or twice-daily administration) may facilitate adherence, some medicines possess short half-lives and may need to be given more frequently. The practitioner should be familiar with the duration of action of regularly encountered medicines to ensure dosage regimens are designed optimally.

Step 4 Providing the medicine

Ensuring that a prescription is legal, legible, accurate and unambiguous contributes in large measure to the right patient receiving the right medicine at the right time. For the majority of pharmacists this involves screening prescriptions written by other professionals, but those acting as supplementary and independent prescribers need to be cognisant of guidance on prescribing, such as that contained within the British National Formulary, when generating their prescriptions.

In providing a medicine for an individual, due account must be taken of the factors that influence the continued availability and supply of the medicine within the hospital or community setting, e.g. formulary and drug tariff status, arrangements for primary/secondary shared care arrangements, and whether the prescribed indication is within the product licence. This is particularly important with unlicensed or non-formulary medicines when information and agreement on continuation of prescribing, recommended monitoring and availability of supply are transferred from a hospital to primary care setting.

Risks in the dispensing process are reduced by attention to products with similar names or packaging, patients with similar names, and when supplying several family members at the same time. Medicines should be labelled accurately, with clear dosage instructions and advisory labels, and presented appropriately for patients with specific needs, for example the visually impaired, those unable to read English or with limited dexterity.

Step 5 Monitoring therapy

Monitoring criteria for the effectiveness of treatment and its potential adverse effects can be drawn from the characteristics of the prescribed medicines used or related to specific patient needs. Close monitoring is required for medicines with narrow therapeutic indices and for the subset of drugs where therapeutic drug monitoring may be beneficial, e.g. digoxin, phenytoin, theophylline and aminoglycosides. Anticoagulant therapy, including warfarin and unfractionated heparin, is associated with much preventable medication-related morbidity and always warrants close scrutiny.

Table 1.11	Pharmaceutical considerations in the administration of medicines
Dose	Is the dose appropriate, including adjustments for particular routes or formulations?
	Examples: differences in dose between intravenous and oral metronidazole, intramuscular and oral chlorpromazine, and digoxin tablets compared with the elixir
Route	Is the prescribed route available (is the patient nil by mouth?) and appropriate for the patient?
	Examples: unnecessary prescription of an intravenous medicine when the patient can swallow, or the use of a solid dosage form when the patient has dysphagia
Dosage form	Is the medicine available in a suitable form for administration via the prescribed route?
Documentation	Is documentation complete? Do nurses or carers require specific information to administer the medicine safely?
	Examples: appropriateness of crushing tablets for administration via nasogastric tubes, dilution requirements for medicines given parenterally, rates of administration and compatibilities in parenteral solutions (including syringe drivers)
Devices	Are devices required, such as spacers for inhalers?

Throughout this textbook details are presented on the monitoring criteria that may be used for a wide range of medicines. Patients with renal or hepatic impairment or an unstable clinical condition need particular attention because of the likely requirement for dosage adjustment or change in therapy.

Step 6 Patient advice and education

There is a vast quantity of information on drug therapy available to patients. The practitioner's contribution in this context is to provide accurate and reliable information in a manner that the patient can understand. This may require the pharmacist to convey the benefits and risks of therapy, as well as the consequences of not taking medicines.

Information about medicines is best provided at the time of, or as soon as possible after, the prescribing decision. In the hospital setting, this means enabling patients to access information throughout their stay, rather than waiting until discharge. With many pharmacy departments providing medicines in patient packs, the patient can be alerted to the presence of information leaflets, encouraged to read them and ask any questions they may have. This approach enables the patient to identify their own information needs and ensures the pharmacist does not create a mismatch between their own agenda and that of the patient. However, there will be a need to explain clearly the limitations of leaflets, particularly when medicines are prescribed for unlicensed indications.

Although the research on adherence indicates the primacy of information that has been tailored to the individual's needs, resources produced by national organizations, such as Diabetes UK (www.diabetes.org.uk) and British Heart Foundation (www. bhf.org.uk), may also be of help to the patient and their family or carers. In addition, patients often require specific information to support their daily routine of taking medicines. All written information, including medicines reminder charts, should be dated and include contact details of the pharmacist to encourage patients to raise further queries or seek clarification.

Step 7 Evaluating effectiveness

The provision of drug therapy for the purpose of achieving definite outcomes is a fundamental objective of pharmaceutical care. These outcomes need to be identified at the outset and form the basis for evaluating the response to treatment. Practitioners delivering pharmaceutical care have a responsibility to evaluate the effectiveness of therapy by reviewing steps 1–6 above and taking appropriate action to ensure the desired outcomes are achieved. Depending on the duration of direct engagement with a patient's care, this may be a responsibility the pharmacist can discharge in person or it may necessitate transfer of care to a colleague in a different setting, where outcomes can be assessed more appropriately.

CASE STUDY

The following case is provided to illustrate the application of several steps in the delivery of pharmaceutical care. It is not intended to be a yardstick against which patient care should be judged.

Case 1.1

Mr JB, a 67-year-old retired plumber, has recently moved to your area and has come to the pharmacy to collect his first prescription. He has a previous medical history of coronary heart disease (CHD) and has recently had a coronary artery stent inserted.

Step 1 Establishing the need for drug therapy

What classes of medicines would you expect to be prescribed for these indications?

Mr JB gives a complete medication history that indicates he takes his medicines as prescribed, he has no medication-related allergies, but does suffer from dyspepsia associated with acute use of nonsteroidal anti-inflammatory agents. He has a summary of his stent procedure from the hospital that indicates normal blood chemistry and liver function tests.

Step 2 Selecting the medicine

What drug–patient, drug–disease and drug–drug interactions can be anticipated (Table 1.12)?

Steps 3 and 4 Administering and providing the medicines

What regimen and individualized doses would you recommend for Mr JB (Table 1.13)?

This predicted regimen can be compared with the prescribed therapy and any discrepancies resolved with the prescriber. Step 4 (provision) in Mr JB's case would be relatively straightforward.

Steps 5, 6 and 7 Monitoring therapy, patient education and evaluation

What criteria would you select to monitor Mr JB's therapy and what information would you share with the patient? What indicators would convey effective management of his condition (Table 1.14)?

Quality assurance of clinical practice

Quality assurance of clinical pharmacy has tended to focus on the review of performance indicators, such as intervention rates, or rely upon senior pharmacists to observe and comment on the practice of others using local measures. The lack of generally agreed or national criteria raises questions about the consistency of these assessments, where they take place, and the overall standard of care provided to patients. Following the Bristol Royal Infirmary Inquiry (2001) into paediatric cardiac surgery there has been much greater emphasis on the need for regulation to maintain the competence of healthcare professionals, the importance of periodic performance appraisal coupled with continuing professional development, and the introduction of revalidation.

The challenges for pharmacists are twofold: first, to demonstrate competence in a range of clinical pharmacy functions and

Table 1.12 The case of Mr JB: potential drug interactions with the patient, the disease or other drugs

	Drug–patient interactions	Drug–disease interactions	Drug–drug interactions
Medicines that should be prescribed for CHD			
Aspirin	Previous history of dyspepsia	Aspirin should be used with caution in asthma	Combination of antiplatelet agents increases risk of bleeding
Clopidogrel	Previous history of dyspepsia		
Statins			Possible increased risk of myopathy if simvastatin given with diltiazem
Nitrates β-blockers		β-blocker contraindicated in asthma	Combination of different agents to control angina may lead to hypotension
Other antianginal therapy			
Medicines that may be prescribed for asthma			
β_2-agonist inhalers	Patient's ability to use inhaler devices effectively	β_2-agonists can cause tachycardia	
Steroid inhalers			
Antimuscarinic inhalers		Antimuscarinic agents can cause tachycardia and atrial fibrillation	Antimuscarinics may reduce effect of sublingual nitrate tablets (failure to dissolve under tongue owing to dry mouth)

CHD, coronary heart disease

Table 1.13 The case of Mr JB: possible therapeutic regimen

	Recommendation	Rationale
Medicines that should be prescribed for CHD		
Aspirin	75 mg daily orally after food	Benefit outweighs risk if used with PPI.
Clopidogrel	75 mg daily orally after food	Benefit outweighs risk if used with PPI. Length of course should be established in relation to previous stent
Omeprazole	20 mg daily orally	Decreases risk of GI bleeds with combination antiplatelets
Simvastatin	20 mg daily orally	Low dose selected due to diltiazem
Nitrates	2 puffs sprayed under the tongue when required for chest pain	
Diltiazem	90 mg m/r twice a day	Used for rate control as β-blockers contraindicated in asthma
Ramipril	10 mg daily	To reduce the progression of CHD and heart failure
Medicines that may have been prescribed		
Salbutamol inhaler	2 puffs (200 µg) to be inhaled when required	Patient should follow asthma treatment plan if peak flow decreases
Beclometasone inhalers	2 puffs (400 µg) twice a day	Asthma treatment plan which may include increasing the dose of inhaled steroids if peak flow decreases

CHD, coronary heart disease; PPI, proton pump inhibitor; GI, gastrointestinal; m/r, modified release

Table 1.14 The case of Mr JB: monitoring criteria and patient advice

	Recommendation
Drugs that should be prescribed for CHD	
Aspirin	Ask patient about any symptoms of dyspepsia or worsening asthma
Clopidogrel	Ask patient about any symptoms of dyspepsia
Omeprazole	
Simvastatin	Cholesterol levels 3 months after any change in dose, or annually if at target
	Liver function tests 3 months after any change in dose, or annually
	Creatinine kinase only if presenting with symptoms of unexplained muscle pain
Nitrates	Frequency of use to be noted. Increasing frequency that results in a resolution of chest pain should be reported to primary care doctor and antianginal therapy may be increased
	ANY use that does not result in resolution of chest pain requires urgent medical attention
Diltiazem	Blood pressure and pulse monitored regularly
Ramipril	Renal function and blood pressure monitored within 2 weeks of any dose change, or annually
Drugs that may have been prescribed for asthma	
Salbutamol inhaler	Salbutamol use should be monitored as any increase in requirements may require increase in steroid dose
Beclometasone inhalers	Monitor for oral candidiasis

second, to engage with continuing professional development in a meaningful way to satisfy the expectations of pharmaceutical care and maintain registration with the professional body. The pragmatic approach to practice and the clinical pharmacy process outlined throughout this chapter has been incorporated into a competency framework that can be used to develop skills, knowledge and other attributes irrespective of the setting of the pharmacist and their patients. This General Level Framework can be accessed at www.codeg.org.

REFERENCES

Barber N D, Batty R, Ridout D A 1997 Predicting the rate of physician-accepted interventions by hospital pharmacists in the United Kingdom. American Journal of Health System Pharmacy 54: 397-405

Bates D W, Cullen D J, Laird N et al 1995 Incidence of adverse drug events and potential adverse drug events in hospitalized patients. Journal of the American Medical Association 274: 29-34

Baumann L J, Leventhal H 1985 'I can tell when my blood pressure is up, can't I?' Health Psychology 4: 203-218

Bond C A, Raehl C L, Franke T 1999 Clinical pharmacy services and hospital mortality rates. Pharmacotherapy 19: 556-564

Bristol Royal Infirmary Inquiry 2001 The report of the public inquiry into children's heart surgery at the Bristol Royal Infirmary 1984–1995. Learning from Bristol. Stationery Office, London

Brodie D C, Parish P A, Poston J W 1980 Societal needs for drugs and drug related services. American Journal of Pharmaceutical Education 44: 276-278

Cipolle R J, Strand L M, Morley P C (eds) 1998 Pharmaceutical care practice. McGraw-Hill, Europe

Cousins D H, Luscombe D K 1995 Forces for change and the evolution of clinical pharmacy practice. Pharmaceutical Journal 255: 771-776

Department of Health 2004 Building a safer NHS for patients: improving medication safety. Department of Health, London

Ernst F R, Grizzle A J 2001 Drug-related morbidity and mortality: updating the cost of illness model. Journal of the American Pharmacy Association 41: 192-199

Hepler C D, Strand L M 1990 Opportunities and responsibilities in pharmaceutical care. American Journal of Hospital Pharmacy 47: 533-543

Horne R 2001 Compliance, adherence and concordance. In: Taylor K, Harding G (eds) Pharmacy practice. Taylor and Francis, London

Howard R L, Avery A J, Howard P D et al 2003 Investigation into the reasons for preventable drug related admissions to a medical admissions unit: observational study. Quality and Safety in Health Care 12: 280-285

Hutchinson R A, Vogel D P, Witte K W 1986 A model for inpatient clinical pharmacy practice and reimbursement. Drug Intelligence and Clinical Pharmacy 20: 989-992

Kucukarslan S N, Peters M, Mlynarek M et al 2003 Pharmacists on rounding teams reduce preventable adverse drug events in hospital general medicine units. Archives of Internal Medicine 163: 2014-2018

Leape L L, Cullen D J, Clapp M D et al 1999 Pharmacist participation on physician rounds and adverse drug events in the intensive care unit. Journal of the American Medical Association 282: 267-270

Ley P 1988 Communicating with patients. Improving communication, satisfaction and compliance. Croom Helm, London

Winterstein A G, Sauer B C, Helper C D et al 2002 Preventable drug-related hospital admissions. Annals of Pharmacotherapy 36: 1238-1248

Zed P J 2005 Drug-related visits to the emergency department. Journal of Pharmacy Practice 18: 329-335

2 Prescribing

B. Strickland-Hodge

To prescribe is to authorize by means of a written prescription the supply of a medicine. Occasionally it may involve advising patients on suitable care or medication that can be bought without a prescription and has also come to mean the act of writing a prescription after all process decisions have been taken.

The factors that motivate an appropriately qualified individual to prescribe are a mix of the rational and the emotional. A rational approach uses evidence and has outcome goals; it evaluates alternatives and matches need to best available medication. However, an emotional element also exists because prescribers, to a greater or lesser extent, are responsive to appeals from patients, the pharmaceutical industry, professional colleagues, their own instincts and an array of other influences. As more pharmacists and other professional groups are authorized to take on a prescribing role alongside more traditional prescribers, it is increasingly important to understand the components of rational and effective prescribing, the factors that influence this process, the need for a systematic approach to prescribing, how to improve the science and art of prescribing and the factors that influence the decision to prescribe a new drug . These issues will be covered in the following sections, mainly, but not exclusively, from the standpoint of a prescriber in primary care.

Rational and effective prescribing

The rational and effective use of medicines saves lives and improves the quality of life for many. It requires the patient to receive medication appropriate to their clinical needs, in doses that meet their individual requirements for an adequate period of time and at the lowest cost to them and their community (WHO 1987). This can be paraphrased as the right drug, in the right place, at the right time, at the right dose for the right duration.

The traditional definitions of what a good prescriber should aim for have been reworked to include the patient dimension (Barber 1995). Good prescribing is now widely accepted to embrace four components:

- maximize effectiveness
- minimize risk
- minimize costs
- respect patient choices.

This definition of what constitutes good prescribing is sufficiently specific to produce outcomes against which prescribing can be monitored.

Inappropriate prescribing

In contrast to appropriate prescribing, inappropriate prescribing can cause distress, ill health, hospitalization and even death. It is characterized by:

- prescribing medicines for self-limiting disease
- prescribing medicines of limited clinical value
- continuing to prescribe a medicine for too long
- prescribing too low a dose of a medicine
- not prescribing a medicine for an adequate duration
- prescribing a medicine that is inappropriate for the disorder to be treated.

Inappropriate prescribing can result in serious morbidity and mortality, particularly when childhood infections or chronic diseases such as hypertension, diabetes, epilepsy and mental disorders are being treated. Inappropriate prescribing also represents a waste of resources and, as in the case of antimicrobials, may present a public health hazard by contributing to increased bacterial resistance. Finally, an overwillingness to prescribe stimulates inappropriate patient demand and fails to help the patient understand when they should seek out support from a healthcare professional.

A systematic approach to prescribing

The decision to prescribe a drug is based, in part, on a desire to do good while minimizing risk to the patient. Although the views of the patient have to be taken into account during the decision-making process, and many patients will try to influence the outcome, ultimately it is the prescriber who is accountable for issuing or withholding a prescription. It is therefore wise to adopt a systematic approach to prescribing to ensure all the relevant issues are taken into account.

Consultation skills and competencies

The consultation is a fundamental part of the prescribing process and the prescriber must understand and utilize this to help them practise effectively. The medical model of disease, diagnosis and prescribing is often central to practice but an understanding of the patient's background together with their medical beliefs and anxieties must not be overlooked as they are also important in helping the prescriber understand their own role and behaviours alongside those of their patients. A broad range of practical skills needs to be utilized in the consultation.

- Interpersonal skills: the ability to communicate and make relationships with patients.
- Reasoning skills: the ability to gather appropriate information, interpret the information and then apply it both in diagnosis and management.
- Practical skills: the ability to perform physical examinations and use clinical instruments.

The style in which the consultation is undertaken is also important. The paternalistic prescriber–patient relationship is generally no longer appropriate and has been replaced by a task-orientated approach that keeps consultation times to a reasonable duration and sets the parameters to ensure a realistic expectation from the consultation. An outline of the elements of a task-orientated consultation and other consultation styles that may need to be used is summarized below.

Task-orientated consultation

The consultation can be broken down into four component tasks.

Task 1 Identification and management of presenting problems. This involves questioning, listening and responding.

Task 2 Management of continuing problems. The consultation is seen as an opportunity to ensure previous medical issues are resolving.

Task 3 Opportunistic anticipatory care. The consultation provides opportunities for education on healthy lifestyles, etc.

Task 4 Modification of the patient's help-seeking behaviour. Prescribers need to ensure patients know when it is advantageous to seek their help (Scott & Davis 1979).

Patient-centred consultation

It is widely recognized by both prescribers and patients that the consultation should be an active dialogue that involves the patient. Prescribers must encourage patients to discuss not only their presenting symptoms but also their feelings and thoughts about the condition and its treatment. This greater involvement of the patient is the cornerstone of the patient-centred consultation.

Evidence-based consultation

The concept of evidence-based practice has become more explicit in recent years. The routine use of the current, relevant evidence base is now essential within the consultation. Even so, there are many concepts taken as evidence based that can be traced back to a more opinion-based decision. The prescriber must therefore always be willing to question the rationale for a given treatment regimen and should not accept the status quo as the evidence-based option. Emerging evidence may at times conflict with the prescriber's own experience and this must be dealt with.

Open consultation

This approach uses a range of consultation styles to meet the needs of the individual patient. The prescriber is aware of, and seeks to understand and respect, patient beliefs and expectations along with the cultural, language and religious implications that may impact upon an individual's ability or willingness to offer certain information or undertake recommended interventions or treatments. Nothing must be taken for granted and the prescriber must remain open-minded. A variety of methods may need to be used depending on need, circumstance and assessment of the patient's ability to be completely involved (Fraser 1999).

The various stages that lead to the eventual writing of a prescription are many and complex (Table 2.1). Symptoms are described by the patient, discussed and investigated to reach a final diagnosis. Factors such as the patient's age, sex and race need to be

Table 2.1 Typical stages in a consultation

Patient

Attend prescriber's clinic

Offer symptoms

Listen and communicate with the prescriber

Influence agenda of consultation

Prescriber

Assess attending patient's symptoms, medical history and medication history

Listen and communicate with patient

Focus on a working diagnosis

Consider the differential diagnosis

Identify and undertake investigations required to aid diagnosis

Make diagnosis

Prescribe medication or non-pharmacological intervention such as diet, lifestyle change, exercise or counselling

Arrange follow-up to confirm diagnosis, ensure prescribed treatment is relieving symptoms, improving quality of life, improving prognosis and not leading to unnecessary risk or side effects

taken into account as appropriate along with co-morbidities and any medication history. Discussions on management can then proceed and suggestions on non-pharmacological options may be offered.

The patient's belief in medicines generally, and in the medicine that may be prescribed, should be discussed. If the patient has had the same symptoms before, this is usually a good starting point for further investigations. If they have had symptoms, what was the treatment and was it successful? The patient who is involved in the decision-making process is more likely to follow the eventual, recommended treatment regimen. Concordance, a therapeutic alliance between prescriber and patient, is essential if the medicine prescribed is to be taken appropriately.

Throughout the consultation, listening to the patient is not a matter of sitting and doing nothing. Active listening is required and this involves paraphrasing, echoing and interpreting statements made by the patient. Neutral facilitative phrases to encourage patients to talk, such as 'um', 'I see', 'yes' are also required along with an appropriately attentive body language. The prescriber must be able to pick up unspoken issues, and may also need to be aware of the perspective of carers, colleagues and other professionals who relate to the patient. An effective relationship with the patient is desirable but not always possible where regular contact is not maintained.

Understanding and accepting professional limitations is sometimes difficult but essential to minimize patient risk. Building up a network of colleagues to contact in difficult circumstances is worthwhile. Likewise, understanding why investigations may not help clarify a given diagnosis and recognizing when to refer a patient are essential skills that need to be acquired.

The consultation may be one of a series for the patient. From the prescriber's perspective it should serve not only to determine the management of the presenting problem but could also be an opportunity to help manage a continuing problem. Each consultation also provides an opportunity for opportunistic health promotion and modification of the patient's health-seeking behaviour.

After the consultation, a follow-up appointment may be required to undertake further investigations or monitor the response to treatment. Pharmacists who prescribe need to ensure they are able to reflect on their actions and not take the consultation in isolation. Discussing issues with patients is essential and studying medical notes can help. The reflection should attempt to draw together the sometimes disparate facts into a whole that can be used to identify whether any change in patient management is required.

Gathering relevant information

Two of the main information-gathering elements of a consultation are the medication history and the medical history. The information revealed by the patient during these elements will invariably influence the selection of the medicine eventually prescribed.

Medication history

For the medication history there is a need to identify the names of medicines taken, their doses, frequency and routes of administration (Table 2.2). Patients may need to be prompted

Table 2.2 Key points to identify when taking a drug history	
Prescribed medicines	
Medication prescribed:	list prescribed medication, dose, frequency and route of administration taken within a relevant timescale, e.g. last 6 months
Duration of treatment:	identify duration of each treatment
Medication knowledge:	explore whether the patient understands what each medicine was prescribed for and how it will help
Adherence:	clarify whether the patient is taking the medication in accordance with the instructions
Side effects:	identify if the patient is experiencing any side effects or adverse reactions
Purchased medicines	
Medication purchased:	identify same information as for prescribed medication, paying attention to medicine taken regularly and intermittently, e.g. for headaches

to reveal details not only of prescribed medicines but also of medicines purchased from a pharmacy, supermarket or other retail outlet, any herbal or homeopathic medicines taken, whether they are taking oral contraceptives, and details of any medicines obtained over the internet or from friends and neighbours. The use of creams or lotions, ear or eye drops, inhalers, patches, suppositories, implants and depot injections may also need to be probed as they are often overlooked by patients. Information about use of illicit drugs is important but often difficult to obtain and unreliable.

At the same time as eliciting the above information, there is need to clarify whether the patient has experienced any allergies or side effects to medicines previously taken. The patient's smoking status and alcohol intake also need to be identified. Both induce liver enzyme activity and therefore, depending on what medicine the patient is taking, caution may be needed before recommending lifestyle changes. Stopping smoking or alcohol, while good for general health, may cause potentially hazardous effects if medicines metabolized by the liver are being taken at the same time.

Medical history

There is a need to obtain a detailed, complete and chronological account of the presenting problem together with the patient's thoughts and feelings about their illness. The mnemonic OLD-CARTS (Table 2.3) is useful to ensure all relevant aspects are considered.

The past medical history of an individual may have a strong influence on what is subsequently prescribed. For example, childhood illnesses such as measles, rubella and chickenpox may have left residual complaints and chronic ailments such as asthma or eczema will all have a bearing on the decision-making process. Likewise, in the adult a history of a medical disorder such as diabetes, hypertension or asthma is important, as

Table 2.3 OLDCARTS mnemonic for medical history taking

Onset: when did it start?

Location: where is it/what part of the body does it affect?

Duration: how long did (does) it last? How often does it occur?

Characteristics: what is it like, how bad is it? Can the context in which symptoms develop or get worse be established, such as environmental factors, personal activities, emotional reactions?

Associated signs and symptoms: does anything else accompany the problem such as headaches, aura, shaking, etc.?

Relieving or aggravating factors: does anything make it better or worse? What treatments have been tried already?

Summarize: repeat your understanding of the situation to ensure all necessary facts have been obtained.

Table 2.4 Issues the prescriber should reflect upon before prescribing a medicine (National Prescribing Centre 1998)

- What is the drug?
  - Is it novel?
  - Is it a line extension?

- What is the drug used for?
  - Licensed indications
  - Any restrictions on initiation
  - Does first line mean first choice?

- How effective is the drug?
  - Is there good evidence for efficacy?
  - How does it compare to existing drugs?

- How safe is the drug?
  - Are there published comparative safety data?
  - Has it been widely used in other countries?
  - Are the details contained in the SPC understood?
  - Are there clinically important drug interactions?
  - Are there monitoring requirements?
  - Can it be used long term?

- Who should not receive this drug?
  - Are there patients in whom it is contraindicated?

- Does the drug provide value for money?
  - Is there good evidence of cost-effectiveness compared to other available interventions?
  - What impact will this drug have on the healthcare budget?

- What is its place in therapy?
  - What advantages are there?
  - Are the benefits worth the cost?
  - Are there some patients that would particularly benefit?

is the date and nature of any surgery. For women an obstetric/gynaecological history that includes details of menstrual history and pregnancies is important. Details of psychiatric disorders with dates, associated hospitalizations and treatments are also essential.

Prescribing

Given all that has been stated above, it may be assumed that the eventual decision to prescribe is always based on the information gathered during the consultation. This has been shown not to be the case. The decision to prescribe may occur for a number of reasons including to:

- cure symptoms
- cure condition
- aid diagnosis
- legitimize the patient in the sick role
- avoid doing anything else
- maintain contact with the patient
- end the consultation.

Reassuringly, to cure symptoms, cure a condition or aid diagnosis are the most frequent reasons for issuing a prescription. The use of a prescription for other purposes, such as to legitimize the sick role is, however, not uncommon. In this particular scenario the issue of a prescription shows the patient that they did not waste the prescriber's time and they did have a condition worthy of diagnosis and treatment.

Medicine selection

When the point of selecting a medicine is reached it is necessary to reflect on the following (see also Table 2.4) before issuing the prescription.

- What is the evidence that the medicine to be prescribed will improve the symptoms or the condition?
- What are the effectiveness, risks and cost of the medicine?
- Are there any contraindications to its use?

- What is the optimal dose and duration of treatment?
- Has the impact of the relevant pathophysiology on the pharmacokinetics and pharmacodynamics of the medicine been taken into account?
- Is there a need for laboratory tests, regular monitoring and follow-up?
- Are there concordance or communication issues with the patient because of language, beliefs, etc.?

Medication review

The value of undertaking a medication review before re-prescribing medicines for long-term treatment is recognized and is an integral part of the prescribing process. The NO TEARS approach (Lewis 2004) is a useful prompt to assist such a review (Table 2.5) and its application is illustrated in Case 2.1.

Need and indication It is necessary to identify if the treatment is still indicated or whether the diagnosis has been confirmed or refuted. For example, an initial, tentative diagnosis of angina may have been subsequently disproved. Medicines may have been inappropriately continued or there may be a need to change the dose of a given drug. It is important to check that the patient

Table 2.5 The NO TEARS approach to medication review

Need and indication

Open questions

Tests and monitoring

Evidence and guidelines

Adverse effects

Risk reduction and prevention

Simplification and switches

knows what their medicines are for and can identify those which must be taken regularly. There is also a need to ensure that the indication for each drug is clearly recorded in the patient's medical notes.

Open questions The prescriber needs to identify what the patient understands about their treatment, and which medicines they are actually taking. Each prescriber will have their own way of asking such questions. It can be helpful to show the patient that the prescriber recognizes some of the drawbacks of therapy by asking questions such as 'I realize a lot of people don't take all their medicines, do you have any problems with any of your tablets?' or 'Can you tell me what you're taking regularly so that I can check that we agree?'.

Tests and monitoring The prescriber should explore whether the disease is under control and symptom relief adequate. Further tests may be required to assess disease control, and for drugs prescribed as part of shared care arrangements between hospital

---

Case 2.1 Application of the NO TEARS approach to medication review

Mr G is 78 years old and attends the clinic because he needs a prescription for three out of five of his repeat medicines and has increasing problems with peripheral oedema. He also suffers from hypertension and visual impairment, and had a hip replacement 6 months ago. He describes his medicines as 'paracetamol for knees, blood pressure tablets and sometimes a stomach tablet'. His blood pressure (BP) was 176/70 mmHg 3 months ago.

Mr G's normal monthly repeat medication is as follows:

Nifedipine   10 mg twice daily

Zoton®   30 mg once a day

Gauze   10 × 10 cm pieces

Paracetamol   500 mg as required

Tramadol   50 mg every 6 h

What aspects of his treatment should be reviewed?

Needs and indication

Mr G's spontaneous comments suggest he is no longer taking Tramadol. Was the dressing also used postoperatively and, if so, can it be removed from his medication list?

Why is Mr G taking a proton pump inhibitor (PPI) and why is he on a treatment dose rather than a maintenance dose?

Open questions

What does Mr G know about his stomach tablet?

Tests and monitoring

Disease monitoring

Does Mr G have adequate pain control?

Does he still get indigestion or abdominal pain?

Should the PPI dose be reduced?

Does he still have high systolic BP?

Blood monitoring

You do not know his blood cholesterol concentration. Should this be checked?

Evidence and guidelines

The PPI dose should be reduced to a maintenance dose after an initial treatment period. Is *H. pylori* eradication appropriate?

The antihypertensive regimen is not ideal as it is not providing adequate BP control and it could be exacerbating peripheral oedema. Thiazide diuretics can be helpful for isolated systolic hypertension and it may be worth considering using one here.

Adverse effects

Mr G complains of uncomfortable ankle swelling in the evenings. Is his peripheral oedema caused by his medication?

Case 2.1 (continued)

Risk reduction and prevention

It transpires that Mr G has trouble differentiating between his tablets because of visual difficulties. Other support agencies may need to be involved.

Simplification and switches

If nifedipine is to be continued, the regimen may be simplified. It could be changed from 10 mg twice daily to 20 mg once daily prescribed by brand name to avoid known product-to-product variation in serum profiles.

---

and primary care it may be necessary to check that monitoring is being undertaken in accordance with agreed protocols. If the patient routinely attends special clinics, e.g. for diabetes, it may be best to focus on other issues to avoid unnecessary duplication and make efficient use of time.

Evidence and guidelines Information on therapeutics is never static and it is useful to pause and reflect on new evidence and recent guidelines. There will be many patients given a diagnosis some years ago who are now on suboptimal treatment. For example, patients with presumed congestive heart failure may need an echocardiogram, dose optimization of an angiotensin converting enzyme (ACE) inhibitor and consideration of other preventive measures. A history of peptic ulcer might prompt *H. pylori* testing.

Adverse effects It is important to recognize when symptoms are the adverse effects of medication. For example, a patient with continuous cough may be spared many investigations if the possibility of ACE inhibitor-induced cough is considered. Related to this is the need to avoid creating a 'prescribing cascade' in which a medicine is prescribed to treat a condition caused by another medicine. The prescribing of an inhaler for wheeze in a patient on a β-blocker is a typical illustration of this.

Risk reduction and prevention If time allows, opportunistic screening for alcohol use, smoking, obesity or family history can be done during the medication review. It can be useful to identify a given patient's risks and establish whether medication is optimized to reduce these. For example, many elderly patients are at risk of falls and this may be exacerbated by medicine-induced postural hypotension.

Simplification and switches Some medication regimens are unnecessarily complicated with, for example, some medicines being given on two or three occasions each day when they could be taken once. Similarly, several low-dose preparations may be better replaced with one higher dose preparation.

Synchronizing treatments by prescribing medicines in quantities that require the patient to request repeat prescriptions for all medicines at the same time is practical and, importantly, reduces waste and may improve compliance.

Strategies to improve prescribing

A number of strategies have emerged to improve prescribing, including the use of formularies, the need to adhere to clinical guidelines, employment of prescribing advisors, use of incentive schemes, setting performance indicators and providing education and prescribing information for prescribers.

Formularies

There are many definitions of a formulary but most suggest that it is a restrictive list from which the medicines to be prescribed and reimbursed must be selected. Generally the medicines in a formulary are deemed to have met rational criteria based on clinical decisions and cost-effectiveness, although the inclusion criteria are not always explicit. Some formularies are developed to cover prescribing in both primary and hospital care but many apply to a single sector. The World Health Organization has set out an essential drug list and its formulary is used widely as a basis from which to create a local or national formulary.

Medicines and prescribing committees in both primary and hospital care can be used to manage the introduction of new medicines and monitor the implementation of formularies in medical practice. Where there is a joint formulary from which hospital doctors must also prescribe, and if this is adhered to, it has a significant influence on prescribing patterns in the area covered by the formulary.

In primary care within the UK formularies are advisory. Hospital formularies are generally more restrictive, with senior staff, such as medical consultants, being the only ones who can prescribe outside the formulary, if anyone is allowed to. Senior hospital staff can, however, normally ask for new drugs to be added to the formulary but this will only occur after evidence gathering and an appraisal of the medicine has been undertaken. Formularies are living documents and regular updating is essential to ensure they continue to meet clinical needs.

Guidelines

Guidelines for the use of a medicine, a group of medicines or the management of a clinical condition may be produced for local or national use.

Local guidelines are often produced to cover areas that are predominantly managed in primary care but where treatment is initiated in the hospital sector, for example the use of anticoagulants following a hospital inpatient episode or the monitoring of disease-modifying antirheumatic drugs (DMARDs) initiated by a specialist hospital clinic.

National guidelines such as those produced by the National Institute for Health and Clinical Excellence (NICE) are used to improve and standardize levels of care and implementation is mandatory.

Guidelines are not produced to replace the knowledge and skills of prescribers but should help to guide and support prescribing decisions. Computerized decision support systems also exist to support prescribers. PRODIGY, for example, has patient information leaflets, helps with differential diagnosis, suggests investigations and referral criteria and gives screens that can be shared between the patient and the prescriber in the surgery.

Prescribing advisors

Prescribing advisors based in primary care organizations and/or within practices are major stakeholders in the prescribing process. Their advice, which is based on current evidence, guidelines or policy, is typically offered at practice meetings. Advice can be followed up with support for specific issues such as use of a particular non-formulary or non-recommended medicine. Prescribing advisors working for a primary care organization and responsible for a given geographical area can sometimes offer financial rewards as an incentive to carry out audits to improve the cost-effective use of medicines. They may also be in a position to impose sanctions if advice is ignored.

The majority of prescribing advisors are pharmacists employed by primary care organizations although some are employed by individual medical practices. They often use techniques gleaned from the pharmaceutical industry such as targeting, information detailing or providing information in a format that is readily digestible and acceptable to prescribers.

Incentives

Incentive schemes to reward good prescribing or modify prescribing patterns may be utilized. The basic concept is that remuneration is offered when targets are achieved. For example, a medical practice might be expected to ensure all prescriptions are computer generated or they may be required to achieve a target level of generic prescribing. Other more sophisticated incentive schemes can have a general component with individualized practice targets. These additional refinements are only feasible where information about prescribing within a practice is readily available. The rewards offered need not be particularly high and usually target both improved quality and cost-effective prescribing.

Performance indicators

By using a set of parameters that in some way define good prescribing, prescribers can be measured against each other at either local or national level. Ideally the indicators used should be evidence based, utilize available data sources such as prescribing data and be both quality and cost orientated (Bateman et al 1996, Campbell et al 2000). Where an issue is specific to a locality, such as the high use of benzodiazepines, this can be incorporated into local indicator targets. The outcome of using indicators is that problematic prescribers can be identified and offered support to improve. Occasionally the problem prescriber may be prevented from receiving associated incentive payments although this decision can be reversed to reward improvements in prescribing that address the areas of concern.

Education

Although a range of educational initiatives is usually available for the prescriber to keep their knowledge up to date, a number may

be sponsored by the pharmaceutical industry. As a consequence attendance at meetings can be a valuable source of information but the influence of the sponsor or the selection of the speaker must not be accepted without question. Ideally all meetings would be organized by the local primary care organization, hospital trust or independent postgraduate education provider but the need to cover the costs of appropriate hospitality and pay speakers usually precludes their sole involvement, thereby opening the door for the involvement of the industry. It is incumbent on the prescriber, therefore, to reflect on the learning points from any educational meeting attended and evaluate whether the message was without bias and worthy of being implemented in day-to-day practice.

Medicines information

There is a perceived risk involved in prescribing any new or existing preparation for a new indication in a given patient. The preferred approach to minimize any risk is to increase the prescriber's knowledge about the new preparation or its use in the new indication. In most cases this involves information processing by reading and reviewing available literature.

National formularies provide healthcare professionals with sound up-to-date information about the use of medicines. Often they include key information about all medicines in use in the country of publication. They discuss drug selection, general notes on prescribing and drug administration. In the UK the British National Formulary (BNF) is supplied to all prescribers and updated every 6 months. It is also available on the web at www.bnf.org and is a valuable source for the key aspects of prescribing including: adverse reactions to drugs; prescribing for children and the elderly; drug interactions; drug use in liver and or kidney disease; drugs used in pregnancy and in breast feeding; intravenous additives; and dressings. Other valuable sources of information for the prescriber can be found on the PRODIGY (www.prodigy.nhs.uk), National Prescribing Centre (www.npc.co.uk) and NICE (www.nice.org.uk) websites.

Factors that influence the prescribing of new medicines

The decision to prescribe a newly marketed medicine does not occur in a vacuum, varies within and between prescribers and is influenced by internal and external factors.

Internal influences

Prescribers differ widely in practice, with some needing very little persuasion to prescribe a new medicine. Those that prescribe early are often classified as innovators or early adopters. This is a subjective term which implies that the prescriber is knowledgeable and up to date. Those that are last to prescribe have been called both laggards and drones, implying they are out of touch and ignoring progress. However, it is just as easy to suggest that the innovator takes too many risks with patients at a time when adverse drug reactions (ADRs) to the new medicines are not fully understood. Conversely, the laggard might be considered the better prescriber, watchfully studying the literature until more is known of the side effects and benefits of the new drug.

In general, prescribers appear more willing to adopt a new drug in a therapeutic class which has few alternatives than in an area where many products already exist and where the perceived risk in prescribing a new medicine is relatively high. A new drug which offers real advantages is taken on through a contagion effect as more information is made available and as more prescribers accept the product and pass on their favourable experiences to others. Preparations that are perceived to be less innovative or where a range of products is already available to treat the same indication take longer to be accepted.

Cognitive stages to prescribing

There are five theoretical cognitive stages (Rogers 2003) that a prescriber must go through before adopting a new drug: awareness, interest, evaluation, trial and adoption.

Awareness This stage marks the period when the prescriber becomes aware of the existence of the new drug and is usually a passive event on their part. The pharmaceutical manufacturer, particularly where an innovative new product is involved, is generally responsible for ensuring awareness is raised and this is usually in the guise of the company representative. This is accompanied by advertisements in the free medical press, professional journals, direct mailings, company-sponsored meetings and other promotional activities. This process has not been without criticism and it has been suggested there should be a reduction in the quantity of promotional material prescribers receive in the first 6 months after the launch of a new product (House of Commons Health Committee 2005). If this approach were adopted it would give more time for professional journals to publish evaluated information on which to base prescribing decisions. For those prescribers not receptive to information from the manufacturer, awareness may take longer and is often raised by colleagues or other professional sources of information.

Interest The second stage in the decision process involves interest. At this point the prescriber begins to ask questions as a perceived need for the product arises and the prescriber starts looking for further information. The prescriber may begin to place the new product, or even old drugs not prescribed before, into the context of their prescribing. If an individual prescriber has a special interest in the clinical area targeted by the new drug, this may invoke interest and a series of questions sooner than for a prescriber not specializing in that area.

Evaluation Evaluation is very closely related to interest and is often referred to as a patient-orientated mental trial. For example, a patient who has not been successfully treated with existing medication may be brought to mind and questions relating to the medicine are necessarily related to that individual. This may also happen when the licence of an existing drug is amended to broaden use to a new group of patients or new indication. Information from peers and colleagues may be sought but the personality or character of the prescriber may mean this stage is very short and dependent on the perceived level of risk associated with the new product. If the prescriber considers the benefits could outweigh the risks, and the perception of this will vary from prescriber to prescriber, then the product will move to the next stage.

Trial The patient who had been brought to mind in the evaluation phase may now be considered as a candidate for a trial of the new product. Routes of administration, dosages for different age groups, etc. will be actively sought. The Summary of Product Characteristics (SPC) may be looked at, and prescribing advisors or practice pharmacists used to obtain further information. The results of this small-scale trial will often determine the outcome of the adoption process.

Adoption Awareness of the new medicine, its evaluation and a successful trial must normally occur before the product becomes part of the prescriber's armamentarium. Some prescribers appear to go through all five stages in a very short time. If the initial outcome of prescribing the new medicine is favourable more prescriptions may follow. A poor outcome reduces the likelihood of this happening. However, even where initial use is successful, subsequent reading of professional, peer-reviewed articles and hospital-based opinion can influence whether the drug will be adopted long term (Prosser et al 2003).

The launch of cimetidine in 1976 serves as a good case history to illustrate the adoption of a new medicine. When first launched, it was a novel molecule and a true innovation. Precursor molecules such as burimamide had been insufficiently potent for oral administration whilst chemical modification had lead to the development of metiamide which, though effective, was associated with unacceptable nephrotoxicity and agranulocytosis. After further work on the molecule, cimetidine was developed. It may have been expected that, because previous molecules in the class had either been ineffective or caused serious problems, caution would have resulted in a slow uptake of cimetidine. However, prescriptions were issued in primary care within the first week of its launch. Within 3 weeks, doses had been amended by prescribers against the recommendations found in the SPC. It is obvious from this that these early prescribers had gone through all stages of the prescribing decision process and overcome any associated perceived risk with the information at their disposal. Whether this decision was entirely based on evidence or on an overconfident belief in the information and its interpretation is not recorded. It is of interest to speculate why this arose. Perhaps the medicine was believed to be an innovation and the risk/benefit was thought to be skewed towards the benefit.

External influences

Pharmaceutical industry

Previous experience of a drug's safety and adverse effect profile is a major influence on a prescriber's choice of medication although this may be tempered by what appears in professional journals and the media. Regardless of this, the pharmaceutical industry, and the pharmaceutical company representative in particular, continue to play a major role in influencing the prescribing of new branded products. One of the major criticisms of using the company representative as a significant source of information on which to base a prescribing decision is that there is rarely any objective discussion of available competitor products. The influence of the pharmaceutical industry is, however, far more diverse than the company representative. Sponsored meetings, direct or unsolicited literature sent to the prescriber, advertisements within medical journals or logos emblazoned on mugs, desk blotters, pens and other office paraphernalia are all part of the promotional armamentarium. Although most prescribers consider themselves sceptical and impervious to approaches from the industry, their influence should not be underrated.

Amongst the documents produced by the pharmaceutical industry when a new medicine is licensed is the SPC. This document is produced in agreement between the company marketing the medicine and the licensing authority. As such, the content cannot be changed except with the agreement of the licensing authority and is the basis of information for health professionals on how to use the medicinal product safely and effectively and is available online (www.medicines.org.uk) .

Colleagues

Colleagues may influence a prescriber to use a new medicine. In particular, senior hospital consultants have been shown to influence the prescribing patterns of prescribers in primary care, although some studies suggest this influence is not as great as might have been thought. The influence of a colleague is often considered only to be a secondary source of information, with its main effect at the evaluation stage of the prescribing process. However, a respected colleague's choice may influence others. Social integration in a primary care group practice may also lead to a tendency to conform to a norm of prescribing a particular medicine within that practice.

Pharmacists

In both hospital and primary care sectors, pharmacists have an influence on prescribing through their roles on wards or as part of their work for primary care organizations. Perhaps the most influential is the pharmacist who works within primary care and provides expert advice and guidance on medicines and their use to prescribers. Likewise specialist clinical and medicines information pharmacists in hospital have an influence on drug choice and patient management in that setting. In whichever sector the pharmacist works, they too need to be aware that their advice and decisions may be influenced by exactly the same factors as the prescriber.

Prescribing budgets

In the early 1990s research in the UK revealed that prescribers were unaware of the cost of the medicines they prescribed. This was thought to be due, in part, to the fact that they did not hold their own prescribing budget and all prescribing costs were met by an open-ended budget administered by a higher body. To overcome this and make prescribers cost sensitive, primary care practices were given their own prescribing budget. If they saved money from this budget they could keep the savings to spend on approved patient care items. If they overspent they could be withdrawn from the fundholding programme. This approach improved medical awareness of cost but raised fears that doctors would be reluctant to prescribe certain expensive medications when they may have been indicated.

Fundholding certainly raised awareness of the economics of prescribing but it came to an end with a change in government. Organizations within primary care again took over responsibility for managing and administering practice budgets.

The reintroduction of a contract for primary care clinicians and a move towards practice-based commissioning will again put some medical practitioners back in control of their prescribing budget. Prescribing data are routinely available to all practices to help them monitor what they are prescribing, in what quantity and at what cost.

In the past hospitals have been guilty of accepting loss leaders to help balance their prescribing budget. As part of this process, a manufacturer tenders an unrealistically low cost to get its product used by the hospital. Following discharge, the patient would be expected to continue on this same medication long term at a different and usually higher price in primary care. This practice has been eliminated mainly by secondary and primary care prescribers discussing these issues more fully and recognizing the adverse impact of this practice on the primary care budget.

Hospital

Working closely with the local hospital when new drugs are requested or when there is a change from one product in a group to another means that primary care prescribers can better manage their introduction. Contracts and tendering need to be open and transparent so implications of specific choices can be discussed. Consultants and those who lecture to primary care practitioners need to be sensitive to the issues around prescribing in the community and the reasons why companies are often willing to sponsor their presentations. More and more primary and secondary care prescribing committees are approving joint formularies where drugs are selected based on evidence and cost. Unfortunately, problems still arise because of the different types of patient seen in each sector. The more difficult to treat or serious conditions are dealt with in hospital. The patient then returns to primary care for continued treatment but with a drug or drug regimen that may not be familiar to the primary care prescriber.

Patient

Studies which have looked at the influence of patients on prescribing show outcomes which vary from country to country. Issues such as whether the patient expects a prescription or whether the prescriber thinks the patient expects a prescription both influence the decision to prescribe. Prescribers have been shown to overestimate when patients expect a prescription. They may then perpetuate the prescribing habit because of the perceived ongoing medical need for a prescription and a wish to maintain a good doctor–patient relationship. This therefore raises the question of whether prescribers should routinely ask patients if they expect a prescription.

Demands to prescribe may not always originate from the individual patient but from organizations supporting patient groups and national campaigns. Some groups receive substantial support from the pharmaceutical industry and campaign to increase access to medicines for their members.

Although direct advertising of medicines to patients is currently only allowed in the USA and New Zealand, there remain many objectors even in these countries. In the UK education for patients may be provided by the manufacturer through sponsored disease awareness campaigns. Some of these campaigns have tackled topics poorly dealt with in the past such as the management of urinary incontinence. Other campaigns, such as one to promote use of blood monitoring strips for frequent blood glucose monitoring in type 2 diabetes, have been suggested as inappropriate. As a consequence there have been calls to control the influence of companies on the production of disease awareness campaigns that impact on the patients, who then exert pressure on the prescriber.

ACKNOWLEDGEMENT

The helpful guidance of WeMeReC (www.wemerec.org) and Dr Tessa Lewis on the application of the NO TEARS approach and permission to reproduce their work is gratefully acknowledged.

REFERENCES

Barber N 1995 What constitutes good prescribing? British Medical Journal 310: 923-925

Bateman D N, Eccles M, Campbell M et al 1996 Setting standards of prescribing performance in primary care: use of a consensus group of general practitioners and application of standards to practices in the north of England. British Journal of General Practice 46: 20-25

Campbell S M, Cantrill J A, Roberts D 2000 Prescribing indicators for UK general practice: Delphi consultation study. British Medical Journal 321: 1-5

Fraser R C (ed) 1999 Clinical method: a general practice approach. Butterworth-Heinemann, Oxford

House of Commons Health Committee 2005 The influence of the pharmaceutical industry. Stationery Office, London

Lewis T 2004 Using the NO TEARS tool for medication review. British Medical Journal 329: 434

National Prescribing Centre 1998 Prescribing new drugs in general practice. MeReC Bulletin 9: 21-24

Prosser H, Almond S, Walley T 2003 Influences on GPs' decision to prescribe new drugs – the importance of who says what. Family Practice 20: 61-68

Rogers E M (ed) 2003 Diffusion of innovations. Simon and Schuster, London

Scott N C H, Davis RH 1979 The exceptional potential in each primary care consultation. Journal of the Royal College of General Practitioners 29:201

WHO 1987 The rational use of drugs. WHO, Geneva

FURTHER READING

Audit Commission 1994 A prescription for improvement: towards more rational prescribing in general practice. HMSO, London

Britten N, Stevenson F, Barry F et al 2000 Misunderstandings in prescribing decisions in general practice: qualitative study. British Medical Journal 320: 484-488

Britten N, Jenkins L, Barber L et al 2003 Developing a measure for the appropriateness of prescribing in general practice. Quality and Safety in Health Care 12: 246-250

Greenhalgh T, Gill P 1997 Pressure to prescribe. British Medical Journal 315: 1482-1483

Lewis D K, Robinson J, Wilkinson E 2003 Factors involved in deciding to start preventive treatment: qualitative study of clinicians' and lay people's attitudes. British Medical Journal 327: 1-6

Strickland-Hodge B, Jepson M H 1980 Usage of information sources by general practitioners. Journal of the Royal Society of Medicine 73: 857-862

Waller D G 2005 Rational prescribing: the principles of drug selection and assessment of efficacy. Clinical Medicine 5: 26-28

3 Practical pharmacokinetics

R. Fitzpatrick

Clinical pharmacokinetics may be defined as the study of the time course of the absorption, distribution, metabolism and excretion of drugs and their corresponding pharmacological response. In practice, pharmacokinetics makes it possible to model what may happen to a drug after it has been administered to a patient. Clearly, this science may be applied to a wide range of clinical situations, hence the term 'clinical pharmacokinetics'. However, no matter how elegant or precise the mathematical modelling, the relationship between concentration and effect must be established before pharmacokinetics will be of benefit to patients.

General applications

Clinical pharmacokinetics can be applied in daily practice for drugs with a low therapeutic index, even if drug level monitoring is not required.

Time to maximal response

By knowing the half-life of a drug, one may estimate the time to reach a steady state (Fig. 3.1), and thus when maximal therapeutic response is likely to occur, irrespective of whether drug level monitoring is needed.

Need for a loading dose

The same type of information can be used to determine whether a loading dose of a drug is necessary, since drugs with longer half-lives are more likely to require loading doses for acute treatment.

Dosage alterations

Clinical pharmacokinetics can be useful in determining dosage alteration if the route of elimination is impaired through end-organ failure (e.g. renal failure) or drug interaction. Using limited pharmacokinetic information such as the fraction excreted unchanged (f_e value), which can be found in most pharmacology textbooks, quantitative dosage changes can be estimated.

Choosing a formulation

An understanding of the pharmacokinetics of absorption may also be useful in evaluating the appropriateness of particular formulations of a drug in a patient.

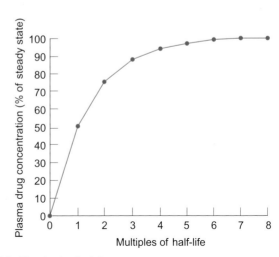

Fig 3.1 Time to steady state.

Application to therapeutic drug monitoring

Clinical pharmacokinetics is usually associated with TDM and its subsequent utilization. When TDM is used appropriately, it has been demonstrated that patients suffer fewer side effects than those who were not monitored (Reid et al 1990). Although TDM is a proxy outcome measure, a study with aminoglycosides (Crist et al 1987) demonstrated shorter hospital stays for patients where TDM was used. Furthermore, a study on the use of anticonvulsants (McFadyen et al 1990) showed better epilepsy control in those patients where TDM was used.

There are various levels of sophistication for the application of pharmacokinetics to TDM. Knowledge of the distribution time and an understanding of the concept of steady state can facilitate determination of appropriate sampling times.

For most drugs that undergo first-order elimination, a linear relationship exists between dose and concentration, which can be used for dose adjustment purposes. However, if the clearance of the drug changes as the concentration changes (e.g. phenytoin) then an understanding of the drug's pharmacokinetics will assist in correct dose adjustments.

More sophisticated application of pharmacokinetics involves the use of population pharmacokinetic data to produce initial dosage guidelines, for example nomograms for digoxin and gentamicin, and to predict drug levels. Pharmacokinetics can also assist in complex dosage individualization using actual patient-specific drug level data.

Given the wide range of clinical situations in which pharmacokinetics can be applied, pharmacists must have a good understanding of the subject and how to apply it in order to maximize their contribution to patient care.

Basic concepts

Volume of distribution

The apparent volume of distribution (V_d) may be defined as the size of a compartment which will account for the total amount of drug in the body (A) if it were present in the same concentration as in plasma. This means that it is the apparent volume of fluid in the body which results in the measured concentration of drug in plasma (C) for a known amount of drug given, i.e.

$$C = \frac{A}{V_d}$$

This relationship assumes that the drug is evenly distributed throughout the body in the same concentration as in the plasma. However, this is not the case in practice, since many drugs are present in different concentrations in various parts of the body. Thus, some drugs which concentrate in muscle tissue have a very large apparent volume of distribution, e.g. digoxin. This concept is better explained in Figure 3.2.

Apparent volume of distribution may be used to determine the plasma concentration after an intravenous loading dose:

$$C = \frac{\text{loading dose}}{V_d} \tag{1}$$

Conversely, if the desired concentration is known, the loading dose may be determined:

$$\text{loading dose} = \text{desired } C \times V_d \tag{2}$$

In the previous discussion, it has been assumed that after a given dose a drug is instantaneously distributed between the various tissues and plasma. In practice this is seldom the case. For practical purposes it is reasonable to generalize by referring to plasma as one compartment and tissue as if it were a single separate compartment. However, in reality there will be many tissue subcompartments. Thus, in pharmacokinetics the body may be described as if it were divided into two compartments: the plasma and the tissues.

Figure 3.3 depicts the disposition of a drug immediately after administration and relates this to the plasma concentration–time graph.

Initially, the plasma concentration falls rapidly, due to distribution and elimination (α phase). However, when an equilibrium is reached between the plasma and tissue (i.e. distribution is complete) the change in plasma concentration is only due to elimination from the plasma (β phase) and the plasma concentration falls at a slower rate. The drug is said to follow a two-compartment model. However, if distribution is completed quickly (within minutes), then the α phase is not seen and the drug is said to follow a one-compartment model.

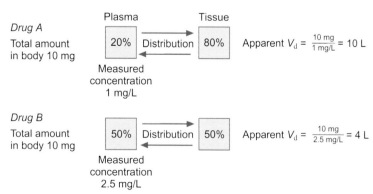

Fig 3.2 Distribution: more of drug A is distributed in the tissue compartment resulting in a higher apparent volume of distribution than drug B, where more remains in the plasma (assumes plasma volume = 2L).

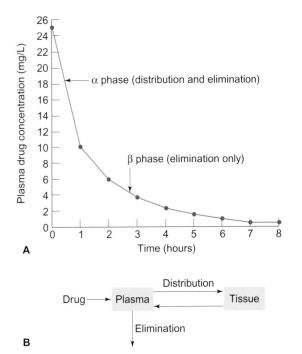

A

B

Fig 3.3 **A** Two-compartment model showing two phases in the plasma concentration–time profile. **B** Representation of a two-compartment model showing distribution of drug between plasma and tissue compartments.

The practical implications of a two-compartment model are that any sampling for monitoring purposes should be carried out after distribution is complete. In addition, intravenous bolus doses are given slowly to avoid transient side effects caused by high peak concentrations.

Elimination

Drugs may be eliminated from the body by a number of routes. The primary routes are excretion of the unchanged drug in the kidneys, or metabolism (usually in the liver) into a more water-soluble compound for subsequent excretion in the kidneys, or a combination of both.

The main pharmacokinetic parameter describing elimination is clearance (CL). This is defined as the volume of plasma completely emptied of drug per unit time. For example, if the concentration of a drug in a patient is 1 g/L and the clearance is 1 L/h, then the rate of elimination will be 1 g/h. Thus, a relationship exists:

$$\text{rate of elimination} = CL \times C \qquad (3)$$

Total body elimination is the sum of the metabolic rate of elimination and the renal rate of elimination. Therefore:

$$\text{total body clearance} = CL \text{ (metabolic)} + CL \text{ (renal)}$$

Thus, if the fraction eliminated by the renal route is known (f_e), then the effect of renal impairment on total body clearance can be estimated.

The clearance of most drugs remains constant for each individual. However, it may alter in cases of drug interactions, changing end-organ function, or autoinduction. Therefore, it is clear from equation (3) that as the plasma concentration changes so

will the rate of elimination. However, when the rate of administration is equal to the rate of elimination, the plasma concentration is constant (C^{ss}) and the drug is said to be at a steady state. At steady state:

$$\text{rate in} = \text{rate out}$$

At the beginning of a dosage regimen the plasma concentration is low. Therefore, the rate of elimination from equation (3) is less than the rate of administration, and accumulation occurs until a steady state is reached (see Fig. 3.1).

$$\text{rate of administration} = \text{rate of elimination} = CL \times C^{ss} \qquad (4)$$

It is clear from equation (3) that as the plasma concentration falls (e.g. on stopping treatment or after a single dose), the rate of elimination also falls. Therefore, the plasma concentration–time graph follows a non-linear curve characteristic of this type of first-order elimination (Fig. 3.4). This is profoundly different from a constant rate of elimination irrespective of plasma concentration, which is typical of zero-order elimination.

For drugs undergoing first-order elimination, there are two other useful pharmacokinetic parameters in addition to the volume of distribution and clearance. These are the elimination rate constant and elimination half-life.

The elimination rate constant (k_e) is the fraction of the amount of drug in the body (A) eliminated per unit time. For example, if the body contains 100 mg of a drug and 10% is eliminated per unit time, then $k_e = 0.1$. In the first unit of time, 0.1×100 mg or 10 mg is eliminated, leaving 90 mg. In the second unit of time, 0.1×90 mg or 9 mg is eliminated, leaving 81 mg. Elimination continues in this manner. Therefore:

$$\text{rate of elimination} = k_e \times A \qquad (5)$$

Combining equations (3) and (5) gives:

$$CL \times C = k_e \times A$$

and since:

$$C = \frac{A}{V_d}$$

then:

$$CL \times \frac{A}{V_d} = k_e \times A$$

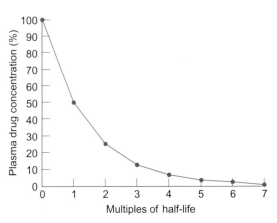

Fig 3.4 First-order elimination.

Therefore:

$$CL = k_e \times V_d \quad (6)$$

Elimination half-life ($t_{1/2}$) is the time it takes for the plasma concentration to decay by half. In five half-lives the plasma concentration will fall to approximately zero (see Fig. 3.4).

The equation which is described in Figure 3.4 is:

$$C_2 = C_1 \times e^{-k_e \times t} \quad (7)$$

where C_1 and C_2 are plasma concentrations and t is time.

If half-life is substituted for time in equation (7), C_2 must be half of C_1. Therefore:

$$0.5 \times C_1 = C_1 \times e^{-k_e \times t_{1/2}}$$

$$0.5 = e^{-k_e \times t_{1/2}}$$

$$\ln 0.5 = -k_e \times t_{1/2}$$

$$0.693 = -k_e \times t_{1/2}$$

$$t_{1/2} = \frac{0.693}{k_e}$$

There are two ways of determining k_e, either by estimating the half-life and applying equation (8) or by substituting two plasma concentrations in equation (7) and applying natural logarithms:

$$\ln C_2 = \ln C_1 - (k_e \times t)$$

$$k_e \times t = \ln C_1 - \ln C_2$$

$$k_e = \frac{\ln C_1 - \ln C_2}{t}$$

In the same way as it takes approximately five half-lives for the plasma concentration to decay to zero after a single dose, it takes approximately five half-lives for a drug to accumulate to the steady state on repeated dosing or during constant infusion (see Fig. 3.1).

This graph may be described by the equation:

$$C = C^{ss}[1 - e^{-k_e \times t}] \quad (9)$$

where C is the plasma concentration at time t after the start of the infusion, and C^{ss} is the steady-state plasma concentration. Thus, if the appropriate pharmacokinetic parameters are known, it is possible to estimate the plasma concentration any time after a single dose or the start of a dosage regimen.

Absorption

In the preceding sections, the intravenous route has been discussed and with this route all the administered drug is absorbed. However, if a drug is administered by any other route it must be absorbed into the bloodstream. This process may or may not be 100% efficient.

The fraction of the administered dose which is absorbed into the bloodstream is the bioavailability (F). Therefore when applying pharmacokinetics for oral administration the dose or rate of administration must be multiplied by F. Bioavailability F is determined by calculating the area under the concentration–time curve (AUC). The rationale for this is described below.

The rate of elimination of a drug after a single dose is given by equation (3). By definition the rate of elimination is amount of drug eliminated per unit time.

The amount eliminated in any one unit of time $dt = CL \times C \times dt$.

The total amount of drug eliminated $= {}^8_0\Sigma\, CL \times C \times dt$

As previously explained, CL is constant Therefore:

Total amount eliminated $= CL \times \Sigma\, C \times dt$ from start until C is zero

$\Sigma\, C \times dt$ from start until zero is actually the AUC (Fig. 3.5)

After a single i.v. dose the total amount eliminated is = the amount administered D i.v. Therefore:

$$D \text{ i.v.} = CL \times AUC \text{ i.v. or } CL = D \text{ i.v.}/AUC \text{ i.v.}$$

However, for an oral dose the amount administered is $F \times D$ p.o. As CL is constant in the same individual:

$$CL = F \times D \text{ p.o.}/AUC \text{ p.o.} = D \text{ i.v.}/AUC \text{ i.v.}$$

Rearranging gives:

$$F = \frac{D \text{ i.v.} \times AUC \text{ p.o.}}{D \text{ p.o.} \times AUC \text{ i.v.}}$$

In this way F can be calculated from plasma concentration time curves.

Dosing regimens

From the preceding sections, it is possible to derive equations which can be applied in clinical practice.

From equation (10) we can determine the change in plasma concentration ΔC immediately after a single dose:

$$\Delta C = \frac{S \times F \times \text{dose}}{V_d} \quad (10)$$

where F is bioavailability and S is the salt factor, which is the fraction of active drug when the dose is administered as a salt (e.g. aminophylline is 80% theophylline, therefore $S = 0.8$).

Conversely, to determine a loading dose:

$$\text{loading dose} = \frac{\text{desired change in } C \times V_d}{S \times F} \quad (11)$$

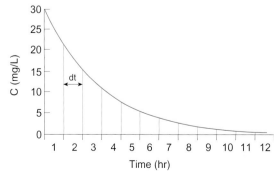

Fig 3.5 The AUC is the sum of $C \times dt$.

At the steady state it is possible to determine maintenance dose or steady-state plasma concentrations from a modified equation (4):

$$\text{rate in} = \frac{S \times F \times \text{dose}}{T} = CL \times \text{average } C^{ss} \quad (12)$$

where T is the dosing interval.

Peak and trough levels

For oral dosing and constant intravenous infusions, it is usually adequate to use the term 'average steady-state plasma concentration' (average C^{ss}). However, for some intravenous bolus injections it is sometimes necessary to determine peak and trough levels (e.g. gentamicin).

At the steady state, the change in concentration due to the administration of an intravenous dose will be equal to the change in concentration due to elimination over one dose interval:

$$\Delta C = \frac{S \times F \times \text{dose}}{V_d} = C_{max} - C_{min}$$

Within one dosing interval the maximum plasma concentration (C^{ss}_{max}) will decay to the minimum plasma concentration (C^{ss}_{min}) as in any first-order process.

Substituting C^{ss}_{max} for C_1 and C^{ss}_{min} for C_2 in equation (7):

$$C^{ss}_{min} = C^{ss}_{max} \times e^{-k_e \times t}$$

where t is the dosing interval. If this is substituted into the preceding equation:

$$\frac{S \times F \times \text{dose}}{V_d} = C^{ss}_{max} - C^{ss}_{max} \times e^{-k_e \times t}$$

Therefore:

$$C^{ss}_{max} = \frac{S \times F \times \text{dose}}{V_d [1 - e^{-k_e \times t}]} \quad (13)$$

$$C^{ss}_{min} = \frac{S \times F \times \text{dose}}{V_d [1 - e^{-k_e \times t}]} \times e^{-k_e \times t} \quad (14)$$

Interpretation of drug concentration data

The availability of the technology to measure the concentration of a drug in serum should not be the reason for monitoring. There are a number of criteria that should be fulfilled before therapeutic drug monitoring is undertaken:

• the drug should have a low therapeutic index
• there should be a good concentration–response relationship
• there are no easily measurable physiological parameters.

In the absence of these criteria being fulfilled, the only other justification for undertaking TDM is to monitor compliance or to confirm toxicity. When interpreting TDM data a number of factors need to be considered.

Sampling times

In the preceding sections, the time to reach the steady state has been discussed. When TDM is carried out as an aid to dose adjustment, the concentration should be at the steady state. Therefore, approximately five half-lives should elapse after initiation or changing a maintenance regimen, before sampling.

The only exception to this rule is when toxicity is suspected. When the steady state has been reached, it is important to sample at the correct time. It is clear from the discussion above that this should be done when distribution is complete (see Fig. 3.3).

Dosage adjustment

Under most circumstances, providing the preceding criteria are observed, adjusting the dose of a drug is relatively simple, since a linear relationship exists between the dose and concentration if a drug follows first-order elimination (Fig. 3.6A). This is the case for most drugs.

Capacity-limited clearance

If a drug is eliminated by the liver, it is possible for the metabolic pathway to become saturated, since it is an enzymatic system. Initially the elimination is first order but once saturation of the system occurs, elimination becomes zero order. This results in the characteristic dose–concentration graph of Figure 3.6B. For the majority of drugs eliminated by the liver, this effect is not seen at normal therapeutic doses and only occurs at very high supratherapeutic levels, which is why the kinetics of some drugs in overdose is different from normal. However, one important exception is phenytoin, where saturation of the enzymatic pathway occurs at therapeutic doses. This will be dealt with in the section on phenytoin.

Increasing clearance

The only other situation in which first-order elimination is not seen is where clearance increases as the plasma concentration increases (Fig. 3.6C). Under normal circumstances, the plasma protein binding sites available to a drug far outnumber the capacity of the drug to fill those binding sites, and the proportion of the total concentration of drug which is protein bound is constant. However, this situation is not seen in one or two instances (e.g. valproate and disopyramide). For these particular drugs, as the concentration increases the plasma protein binding sites become saturated, and the ratio of unbound drug to bound drug increases. The elimination of these drugs increases disproportionately to

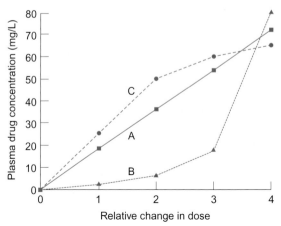

Fig 3.6 Dose–concentration relationships. **A** First-order elimination. **B** Capacity-limited clearance. **C** Increasing clearance.

the total concentration, since elimination is dependent on the unbound concentration.

Therapeutic range

Wherever TDM is carried out, a therapeutic range is usually used as a guide to the optimum concentration. The limits of these ranges should not be taken as absolute. Some patients may respond to levels above or below these ranges, whereas others may experience toxic effects within the so-called therapeutic range. These ranges are only adjuncts to dose determination, which should always be undertaken in the light of clinical response.

Clinical applications

Estimation of creatinine clearance

Since many drugs are renally excreted, and the most practical marker of renal function is creatinine clearance, it is often necessary to estimate this in order to undertake dosage adjustment in renal impairment. The usual method is to undertake a 24-hour urine collection coupled with a serum creatinine measurement. The laboratory then estimates the patient's creatinine clearance. The formula used to determine creatinine clearance is based upon the pharmacokinetic principles in equation (3).

The rate of elimination is calculated from the measurement of the total amount of creatinine contained in the 24-hour urine sample divided by 24:

$$\frac{\text{amount of creatinine}}{24} = \text{rate of excretion (mg/h)}$$

Using this rate of excretion and substituting the measured serum creatinine for C^{ss} in equation (4), the creatinine clearance can be calculated.

However, there are practical difficulties with this method. The whole process is cumbersome and there is an inevitable delay in obtaining a result. The biggest problem is the inaccuracy of the 24-hour urine collection.

An alternative approach is to estimate the rate of production of creatinine (i.e. rate in) instead of the rate of elimination (rate out). Clearly this has advantages, since it does not involve 24-hour urine collections and requires only a single measure of serum creatinine. There are data in the literature relating creatinine production to age, weight and sex, since the primary source of creatinine is the breakdown of muscle. Therefore, equations have been produced which are rearrangements of equation (4), i.e.:

$$\text{creatinine clearance} = \frac{\text{rate of production}}{C^{ss}}$$

Rate of production is replaced by a formula which estimates this from physiological parameters of age, weight and sex.

The equation produced by Cockcroft & Gault (1976) has traditionally been used to measure creatinine clearance. A modified version using SI units is shown below:

$$\frac{\text{creatinine clearance}}{\text{(mL/min)}} = \frac{F \times [(140 - \text{age in years}) \times \text{weight (kg)}]}{\text{serum creatinine (µmol/L)}}$$

where $F = 1.04$ (females) or 1.23 (males).

However, there are limitations using only serum creatinine to estimate renal function. The Modification of Diet in Renal Disease (MDRD) formula is now routinely used to estimate glomerular filtration rate (eGFR). This formula uses serum creatinine, age, sex and ethnicity (DH 2006).

$$eGFR = 175 \times [\text{serum creatinine (µmol/L)} \times 0.011312]^{-1.154} \\ \times [\text{age in years}]^{-0.203} \times [1.212 \text{ if patient is black}] \\ \times [0.742 \text{ if female}]$$

eGFR = glomerular filtration rate (mL/min per 1.73 m²)

Digoxin

Action and uses

Digoxin is the most widely used of the digitalis glycosides. Its primary actions on the heart are increasing the force of contraction and decreasing conduction through the atrioventricular node. Currently, its main role is in the treatment of atrial fibrillation by slowing down the ventricular response although it is also used in the treatment of heart failure in the presence of sinus rhythm. The primary method of monitoring its clinical effect in atrial fibrillation is by measurement of heart rate but knowledge of its pharmacokinetics can be helpful in predicting a patient's dosage requirements.

Serum concentration–response relationship

- <0.5 µg/L: no clinical effect
- 0.7 µg/L: some positive inotropic and conduction blocking effects
- 0.8–2 µg/L: optimum therapeutic range
- 2–2.5 µg/L: increased risk of toxicity, although tolerated in some patients
- >2.5 µg/L: gastrointestinal, cardiovascular system and central nervous system toxicity

Distribution

Digoxin is widely distributed and extensively bound in varying degrees to tissues throughout the body. This results in a high apparent volume of distribution. Digoxin volume of distribution can be estimated using the equation 7.3 L/kg (lean body weight (BWt)) which is derived from population data. However, distribution is altered in patients with renal impairment, and a more accurate estimate in these patients is given by:

$$V_d = 3.8 \times \text{lean BWt} + (3.1 \times \text{creatinine clearance (mL/min)})$$

A two-compartment model best describes digoxin disposition (see Fig. 3.3) with a distribution time of 6–8 hours. Clinical effects are seen earlier after intravenous doses, since the myocardium has a high blood perfusion and affinity for digoxin. Sampling for TDM must be done no sooner than 6 hours post dose, otherwise an erroneous result will be obtained.

Elimination

Digoxin is eliminated primarily by renal excretion of unchanged drug (60–80%), but some hepatic metabolism occurs (20–40%).

The population average value for digoxin clearance is:

$$\text{digoxin clearance (mL/min)} = 0.8 \times \text{BWt} + \\ (\text{creatinine clearance (mL/min)})$$

However, patients with severe congestive heart failure have a reduced hepatic metabolism and a slight reduction in renal excretion of digoxin:

$$\text{digoxin clearance (mL/min)} = 0.33 \times \text{BWt} + \\ (0.9 \times \text{clearance (mL/min)})$$

Lean body weight should be used in these equations.

Absorption

Digoxin is poorly absorbed from the gastrointestinal tract and dissolution time affects the overall bioavailability. The two oral formulations of digoxin have different bioavailabilities:

F (tablets) = 0.65
F (liquid) = 0.8

Practical implications

Using population averages it is possible to predict serum concentrations from specific dosages, particularly since the time to reach the steady state is long. Population values are only averages and individuals may vary. In addition, a number of diseases and drugs affect digoxin disposition.

As can be seen from the preceding discussion, congestive heart failure, hepatic and renal disease all decrease the elimination of digoxin. In addition, hypothyroidism increases the serum concentration (decreased metabolism and renal excretion) and increases the sensitivity of the heart to digoxin. Hyperthyroidism has the opposite effect. Hypokalaemia, hypercalcaemia, hypomagnesaemia and hypoxia all increase the sensitivity of the heart to digoxin. There are numerous drug interactions reported of varying clinical significance. The usual cause is either altered absorption or clearance.

Theophylline

Theophylline is an alkaloid related to caffeine. It has a variety of clinical effects including mild diuresis, central nervous system stimulation, cerebrovascular vasodilation, increased cardiac output and bronchodilation. It is the latter which is the major therapeutic effect of theophylline. Theophylline does have some serious toxic effects but there is a good serum concentration–response relationship.

Serum concentration–response relationship

- <5 mg/L: no bronchodilation*
- 5–10 mg/L: some bronchodilation and possible anti-inflammatory action
- 10–20 mg/L: optimum bronchodilation, minimum side effects
- 20–30 mg/L: increased incidence of nausea, vomiting** and cardiac arrhythmias
- >30 mg/L: cardiac arrhythmias, seizures

Distribution

Theophylline is extensively distributed throughout the body, with an average volume of distribution based on population data of 0.48 L/kg.

Theophylline does not distribute very well into fat and estimations should be based on lean body weight. A two-compartment model best describes theophylline disposition, with a distribution time of approximately 40 minutes.

Elimination

Elimination is a first-order process primarily by hepatic metabolism to relatively inactive metabolites.

The population average for theophylline clearance is 0.04 L/h/kg, but this is affected by a number of diseases/drugs/pollutants. Therefore, this value should be multiplied by:

- 0.5 where there is cirrhosis, or when cimetidine, erythromycin or ciprofloxacin is being taken concurrently
- 0.4 where there is congestive heart failure with hepatomegaly
- 0.8 where there is severe respiratory obstruction (FEV_1 <1 L)
- 1.6 in patients who smoke (defined as more than 10 cigarettes per day), since they metabolize theophylline more quickly.

Neonates metabolize theophylline differently, with 50% being converted to caffeine. Therefore, when it is used to treat neonatal apnoea of prematurity a lower therapeutic range is used (usually 5–10 mg/L), since caffeine contributes to the therapeutic response.

Product formulation

Aminophylline (the ethylenediamine salt of theophylline) is only 80% theophylline. Therefore, the salt factor (S) is 0.8. Most sustained-release (SR) preparations show good bioavailability but not all SR preparations are the same.

Practical implications

Intravenous bolus doses of aminophylline need to be given slowly (preferably by short infusion) to avoid side effects due to transiently high blood levels during the distribution phase. Oral doses with slow-release preparations can be estimated using population average pharmacokinetic values and titrated proportionately according to blood levels and clinical response. In most circumstances, the available modified-release preparations may be assumed to provide 12 hours' cover. However, more marked peaks and troughs are seen with fast metabolizers (smokers and children) and an increase in dose or frequency of administration may be required.

*Some patients exhibit a clinical effect at these levels which has been attributed to possible anti-inflammatory effects.

** Nausea and vomiting can occur within the therapeutic range.

Gentamicin

Clinical use

The spectrum of activity of gentamicin is similar to other aminoglycosides but its most significant activity is against *Psuedomonas aeruginosa*. It is still regarded by many as first choice for this type of infection.

Therapeutic range

Gentamicin has a low therapeutic index, producing dose-related side effects of nephro- and ototoxicity. The use of TDM to aid dose adjustment is essential if these toxic effects, which appear to be related to peak and trough serum levels, are to be avoided. It is generally accepted that the peak level (drawn 1 hour post dose after an intravenous bolus or intramuscular injection) should not exceed 12 mg/L and the trough level (drawn immediately pre-dose) should not exceed 2 mg/L.

The above recommendations relate to multiple-daily dosing of gentamicin. If once-daily dosing is used, then different monitoring and interpretation parameters apply as described at the end of this section.

Distribution

Gentamicin is relatively polar and distributes primarily into extracellular fluid. Thus, the apparent volume of distribution is only 0.25 L/kg. Gentamicin follows a two-compartment model with distribution being complete within 1 hour.

Elimination

Elimination is by renal excretion of the unchanged drug. Gentamicin clearance is approximately equal to creatinine clearance.

Practical implications

Since the therapeutic range is based on peak (1 hour post dose to allow for distribution) and trough (pre-dose) concentrations, it is necessary to be able to predict these from any given dosage regimen.

Initial dosage This may be based on the patient's physiological parameters. Gentamicin clearance may be determined directly from creatinine clearance. The volume of distribution may be determined from lean body weight. The elimination constant k_e may then be estimated using these parameters in equation (6). By substituting k_e and the desired peak and trough levels into equation (7), the optimum dosage interval can be determined (add on 1 hour to this value to account for sampling time). Using this value (or the nearest practical value) and the desired peak or trough value substituted into equations (13) or (14), it is possible to determine the appropriate dose.

Changing dosage This is not as straightforward as for theophylline or digoxin, since increasing the dose will increase the peak and trough levels proportionately. If this is not desired, then use of pharmacokinetic equations is necessary. By substituting the measured peak and trough levels and the time between them into equation (7), it is possible to determine k_e (and the

half-life from equation (8) if required). To estimate the patient's volume of distribution from actual blood level data, it is necessary to know the C^{ss}_{max} immediately after the dose (time zero), not the 1 hour value which is measured. To obtain this, equation (7) may be used, this time substituting the trough level for C_2 and solving for C_1. Subtracting the trough level from this C^{ss}_{max} at time zero, the volume of distribution may be determined from equation (10). Using these values for k_e and V_d, derived from actual blood level data, a new dose and dose interval can be determined as before.

Once-daily dosing There are theoretical arguments for once-daily dosing of gentamicin, since aminoglycosides display concentration-dependent bacterial killing, and a high enough concentration to minimum inhibitory concentration (MIC) ratio may not be achieved with multiple dosing. Furthermore, aminoglycosides have a long postantibiotic effect. Aminoglycosides also accumulate in the kidneys, and once-daily dosing could reduce renal tissue accumulation.

There have been a number of clinical trials comparing once-daily administration of aminoglycosides with conventional administration. A small number of these trials have shown less nephrotoxicity, no difference in ototoxicity, and similar efficacy with once-daily administration. Initial dosage for a once-daily regimen is 5–7 mg/kg/day for patients with a creatinine clearance of >60 mL/min. This is subsequently adjusted on the basis of blood levels. However, monitoring of once-daily dosing of gentamicin is different from that of multiple dosing. One approach is to take a blood sample 6–14 hours after the first dose and plot the time and result on a standard concentration–time plot (the Hartford nomogram, Nicolau et al 1995; Fig. 3.7). The position of the individual patient's point in relation to standard lines on the nomogram indicates what the most appropriate dose interval should be (24, 36 or 48 hours). Once-daily dosing of gentamicin has not been well studied in children, pregnant or breast-feeding women, patients with major burns, renal failure, endocarditis or cystic fibrosis. Therefore, it cannot be recommended in these groups and multiple-daily dosing should be used.

Lithium

Lithium is effective in the treatment of acute mania and in the prophylaxis of manic depression. The mechanism of action is not fully understood but it is thought that it may substitute for sodium or potassium in the central nervous system. Lithium is toxic, producing dose-dependent and dose-independent side effects. Therefore, TDM is essential in assisting in the management of the dosage.

Dose-dependent effects

The serum concentration–response relationship derived on the basis of the 12-hour standardized lithium level (measured 12 hours after the evening dose of lithium) is shown below:

- <0.4 mmol/L: little therapeutic effect
- 0.4–1.0 mmol/L: optimum range for prophylaxis
- 0.8–1.2 mmol/L: optimum range for acute mania
- 1.2–1.5 mmol/L: causes possible renal impairment

If result available within 24 h
- Use graph below to select dose interval. Use serum concentration and time interval between start of infusion and sample to plot intercept (see example given on graph).
- Give next dose (7 mg/kg by infusion as above) after interval indicated by graph.
  If result falls above upper limit for Q48 h, abandon once daily regimen. Measure gentamicin concentration after another 24 h and adopt multiple daily dose regimen if result <2 mg/L
  If result falls on Q24 h sector it is not necessary to recheck gentamicin concentration within 5 days unless patient's condition suggests renal function may be compromised.

- **Graph:** Use values of plasma concentration and time interval to find intercept
  (Example given of 6 mg/L after 10 h yields dose interval of 36 h)

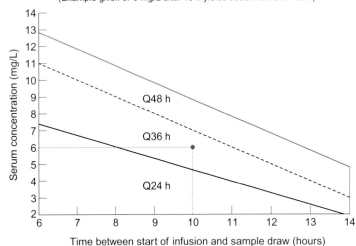

MONITORING
- Repeat U&E daily. Calculate creatinine clearance from serum creatinine to check dose interval has not changed.
- If dose interval has to be changed, check gentamicin concentration 6–14 h after start of next infusion note time of start of infusion and time of sampling and use graph to verify correct dose interval.

Fig 3.7 Nomogram for adjustment of once-daily gentamicin dosage (Nicolau et al 1995).

- 1.5–3.0 mmol/L: causes renal impairment, ataxia, weakness, drowsiness, thirst, diarrhoea
- 3.0–5.0 mmol/L: causes confusion, spasticity, dehydration, convulsions, coma, death (levels above 3.5 mmol/L are regarded as a medical emergency)

Dose-independent effects

These include tremor, hypothyroidism (approximately 10% of patients on chronic therapy), nephrogenic diabetes insipidus, gastrointestinal upset, loss in bone density, weight gain (approximately 20% of patients gain more than 10 kg) and lethargy.

Distribution

Lithium is unevenly distributed throughout the body, with a volume of distribution of approximately 0.5–1 L/kg. Lithium follows a two-compartment model (see Fig. 3.3) with a distribution time of 8 hours (hence, 12-hour sampling criterion).

Elimination

Lithium is excreted unchanged by the kidneys. Lithium clearance is approximately 20% of creatinine clearance, since there is extensive reabsorption in the renal tubules.

In addition to changes in renal function, dehydration, diuretics (particularly thiazides), angiotensin-converting enzyme (ACE) inhibitors and non-steroidal anti-inflammatory drugs (NSAIDs) (except aspirin and sulindac) all decrease lithium clearance. Conversely, aminophylline and sodium loading increase lithium clearance.

Notwithstanding the above factors, there is a wide interindividual variation in clearance and the lithium half-life in the population varies between 8 and 35 hours, with an average of approximately 18 hours. Lithium clearance shows a diurnal variation, being slower at night than during the day.

Practical implications

In view of the narrow therapeutic index, lithium should not be prescribed unless facilities for monitoring serum lithium concentrations are available. Since lithium excretion is a first-order process, changes in dosage result in a proportional change in blood levels. Blood samples should be drawn 12 hours after the evening dose, since this will allow for distribution and represent the slowest excretion rate. Population pharmacokinetic data (particularly the volume of distribution) cannot be relied upon to make initial dosage predictions, although renal function may give an approximate guide to clearance. Blood level measurements are reported in SI units and therefore it is useful to know the conversion factors for the various salts.

- 100 mg of lithium carbonate is equivalent to 2.7 mmol of lithium ions
- 100 mg of lithium citrate is equivalent to 1.1 mmol of lithium ions

Phenytoin

Phenytoin is effective in the treatment of generalized tonic–clonic and partial seizures. It is associated with dose-independent side effects which include hirsutism, acne, coarsening of facial features, gingival hyperplasia, hypocalcaemia and folic acid deficiency. However, phenytoin has a narrow therapeutic index and has serious concentration-related side effects.

Serum concentration–response relationship

- <5 mg/L: generally no therapeutic effect
- 5–10 mg/L: some anticonvulsant action
- 10–20 mg/L: optimum concentration for anticonvulsant effect
- 20–30 mg/L: nystagmus, blurred vision
- >30 mg/L: ataxia, dysarthria, drowsiness, coma

Distribution

Phenytoin follows a two-compartment model with a distribution time of 30–60 minutes. The apparent volume of distribution is 1 L/kg.

Elimination

The main route of elimination is via hepatic metabolism. However, this metabolic route can be saturated at normal therapeutic doses. This results in the characteristic non-linear dose–concentration curve seen in Figure 3.6B. Therefore, instead of the usual first-order pharmacokinetic model, a Michaelis-Menten model, used to describe enzyme activity, is more appropriate. Using this model, the daily dosage of phenytoin can be described by:

$$\frac{S \times F \times dose}{T} = \frac{V_{max}\, C^{ss}}{K_m + C^{ss}} \qquad (15)$$

K_m is the serum concentration at which metabolism proceeds at half the maximal rate. The population average for this is 6 mg/L, although this value varies greatly with age and race.

V_{max} is the maximum rate of metabolism of phenytoin and is more predictable, at approximately 7 mg/kg/day.

Elimination half-life

Since clearance changes with blood concentration, the half-life also changes. The usual reported value is 22 hours but this increases as concentration increases. Therefore, it is difficult to predict when the steady state will be reached; however, as a rule of thumb, 1–2 weeks should be allowed to elapse before sampling after a dosage change.

In overdose, it can be assumed that metabolism of the drug is occurring at the maximum rate of V_{max}. Therefore, the decline in serum concentration is linear (zero order) at approximately 7 mg/L/day.

Practical applications

Since the dose–concentration relationship is non-linear, changes in dose do not result in proportional changes in serum concentration (see Fig. 3.6B). Using the Michaelis-Menten model, if the serum concentration is known at one dosage, then V_{max} may be assumed to be the population average (7 mg/kg/day), since this is the more predictable parameter, and K_m calculated using equation (15). The revised values of K_m can then be used in equation (15) to estimate the new dosage required to produce a desired concentration. Alternatively, a nomogram may be used to assist in dose adjustments (Fig. 3.8).

Care is needed when interpreting TDM data and making dosage adjustments when phenytoin is given concurrently with other anticonvulsants, since these affect distribution and metabolism of phenytoin. Since phenytoin is approximately 90% protein bound, hypoalbuminaemia and renal failure will affect this, and care is needed when estimating doses in these clinical situations.

The oral formulations of phenytoin show good bioavailability. However, tablets and capsules contain the sodium salt ($S = 0.9$), whereas the suspension is phenytoin base ($S = 1$). Intramuscular phenytoin is slowly and unpredictably absorbed, due to crystallization in the muscle tissue, and is therefore not

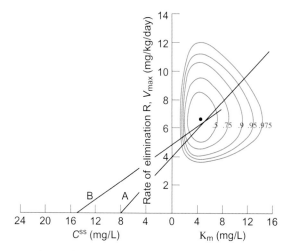

Fig 3.8 Orbit graph. The most probable values of V_{max} and k_m for a patient may be estimated using a single steady-state phenytoin concentration and a known dosing regimen. The eccentric circles or 'orbits' represent the fraction of the sample patient population whose k_m and V_{max} values are within that orbit. (1) Plot the daily dose of phenytoin (mg/kg/day) on the vertical line (rate of elimination). (2) Plot the steady-state concentration (C^{ss}) on the horizontal line. (3) Draw a straight line connecting C^{ss} and daily dose through the orbits (line A). (4) The co-ordinates of the midpoint of the line crossing the innermost orbit through which the line passes are the most probable values for the patient's V_{max} and k_m. (5) To calculate a new maintenance dose, draw a line from the point determined in Step 4 to the new desired C^{ss} (line B). The point at which line B crosses the vertical line (rate of elimination) is the new maintenance dose (mg/kg/day). The line A represents a C^{ss} of 8 mg/L on 276 mg/day of phenytoin acid (300 mg/day of sodium phenytoin) for a 70 kg patient. Line B has been drawn assuming the new desired steady-state concentration was 15 mg/L (μg/mL). The original figure is modified so that R and V_{max} are in mg/kg/day of phenytoin acid (modified from Evans et al 1992).

recommended. Fosphenytoin, a pro-drug of phenytoin, is better absorbed from the intramuscular site. Doses should be expressed as phenytoin equivalent. Fosphenytoin sodium 1.5 mg is equivalent to phenytoin sodium 1 mg.

Carbamazepine

Carbamazepine is a drug of choice for simple and complex partial seizures, and for tonic–clonic seizures secondary to a focal discharge. There are a number of dose-independent side effects, including various dermatological reactions and, more rarely, aplastic anaemia and the Stevens–Johnson syndrome. However, the more common side effects are concentration related.

Serum concentration–response relationship

- <4 mg/L: little therapeutic benefit
- 4–12 mg/L: optimum therapeutic range for monotherapy
- >9 mg/L: possible side effects of nystagmus, diplopia, drowsiness and ataxia, particularly if patients are on other anticonvulsant therapy
- >12 mg/L: side effects common, even on monotherapy

Distribution

Carbamazepine is distributed widely in various organs, with the highest concentration found in liver and kidneys. It is 70–80% protein bound and shows a wide variation in the population average apparent volume of distribution (0.8–1.9 L/kg). This wide variation is thought to be due to variations in absorption (since there is no parenteral form) and protein binding.

Elimination

Carbamazepine is eliminated almost exclusively by metabolism, with less than 2% being excreted unchanged in the urine. Elimination is a first-order process but carbamazepine induces its own metabolism. Therefore, at the beginning of therapy, clearance is 0.01–0.03 L/h/kg, rising to 0.05–0.1 L/h/kg on chronic therapy. Autoinduction begins in the first few days of commencing therapy and is maximal at 2–4 weeks.

Since clearance changes with time, so does half-life, with reported values as long as 35 hours after a single dose, decreasing to 5–7 hours on regular dosing.

Absorption

Absorption after oral administration is slow, with peak concentrations being reached 2–24 hours post dose (average 6 hours). Absorption is incomplete, with bioavailability estimated at approximately 80% ($F = 0.8$).

Practical implications

Use of pharmacokinetic equations is limited, due to the autoinduction effect. However, there are a number of important practical points.

- Blood samples should not be drawn before steady state, which will not be achieved until 2–4 weeks after starting therapy or 3–4 days after subsequent dose adjustments.
- When sampling, the trough level should be measured because of the variable absorption pattern.
- Complex calculations are not helpful but as a rule of thumb, each 100 mg dose will increase the plasma concentration at the steady state by approximately 1 mg/L in adults.
- A number of other drugs (including phenytoin) when given concurrently will affect carbamazepine metabolism and subsequent blood levels.

Phenobarbital

Phenobarbital is effective in the treatment of tonic–clonic and partial seizures, and is also useful in the treatment of febrile seizures. Although there is a clear concentration–response relationship, routine serum concentration monitoring is less useful than for other drugs, since tolerance occurs.

Serum concentration–response relationship

- <15 mg/L: little therapeutic effect
- 15–40 mg/L: optimum range
- 40–50 mg/L: sedation, confusion (elderly), although may be tolerated by some patients
- >60 mg/L: serious toxic effects of ataxia, lethargy, stupor, coma

The sedation which commonly manifests early on in therapy becomes less with continued treatment.

Distribution

Phenobarbital readily distributes into most body tissues and is 50% protein bound. The population average volume of distribution is 0.7–1 L/kg.

Elimination

Phenobarbital is primarily (80%) metabolized by the liver, with approximately 20% being excreted unchanged in the urine. Elimination is a first-order process but is relatively slow, with a population average clearance of approximately 0.004 L/h/kg. However, as with theophylline, clearance in children is increased. In the case of phenobarbital, the adult clearance value is doubled in children. Applying equations (6) and (8) to these population values gives an estimate of the half-life of the order of 5 days. This is much shorter in children and longer in the elderly.

Practical application

In view of the long half-life, single daily dosage is possible with phenobarbital. Samples for therapeutic monitoring may be drawn any time during a dose interval, since concentration fluctuation between doses is minimal. However, the patient should be at steady state, which takes 2–4 weeks (1–2 weeks in children). The pharmacokinetics of phenobarbital may be altered by liver and (less markedly) renal disease, but is not affected by the concurrent administration of other anticonvulsants.

Primidone

Like phenobarbital, primidone is effective in the treatment of tonic–clonic and partial seizures. Much of the anticonvulsant activity of primidone is due to the metabolites phenobarbital and phenylethylmalonamide. Therefore, primidone serum concentrations are only useful to confirm transient toxicity. Toxic manifestations such as sedation, nausea and ataxia are seen at concentrations greater than 15 mg/L. The plasma concentration should be drawn approximately 3 hours post dose, which corresponds to the peak concentration.

Phenylethylmalonamide assays are not available routinely, although this metabolite probably contributes to anticonvulsant activity. Measurement of phenobarbital levels is of limited value, since conversion of primidone to phenobarbital is variable between individuals. However, phenobarbital levels may be helpful in dosage selection, where seizures are not adequately controlled despite regular dosage or where there is suspected toxicity.

Valproate

Sodium valproate as valproic acid in the bloodstream has a broad spectrum of anticonvulsant activity, being useful in generalized absence, generalized tonic–colonic and partial seizures.

Serum concentration–response relationship

There is no clear concentration–response relationship for valproate, although a range of 50–100 mg/L is often quoted as being optimal. Levels exceeding this range do not confer any additional therapeutic benefits. Although there is no clear relationship between serum levels and toxic effects, the rare hepatotoxicity associated with valproate appears to be related to very high levels of over 150 mg/L.

Distribution

Valproate is extensively bound to plasma protein (90–95%) and, unlike other drugs, it can saturate protein binding sites at concentrations greater than 50 mg/L, altering the free fraction of drug. Therefore, the apparent volume of distribution of valproate varies from 0.1 to 0.5 L/kg.

Elimination

Elimination of valproate is almost entirely by hepatic metabolism, with less than 5% being eliminated by the kidneys.

As a result of the saturation of protein binding sites and the subsequent increase in the free fraction of the drug, clearance of the drug increases at higher concentrations. Therefore, there is a non-linear change in plasma concentration with dose (illustrated in Fig. 3.6C).

Practical implications

In view of the lack of a clear concentration–response relationship and the variable pharmacokinetics, there are limited indications for the measurement of valproate levels. In most cases, dosage should be based on clinical response. However, in a few cases where seizures are not controlled at high dosage, a serum level may be helpful in confirming treatment failure. If monitoring is to be undertaken, levels should be drawn at steady state (2–3 days). A trough sample will be the most useful, since wide fluctuations of blood levels may occur during a dose interval.

Lamotrigine, vigabatrin, gabapentin, tiagabine and topiramate

These newer anticonvulsants are indicated for the treatment of a range of types of epilepsy. All are used as adjunctive treatment with other anticonvulsants, with lamotrigine, vigabatrin and topiramate also indicated for monotherapy.

Serum concentration–response relationship

There is no clear relationship between serum concentration and response for these newer anticonvulsants. The situation is further complicated by the fact that these preparations are usually used as an add-on therapy with other anticonvulsants.

Practical implications

While these newer anticonvulsants have narrow therapeutic indices and inter- and intraindividual variations in pharmacokinetics, there is not enough evidence to support routine TDM, and dosage should be titrated to clinical response.

Ciclosporin

Ciclosporin is a neutral lipophilic cyclic endecapeptide extracted from the fungus *Tolypocladium inflatum gams*. It is a potent immunosuppressive agent, used principally to reduce graft rejection after kidney, heart, heart–lung, liver, pancreas and bone marrow transplants. The drug has a low therapeutic index, with a number of toxic effects including nephrotoxicity, hepatotoxicity, gastrointestinal intolerance, hypertrichosis and neurological problems. Efficacy in reducing graft rejection as well as the main toxic effect of nephro- and hepatotoxicity appear to be concentration related.

Serum concentration–response relationship

With all drugs that are monitored the therapeutic range is a window with limits, which are not absolute. It is even more difficult to define a therapeutic range for ciclosporin, since there are a number of influencing factors. First, the measured concentration varies depending on sampling matrix (i.e. whole blood, plasma or serum). Second, it depends on whether the assay is specific for ciclosporin alone or non-specific to include metabolites. A target concentration range of 200–400 μg/L is generally accepted for the immediate postoperative phase following renal transplants. Levels below the lower limit of this window are associated with an increased incidence of graft rejection. Levels above the upper limit are associated with an increased incidence of nephrotoxicity and hepatotoxicity, although an upper limit of 800 μg/L has also been suggested. This target range can be reduced to 100–200 μg/L 3–6 months post transplant. These target ranges are based on assays specific for the ciclosporin parent compound.

Distribution

Ciclosporin is highly lipophilic and is distributed widely throughout the body with a volume of distribution of 4–8 L/kg. There is variable distribution of ciclosporin within blood, since the whole blood concentration is approximately twice the plasma concentration. Within plasma, ciclosporin is 98% protein bound.

Elimination

Ciclosporin is eliminated primarily by hepatic metabolism, with wide interindividual variation in clearance (0.1–2 L/h/kg). In children these values are approximately 40% higher, with a resulting increased dosage requirement on a milligram per kilogram basis. In elderly patients or patients with hepatic impairment a lower clearance rate has been observed.

Practical implications

In addition to the wide interpatient variability in distribution and elimination pharmacokinetic parameters, absorption of standard formulations of ciclosporin is variable and incomplete (F = 0.2–0.5 in normal subjects). In transplant patients this variation in bioavailability is even greater, and increases during the first few months after transplant. Furthermore, a number of drugs are known to interact with ciclosporin. All these factors suggest that TDM will assist in optimum dose selection but the use of population averages in dose prediction is of little benefit, due to wide interpatient variation. When using TDM with ciclosporin, a number of practical points need to be considered.

- The sampling matrix should be whole blood, since there is a variable distribution of ciclosporin between blood and serum.
- Samples should represent trough levels and be drawn at steady state, which is achieved 2–3 days after initiating or changing the dosage (average half-life is 9 hours).
- Ciclosporin concentration monitoring should be undertaken every 2–3 days in the immediate postoperative phase until the patient's clinical condition is stable. Thereafter, monitoring can be undertaken every 1–2 months.
- TDM should be performed when changing brands of ciclosporin, since there are marked differences in the bioavailability of different brands.

Summary pharmacokinetic data for drugs with therapeutic serum concentrations are listed in Table 3.1.

CASE STUDIES

Case 3.1

You are reviewing a formulary submission for a new formulation of a product, which reportedly has an improved side effect profile due to better absorption characteristics. However, there is conflicting

Table 3.1 Summary of pharmacokinetic data

Drug	Therapeutic range of serum concentrations	V_d(L/kg)	CL(L/h/kg)	Half-life (h)
Digoxin	0.8–2.0 µg/L 1–2.6 nmol/L	7.3	See text	36
Theophylline	10–20 mg/L 55–110 µmol/L	0.48	0.04	8
Gentamicin	Peak 5–12 mg/L, trough <2 mg/L	0.25	$1 \times CL$ (creatinine)	2
Lithium	0.4–0.8 mmol/L	0.5–1	$0.2 \times CL$ (creatinine)	18
Phenytoin	10–20 mg/L 40–80 µmol/L	1	$K_m = 6$ mg/L $V_{max} = 7$ mg/kg/day	
Carbamazepine	4–12 mg/L 17–50 µmol/L	0.8–1.9	0.05–1	
Phenobarbital	15–40 mg/L 65–172 µmol/L	0.7–1	0.004	120
Primidone	< 15 mg/L < 69 µmol/L	0.6		
Valproate	< 100 mg/L < 693 µmol/L			
Ciclosporin	200–400 µg/L			9

evidence in the literature over the absorption of the new preparation. One paper, which is available to you, shows a concentration–time profile for the oral formulation after a single oral dose of 250 mg as:

Time after administration	1h	2h	3h	4h	5h	6h	7h	8h	9h	10h	11h	12h
Concentration (mg/L)	10	18	12.7	9	6.4	4.5	3.2	2.25	1.6	1.1	0.78	0.55

The paper also quotes an AUC after a single i.v. dose of 200 mg as 87 mg/L/h.

Questions

1. What is the AUC after the single oral dose of 250 mg?
2. What is the bioavalability of the new formulation?

Answers

1. Draw the concentration time profile on a piece of paper; try to do it reasonably accurately but it does not have to be exact. Draw down vertical lines from the curve at each 1-hour time interval to create a series of trapeziums (the first one is actually a triangle). Calculate the area of each trapezium from the formula:

    area of trapezium = (sum of the height of each side/2) × width (1 h)

    Then add all the areas together (assume a value of 0 after 12 hours):

$$\text{AUC p.o.} = 69.99 \text{ mg/L/h}$$

2. From the equation $F = \dfrac{D\ i.v. \times AUC\ p.o}{D\ p.o. \times AUC\ i.v.}$

$$F = 200 \times 69.99/\ 250 \times 87$$
$$F = 0.64$$

Case 3.2

Miss JM is a 60 kg woman taking phenytoin at a dose of 100 mg three times a day for the last 6 months. She is seen at outpatient clinic and complains she is still having fits, despite taking her medication regularly. A sample is taken for phenytoin levels which is reported as 10 mg/L.

Questions

1. Using pharmacokinetic equations, what dose is required to achieve a level of 15 mg/L?
2. Check your answer using the orbit graph.
3. If phenytoin needed to be administered as a suspension would the dose need to be changed?

Answers

1. From population data V_{max} = 7 mg/day/kg × 60 kg = 420 mg/day. Substitute this together with the dose (remember S = 0.9) and the measured concentration into equation (15) to estimate k_m (since k_m is more variable than V_{max}). Substitute this estimated k_m (5.5 mg/L) together with V_{max} and a target concentration of 15 mg/L into equation (15) to determine a new dose (341 mg per day). Rework the calculation using the most practical dose of 350 mg per day to check the estimated level is still in the therapeutic range (16.5 mg).

2. Using the orbit graph (Fig. 3.8) the new dosage would be 366 mg/day after correcting for S.
3. Rearranging equation (15) to solve for C^{ss}

$$\frac{S \times F \times D/T \times K_m}{V_{max} - (S \times F \times D/T)}$$

Substituting S = 1 for the suspension gives a new C^{ss} of 27.5 mg. Therefore, yes, the dose would definitely need to be changed.

Case 3.3

Mr B is a 55-year-old, 65 kg man with chronic obstructive airways disease (COAD). He has been taking Nuelin SA 250 mg tablets in a dose of two tablets twice a day for many years. He has been admitted to hospital with congestive heart failure (CHF). On examination he has ankle oedema, hepatomegaly and raised jugular venous pressure (JVP).

Three days after admission Mr B starts fitting and theophylline toxicity is considered. A theophylline level is taken just before the next dose is due, although this is not given and theophylline is discontinued. This theophylline level is reported as 33 mg/L and a level taken 12 hours later reported as 20 mg/L.

Questions

1. What is the half-life of theophylline in this patient?
2. How long will it take for the theophylline level to fall to 15 mg/L?
3. How long will it take for the theophylline to be cleared from his body?
4. Should the patient be restarted on theophylline at a lower dose?

Answers

1. As the first level was taken just before the next dose was due you may assume no more theophylline is going into his body. Therefore, use the two blood levels to estimate his k_e and half-life by substituting into equation (7) and solve for k_e.

$$20 \text{ mg/L} = 33 \text{ mg/L} \times e^{-k_e \times 12}$$
$$\ln 20 = \ln 33 - k_e \times 12$$
$$3.0 = 3.5 - (k_e \times 12)$$
$$k_e = 0.0416 \text{ h}^{-1}$$

Substituting this into equation (8) gives a half-life of 16.65 hours.

2. To calculate how long it will take for the theophylline level to fall to 15 mg/L, apply equation (7) again this time using the 20 mg/L and the target concentration of 15 mg/L.

$$15 \text{ mg/L} = 20 \text{ mg/L} \times e^{-0.0416 \times t}$$
$$\ln 15 = \ln 20 - (0.0416 \times t)$$
$$2.7 = 3 - (0.0416 \times t)$$
$$0.3 = 0.0416 \times t$$
$$t = 7.2 \text{ hours}$$

Therfore, it will take a further 7.2 hours to fall to 15 mg/L.

3. As it takes five half-lives for a medicine to be completely eliminated from the body it will take 5 × 16.65 hours (83.25) or 3.5 days for the theophylline to be completely cleared from his body.
4. It would be unwise to restart this patient's theophylline, as his clearance is changing as his heart failure status changes. If treatment improves his heart failure then his theophylline clearance will increase. Although it is possible to calculate pharmacokinetic variables from population data, this would be unreliable in an unstable situation.

Case 3.4

A 74-year-old 60 kg man is commenced on gentamicin i.v. in a dose of 80 mg every 8 hours. However, his serum creatinine is raised at 220 μmol/L and the doctor is worried about toxicity. He asks you what levels this dosage is likely to produce

....

Questions

1. Calculate the patient's pharmacokinetic parameters of k_e, V_d and CL from population data using the Cockcroft & Gault equation and MDRD formula.
2. Predict steady-state peak and trough levels likely to be achieved with this dosage regimen.
3. What would your advice be to the doctor based on these predicted levels?

....

Answers

1. Using the Cockcroft & Gault equation:

$$CL \text{ (creatinine)} = \frac{1.23 \times (140-74) \times 60}{220}$$

$$CL \text{ creatinine} = 22.14 \text{ mL/min}$$

Using the MDRD formula:

$$eGFR = 175 \times [220 \times 0.011312]^{-1.154} \times [74]^{-0.203}$$

$$eGFR = 25.47 \text{ glomerular filtration rate (mL/min per 1.73 m}^2)$$

As gentamicin clearance is the same as creatinine clearance, gentamicin clearance is also:

22.14 mL/min or 1.33 L/h (Cockcroft & Gault equation)

25.45 mL/min per 1.73 m² or 1.53 L/h per 1.73 m² (MDRD formula)

From population averages $V_d = 15.6$ l

Cockcroft & Gault equation:

Using equation (6) $k_e = 0.085$ h^{-1} and equation (8) half-life = 8.12 hours

MDRD formula:

Using equation (6) $k_e = 0.111$ h^{-1} and equation (8) half-life = 6.25 hours

2. Substituting the parameters (Cockcroft & Gault) into equation (13):

$$Cp^{ss}_{max} = 80/15.61 \ (1 - e^{-0.085 \times 8})$$

$$Cp^{ss}_{max} = 10.39 \text{ mg/L}$$

Substituting this estimated Cp^{ss}_{max} into equation (7):

The peak at 1 hour, $C^{ss}_{max} \ 1 = 10.39 \times e^{-0.085 \times 1}$

$$= 9.54 \text{ mg/L}$$

The trough at 8 hours, $C^{ss}_{min} = 10.39 \times e^{-0.085 \times 8}$

$$= 5.26 \text{ mg/L}$$

3. The trough levels are too high, indicating that the dosage interval is too short. Substitute the desired peak and trough (9 and 1) into equation (7) with k_e estimated in the previous section (0.085 h^{-1}) and solve for t.

$$1 = 9 \times e^{-0.085 \times t}$$

$$Ln \ 1 = Ln \ 9 - 0.085 \times t$$

$$0 = 2.19 - 0.085 \times t$$

$$t = 25.8 \text{ hours}$$

A practical dose interval will be 24 hours.

Since the target peak level of 9 mg/L represents what would be measured 1 hour post dose we now need to calculate the actual C^{ss}_{max} immediately after the dose is given.

Substitute 9 mg/L (the desired 1 h post-dose level) as C_2 in equation (7) where $t = 1$ and solve for C_1. This will give a C^{ss}_{max} of 9.78 mg/L.

Substitute this into equation (13) with a dose interval of 24 h and solve for dose

$$9.78 = \text{dose}/15.61 \ (1 - e^{-0.085 \times 24})$$

$$\text{Dose} = 132 \text{ mg}$$

Check C^{ss}_{min} using equation (14).

$$C^{ss}_{min} = \frac{132 \times e^{-0.085 \times 24}}{15.61 \ (1 - e^{-0.085 \times 24})}$$

$$C^{ss}_{min} = 1.3 \text{ mg/L}$$

A practical dose would be 130 mg once a day.

REFERENCES

Cockroft D W, Gault M H 1976 Prediction of creatinine clearance from serum creatinine. Nephron 16: 31-41

Crist K D, Nahata M C, Ety J 1987 Positive impact of a therapeutic drug monitoring program on total aminoglycoside dose and hospitalisation. Therapeutic Drug Monitoring 9: 306-310

Department of Health 2006 Estimated glomerular filtration rate (eGFR). Department of Health Publications, London. Available online at: www.dh.gov.uk/PolicyAndGuidance/HealthAndSocialCareTopics/Renal/ RenalInformation/RenalInformationArticle/fs/en?CONTENT_ID=4133073&chk=RU5tge

Evans W E, Shentag J J, Jusko W J (eds) 1992 Applied pharmacokinetics, 3rd edn. Applied Therapeutics series. Lippincott Williams and Wilkins, Baltimore, pp. 586-617

McFadyen M L, Miller R, Juta M et al 1990 The relevance of a first world therapeutic drug monitoring service to the treatment of epilepsy in third world conditions. South African Medical Journal 78: 587-590

Nicolau D P, Freeman C D, Belliveau P P et al 1995 Experience with a once daily aminoglycoside program administered to 2,184 adult patients. Antimicrobial Agents and Chemotherapy 39: 650-655

Reid L D, Horn J R, McKenna D A 1990 Therapeutic drug monitoring reduces toxic drug reactions: a meta-analysis. Therapeutic Drug Monitoring 12: 72-78

FURTHER READING

Bauer L 2005 Clinical pharmacokinetics handbook. McGraw-Hill, Maidenhead

Begg E J, Barclay M L, Duffull S B 1995 A suggested approach to once daily aminoglycoside dosing. British Journal of Clinical Pharmacology 39: 605-609

Burton M E, Shaw L M, Schentag J J 2006 Applied pharmacokinetics and pharmacodynamics: principles of therapeutic drug monitoring, 4th edn, Lippincott Williams and Wilkins, Baltimore

Dhillon S, Kostrzewski A 2006 Clinical pharmacokinetics. Pharmaceutical Press, London

Luke D R, Halstenson C E, Opsahl J A et al 1990 Validity of creatinine clearance estimates in the assessment of renal function. Clinical Pharmacology and Therapeutics 48: 503-508

Rambeck B, Boenigk H E, Dunlop A et al 1980 Predicting phenytoin dose: a revised nomogram. Therapeutic Drug Monitoring 1: 325-354

Tserng K, King K C, Takieddine F N 1981 Theophylline metabolism in premature infants. Clinical Pharmacology and Therapeutics 29: 594-600

Winter M E 2003 Basic clinical pharmacokinetics. Lippincott Williams and Wilkins, Baltimore

4 Drug interactions

A. Lee   I. H. Stockley

KEY POINTS

- Drug interactions can cause significant patient harm and are an important cause of morbidity.
- Most clinically important drug interactions occur as a result of either decreased drug activity with diminished efficacy or increased drug activity with exaggerated or unusual effects. Drugs with a narrow therapeutic range, such as theophylline, lithium and digoxin, or a steep dose–response curve, such as anticoagulants, oral contraceptives and antiepileptics, are often implicated.
- The most important pharmacokinetic interactions involve drugs that can induce or inhibit enzymes in the hepatic cytochrome P450 system.
- Pharmacodynamic interactions are difficult to classify but their effects can often be predicted when the pharmacology of co-administered drugs is known.
- In many cases, potentially interacting drugs can be given concurrently provided the possibility of interaction is kept in mind and any necessary changes to dose or therapy are initiated promptly. In some situations, however, concurrent use of potentially interacting drugs should be avoided altogether.
- Suspected adverse drug interactions should be reported to the appropriate regulatory authority as for other adverse drug reactions.

Drug interactions are an increasingly important cause of adverse drug reactions (ADR). This was recognized over 100 years ago, when it was noted that an adrenal extract, when given to a dog anaesthetized with chloroform, could cause arrhythmias. Today, with the increasing availability of complex therapeutic agents and widespread polypharmacy, the potential for drug interactions is enormous. Despite rigorous attempts to ensure that the safety profile of new medicines is as fully defined as possible at the time they are marketed, the potential for adverse interactions is not always evident. This was illustrated by the worldwide withdrawal of the calcium channel blocker mibefradil, within months of launch, following reports of serious drug interactions (Li Wan Po & Zhang 1998). In the past decade, a number of medicines have been either withdrawn from the market or had their use restricted because of prolongation of the QT interval on the electrocardiogram, which incurs a risk of life-threatening ventricular arrhythmias (Roden 2004). Drug interactions are an important cause of QT prolongation and the arrhythmia known as torsades de pointes.

Patients are now more likely to self-treat with herbal and other complementary preparations and awareness of their involvement in drug interactions is increasing. For example, there is good evidence implicating St John's wort as a cause of serious interactions due to its ability to induce CYP3A4 and P-glycoprotein.

Drug interactions with food and drink are known to occur, exemplified by the well-known interaction between monoamine oxidase inhibitor antidepressants and tyramine containing foodstuffs. Currently, however, grapefruit juice causes the most clinically relevant of these interactions. For example, patients prescribed simvastatin should be advised not to drink grapefruit juice due to the increased risk of statin-induced adverse effects such as myopathy. Grapefruit juice inhibits cytochrome P450 3A4, which is involved in simvastatin's metabolism.

Although the medical literature is awash with case reports of adverse drug interactions, only a relatively small number are clinically significant. It is therefore important to anticipate when a potential drug interaction might have clinically significant consequences for the patient. In these situations advice should be given on how to minimize the risk of harm, for example by recommending an alternative treatment to avoid the combination of risk, by making a dose adjustment or by monitoring the patient closely. To do this, a practical knowledge of the pharmacological mechanisms involved in drug interactions is required as well as a good understanding of high-risk drugs and the most vulnerable patient groups.

Definition

An interaction is said to occur when the effects of one drug are changed by the presence of another drug, herbal medicine, food, drink or some environmental chemical agent (Baxter 2005). The net effect of the combination may manifest as, for example, an additive or enhanced effect of one or more drugs, antagonism of the effect of one or more drugs, or any other alteration in the effect of one or more drugs.

When a therapeutic combination could lead to an unexpected change or complication in the condition of the patient, this would be described as an interaction of potential clinical significance. Although recognized drug interactions are sometimes used with the aim of therapeutic benefit, in this chapter we are concerned only with drug–drug interactions which have the potential for undesirable effects on patient care.

Epidemiology

It is difficult to give an accurate estimate of the incidence of drug interactions mainly because published studies have frequently used different criteria for defining a drug interaction, particularly in distinguishing between clinically significant and non-significant interactions. Some of the early studies uncritically compared prescribed drugs with lists of possible drug interactions without taking into account their potential clinical significance. A review of nine studies of the epidemiology of drug–drug interactions in hospital admissions found that the reported incidence ranged from 0% to 2.8% (Jankel & Fitterman 1993). However, the authors considered all studies reviewed to be flawed to some extent. In the Harvard Medical Practice Study of adverse events, 20% of events in acute hospital inpatients were drug related. Of these, 8% were considered to be due to a drug interaction, suggesting that interactions are responsible for less than 2% of adverse events in this patient group (Leape et al 1992). In a recent UK study carried out to assess adverse drug reactions as a cause of hospital admission, drug interactions were involved in 16.6% of adverse reactions identified (Pirmohamed et al 2004). Few studies have attempted to quantify the incidence of drug–drug interactions in the community. In the early 1990s a USA community pharmacy study revealed a 4.1% incidence of interactions, while a Swedish study reported an incidence of 1.9%.

Even if the overall incidence of adverse drug interactions is low, as some studies suggest, they are still a considerable problem in terms of the global number of patients at risk and the potential for morbidity and mortality.

Susceptible patients

Certain patients are at increased risk of drug interactions. Polypharmacy is common and often unavoidable. However, the more drugs a patient takes, the greater is the likelihood of an ADR. One hospital study found an ADR rate of 7% in patients taking 6–10 drugs, increasing to 40% in those taking 16–20 drugs (Smith et al 1969). This exponential rise is partly due to drug interactions, which are more likely to have serious consequences when they affect elderly or seriously ill patients. Patients at particular risk include those with hepatic or renal disease, those on long-term therapy for chronic disease (e.g. HIV infection, epilepsy, diabetes), patients in intensive care, transplant recipients, patients undergoing complicated surgical procedures and those with more than one prescribing doctor. Critically ill and elderly patients are at increased risk not only because they take more medicines but also because of impaired homeostatic mechanisms that might otherwise counteract some of the unwanted effects. Interactions may occur in some individuals but not in others. The effects of interactions involving drug metabolism may vary greatly in individual patients because of differences in the rates of drug metabolism and in susceptibility to microsomal enzyme induction. Certain drugs are frequently implicated in drug interactions and require careful attention (Table 4.1).

Mechanisms of drug interactions

Drug interactions are conventionally discussed according to the mechanisms involved. There are some situations where drugs interact by unique mechanisms, but certain mechanisms are encountered time and time again. These mechanisms can be conveniently divided into those with a pharmacokinetic basis and those with a pharmacodynamic basis. Drug interactions often involve more than one mechanism.

Table 4.1 Some drugs with high risk of interaction

Concentration-dependent toxicity
Digoxin
Lithium
Aminoglycosides
Cytotoxic agents
Warfarin

Steep dose–response curve
Verapamil
Sulphonylureas
Levodopa

Patient dependent on therapeutic effect
Immunosuppressives, e.g. ciclosporin, tacrolimus
Glucocorticoids
Oral contraceptives
Antiepileptics
Antiarrhythmics
Antipsychotics
Antiretrovirals

Saturable hepatic metabolism
Phenytoin
Theophylline

Pharmacokinetic interactions

Pharmacokinetic interactions are those that can affect the processes by which drugs are absorbed, distributed, metabolized or excreted. Due to marked interindividual variability in these processes, these interactions may be expected but their extent cannot easily be predicted. Such interactions may result in a change in the drug concentration at the site of action with subsequent toxicity or decreased efficacy.

Absorption

Most drugs are given orally for absorption through the mucous membranes of the gastrointestinal tract. Most of the interactions that occur within the gut result in reduced rather than increased absorption. It is important to recognize that the majority result in changes in absorption rate, although in some instances the total amount (i.e. extent) of drug absorbed is affected. For drugs that are given chronically on a multiple dose regimen, such as the oral anticoagulants, the rate of absorption is usually unimportant provided the total amount of drug absorbed is not markedly altered. On the other hand, delayed absorption can be clinically significant where the drug affected has a short half-life or where it is important to achieve high plasma concentrations rapidly, as may be the case with analgesics or hypnotics. Often these interactions can be avoided if an interval of 2–3 hours is allowed between doses of the interacting drugs.

Changes in gastrointestinal pH. The absorption of a drug across mucous membranes depends on the extent to which it exists in the non-ionized, lipid-soluble form. The ionization state depends on the pH of its milieu, the pKa of the drug and formulation factors. Weakly acidic drugs, such as the salicylates, are better absorbed at low pH because the non-ionized form predominates. An alteration in gastric pH due to antacids, histamine H_2 antagonists or proton pump inhibitors therefore has the potential to affect the absorption of other drugs. The clinical significance of antacid-induced changes in gastric pH is not certain, particularly since relatively little drug absorption occurs in the stomach. Changes in gastric pH tend to affect the rate of absorption rather than the total bioavailability, provided that the drug is acid labile. Theoretically antacids could be expected to markedly influence the absorption of other drugs via this mechanism, but in practice there are very few clinically significant examples. Antacids, histamine H_2 antagonists and omeprazole can significantly decrease the bioavailability of ketoconazole and itraconazole, as both require gastric acidity for optimal absorption. The absorption of fluconazole and voriconazole, however, is not significantly altered by changes in gastric pH. The alkalinizing effects of antacids on the gastrointestinal tract are transient and the potential for interaction may be minimized by leaving an interval of 2–3 hours between the antacid and the potentially interacting drug.

Adsorption, chelation and other complexing mechanisms Certain drugs react directly within the gastrointestinal tract to form chelates and complexes which are not absorbed. The drugs most commonly implicated in this type of interaction include tetracyclines and the quinolone antibiotics which can complex with iron, and antacids containing calcium, magnesium and aluminium. Tetracyclines can chelate with divalent or trivalent metal cations such as calcium, aluminium, bismuth and iron to form insoluble complexes, resulting in greatly reduced plasma tetracycline concentrations.

Bisphosphonates are often co-prescribed with calcium supplements in the treatment of osteoporosis. If these are taken concomitantly, however, the bioavailability of both is significantly reduced, with the possibility of therapeutic failure .

The absorption of some drugs may be reduced if they are given with adsorbents such as charcoal or kaolin, or anionic exchange resins such as colestyramine or colestipol. The absorption of propranolol, digoxin, warfarin, tricyclic antidepressants, ciclosporin and levothyroxine is reduced by colestyramine. Most chelation and adsorption interactions can be avoided if an interval of 2–3 hours is allowed between doses of the interacting drugs.

Effects on gastrointestinal motility Since most drugs are largely absorbed in the upper part of the small intestine, drugs that alter the rate at which the stomach empties its contents can affect absorption. Drugs with anticholinergic effects, such as tricyclic antidepressants, phenothiazines and some antihistamines, decrease gut motility and delay gastric emptying. The outcome of the reduced gut motility can either be an increase or a decrease in drugs given concomitantly. For example, tricyclic antidepressants can increase dicoumarol absorption, probably as a result of increasing the time available for its dissolution and absorption. Anticholinergic agents used in the management of movement disorders have been shown to reduce the bioavailability of levodopa by as much as 50%, possibly as a result of increased metabolism in the intestinal mucosa.

Opioids such as diamorphine and pethidine strongly inhibit gastric emptying and greatly reduce the absorption rate of paracetamol. Codeine, however, has no significant effect on paracetamol absorption. Metoclopramide increases gastric emptying and increases the absorption rate of paracetamol, an effect which is used to therapeutic advantage in the treatment of migraine. It also accelerates the absorption of propranolol, mefloquine, lithium and ciclosporin. In general, this type of interaction is rarely clinically significant.

Induction or inhibition of drug transport proteins The oral bioavailability of some drugs is limited by the action of drug transporter proteins, which eject drugs that have diffused across the gut lining back into the gut. At present, the most well-characterized drug transporter is P-glycoprotein. Digoxin is a substrate of P-glycoprotein and drugs that inhibit P-glycoprotein, such as verapamil, may increase digoxin bioavailability with the potential for digoxin toxicity (DuBuske 2005).

Drug distribution

Once absorbed, a drug is distributed to its site of action and during this process it may interact with other drugs. In practice, the main mechanism behind such interactions is displacement from protein-binding sites. A drug displacement interaction is defined as a reduction in the extent of plasma protein binding of one drug caused by the presence of another drug, resulting in an increased free or unbound fraction of the displaced drug. Many drugs and their metabolites are highly bound to plasma proteins. Albumin is the main plasma protein to which acidic drugs such as warfarin are bound, while basic drugs, such as tricyclic antidepressants, lidocaine, disopyramide and propranolol are generally bound to α_1-acid glycoprotein. Displacement from these proteins can be demonstrated in vitro for many drugs and in the past it was thought to be an important mechanism underlying many interactions. Current evidence suggests that, for most drugs, if displacement occurs, then the concentration of free drug will rise temporarily, but metabolism and distribution will return the free concentration to its previous level. The time this takes will depend on the half-life of the displaced drug. The biological significance of the short-term rise of free concentration is generally of minor importance but may need to be taken into account in therapeutic drug monitoring. For example, if a patient taking phenytoin is given a drug which displaces some phenytoin from its binding sites, the total (i.e. free plus bound) plasma phenytoin concentration will fall even though the free (active) concentration remains the same.

There are few examples of clinically important interactions which are entirely due to protein-binding displacement. It has been postulated that a sustained change in steady-state free plasma concentration could arise with the parenteral administration of some drugs which are extensively bound to plasma proteins and non-restrictively cleared (i.e. the efficiency of the eliminating organ is high). Lidocaine has been given as an example of a drug fitting these criteria.

Drug metabolism

Most clinically important interactions involve the effect of one drug on the metabolism of another. Metabolism refers to the process by which drugs and other compounds are biochemically modified to facilitate their degradation and subsequent removal from the body. The liver is the principal site of drug metabolism although other organs such as the gut, kidneys, lung, skin and placenta are involved. Drug metabolism consists of phase I reactions, such as oxidation, hydrolysis and reduction, and phase II reactions, which primarily involve conjugation of the drug with substances such as glucuronic acid and sulphuric acid. Phase I metabolism generally involves the cytochrome P450 mixed function oxidase system. The liver is the major site of CYP450-mediated metabolism, but the enterocytes in the small intestinal epithelium are also potentially important.

Cytochrome P450 isoenzymes The cytochrome P450 system comprises 57 isoenzymes, each derived from the expression of an individual gene. As there are many different isoforms of these enzymes, a classification for nomenclature has been developed, comprising a family number, a subfamily letter and a number for an individual enzyme within the subfamily (Schwarz 2003, Wilkinson 2005). Four main subfamilies of P450 isoenzymes are thought to be responsible for most (about 90%) of the metabolism of commonly used drugs in humans: CYP1, CYP2, CYP3 and CYP4. The most extensively studied isoenzyme is CYP2D6, also known as debrisoquine hydroxylase. Although there is overlap, each CYP isoenzyme tends to metabolize a discrete range of substrates. Of the many isoenzymes, just a few (CYP1A2, CYP2C9, CYP2C19, CYP2D6, CYP2E1 and CYP3A4) seem to be responsible for the metabolism of most commonly used drugs.

The genes that encode specific CYP isoenzymes can vary between individuals and, sometimes, ethnic groups. These variations (polymorphisms) may affect metabolism of substrate drugs. Interindividual variability in CYP2D6 activity is well recognized (see Chapter 5). It shows a polymodal distribution and people may be described according to their ability to metabolize debrisoquine. Poor metabolizers tend to have reduced

first-pass metabolism, increased plasma levels and exaggerated pharmacological response to this drug, resulting in postural hypotension. By contrast, ultra-rapid metabolizers may require considerably higher doses for a standard effect. The antidepressants nortriptyline and desipramine are metabolized by similar mechanisms to those of debrisoquine and as a result the steady-state plasma levels reached with these drugs are dependent on the individual's phenotype. About 5–10% of white caucasians and up to 2% of Asians and black people are poor metabolizers.

The CYP3A family of P450 enzymes comprises two isoenzymes, CYP3A4 and CYP3A5, so similar that they cannot easily be distinguished. CYP3A is probably the most important of all drug-metabolizing enzymes because it is abundant in both the intestinal epithelium and the liver and it has the ability to metabolize a multitude of chemically unrelated drugs from almost every drug class. It is likely that CYP3A is involved in the metabolism of more than half the therapeutic agents that undergo alteration by oxidation. In contrast to other CYP450 enzymes, CYP3A shows continuous unimodal distribution, suggesting that genetic factors play a minor role in its regulation. Nevertheless, the activity of the enzyme can vary markedly among members of a given population.

The effect of a CYP isoenzyme on a particular substrate can be altered by interaction with other drugs. Drugs may be themselves substrates for a CYP isoenzyme and/or may inhibit or induce the isoenzyme. In most instances, oxidation of a particular drug is brought about by several CYP isoenzymes and results in the production of several metabolites. So, inhibition or induction of a single isoenzyme would have little effect on plasma levels of the drug. However, if a drug is metabolized primarily by a single CYP isoenzyme, inhibition or induction of this enzyme would have a major effect on the plasma concentrations of the drug. For example, if erythromycin (an inhibitor of CYP3A4) is taken by a patient being given carbamazepine (which is extensively metabolized by CYP3A4), this may lead to toxicity due to

Table 4.2 Some drug substrates, inducers and inhibitors of the major cytochrome P450 enzymes

P450 isoform	Substrate	Inducer	Inhibitor
CYP1A2	Caffeine Clozapine Imipramine Olanzapine Theophylline Tricyclic antidepressants R-warfarin	Omeprazole Lansoprazole Phenytoin Tobacco smoke	Amiodarone Cimetidine Fluoroquinolones Fluvoxamine
CYP2C9	Diazepam Diclofenac Losartan Statins S-warfarin	Barbiturates Rifampicin	Amiodarone Azole antifungals Isoniazid SSRIs
CYP2C19	Cilostazol Diazepam Lansoprazole Omeprazole	Carbamazepine Rifampicin	Cimetidine Fluoxetine Lansoprazole Omeprazole Tranylcypromine

continued

Table 4.2 (continued)

P450 isoform	Substrate	Inducer	Inhibitor
CYP2D6	Amitriptyline Codeine Dihydrocodeine Flecainide Fluoxetine Haloperidol Imipramine Nortriptyline Olanzapine Ondansetron Opioids Paroxetine Propranolol Risperidone Thioridazine Tramadol Venlafaxine	Dexamethasone Rifampicin	Amiodarone Bupropion Celecoxib Duloxetine Fluoxetine Paroxetine Ritonavir Sertraline
CYP2E1	Enflurane Halothane	Alcohol (chronic) Isoniazid	Disulfiram
CYP3A4	Amiodarone Terfenadine Ciclosporin Corticosteroids Oral contraceptives Tacrolimus R-warfarin Calcium channel blockers Donepezil Benzodiazepines Cilostazol	Carbamazepine Phenytoin Barbiturates Dexamethasone Primidone Rifampicin St John's wort Bosentan Efavirenz Nevirapine	Cimetidine Clarithromycin Erythromycin Itraconazole Ketoconazole Grapefruit juice Aprepitant Diltiazem Protease inhibitors Imatinib Verapamil

higher concentrations of carbamazepine. Table 4.2 gives examples of some drug substrates, inducers and inhibitors of the major CYP450 isoenzymes.

Enzyme induction The most powerful enzyme inducers in clinical use are the antibiotic rifampicin and antiepileptic agents such as barbiturates, phenytoin and carbamazepine. Some enzyme inducers, notably barbiturates and carbamazepine, can induce their own metabolism (autoinduction). Cigarette smoking, chronic alcohol use and the herbal preparation St John's wort can also induce drug-metabolizing enzymes. Since the process of enzyme induction requires new protein synthesis, the effect usually develops over several days or weeks after starting an enzyme-inducing agent. Similarly, the effect generally persists for a similar period following drug withdrawal. Enzyme-inducing drugs with short half-lives such as rifampicin will induce metabolism more rapidly than inducers with longer half-lives, e.g. phenytoin, because they reach steady-state concentrations more rapidly. Enzyme induction usually results in a decreased pharmacological effect of the affected drug, except perhaps in the case of drugs with active metabolites. The effects of enzyme induction vary considerably between patients and are dependent upon age, genetic factors, concurrent drug treatment and disease state. There is evidence that the enzyme induction process is dose dependent, although some drugs may induce enzymes at any dose. St John's wort is now known to be a potent inducer

of CYP3A (Mannel 2004). Thus, when a patient receiving ciclosporin, tacrolimus, HIV-protease inhibitors, irinotecan or imatinib takes St John's wort, there is a risk of therapeutic failure with the affected drug. Some examples of interactions due to enzyme induction are shown in Table 4.3.

Enzyme inhibition Enzyme inhibition is an extremely common mechanism behind drug interactions. Just as some drugs can stimulate the activity of CYP450 enzymes, there are many which have the opposite effect and act as inhibitors. The rate of metabolism of drugs given concurrently can be reduced and they begin to accumulate within the body. Some enzyme inhibitors are shown in Table 4.4. Enzyme inhibition appears to be dose related; inhibition of metabolism of the affected drug begins as soon as sufficient concentrations of the inhibitor appear in the liver, and the effects are usually maximal when the new steady-state plasma concentration is achieved. Thus, for drugs with a short half-life, the effects may be seen within a few days of administration of the inhibitor. The effects are not seen until later for drugs with a long half-life.

The clinical significance of this type of interaction depends on various factors, including dosage (of both drugs), alterations in pharmacokinetic properties of the affected drug, such as half-life, and patient characteristics such as disease state. Interactions of this type are again most likely to affect drugs with a narrow therapeutic range, such as theophylline, ciclosporin, oral anti-

Table 4.3 Some examples of interactions due to enzyme induction

Drug affected	Inducing agent	Clinical outcome
Oral contraceptives	Rifampicin	Therapeutic failure of contraceptive
	Rifabutin	Additional contraceptive precautions required
	Modafinil	Increased oestrogen dose required
Ciclosporin	Phenytoin Carbamazepine St John's wort	Decreased ciclosporin levels with possibility of transplant rejection
Paracetamol	Alcohol (chronic)	In overdose, hepatotoxicity may occur at lower doses
Corticosteroids	Phenytoin Rifampicin	Increased metabolism with possibility of therapeutic failure

Table 4.4 Some enzyme inhibitors frequently implicated in interactions

Antibacterials
Ciprofloxacin
Clarithromycin
Erythromycin
Isoniazid
Metronidazole

Antidepressants
Duloxetine
Fluoxetine
Fluvoxamine
Nefazodone
Paroxetine
Sertraline

Antifungals
Fluconazole
Itraconazole
Ketoconazole
Miconazole
Voriconazole

Antivirals
Amprenavir
Indinavir
Nelfinavir
Ritonavir
Saquinavir

Cardiovascular drugs
Amiodarone
Diltiazem
Quinidine
Verapamil

Gastrointestinal drugs
Cimetidine
Esomeprazole
Omeprazole

Antirheumatic drugs
Allopurinol
Azapropazone
Phenylbutazone

Other
Aprepitant
Bupropion
Disulfiram
Grapefruit juice
Imatinib
Propoxyphene
Sodium valproate

coagulants and phenytoin. For example, starting treatment with an enzyme inhibitor such as ritonavir in a patient taking sildenafil could result in a marked increase in sildenafil plasma concentrations. Some examples of interactions due to enzyme inhibition are shown in Table 4.5.

The isoenzyme CYP3A4, in particular, is present in the enterocytes. Thus, after oral administration of a drug, CYP450 enzymes in the intestine and the liver may reduce the portion of a dose that reaches the systemic circulation (i.e. the bioavailability). Drug interactions resulting in inhibition or induction of enzymes in the intestinal epithelium can have significant consequences. For example, by selectively inhibiting CYP3A4 in the enterocyte, grapefruit juice can markedly increase the bioavailability of some oral calcium channel blockers, including felodipine (Wilkinson 2005). Such an interaction is usually considered to be a drug metabolism interaction, even though the mechanism involves an alteration in drug absorption. A single glass of grapefruit juice can cause CYP3A inhibition for 24–48 hours and regular consumption may continuously inhibit enzyme activity. For this reason, the consumption of grapefruit juice is not recommended in patients receiving drugs that are extensively metabolized by CYP3A such as simvastatin, tacrolimus and vardenafil.

Predicting interactions involving metabolism Predicting drug interactions is not easy for many reasons. First, individual drugs within a therapeutic class may have different effects on an isoenzyme. For example, the quinolone antibiotics ciprofloxacin and norfloxacin inhibit CYP1A2 and have been reported to increase plasma theophylline levels, whereas moxifloxacin is a much weaker inhibitor and appears not to interact in this way. While atorvastatin and simvastatin are metabolized predominantly by the CYP3A4 enzyme, fluvastatin is metabolized by CYP2C9 and pravastatin is not metabolized by the CYP450 system to any significant extent.

The relationship between drugs and the cytochrome P450 system is often tested early in drug development using in vitro techniques. This is an increasingly important area of drug

Table 4.5 Some examples of interactions due to enzyme inhibition

Drug affected	Inhibiting agent	Clinical outcome
Anticoagulants (oral)	Ciprofloxacin Clarithromycin	Anticoagulant effect increased and risk of bleeding
Azathioprine	Allopurinol	Enhancement of effect with increased toxicity
Carbamazepine Phenytoin Sodium valproate	Cimetidine	Antiepileptic levels increased with risk of toxicity
Sildenafil	Ritonavir	Enhancement of sildenafil effect with risk of hypotension

development as it may allow early identification of potential interactions that can be studied further in people. However, the findings of in vitro studies are not always replicated in vivo. Some interactions affect only a small subset of individuals and consequently a large numbers of patients or volunteers would need to be studied before a significant effect could be demonstrated.

Suspected drug interactions are often described initially in published case reports and are then subsequently evaluated in formal studies. For example, published case reports indicate that some antibiotics reduce the effect of oral contraceptives although this interaction has not been demonstrated in formal studies. Another factor complicating the understanding of metabolic drug interactions is the finding that there is a large overlap between the inhibitors/inducers and substrates of the drug transporter protein P-glycoprotein and those of CYP3A4. Therefore, both mechanisms may be involved in many of the drug interactions previously thought to be due to effects on CYP3A4.

Elimination interactions

Most drugs are excreted in either the bile or urine. Blood entering the kidneys is delivered to the glomeruli of the tubules where molecules small enough to pass across the pores of the glomerular membrane are filtered through into the lumen of the tubules. Larger molecules, such as plasma proteins and blood cells, are retained. The blood then flows to other parts of the kidney tubules where drugs and their metabolites are removed, secreted or reabsorbed into the tubular filtrate by active and passive transport systems. Interactions can occur when drugs interfere with kidney tubule fluid pH, active transport systems or blood flow to the kidney, thereby altering the excretion of other drugs.

Changes in urinary pH   As with drug absorption in the gut, passive reabsorption of drugs depends on the extent to which the drug exists in the non-ionized lipid-soluble form. Only the non-ionized form is lipid soluble and able to diffuse back through the tubule cell membrane. Thus at alkaline pH, weakly acidic drugs (pKa 3.0–7.5) largely exist as ionized lipid-insoluble molecules which are unable to diffuse into the tubule cells and will therefore be lost in the urine. The renal clearance of these drugs is increased if the urine is made more alkaline. Conversely, the clearance of weak bases (pKa 7.5–10) is higher in acid urine. Strong acids and bases are virtually completely ionized over the physiological range of urinary pH and their clearance is unaffected by pH changes.

This mechanism of interaction is of very minor clinical significance because most weak acids and bases are inactivated by hepatic metabolism rather than renal excretion. Furthermore, drugs that produce large changes in urine pH are rarely used clinically. Urine alkalinization or acidification has been used as a means of increasing drug elimination in poisoning with salicylates and amphetamines respectively.

Changes in active renal tubule excretion   Drugs that use the same active transport system in the kidney tubules can compete with one another for excretion. Such competition between drugs can be used to therapeutic advantage. For example, probenecid may be given to increase the plasma concentration of penicillins by delaying renal excretion. With the increasing understanding of drug transporter proteins in the kidneys, it is now known that probenecid inhibits the renal secretion of many other anionic drugs via organic anion transporters (OATs) (Lee & Kim 2004). Increased methotrexate toxicity, sometimes life-threatening, has been seen in some patients concurrently treated with salicylates and some other NSAIDs. The development of toxicity is more likely in patients treated with high-dose methotrexate and those with impaired renal function. The mechanism of this interaction may be multifactorial but competitive inhibition of methotrexate's renal tubular secretion is likely to be involved. If patients taking methotrexate are given salicylates or NSAIDs concomitantly, the dose of methotrexate should be closely monitored.

Changes in renal blood flow   Blood flow through the kidney is partially controlled by the production of renal vasodilatory prostaglandins. If the synthesis of these prostaglandins is inhibited, e.g. by indometacin, the renal excretion of lithium is reduced with a subsequent rise in plasma levels. The mechanism underlying this interaction is not entirely clear, as plasma lithium levels are unaffected by some potent prostaglandin synthetase inhibitors, e.g. aspirin. If an NSAID is prescribed for a patient taking lithium the plasma levels should be closely monitored.

Biliary excretion and the enterohepatic shunt   A number of drugs are excreted in the bile, either unchanged or conjugated, e.g. as the glucuronide, to make them more water soluble. Some of the conjugates are metabolized to the parent compound by the gut flora and are then reabsorbed. This recycling process prolongs the stay of the drug within the body but if the gut flora are diminished by the presence of an antibacterial, the drug is not recycled and is lost more quickly. This mechanism has been postulated as the basis of an interaction between broad-spectrum antibiotics and oral contraceptives. Antibiotics may reduce the enterohepatic circulation of ethinyloestradiol conjugates, leading to reduced circulating oestrogen levels with the potential for therapeutic failure. There is considerable debate about the nature of this interaction as the evidence from pharmacokinetic studies is not convincing. However, due to the potential adverse consequences of pill failure, most authorities recommend a conservative approach, including the use of additional contraceptive precautions to cover the short-term use of broad-spectrum antibiotics.

Drug transporter proteins Drugs and endogenous substances are now known to cross biological membranes not just by passive diffusion but by carrier-mediated processes, often known as transporters. Significant advances in the identification of various transporters have been made and although their contribution to drug interactions is not yet clear, they are now thought to play a role in many interactions formerly attributed to CYP450 enzymes (DuBuske 2005).

P-glycoprotein (P-gp) is a large cell membrane protein that is responsible for the transport of many substrates, including drugs. It is a product of the ABCB1 gene (previously known as the multidrug resistance gene, MDR1) and a member of the adenosine triphosphate (ATP)-binding cassette family of transport proteins (ABC transporters). P-gp is found in high levels in various tissues including the renal proximal tubule, hepatocytes, intestinal mucosa, the pancreas and the blood–brain barrier. P-gp acts as an efflux pump, exporting substances into urine, bile and the intestinal lumen. Its activity in the blood–brain barrier limits drug accumulation in the CNS. Examples of some possible inhibitors and inducers of P-gp are shown in Table 4.6. The pumping actions of P-gp can be induced or inhibited by some drugs. For example, concomitant administration of digoxin and verapamil, a P-gp inhibitor, is associated with increased digoxin levels with the potential for digoxin toxicity. There is an overlap between CYP3A4 and P-glycoprotein inhibitors, inducers and substrates. Many drugs that are substrates for CYP3A4 are also substrates for P-gp. Therefore both mechanisms may be involved in many of the drug interactions initially thought to be due to changes in CYP3A4. Digoxin is an example of the few drugs that are substrates for P-glycoprotein but not CYP3A4.

Pharmacodynamic interactions

Pharmacodynamic interactions are those where the effects of one drug are changed by the presence of another drug at its site of action. Sometimes these interactions involve competition for specific receptor sites but often they are indirect and involve interference with physiological systems. They are much less easy to classify than interactions with a pharmacokinetic basis.

Antagonistic interactions

It is to be expected that a drug with an agonist action at a particular receptor type will interact with antagonists at that receptor. For example, the bronchodilator action of a selective β_2-adrenoreceptor agonist such as salbutamol will be antagonized by β-adrenoreceptor antagonists. There are numerous examples of interactions occurring at receptor sites, many of which are used to therapeutic advantage. Specific antagonists may be used to reverse the effect of another drug at receptor sites; examples include the opioid antagonist naloxone and the benzodiazepine antagonist flumazenil. α-Adrenergic agonists such as metaraminol may be used in the management of priapism induced by α-adrenergic antagonists such as phentolamine. There are many other examples of drug classes that have opposing pharmacological actions, such as anticoagulants and vitamin K and levodopa and dopamine antagonist antipsychotics.

Additive or synergistic interactions

If two drugs with similar pharmacological effects are given together, the effects can be additive (see Table 4.7). Although not strictly drug interactions, the mechanism frequently contributes to adverse drug reactions. For example, the concurrent use of drugs with CNS depressant effects such as antidepressants, hypnotics, antiepileptics and antihistamines may lead to excessive drowsiness, yet such combinations are frequently encountered. Combinations of drugs with arrhythmogenic potential such as antiarrhythmics, neuroleptics, tricyclic antidepressants and those producing electrolyte imbalance (e.g. diuretics) may lead to ventricular arrhythmias and should be avoided. Another example which has assumed greater importance of late is the risk of ventricular tachycardia and torsade de pointes associated with the concurrent use of more than one drug with the potential to prolong the QT interval on the electrocardiogram (Roden 2004).

Table 4.6 Examples of inhibitors and inducers of P-glycoprotein

Inhibitors	Atorvastatin
	Clarithromycin
	Dipyramidole
	Erythromycin
	Itraconazole
	Ketoconazole
	Propafenone
	Quinidine
	Valspodar
	Verapamil
Inducers	Rifampicin
	St John's wort

Table 4.7 Some additive or synergistic interactions

Interacting drugs	Pharmacological effect
NSAID, warfarin, clopidogrel	Increased risk of bleeding
ACE inhibitors and K-sparing diuretic	Increased risk of hyperkalaemia
Verapamil and β-adrenergic antagonists	Bradycardia and asystole
Neuromuscular blockers and aminoglycosides	Increased neuromuscular blockade
Alcohol and benzodiazepines	Increased sedation
Thioridazine and sotalol	Increased risk of QT interval prolongation
Clozapine and co-trimoxazole	Increased risk of bone marrow suppression

Serotonin syndrome

Serotonin syndrome (SS) is associated with an excess of serotonin that results from therapeutic drug use, overdose or inadvertent interactions between drugs. Although uncommon, it is becoming increasingly well recognized in patients receiving combinations of serotonergic drugs (Boyer & Shannon 2005). It can occur when two or more drugs affecting serotonin are given at the same time or after one serotonergic drug is stopped and another started. The syndrome is characterized by symptoms including confusion, disorientation, abnormal movements, exaggerated reflexes, fever, sweating, diarrhoea and hypotension or hypertension. Diagnosis is made when three or more of these symptoms are present and no other cause can be found. Symptoms usually develop within hours of starting the second drug but occasionally they can occur later. Drug-induced serotonin syndrome is generally mild and resolves when the offending drugs are stopped. However, it can be severe and deaths have occurred.

Serotonin syndrome is best prevented by not using serotonergic drugs in combination. Special care is needed when changing from an SSRI to an MAOI and vice versa. The SSRIs, particularly fluoxetine, have long half-lives and serotonin syndrome may occur if a sufficient wash-out period is not allowed before switching from one to the other. When patients are being switched between these two groups of drugs the guidance in manufacturers' Summaries of Product Characteristics should be followed.

Drug or neurotransmitter uptake interactions

Monoamine oxidase inhibitors Although seldom prescribed nowadays, the monoamine oxidase inhibitor antidepressants (MAOIs) have significant potential for interactions with other drugs and foods. MAOIs reduce the breakdown of noradrenaline in the adrenergic nerve ending. Large stores of noradrenaline can then be released into the synaptic cleft in response to either a neuronal discharge or an indirectly acting amine. The action of the directly acting amines adrenaline, isoprenaline and noradrenaline appears to be only moderately increased in patients taking MAOIs. In contrast, the concurrent use of MAOIs and indirectly acting sympathomimetic amines such as amphetamines, tyramine, MDMA (ecstasy), phenylpropanolamine and pseudoephedrine can result in a potentially fatal hypertensive crisis. Some of these compounds are contained in proprietary cough and cold remedies. Tyramine, contained in some foods, e.g. cheese and red wine, is normally metabolized in the gut wall by MAO to inactive metabolites. In patients taking MAOI, however, tyramine will be absorbed intact. If patients taking MAOIs also take these amines there may be a massive release of noradrenaline from adrenergic nerve endings, causing a sympathetic overactivity syndrome, characterized by hypertension, headache, excitement, hyperpyrexia and cardiac arrhythmias. Fatal intracranial haemorrhage and cardiac arrest may result. The risk of interactions continues for several weeks after the MAOI is stopped as new MAO enzyme must be synthesized. Patients taking irreversible MAOIs should not take any indirectly acting sympathomimetic amines. All patients must be strongly warned about the risks of cough and cold remedies, illicit drug use and the necessary dietary restrictions.

Drug–food interactions

It is well established that food can cause clinically important changes in drug absorption through effects on gastrointestinal motility or by drug binding. Two examples already outlined in this chapter include the interaction between tyramine in some foods and MAOIs, and the interaction between grapefruit juice and the calcium channel blocker felodipine. With improved understanding of drug metabolism mechanisms, there is greater recognition of the effects of some foods on drug metabolism. There have been recent reports of an interaction between cranberry juice and warfarin, prompting regulatory advice that the international normalized ratio (INR) should be closely monitored in patients taking this combination. Drug interactions with grapefruit juice continue to attract considerable interest.

Cruciferous vegetables and charcoal-grilled meats

Cruciferous vegetables, such as brussels sprouts, cabbage and broccoli, contain substances that are inducers of the cytochrome P450 isoenzyme CYP1A2. Chemicals formed by 'burning' meats additionally have these properties. These foods do not appear to cause any clinically important drug interactions in their own right, but their consumption may add another variable to drug interaction studies, so complicating interpretation.

Grapefruit juice

By chance, grapefruit juice was chosen to mask the taste of ethanol in a study of the effect of ethanol on felodipine, which led to the discovery that grapefruit juice itself markedly increased felodipine levels. Grapefruit juice mainly inhibits intestinal CYP3A4, with only minimal effects on hepatic CYP3A4. This is demonstrated by the fact that intravenous preparations of drugs metabolized by CYP3A4 are not much affected, whereas oral preparations of the same drugs are. Some drugs that are not metabolized by CYP3A4 show decreased levels with grapefruit juice, such as fexofenadine. The probable reason for this is that grapefruit juice inhibits some drug transporter proteins and possibly affects organic anion-transporting polypeptides (OATPs), although inhibition of P-glycoprotein has also been suggested.

The active constituent of grapefruit juice is uncertain. Grapefruit contains naringin, which degrades during processing to naringenin, a substance known to inhibit CYP3A4. Because of this, it has been assumed that whole grapefruit will not interact, but that processed grapefruit juice will. However, some reports have implicated the whole fruit. Other possible active constituents in the whole fruit include bergamottin and dihydroxybergamottin.

Conclusion

It is impossible to remember all drug interactions of potential clinical significance. Healthcare staff should be continually alert to the possibility of drug interactions and take appropriate steps to minimize their occurrence. In general, where the combination of potentially interacting drugs is unavoidable, the dose of any drug likely to have increased effects as a result of the interaction should be reduced, e.g. by one-third to one-half, and the patient monitored for toxic effects using clinical variables or plasma drug levels for at least 2 weeks or until these are stable. For drugs that are likely to have reduced effects as a result of the interaction, the patient should be monitored similarly for therapeutic failure for at least 2 weeks or until stable, and the dose increased if necessary. Alternatively, it may be appropriate to switch one of the treatments to one which does not interact. Patients should be advised to seek guidance about their medication if they plan to stop smoking, or start a herbal remedy, as they may need close monitoring during the transition.

CASE STUDIES

Case 4.1

Mrs C is a 62-year-old woman with a history of hypertension, atrial fibrillation and type 2 diabetes. She is a non-smoker and obese. Her current medication comprises flecainide 100 mg twice a day, aspirin 75 mg daily, simvastatin 40 mg, and diltiazem 180 mg daily. Mrs C is suffering from a respiratory tract infection and her GP has prescribed a 5-day course of clarithromycin.

Questions

1. Are there likely to be any clinically significant drug interactions?
2. What advice do you give?

Answers

1. There is a potential interaction between simvastatin and diltiazem and between simvastatin and clarithromycin. Some statins, particularly simvastatin and atorvastatin, are metabolized by cytochrome P450 (CYP3A4) and co-administration of potent inhibitors of this enzyme may particularly increase plasma levels of these statins and so increase the risk of dose-related side effects, including rhabdomyolysis. Clarithromycin is a potent inhibitor of CYP3A4 and diltiazem is a less potent inhibitor.
2. Current advice is that diltiazem and simvastatin may be given together provided the simvastatin dose does not exceed 40 mg daily, so it is reasonable for this therapy to be continued. However, clarithromycin should not be given together with simvastatin. Myopathy and rhabdomyolysis have been reported in patients taking the combination. Mrs C should be advised not to take her simvastatin while she is taking clarithromycin and to start taking it again after she has completed the course of antibiotic.

Case 4.2

A 19-year-old woman is on long-term treatment with minocycline 100 mg daily for acne. She wishes to start using the combined oral contraceptive and her doctor has prescribed a low-strength pill (containing ethinyloestradiol 20 μg with norethisterone 1 mg). The doctor contacts the pharmacist for advice on whether the tetracycline will interfere with the efficacy of the oral contraceptive.

Question

Is there a clinically significant interaction in this situation?

Answer

Contraceptive failure has been attributed to doxycycline, lymecycline, oxytetracycline, minocycline and tetracycline in about 40 reported cases, seven of which specified long-term antibacterial use. There is controversy about whether or not a drug interaction occurs but if there is one it appears to be very rare. Controlled trials have not shown any effect of tetracycline or doxycycline on contraceptive steroid levels. The postulated mechanism is suppression of intestinal bacteria resulting in a fall in enterohepatic recirculation of ethinyloestradiol. Overall there is no evidence that this is clinically important.

In the case of long-term use of tetracyclines for acne, a small number of cases of contraceptive failure have been reported. Nevertheless, the only well-designed, case–control study in dermatological practice indicated that the incidence of contraceptive failure due to this interaction could not be distinguished from the general and recognized failure rate of oral contraceptives. The UK Family Planning Association advises that women on long-term antibiotic therapy need only take extra precautions for the first 3 weeks of oral contraceptive use because, after about 2 weeks, the gut flora becomes resistant to the antibiotic. In addition, there is some evidence that ethinyloestradiol may accentuate the facial pigmentation that can be caused by minocycline.

Case 4.3

A 48-year-old man with a history of epilepsy is admitted to hospital with tremor, ataxia, headache, abnormal thinking and increased partial seizure activity. His prescribed medicines are phenytoin 300 mg daily, clonazepam 6 mg daily and fluoxetine 20 mg daily. It transpires that fluoxetine therapy had been initiated 2 weeks previously. The patient's phenytoin level is found to be 35 mg/L; at the last outpatient clinic visit 4 months ago, it was 18 mg/L.

Question

What is the proposed mechanism of interaction between fluoxetine and phenytoin and how should it be managed?

Answer

Fluoxetine is believed to inhibit the metabolism of phenytoin by the cytochrome P450 isoenzyme CYP2C9, potentially leading to increased plasma phenytoin levels. There are a number of published case reports and anecdotal observations of phenytoin toxicity occurring with the combination, but the available evidence is conflicting. A review by the US Food and Drug Administration suggested that a marked increase in plasma phenytoin levels, with accompanying toxicity, can occur within 1–42 days (mean onset time of 2 weeks) after starting fluoxetine. If fluoxetine is added to treatment with phenytoin, the patient should be closely monitored. Ideally the phenytoin plasma levels should be monitored and there may be a need to reduce the phenytoin dosage.

Case 4.4

A 79-year-old man presented to hospital with a 3-day history of increasing confusion and collapse. He had a history of chronic lumbosacral pain, treated with oxycodone 10 mg twice daily and amitriptyline 75 mg daily. Five days before hospital admission he had been prescribed tramadol 100 mg four times daily for worsening sciatica. On admission the patient had a Glasgow Coma Scale of 11 and he was delirious and hallucinating. There were no focal neurological signs. Over the next 2 days he became increasingly unwell, confused and sweaty with pyrexia and muscular rigidity. Biochemical tests showed a metabolic acidosis (base deficit of 10.7) and an elevated creatine kinase level of 380 IU/L. There was no evidence of infection. At this stage a diagnosis of probable serotonin syndrome was made.

Questions

1. What is serotonin syndrome and what drugs are most commonly associated with it?
2. How is serotonin syndrome managed?

Answers

1. Serotonin syndrome is often described as a clinical triad of mental status changes, autonomic hyperactivity and neuromuscular abnormalities. However, not all these features are consistently present in all patients with the disorder. Symptoms arising from a serotonin excess range from diarrhoea and tremor in mild cases to delirium, neuromuscular rigidity, rhabdomyolysis and hyperthermia in life-threatening cases. Disturbance of electrolytes, transaminases and creatine kinase may occur. Clonus is the most important finding in establishing the diagnosis of the serotonin syndrome. The differential diagnosis includes neuroleptic malignant syndrome, sepsis, hepatic encephalopathy, heat stroke, delirium tremens and anticholinergic reactions. Serotonin syndrome may not be recognized in some cases because of its protean manifestations. A wide range of drugs and drug combinations has been associated with the serotonin syndrome, including MAOIs, tricyclic antidepressants, SSRIs, opioids, linezolid and $5HT_1$-agonists. Tramadol is an atypical opioid analgesic with partial μ antagonism and central reuptake inhibition of serotonin (5HT) and noradrenaline. At high doses it may also induce serotonin release. Tramadol is reported as causing serotonin syndrome alone (in a few case reports) and in combination with SSRIs, venlafaxine and atypical antipsychotics.

2. Management of the serotonin syndrome involves removal of the precipitating drugs and supportive care. Many cases typically resolve within 24 hours after serotonergic drugs are stopped but symptoms may persist in patients taking medicines with long half-lives or active metabolites. The $5HT_{2A}$-antagonist cyproheptadine and atypical antipsychotic agents with $5HT_{2A}$-antagonist activity, such as olanzapine, have been used to treat serotonin syndrome, although their efficacy has not been conclusively established.

REFERENCES

Baxter K 2005 (ed) Stockley's drug interactions, 7th edn. Pharmaceutical Press, London

Boyer E W, Shannon M 2005 Current concepts: the serotonin syndrome. New England Journal of Medicine 352: 1112-1120

DuBuske L M 2005. The role of P-glycoprotein and organic anion-transporting polypeptides in drug interactions. Drug Safety 28: 789-801

Jankel C A, Fitterman L K 1993 Epidemiology of drug–drug interactions as a cause of hospital admissions. Drug Safety 9: 55-59

Leape L L, Brennan T A, Laird N et al 1992 The nature of adverse events in hospitalised patients: results of the Harvard Medical Practice Study II. New England Journal of Medicine 324: 377-384

Lee W, Kim R B 2004 Transporters and renal drug elimination. Annual Reviews in Pharmacology and Toxicology 44: 137-166

Li Wan Po A, Zhang W Y 1998 What lessons can be learnt from withdrawal of mibefradil from the market? Lancet 351: 1829-1830

Mannel M 2004 Drug interactions with St John's wort: mechanisms and clinical implications. Drug Safety 27: 773-797

Pirmohamed M, James S, Meakin S et al 2004 Adverse drug reactions as cause of admission to hospital: prospective analysis of 18820 patients. British Medical Journal 329:15-19

Roden D M 2004 Drug-induced prolongation of the QT interval. New England Journal of Medicine 350: 1013-1022

Schwarz U I 2003 Clinical relevance of genetic polymorphisms in the human CYP2C9 gene. European Journal of Clinical Investigation 33(suppl 2): 23-30

Smith J W, Seidl L G, Cluff L E 1969 Studies on the epidemiology of adverse drug reactions. V. Clinical factors influencing susceptibility. Annals of Internal Medicine 65: 629

Wilkinson G R 2005 Drug therapy: drug metabolism and variability among patients in drug response. New England Journal of Medicine 352: 2211-2221

FURTHER READING

Fugh-Berman A 2000 Herb–drug interactions. Lancet 355: 134-138

Pirmohamed M, Orme M L'E 1998 Drug interactions of clinical importance. In: Davies D M, Ferner R E, de Glanville H (eds) Davies's textbook of adverse drug reactions, 5th edn. Chapman and Hall Medical, London

Adverse drug reactions 5

A. Lee   S. H. L. Thomas

KEY POINTS

- Adverse drug reactions are an important cause of morbidity and mortality. They are responsible for a considerable number of hospital admissions and significantly increase healthcare costs.
- An adverse drug reaction is an unwanted or harmful reaction experienced after the administration of a drug or combination of drugs under normal conditions of use and suspected to be related to the drug.
- Adverse drug reactions can be classified as type A or type B. Type A (augmented) reactions are normal pharmacological effects which are undesirable. They are usually dose dependent and often predictable. They are an important cause of morbidity but death is unusual.
- Type B (bizarre) reactions are effects unrelated to the known pharmacology of a drug. These reactions are rare, unpredictable and generally unrelated to dose. Reactions are often severe or fatal.
- Important predisposing factors to adverse drug reactions include extremes of age, polypharmacy, intercurrent disease and genetic factors. Mechanisms of reactions may be pharmaceutical, pharmacokinetic or pharmacodynamic.
- Early recognition of potential adverse drug reactions is critical. Type B reactions and uncommon type A reactions are unlikely to be detected during clinical trials. Postmarketing surveillance, including spontaneous reporting of suspected adverse drug reactions, is essential for monitoring drug safety.

An adverse drug reaction (ADR) is any undesirable effect of a drug beyond its anticipated therapeutic effects occurring during clinical use. Drug therapy has been recognized as a significant cause of harm since the earliest times. Around 400 BC Hippocrates warned about the dangers of drugs, recommending that they should never be prescribed unless the patient had been thoroughly examined. In 1785 when William Withering described the benefits of digitalis, he also described the vomiting, alteration of vision, bradycardia, convulsions and death it could cause. In the 20th century great therapeutic advances were accompanied by a growing awareness of the problems of adverse reactions to medicines among both healthcare professionals and consumers. In particular, the thalidomide tragedy in the early 1960s was the seminal event leading to the development of modern drug regulation. Thalidomide, prescribed as a 'safe' hypnotic to many thousands of pregnant women, caused a severe form of limb abnormality known as phocomelia in many of the babies born to these women.

Drug-induced disease is rarely specific and almost invariably mimics naturally occurring disease. Few adverse drug reactions are associated with diagnostic clinical or laboratory findings which demarcate them from the features of a spontaneous disease. Moreover, many of the subjective effects frequently attributed to medicines, such as headache, nausea and dizziness, occur commonly in healthy individuals taking no medication and in patients taking a placebo. Pharmacists have a key role in minimizing the occurrence of adverse drug reactions. This requires knowledge of the adverse effects of medicines, including their frequency and severity, the most common predisposing factors, and the relationship to dosage and duration of treatment. There is a huge literature on adverse drug reactions. This chapter will concentrate on the epidemiology, mechanisms and classification of adverse drug reactions, important predisposing factors, and how adverse reactions are identified and evaluated.

Epidemiology

Many studies have attempted to determine the incidence of adverse drug reactions in a variety of settings. The estimates of incidence vary widely and this reflects differences in the methods used to detect and define suspected reactions. Some key studies only are described here. In the 1960s the Boston Collaborative Drug Surveillance Program was pivotal in establishing the epidemiological basis of drug-induced disease. Data were collected on over 50 000 consecutive patients admitted to medical wards over a 10-year period, allowing much original research on the association between short-term drug exposures and acute ADRs. In an interim analysis of 19 000 patients monitored, the adverse reaction rate was 30%. Many ADRs were, however, minor and it was concluded that drugs were 'remarkably non-toxic'. Detailed analysis of the data provided much information on patient characteristics predisposing to ADRs and allowed some established adverse effects of drugs, such as excessive drowsiness with flurazepam, to be quantified.

The Harvard Medical Practice Study found a 3.7% incidence of adverse drug events (a categorization that included overdose and medication error) in 30 195 acute hospital inpatients (Brennan et al 1991). In a further 6-month study of 4031 medical and surgical admissions the investigators found a 6% incidence of adverse drug events and a 5% incidence of potential adverse drug events (or near misses). Of all adverse drug events observed, 1% were fatal, 12% life-threatening, 30% serious and 57% significant. Twenty-eight percent were considered preventable, with a greater proportion of the life-threatening and serious reactions in that category. The classes of medicine implicated most frequently in serious reactions were analgesics, antibiotics, sedatives, cytotoxics, cardiovascular drugs, anticoagulants, antipsychotics, antidiabetics and electrolytes.

Another US study of hospital inpatients in 1992 found a similar frequency and type of adverse events to those observed in the Harvard study. A review of data on nearly 15 000 patients discharged from 28 hospitals suggested a 2.9% rate of adverse events (not necessarily drug related). Adverse drug reactions were the second most common type of adverse event, accounting for 19.3% of those identified. Antibiotics, cardiovascular drugs, analgesics and anticoagulants again featured among the classes of medicine implicated most frequently. More than a third of the ADRs were considered avoidable and nearly 1 in 10 caused irreversible harm. UK data on morbidity in hospital inpatients as a consequence of adverse drug reactions are lacking. One study suggested that 7% of over 20 000 medical inpatients experienced an ADR during their hospital stay .

Adverse drug reactions are responsible for a significant number of hospital admissions, with reported rates ranging from 0.3% to 11%. Data from meta-analyses and systematic review suggest that the rate of admissions directly due to ADRs is 5% (Einarson et al 1993, Wiffen et al 2002). Recent work has suggested that many of these reactions are predictable and preventable. A prospective analysis of admissions caused by ADRs in two large UK hospitals was undertaken by Pirmohamed at al (2004). All adult patients admitted over a 6-month period were assessed to determine if the admission had been caused by an ADR. Patients were categorized as having an ADR if the cause of admission was consistent with the known adverse effect profile of the drug, if there was a plausible temporal relationship with the drug therapy and if, after appropriate investigations, other causes were excluded. The main outcome measures were the prevalence of admissions due to an ADR, length of stay, avoidability and patient outcome.

There were 18 820 admissions over the 6-month period; 1225 of these were related to an ADR, giving a prevalence of 6.5%. Eighty percent of the ADRs were judged to have been directly responsible for the admission (termed causal) while 20% were identified through screening (termed coincidental). Patients admitted with ADRs (median age 76 years) were significantly older than those without ADRs (median age 66 years). Although most patients recovered, 28 (2.3%) died as a result of the ADR. The overall fatality rate was 0.15%. Only 340 (28%) of the 1225 ADR-related admissions were assessed as unavoidable, while 107 (9%) and 773 (63%) were classified as 'definitely avoidable' and 'possibly avoidable' respectively. Drug interactions accounted for 16.6% of ADRs. The most common reaction was gastrointestinal bleeding. The majority of the drugs commonly implicated as a cause of ADRs in this study (non-steroidal anti-inflammatory agents, diuretics, warfarin, digoxin, opioids) are consistent with the results of previous studies.

For ADRs occurring in the community, the reported incidence ranges from 2.6% to 41% of patients, but this is a more complex area to study and there are fewer well-designed studies. A prospective cohort study in an ambulatory primary care setting in four primary care practices in Boston, USA (Gandhi et al 2003), revealed that of 661 patients who responded to a telephone survey (response rate, 55%), 162 (25%) described experiencing adverse drug events, with a total of 181 events. Twenty-four of the events (13%) were serious, 51 (28%) were ameliorable, and 20 (11%) were preventable. None was fatal or life-threatening. Of the 51

ameliorable events, 32 (63%) were attributed by independent physicians to the prescriber's failure to respond to medication-related symptoms and 19 (37%) to the patient's failure to inform the prescriber of the symptoms. The most frequent types of adverse drug event were central nervous system, gastrointestinal and cardiovascular events. The classes of medicine implicated most frequently were selective serotonin reuptake inhibitors (SSRIs) (10%), β-blockers (9%), angiotensin converting enzyme inhibitors (8%), and non-steroidal anti-inflammatory agents (8%). The authors concluded that adverse drug events in primary care are common and many are preventable or ameliorable. Acting on early signs or symptoms and improving communication were identified as important issues.

A cohort study assessed the incidence and preventability of adverse drug events in elderly people aged 65 years and over in the ambulatory care setting (equivalent to 30 397 person-years of observation) in the USA (Gurwitz et al 2003). Over a 1-year period there were 1523 identified adverse events, of which 421 (27.6%) were considered preventable and 578 (38%) were categorized as serious, life-threatening or fatal. The classes of medicine implicated most frequently were cardiovascular drugs, diuretics, non-opioid analgesics, antidiabetics and anticoagulants.

Adverse drug reactions also have a significant impact on healthcare costs. Two US case–control studies found a significantly greater length of hospital stay in patients who experienced an ADR while in hospital. Both studies estimated direct costs associated with ADRs and, not surprisingly, concluded that such costs may be substantial. The occurrence of an ADR was estimated to increase the cost of care by $2262 per patient (Classen et al 1997) and the cost of preventable ADRs in a 700-bed hospital was estimated at $2.8 million per annum (Bates et al 1997). In the UK the median bed stay in patients with drug-related admissions was 8 days (Pirmohamed et al 2004). The authors estimated that if these findings were extrapolated across the NHS in England, at any one time the equivalent of up to seven 800-bed hospitals would be occupied by patients admitted with ADRs. The projected annual cost of such admissions to the NHS was £466m (€706m).

These studies demonstrate that adverse drug reactions remain a significant cause of patient harm. The associated burden on healthcare is clearly high, accounting for considerable morbidity, mortality and extra costs. The high proportion of ADRs categorized as avoidable in recent studies suggests that inappropriate prescribing is a common problem. Strategies are needed to reduce the impact of ADRs and further improve the benefit:harm ratio of medicines. The imperative to reduce the occurrence of adverse drug reactions is a shared responsibility, presenting a considerable challenge to all health professionals.

Definition and classification

The World Health Organization definition of an adverse drug reaction is 'a response to a drug which is noxious, unintended and occurs at doses used in man for prophylaxis, diagnosis or therapy'. Although widely accepted, this definition has limitations and others have been suggested. The UK Commission on Human Medicines defines an adverse drug reaction as 'an unwanted or harmful reaction experienced after the administration of a drug or combination of drugs under normal conditions of use and suspected to be related to the drug'.

There are several ways of classifying adverse reactions. The simplest is to separate them into types A and B (Rawlins & Thompson 1977) (Table 5.1). Type A (or augmented) reactions are the result of an exaggerated, but otherwise normal, pharmacological action of a drug given in the usual therapeutic doses. Examples include orthostatic hypotension with a phenothiazine or hypoglycaemia with a sulphonylurea. Type A reactions are predictable from a drug's known pharmacology and usually dose dependent. Because they are common the associated morbidity is generally high but fatal outcomes are rare. Some type A reactions have a long latency. Examples include teratogenicity, chloroquine retinopathy and vaginal adenocarcinoma which may occur in the daughters born to women who received diethylstilboestrol during the pregnancy.

Type B reactions, in contrast, are bizarre effects that are not predictable on the basis of a drug's pharmacology. Examples include malignant hyperthermia of anaesthesia, acute porphyria and many immunological reactions. Type B reactions are generally unrelated to dosage and, although comparatively rare, they are more likely to result in serious illness and death. This type of reaction is often not observed during the pre-marketing clinical trial programme for a medicine and consequently accounts for many drug withdrawals from the market.

Although this classification is simple, some adverse reactions do not fit neatly into one type (Aronson & Ferner 2003). Additional categories of ADR have subsequently been suggested to include type C (chronic), type D (delayed), type E (end of use), type F (therapeutic failure) and type G (genetic/genomic) reactions. Use of this extended classification does not mitigate all difficulties, however, and a new system of classification has recently been proposed (Aronson & Ferner 2003). This takes into account properties of both the reaction and the affected individual as well as those of the drug itself. The three-dimensional classification system, known as DoTS, is based on dose-relatedness, time course and susceptibility. It may have some advantages over previous classifications.

Predisposing factors

The main factors known to predispose patients to ADRs include the following.

Multiple drug therapy

The incidence of adverse drug reactions and interactions has been shown to increase sharply with the number of drugs taken. This suggests that the effects of multiple drug use are not simply additive. There is likely to be a synergistic effect, but the concept of confounding by multiple disease states must be borne in mind.

Age

The very old and the very young are more susceptible to ADRs. The elderly often have multiple and chronic diseases and so are more likely than younger people to be taking several medicines at any one time. They are particularly vulnerable to the adverse effects of drugs because of the physiological changes that accompany ageing. Most studies have shown a positive correlation between age and the number of ADRs but this is a complex issue. It is difficult to determine whether age alone renders these patients more susceptible to ADRs or whether this simply reflects increased drug exposure, multiple disease states and age-related pharmacokinetic changes. Drug metabolism is impaired in the elderly. In fit elderly people, changes in the rates of drug metabolism are mainly due to the age-related decrease in liver blood flow and liver size (Wynne 2005). Consequently there is greater systemic exposure to drugs that are avidly cleared by the liver. In normal ageing, in general, activity of the cytochrome P450 enzymes is preserved, although a decline in frail older people has been noted. There is also evidence that age-related pharmacodynamic changes make the elderly more sensitive to the effects of some medicines. Adverse reactions in elderly patients often have a vague, non-specific presentation. Mental confusion, constipation, hypotension and falls may be the presenting features of illness but may also suggest ADRs. Drugs that commonly cause problems in elderly patients include hypnotics, diuretics, non-steroidal anti-inflammatory drugs, antihypertensives, psychotropics and digoxin.

All children, and particularly neonates, differ from adults in the way they handle and respond to drugs. In studies that have investigated the characteristics of ADRs specifically in children, the reported incidence has varied considerably. This partly reflects the limited amount of high-quality research in children but also the variation in study methodologies. A meta-analysis of observational studies on the incidence of ADRs in children in different healthcare settings found an overall incidence of ADRs of 9.53% in hospitalized children; severe reactions accounted for 12.29% of the total (Impicciatore et al 2001). The overall rate of hospital admissions due to ADRs was 2.09%; 39.3% of these were life-threatening reactions. For outpatients the overall incidence of ADRs was 1.46%.

These rates are broadly similar to the findings of systematic reviews and meta-analyses of studies in adults, although the rate of drug-induced hospital admissions is somewhat lower than in

Table 5.1 Characteristics of type A and type B adverse drug reactions (after Rawlins & Thompson 1977)

	Type A (augmented response)	Type B (bizarre response)
Pharmacologically predictable	Yes	No
Dose dependent	Yes	No
Incidence	High	Low
Morbidity	High	Low
Mortality	Low	High
Management	Dosage adjustment often appropriate	Stop

adult studies. However, the high proportion of severe ADRs in the hospital setting gives cause for concern as these are higher than the corresponding figures in studies in adults. Some studies have suggested the risk of ADRs associated with unlicensed or off-label use (and this applies to many paediatric medicines) may be greater than the corresponding risks for licensed medicines. As in adults, polypharmacy was found to be a consistent risk factor for ADRs.

A review of all reports of suspected ADRs with a fatal outcome in children under 16 years from 1964 to 2000 showed that 331 deaths had been reported with 390 suspected medicines (Clarkson & Choonara 2002). Limited conclusions can be drawn from this study as it was based on data from a voluntary reporting scheme, but the study provides some insight into the medicines suspected of having caused deaths in children. The classes of medicine most frequently associated with fatalities were antiepileptics, cytotoxic agents, anaesthetic gases and antibiotics. The nature of the reported ADRs was diverse, with hepatic failure the most frequent.

Some medicines are particularly likely to cause problems in neonates but are generally well tolerated in older children, e.g. morphine. Others are associated with an increased risk of problems in children of any age, e.g. sodium valproate. Hazardous drugs for neonates include chloramphenicol, morphine and antiarrhythmics. Specific examples of concern in children are Reye's syndrome with aspirin and hepatotoxicity with sodium valproate.

Gender

Women are thought to be at greater risk of ADRs than men. Females appear to have a 1.5- to 1.7-fold greater risk of developing an ADR. The reasons for this are not entirely clear but may include gender-related differences in pharmacokinetic, immunological and hormonal factors. Women are reputed to be more susceptible to blood dyscrasias with phenylbutazone and chloramphenicol, histaminoid reactions to neuromuscular blocking drugs, and to drug-induced prolongation of the QT interval on the electrocardiogram.

Intercurrent disease

Patients with impaired renal or hepatic function are at substantially increased risk of developing ADRs to drugs eliminated by these organs. There are, however, specific disease states which may predispose to adverse drug reactions, such as HIV infection, critical illness and trauma. For example, HIV-infected patients are more likely to experience severe skin reactions with co-trimoxazole. Immune deficiency is a complex clinical area with multiple drug exposures, multiple illness events and consequent difficulty in interpreting drug toxicity data.

Race and genetic polymorphism

Inherited factors that affect the pharmacokinetics and pharmacodynamics of numerous drugs are of great importance in determining an individual's risk of ADR. The discipline of pharmacogenetics deals with variability in drug response that is under hereditary control. Genetic variations in genes for drug-

metabolizing enzymes, drug receptors and drug transporters have been associated with individual variability in the efficacy and toxicity of drugs (Pirmohamed & Atuah 2006). These genetic polymorphisms of drug metabolism produce the phenotypes of 'poor metabolizers', 'extensive metabolizers' and 'ultra-rapid metabolizers' of many drugs. Polymorphisms in the cytochrome P450 enzymes in the liver can have a profound effect on drug efficacy. In 'poor metabolizers' the genes encoding specific cytochrome P450 enzymes often contain inactivating mutations, which result in a complete lack of active enzyme and a severely compromised ability to metabolize drugs.

The ultimate aim of pharmacogenetics is to individualize drug therapy, where the choice of medicine is determined by the genetic status of the patient. In this scenario, genetically determined varations in drug response will be identified prior to prescription, and the potential for reduced efficacy and/or increased toxicity reduced. New genetic polymorphisms are being discovered at an increasing rate, but not all have pharmacokinetic or pharmacodynamic consequences. There is some evidence that prior knowledge of a patient's pharmacogenetic profile may prevent some ADRs. For example, determination of the genotype may reduce the adverse effects of warfarin and azathioprine in patients lacking the enzymes responsible for metabolism of these drugs. An important challenge facing pharmacogenetics is the need for evidence of the clinical and cost-effectiveness of the technology, particularly in relation to the prevention and management of ADRs.

Mechanisms of dose-related (type A) adverse drug reactions

There is great variability in the individual response to drug therapy. This is manifest either as different doses being required to produce the pharmacological effect or different responses to a defined dose. Such interindividual variation is the basis of many dose-related adverse reactions (Wilkinson 2005). Such reactions may occur because of variations in the pharmaceutical, pharmacokinetic or pharmacodynamic properties of a drug, and are often due to the underlying disease state or pharmacogenetic characteristics of the patient. In some cases a combination of these causes may be responsible.

Pharmaceutical causes

Adverse reactions can occur due to pharmaceutical aspects of a dosage form because of alterations in either the quantity of drug present or its release characteristics. As a result of the stringent requirements of regulatory authorities, such reactions are now rare in developed countries. In 1983 a rate-controlled preparation of indometacin (Osmosin) was withdrawn following reports of gastrointestinal bleeding and haemorrhage. This was probably due to the irritant effects of a very high concentration of the active ingredient on a localized area of intestinal mucosa.

Pharmacokinetic causes

Quantitative alterations in the absorption, distribution, metabolism and elimination of drugs may lead to alterations in the concentration of a drug at its site of action with corresponding changes in its pharmacological effects. Such alterations may produce either an exaggerated response or therapeutic failure as a consequence of abnormally low drug concentrations.

Absorption

The rate and magnitude of the oral absorption of a drug are key determinants of its bioavailability. Factors which can influence these include dosage, pharmaceutical factors, gastrointestinal tract motility, the absorptive capacity of the gastrointestinal mucosa, and first-pass metabolism in the liver and gut wall before the drug reaches the systemic circulation. The rate of absorption of orally administered drugs is largely determined by the rate of gastric emptying, which is influenced by factors including the nature of the gastric contents, disease and concomitant drugs. The majority of adverse reactions resulting from changes in drug absorption are reduced therapeutic efficacy or therapeutic failure.

Distribution

The distribution of drugs to various tissues and organs is dependent on factors such as regional blood flow, plasma protein and tissue binding. Changes in how a drug is distributed may, theoretically, predispose to adverse effects although the clinical importance of such mechanisms is unclear.

Elimination

Most drugs are excreted in the urine or bile or metabolized by the liver to yield metabolites that are then excreted by the kidneys. Changes in drug elimination rates are probably the most important cause of type A adverse drug reactions. Reduced elimination leads to drug accumulation, with potential toxicity due to increased plasma and tissue levels. Conversely, enhanced elimination leads to reduced plasma and tissue drug levels, resulting in therapeutic failure.

Renal excretion Impaired glomerular filtration leads to reduced elimination of drugs that undergo renal excretion. Individuals with reduced glomerular filtration, such as patients with renal disease, the elderly and neonates, are liable to develop type A adverse reactions to standard therapeutic doses of drugs that are mainly excreted by the kidney. Some of the most potentially toxic drugs in this respect are digoxin, ACE inhibitors, aminoglycoside antibiotics, some class I antiarrhythmic agents (disopyramide, flecainide) and many cytotoxic agents. The occurrence of these ADRs may be minimized by adjusting the dosage given to individual patients on the basis of their renal function.

Drug metabolism

Lipid-soluble agents are frequently metabolized to water-soluble compounds that can be excreted by the kidney. Metabolism occurs predominantly in the liver, although the kidney, lungs, skin and gut also have some metabolizing capacity. In man, drug metabolism can be divided into two phases. Phase I (oxidation, reduction or hydrolysis) exposes functionally reactive groups or

adds them to the molecule. Phase II (sulphation, glucuronidation, acetylation or methylation) involves conjugation of the drug at a reactive site produced during phase I. Drugs that already have reactive groups undergo phase II reactions only. Others are sufficiently water soluble after phase I metabolism to be eliminated by renal excretion.

Interindividual differences or alterations in the rate at which drugs are metabolized result in appropriate variations in elimination rates. Reduced rates of metabolism may lead to drug accumulation and an increased risk of type A adverse drug reactions, while enhanced rates of metabolism may result in therapeutic failure. There is wide interindividual variation in some routes of metabolism, even among normal individuals, because of genetic and environmental influences. This particularly applies to oxidation, hydrolysis and acetylation. Competition for glucuronidation may occur when two drugs metabolized by this pathway are given concurrently.

Microsomal oxidation Drug oxidation occurs mainly in the smooth endoplasmic reticulum of the liver by the cytochrome P450 enzyme system. It is mediated by a group of enzymes known as the cytochrome P450 superfamily. Four main subfamilies of P450 isoenzymes are thought to be responsible for most (about 90%) of the metabolism of commonly used drugs in humans: CYP1, CYP2, CYP3 and CYP4. Individual isoenzymes that have been specifically identified are given a further number (e.g. CYP2D6, which is the most extensively studied isoenzyme, debrisoquine hydroxylase). Although there is overlap, each CYP isoenzyme tends to metabolize a discrete range of substrates. Of the many isoenzymes, just a few (CYP1A2, CYP2C9, CYP2C19, CYP2D6, CYP2E1 and CYP3A4) seem to be responsible for the metabolism of most commonly used drugs. As previously discussed, the genes that encode specific CYP isoenzymes can vary between individuals and, often, ethnic groups (Wilkinson 2005).

Interindividual variability in debrisoquine metabolism is well recognized. Poor metabolizers tend to have reduced first-pass metabolism, increased plasma levels and exaggerated pharmacological response to this drug, resulting in postural hypotension. By contrast, ultra-rapid metabolizers may require considerably higher doses for a standard effect. The enzyme showing polymorphism in this situation is debrisoquine hydroxylase or CYP2D6. About 5–10% of Europeans have a poor ability to metabolize drugs by this route and are thus at risk of compromised metabolism or ADRs when prescribed drugs that are CYP2D6 substrates. More than 65 commonly used drugs are metabolized by CYP2D6, many of which are used in the treatment of psychiatric, neurological and cardiovascular diseases. Studies with several antipsychotics metabolized by CYP2D6 have demonstrated a higher incidence of adverse effects, such as extrapyramidal symptoms, in poor metabolizers. However, data in the literature are equivocal and at present no firm recommendations can be given with regard to genotyping patients for CYP2D6 status before starting antipsychotic therapy.

The CYP2C subfamily accounts for around 18% of the CYP protein content in human hepatocytes. It is now known that there are about 12 genotypes of the CYP2C9 gene. One of the important drugs metabolized by CYP2C9 is warfarin (specifically the more active S-enantiomer), which has been the subject of numerous pharmacogenetic studies. It is well recognized that many patients, despite frequent monitoring of the International Normalized Ratio (INR), fail to consistently achieve an INR within the therapeutic range, and the required dose can vary from 0.5 mg to 15 mg per day.

A review of several retrospective studies among outpatients receiving long-term warfarin therapy indicates that the mean maintenance dose depends on the CYP2C9 genotype. Thus, individuals homozygous for the *1 allele (CYP2C9*1/*1) have 'normal' warfarin metabolic rates, while the CYP2C9*3/*3 genotype is associated with the lowest metabolic clearance rate. Patients with variant CYP2C9 genotypes are more likely to have INRs above the therapeutic range, and consequently a greater risk of serious and life-threatening bleeding complications, during both induction and maintenance of anticoagulation, compared with the wild-type genotypes (4.89 and 0.7 per 100 patient years, respectively) (Higashi et al 2002). Thus, genotyping may identify a subpopulation of individuals who may require extra monitoring during the initiation phase of warfarin therapy. However, the predictive value of CYP2C9 genotyping for the individual is low, and at present it cannot be used to indicate the final maintenance dose.

The potential effects of enzyme induction and inhibition on other drugs are discussed in Chapter 4.

Hydrolysis Suxamethonium apnoea is the best-known example of altered drug response due to individual variation in drug hydrolysis. The neuromuscular blocking effects of suxamethonium are usually short-lived, as it is rapidly inactivated in plasma by hydrolysis. The hydrolysis is catalysed by plasma pseudocholinesterase which exists in several different genetically determined forms. Individuals homozygous for the atypical gene (about 1 in 2500 of the UK population) may develop prolonged neuromuscular blockade. Suxamethonium apnoea may also be somewhat prolonged in individuals who are heterozygous for the gene, i.e. who possess both the usual and the atypical gene. The frequency of the atypical genes shows marked racial variation. Phenotypic studies of patients who develop prolonged neuromuscular blockade after suxamethonium do not always reveal recognizable genetic abnormalities. In some instances this reaction is secondary to liver or renal disease, both of which can influence the activity of plasma cholinesterase.

Acetylation A number of drugs are metabolized by acetylation including dapsone, isoniazid, hydralazine, phenelzine, procainamide and many sulphonamides. Acetylation is under genetic control and shows a polymorphism, such that individuals may be phenotyped as either 'slow' or 'rapid' acetylators. The variability is due to differences in the activity of the liver enzyme N-acetyltransferase. In the UK about half the population are rapid acetylators, but there are considerable differences among ethnic groups. The incidence of rapid acetylation is highest amongst the Japanese and Canadian Inuit.

Slow acetylators are at increased risk of developing type A adverse reactions. Thus, isoniazid-induced peripheral neuropathy, the haematological adverse effects of dapsone and the adverse effects of sulphapyridine are more likely to occur in these individuals. Slow acetylators of hydralazine and procainamide are also at greater risk of developing systemic lupus erythematosus than fast acetylators.

Glucuronidation Several drugs commonly used in clinical practice (e.g. morphine, paracetamol and ethinyloestradiol) are eliminated at least partly by glucuronide conjugates. There is evidence that, like the CYP450 enzyme system, glucuronyltransferases exist in multiple forms with many drugs acting as substrates for more than one isoenzyme. Glucuronyltransferases are also inducible and the administration of an inducing drug can lead to loss of efficacy of combined oral contraceptives.

Pharmacodynamic causes

Many dose-related ADRs have a pharmacokinetic basis but some are due to altered sensitivity of target organs or tissues. Moreover, in some individuals, ADRs may result from a combination of the two mechanisms. Much recent research has attempted to determine why tissues from different individuals should respond differently to drugs. Evidence is accumulating to show that target organ sensitivity is influenced by pharmacogenetic factors as well as by physiological homeostatic mechanisms and by disease.

Mechanisms of non dose-related (type B) adverse drug reactions

Type B reactions have historically been regarded as those that are inexplicable in terms of the normal pharmacology of the drug. The cause may be pharmaceutical or pharmacokinetic, or may lie in target organ response (pharmacodynamic). As a result of increased research in pharmacogenetics, there is an improved understanding of the proposed mechanism for several type B reactions.

Pharmaceutical causes

Pharmaceutical aspects of the dosage form may be the cause of type B adverse reactions. Such reactions can occur due to the presence of degradation products of the active constituents, the effects of the non-drug components of the formulation, such as excipients and other compounds, e.g. colourings, preservatives and antioxidants, or the actions of synthetic by-products of the active constituents. In most cases the administration of a decomposed drug will result in therapeutic failure, but in some cases the decomposition product may be toxic and potentially lethal, e.g. early formulations of tetracycline. Adverse reactions have resulted from the incorporation of clearly toxic substances such as diethylene glycol, which caused 105 deaths in the USA in 1937 when it was used as a solvent in sulphanilamide elixir; the use of certain excipients in susceptible patient groups, such as asthmatics or neonates; and the alteration of an excipient mixture resulting in changes in the bioavailability of drugs such as digoxin and phenytoin. A number of adverse reactions due to pharmaceutical excipients are recognized.

Nowadays, with stringent controls by manufacturers and monitoring by regulatory authorities, it is extremely unusual for pharmaceutical preparations to be adulterated with synthetic by-products. An example from some years ago is the potentially fatal syndrome of eosinophilia and myalgia associated with L-tryptophan, which was probably due to a contaminant, although genetic factors may have also been involved.

Pharmacokinetic causes

Recent research has shown that some adverse reactions may result from differences in oral bioavailability due to genetic polymorphism in drug transporters. The best studied of these transport proteins is a protein named P-glycoprotein (P-gp), also termed MDR1, found within the cells of the gut wall and the surfaces of hepatocytes and renal tubular cells. The activity of MDR1 in the gut has been shown to be subject to a genetic polymorphism. The cardiac glycoside digoxin is an MDR1 substrate and preliminary research suggests that this polymorphism influences digoxin plasma levels (Marzolini et al 2004).

Pharmacodynamic causes

Individual patients vary widely in their response to drugs. Even if allowance has been made for the patient's age, gender, bodyweight, disease state and concurrent drug regimens, there is still variation between individuals. Qualitative differences in the target organ response to drugs may be considered as genetic, immunological, neoplastic or teratogenic.

Genetic causes for abnormal response

Until recently, many adverse reactions that could not be easily classified were termed 'idiosyncratic'. This situation is changing slowly as the underlying mechanisms become clearer and it is apparent that many have a genetic basis (see Table 5.2).

Erythrocyte glucose-6-phosphate dehydrogenase (G6PD) deficiency

A well-known example of qualitative difference in the response to drugs is G6PD deficiency, which affects about 100–400 million people worldwide. G6PD is an enzyme required for the stability of red blood cells. Individuals with a sex-linked inherited deficiency in this enzyme have weakened red cell membranes and are predisposed to haemolysis due to oxidant drugs such as primaquine, sulphonamides and sulphones, and nitrofurantoin. There are many variants of G6PD and not all are associated with drug-induced haemolysis. The frequency of the enzyme deficiency also varies widely between and within various populations. The African type G6PD (A-) is characterized by mild enzyme deficiency with a mean activity of 8–20% of normal. The Mediterranean type, on the other hand, is characterized by severe enzyme deficiency (0–4% enzyme activity). Consequently, a potentially haemolytic drug is likely to produce only mild haemolysis in people with the African type, but it may have severe and potentially fatal effects in people with the Mediterranean type.

Many medicines have been associated with haemolysis in G6PD deficiency, but the severity of the reaction varies between drugs and also depends on the type of enzyme deficiency. Haemolytic episodes can be provoked by drugs or illness in G6PD-deficient individuals and some drugs have been wrongly implicated as a cause of haemolysis. The number of currently available medicines with proven haemolytic potential in G6PD-deficient individuals is relatively small; primaquine is probably the best-known example. Drugs that should be avoided in G6PD deficiency are shown in Table 5.3. The British National Formulary contains an up-to-date list of drugs with a definite and possible risk of haemolysis in G6PD deficiency.

Hereditary methaemoglobinaemias

An inherited deficiency of methaemoglobin reductase in erythrocytes renders affected individuals susceptible to the development of methaemoglobinaemia and cyanosis in response to oxidant drugs. Drugs that are oxidizing agents, nitrites and all the drugs listed in Table 5.3 may cause this effect.

Table 5.2 Examples of genetically determined adverse drug reactions

Condition	Drug	Effects
Erythrocyte enzyme deficiencies • Glucose-6-phosphate dehydrogenase • Methaemoglobin reductase	Oxidant drugs (Table 5.3) Oxidant drugs (Table 5.3)	Haemolytic anaemia Methaemoglobinaemia
Haemoglobin variants • Haemoglobin H, Zurich, Torino • Haemoglobin Zurich	Oxidant drugs (Table 5.3) Sulphonamides	Haemolytic anaemia Haemolytic anaemia
Porphyria (hepatic)	Barbiturates, sulphonamides, griseofulvin	Preciptate attack of porphyria
Malignant hyperthermia	General anaesthetics (halothane) Muscle relaxants	Hyperthermia with prolonged muscle rigidity, acidosis
Genetic predisposition to raised intraocular pressure	Topical corticosteroids	Increased intraocular pressure
Familial dysautonomia (Riley–Day syndrome)	General anaesthetics Parasympathomimetics	Exaggerated response

Table 5.3 Drugs to be avoided in G6PD deficiency
Dapsone
Niridazole
Methylene blue (methylthioninium chloride)
Primaquine
Quinolones (including ciprofloxacin, nalidixic acid, norfloxacin and ofloxacin)
Sulphonamides (including co-trimoxazole)

Porphyrias

The porphyrias are a heterogeneous group of inherited disorders of haem biosynthesis. The disorders are transmitted as autosomal dominants, with the exception of the rare congenital porphyria, which is recessive. The effects of drugs are of most importance in patients with acute porphyrias, in whom certain commonly prescribed agents may precipitate life-threatening attacks. Other trigger factors include alcohol and changes in sex hormone balance. In the acute porphyrias, patients develop abdominal and neuropsychiatric disturbances, and they excrete in their urine excessive amounts of the porphyrin precursors 5-aminolaevulinic acid (ALA) and porphobilinogen.

A number of drugs may induce excess porphyrin synthesis. However, it is extremely difficult to predict whether or not a drug may cause problems in patients with porphyria and the only factors shown to be clearly linked with porphyrinogenicity are lipid solubility and membrane fluidization, i.e. the ability to disrupt the phospholipid bilayer of the cell membrane. A number of commonly used drugs induce ALA synthase in the liver, but there is wide variation between porphyric patients in their sensitivity to drugs which may trigger attacks. Thus, whereas a single dose of a drug may be sufficient to trigger an acute attack in one patient, another may require a number of relatively large doses of the same drug to produce any clinically significant effect. Lists of drugs which are known to be unsafe and drugs which are thought to be safe for use in acute porphyria are available in the British National Formulary.

Malignant hyperthermia

Malignant hyperthermia is a rare but potentially fatal condition in which there is a rapid rise in body temperature (at least 2°C per hour) occurring without obvious cause after administration of anaesthetics or muscle relaxants. The condition usually follows the administration of an inhalational general anaesthetic, often halothane, in combination with suxamethonium. In addition to the temperature rise, the syndrome is characterized by stiffness of skeletal muscles, hyperventilation, acidosis, hyperkalaemia, and signs of increased activity of the sympathetic nervous system. It is likely that the condition is triggered by an abnormal release of intracellular ionized calcium, which may be due to an inherited defect of cellular membranes. When the condition was first identified it was associated with a mortality rate of up to 80% but this has now decreased to around 10%. Dantrolene has become the gold standard treatment of this condition; it is thought to act by inhibition of calcium release into the muscle tissue.

Glucocorticoid glaucoma

In genetically predisposed individuals glucocorticoids can cause a rise in intraocular pressure leading to blindness. Development of increased intraocular pressure appears to be correlated with dosage, and may persist for several months after stopping steroid treatment. It is important to remember that this complication may arise in patients treated with glucocorticoid eye drops.

Cholestatic jaundice induced by oral contraceptives

Oral contraceptives are known to cause jaundice in some women, especially during the first month of medication, which recovers rapidly on discontinuation of treatment. Available evidence suggests that a genetic component is important for the development of the reaction. The underlying mechanism for this reaction is unclear, but it is likely that oestrogen-induced changes in the composition of the hepatocyte membrane are involved.

Immunological reasons for abnormal response

Many adverse drug reactions have an immunological basis. Some drugs, e.g. peptides of foreign origin such as streptokinase, are immunogenic and may cause immunological reactions in their own right. True allergic reactions are immunologically mediated effects. The features of these reactions are:

- they have no relation to the usual pharmacological effects of the drug
- there is often a delay between the first exposure to the drug and the occurrence of the subsequent adverse reaction
- very small doses of the drug may elicit the reaction once allergy is established
- the reaction disappears on withdrawal
- the illness is often recognizable as a form of immunological reaction.

Allergic reactions vary from rash, serum sickness and angio-oedema to life-threatening bronchospasm and hypotension associated with anaphylaxis. Many factors influence the development of allergic reactions. Patients with a history of atopic or allergic disorders are at greatest risk. Table 5.4 lists some examples of adverse reactions with an immunological basis.

There is mounting evidence that many drug hypersensitivity reactions have a pharmacogenetic basis (Pirmohamed & Atuah 2006). Human chromosome 6 contains a region known as the major histocompatibility complex (MHC); about 60% of the genes in this region code for proteins that regulate the immune response. The human leucocyte antigen system (HLA), which resides within the MHC, is a vital system that governs our ability to fight off infections and other harmful substances within the environment. The HLA system encodes proteins that bind peptides and presents them as antigens that interact with T-cell receptors. There are two forms of antigen, in terms of protein structure and function, namely HLA class I and class II. Given the need to recognize a large array of infecting organisms, the

Table 5.4 Classification of immunological (hypersensitivity) reactions

Type I reactions are caused by the formation of drug/antigen-specific IgE that cross-links with receptors on mast cells and basophils. This leads to immediate release of chemical mediators, including histamine and leukotrienes. Clinical features include pruritus, urticaria, angio-oedema and, less commonly, bronchoconstriction and anaphylaxis. The drugs most commonly responsible for type I hypersensitivity are aspirin, opioids, penicillins and some vaccines.

Type II or cytotoxic reactions are based on IgG- or IgM-mediated mechanisms. These involve binding of antibody to cells with subsequent binding of complement and cell rupture. This mechanism accounts for blood cell dyscrasias such as haemolytic anaemia and thrombocytopenia.

Type III reactions are mediated by intravascular immune complexes. These arise when drug antigen and antibodies, usually of IgG or IgM class, are both present in the circulation, with the antigen present in excess. Slow removal of immune complexes by phagocytes leads to their deposition in the skin and the microcirculation of the kidneys, joints and gastrointestinal system. Serum sickness and vasculitis are examples of type III reactions.

Type IV reactions are mediated by T-cells causing 'delayed' hypersensitivity reactions. Typical examples include contact dermatitis or delayed skin tests to tuberculin. Drug-related, delayed-type hypersensitivity reactions include Stevens–Johnson syndrome and toxic epidermal necrolysis (TEN). Recent work has proposed that type IV reactions be divided into four subtypes based on the T-lymphocyte subset and cytokine expression profile involved.

Table 5.5 Examples of HLA alleles and haplotypes associated with ADRs (adapted from Pirmohamed & Atuah 2006)

HLA allele or haplotype	Drug	ADR associated with HLA
HLA-B*1502	Carbamazepine	Stevens–Johnson syndrome
HLA-DRB1*1501, HLA-DQB1*0602, HLA-DRB5*0101	Amoxicillin – clavulanic acid	Hepatitis
HLA-DQ7	Pyrazolone	Pyrazolone hypersensitivity
HLA-A29, HLA-B12, HLA-DR7	Sulphonamides	Toxic epidermal necrolysis
HLA-B38, HLA-DR4, HLA-DQ3, HLA-Cw*7, HLA-DQB*0502, HLA-DRB*0101, HLA-DRB3*0202	Clozapine	Agranulocytosis
HLA-B*5701, HLA-DR7, HLA-DQ3	Abacavir	Abacavir hypersensitivity reaction
HLA-DR4	Hydralazine	Systemic lupus erythematosus

HLA system has evolved to be the most polymorphic system in the human genome. This huge degree of variability unfortunately also leads to the development of aberrant immune responses in certain individuals leading to autoimmune diseases and, in the case of drugs, to allergic reactions (see Table 5.5).

Delayed adverse effects of drugs

A number of adverse effects may only become apparent after long-term treatment, such as the relatively harmless melanin deposits in the lens and cornea that are seen after years of phenothiazine treatment, and which should be distinguished from pigmentary retinopathy, a dose-related adverse effect occurring within several months of initiation of treatment. Other examples include the development of vaginal carcinoma in the daughters of women given stilboestrol during pregnancy for the treatment of threatened abortion, and immunosuppressives and chemotherapeutic agents which can induce malignancies that may not be apparent until years after treatment has been given.

Adverse effects associated with drug withdrawal

Some drugs cause symptoms when treatment is stopped abruptly, for example the benzodiazepine withdrawal syndrome, rebound hypertension following discontinuation of antihypertensives such as clonidine, and the acute adrenal insufficiency that may be precipitated by the abrupt withdrawal of corticosteroids.

Detection and monitoring of adverse drug reactions

By the time a drug receives a marketing authorization it will usually have been given to about 1500 people on average, and it is likely that clinical trials will have detected only the most common adverse drug reactions. It follows that infrequent or rare reactions, particularly those with an incidence of 1 in 500 or less, are unlikely to have been identified before this. It is only after much wider use that rare reactions, or those which occur predominantly in certain subgroups within the populations, such as the elderly, are detected and it is therefore essential to monitor safety once a drug has been marketed (Stricker & Psaty 2004). Some methods used commonly in postmarketing surveillance are described below.

Case reports

The publication of single case reports, or case series, of adverse drug reactions in the medical literature is an important means of detecting new and serious reactions, particularly infrequent reactions. Case reports have, in the past, been vital in alerting the professions to several serious adverse reactions, such as the oculomucocutaneous syndrome associated with practolol, and halothane-induced hepatitis. In recent years, published single case reports have become less important with the emergence of formalized spontaneous reporting systems.

Cohort studies

Cohort studies are prospective studies that monitor a large group of patients taking a particular drug. The best studies compare adverse event rates in groups of patients taking the index drug with a comparative group. Cohort studies include ad hoc investigations set up to investigate specific problems, e.g. the Royal College of General Practitioners' oral contraceptive study, studies sponsored by pharmaceutical companies, prescription event monitoring (PEM), and a variety of record linkage schemes.

Case–control studies

Case–control studies compare drug usage in a group of patients with a particular disease with use among a matched control group who are similar in potentially confounding factors, but who do not have the disease. The prevalence of drug taking is then compared between the groups, and a significant excess of drug takers in the disease group may be evidence of an association with the drug. This is a useful retrospective method which can provide valuable information on the incidence of type B reactions and the association between drugs and disease. Examples of associations which have been established by case control studies are Reye's syndrome and aspirin, and the relationship between maternal diethylstilboestrol ingestion and vaginal adenocarcinoma in female offspring. The case–control method is an effective means for confirming whether or not a drug causes a given reaction once a suspicion has been raised. It is not capable of detecting previously unsuspected adverse reactions.

Spontaneous reporting schemes

The thalidomide tragedy led to the establishment, in many countries, of national schemes for the voluntary collection of adverse drug reaction reports. In the UK the Commission on Human Medicines (formerly the Committee on Safety of Medicines; CSM) adverse reactions reporting scheme, often referred to as the yellow card scheme, has been operating for more than 30 years. The scheme has received over 500 000 reports of suspected adverse reactions. Doctors, pharmacists and nurses are asked to report all suspected serious adverse reactions, and all suspected reactions to newer products (marked with an inverted black triangle symbol in product information and in the British National Formulary). Direct reporting of suspected adverse drug reactions by patients has also been introduced recently.

Spontaneous reporting schemes cannot provide estimates of risk because the true number of cases is invariably underestimated, and the denominator (i.e. total number of patients treated with the drug in question) is not known. However, the yellow card reporting scheme has been shown to provide valuable early warnings or signals of possible adverse drug reactions, and to enable the study of associated factors. The main advantages of the scheme are:

- its accessibility for all doctors, pharmacists and nurses to report
- it covers all therapeutic agents, including vaccines and herbal medicines
- it is capable of detecting both rare and common reactions
- it is relatively inexpensive to operate.

The main disadvantage of the scheme is the level of underreporting of reactions; it is likely that less than 10% of serious reactions are notified. The scheme operates on the basis that reports should be made despite uncertainty about a causal relationship, irrespective of whether or not the reaction is well recognized, and regardless of other drugs having been given concurrently.

Identification of adverse drug reactions

The establishment of a causal relationship between a specific drug and a clinical event is a fundamental problem in adverse reaction assessment. First, adverse drug reactions frequently mimic other diseases and second, many of the symptoms attributed to them occur commonly in healthy individuals taking no medication. Clinicians may thus fail to recognize the features of an adverse drug reaction because they do not fit into a clearly defined pattern.

When a suspected adverse reaction has occurred, it may be helpful to try to assess whether it is definitely, probably or possibly due to the drug. This process, known as causality assessment, is fraught with difficulties, although some decision on the likelihood that a drug caused a particular reaction is usually taken, perhaps subconsciously in some cases. Various systematic approaches, or algorithms, have been developed in an attempt to rationalize causality assessment of adverse reactions, but these are of limited value.

Factors taken into account when assessing the likelihood of an adverse drug reaction

Where an adverse drug reaction is suspected, a full history is important, particularly details of other drugs taken by the patient, including over-the-counter and herbal medicines. The patient should be asked about the nature and timing of the symptom or event, and whether such effects have occurred in the past. The temporal relationship of a suspected adverse drug reaction is important. It is relatively easy to recognize an adverse reaction that occurs soon after drug administration and an event predating prescription is clearly unlikely to be drug related. However, when more than a few weeks have elapsed, the association between the drug and the event is more difficult. There are very few cases where it is certain that a given drug caused a particular reaction in a specific patient, even though the drug is known to cause the reaction, or increase the risk of an adverse event, in some recipients. Although there is evidence that COX-II selective inhibitors increase the risk of cardiovascular events, for example, it is exceptionally difficult to establish the involvement of such drug therapy in an individual exposed patient who has experienced a myocardial infarction. Unlike other conditions in medicine, adverse drug reactions rarely produce characteristic physical signs and laboratory investigations. It is reassuring to find that an adverse reaction resolves once a drug is stopped, but this may take time. Occasionally the adverse reaction is irreversible, as in tardive dyskinesia which may actually deteriorate when the offending drug is withdrawn. Rechallenge sometimes occurs inadvertently but is very seldom justified clinically to confirm a diagnosis. Positive rechallenge is often taken as proof of a causal relationship, but this may not always be the case, particularly where the suspected reaction is subjective in nature.

Patients and adverse drug reactions

There are three main reasons why people taking medicines need to know about adverse reactions.

- It is their right to have understandable information about the harm that medicines might do to them.
- To make informed decisions about medicines, including their benefits and harms, people must be able to understand information about side effects and their frequency and apply it to their own circumstances.
- Minimizing the impact of side effects depends crucially on the patient identifying a possible side effect early, and knowing what action to take.

There is some evidence that patients themselves are capable of correctly distinguishing probable adverse drug reactions from other types of adverse clinical event (Raynor et al 2006). There has been an increasing recognition of the need to provide people with information about their medicines. However, the extent to which people should be told about medication adverse reactions has been a particular area of debate. This is despite several studies which show that people always rank side effect information highly when asked about their medicine information needs.

In an investigation of the attitudes of patients with ankylosing spondylitis, 47% reported serious adverse drug reactions associated with their medication. They regarded insufficient information and inadequate monitoring by the doctor as important causes of adverse drug reactions. A US study in 2500 hospital outpatients attempted to determine whether patients believed the physician should use discretion in the amount of information given to them on potential adverse drug reactions. It found that most individuals wished to be told of all possible adverse effects and did not favour physician discretion. More recent research investigating what people wanted to know about their medicines found that information about side effects was the most sought-after type of information, and that its provision was highly rated in terms of satisfaction. However, when doctors were asked about their perception of patient needs, the investigators found that there was almost no relationship between the patients' and the doctors' ratings of the information categories. The most noticeable difference was in terms of the patients' top two categories (namely, information about side effects and what the medicine actually does), as both these categories were given low rankings by doctors.

When considering the provision of information on side effects to patients, two possible implications are often raised. The first is the potential impact of the information on patient compliance and the second is whether side effect information leads to spurious reporting of adverse effects by patients. It is known that access to understandable and useable information about side effects can affect people's decisions on whether to take their medicine, and how much of it to take. Research has shown that the inclusion of negative information affected ratings of likely compliance. If healthcare professionals are to accept the concept of partnership in medicine taking, then we should aim

for the situation where patients, when fully informed about the benefits and harm of their medicines, can appropriately decide not to take a medicine. Studies on the effects of written patient information on patient compliance and awareness of side effects have shown equivocal findings. However, in general it seems that information on side effects has an attributing, rather than a suggesting, effect.

Pharmacists' role

Ensuring that medicines are used safely is fundamental to the pharmacist's role. Pharmacist involvement in patient care should result in prevention of some and early detection of other ADRs. Studies have demonstrated that pharmacist involvement with patients averted a large number of potential adverse reactions. Based on knowledge of relevant patient and medication factors, pharmacists can ensure that prescribing is as safe as reasonably possible. The pharmacist also has a significant role in the education of other healthcare professionals about the prevention, detection and reporting of ADRs. Regulatory authorities in many countries accept reports of adverse reactions from pharmacists. The involvement of UK hospital pharmacists has been shown to increase the number of yellow cards submitted with no discernible difference in the quality of reports when compared to hospital doctors. Similarly, yellow card reports from community pharmacists have been shown to be comparable to those received from primary care doctors. All pharmacists in the UK are now able to contribute to yellow card reporting. Community pharmacists are well placed to assist in monitoring problems with over-the-counter medicines, complementary therapies and new medicines.

CASE STUDIES

Case 5.1

Mrs T, aged 78, has a history of coronary heart disease, for which she has recently undergone coronary angioplasty and stenting. She is currently taking clopidogrel 75 mg, aspirin 75 mg, atorvastatin 80 mg, nicorandil 30 mg, and atenolol 50 mg. She stopped smoking a year ago. Mrs T presents to the community pharmacist complaining of black, bloody stools. The problem has gradually worsened over the last day or two. She has no previous history of gastrointestinal problems.

Questions

1. What risk factors does Mrs T have for drug-induced gastric ADR?
2. What advice should the community pharmacist give?

Answers

1. Mrs T is currently taking both aspirin and clopidogrel, which is standard practice after percutaneous coronary intervention, as there is evidence that the addition of clopidogrel to aspirin reduces the risk of reinfarction, stroke and death by a further 20%. However, the benefit comes at the cost of increased gastrointestinal complications. Major complications include gastroduodenal ulcerations that can lead to gastrointestinal haemorrhage, perforation and death. Minor complications include dyspepsia, oesophagitis and erosions or

ulceration in the stomach and duodenum. Mrs T's age (>60 years) is an additional risk factor. Other possible risk factors are a history of gastrointestinal problems, gastric or duodenal ulcer, smoking and concomitant use of corticosteroids or NSAIDs.

The suppression of gastroduodenal mucosal prostaglandin synthesis is one of the important mechanisms of mucosal damage by aspirin. Serious gastrointestinal ulcer complications are 2- to 4-fold more common in patients who take 75–300 mg aspirin compared with controls. Clopidogrel is an antiplatelet drug that irreversibly inhibits adenosine diphosphate receptor function. The findings of recent studies show that it is associated with a greater risk of gastrointestinal bleeding than a combination of low-dose aspirin plus a proton pump inhibitor. Although evidence is currently lacking on the protective benefits of acid suppressive therapy in addition to clopidogrel and aspirin, its use in high-risk patients is reasonable.

2. Black stool or melaena indicates the presence of denatured blood after upper gastrointestinal loss and passage through the intestine. It is an important condition because it can be a life-threatening emergency requiring urgent specialist intervention. Upper gastrointestinal bleeding is especially threatening in the elderly in whom there is a substantially increased risk of complications and mortality. This is due to frailty and to the increased presence of concurrent health problems contributing to serious complications. NSAID- and aspirin-induced ulcers are the major cause of upper gastrointestinal bleeding in the elderly. Mrs T should be advised to contact her doctor immediately.

Case 5.2

Mr B is a 71-year-old man who recently completed a 10-day course of flucloxacillin 500 mg three times a day for cellulitis. Three weeks later he presents to his doctor complaining of lethargy and increasing nausea. Several days ago he noted slight yellowing of his eyes and that his urine was dark in colour. Over the last 2 days he has suffered from an itch all over his trunk and legs which is interfering with sleep.

Questions

1. What form of liver disease is suggested by this presentation?
2. The patient was admitted to hospital. LFTs on admission were as follows.

- Albumin 37 g/L (normal 35–55)
- Aspartate transaminase (AST) 172 units/L (<35)
- Alanine transaminase (ALT) 211 units/L (<50)
- Alkaline phosphatase 1975 units/L (70–290)
- Bilirubin 172 μmol/L (3–17)

What type of liver dysfunction is indicated by these results?
3. How would you treat the symptoms?

Answers

1. General malaise, tiredness and gastrointestinal symptoms of nausea and vomiting are common signs of drug-induced liver disease. Pruritus in particular is associated with liver dysfunction of cholestatic origin. The cause of the pruritus is unknown but is now thought to involve endogenous opioids as well as the accumulation of bile salts in plasma.
2. The liver function tests reveal a predominantly cholestatic picture, as evidenced by the much larger increase in alkaline phosphatase compared with the transaminases AST and ALT. The cholestasis appears to predominate, suggesting that this is a cholestatic hepatitis. The albumin is in the normal reference range which indicates that the liver injury is acute rather than chronic or is not sufficiently severe to affect hepatic synthetic function. Liver function tests can only provide a crude guide to the type of liver disease, and changes do not always accurately indicate the extent of liver damage.

Flucloxacillin is associated with cholestatic liver disease, consisting of prolonged painless jaundice with elevation of cholestatic liver enzymes diagnosed within 2–6 weeks after prescription and as much as 3 weeks after the drug was stopped. Most patients recover fully within several months but a chronic vanishing bile duct syndrome has been reported in some patients. In rare cases the outcome has been fatal. The risk is estimated at 7–8.5 per 100 000 users. The risk of this complication is greater in people aged over 55 years and where the duration of treatment is greater than 14 days.

3. Pruritus is a common and debilitating effect of cholestatic injury and will probably be the main symptomatic complaint. Once the patient has been assessed, treatment with antihistamines, colestyramine and/or topical therapy with menthol in aqueous cream may be considered. Sedating antihistamines, such as chlorphenamine, are often used because of their longer term safety record and because lack of sleep is a debilitating feature of pruritus. However, they should only be used in patients with stable liver disease. Non-sedating antihistamines, such as loratadine and cetirizine, are increasingly used. Resolution of the underlying condition will provide the most effective relief from the pruritus.

Case 5.3

A 58-year-old woman was admitted to hospital for investigation after several episodes of syncope. On admission she was taking tibolone 2.5 mg daily, indapamide 2.5 mg daily, sumatriptan and co-codamol prn for migraine and mizolastine 10 mg daily for hayfever. The ECG showed a prolonged QT interval (the corrected QT interval, QTc, measured 550 milliseconds). All electrolyte levels were normal.

Questions

1. Could any of the current medication have contributed to the patient's problem?
2. How should QT interval prolongation be managed?

Answers

1. A number of drugs have the potential to prolong the QT interval on the electrocardiogram (ECG). The QT interval is an indirect measure of the duration of the ventricular action potential and ventricular repolarization. Prolongation of ventricular repolarization can cause arrhythmias, the most characteristic of which is torsade de pointes (twisting of the points), a specific form of ventricular tachycardia. The name describes the characteristic 'twisting' of the QRS complexes around the electrical axis on the ECG, which can appear as an intermittent series of rapid spikes lasting a few seconds during which the heart fails to pump effectively. This is usually a self-limiting arrhythmia that may cause dizziness or syncope, but it can lead to ventricular fibrillation which can cause sudden death. The cause of malfunction may be genetic (congenital LQTS) or related to metabolic disturbance or drug therapy (acquired LQTS). Drugs are thought to prolong repolarization either by blocking potassium channels, and thus delaying potassium outflow, or by enhancing inward sodium or calcium currents. QT prolongation is usually assumed to be present when the QT interval corrected for changes in the heart rate (QTc) is greater than 450 milliseconds (ms), although arrhythmias are most often associated with values of 550 ms or more.

The antihistamine mizolastine has a weak potential to prolong the QT interval in a few individuals. The degree of prolongation is described as modest and cardiac arrhythmias have not been reported. This patient is also taking the diuretic indapamide; diuretic use, independent of electrolyte concentrations, is a known risk factor for torsade de pointes.

2. If a patient is suspected of having drug-induced prolongation of the QT interval, the implicated drug(s) should be stopped immediately. In this case, the patient's syncope episodes may have been related to an arrhythmia. Some patients with torsade de pointes may be asymptomatic while others experience dizziness, light-headedness, syncope, collapse, irregular heart beat and palpitations. The arrhythmia should be controlled by accelerating the heart rate, either by atrial pacing or by an isoprenaline infusion. Electrolyte abnormalities should be corrected and magnesium sulphate infusion may effectively terminate the arrhythmia, even in the presence of normal magnesium levels. Antiarrhythmic drugs may worsen the problem and should be avoided. Torsade de pointes that degenerates to ventricular fibrillation requires DC shock for termination.

Case 5.4

A consultant psychiatrist asks your advice about a 49-year-old woman who is taking olanzapine 10 mg daily for schizophrenia. The patient has type 2 diabetes which is managed by diet only. Within 6 weeks of starting olanzapine, the patient noted a deterioration in her blood glucose control. Her fasting blood glucose levels before treatment was started were generally in the range 6–9 mmol/L but have now increased to around 12 mmol/L. The patient has gained 2.5 kg in weight since olanzapine was started.

Questions

1. Is olanzapine likely to have worsened diabetic control in this patient?
2. If so, which alternative antipsychotics may be used?

Answers

1. All atypical antipsychotics are associated with weight gain. Olanzapine has been reported to cause or exacerbate diabetes in several published case reports. The exact cause of glucose dysregulation with olanzapine is unclear, but weight gain does not seem to be the sole aetiology.

It has been postulated that serotonin ($5HT_{IA}$) antagonism may decrease the responsiveness of the pancreatic β-cells. This would result in inappropriately low insulin secretion and hyperglycaemia. Further examination of the incidence and aetiology of this problem is needed.

2. Olanzapine is not contraindicated in patients with diabetes, but should be used with careful monitoring of blood glucose control. In this case, where the patient's diabetic control has worsened during therapy, it would be reasonable to discontinue olanzapine and switch to another antipsychotic. Risperidone and quetiapine are alternative atypical antipsychotics not associated with problems in diabetic patients.

REFERENCES

Aronson J K, Ferner R E 2003 Joining the DoTS: new approach to classifying adverse drug reactions. British Medical Journal 327: 1222-1225

Bates D W, Spell N, Cullen D J et al 1997 The costs of adverse drug events in hospitalized patients. Journal of the American Medical Association 277: 307-311

Brennan T A, Leape L L, Laird N et al 1991 The nature of adverse events in hospitalized patients. The results of the Harvard Medical Practice Study II. New England Journal of Medicine 324: 377-384

Clarkson A, Choonara I 2002 Surveillance for fatal suspected adverse drug reactions in the UK. Archives of Diseases in Childhood 87: 462-467

Classen D C, Pestotnik S L, Evans R S et al 1997 Adverse drug events in hospitalized patients: excess length of stay, extra costs, and attributable mortality. Journal of the American Medical Association 277: 301-306

Einarson T R, Gutierrez L M, Rudis M 1993 Drug-related hospital admissions. Annals of Pharmacotherapy 27(7-8): 832-840

Gandhi T K, Weingart S N, Borus J et al 2003 Adverse drug events in ambulatory care. New England Journal of Medicine 348(16): 1556-1564

Gurwitz J H, Filed T S, Harrold L R et al 2003 Incidence and preventability of adverse drug events among older persons in the ambulatory setting. Journal of the American Medical Association 289(9): 1107-1116

Higashi M K, Veenstra D L, Kondo L M et al 2002 Association between CYP2C9 genetic variants and anticoagulation-related outcomes during warfarin therapy. Journal of the American Medical Association 287(13): 1690-1698

Impicciatore P, Choonara I, Clarkson A et al 2001 Incidence of adverse drug reactions in paediatric in/out-patients: a systematic review and meta-analysis of prospective studies. British Journal of Clinical Pharmacology 52(1): 77-83

Marzolini C, Paus E, Buclin T et al 2004 Polymorphisms in human MDR1 (P-glycoprotein): recent advances and clinical relevance. Clinical Pharmacology and Therapeutics 75: 13-33

Pirmohamed M, Atuah K 2006 Pharmacogenetics and adverse drug reactions. In: Lee A (ed) Adverse drug reactions, 2nd edn. Pharmaceutical Press, London, pp 43-73

Pirmohamed M, James S, Meakin S et al 2004 Adverse drug reactions as cause of admission to hospital: prospective analysis of 18 820 patients. British Medical Journal 329: 15-19

Rawlins M D, Thompson J W 1977 Pathogenesis of adverse drug reactions. In: Davies D M (ed) Textbook of adverse drug reactions. Oxford University Press, Oxford

Raynor T, Knapp P, Berry D 2006 Side effects and patients. In: Lee A (ed) Adverse drug reactions, 2nd edn. Pharmaceutical Press, London, pp 23-41

Stricker B H, Psaty B M 2004 Detection, verification and quantification of adverse drug reactions. British Medical Journal 329: 44-47

Wiffen P, Gill M, Edwards J, Moore A 2002 Adverse drug reactions in hospital patients. A systematic review of the prospective and retrospective studies. Bandolier Extra June: 1-16

Wilkinson G R 2005 Drug therapy: drug metabolism and variability among patients in drug response. New England Journal of Medicine 352(21): 2211–2221

Wynne H 2005 Drug metabolism and ageing. Journal of the British Menopause Society 11: 51-56

FURTHER READING

Aronson J K, Ferner R E 2005 Clarification of terminology in drug safety. Drug Safety 28: 851-870

Coleman J J, McDowell S E 2005 Ethnicity and adverse drug reactions. Adverse Drug Reaction Bulletin 234: 899-902

Davies D M, Ferner R E, de Glanville H (eds) 1998 Davies's textbook of adverse drug reactions, 5th edn. Chapman and Hall Medical, London

Edwards I R, Aronson J K 2000 Adverse drug reactions: definitions, diagnosis, and management. Lancet 356: 1255-1259

Gruchalla R S 2000 Clinical assessment of drug-induced disease. Lancet 356: 1505-1510

Lee A (ed) 2006 Adverse drug reactions. Pharmaceutical Press, London

Pirmohamed M, Park B K 2003 Cytochrome P450 enzyme polymorphisms and adverse drug reactions. Toxicology 192: 23-32

6 Laboratory data

H. Wynne   C. Edwards

This chapter will consider the common biochemical and haematological tests that are of clinical and diagnostic importance. For convenience, each individual test will be dealt with under a separate heading and a brief review of the physiology and pathophysiology will be given where appropriate to explain the basis of biochemical and haematological disorders.

It is usual for a reference range to be quoted for each individual test (see Tables 6.1 and 6.8). This range is based on data obtained from a sample of the general population which is assumed to be disease free. Many test values have a normal distribution and the reference values are taken as the mean ± 2 standard deviations (SD). This includes 95% of the population. The 'normal' range must always be used with caution since it takes little account of an individual's age, sex, weight, height, muscle mass or disease state, many of which variables can influence the value obtained. Although reference ranges are valuable guides, they must not be used as sole indicators of health and disease. A series of values rather than a simple test value may be required to ensure clinical relevance and to eliminate erroneous values caused, for example, by spoiled specimens or interference from diagnostic or therapeutic procedures. Furthermore, a disturbance of one parameter often cannot be considered in isolation without looking at the pattern of other tests within the group.

Further specific information on the clinical and therapeutic relevance of each test may be obtained by referral to the relevant chapter in this book.

Table 6.1 Biochemical data: typical normal adult reference values measured in serum

Laboratory test	Reference range
Urea & electrolytes	
Sodium	135–145 mmol/L
Potassium	3.4–5.0 mmol/L
Calcium (total)	2.12–2.60 mmol/L
Calcium (ionized)	1.19–1.37 mmol/L
Phosphate	0.80–1.44 mmol/L
Creatinine	75–155 µmol/L
Urea	3.1–7.9 mmol/L
Glucose	
Fasting	3.3–6.0 mmol/L
Non-fasting	<11.1 mmol/L
Glycated haemoglobin	<5.5%
Liver function tests	
Albumin	34–50 g/L
Bilirubin (total)	<19 µmol/L
Bilirubin (conjugated)	<4 µmol/L
Enzymes	
Alanine transaminase	<45 U/L
Aspartate transaminase	<35 U/L
Alkaline phosphatase	35–120 U/L
γ-Glutamyl transpeptidase	<70 U/L
Ammonia	
Men	15–50 µmol/L
Female	10–40 µmol/L
Amylase	<100 U/L
Cardiac markers	
Cardiac troponin (cTnT)	<0.1 µg/L
Other tests	
Osmolality	282–295 mosmol/kg
Uric acid	0.15–0.47 mmol/L
Parathyroid hormone (adult with normal calcium)	10–65 ng/L
25-Hydroxyvitamin D	10–75 nmol/L

Biochemical data

The homeostasis of various elements, water and acid–base balance are closely linked, both physiologically and clinically. Standard biochemical screening includes several measurements which provide a picture of fluid and electrolyte balance and renal function. These are commonly referred to colloquially as 'Us and Es' (urea and electrolytes) and the major tests are described below.

Sodium and water balance

Sodium and water metabolism are closely interrelated both physiologically and clinically, and play a major role in determining the osmolality of serum.

Water constitutes approximately 60% of body weight in men and 55% in women (women have a greater proportion of fat tissue which contains little water). Approximately two-thirds of body water is found in the intracellular fluid (ICF) and one-third in the extracellular fluid (ECF). Of the ECF, 75% is found within interstitial fluid and 25% within serum (Fig. 6.1).

In general, water permeates freely between the ICF and ECF. Cell walls function as semipermeable membranes, with water movement from one compartment to the other being controlled by osmotic pressure: water moves into the compartment with the higher osmotic concentration. The osmotic content of the two compartments is generally the same, i.e. they are isotonic. However, the kidneys are an exception to the rule.

The osmolality of the ECF is largely determined by sodium and its associated anions, chloride and bicarbonate. Glucose and urea have a lesser, but nevertheless important, role in determining ECF osmolality. Protein (especially albumin) makes only a small (0.5%) contribution to the osmolality of the ECF but is a major factor in determining water distribution between the two compartments. The contribution of proteins to the osmotic pressure of serum is known as the colloid osmotic pressure, or oncotic pressure.

The major contributor to the osmolality of the ICF is potassium.

The amount of water taken in and lost by the body depends on intake, diet, activity and the environment. Over time the intake of water is normally equal to that lost (Table 6.2). The minimum daily intake necessary to maintain this balance is approximately 1100 mL. Of this, 500 mL is required for normal excretion of waste products in urine, whilst the remaining volume is lost via the skin in sweat, via the lungs in expired air, and in faeces.

Water depletion

Water depletion will occur if intake is inadequate or loss excessive. Excessive loss of water through the kidney is unusual except in diabetes insipidus or following the overuse of diuretics.

Patients with fever will lose water through the skin and ventilated patients will lose it through the lungs. Diarrhoea causes water depletion. Water loss is usually compensated for if the thirst mechanism is intact or can be responded to, but this may not occur in patients who are unconscious, have swallowing difficulties or are disabled. Severe water depletion may induce cerebral dehydration causing confusion, fits and coma and circulatory failure.

The underlying cause for the water depletion should be identified and treated. Replacement water should be given orally, where possible, or by nasogastric tube, intravenously or subcutaneously as necessary with 5% dextrose in water or, in patients with associated sodium deficits, isotonic saline. Hypotonic saline is sometimes used, but with great caution, where neurological effects of hypertonicity predominate. Hypernatraemia should be corrected slowly: not more than half of the water deficit should be corrected in the first 12–24 hours.

Water excess

Water excess is usually associated with an impairment of water excretion such as that caused by renal failure or the syndrome of inappropriate secretion of antidiuretic hormone (SIADH). This syndrome has several causes including chest infections and some tumours, particularly small cell carcinoma of the lung. Excess intake is rarely a cause of water excess since the healthy adult kidney can excrete water at a rate of up to 2 mL/min. Patients affected usually present with signs consistent with cerebral overhydration, although if it is of gradual onset, over several days, they may be asymptomatic. Hyponatraemia is usually present.

Water and ECF osmolality

If the body water content changes independently of the amount of solute, osmolality will be altered (the normal range is

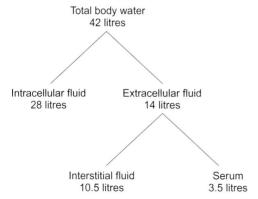

Fig 6.1   Approximate distribution of water in a 70 kg man.

Total body water
42 litres

Intracellular fluid
28 litres

Extracellular fluid
14 litres

Interstitial fluid
10.5 litres

Serum
3.5 litres

Table 6.2 Typical daily water balance for a healthy 70 kg adult			
	Input (mL)		Output (mL)
Oral fluids	1400	Urine	1500
Food	700	Lung	400
Metabolic oxidation	400	Skin	400
		Faeces	200
Total	2500		2500

282–295 mmol/kg of water). A loss of water from the ECF will increase its osmolality and result in the movement of water from the ICF to the ECF. This increase in ECF osmolality will stimulate the hypothalamic thirst centres to promote a desire to drink while also stimulating the release of vasopressin or antidiuretic hormone (ADH). ADH increases the permeability of the renal collecting ducts to water and promotes water reabsorption with consequent concentration of urine.

If the osmolality of the ECF falls, there is no desire to drink and no secretion of ADH. Consequently a dilute urine is produced which helps restore ECF osmolality to normal.

The secretion of ADH is also stimulated by angiotensin II, arterial and venous baroreceptors, volume receptors, stress (including pain), exercise and drugs such as morphine, nicotine, tolbutamide, carbamazepine and vincristine. If blood volume decreases by more than 10%, the hypovolaemia stimulates ADH release and overrides control based on osmolality.

Sodium distribution

The body of an average 70 kg man contains approximately 3000 mmol of sodium. Most of this sodium is freely exchangeable and is extracellular. The normal serum range is 135–145 mmol/L. In contrast, the ICF concentration of sodium is only about 10 mmol/L.

Each day approximately 1000 mmol of sodium is secreted into the gut and 25 000 mmol filtered by the kidney. The bulk of this is recovered by reabsorption from the gut and renal tubules. It should be clear therefore that partial failure of homeostatic control can potentially have major consequences.

Sodium and ECF volume

The ECF volume is dependent upon total body sodium since sodium is almost entirely restricted to the ECF, and water intake and loss are regulated to maintain a constant concentration of sodium in the ECF compartment.

Sodium balance is maintained by renal excretion. Normally, 70% of filtered sodium is actively reabsorbed in the proximal tubule, with further reabsorption in the Loop of Henle. Less than 5% of the filtered sodium load reaches the distal tubule where aldosterone can stimulate further sodium reabsorption.

Other factors such as natriuretic peptide hormone can also affect sodium reabsorption. This hormone is secreted by the cardiac atria in response to atrial stretch following a rise in atrial pressure associated with, perhaps, volume expansion. It is natriuretic (increases sodium excretion in urine) and, amongst other actions, reduces aldosterone concentration.

Sodium depletion

Inadequate oral intake of sodium is rarely the cause of sodium depletion although inappropriate parenteral treatment may occasionally be implicated. Sodium depletion commonly occurs with water depletion, resulting in dehydration or volume depletion. The normal response of the body to the hypovolaemia includes an increase in aldosterone secretion, which stimulates renal sodium reabsorption, and an increase in ADH secretion if ECF volume depletion is severe.

The serum sodium level can give an indication of depletion, but it must be borne in mind that the serum sodium may be:

- increased, e.g. where there is sodium and water loss but with predominant water loss, as occurs in excessive sweating
- normal, e.g. where there is isotonic sodium and water loss, as occurs from burns or a haemorrhage
- decreased, e.g. sodium loss with water retention as would occur if an isotonic sodium depletion were treated with a hypotonic sodium solution.

Sodium excess

Sodium excess can be due to either increased intake or decreased excretion. Excessive intake is not a common cause although iatrogenic hypernatraemia can be associated with excessive intravenous saline infusion.

Sodium excess is usually due to impaired excretion. It may also be caused by a primary mineralocorticoid excess, for example Cushing's syndrome or Conn's syndrome, but is often due to a secondary hyperaldosteronism associated with disorders such as congestive cardiac failure, nephrotic syndrome, hepatic cirrhosis with ascites, or renal artery stenosis. Sodium and water retention causes oedema.

Hypernatraemia

The signs and symptoms of hypernatraemia include muscle weakness and confusion.

Drug-induced hypernatraemia is often the result of a nephrogenic diabetes insipidus-like syndrome whereby the renal tubules are unresponsive to ADH. The affected patient presents with polyuria, polydipsia or dehydration. Lithium and phenytoin are the most commonly implicated drugs.

- The diabetes insipidus-like syndrome with lithium has been reported after only 2 weeks of therapy. The syndrome is usually reversible on discontinuation. Whilst affected, however, many patients are unresponsive to exogenous ADH.
- Demeclocycline can also cause diabetes insipidus and can be used in the management of patients with the syndrome of inappropriate ADH secretion (SIADH).
- Phenytoin generally has a less pronounced effect on urinary volume than lithium or demeclocycline, and does not cause nephrogenic diabetes insipidus. It inhibits ADH secretion at the level of the central nervous system.

Hypernatraemia can be caused by a number of other drugs (Table 6.3) and by a variety of mechanisms; for example, hypernatraemia secondary to sodium retention is known to occur with corticosteroids whilst the administration of sodium-containing drugs parenterally in high doses also has the potential to cause hypernatraemia.

Hyponatraemia

A fall in the serum sodium level can be the result of sodium loss, water retention in excess of sodium, or a combination of both factors. A number of drugs have also been implicated as causing hyponatraemia (Table 6.4).

Table 6.3 Examples of drugs known to cause hypernatraemia
Adrenocorticotropic hormone
Anabolic steroids
Androgens
Carbenoxolone
Clonidine
Corticosteroids
Diazoxide
Lactulose
Methyldopa
Oestrogens
Oral contraceptives
Sodium bicarbonate

Table 6.4 Examples of drugs known to cause hyponatraemia
Aminoglutethimide
Amitriptyline and other tricyclic antidepressants
Amphotericin
Angiotensin-converting enzyme (ACE) inhibitors
Carbamazepine
Chlorpropamide
Cisplatin
Clofibrate
Cyclophosphamide
Diuretics
Heparin
Lithium
Miconazole
Non-steroidal anti-inflammatory agents
Opiates
Oxcarbazepine
Tolbutamide
Vasopressin
Vincristine

The inappropriate secretion of ADH is the mechanism underlying many drug-induced hyponatraemias. In this syndrome the drug may augment the action of endogenous ADH, e.g. chlorpropamide, increase the release of ADH, e.g. carbamazepine, or have a direct ADH-like action on the kidney, e.g. oxytocin. Hyponatraemia can also be induced by mechanisms different from those described above. Lithium may cause renal damage and a failure to conserve sodium. Likewise the natriuretic action of diuretics can predispose to hyponatraemia.

Potassium

The total amount of potassium in the body, like sodium, is 3000 mmol. About 10% of the body potassium is bound in red blood cells, bone and brain tissue and is not exchangeable. The remaining 90% of total body potassium is free and exchangeable, with the vast majority having an intracellular location. Only 2% of the exchangeable total body potassium is in the ECF, the compartment from where the serum concentration is sampled and measured. Consequently, the measurement of serum potassium is not an accurate index of total body potassium, but together with the clinical status of a patient it permits a sound practical assessment of potassium homeostasis.

The serum potassium concentration is controlled mainly by the kidney with the gastrointestinal tract normally having a minor role. The potassium filtered in the kidney is almost completely reabsorbed in the proximal tubule. Potassium secretion is largely a passive process in response to the need to maintain membrane potential neutrality associated with active reabsorption of sodium in the distal convoluted tubule and collecting duct. The extent of potassium secretion is determined by a number of factors including:

- the amount of sodium available for exchange in the distal convoluted tubule and collecting duct

- the availability of hydrogen and potassium ions for exchange in the distal convoluted tubule or collecting duct
- the ability of the distal convoluted tubule or collecting duct to secrete hydrogen ions
- the concentration of aldosterone
- tubular fluid flow rate.

As described above, both potassium and hydrogen can neutralize the membrane potential generated by active sodium reabsorption and, consequently, there is a close relationship between potassium and hydrogen ion homeostasis. In acidosis, hydrogen ions are normally secreted in preference to potassium, i.e. hyperkalaemia is often associated with acidosis, except in renal tubular acidosis. In alkalosis, fewer hydrogen ions will be present and potassium is excreted, i.e. hypokalaemia is often associated with alkalosis.

The normal daily dietary intake of potassium is of the order of 60–200 mmol, which is more than adequate to replace that lost from the body. It is unusual for a deficiency of normal intake to account for hypokalaemia. A transcellular movement of potassium into cells, loss from the gut or excretion in the urine are the main causes of hypokalaemia.

Hypokalaemia

Transcellular movement into cells The shift of potassium from the serum compartment of the ECF into cells accounts for the hypokalaemia reported following intravenous or, less frequently, nebulized administration of β-adrenoreceptor agonists such as salbutamol. Parenteral insulin also causes a shift of potassium into cells, and is used for this purpose in the acute management of patients with hyperkalaemia.

Loss from the gastrointestinal tract Although potassium is secreted in gastric juice, much of this, together with potassium ingested in the diet, is reabsorbed in the small intestine. Stools do contain some potassium but in a patient with chronic diarrhoea or a fistula, considerable amounts of potassium may be lost and precipitate hypokalaemia. Likewise, the abuse of laxatives increases gastrointestinal potassium loss and may precipitate hypokalaemia. Analogous to the situation with diarrhoea, the potassium secreted in gastric juice may be lost following persistent vomiting and can also contribute to hypokalaemia.

Loss from the kidneys Mineralocorticoid excess, whether it be due to primary or secondary hyperaldosteronism or Cushing's syndrome, can increase urinary potassium loss and cause hypokalaemia. Likewise, increased excretion of potassium can result from renal tubular damage. Nephrotoxic antibiotics such as gentamicin have also been implicated.

Many drugs which can induce hypokalaemia do so by affecting the regulatory role of aldosterone upon potassium–sodium exchange in the distal tubule and collecting duct. Administered corticosteroids mimic aldosterone and can therefore increase potassium loss.

The most commonly used groups of drugs that can cause hypokalaemia are thiazide and loop diuretics. Both groups increase the amount of sodium delivered and available for reabsorption at the distal convoluted tubule and collecting duct. Consequently, this will increase the amount of potassium excreted from the kidneys. Some of the drugs known to cause hypokalaemia are shown in Table 6.5.

Clinical features The patient with moderate hypokalaemia may be asymptomatic, but the symptoms of more severe hypokalaemia include muscle weakness, hypotonia, paralytic ileus, depression and confusion. Arrhythmias may occur. Typical changes on the electrocardiogram (ECG) are of ST depression, T-wave depression/inversion and prolonged P–R interval. Insulin secretion in response to a rising blood glucose concentration requires potassium and this mechanism may be impaired in hypokalaemia. Rarely there may be impaired renal concentrating ability with polyuria and polydipsia.

Hypokalaemia is managed by giving either oral potassium or intravenous suitably dilute potassium, depending on its severity and the clinical state of the patient.

Hyperkalaemia

Hyperkalaemia may arise from excessive intake, decreased elimination or shift of potassium from cells to the ECF. It is rare for excessive oral intake to be the sole cause of hyperkalaemia. The inappropriate use of parenteral infusions containing potassium is probably the most common iatrogenic cause of excessive intake. Hyperkalaemia is a common problem in patients with renal failure due to their inability to excrete a potassium load.

The combined use of potassium-sparing diuretics such as amiloride, triamterene or spironolactone with an angiotensin-converting enzyme (ACE) inhibitor, which will lower aldosterone, is a recognized cause of hyperkalaemia, particularly in the elderly. Mineralocorticoid deficiency states such as Addison's disease where there is a deficiency of aldosterone also decrease renal potassium loss and contribute to hyperkalaemia. Those at risk of hyperkalaemia should be warned not to take salt (NaCl) substitutes in the form of potassium chloride.

The majority of body potassium is intracellular. Severe tissue damage, catabolic states or impairment of the energy-dependent sodium pump, caused by hypoxia or diabetic ketoacidosis, may result in apparent hyperkalaemia due to potassium moving out of and sodium moving into cells. Table 6.6 gives examples of some drugs known to cause hyperkalaemia.

Haemolysis during sampling or a delay in separating cells from plasma will result in potassium escaping from blood cells into plasma and causing an artefactual hyperkalaemia.

Clinical features Hyperkalaemia can be asymptomatic but fatal. An elevated potassium level has many effects on the heart: notably the resting membrane potential is lowered and the action potential shortened. Characteristic changes of the ECG precede ventricular fibrillation and cardiac arrest.

In emergency management of a patient with hyperkalaemia (>6.5 mmol/L ± ECG changes), intravenous calcium gluconate

Table 6.5 Examples of drugs known to cause hypokalaemia

| Amphotericin |
| Aspirin |
| Corticosteroids |
| Diuretics |
| Gentamicin |
| Glucose |
| Insulin |
| Laxatives |
| Penicillin G (sodium salt) |
| Piperacillin + tazobactam |
| Salicylates |
| Sodium bicarbonate |
| Sodium chloride |
| Terbutaline |
| Ticarcillin + clavulanic acid |

Table 6.6   Examples of drugs known to cause hyperkalaemia

Angiotensin-converting enzyme inhibitors

Antineoplastic agents (e.g. cyclophosphamide, vincristine)

Non-steroidal anti-inflammatory drugs

β-adrenoreceptor blocking agents

Ciclosporin

Digoxin (in acute overdose)

Diuretics, potassium sparing (amiloride, triamterene, spironolactone)

Heparin

Isoniazid

Lithium

Penicillins (e.g. potassium salt)

Potassium supplements

Tetracycline

(or chloride) at a dose of 10 mL of 10% solution is given intravenously over 5 minutes. This does not reduce the potassium concentration but antagonizes the effect of potassium on cardiac tissue. Immediately thereafter, glucose 50 g with 20 units soluble insulin, for example, by intravenous infusion will lower serum potassium levels within 30 minutes by increasing the shift of potassium into cells.

If acidosis is present, bicarbonate administration may be considered.

The long-term management of hyperkalaemia may involve the use of oral or rectal polystyrene cation-exchange resins which remove potassium from the body. Chronic hyperkalaemia in renal failure is managed by a low potassium diet.

Calcium

The body of an average man contains about 1 kg of calcium and 99% of this is bound within bone. Calcium is present in serum bound mainly to the albumin component of protein (46%), complexed with citrate and phosphate (7%), and as free ions (47%). Only the free ions of calcium are physiologically active. Calcium metabolism is regulated by parathyroid hormone (PTH) which is inhibited by increased serum concentrations of calcium ions. PTH is secreted in response to low calcium concentrations and increases serum calcium by actions on osteoclasts, kidney and gut.

The serum calcium level is often determined by measuring total calcium, i.e. that which is free and bound, but the measurement of free or ionized calcium offers advantages in some situations.

In alkalosis, hydrogen ions dissociate from albumin, and calcium binding to albumin increases, together with an increase

in complex formation. If the concentration of ionized calcium falls sufficiently, clinical symptoms of hypocalcaemia may occur despite the total serum calcium concentration being unchanged. The reverse effect, i.e. increased ionized calcium, occurs in acidosis.

Changes in serum albumin also affect the total serum calcium concentration independently of the ionized concentration. A variety of equations is available to estimate the calcium concentration. A commonly used formula is shown in Figure 6.2. Caution must be exercised when using such a formula in the presence of disturbed blood hydrogen ion concentrations.

Hypercalcaemia

Hypercalcaemia may be caused by a variety of disorders, the most common being hyperparathyroidism and malignancy. Hypercalcaemia of malignancy is seen in multiple myeloma and carcinomas which metastasize in bone. It is also seen in squamous carcinoma of the bronchus, as a result of a peptide with PTH-like activity, produced by the tumour. Hypercalcaemia also occurs in thyrotoxicosis, vitamin A and D intoxication, renal transplantation and acromegaly.

Thiazide diuretics, lithium, tamoxifen and calcium supplements used in the management of osteoporosis are examples of some of the drugs which can cause hypercalcaemia.

An artefactual increase in total serum calcium may sometimes be seen as a result of a tourniquet being applied during venous sampling. The resulting venous stasis may cause redistribution of fluid from the vein into the extravascular space, and the temporary haemoconcentration will affect albumin levels.

Management of hypercalcaemia involves correction of any dehydration with normal saline followed by furosemide which inhibits tubular reabsorption of calcium. Bisphosphonates are used to inhibit bone turnover.

Hypocalcaemia

Hypocalcaemia can be caused by a variety of disorders including hypoalbuminaemia, hypoparathyroidism, pancreatitis and those that cause vitamin D deficiency, e.g. malabsorption, reduced exposure to sunlight, liver disease and renal disease. In alkalaemia, for instance as may occur when a patient is hyperventilating, there is an increase in protein binding of calcium, which can result in a fall in plasma levels of ionized calcium, manifesting itself as paraesthesiae or tetany.

For albumin < 40 g/L:

Corrected calcium = [Ca] + 0.02 × (40 − [alb]) mmol/L

For albumin > 45 g/L:

Corrected calcium = [Ca] − 0.02 ([alb] − 45) mmol/L

Fig 6.2   Formula for correction of total plasma calcium concentration for changes in albumin concentration: albumin concentration = [alb] (albumin units = g/L); calcium concentration = [Ca] (total calcium units = mmol/L).

Drugs that have been implicated as causing hypocalcaemia include phenytoin, phenobarbital, aminoglycosides, phosphate enemas, calcitonin, mithramycin and furosemide.

Biochemical measurements of serum calcium, phosphate and alkaline phosphatase can be normal in some patients with vitamin D deficiency and osteomalacia. The recent development of non-radioactive automated assays for serum PTH and 25-hydroxyvitamin D (25 OHD) has made measurement of these two hormones possible in many laboratories. There is a lack of consensus regarding a specific level of 25-hydroxyvitamin D that is indicative of vitamin D deficiency, but this has usually been established by assessing the point at which serum PTH starts to rise. This, together with methodological and technical issues, prevents direct comparison of values across laboratories. Clinical decision limits for PTH and 25 OHD are laboratory specific and must be interpreted within the clinical context of each patient.

Phosphate

About 80% of body phosphate is in bone, 15% in intracellular fluid and only 0.1% in ECF. Its major function is in energy metabolism. Plasma levels are regulated by absorption from the diet, which is partly under the control of vitamin D, and PTH which controls its excretion by the kidney.

Hypophosphataemia

Severe hypophosphataemia can cause muscle weakness and wasting and some skeletal wasting.

Hyperphosphataemia

Hyperphosphataemia occurs in chronic renal failure and hypo-parathyroidism.

Creatinine

Serum creatinine concentration is largely determined by its rate of production, rate of renal excretion and volume of distribution. It is frequently used to evaluate renal function.

Creatinine is produced at a fairly constant rate from creatine and creatine phosphate in muscle. Daily production is a function of muscle mass and declines with age from 24 mg/kg/day in a healthy 25 year old to 9 mg/kg/day in a 95 year old. Creatinine undergoes complete glomerular filtration with little reabsorption by the renal tubules. Its clearance is therefore usually a good indicator of the glomerular filtration rate (GFR). As a general rule, and only at the steady state, if the serum creatinine doubles this equates to a 50% reduction in the GFR and consequently renal function. The serum creatinine level can be transiently elevated following meat ingestion, but less so than urea, or strenuous exercise. Individuals with a high muscle bulk produce more creatinine and therefore have a higher serum creatinine level compared to an otherwise identical but less muscular individual.

The value for creatinine clearance is higher than the true GFR due to the active tubular secretion of creatinine. In a patient with a normal GFR this is of little significance. However, in an individual in whom the GFR is low (<10 mL/min) the tubular secretion may make a significant contribution to creatinine elimination and overestimate the GFR. In this type of patient, the breakdown of creatinine in the gut can also become a significant source of elimination.

Urea

The catabolism of dietary and endogenous amino acids in the body produces large amounts of ammonia. Ammonia is toxic and its concentration is kept very low by conversion in the liver to urea. Urea is eliminated in urine and represents the major route of nitrogen excretion. The urea is filtered from the blood at the renal glomerulus and undergoes significant tubular reabsorption. This tubular reabsorption is pronounced at low rates of urine flow. Moreover, urea levels vary widely with diet, rate of protein metabolism, liver production and the GFR. A high protein intake from the diet or following haemorrhage in the gut, and consequent absorption of the protein from the blood, may produce elevated serum urea levels (up to 10 mmol/L). Urea concentrations of more than 10 mmol/L are usually due to renal disease or decreased renal blood flow following shock or dehydration. As with serum creatinine levels, serum urea levels do not begin to increase until the GFR has fallen by 50% or more.

Production is decreased in situations where there is a low protein intake and in some patients with liver disease. Thus non-renal as well as renal influences should be considered when evaluating changes in serum urea concentrations.

Arterial blood gases

Arterial blood gas analysis provides a rapid and accurate assessment of oxygenation, alveolar ventilation and acid–base status, the three processes which maintain pH homeostasis. The maintenance of arterial CO_2 tension ($PaCO_2$) depends on the quantity of CO_2 produced in the body and its removal through alveolar ventilation. High $PaCO_2$ (>6.1 kPa) indicates alveolar hypoventilation and low $PaCO_2$ (<4.5 kPa) implies alveolar hyperventilation.

The adequate delivery of oxygen to the tissues depends upon the cardiopulmonary system, arterial oxygen tension (PaO_2), oxygen concentration in inspired air and haemoglobin content and its affinity for oxygen. Oxygen saturation is measured by pulse oximetry or by arterial blood gas analysis. Hypoxaemia is defined as a PaO_2 of less than 12 kPa at sea level in an adult patient breathing room air.

Bicarbonate and acid–base

Bicarbonate acts as part of the carbonic acid–bicarbonate buffer system and is important in the maintenance of acid–base balance and thus the pH of the blood. The partial pressure of CO_2 ($PaCO_2$) is measured in blood and is directly proportional to blood CO_2. As a consequence, $PaCO_2$ is used to represent the concentration of acid in the system whilst measurement of bicarbonate (HCO_3^-) indicates the concentration of base. Plasma bicarbonate, CO_2 concentrations and pH are chemically related to each other by the Henderson–Hasselbalch equation:

$$pH = pKa + \log \frac{HCO_3^-}{0.03 \times PaCO_2}$$

where the pKa is the negative logarithm of the dissociation constant for carbonic acid, and 0.03 relates PaCO2 to the amount of CO2 dissolved in plasma. This equation is important because it predicts that the ratio of HCO3– to dissolved CO2 determines blood pH. This is of physiological significance because pulmonary and renal mechanisms regulate pH by adjusting this ratio. The PaCO2 can be altered quickly by changes in respiratory minute volume while plasma bicarbonate can be altered by changes in excretion from the kidneys

In metabolic acidosis such as occurs in renal failure, diabetic ketoacidosis or salicylate poisoning, bicarbonate levels fall. In metabolic alkalosis, the plasma bicarbonate concentration is high. This can occur, for instance, when there is a loss of hydrogen ions from the stomach, as in severe vomiting, or loss through the kidneys, as in mineralocorticoid excess or severe potassium depletion. In the latter situation an increase in sodium reabsorption in the kidney results in bicarbonate retention and a loss of hydrogen ions. The blood buffer system of carbonic acid–bicarbonate base can act immediately to prevent excessive change in pH. The respiratory system takes a few minutes but the kidneys can take up to several days to readjust H^+ ions concentration.

Glucose

The serum glucose concentration is largely determined by the balance of glucose moving into, and leaving, the extracellular compartment. In a healthy adult, this movement is capable of maintaining serum levels below 10 mmol/L, regardless of the intake of meals of varying carbohydrate content.

The renal tubules have the capacity to reabsorb glucose from the glomerular filtrate, and little unchanged glucose is normally lost from the body. Glucose in the urine (glycosuria) is normally only present when the concentration in serum exceeds 10 mmol/L, the renal threshold for total reabsorption.

Normal ranges for serum glucose concentrations are often quoted as non-fasting (<11.1 mmol/L) or fasting (3.3–6.0 mmol/L) concentration ranges. Fasting blood glucose levels between 6.1 and 7.0 mmol/L indicate impaired glucose tolerance and levels above 7.0 mmol/L are consistent with a diagnosis of diabetes. Other signs and symptoms, notably those attributable to an osmotic diuresis, will suggest clinically the diagnosis of diabetes mellitus.

Glycated haemoglobin

Glucose binds to a part of the haemoglobin molecule to form a small glycated fraction. Normally about 5% of haemoglobin is glycated, but this amount is dependent on the average blood glucose concentration over the lifespan of the red cells (about 120 days). The major component of the glycated fraction is referred to as HbA_{1C}.

Measurement of HbA_{1C} is well established as an indicator of chronic glycaemic control in patients with diabetes. Several methods exist for its determination and until standardization is achieved, clinicians should be aware that the ranges indicating good or poor glycaemic control can vary between different assays and laboratories.

Uric acid

Uric acid is the end-product of purine metabolism. The purines, which are used for nucleic acid synthesis, are produced by the breakdown of nucleic acid from ingested meat or synthesized within the body.

Monosodium urate is the form in which uric acid usually exists at the normal pH of body fluids. The term urate is used to represent any salt of uric acid.

Two main factors contribute to elevated serum uric acid levels: an increased rate of formation and reduced excretion. Uric acid is poorly soluble and an elevation in serum concentration can readily result in deposition, as monosodium urate, in tissues or joints. Deposition usually precipitates an acute attack of gouty arthritis. The aim of treatment is to reduce the concentration of uric acid and prevent further attacks of gout. Low serum uric acid levels appear to be of no clinical significance.

Liver function tests

Routine liver function tests (LFTs) give information mainly about the activity or concentrations of enzymes and compounds in serum rather than quantifying specific hepatic functions. Results are useful in confirming or excluding a diagnosis of clinically suspected liver disease, and monitoring its course.

Serum albumin levels and prothrombin time indicate hepatic protein synthesis; bilirubin is a marker of overall liver function.

Transaminase levels indicate hepatocellular injury and death, while alkaline phosphatase levels estimate the amount of impedance of bile flow.

Albumin

Albumin is quantitatively the most important protein synthesized in the liver, with 10–15 g per day being produced in a healthy man. About 60% is located in the interstitial compartment of the ECF, the remainder in the smaller, but relatively impermeable, serum compartment where it is present at a higher concentration. The concentration in the serum is important in maintaining its volume since it accounts for approximately 80% of serum colloid osmotic pressure. A reduction in serum albumin concentration often results in oedema.

Albumin has an important role in binding, among others, calcium, bilirubin and many drugs. A reduction in serum albumin will increase free levels of agents which are normally bound and adverse effects can result if the 'free' entity is not rapidly cleared from the body.

The serum concentration of albumin depends on its rate of synthesis, volume of distribution and rate of catabolism. Synthesis falls in parallel with increasing severity of liver disease or in malnutrition states where there is an inadequate supply of amino acids to maintain albumin production or in response to inflammatory mediators such as interleukin. A low serum albumin concentration will occur when the volume of distribution of albumin increases, as happens for example in cirrhosis with ascites, in fluid retention states such as pregnancy or where a shift of albumin from serum to interstitial fluid causes dilutional hypoalbuminaemia after parenteral infusion of excess protein-free fluid. The movement of albumin from serum into interstitial fluid is often associated with increased capillary permeability in postoperative patients or those with septicaemia. A shift of protein is known to occur physiologically when moving from lying down to the upright position. This can account for an increase in the serum albumin level of up to 10 g/L and can contribute to the variation in serum concentration of highly bound drugs which are therapeutically monitored.

Other causes of hypoalbuminaemia include catabolic states associated with a variety of illnesses and increased loss of albumin, either in urine from damaged kidneys, as occurs in the nephrotic syndrome, or via the skin following burns or a skin disorder such as psoriasis, or from the intestinal wall in a protein-losing enteropathy.

Albumin's serum half-life of approximately 20 days precludes its use as an indicator of acute change in liver function but levels are of prognostic value in chronic disease.

An increase in serum albumin is rare and can be iatrogenic, for example inappropriate infusion of albumin, or the result of dehydration or shock.

Bilirubin

At the end of their life, red blood cells are broken down by the reticuloendothelial system, mainly in the spleen. The haemoglobin molecules, which are subsequently liberated, are split into globin and haem. The globin enters the general protein pool, the iron in haem is reutilized, and the remaining tetrapyrrole ring of haem is degraded to bilirubin. Unconjugated bilirubin, which is water insoluble and fat soluble, is transported to the liver tightly bound to albumin; there it is actively taken up by hepatocytes, conjugated with glucuronic acid and excreted into bile. The conjugated bilirubin is water soluble and secreted into the gut where it is broken down by bacteria into urobilinogen, a colourless compound, which is subsequently oxidized in the colon to urobilin, a brown pigment excreted in faeces. Some of the urobilinogen is absorbed and most is subsequently re-excreted in bile (enterohepatic circulation). A small amount is absorbed into the systemic circulation and excreted in urine, where it too may be oxidized to urobilin.

The liver produces 300 mg of bilirubin each day. However, because the mature liver can metabolize and excrete up to 3 g daily, serum bilirubin concentrations are not a sensitive test of liver function. As a screening test they rarely do other than confirm the presence or absence of jaundice. In chronic liver disease, however, changes in bilirubin concentrations over time do convey prognostic information.

An elevation of serum bilirubin concentration above 50 μmol/L, i.e. approximately 2.5 times the normal upper limit, will reveal itself as jaundice, seen best in the skin and sclerae. Elevated bilirubin levels can be caused by increased production of bilirubin, e.g. haemolysis, ineffective erythropoiesis, impaired transport into hepatocytes, e.g. interference with bilirubin uptake by drugs such as rifampicin or hepatitis, decreased excretion, e.g. with drugs such as rifampicin and methyltestosterone, intrahepatic obstruction due to cirrhosis, tumours, etc. or a combination of the above factors.

The bilirubin in serum is normally unconjugated, bound to protein, not filtered by the glomeruli and does not normally appear in the urine. Bilirubin in the urine (bilirubinuria) is usually the result of an increase in serum concentration of conjugated bilirubin and indicates an underlying pathological disorder.

Enzymes

The enzymes measured in routine liver function tests are listed in Table 6.1. Enzyme concentrations in the serum of healthy individuals are normally low. When cells are damaged, increased amounts of enzymes are detected as the intracellular contents are released into the blood.

It is important to remember that the assay of 'serum enzymes' is a measurement of catalytic activity and not actual enzyme concentration and that activity can vary depending on assay conditions. Consequently the reference range may vary widely between laboratories.

While the measurement of enzymes may be very specific, the enzymes themselves may not be specific to a particular tissue or cell. Many enzymes arise in more than one tissue and an increase in the serum activity of one enzyme can represent damage to any one of the tissues which contain the enzymes. In practice, this problem may be clarified because some tissues contain two or more enzymes in different proportions which are released on damage. For example, alanine and aspartate transaminase both occur in cardiac muscle and liver cells but their site of origin can often be differentiated, because there is more alanine transaminase in the liver than in the heart. In those situations where it is not possible to look at the relative ratio of enzymes, it is sometimes possible to differentiate the same enzyme from different tissues. Such enzymes have the same catalytic activity but differ in some other measurable property, and are referred to as isoenzymes.

The measured activity of an enzyme will be dependent upon the time it is sampled relative to its time of release from the cell. If a sample is drawn too early after a particular insult to a tissue there may be no detectable increase in enzyme activity. If it is drawn too late, the enzyme may have been cleared from the blood.

Alkaline phosphatase

Alkaline phosphatases are found in the canalicular plasma membrane of hepatocytes, in bone where they reflect bone building or osteoblastic activity, and in the intestinal wall and placenta. Each site of origin produces a specific isoenzyme of alkaline phosphatase, which can be electrophoretically separated if concentrations are sufficiently high.

Disorders of the liver which can elevate alkaline phosphatase include intra- or extrahepatic cholestasis, space-occupying lesions such as a tumour or abscess, and hepatitis.

Physiological increases in serum alkaline phosphatase activity also occur in pregnancy due to release of the placental isoenzyme and during periods of growth in children and adolescents when the bone isoenzyme is released.

Pathological increases in serum alkaline phosphatase of bone origin may arise in disorders such as osteomalacia and rickets, Paget's disease of bone, bone tumours, renal bone disease, osteomyelitis and healing fractures. Alkaline phosphatase is also raised as part of the acute phase response; for example, intestinal alkaline phosphatase may be raised in active inflammatory bowel disease.

Transaminases

The two transaminases of diagnostic use are aspartate transaminase (AST; also known as aspartate aminotransferase) and alanine transaminase (ALT; also known as alanine aminotransferase). These enzymes are found in many body tissues, with the highest concentration in hepatocytes and muscle cells.

Serum AST levels are increased in a variety of disorders including liver disease, crush injuries, severe tissue hypoxia, myocardial infarction, surgery, trauma, muscle disease and pancreatitis. ALT is elevated to a similar extent in the disorders listed which involve the liver, though to a lesser extent, if at all, in the other disorders. In the context of liver disease, increased transaminase activity indicates deranged integrity of hepatocyte plasma membranes and/or hepatocyte necrosis. They may be raised in all forms of viral, non-viral, acute and chronic liver disease. They are most markedly raised in acute viral, drug-induced (e.g. paracetamol poisoning), alcohol-related conditions and ischaemic liver damage.

γ-Glutamyl transpeptidase

γ-Glutamyl transpeptidase (γ-GT; also known as γ-glutamyl transferase) is present in high concentrations in the liver, kidney and pancreas, where it is found within the endoplasmic reticulum of cells. It is a sensitive indicator of hepatobiliary disease but does not differentiate a cholestatic disorder from hepatocellular disease. It can also be elevated in alcoholic liver disease, hepatitis, cirrhosis, pancreatitis and congestive cardiac failure.

Serum levels of γ-glutamyl transpeptidase activity can be raised by enzyme induction by certain drugs such as phenytoin, phenobarbital and rifampicin.

Serum γ-glutamyl transpeptidase activity is usually raised in an individual with alcoholic liver disease. However, it can also be raised in heavy drinkers of alcohol who do not have liver damage, due to enzyme induction. Its activity can remain elevated for up to 4 weeks after stopping alcohol intake.

Ammonia

The concentration of free ammonia in the blood is very tightly regulated and is exceeded by two orders of magnitude by its derivative, urea. The normal capacity for urea production far exceeds the rate of free ammonia production by protein catabolism under normal circumstances, such that any increase in free blood ammonia concentration is a reflection of either biochemical or pharmacological impairment of urea cycle function or fairly extensive hepatic damage. Clinical signs of hyperammonaemia occur at concentrations >60 mmol/L and include anorexia, irritability, lethargy, vomiting, somnolence, disorientation, asterixis, cerebral oedema, coma and death; appearance of these findings is generally proportional to free ammonia concentration. Causes of hyperammonaemia include genetic defects in the urea cycle and disorders resulting in significant hepatic dysfunction. Ammonia plays an important role in the increase in brain water which occurs in acute liver failure. Measurement

of the blood ammonia concentration in the evaluation of patients with known or suspected hepatic encephalopathy can help in diagnosis and assessing the effect of treatment. Valproic acid can induce hyperammonaemic encephalopathy as one of its adverse neurological effects.

Amylase

The serum amylase concentration rises within the first 24 hours of an attack of pancreatitis and then declines to normal over the following week. Although a number of abdominal and extra-abdominal conditions can result in a high amylase activity, in patients with the appropriate clinical picture of severe upper abdominal symptoms, the specificity and sensitivity of an amylase level over 1000 U/L a diagnosis of pancreatitis is over 90%.

Cardiac markers

Troponins

Cardiac troponin I (cTnI) and cardiac troponin T (cTnT) are component proteins of the contractile apparatus in cardiac muscle cells. The cardiac specific isoforms are released into plasma as a result of myocardial damage, when raised levels can be detected. They are the preferred marker for the detection of myocardial damage, and they contribute significantly to stratification of individuals with acute coronary syndromes, either alone or in combination with admission ECG or a predischarge exercise stress test. The decision as to whether to monitor cTnT or cTnI in a given laboratory is a balance between cost, availability of automated instrumentation and assay performance. Cardiac troponins offer extremely high tissue specificity and sensitivity but do not discriminate between ischaemic and non-ischaemic mechanisms of myocardial injury.

Creatine kinase

Creatine kinase (CK) is an enzyme which is present in relatively high concentrations in heart muscle, skeletal muscle and in brain in addition to being present in smooth muscle and other tissues. Levels are markedly increased following shock and circulatory failure, myocardial infarction and muscular dystrophies. Less marked increases have been reported following muscle injury, surgery, physical exercise, muscle cramp, an epileptic fit, intramuscular injection and hypothyroidism. The most important adverse effects associated with statins are myopathy and an increase in hepatic transaminases, both of which occur infrequently. Statin-associated myopathy represents a broad clinical spectrum of disorders, from mild muscle aches to severe pain and restriction in mobility, with grossly elevated creatine kinase levels. In rhabdomyolysis, a potentially life-threatening syndrome resulting from the breakdown of skeletal muscle fibres, large quantities of creatine kinase are measurable in the blood. Medications and toxic substances that increase the risk of rhabdomyolysis are shown in Table 6.7.

Creatine kinase has two protein subunits, M and B, which combine to form three isoenzymes, BB, MM and MB. BB is found in high concentrations in the brain, thyroid and some smooth muscle tissue. Little of this enzyme is present in the

Table 6.7 Medications and toxic substances that increase the risk of rhabdomyolysis

Direct myotoxicity	Indirect muscle damage
HMG-CoA reductase inhibitors, especially in combination with fibrates	Alcohol
Corticosteroids	Central nervous system depressants
Ciclosporin	Cocaine
Itraconazole	Amphetamine
Erythromycin	Ecstasy (MDMA)
Colchicine	LSD
Zidovudine	Neuromuscular blocking agents

HMG-CoA, 3-hydroxy-3-methylglutaryl coenzyme A; LSD, lysergic acid diethylamide; MDMA, methylene dioxymethamphetamine

serum, even following damage to the brain. The enzyme found in serum of normal subjects is the MM isoenzyme which originates from skeletal muscle.

Cardiac tissue contains more of the MB isoenzyme than skeletal muscle. Following a myocardial infarction there is a characteristic increase in serum creatine kinase activity. Although measurement of activity of the MB isoenzyme was used in the past to detect myocardial damage, cardiac troponin measurement has now replaced this as the preferred biomarker for establishing the diagnosis of myocardial infarction.

Lactate dehydrogenase

Lactate dehydrogenase has five isoenzymes (LD1–LD5). Total lactate dehydrogenase activity is rarely measured because of the lack of tissue specificity. Levels of activity are elevated following damage to the liver, skeletal muscle and kidneys and in both megaloblastic and haemolytic anaemias. In lymphoma, a high LD activity indicates a poor prognosis. Elevation of LD1 and LD2 occurs after myocardial infarction, renal infarction or megaloblastic anaemia; LD2 and LD3 are elevated in acute leukaemia; LD3 is often elevated in some malignancies; and LD5 is elevated after damage to liver or skeletal muscle.

Tumour markers

While only a few markers contribute to the diagnosis of cancer, serial measurements can be useful in assessing the presence of residual disease and response to treatment. A detailed discussion of markers such as prostate-specific antigen, human chorionic gonadotropin, α-fetoprotein, carcinoembryonic antigen, cancer antigen (CA125 and CA19) is outside the scope of this chapter.

Prostate-specific antigen (PSA) is a serine protease produced by normal and malignant prostatic epithelium and secreted into seminal fluid. Only minor amounts leak into the circulation from the normal prostate, but the release is increased in prostatic disease. It is involved not only in screening for early detection of prostatic cancer but also in the detection of recurrence, disease progression and response to therapies. In order to improve the specificity of PSA testing, a number of refinements

to measurement have been proposed, including free to total PSA ratio, PSA density, and age-specific reference ranges.

Immunoglobulins

Immunoglobulins are antibodies which are produced by B-lymphocytes. They are detected on electrophoresis as bands in three regions: α, β and γ, most occurring in the γ region. Hypergammaglobulinaemia may result from stimulation of B-cells and produces an increased staining of bands in the γ region on electrophoresis. This occurs in infections, chronic liver disease and autoimmune disease.

In some diseases such as chronic lymphatic leukaemia, lymphoma and multiple myeloma, a discrete, densely staining band (paraprotein) can be seen in the γ region. In multiple myeloma, abnormal fragments of immunoglobulins are produced (Bence-Jones protein) which clear the glomerulus and are found in the urine.

Haematology data

The haematology profile is an important part of the investigation of many patients and not just those with primary haematological disease.

Typical measurements reported in a haematology screen, with their normal values, are shown in Table 6.8, whilst a list of the common descriptive terms used in haematology is presented in Table 6.9.

Red blood cell count (RBC)

Red blood cells are produced in the bone marrow by the process of erythropoiesis. One of the major stimulants of this process is erythropoietin, produced mainly in the kidney. Immature erythroblasts develop into mature erythrocytes which are then released into the circulation:

erythroblasts

↓

normoblasts

(nucleated)

↓

reticulocytes

(non-nucleated)

↓

erythrocytes

Normally only reticulocytes and non-nucleated mature erythrocytes are seen in the peripheral blood.

The lifespan of a mature red cell is usually about 120 days. If this is shortened, as for instance in haemolysis, the circulating mass of red cells is reduced and with it the supply of oxygen to tissues is decreased. In these circumstances, red cell production

Table 6.8 Haematology data: typical normal adult reference values

Haemoglobin	13.0–18.0 g/dL males 11.5–16.5 g/dL females
Red blood cell count (RBC)	$4.5–5.9 \times 10^{12}$/L males $3.8–5.2 \times 10^{12}$/L females
Reticulocyte count	$50–100 \times 10^9$/L
Packed cell volume (PCV)	0.40–0.52 males 0.37–0.47 females
Mean cell volume (MCV)	83–101 fL
Mean cell haemoglobin (MCH)	27–34 pg
Mean cell haemoglobin concentration (MCHC)	31.5–34.5 g/dL
White cell count (WBC)	$4.0–11.0 \times 10^9$/L
Differential white cell count: Neutrophils (30–75%) Lymphocytes (5–15%) Monocytes (2–10%) Basophils (<1%) Eosinophils (1–6%)	$2.0–7.0 \times 10^9$/L $1.5–4.0 \times 10^9$/L $0.2–0.8 \times 10^9$/L $<0.1 \times 10^9$/L $0.04–0.4 \times 10^9$/L
Platelets	$150–450 \times 10^9$/L
Erythrocyte sedimentation rate (ESR)	<10 mm/h (rises with age)
Serum iron	13–32 μmol/L
Transferrin	1.2–2.0 μmol/L
Ferritin	21–300 μg/L males 15–150 μg/L females
Total iron binding capacity (TIBC)	47–70 μmol/L
Serum B$_{12}$	170–700 ng/L
Red cell folate	160–600 μg/L
Iron	11–29 μmol/L
Transferrin	1.7–3.4 g/L

Table 6.9 Descriptive terms in common use in haematology

Anisocytosis	Abnormal variation in cell size (usually refers to RBCs)
Agranulocytosis	Lack of granulocytes (principally neutrophils)
Aplastic	Depression of synthesis of all cell types in bone marrow
Basophilia	Increased number of basophils
Hypochromic	MCHC low, red cells appear pale microscopically
Leucocytosis	Increased white cell count
Leucopenia	Reduced white cell count
Macrocytic	Large cells
Microcytic	Small cells
Neutropenia	Reduced neutrophil count
Neutrophilia	Increased neutrophil count
Normochromic	MCHC normal; red cells appear normally pigmented
Pancytopenia	Decreased number of all cell types: it is synonymous with aplastic anaemia
Poikilocytosis	Abnormal variation in cell shape, e.g. some red cells appear pear shaped in macrocytic anaemias
Thrombocytopenia	Lack of platelets

Reticulocytes

Reticulocytes are the earliest non-nucleated red cells. They owe their name to the fine net-like appearance of their cytoplasm which can be seen, after appropriate staining, under the microscope and contains fine threads of ribonucleic acid (RNA) in a reticular network. Reticulocytes normally represent between 0.5% and 1.0% of the total RBC and do not feature significantly in a normal blood profile. However, increased production (reticulocytosis) can be detected in times of rapid red cell regeneration as occurs in response to haemorrhage or haemolysis. At such times the reticulocyte count may reach 40% of the RBC. The reticulocyte count may be useful in assessing the response of the marrow to iron, folate or vitamin B$_{12}$ therapy. The count peaks at about 7–10 days after starting such therapy and then subsides.

Mean cell volume (MCV)

The mean cell volume (MCV) is the average volume of a single red cell. It is measured in femtolitres (10^{-15} L). Terms such as 'microcytic' and 'macrocytic' are descriptive of a low and high MCV, respectively. They are useful in the process of identification of various types of anaemias such as those caused

is enhanced in healthy bone marrow by an increased output of erythropoietin by the kidneys. Under normal circumstances red cells are destroyed by lodging in the spleen due to decreasing flexibility of the cells. They are removed by the reticuloendothelial system.

A high RBC (erythrocytosis or polycythaemia) indicates increased production by the bone marrow and may occur as a physiological response to hypoxia, as in chronic airways disease, or as a malignant condition of red cells such as in polycythaemia rubra vera.

by iron deficiency (microcytic) or vitamin B_{12} or folic acid deficiency (megaloblastic or macrocytic).

Packed cell volume (PCV)

The packed cell volume (PCV) or haematocrit is the ratio of the volume occupied by red cells to the total volume of blood. It can be measured by centrifugation of a capillary tube of blood and then expressing the volume of red cells packed in the bottom as a percentage of the total volume. It is reported as a fraction of unity or as a percentage (e.g. 0.45 or 45%). The PCV is calculated nowadays as the product of the MCV and RBC. The PCV often reflects the RBC and will therefore be decreased in any sort of anaemia. It will be raised in polycythaemia. It may, however, be altered irrespective of the RBC, when the size of the red cell is abnormal, as in macrocytosis and microcytosis.

Mean cell haemoglobin (MCH)

The mean cell haemoglobin (MCH) is the average weight of haemoglobin contained in a red cell. It is measured in picograms (10^{-12} g) and is calculated from the relationship:

$$MCH = \frac{Haemoglobin}{RBC}$$

The MCH is dependent on the size of the red cells as well as the concentration of haemoglobin in the cells. Thus it is usually low in iron deficiency anaemia when there is microcytosis and there is less haemoglobin in each cell, but it may be raised in macrocytic anaemia.

Mean cell haemoglobin concentration (MCHC)

The mean cell haemoglobin concentration (MCHC) is a measure of the average concentration of haemoglobin in 100 mL of red cells. It is usually expressed as grams per litre but may be reported as a percentage. The MCHC will be reported as low in conditions of reduced haemoglobin synthesis, such as in iron deficiency anaemia. In contrast, in macrocytic anaemias the MCHC may be normal or only slightly reduced because the large red cells may contain more haemoglobin, thus giving a concentration approximating that of normal cells. The MCHC can be raised in severe prolonged dehydration. If the MCHC is low, the descriptive term 'hypochromic' may be used as in a hypochromic anaemia, whereas the term 'normochromic' describes a normal MCHC.

Haemoglobin

The haemoglobin concentration in men is normally greater than in women, reflecting in part the higher RBC in men. Lower contrations in women are due, at least in part, to menstrual loss.

Haemoglobin is most commonly measured to detect anaemia. In some relatively rare genetic diseases, the haemoglobinopathies, alterations in the structure of the haemoglobin molecule can be detected by electrophoresis. Abnormal haemoglobins which can be detected in this manner include HbS (sickle haemoglobin in sickle cell disease) and HbA_2 found in β-thalassaemia carriers.

Platelets (thrombocytes)

Platelets are formed in the bone marrow. A marked reduction in platelet number (thrombocytopenia) may reflect either a depressed synthesis in the marrow or destruction of formed platelets.

Platelets are normally present in the circulation for 8–12 days. This is useful information when evaluating a possible drug-induced thrombocytopenia, since recovery should be fairly swift when the offending agent is withdrawn.

A small fall in the platelet count may be seen in pregnancy and following viral infections. Severe thrombocytopenia may result in spontaneous bleeding. A reduced platelet count is also found in disseminated intravascular coagulation, which manifests clinically as severe haemorrhages, particularly in the skin and results in rapid consumption of clotting factors and platelets.

An increased platelet count (thrombocytosis) occurs in malignancy, inflammatory disease and in response to blood loss.

White blood cell count (WBC)

White cells (leucocytes) comprise two types of cell: granulocytes and agranular cells. They are made up of various types of cells (Fig. 6.3) with different functions and it is logical to consider them separately. A haematology profile often reports a total white cell count and a differential count, the latter separating the composition of white cells into the various types.

Neutrophils

Neutrophils or polymorphonucleocytes (PMNs) are the most abundant type of white cell. They have a phagocytic function, with many enzymes contained in the lysosomal granules. They are formed in the bone marrow from the stem cells which form myoblasts and these develop through a number of stages into the neutrophil with a multiple-segmented nucleus. Neutrophils constitute approximately 40–70% of circulating white cells in normal healthy blood. Their lifespan is 10–20 days. The

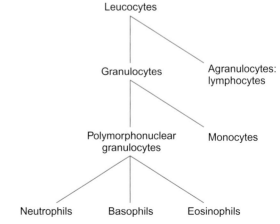

Fig 6.3 Types of white cells.

neutrophil count increases in the presence of infection, tissue damage, e.g. infarction, and inflammation, e.g. rheumatoid arthritis, acute gout. Neutropenia, also described as agranulocytosis in its severest forms, is associated with malignancy and drug toxicity, but may also occur in viral infections such as influenza, infectious mononucleosis and hepatitis.

Basophils

Basophils normally constitute a small proportion of the white cell count. Their function is poorly understood but basophilia occurs in various malignant and premalignant disorders such as leukaemia and myelofibrosis.

Eosinophils

Eosinophils constitute normally less than 6% of white cells. Their function appears to be concerned with inactivation of mediators released from mast cells, and eosinophilia is therefore apparent in many allergic conditions such as asthma, hay fever and drug sensitivity reactions as well as some malignant diseases.

Lymphocytes

Lymphocytes are the second most abundant white cells in the circulating blood, but the majority of them are found in the spleen and other lymphatic tissue. They are formed in the bone marrow. An increase in lymphocyte numbers occurs particularly in viral infections such as rubella, mumps, infectious hepatitis and infectious mononucleosis.

Monocytes

Monocytes are macrophages. Their numbers increase in some infections such as typhoid, subacute bacterial endocarditis, infectious mononucleosis and tuberculosis.

Monitoring anticoagulant therapy

One-stage prothrombin time

Measuring the prothrombin time (PT) is the most commonly used method for monitoring oral anticoagulation therapy. The PT is responsive to a reduction of three of the four vitamin K-dependent factors (factors II, VII and X). The PT is measured by adding calcium and thromboplastin (a phospholipid-protein extract of tissue that promotes the activation of factor X by factor VIII) to citrated plasma.

International normalized ratio (INR)

The results of the test are commonly expressed as a ratio of the PT time of the patient compared with that of the normal control. This is known as the International Normalized Ratio (INR), a system used to standardize reporting worldwide.

$$INR = \left[\frac{\text{Patient's PT}}{\text{Control PT}}\right]^{ISI}$$

The ISI is the international sensitivity index and represents the responsiveness of a given thromboplastin to the reduction of vitamin K-dependent clotting factors and is allocated to commercial preparations of thromboplastin to standardize them. More responsive thromboplastins have lower ISI values.

The target value varies according to the indication for the anticoagulant but for most, including for thromboembolic prophylaxis in atrial fibrillation, it is 2.5. For some indications including recurrent deep vein thrombosis and pulmonary embolism whilst on warfarin, the target is higher at 3.5.

The most common use of the PT and INR is to monitor oral anticoagulant therapy, but the prothrombin time is also useful in assessing liver function.

Activated partial thromboplastin time (APTT)

The activated partial thromboplastin time (APTT) is the most common method for monitoring unfractionated heparin therapy.

A thromboplastic reagent is added to an activator such as activated silicone or kaolin. If the activator is kaolin, the test may be referred to as the PTTK (partial thromboplastin time kaolin) or the KCCT (kaolin–cephalin clotting time). Cephalin is a brain extract supplying the thromboplastin.

The mixture of thromboplastin and activator is combined with citrated plasma to which calcium is added, and the time for the mixture to clot is recorded. The desirable APTT for optimal heparin therapy is between 1.5 and 2.5 times the normal control.

Low molecular weight heparins are effective and safe for the prevention and treatment of venous thromboembolism, and because they provide more predictable anticoagulant activity than unfractionated heparin it is usually not necessary to monitor the APTT during treatment. Laboratory monitoring using an anti-factor Xa assay may be of value in certain clinical settings, including patients with renal insufficiency, and use of fractionated heparin for prolonged periods in pregnancy or in newborns and children.

D-dimers

D-dimers are degradation products of cross-linked fibrins, formed when plasmin degrades fibrin clots. Several methods for their analysis are available. There is no standard unit of measurement. Levels of D-dimers in the blood are raised in conditions associated with coagulation and are used to detect venous thromboembolism, although they are influenced by the presence of co-morbid conditions such as cancer, surgery and infectious diseases. Rapid tests have been developed, feasible for use in emergency conditions. D-dimers are not specific to venous thromboembolism and there is no consensus as to a critical cut-off value for screening for deep vein thrombosis (DVT) or pulmonary embolism (PE), but a cut-off level of around 0.3–0.5 mg/L is often used. Diagnosis of DVT or PE should include a clinical probability assessment as well as D-dimer measurements. In patients with a low or moderate clinical probability of pulmonary embolism, the condition can be excluded by a negative quantitative D-dimer test result, a normal or near normal ventilation–perfusion lung scan, or normal findings on spiral computed tomography of the thorax and leg vein ultrasonography.

Other blood tests

Erythrocyte sedimentation rate (ESR)

The erythrocyte sedimentation rate (ESR) is a measure of the settling rate of red cells in a sample of anticoagulated blood, over a period of 1 hour, in a cylindrical tube.

In youth the normal value is less than 10 mm/h, but normal values do rise with age. The Westergren method, performed under standardized conditions, is commonly used in haematology laboratories. The ESR is strongly correlated with the ability of red cells to aggregate into orderly stacks or rouleaux. In disease, the most common cause of a high ESR is an increased protein level in the blood, such as the increase in acute phase proteins seen in inflammatory disease. Proteins are thought to affect the repellent surface charges on red cells and cause them to aggregate into rouleaux and hence the sedimentation rate increases.

Although some conditions may cause a low ESR, the test is principally used to monitor inflammatory disease. The ESR may be raised in the active phase of rheumatoid arthritis, inflammatory bowel disease, malignant disease and infection. The ESR is non-specific and therefore of little diagnostic value, but serial tests are helpful in following the progress of disease and its response to treatment.

C-reactive protein

Although C-reactive protein is measured by clinical biochemistry laboratories rather than the haematology laboratory, it is described here since it is an acute phase reactant which is used for a similar purpose to the ESR.

C-reactive protein is secreted by the liver in response to a variety of inflammatory cytokines. It recognizes altered self and foreign molecules, as a result of which it activates complement and generates proinflammatory cytokines and activation of the adaptive immune system. Raised levels are a non-specific indicator of inflammation, trauma and infection and serial measurements can be used to monitor response to treatment and resolution of the condition.

Haptoglobin

Haptoglobin is an acute phase protein that binds free haemoglobin and removes it from the circulation, suppressing the inflammatory response associated with free haemoglobin, and preventing kidney damage and iron loss following haemolysis by facilitating hepatic recycling of haem iron. In this way it functions as an antioxidant. Changes in the measured concentration of haptoglobin in serum may help to assess the disease status of patients with inflammatory conditions such as infections and malignancy where it will increase, in contrast to haemolytic conditions where it will decrease.

Coagulation

Coagulation is the process by which a thrombus is formed. The current model of a 'coagulation network' differs from the previous popular cascade scheme. It proposes that blood coagulation is localized on the surfaces of activated cells in three overlapping steps: initiation, amplification and propagation. Coagulation is initiated when a tissue factor (TF)-bearing cell is exposed to blood flow, following either damage of endothelium such as by perforation of a vessel wall or activation by chemicals, cytokines or the inflammatory process. The formation of a clot then involves a complex interaction between endothelium, platelets, von Willebrand factor and numerous clotting proteins. The coagulation process ends with the generation of thrombin, which leads to the formation of a stable fibrin clot. To prevent inappropriate propagation of the thrombus, the process is controlled by naturally occurring anticoagulants and the fibrinolytic system. The interaction between tissue factor and factor VII is the most important in the initiation of coagulation and many of the coagulation reactions occur on the surface of cells, particularly platelets.

The cellular model of normal haemostasis is shown in Figure 6.4. Despite the complexity of this model, the basic coagulation tests can still be interpreted in relation to the 'intrinsic', 'extrinsic' and 'final common pathway' components of the traditional and previously held cascade (Fig. 6.5).

Coombs' test

Coombs' reagent is a mixture of anti-human immunoglobulin antibody and anticomplement antibody. When added to washed red blood cells, it will detect antibody or complement on the cell surface and cause agglutination of the red cells. The test is positive, i.e. agglutination occurs in cases of autoimmune anaemia.

Xanthochromia

Xanthochromia is a yellow discolouration of cerebrospinal fluid caused by haemoglobin catabolism. It is thought to arise within several hours of subarachnoid haemorrhage (SAH) and can help to distinguish the elevated red cell count observed after traumatic lumbar puncture from that observed following SAH, particularly if few red cells are present. Although some hospitals rely on visual inspection, spectrophotometry to detect the presence of both oxyhaemoglobin and bilirubin, which both contribute to xanthochromia following SAH, is becoming more established.

Iron, transferrin and iron binding

Iron circulating in the serum is bound to transferrin. It leaves the serum pool and enters the bone marrow where it becomes incorporated into haemoglobin in developing red cells. Serum iron levels are extremely labile and fluctuate throughout the day and therefore provide little useful information about iron status.

Transferrin, a simple polypeptide chain with two iron binding sites, is the plasma iron binding protein. Measurement of total iron binding capacity (TIBC), from which the percentage of transferrin saturation with iron may be calculated, gives more information. Saturation of 16% or lower is usually taken to indicate an iron deficiency, as is a raised TIBC of greater than 70 μmol/L.

Ferritin is an iron store protein found in cell cytosol. Serum ferritin measurement is the test of choice in patients suspected of having iron deficiency anaemia.

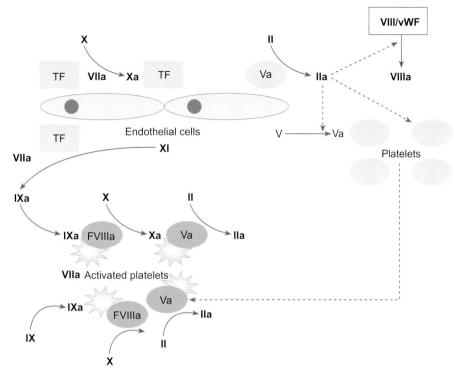

Fig 6.4 Cellular model for normal haemostasis

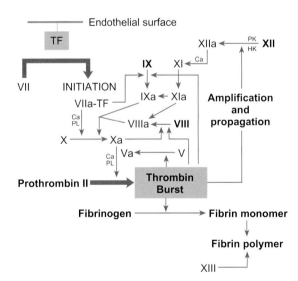

Fig 6.5 Coagulation network.

In normal individuals, the serum ferritin concentration is directly related to the available storage iron in the body. The serum ferritin level falls below the normal range in iron deficiency anaemia, and its measurement can provide a useful monitor for repletion of iron stores after iron therapy. Ferritin is an acute phase protein and levels may be normal or high in the anaemia of chronic disease, such as occurs in rheumatoid arthritis or chronic renal disease.

Iron overload causes high concentrations of serum ferritin, as can liver disease and some forms of cancer.

Free protoporphyrin concentration increases in red blood cells in iron deficiency. These can be estimated with an assay which measures the fluorescence of zinc protoporphyrin (ZPP). ZPP is increased in iron deficiency, but also in chronic disease. In general, ZPP levels provide less information about iron storage in anaemic patients than does serum ferritin.

Vitamin B12 and folate

In the haematology literature, B_{12} refers not only to cyanocobalamin but also to several other cobalamins with identical nutritional properties. Folic acid, which can designate a specific compound, pteroylglutamic acid, is also more commonly used as a general term for the folates. Deficiency of cobalamin can result both in anaemia, usually macrocytic, and neurological disease, including neuropathies, dementia and psychosis. Folate deficiency produces anaemia, macrocytosis, depression, dementia and neural tube defects.

There is some controversy about the definition of the lower limit of normal for serum B_{12}. Liver disease tends to increase B_{12} levels, and they may be reduced in folate-deficient patients. Serum folate levels tend to increase in B_{12} deficiency, and alcohol can reduce levels. Red blood cell folate is a better measure of folate tissue stores.

CASE STUDIES

Case 6.1

Mrs A is a 70-year-old lady who presents with diffuse pains in her arms and legs. Her recent drug history is paracetamol and codeine. She has the following biochemical test results.

Alkaline phosphatase	353 U/L
Urea	4.6 mmol/L
Ionized calcium	1.10 mmol/L
Creatinine	63 µmol/L
Phosphate	0.97 mmol/L
25-hydroxyvitamin D	9 nmol/L
Parathyroid hormone	120 ng/L

All other results are normal.

Questions

1. With respect to Mrs A's blood results, what is the diagnosis?
2. How should she be treated?
3. How should she be monitored?

Answers

1. Osteomalacia
2. In osteomalacia due to dietary absence of vitamin D or inadequate exposure to sunlight, vitamin D_2 (cholecalciferol) or vitamin D_3 (ergocalciferol) is given orally in doses of 2000–4000 iu (0.05–0.1 mg) daily for 6–12 weeks, followed by daily supplements of 200–400 iu. Where osteomalacia is due to intestinal malabsorption, higher doses of vitamin D and large doses of calcium may be required. In some instances oral vitamin D is ineffective and the parenteral (intramuscular) route is required.
3. Serum calcium should be monitored frequently during the first 1–2 months of therapy and less frequently once a stable dose has been established which has ensured return to normal of calcium, alkaline phosphatase and parathyroid hormone levels.

Case 6.2

A 50-year-old man on a hospital medical ward has a fast pulse rate and falling blood pressure. His recent drug history is bendroflumethiazide and aspirin. He has the following blood results.

Haematology results	Hb 8.8 g/dL
	RBC 4.7×10^{12}/L
Platelets	570×10^9/L

MCV, MCH and the rest of the blood profile are normal

Clinical biochemistry	Urea 11.6 mmol/L

Creatinine is normal and sodium and potassium concentrations are normal.

Questions

1. What cause of this patient's low haemoglobin should be considered and investigated?
2. What is the likely cause of his raised urea level?
3. What terms describe this type of anaemia?

Answers

1. The most likely cause of a low haemoglobin in a man with this clinical picture is haemorrhage, particularly a gastrointestinal bleed. The picture is one of blood loss, manifested by a loss of red cells and haemoglobin. The red cells are of normal size and colour. As, initially after a bleed, haemoglobin is normal, the bleed must have begun sufficiently long ago for haemodilution, through ingestion of fluid, to have occurred.
2. A raised urea in the presence of a normal creatinine may signify dehydration or gastrointestinal bleeding. In this case, given the blood

picture, the latter is more likely. Blood in the gastrointestinal tract is a source of protein which will be absorbed into the hepatic portal system and converted to urea in the liver.
3. The blood picture is one of normocytic, normochromic anaemia, typically seen in haemorrhage.

Case 6.3

A 75-year-old lady who had been treated by her primary care doctor with amoxicillin for a chest infection 1 week previously is admitted to hospital with confusion. She has a past history of peptic ulcer. Her only medication is omeprazole. Her biochemistry profile shows the following abnormalities.

Sodium	110 mmol/L
Urine sodium	114 mmol/L
Potassium	3.7 mmol/L
Urine potassium	455 mmol/L
Urea	5.1 mmol/L
Creatinine	71 µmol/L
Serum osmolality	233 mosmol/kg
Urine osmolality	476 mosmol/kg
Random cortisol	1943 nmol/L

Questions

1. What is the diagnosis?
2. What are the possible causes of this condition?
3. How should she be treated?

Answers

1. SIADH (syndrome of inappropriate secretion of vasopressin; also known as antidiuretic hormone).
2. Malignant neoplasms with autonomous vasopressin release, most commonly small cell carcinoma of the lung. Non-malignant pulmonary disease such as tuberculosis or, in this lady, her recent pneumonia. Central nervous system disorders such as skull fracture, subdural haematoma, stroke, encephalitis or meningitis. Several drugs can cause SIADH, including carbamazepine, antidepressants, some cytotoxics and, possibly relevant in her case, omeprazole.
3. Restriction of fluid to 800–1000 mL daily is essential treatment together with treatment of the underlying condition. Drugs that block the effect of vasopressin on the renal tubule may occasionally be useful in this syndrome, of which demeclocycline is the most potent inhibitor that is available for chronic administration.

Case 6.4

An 88-year-old man presented with a 3-week history of increasing weakness and pain in his muscles. Four weeks previously he had been in hospital with a bleeding, *H. pylori* associated duodenal ulcer, as a result of which his aspirin therapy had been stopped and he had been given a course of *H. pylori* eradication. One year previously he had had a myocardial infarction. His current medication was furosemide, lisinopril, simvastatin and lansoprazole.

Biochemical tests of urea and electrolytes, liver function, creatine kinase, full blood count and clotting revealed the following.

Sodium	136 mmol/L
Potassium	5.8 mmol/L
Urea	21.3 mmol/L
Creatinine	190 µmol/L
Creatine kinase	92 300 u/L

Questions

1. What is the most likely diagnosis?
2. What investigation would support the diagnosis?
3. What are the possible causes of his raised creatine kinase level?

Answers

1. Rhabdomyolysis.
2. Testing urine for myoglobin: myoglobinuria causes a positive urine test for blood in the absence of urinary erythrocytes. Confimatory testing for myoglobin uses a specific immunoassay.
3. Acute muscle destruction, rhabdomyolysis associated with myoglobinuria occurs with acute toxic, metabolic, inflammatory, infectious and traumatic muscle damage. HMG-CoA reductase inhibitors such as simvastatin increase the risk of rhabdomyolysis, which may occur several months or years after commencement of therapy. Medications and toxic substances that increase the risk of rhabdomyolysis are shown in Table 6.7.

Case 6.5

An 80-year-old lady presents with a 2-day history of swelling of her left leg. She is thin and frail, residing in a nursing home. She is taking furosemide and lisinopril for congestive cardiac failure, which is not well controlled. Biochemical tests of liver function and D-dimers reveal the following.

Alanine transaminase	67 U/L
Alkaline phosphatase	94 U/L
Bilirubin	28 µmol/L
D-dimers	2.7 mg/L
Clotting	PT 13.5 seconds/INR 1.0

Questions

What are the likely diagnoses?

Answers

Deep vein thrombosis (DVT) in the left leg and hepatic congestion secondary to congestive cardiac failure.

Ultrasound of her left leg confirms DVT. Ultrasound of her liver suggests inferior vena caval and hepatic congestion. She is given 5 mg of warfarin each day for the next 2 days. Her INR on the third day is 9.0.

Questions

Outline possible contributory causes to her extreme sensitivity to warfarin.

Answers

Sensitivity to warfarin increases with age and is inversely related to body mass. Her hepatic congestion may be interfering with her ability to produce clotting factors. She is thin and frail and is likely to have a low oral intake, particularly of dietary vitamin K. The rate of warfarin metabolism is under genetic control and the lady in question may be a slow metabolizer.

Case 6.6

A patient with a history of insulin-dependent diabetes, heart failure and ischaemic heart disease is admitted to hospital after vomiting. His medication includes lisinopril, furosemide with potassium, nifedipine and isosorbide mononitrate. Biochemistry results show:

Potassium	5.5 mmol/L
Urea	15 mmol/L
Creatinine	150 µmol/L
Random blood glucose	23 mmol/L

Arterial blood gases:	
pH	7.25
$PaCO_2$	2.8 kPa
Actual bicarbonate	9.5 mmol/L
PaO_2	12.7 kPa

Questions

1. What is the likely cause of this patient's raised serum potassium level?
2. Why are the urea and creatinine raised?
3. What do his blood gases suggest?

Answers

1. Insulin deficiency causes a reduction in absorption of potassium into the tissues. The patient has metabolic ketoacidosis, evidenced by his raised blood glucose and reduced pH and bicarbonate. Hyperkalaemia may also be caused by renal failure. The potassium supplements and lisinopril will also have contributed.
2. Renal failure is a complication of diabetes. The patient will be dehydrated because of vomiting, furosemide and the osmotic diuresis caused by hyperglycaemia.
3. An acid plasma pH together with a low plasma bicarbonate concentration suggests a metabolic acidosis. The low $PaCO_2$ reflects the body's attempt to blow off CO_2 from the lungs (Kussmaul respiration) in order to restore the plasma pH to normal. This is a typical picture seen in metabolic ketoacidosis in diabetic patients, but may also occur as a result of diarrhoea because of loss of bicarbonate-rich intestinal fluid or renal failure.

FURTHER READING

Cowan R, O'Reilly D, Stewart M et al 2004 Clinical biochemistry, 3rd edn. Churchill Livingstone, Edinburgh.

Henson A 2002 ABC of clinical haematology, 2nd edn. BMJ Books, London

Howard M R, Hamilton P J 1997 Haematology: an illustrated colour text. Harcourt Brace, Edinburgh

Marshall W J 2000 Clinical chemistry, 4th edn. Mosby, London

Swaminathan R 2004 Handbook of clinical biochemistry. OUP, New Delhi

7 Parenteral nutrition

S. J. Dunnett

KEY POINTS

- Parenteral nutrition is indicated when the gastrointestinal tract is inaccessible, inadequate or inappropriate to meet the patient's ongoing nutritional needs.
- Combinations of oral diet, enteral feeding and parenteral nutrition, either peripherally or centrally, may be appropriate.
- Regimens, tailored to the nutritional needs of the patient, should contain a balance of seven essential components: water, L-amino acids, glucose, lipid with essential fatty acids, vitamins, trace elements and electrolytes.
- Advances in technology alongside expertise in pharmaceutical stability often permit the required nutrients to be administered from a single container. Increasingly, standard formulations are used, including licensed presentations.
- Parenteral nutrition must be compounded under validated aseptic conditions by trained specialists.
- Prescriptions are guided by baseline nutritional assessment, calculation of requirements using a range of algorithms, knowledge of the patient's disease status and ongoing monitoring.
- The incidence of complications with parenteral nutrition is reducing; knowledge of management is improving.

Introduction

Malnutrition

Malnutrition can be described as 'a deficiency or excess (or imbalance) of energy, protein, and other nutrients that causes measurable adverse effects on the tissue/body size, shape, composition and function and clinical outcome'.

In UK hospitals, most malnutrition appears to be a general undernutrition of all nutrients (protein, energy and micro-nutrients) rather than marasmus (insufficient energy provision) or kwashiorkor (insufficient protein provision). Alternatively, there may be a specific deficiency, such as thiamine in severe hepatic disease.

Multiple causes may contribute to malnutrition. They may include inadequate or unbalanced food intake, increased demand due to clinical disease status, defects in food digestion or absorption, or a compromise in nutritional metabolic pathways. Onset may be acute or insidious.

Even mild malnutrition can result in problems with normal body form and function, with adverse effects on clinical, physical and psychosocial status. Symptoms may include impaired immune response, reduced skeletal muscle strength and fatigue, reduced respiratory muscle strength, impaired thermoregulation, impaired skin barrier and wound healing. In turn, these predispose the patient to a wide range of problems including infection, delayed clinical recovery, increased clinical complications, inactivity, psychological decline and reduced quality of life. As symptoms may be non-specific, the underlying malnutrition may be left undiagnosed. Early nutrition intervention is associated with reduced average length of hospital stay and linked cost savings.

Nutrition screening

Routine screening is recommended by the Malnutrition Advisory Group of the British Association of Parenteral and Enteral Nutrition (BAPEN). This group has worked to promote awareness of the clinical significance of malnutrition and has produced guidelines to monitor and manage malnutrition. A range of screening criteria and tools has been developed and refined to assess nutritional status. Examples include the relatively simple and reproducible body mass index tool with consideration of other key factors (Table 7.1). and the BAPEN 'MUST' tool (Malnutrition Universal Screening Tool; BAPEN 2003). Body weight should not be used in isolation; significant weight fluctuations may reflect fluid disturbances, and muscle wasting may be due to immobility rather than undernutrition. More complex anthropometry measurements are sometimes indicated to track changes.

Incidence of undernutrition

The incidence of undernutrition in hospitalized patients is not accurately known although it is estimated as being between 20% and 40%.

Table 7.1 Body mass index as a screening tool

Body mass index (BMI) = $\dfrac{\text{weight (kg)}}{\text{height (m)}^2}$	
BMI category	Likelihood of chronic protein-energy undernutrition
<18.5 kg/m^2	Probable
18.5–20 kg/m^2	Possible
>20 kg/m^2	Unlikely

Indications for parenteral nutrition

Parenteral nutrition (PN) is the intravenous administration of a nutritionally balanced and physicochemically stable sterile emulsion or solution. It is indicated whenever the gastrointestinal tract is inaccessible, inadequate or inappropriate to meet the patient's ongoing nutritional needs. PN may fulfil the total nutritional requirements or may be supplemental to an enteral feed or diet.

The simplest way to correct or prevent undernutrition is through conventional balanced food. However, this is not always possible. Nutritional support may then require oral supplements or enteral feeding. Assuming the gut is functioning normally, the patient will be able to digest and absorb their required nutrients. These include water, protein, carbohydrate, fat, vitamins, minerals and electrolytes. However, if the gut is not accessible or functioning adequately to meet the patient's needs, or gut rest is indicated, then PN is used. While the enteral route is the first choice, this may still fail to provide sufficient nutrient intake in a number of patients (Woodcock et al 2001). Complications and limitations of enteral nutrition need to be recognized.

A decision pathway can be followed to guide initial and ongoing nutritional support. While many are published, a locally tailored and regularly updated pathway is favoured. Figure 7.1 may provide a useful starting point.

Close monitoring should ensure the patient's needs are met; a combination of nutrition routes is sometimes the best course. Where possible, PN patients should also receive enteral intake. Even minor gut stimulation has been linked with a reduction in the incidence of bacterial translocation through maintaining gut integrity and preventing overgrowth and cholestatic complications. PN should not be stopped abruptly but should be gradually reduced in line with the increasing enteral diet.

Nutrition support teams

Multidisciplinary nutrition teams have been formed in many of the larger hospitals. They function in a variety of ways, depending on the patient populations and resources. In general, they adopt either a consultative or an authoritative role in nutrition management. Many studies have shown their positive contribution to the total nutritional care of the patient through efficient and appropriate selection and monitoring of feed and route. The British Pharmceutical Nutrition Group (BPNG) has developed a patient information leaflet which is available through its website.

Components of a parenteral nutrition regimen

In addition to water, six main groups of nutrients need to be incorporated in a PN regimen (Table 7.2). The aim is to provide appropriate sources and amounts of all the equivalent building blocks in a single daily admixture.

Water volume

Water is the principal component of the body and accounts for approximately 60% and 55% of total body weight in men and women, respectively. Usually, homeostasis maintains appropriate fluid levels and electrolyte balance, and thirst drives the healthy person to drink. However, some patients are not able physically to respond by drinking and so this homeostasis is ineffective. There is risk of over- or underhydration if the range of factors affecting fluid and electrolyte balance is not fully understood and monitored (see Chapter 6). In general, an adult patient will

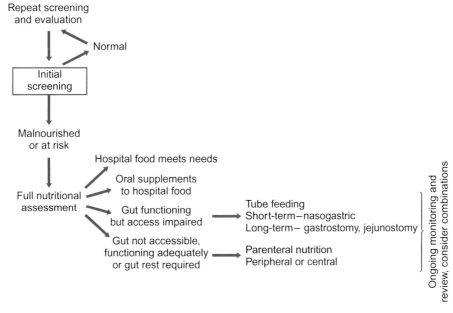

Fig 7.1 Decision pathway to guide initial and ongoing nutritional support.

Table 7.2 Oral and equivalent parenteral nutrition source

Oral diet	Parenteral nutrition source
Water/volume	Water/volume
Protein	L-amino acids mixture
Carbohydrate	Glucose
Fat with essential fatty acids	Lipid emulsions with essential fatty acids
Vitamins	Vitamins
Minerals	Trace elements
Electrolytes	Electrolytes

require 20–40 mL/kg/day fluid. However, Table 7.3 describes other factors that should be considered in tailoring input to needs.

Amino acids

Twenty L-amino acids are required for protein synthesis and metabolism. A majority of these can be synthesized endogenously. Eight are called 'essential' amino acids because they cannot be synthesized (isoleucine, leucine, lysine, methionine, phenylalanine, threonine, tryptophan and valine). A further group of 'conditionally essential' amino acids, arginine, choline, glutamine, taurine and S-adenosyl-L-methionine, are defined as the patient's needs exceed the synthesis in clinically stressed conditions. Also, due to the immature metabolic pathways of neonates, infants and children, some other amino acids are essential in the young patient, and these include histidine, proline, cysteine, tyrosine and taurine. Immature neonatal metabolism does not fully metabolize glycine, methionine, phenylalanine and threonine and so requirements are reduced.

To balance the patient's amino acid requirements and the chemical characteristics of the amino acids (solubility, stability and compatibility), a range of commercially available licensed solutions has been formulated containing a range of amino acid profiles (Table 7.4). Aminoplex, Intrafusin, Synthamin and Vamin are designed for adult patients. The amino acid profiles of Primene and Vaminolact are specifically tailored to neonates, infants and children (reflecting the amino acid profile of maternal cord blood and breast milk, respectively).

L-glutamine was initially excluded from formulations due to its low solubility and relatively poor stability in the aqueous environment. However, it is recognized that there is a clinical need for this amino acid in catabolic stress, and it is now available as a free L-glutamine additive and as a dipeptide (with alanine and lysine; the peptide bond cleaves in the blood, releasing free L-glutamine). Research is also considering the rationale and merits of supplementing arginine, glutathione and ornithine α-ketoglutarate.

For adults, PN solutions are generally prescribed in terms of the amount of nitrogen they provide, rounding to the nearest gram; for example, 9 g, 11 g, 14 g or 18 g nitrogen regimens may be prescribed. Assuming adequate energy is supplied, most adult patients achieve nitrogen balance with approximately 0.2 g nitrogen/kg/day, although care should be taken with overweight patients.

A 24-hour urine collection can be used as an indicator of nitrogen loss, assuming all urine is collected and urea or volume output is not compromised by renal failure. However, a true nitrogen output determination requires measurement of nitrogen output from all body fluids, including urine, sweat, faeces, skin and wounds. Nitrogen balance studies can indicate the metabolic state of the patient (positive balance in net protein synthesis, negative balance in protein catabolism). Urinary urea constitutes approximately 80% of the urinary nitrogen. A number of predictive equations have been developed to estimate the nitrogen output from urinary urea. For example:

$$\text{nitrogen loss} = \text{urea (micrograms/24 h)} \times 0.035$$

or

$$\text{nitrogen loss} = \text{urea (mmol/24 h)} \times 0.028 + 2.$$

In paediatrics, the term 'amino acid' is preferred when formulating PN solutions. The term 'protein content' is no longer favoured as the solutions contain amino acids, not protein. The conversion factor for g of protein to g of nitrogen varies depending on the amino acid profile, with different amino acid profiles releasing

Table 7.3 Factors affecting fluid requirements

Consider increasing the fluid input	Consider reducing the fluid input
• Signs/symptoms of dehydration • Fever: increased insensible losses from lungs in hyperventilation and from skin in sweating. Allow 10–15% extra water per 10°C above normal • Acute anabolic state: increased water required for increased cell generation • High environmental temperature or low humidity: increased rate of evaporation • Abnormal GI loss (vomiting, ostomies, diarrhoea): consider both volume loss and electrolyte content • Burns or open wound(s): increased water evaporation • Blood loss: assess volume lost and whether replaced by transfusion, colloid, crystalloid	• Signs/symptoms of fluid overload • High humidity: reduced rate of evaporation • Blood transfusion: volume input • Drug therapy: assess volume and electrolyte content of infused drug • Cardiac failure: may limit tolerated blood volume • Renal failure: fluid may accumulate so reduce input accordingly or provide artificial renal support

Table 7.4 Amino acid and consequential nitrogen content of licensed amino acid solutions available in the UK (alphabetical)

		Amino acid content (g/L)	Nitrogen content (g/L)
Paediatric	Primene 10%	100	15
	Vaminolact	65.3	9.3
Adult	Glamin	134 g (inc. dipeptide)	22.4 (total)
	Hyperamine 30	179	30
	Intrafusin 11	73.28	11.4
	Intrafusin 22	152.3	22.8
	Synthamin 9/9EF	55	9.1
	Synthamin 14/14EF	85	14
	Synthamin 17/17EF	100	16.5
	Vamin 9/9 Glucose	70.2	9.4
	Vamin 14/14EF	85	13.5
	Vamin 18EF	114	18.0

a different proportion of water molecules as the peptide bonds are formed. However, some publications refer to a conversion factor of 1 g of nitrogen per 6.25 g of protein. This should be used with caution.

Amino acid solutions are hypertonic to blood and should not be administered alone into the peripheral circulation.

Energy

Many factors affect the energy requirement of individual patients. These include age, activity and illness (both severity and stage). Predictive formulae can be applied to estimate the energy requirement, for example the Harris Benedict equation or the more commonly used Schofield equation. Alternatively, calorimetry techniques can be used. However, no single method is ideal or suits all scenarios. Often it is found that two methods result in different recommendations. The majority of adults can be appropriately maintained on 25–35 non-protein kcal/kg/day. There is debate over whether to include amino acids as a source of calories since it is simplistic to assume they are either all spared for protein synthesis or fed into the metabolic pathways (Krebs cycle) and contribute to the release of energy-rich molecules. In general, we refer to 'non-protein energy' and sufficient lipid and glucose energy is supplied to spare the amino acids. As a rough guide, the non-protein energy-to-nitrogen ratio is approximately 150:1 although an ideal ratio for all patients has not been absolutely defined. A lower ratio is considered for critically ill patients while higher ratios are considered for less catabolic patients.

Dual energy

In general, energy should be sourced from a balanced combination of lipid and glucose. This is termed 'dual energy' and is more physiological than an exclusive glucose source. Typically, the fat-to-glucose ratio remains close to the 60:40 to 40:60 range.

Dual energy can minimize the risk of giving too much lipid or glucose since complications increase if the metabolic capacity of either is exceeded. A higher incidence of acute adverse effects is noted with faster infusion rates and higher total daily doses,

especially in patients with existing metabolic stress. It is therefore essential that the administered dose complements the energy requirements and the infusion rate does not exceed the metabolic capacity.

While effectively maintaining nitrogen balance, lipid inclusion is seen to confer a number of advantages (Table 7.5).

Some patients, notably long-term home patients, do not tolerate daily lipid infusions and need to be managed on an individual basis. Depending on the enteral intake and nutritional needs, lipids are prescribed for a proportion of the days. A trial with the newer generation lipid emulsions may be appropriate.

Glucose

Glucose is the recommended source of carbohydrate (1 g anhydrous glucose provides 4 kcal). Table 7.6 indicates the energy provision and tonicity for a range of concentrations. Glucose 5% is regarded as isotonic with blood. The higher concentrations cause phlebitis if administered directly to peripheral veins and should therefore be given by a central vein or in combination with compatible solutions to reduce the tonicity.

Table 7.5 Examples of the advantages of dual energy systems over glucose-only energy systems

Minimize risk of hyperglycaemia and related complications
Prevent and reverse fatty liver (steatosis)
Reduce carbon dioxide production and respiratory distress
Meet higher calorie requirements of septic and trauma patients when glucose oxidation reduced and lipid oxidation increased
Reduce metabolic stress
Support immune function
Improve lean body mass and reduce water retention
Permit peripheral administration, through reduced tonicity
Facilitate fluid restriction, as lipid is a concentrated source of energy
Source of essential fatty acids, preventing and correcting deficiency

Table 7.6 Energy provision and tonicity of glucose solutions

Concentration (w/v)	Energy content (kcal/L)	Approximate osmolarity (mOsmol/L)
5%	200	278
10%	400	555
20%	800	1110
50%	2000	2775
70%	2800	3885

PN formulations classically contain one or more concentrations of glucose, selected both to provide the required glucose calories and to meet total volume requirement.

The glucose infusion rate should generally be between 2 and 4 mg/kg/min. An infusion of 2 mg/kg/min (equating to approximately 200 g (800 kcal) per day for a 70 kg adult) represents the basal glucose requirement, whereas 4 mg/kg/day is regarded as the physiological optimal rate. Higher levels (up to 7 mg/kg/min) are tolerated by some patients but are not generally recommended; glucose oxidation occurs but there is an increased conversion to glycogen and fat. If excess glucose is infused and the glycogen storage capacity exceeded, the circulating glucose level rises, de novo lipogenesis occurs (production of fat from glucose) and there is an increased incidence of metabolic complications.

Lipid emulsions

Lipid emulsions are used as a source of energy and for the provision of the essential fatty acids, linoleic and α-linolenic acid. Supplying 10 kcal energy per gram of oil, they are energy rich and can be infused directly into the peripheral veins since they are relatively isotonic with blood.

Typically, patients receive up to 2.5 g lipid/kg/day. For practical compounding reasons, and assuming clinical acceptance, this tends to be rounded to 100 g or 50 g. Table 7.7 gives details of the lipid emulsions available within the UK.

Lipid emulsions are oil-in-water formulations. Figure 7.2 shows the structure of triglycerides (three fatty acids on a glycerol backbone) and a lipid globule, stabilized at the interface by phospholipids. Ionization of the polar phosphate group of the phospholipid results in a net negative charge of the lipid globule and an electromechanically stable formulation. The lipid globule size distribution is similar to that of the naturally occurring chylomicrons (80–500 nanometers), as indicated in Figure 7.3.

The first-generation lipid emulsions have been in use since the 1970s and utilize soybean oil as the source of long chain fatty acids. More recent research on lipid metabolic pathways and clinical outcomes has indicated that the fatty acid profile of soybean oil alone is not ideal. For example, it is now recognized that these lipid emulsions presented excess essential polyunsaturated fatty acids, resulting in a qualitative and quantitative compromise to the eicosanoid metabolites that have important roles in cell structure, haemodynamics, platelet function, inflammatory response and immune response.

Table 7.7 Licensed lipid emulsions available in the UK	
Lipid emulsion type	Details of products with kcal per litre
Soybean oil (egg phospholipids)	Intralipid 10% (1100 kcal), 20% (2000 kcal), 30% (3000 kcal) Ivelip 10% (1100 kcal), 20% (2000 kcal)
Olive oil (80%)/soybean oil (20%) (egg phospholipids)	ClinOleic 20% (2000 kcal)
MCT (50%)/LCT (50%) (egg phospholipids)	Lipofundin MCT/LCT 10% (1054 kcal), 20% (1904 kcal)
Structured triglyceride (egg phospholipids)	Structolipid 20% (1960 kcal)

MCT, medium chain triglyceride; LCT, long chain triglyceride

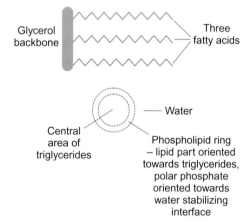

Fig 7.2 Triglyceride structure and composition of lipid emulsion globule.

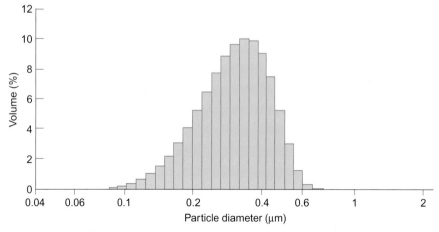

Fig 7.3 Lipid globule size distribution curve of Ivelip 20%.

The molecular structure of the fatty acids has an important impact on the patient's oxidative stress. Two strategies have been applied to overcome this: a reduction in the polyunsaturated fatty acid content through an improved balance of fatty acids or the inclusion of medium chain fatty acids. This has resulted in the development of lipid emulsions that include olive oil (rich in monounsaturated oleic acid and antioxidant α-tocopherol with an appropriate level of essential polyunsaturated fatty acids), fish oil, (rich in omega 3 fatty acids) and medium chain triglycerides or structured triglycerides (reduced long chain fatty acid content). Clinical application of these newer lipid emulsions depends upon good clinical studies within the relevant patient population. Such studies should evaluate the efficacy of energy provision and clinical tolerance and report improvements in the eicosanoid-dependent functions or oxidative stress (see Göbel et al 2003).

Both egg and soybean phospholipids include a phosphate moiety. There is a debate as to whether this is bioavailable. Therefore some manufacturers include the phosphate content in their stability calculations while others do not.

The 20% lipid emulsions are favoured, especially in paediatrics, as they contain less phospholipid than the 10% emulsions in relation to triglyceride provision. If there is incomplete clearance of the infused phospholipids, lipoprotein X, an abnormal phospholipid-rich low-density lipoprotein, is generated and a raised blood cholesterol observed. The incidence of raised lipoprotein X levels is greater with the 10% emulsions as they present proportionally more phospholipid.

Lipid clearance monitoring is particularly important in patients who are at risk of impaired clearance, including those who are hyperlipidaemic, diabetic, septic, have impaired renal or hepatic function, or are critically ill (Crook 2000).

Micronutrients

Micronutrients have a key role in intermediary metabolism, as both co-factors and co-enzymes. For example, zinc is required by over 200 enzyme systems and affects many diverse body functions including acid–base balance, immune function and nucleic acid synthesis. It is evident, therefore, that the availability of micronutrients can affect enzyme activity and total metabolism. When disease increases the metabolism of the major substrates, the requirement for micronutrients is increased. Some of the micronutrients also play an essential role in the free radical scavenging system. These include:

- copper, zinc and manganese: in the form of superoxide dismutase, dispose of superoxide radicals
- selenium: in the form of glutathione peroxidase, removes hydroperoxyl compounds
- vitamin C: a strong reducing agent
- vitamins A, E and β-carotene: react directly with free radicals.

By the time a patient starts parenteral nutrition, they may have already developed a deficiency of one or more essential nutrients. By the time a specific clinical deficiency is observed, for example depigmentation of hair in copper deficiency or skin lesions in zinc deficiency, the patient will already have tried to compensate to maintain levels, compromised intracellular enzyme activity and antioxidant systems and expressed non-specific symptoms such as fatigue and impaired immune response. A summary of factors that affect micronutrient needs is presented in Table 7.8.

Micronutrient monitoring can be costly and complex. Results require careful interpretation alongside clinical symptoms (Misra & Kirby 2000). Deficiency states are clinically significant but, with non-specific symptoms, they are often difficult to diagnose.

Micronutrient experts prefer to prevent a deficit developing and compromising the clinical state, rather than perform regular monitoring of blood results.

Vitamins and trace elements should be included daily from the start of the parenteral nutrition. The requirements are increased during critical illness and in chronically depleted patients. Major burns and trauma or patients with artificial renal support can quickly become depleted. Their supplementation may influence the outcome of the disease. Even if the patient has reasonable levels and reserves initially, they can quickly become depleted if they are not supported by daily administration. Additional oral or enteral supplements may be considered if there is some intestinal absorption. However, copper deficiency can increase iron absorption and zinc intake can decrease copper absorption.

The micronutrients naturally fall into two groups: the trace elements and vitamins.

Trace elements

Trace elements are generally maintained at a relatively constant tissue concentration and are present to a level of less than 1 mg/kg body weight. They are essential; deficiency results in structural and physiological disorders which, if identified early enough, can be resolved by readministration. Ten essential trace elements are known: iron, copper, zinc, fluorine, manganese, iodine, cobalt (or as hydroxycobalamin), selenium, molybdenum and chromium.

Table 7.8 Factors affecting micronutrient requirements

Baseline nutritional state on starting parenteral nutrition
- Acute or chronic onset of illness
- Dietary history
- Duration and severity of inadequate nutritional intake

Increased loss
- Small bowel fistulae/aspirate – rich in zinc
- Biliary fluid loss – rich in copper
- Burn fluid loss – rich in zinc, copper, selenium

Increased requirement
- Increased metabolism – acute in anabolic phase following catabolic phase of critically ill
- Active growth

Organ function
- Liver failure – copper and manganese clearance reduced
- Renal failure – aluminium, chromium, zinc and nickel clearance reduced

Various recommended baseline doses have been published but no single licensed preparation provides all trace elements at the dose required (Table 7.9). Concern over neurotoxicity with accumulated manganese, especially in liver failure, led to a reduction in the advised daily dose and recommendations for plasma monitoring. Recognizing the benefits of zinc and selenium on the free radical scavenging system, some specialists advise an increase in the administered dose. Some patients, notably those with burns, renal replacement therapy and/or multiple trauma, as well as long-term patients, may require extra trace elements.

Vitamins

There are two groups of vitamins: the water-soluble vitamins and the fat-soluble vitamins. Fat-soluble vitamins are stored in the body whereas excess water-soluble vitamins are renally cleared. Therefore, if there is inadequate provision, deficiency states for the water-soluble vitamins reveal themselves first.

Table 7.10 indicates the recommended (FDA 2000) daily requirements of vitamins and the formulation of commercial licensed preparation. No preparation meets the guideline requirements, therefore it is common practice for preparations to be used in combination. For example, daily Cernevit is frequently used in combination with weekly doses of Konakion MM and Solivito N is frequently used with Vitlipid N Adult. Vitamins should be included in the daily parenteral nutrition bag.

Electrolytes

Electrolytes are included to meet the patient's needs. Typical daily parenteral requirements are:

- sodium (1–1.5 mmol/kg)
- potassium (1–1.5 mmol/kg)
- calcium (0.1–0.15 mmol/kg)
- magnesium (0.1–0.2 mmol/kg)
- phosphate (0.5–0.7 mmol/kg).

Depending upon the stability of the patient's clinical state, they are kept relatively constant or adjusted on a near daily basis, reflecting changes in blood biochemistry. Tables (e.g. British National Formulary) can be used to guide electrolyte replacement if there is excessive gastrointestinal waste or high losses through burns. Hypophosphataemia should be corrected before starting parenteral or enteral nutrition to avoid the refeeding syndrome.

To prevent frequent minor adjustments in electrolyte prescriptions, many practitioners define the minimum prescription dose change, for example 15 mmol for potassium in an adult bag.

Table 7.9 Trace element requirements and content of UK licensed products (adapted from data in Okada et al 1995)

	Units	American Medical Association 1979	Shenkin 1995	Fleming 1989	Additrace 1 ampoule	Decan 1 vial
Iron	µmol		17.5–70		20	17.9
	mg		1–4		1.12	1.000
Zinc	µmoL	38–61.5	49–210	38.5–61.5	100	153
	mg	2.5–4	3–14	2.4–4	6.54	10.00
Copper	µmol	9.1–27.3	5–30	5–9.1	20	7.55
	mg	0.5–1.6	0.3–1.8	0.3–0.5	1.27	0.480
Manganese	µmol	2.7–14.5	6–36		5	3.64
	mg	0.15–0.8	0.3–2		0.275	0.200
Fluorine	µmol		49		50	76.3
	mg		0.9		0.95	1.450
Cobalt	µmol					0.025
	mg					1.470
Iodine	µmol		1		1	0.012
	mg		130		126.9	1.520
Selenium	µmol		0.4	0.5–1	0.4	0.887
	mg		0.03	0.04–0.08	0.032	0.070
Molybdenum	µmol		0.2	1–2	0.2	0.261
	mg		0.02	0.1–0.2	0.019	0.025
Chromium	µmol	0.19–0.29	1	0.19–0.38	0.2	0.289
	mg	0.01–0.015	0.05	0.01–0.02	0.01	0.015

Table 7.10 Vitamin requirements and UK licensed products (alphabetical)

	Vitamin	Recommended daily parenteral dose	Cernevit 1 vial	Konakion MM 10 mg/mL	Solivito N 1 vial		Vitlipid N Adult 10 mL
Fat-soluble	A (retinol)	1 mg (3330 IU)	3500 IU	–	–		3300 IU
	D	5 µg	(D3) 220 IU	–	–		(D2) 200 IU
	E (α-tocopherol)	10 mg (15 IU)	11.2 IU	–	–		10 IU
	K₁	150 µg	–	Flexibility from 10 µg/mL presentation	–		150 µg
Water-soluble	B₁ (thiamine)	6.0 mg	3.51 mg	–	2.5 mg		–
	B₂ (riboflavin)	3.6 mg	4.14 mg	–	3.6 mg		–
	B₆ (pyridoxine)	4.0 mg	4.53 mg	–	4.0 mg		–
	B₁₂	5 µg	6 µg	–	5 µg		–
	C	200 mg	125 mg	–	100 mg		–
	Folic acid	600 µg	414 µg	–	400 mg		–
	Pantothenic acid	15 mg	17.25 mg	–	15 mg		–
	Biotin	60 µg	69 µg	–	60 µg		–
	Niacin	40 mg	46 mg	–	40 mg nicotinamide		–

Some crystalloid and amino acid solutions contain electrolytes, whereas others are electrolyte free. Table 7.11 indicates the electrolyte content of a selection of concentrated sources that may be added to PN formulations, assuming stability is confirmed.

Administration of parenteral nutrition

Routes of administration

PN can be administered peripherally or centrally.

Peripheral route

Peripheral administration should be considered the first choice for short-term parenteral feeding. Supported by good techniques, line care and low tonicity feeds, patients can be successfully maintained with this route for many weeks. Peripheral lines are less costly than central lines, they can be inserted by less specialized staff, there is no requirement for a chest X-ray to confirm placement, and line care protocols are simpler. A midline should be considered as a peripheral line as it does not reach the central circulation.

Some indications and contraindications to the use of the peripheral route are summarized in Table 7.12.

Peripheral administration is sometimes complicated or delayed by phlebitis, where an insult to the endothelial vessel wall causes inflammation, redness, pain and possible extravasation. Peripheral tolerance can be influenced by a range of factors (Table 7.13).

Many consider that the tonicity of the infused solution or emulsion is a key factor defining peripheral infusion tolerance. The total number of osmotically active particles in the intracellular and extracellular fluids is essentially the same, approximately 290–310 mOsmol/L. When a lipid emulsion is included, infusions of approximately three times this osmolarity are generally well tolerated via the peripheral route and there are reports of success with higher levels. However, other factors should also be considered. Patient factors, such as vein fragility and blood flow, may mean that some infusion episodes are better tolerated than others. One administration of a high tonicity value may indeed be more successful than another with a lower value.

The osmolarity of a PN formulation can be estimated by applying the following equation:

$$= \frac{\Sigma\,[\text{osmolarity}_n\,(\text{mOsmol/L}) \times \text{volume}_n\,(\text{L})]}{\text{Total volume (L)}}$$

where n indicates the component.

By considering the macronutrients included in the regimen, i.e. the amino acids, glucose and lipid, an estimation of the osmolarity can be made. The value will be increased by electrolyte or micronutrient additions. However, since the peripheral tolerance is affected by so many factors, including tonicity, and because the limit is only an estimate, the effect of these additions is relatively low unless high levels of monovalent ions are included.

Table 7.11 Electrolyte and micronutrient content of additives used in parenteral nutrition compounding

	Content per mL									
	Sodium (mmol)	Potassium (mmol)	Magnesium (mmol)	Calcium (mmol)	Phospate HPO4–(mmol)	Chloride (mmol)	Acetate (mmol)	Iron (μmol)	Selenium (μmol)	Zinc (μmol)
Sodium chloride 10%	1.7	–	–	–	–	1.7	–	–	–	–
Sodium chloride 23.5%	4	–	–	–	–	4	–	–	–	–
Sodium chloride 30%	5.1	–	–	–	–	5.1	–	–	–	–
Sodium acetate 40 mmol/10 mL	4	–	–	–	–	–	4	–	–	–
Sodium glycero–phosphate 21.6%	2	–	–	–	1	–	–	–	–	–
Potassium chloride 15%	–	2	–	–	–	2	–	–	–	–
Potassium acid phosphate 13.6%	–	1	–	–	1	–	–	–	–	–
Calcium chloride 1 mmol/mL	–	–	–	1	–	2	–	–	–	–
Calcium chloride 0.5 mmol/1 mL	–	–	–	0.5	–	1	–	–	–	–
Calcium chloride 13.4%	–	–	–	0.91	–	1.82	–	–	–	–
Calcium gluconate 10%	–	–	–	0.22	–	–	–	–	–	–
Magnesium sulphate 10%	–	–	0.4	–	–	–	–	–	–	–
Magnesium sulphate 50%	–	–	2	–	–	–	–	–	–	–
Addiphos	1.5	1.5	–	–	2	–	–	–	–	–
Glycophos	2	–	–	–	1	–	–	–	–	–
Iron chloride 100 μg/mL	–	–	–	–	–	–	–	1.79	–	–
Iron chloride 300 μg/mL	–	–	–	–	–	–	–	5.37	–	–
Sodium selenite 16 μg/mL	–	–	–	–	–	–	–	–	0.2	–

Central route

The central venous route is indicated when longer term feeding is anticipated, high tonicity formulations are required or the peripheral route is inaccessible. The rapid and turbulent blood flow in the central circulation and the constant movement of the heart ensure rapid mixing and reduce the risk of osmotically induced injury to the endothelium.

A range of single-, double-, triple- and quadruple-lumen central lines are available and one lumen must be dedicated for the nutrition. These lines require skilful insertion, usually into the jugular or subclavian vein, and confirmation of their position by X-ray. This relatively invasive and costly procedure is performed by trained medical staff. Tunnelling of the line to an appropriate exit site facilitates line care and may reduce the incidence of significant line sepsis. The femoral route is not favoured due to a higher incidence of sepsis.

PICCs

Peripherally inserted central catheters (PICCs) are typically inserted into a peripheral vein, usually the cephalic or basilic in the upper arm, with the exit tip in the superior vena cava just above the right atrium. As the name suggests, they are used for the central administration of infusions. Single- and double-lumen

Table 7.12   Indications and contraindications to the use of peripheral parenteral nutrition

Indications

- Duration of feed likely to be short term
- Supplemental feeding
- Compromised access to central circulation, e.g. local trauma, surgery or thrombosis
- No immediate facilities or trained staff to insert central catheter
- High risk of fungal or bacterial sepsis, e.g. patients with purulent tracheostomy secretions, immune deficiency state, history of repeated sepsis
- Contraindication to central venous catheterization

Contraindications

- Inadequate or inaccessible peripheral veins
- High calorie/nitrogen requirements alongside fluid restrictions (admixture osmolarity too high)

Table 7.13   Factors that improve tolerance to peripheral lines

- Aseptic insertion and line care
- Selection of large vessel with good blood flow and direct path, e.g. cephalic vein
- Fine-bore catheter (22 G) for minimal trauma on insertion and disturbance of blood flow
- Fine polyurethane catheter
- Secure catheter to minimize physical trauma
- Glyceryl trinitrate patch distal to insertion site, over tip to vasodilate vein
- Regular replacement of catheter, using alternate arms (12 hourly)
- Flushing of lines not in use
- Low-tonicity infusions
- Inclusion of lipid emulsion; venoprotective and isotonic with blood
- Inclusion of heparin and/or hydrocortisone where stability confirmed

versions are available. Some also have a one-way valve to prevent backflow. Insertion is less invasive than for conventional central lines and can be undertaken by trained nurse practitioners.

Infusion control

Pumps

PN must always be administered under the control of an infusion pump. Acute overload of fluid, nutrition and electrolytes can have morbid consequences.

Infusion pumps should be used with an appropriate infusion or giving set which is compatible with both the infusion pump and the PN admixture. For home patients, small, simple battery-powered ambulatory pumps are favoured.

Temperature

PN should be at room temperature when it is infused. It must, therefore, be removed from the refrigerator in which it is stored approximately 3 hours before connection and left to warm naturally to room temperature (for a $2\frac{1}{2}$ litre regimen). No external heat should be applied, although intermittent inversion of the bag may help.

If a cold admixture is infused, the patient may experience infusion discomfort, and the acute release of gas from where it was dissolved in the admixture may cause the pump to alarm 'air in line'.

Compounded formulations

Historically, PN was administered from a series of separate bottles. Healthcare staff had to accurately and safely manage a combination of giving sets, infusion rates and total infusion times. Most patients now receive their complete nutrition from a single daily bag of a pharmaceutically stable PN formulation. The advantages of such a system far outweigh the disadvantages, as indicated in Table 7.14.

Various terms are used to describe the PN formulation, depending on whether lipid is included. If it contains lipid, it is called a 3-in-1, ternary or all-in-one admixture. If no lipid is present, the terms 2-in-1, binary or aqueous admixture are used.

Standardized formulations

It is estimated that up to 80% of adult patient needs can be met with standard PN formulations.

Table 7.14   Advantages and disadvantages of compounded PN formulations compared to bottle systems

Advantages

- Convenience and time saving for care staff and patient; single bag, single pump and rate, single line
- Simultaneous infusion of all nutrients, permitting optimal utilization
- Reduced infection risk; fewer connections and disconnections at ward level
- Reduced risk of error; pharmacy compounding in controlled environment with controlled procedures, single infusion managed at ward level
- Home management possible
- Storage and stock management of single item, rather than multiple nutrition sources
- Reduced scope for incompatible formulations to be compounded

Disadvantages

- Physical and chemical stability needs to be known for both the storage and infusion time (separate bottle system offers an informed practitioner the scope to infuse incompatible parts separately, in contact for a shorter time)
- Potential time delay in compounding to unique specification
- Potential wastage of original admixture if patient's needs change
- Fridge storage required

Depending on the type (size and specialty) of the hospital, a range of standard formulations are maintained and supported with prescribing guidelines. These may be compounded from scratch, compounded from 'base-bags' locally or by a licensed unit, or purchased as licensed ready-to-use presentations.

The range is specifically selected to meet the needs of the patients managed by the hospital and will typically include a low-tonicity regimen suitable for peripheral administration, a higher calorie and nitrogen regimen for central administration to catabolic patients and a high-tonicity regimen for fluid-restricted patients. Baseline electrolytes will generally be included although the flexibility for reduced levels is usually offered.

Licensed ready-to-use products

A range of licensed ready-to-use preparations is available. For convenience, baseline electrolyte levels are included in many formulations and meet the needs of most patients. Electrolyte-free options are becoming more readily available. Some are licensed in paediatrics and/or for peripheral use. Manufacturers advise on stability and shelf-life for electrolyte and micronutrient additions. The range of ready-to-use products includes:

- triple chamber bags (OliClinomel, Compleven, Kabiven, StructoKabiven and Nutriflex Lipid ranges): chambers separately pre-filled with lipid, amino acid and glucose and terminally sterilized. Activated by applying external pressure so weak seal peels open, mixing the contents to a 3-in-1 formulation
- dual chamber bags (Clinimix and Nutriflex ranges): chambers separately pre-filled with amino acid and glucose and terminally sterilized. Activated to a 2-in-1 formulation. Flexibility to omit or add a compatible lipid
- two-bottle system (Vitrimix-KV): transfer set and vacuum used to transfer lipid emulsion into the amino acid and glucose mix.

Cyclic infusions

Cyclic PN is when the daily requirements are administered over a short period. A classic example is the stable home patient who administers their feed overnight, freeing themselves from the constraints of an infusion during the day. This enables them to have more physical freedom and improves their quality of life.

Since cyclic feeding more closely simulates the human feeding pattern and is a closer match to normal hormonal and metabolic cycles, it also offers a range of metabolic and clinical advantages. Steatosis, fatty infiltration of the liver, is less common and may be corrected by employing cyclic feeding because the feed-free period facilitates lipolysis and fat mobilization. Peripheral tolerance may be improved as the endothelia recover between infusion periods.

Initially, the patient should receive the PN infusion slowly over the full 24 hours. As tolerated, the rate of infusion can be increased slowly to decrease the infusion time. This should be done over a series of days. During this period, the patient must be monitored closely for any signs of fluid, electrolyte or acid–base imbalance and hyper/hypoglycaemia. For example,

on stopping the infusion, rebound hypoglycaemia may occur. The patient should also be monitored for the recognized potential adverse events of lipid and amino acid infusions such as nausea, vomiting, sweating and flushing which occur more frequently when infused at faster rates.

Pharmaceutical issues

Having identified the balance of nutrients required for a patient in a single day, it is necessary to formulate a physically and chemically stable sterile admixture.

PN admixtures contain over 50 chemical entities and, as such, are extremely complex. Professional advice or reference material should be used before compounding and administering PN. Manufacturers and third party experts can advise on stability issues

Physical stability

Physical instability takes a number of forms including precipitation of solids and cracking of the lipid emulsion.

Precipitation

Precipitation carries two key risks. First, the potential to infuse solid particles to the narrow pulmonary capillaries may result in fatal emboli. Second, the prescribed nutrients may not be infused.

Clinically dangerous precipitates may not always be visible to the naked eye, especially if lipid emulsion is present. They may also develop over time, and an apparently 'safe' admixture may develop a fatal precipitate in use.

Precipitation of solid is epitomized by the formation of calcium phosphate. This is of special concern in neonatal admixtures where the requirements to prevent hypophosphataemic rickets and severe osteopenia may exceed the safe concentrations. Such concentrations are rarely seen in adult regimens.

It is known that calcium and phosphate can form a number of different salt forms with different solubility profiles, for example $Ca(H_2PO_4)_2$ which is highly soluble in comparison to $CaHPO_4$ and $Ca_3(PO_4)_2$. $Ca_3(PO_4)_2$ precipitation is relatively immediate, and has a white, fluffy amorphous appearance. However, $CaHPO_4.2H_2O$ precipitation is time mediated and has a more crystalline appearance.

Factors affecting calcium phosphate precipitation are shown in Table 7.15. Practical measures can be taken to minimize the risks; these include accurate calculation of the proposed formulation, comparison against professionally defined comprehensive matrices and thorough mixing. Solubility curves and algorithms should be used with extreme caution, even if they are quoted for a specific amino acid source. This is because they do not consider all the factors and do not consistently identify risk. Assuming the sodium content can be tolerated, use of an organic phosphate salt form may be beneficial.

Trace elements have also been associated with clinically significant precipitation. These include iron phosphate and copper sulphide (hydrogen sulphide from the minor degradation of cysteine/cystine).

Table 7.15 Factors affecting calcium phosphate precipitation

	Mechanism and effect
pH	Low pH supports solubility, whereas a higher pH supports precipitation. Depending on the amount and buffering capacity of the amino acids, this can be affected by different concentrations and sources of glucose solution and acetate salt forms
Temperature	Higher temperatures associated with greater precipitation – increased availability of free calcium to interact and a shift to the more insoluble salt forms
Amino acids	Buffer pH changes Complex with calcium so less available to react with phosphate Both the source of amino acid and the relative content are important
Magnesium	Complex with phosphate forming soluble salts rather than less soluble calcium salts
Calcium salt form	Calcium chloride dissociates more readily than calcium gluconate, releasing it to react with the phosphate
Phosphate salt form	Monobasic salts, e.g. dipotassium phosphate, dissociate more readily than dibasic salts, e.g. potassium acid phosphate, releasing phosphate to react with the calcium Organic salts, such as sodium glycerophosphate and glucose-1-phosphate, are more stable
Mixing order	Optimum stability achieved by only permitting calcium and phosphate to come together in a large volume admixture Agitate between additions to avoid pockets of concentration

Lipid destabilization

The oil-in-water lipid emulsions are sensitive to destabilization by a range of factors including the presence of positively charged ions and heat. The lipid globules may come together and coalesce to form larger globules and release free oil. This could occlude the lung microvasculature and cause respiratory and circulatory compromise and lead to death.

Positively charged ions destabilize the admixture by drawing the negatively charged lipid globules together, overwhelming the electromechanical repulsion of the charged phospholipids and increasing their tendency to join or coalesce. The divalent and trivalent ions have a more significant effect. Therefore, there are tightly defined limits for the amount of Ca^{2+} and Mg^{2+} that can be added to a 3-in-1 admixture. Although the limits for the other

polyvalent ions (such as zinc and selenium) are also controlled, because they are given in micromolar or nanomolar quantities they are less of a problem.

Low concentrations of amino acids and glucose also reduce the stability of the emulsion and increase the tendency for creaming.

The naked eye can identify large-scale destabilization, as shown in Table 7.16. However, the limitations of this method need to be recognized; clinically significant destabilization might not be visible to the naked eye. In practice, stability laboratories apply specific technical equipment and defined criteria to establish the physical stability of a formulation. These include assessing changes in lipid globule size distribution with the optical microscope and particle size counters applying defined limits of pharmaceutical acceptance. A wide safety margin is applied.

Table 7.16 Lipid instability

	Description	Visual observation
Stable, normal emulsion	Lipid globules equally dispersed Suitable for administration	Normal emulsion
Light creaming	Lipid globules rising to the top of the bag. Slight layering visible. Readily redisperses on inverting the bag. Suitable for administration	Light creaming
Heavy creaming, flocculation	Lipid globules coming together but not joining. Rising to the top of the bag. More obvious layering visible. Readily redisperses on inverting the bag. Acceptable for administration	Heavy creaming
Coalescence	Lipid globules come together, coalesce to form larger globules and rise to the surface. Larger globules join, releasing free oil. Irreversible destabilization of the lipid emulsion. Not suitable for administration	Cracked Oil layer viewed close up

Chemical stability

Chemical stability takes many forms, notably chemical degradation of the vitamins and amino acids.

Vitamin stability

Many vitamins readily undergo chemical degradation, and vitamin stability often defines the shelf-life of the formulation.

Vitamin C (ascorbic acid), the least stable, is generally regarded as the marker for vitamin degradation. Vitamin C oxidation is accelerated by heat, oxygen and certain trace elements, including copper. Other examples include vitamin A photolysis and vitamin E photo-oxidation. Measures that minimize oxygen presence, such as minimal aeration during compounding, evacuation of air at the end of compounding and use of oxygen barrier bags, and light protection are recommended.

Amino acid stability

The amino acid profile should be maintained for the shelf-life of the formulation and manufacturers perform assays to confirm this prior to issuing stability reports.

Maillard reaction

The Maillard reaction is a complex pathway of chemical reactions that starts with a condensation of the carbonyl group of the glucose and the amino group of the amino acid. At present, relatively little is known about the clinical effects of these Maillard reaction products; however, it is prudent to minimize their presence by protecting from light and avoiding high temperatures.

Microbial stability

PN is a highly nutritious medium although hypertonicity will partially limit microbial growth potential. Growth in lipid alone is greater.

Pharmaceutical developments have enabled terminal sterilization of many of the components, including the multichamber bag presentations. Manipulations should only be performed using validated aseptic techniques. Nurses, patients and carers must be trained to apply aseptic methods when connecting and disconnecting infusions. Many centres have documented line care and PN protocols.

Shelf-life and temperature control

The manufacturer may be able to provide physical and chemical stability data to support a formulation for a shelf-life of up to 90 days at 2–8°C followed by 24 hours at room temperature for infusion. This assumes that a strict aseptic technique is used during compounding. Units holding a manufacturing licence covering aseptic compounding of PN are able to assign this full shelf-life. Unlicensed units are limited to a maximum shelf-life of 7 days.

PN must be stored and transported within the defined temperature limits. A validated cold-chain must be employed. The formulations must not freeze. Pharmaceutical-grade fridges should be used and monitored to ensure appropriate air cycling and temperature maintenance. The temperature during the infusion period should be known; neonatal units and incubators are classically maintained at higher temperatures, and formulations used must have been validated at these temperatures.

Drug stability

The addition of drugs to PN admixtures, or Y-site co-administration, is actively discouraged unless the compatibility has been formally confirmed. Wherever possible, the nutrition should be administered through a dedicated line. Multilumen catheters can be used to infuse PN separately from other infusion(s).

However, extreme competition for i.v. access may prompt consideration of drug and PN combinations. Many factors need to be considered: the physical and chemical stability of the PN, the physical and chemical stability of the drug, the bioavailability of the drug and the effect of stopping and starting Y-site infusions on the actual administration rates. It is not possible to reliably extrapolate data from a specific PN composition, between brands of solutions and salt forms or between brands or doses of drugs. A range of studies has been performed and published; however, these should be used with caution.

In practice, drugs should only be infused with PN when all other possibilities have been exhausted. These may include gaining further i.v. access and changing the drug(s) to clinically acceptable non-i.v. alternatives.

The relative risks of stopping and starting the PN infusion and repeatedly breaking the infusion circuit should be fully considered before sharing a line for separate infusions of PN and drug. In most cases, the risks outweigh the benefits. However, if this option is adopted, the line must be flushed before and after with an appropriate volume of solution known to be stable with both the PN and the drug. Strict aseptic technique should be adopted to minimize the risk of contaminating the line and infusions.

Filtration

All intravenous fluids pass through the delicate lung microvasculature with its capillary diameter of 8–12 μm. The presence of particulate matter has been demonstrated to cause direct embolization, direct damage to the endothelia, formation of granulomata and formation of foreign body giant cells, and to have a thrombogenic effect. In addition, the presence of microbial and fungal matter can cause a serious infection or inflammatory response.

Precautions taken to minimize the particulate load of the compounded regimen must include:

- use of in-line filters (25 μm) and filter needles or straws (5 μm) during compounding to catch larger particles such as cored rubber from bottles and glass shards from ampoules
- air particle levels kept within defined limits in aseptic rooms by the use of air filters and non-shedding clothing and wipes
- use of quality raw materials with minimal particulate presence, including empty bags and leads

- confirmation of physical and chemical stability of the formulation prior to aseptic compounding applying approved mixing order (stability for the required shelf-life time and conditions).

There is ongoing debate as to whether in-line filters should be used routinely during PN infusion. Guidelines have been published that endorse their use, especially for patients requiring intensive or prolonged parenteral therapy, including home patients, the immunocompromised, neonates and children (Bethune et al 2001). The filter should be placed as close to the patient as possible and validated for the PN to be used. For 2-in-1 formulations, 0.2 µm filters may be used. For 3-in-1 formulations, validated 1.2 µm filters may be used.

Light protection

It is widely recognized that exposure to light, notably phototherapy light and intense sunlight, may increase the degradation rate of certain constituents such as vitamins A and E. It is recommended that all regimens should be protected from light both during storage and during infusion, since:

- lipid does not totally protect against vitamin photodegradation
- the Maillard reaction is influenced by light exposure
- ongoing research suggests lipid peroxidation is accelerated by a range of factors, including exposure to certain wavelengths of light and in order to minimize confusion.

Validated bag covers should always be used.

Nutritional assessment and monitoring

Initial assessment

Once screening has identified that a patient is in need of nutritional intervention, a more detailed assessment is performed. This will include an evaluation of nutritional requirements, the expected course of the underlying disease, consideration of the enteral route and, where appropriate, identification of access routes for parenteral nutrition. This will be supported by a clinical assessment that will include:

- clinical history
- dietary history
- physical examination
- anthropometry including muscle function tests
- biochemical, haematological and immunological review.

Monitoring

PN monitoring has a number of objectives. It should:

- evaluate ongoing nutritional requirements, including fluid and electrolytes
- determine the effectiveness of the nutritional intervention
- facilitate early recognition of complications
- identify any deficiency, overload or toxicity to individual nutrients
- determine discrepancies between prescribed, delivered and received dose.

Regular monitoring contributes to the success of the PN and a monitoring protocol should be in place for each individual patient. Baseline data should be recorded so deviations can be recognized and interpreted. In the early stages, while the patient is in the acute stage of their illness and the nutritional requirements are being established, the frequency of monitoring will be greatest. Some tests may be defined by the underlying disease state, rather than by the presence of PN per se. As the patient's status stabilizes, the frequency of monitoring will reduce although the range of parameters monitored is likely to increase. Examples of parameters monitored include the following.

- *Clinical symptoms or presentation.* May be specific, e.g. thrombophlebitis, or non-specific, e.g. confusion.
- *Temperature, blood pressure and pulse.* Vigilance for the risk of sepsis.
- *Fluid balance and weight.* Acute weight changes reflect fluid gain or loss and prompt review of the volume of the PN. Slow, progressive changes more likely to reflect nutritional status.
- *Nitrogen balance.* An assessment of urine urea and insensible loss and their relation to nitrogen input. Difficult to obtain accurate figures.
- *Visceral proteins.* While albumin levels may indicate malnutrition, the long half-life limits its sensitivity to detect acute changes in nutritional status. Other markers with a shorter half-life may be more useful, e.g. transferrin.
- *Haematology.* For example, platelet counts and clotting studies for thrombocytopenia.
- *C-reactive protein.* Trends to monitor the inflammatory process.
- *Blood glucose.* Hyperglycaemia is a relatively frequent complication that prompts reduction in the infused dose. Insulin is not routinely recommended. May indicate sepsis. Hypoglycaemia may be rebound to a reduction in the input.
- *Lipid tolerance.* Turbidity, cholesterol and triglyceride profiles required.
- *Electrolyte profile.* Indicates appropriate provision or other complicating clinical activity. In the first few days, low potassium, magnesium and/or phosphate with or without clinical symptoms may reflect the refeeding syndrome (see below).
- *Liver function tests.* An abnormal liver profile may be observed and it is often difficult to identify a single cause. PN and other factors such as sepsis, drug therapy and underlying disease may all interplay. In adults, PN-induced abnormalities tend to be mild, reversible and self-limiting. In the early stages, fatty liver (steatosis) is seen. In longer-term patients, a cholestatic picture tends to present.
- *Anthropometry.* Assesses longer-term status.
- *Acid–base profile.* Indicative of respiratory or metabolic compromise and may require review of PN formulation.
- *Vitamin and trace element screen.* A range of single compounds or markers to consider tolerance and identify deficiencies, although of limited value as some tests are non-specific and inaccurate.
- *Catheter entry site.* Vigilance for phlebitis, erythema, extravasation, infection, misplacement.

Complications

Complications of PN fall into two main categories: catheter related and metabolic (Table 7.17). Overall, the incidence of such complications has reduced because of increased knowledge and skills together with more successful management (Maroulis & Kalfarentoz 2000).

Line sepsis

This is a serious and potentially life-threateening condition. Monitoring protocols should ensure that signs of infection are identified early and a local decision pathway should be in place to guide efficient diagnosis and management. Management will depend upon the type of line and the source of infection. Alternative sources of sepsis should be considered. Initially, the PN is usually stopped.

Line blockage

Line occlusion may be caused by a number of factors, including:

- fibrin sheath forming around the line, or a thrombosis blocking the tip
- internal blockage of lipid, blood clot or salt and drug precipitates
- line kinking
- particulate blockage of a protective line filter.

Management will depend on the cause of the occlusion. In general, the aim is to save the line and resume feeding with minimum risk for the patient. The use of locks and flushes with urokinase (for fibrin and thrombosis), ethanol (for lipid deposits) and dilute hydrochloric acid (for salt and drug precipitates) may be considered. In some cases, the lines may need to be replaced.

Refeeding syndrome

This metabolic complication occurs when the infused nutrition exceeds the tolerance of a previously malnourished patient. High glucose infusions result in hyperinsulinaemia and an anabolic effect with the intracellular shift of magnesium, potassium and phosphate. Acute hypophosphataemia, hypokalaemia and hypomagnesaemia may present with cardiac, haematological and neurological dysfunction; death has been reported.

Some centres selectively increase to the full nutritional regimen over 2 days to avoid this acute refeeding syndrome. Thiamine affords some protection and may be administered before the nutrition is started and over the first few days of infusion.

Specific disease states

Liver

Due to the complexity of liver function, the range of potential disorders and its role in metabolism, the use of PN in liver disease is not without problems. The European Society for Clinical Nutrition and Metabolism (ESPEN) has published consensus guidelines for the use of PN in liver disease (Plauth et al 1997). Nutritional intervention may be essential for recovery, although care must be exercised with amino acid input and the risk of encephalopathy, calorie input and metabolic capacity, and the reduced clearance of trace elements such as copper and manganese (Maroulis & Kalfarentoz 2000). Low-sodium, low-volume feeds are indicated if there is ascites. Cyclic feeding appears useful, especially in steatosis. Lipid-soluble vitamins plus zinc and selenium should be considered.

Renal

Fluid and electrolyte balance demand close attention. A low-volume and poor-quality urine output may necessitate a concentrated PN formulation with a reduction in electrolyte content, particularly potassium and phosphate. In the polyuric phase or the nephrotic syndrome, a higher volume formulation may be required. If there is fluid retention, ideal body weight should be used for calculating requirements rather than the actual body weight.

The metabolic stress of acute renal failure and the malnutrition of chronic renal failure may initially demand relatively high nutritional requirements. However, nitrogen restriction may be necessary to control uraemia in the absence of dialysis or filtration and avoid uraemia-related impaired glucose tolerance, because of peripheral insulin resistance, and lipid clearance.

Micronutrient requirements may also change in renal disease. For example, renal clearance of zinc, selenium, fluoride and chromium is reduced and there is less renal 1α-hydroxylation of vitamin D.

Table 7.17   Examples of complications during parenteral nutrition

Catheter related
- Thrombophlebitis (peripheral)
- Catheter-related infection, local or systemic
- Venous thrombosis
- Line occlusion (lipid, thrombus, particulate)
- Pneumothorax, catheter malposition, vessel laceration, embolism, hydrothorax, dysrhythmias, incorrect placement (central)

Metabolic
- Hyperglycaemia or hypoglycaemia
- Electrolyte imbalance
- Lipid intolerance
- Refeeding syndrome
- Dehydration or overhydration
- Specific nutritional deficiency or overload
- Liver disease or biliary disease
- Gastrointestinal atrophy
- Metabolic bone dysfunction (in long term)
- Thrombocytopenia
- Adverse events with PN components
- Essential fatty acid deficiency

Lipid emulsions can usually be administered at the same time as dialysis and filtration procedures. Chronic renal failure patients are predisposed to malnutrition and an enteral diet may be supplemented with intradialytic parenteral nutrition (IDPN) during the dialysis session (Foulks 1999).

A working group has published guidance on nutritional management in renal insufficiency (Toigo et al 2000).

Pancreatitis

Acute pancreatitis is a metabolic stress that requires high-level nutritional support and pancreatic rest to recover. ESPEN has published guidelines for nutrition in acute pancreatitis (Meiier et al 2002).

While enteral nutrition stimulates the pancreas, parenteral amino acids and glucose do not appear to. There is some concern that parenteral lipids may induce or exacerbate pancreatitis. However, so long as there is no familial hyperlipidaemia and the pancreatitis is not secondary to a lipid disorder, lipid can generally be beneficially administered. A test dose and gradual increase from 100 mL of lipid 20% may be considered. Lipid clearance and the clinical state of the pancreas should be monitored.

Hyperglycaemia may occur and require exogenous insulin.

Sepsis and injury

Significant fluctuations in macronutrient metabolism are seen during sepsis and injury. There are two metabolic phases: the 'ebb' phase of 24–48 hours and the following 'flow' phase. The initial hyperglycaemia, reflecting a reduced utilization of glucose, is followed by a longer catabolic state with increased utilization of lipid and amino acids. The effect of the different lipid emulsions on immune function is the subject of much research. It is important not to overfeed and also to consider the reduced glucose tolerance during the critical days. This is due to increased insulin resistance and incomplete glucose oxidation. Exogenous insulin may be required.

Respiratory

While underfeeding and malnutrition can compromise respiratory effort and muscle function, overfeeding can equally compromise respiratory function due to increased carbon dioxide and lipid effects on the circulation. While chronic respiratory disease may be linked with a long-standing malnutrition, the patient with acute disease will generally be hypermetabolic.

Cardiac

Cardiac failure and multiple drug therapy may limit the volume of PN that can be infused. Concentrated formulations are used and, as a consequence of the high tonicity, administered via the central route.

Close electrolyte monitoring and adjustment is required. Cardiac drugs may affect electrolyte clearance.

Although central lines may already be in use for other drugs or cardiac monitoring, it is essential to maintain a dedicated lumen or line for the feed.

Diabetes mellitus

Diabetic patients can generally be maintained with standard dual-energy regimens. It is important to use insulin to manage blood glucose rather than reduce the nutritional provision of the feed.

Close glucose monitoring will guide exogenous insulin administration. This should be given as a separate infusion (sliding scale) or, if the patient is stable, in bolus doses. Insulin should not be included within the PN formulation due to stability problems and variable adsorption to the equipment. Y-site infusion with the PN should be avoided as changes in insulin rates will be delayed and changes in feed rates will result in significant fluctuations in insulin administration. Extra potassium and phosphate may be required due to the impact of the glucose and insulin.

Cancer and palliative care

Nutritional support in cancer and palliative care is guided by the potential risks and benefits of the intervention, alongside the wishes of the patient and their carers. Further research is required to evaluate the effects of PN on length and quality of life.

Standard PN may be useful during prolonged periods of gastrointestinal toxicity, as in bone marrow transplant patients. The use of PN is not thought to stimulate tumour growth (Nitenberg & Raynard 2000).

Short bowel syndrome

The small intestine is defined as 'short' if it is less than 200 cm. Treatment options depend upon which part of the gut has been removed and the functional state of the remaining organ. The surface area for absorption of nutrition and reabsorption of fluid and electrolytes is significantly compromised. Fluid and electrolyte balance needs to be managed closely due to the high-volume losses. High-volume PN formulations with raised electrolyte content (notably sodium and magnesium) may be required. Vitamin and trace element provision is very important.

Long-term parenteral nutrition

Home care is well established in the UK, with some patients successfully supported for over 20 years. Total or supplemental PN may be appropriate. Trace elements, notably selenium, should be managed closely as requirements may be increased.

Most patients are extremely well informed about their underlying disease and their PN; many also benefit from the PINNT (Patients on Intravenous and Nasogastric Nutrition Therapy) and LITRE (Looking Into The Requirements for Equipment) support groups.

Paediatric parenteral nutrition

Nutritional requirements

Early nutritional intervention is required in paediatric patients due to their low reserve, especially in neonates. Where possible, premature neonates should commence feeding from day 1. In addition to requirements for the maintenance of body tissue, function and repair, it is also important to support growth, especially in the infant and adolescent.

Typical guidelines for average daily requirements of fluid, energy and nitrogen are shown in Table 7.18. The dual-energy approach is favoured in paediatrics. Approximately 30% of the non-protein calories are provided as lipid using a 20% emulsion. Most centres gradually increase the lipid provision from day 1 from 1 g/kg/day to 2 g/kg/day and then 3 g/kg/day, monitoring lipid clearance through the serum triglyceride level. This ensures the essential fatty acid requirements of premature neonates are met.

Formulation and stability issues

Many centres use standard PN formulations including the specific paediatric amino acid solutions (Primene or Vaminolact). Prescriptions and formulations are tailored to reflect clinical status, biochemistry and nutritional requirements.

Micronutrients are included daily. Paediatric licensed preparations are available and are included on a mL/kg basis up to a maximum total volume (Peditrace, Solivito N and Vitlipid N Infant). Electrolytes are also monitored and included in all formulations on a mmol/kg basis. Acid–base balance should be considered. Potassium and sodium acetate salt forms are used in balance with the chloride salt forms in neonatal formulae. This is to avoid excessive chloride input contributing to acidosis. Acetate is metabolized to bicarbonate, an alkali. In the initial stages, neonates tend to hypernatraemia due to relatively poor renal clearance. This should be reflected in the standard formulae used.

Due to the balance of nutritional requirements, a relatively high glucose requirement with high calcium and phosphate provision, the neonatal and paediatric prescription may be supplied by a separate 2-in-1 bag of amino acids, glucose, trace elements and electrolytes and a lipid syringe with vitamins. These are generally given concurrently, joining at a Y-site. Older children can sometimes be managed with 3-in-1 formulations. A single infusion is particularly useful in the home care environment. Some ready-to-use formulations are licensed for use in paediatrics and include Kabiven Peripheral and the OliClinomel range.

Improved stability profiles with the new lipid emulsions, and increasing stability data, may support 3-in-1 formulations that meet the nutritional requirements of younger children.

Concerns over the contamination of calcium gluconate with aluminium, and the association between aluminium contamination of neonatal PN and impaired neurological development have favoured the use of calcium chloride over gluconate.

Heparin

Historically, low concentrations of heparin were included in 2-in-1 formulations in an attempt to improve fat clearance through enhanced triglyceride hydrolysis, prevent the formation of fibrin around the infusion line, reduce thrombosis and reduce thrombophlebitis during peripheral infusion. However, this is no longer recommended. It is recognized that when the 2-in-1 formulation comes into contact with the lipid phase, calcium–heparin bridges form between these lipid globules, destabilizing the formulation. Also, there is limited evidence of clinical benefit of the heparin inclusion.

Route of administration

Peripheral administration is less common in neonates and children due to the risk of thrombophlebitis. However, it is useful when low-concentration, short-term PN is required and there is good peripheral access. The maximum glucose concentration for peripheral administration in paediatrics is generally regarded to be 12%. However, considering all the other factors that can affect the tonicity of a regimen and peripheral tolerance, it is clear that this is a relatively simplistic perspective. Many centres favour a limit of 10% with close clinical observation.

Central administration is via long line (peripheral long line or peripherally inserted central catheters), Broviac or Hickman catheter. There is limited experience with the Port-a-Cath devices in paediatric PN.

The Cochrane Collaboration has compared percutaneous central venous catheters with peripheral cannulae for neonates but the results were inconclusive (Ainsworth et al 2005).

Prepared with Rebecca White, Lead Pharmacist – Nutrition and Surgery, John Radcliffe Hospital, Oxford.

Table 7.18 Typical average daily parenteral nutrition requirements

Age (years)	Fluid (mL/kg/day)	Energy (kcal/kg/day)	Nitrogen (g/kg/day)
Preterm	200–150	130–150	0.5–0.65
0–1	150–110	130–110	0.34–0.46
1–6	100–80	100–70	0.22–0.38
6–12	80–75	70–50	0.2–0.33
12–18	75–50	50–40	0.16–0.2

CASE STUDY

Case 7.1

Mrs B, aged 47, was admitted for investigation of chronic diarrhoea and 6 kg weight loss in 2 months.

Questions

1. Why were the calories provided in the initial bags less than Mrs B's requirements?
2. Why should potassium, magnesium and phosphate levels be monitored closely?
3. Why was no extra magnesium given in the PN on day 5?
4. How much nutrition can be provided to promote weight gain and how could this be provided?

Day	Clinical observation/event	PN changes
1	Admitted to gastroenterology ward from clinic for investigation of chronic diarrhoea and weight loss. Weight 49 kg, height 1.65 m, BMI 18 kg/m^2, BMR 1250 kcal approx, EER 1500 kcal	
2	Contrast study revealed intestinal fistula between small bowel and transverse colon. Diarrhoea approx 1.5 L/day	
3	Case discussed with surgeons. For parenteral nutrition for 2–3 weeks prior to surgery to improve nutritional status. Patient made 'nil by mouth'. Peripherally inserted central catheter (PICC) inserted for PN use only	PN prescribed (considering both fluid and electrolytes from other therapies, and potassium loss from diarrhoea of approx 30–70 mmol/L): Volume 2 L Nitrogen 4.5 g Carbohydrate 400 kcal Lipid 550 kcal Na$^+$ 100 mmol, K$^+$ 80 mmol, Ca^{2+} 5 mmol, Mg^{2+} 15 mmol, phosphate 40 mmol
4	Biochemistry results: Na$^+$ 142, K$^+$ 3.2, Ur 1.3, Cr 86, Corr Ca^{2+} 2.3, Mg^{2+} 0.75, phosphate 0.85 TPR (temperature/pulse/respiration) normal, diarrhoea losses reduced to 800 mL/day	Regimen unchanged
5	Biochemistry results: Na$^+$ 140, K$^+$ 3.1, Ur 1.4, Cr 85, Corr Ca^{2+} 2.2, Mg^{2+} 0.35, phosphate 0.60	Regimen unchanged. Additional 20 mmol magnesium prescribed in 500 mL of saline infused over 6 hours
6	Biochemistry results: Na$^+$ 138, K$^+$ 3.4, Ur 1.6, Cr 86, Corr Ca 2.2, Mg^{2+} 0.78, phosphate 0.9 Diarrhoea reduced to 500 mL/day	PN regimen changed to: Volume 2 L Nitrogen 9 g Carbohydrate 800 kcal Lipid 800 kcal Na$^+$ 100 mmol, K$^+$ 80 mmol, Ca^{2+} 5 mmol, Mg 15 mmol, phosphate 40 mmol
7	Biochemistry results: Na$^+$ 139, K$^+$ 4.1, Ur 1.8, Cr 78, Mg^{2+} 0.95, phosphate 1.3	Potassium reduced to 60 mmol Magnesium reduced to 10 mmol Phosphate reduced to 30 mmol

Answers

1. Mrs B's significant weight loss and likely malabsorption place her at risk of refeeding syndrome. To avoid a hyperinsulinaemic response to her parenteral nutrition, the quantity of glucose is kept low for the first few days until the risk of refeeding syndrome has passed. An initial maximum rate of 10–20 kcal/kg is recommended. In practice this is often achieved by administering half the patient's nutritional requirements over 24 hours; however, the provision of adequate quantities of magnesium, potassium and phosphate can be problematic unless a 2 litre bag is used. It is also essential that sufficient micronutrients are provided, especially thiamine, to ensure effective metabolism of the macronutrients provided.

2. Potassium, magnesium and phosphate are all driven intracellularly during the refeeding response to glucose infusion.

3. Extra magnesium could not be added to the regimen on day 5 due to the stability limits for the regimen prescribed. The lipid content of the regimen places tight limits on the divalent ion content. This can be overcome by using lipid-free regimens but this must be considered in the context of the patient's long-term nutritional plan.

4. Mrs B's predicted basic metabolic rate is only 1250 kcal. Allowing for activity, energy expenditure can be expected to increase to 1500 kcal. The provision of additional calories to promote weight gain is only appropriate if the patient is in an anabolic state and able to utilize the additional energy and nitrogen effectively to gain functional tissue. Excessive calorie intake in the face of ongoing catabolism is most likely to increase metabolic stress and increase the risk of complications such as abnormal LFTs. An additional 400–1000 kcal per day is considered sufficient to promote weight gain. The increased calories can be provided within a 3-in-1 regimen but care should be taken not to exceed the predicted glucose oxidation rate or lipid intake of 1.5 g/kg/day.

REFERENCES

Ainsworth S B, Clerihew L, McGuire W 2005 Percutaneous central venous catheters versus peripheral cannulae for delivery of parenteral nutrition in neonates. The Cochrane Database of Systematic Reviews, Issue 4, Oxford

American Medical Association 1979 Guidelines for essential trace element preparations for parenteral use. Journal of the American Medical Association 241: 2051

Bethune K, Allwood M, Grainger C et al 2001 Use of filters during the preparation and administration of parenteral nutrition: position paper and guidelines prepared by a British Pharmaceutical Nutrition Group Working Party. Nutrition 17: 403-408

British Association of Parenteral and Enteral Nutrition 2003 Malnutrition Universal Screening Tool. Available online at: www.bapen.org.uk/the-must.htm

Crook M A 2000 Lipid clearance and total parenteral nutrition: the importance of monitoring of plasma lipids. Nutrition 16: 774-775

Fleming C R 1989 Trace element metabolism in adult patients requiring total parenteral nutrition. American Journal of Clinical Nutrition 49: 573

Food and Drug Administration 2000 Parenteral multivitamin products. Reference DESI 2847. Federal Register 65: 21200-21201

Foulks C J 1999 An evidence-based evaluation of intradialytic parenteral nutrition. American Journal of Kidney Disease 33: 186-192

Göbel Y, Koletzko B, Bohles H J et al 2003 Parenteral fat emulsions based on olive and soybean oils: a randomized clinical trial in preterm infants. Journal of Paediatric Gastroenterology and Nutrition 37(2): 161-167

Maroulis J, Kalfarentoz F 2000 Complications of parenteral nutrition at the end of the century. Clinical Nutrition 19: 299-304

Meiier R, Beglinger C, Layer P et al 2002 ESPEN guidelines on nutrition in acute pancreatitis. Clinical Nutrition 21(2): 173-183

Misra S, Kirby D F 2000 Micronutrient and trace element monitoring in adult nutrition support. Nutrition in Clinical Practice 15: 120-126

Nitenberg G, Raynard B 2000 Nutritional support of the cancer patient: issues and dilemmas. Critical Reviews in Oncology/Haematology 34: 137-168

Okada A, Takagi Y, Nezu K et al 1995 Trace element metabolism in parenteral and enteral nutrition. Nutrition 11(1 suppl): 106-113

Plauth M, Merli M, Kondrup J et al 1997 ESPEN guidelines for nutrition in liver disease and transplantation. Clinical Nutrition 16: 43-55

Shenkin A 1995 Trace elements and inflammatory response: implications for nutritional support. Nutrition 11: 100-105

Toigo G, Aparico M, Attman P O et al 2000 Expert working group report on nutrition in adult patients with renal insufficiency (part 1 and part 2). Clinical Nutrition 19: 197-207, 281-291

Woodcock N P, Zeigler D, Palmer M D et al 2001 Enteral vs parenteral nutrition: a pragmatic study. Nutrition 17: 1-12

FURTHER READING

Bowling T (ed) 2004 Nutritional support for adults and children – a handbook for hospital practice. Radcliffe Medical Press, Abingdon

British Pharmaceutical Nutrition Group. Available online at: www.bpng.co.uk

Rombeau J L, Rolandelli R H (eds) 2000 Clinical nutrition – parenteral nutrition. W B Saunders, Philadelphia

Sobotka L, Allison S P, Fürst P et al (eds) 2004 Basics in clinical nutrition, 3rd edn. Galén, Prague

Pharmacoeconomics 8

J. Cooke

KEY POINTS

- Expenditure on medicines is increasing at a greater rate than other healthcare costs.
- Increasingly governments are employing health economics to help prioritize between different medicines.
- In health economics consequences of a treatment can be expressed in monetary terms (cost–benefit), natural units of effectiveness (cost–effectiveness) and in terms of patient preference or utility (cost–utility).
- Head-to-head studies offer the best way of determining overall effectiveness and cost–effectiveness.
- Sensitivity analysis can be used to address areas of uncertainty.
- Medication non-concordance, medication errors and unwanted drug effects place a considerable burden on societal healthcare costs.
- Decision analysis techniques offer a powerful tool for comparing alternative treatment options.

The demand for and hence the cost of healthcare are growing in all countries in the world as the improvement and sophistication of health technologies increase. Many governments are focusing their activities on promoting the effective and economic use of resources allocated to healthcare. The increased use of evidence-based programmes not only concentrates on optimizing health outcomes but also utilizes health economic evaluations.

While there have been marked gains in longevity in those countries which make up the Organization for Economic Co-operation and Development (OECD), health costs have also risen. In most countries health expenditure has increased at a faster rate than overall economic growth with, in 2003, the OECD countries spending an average 8.8% of their gross domestic product (GDP) on health, up from 7.1% in 1990 and just over 5% in 1970. Interestingly, there is a wide variation of spending on health ranging from 15% of GDP in the United States to less than 6% in the Slovak Republic and Korea. Per capita expenditure on health ranges from around £1400 in the UK to £3200 in the USA (OECD 2005).

Medicines form a small but significant proportion of total healthcare costs and one that has been increasing consistently as new medicines are marketed. The writing of a prescription is the most common therapeutic intervention in medicine, with more than 676 million prescriptions being dispensed in primary care in England in 2004.

Expenditure on medicines has seen a considerable rise over recent years with more than 5% per year growth on average since 1997. This has contributed to the overall rise in expenditure on health. Most OECD countries have seen growth in spending on medicines outstrip growth in total health spending over this period. In the United States and Australia, pharmaceutical spending has increased at more than double the rate of growth in total health spending (OECD 2005).

In England over £8 billion was spent on medicines in 2004, which represents approximately £160 per person. Seventy-eight percent of the costs are incurred in primary care and constitute up to 50% of the primary care revenue costs. Within an average general hospital, at least 5% of the total revenue expenditure is spent on medicines. In cancer hospitals this can rise to as much as one-third of the total costs of running the hospital.

There are a number of reasons why prescribing costs are increasing.

- Demographic changes have resulted in an ageing population which is living longer and has greater needs for therapeutic interventions.
- Health screening programmes and improved diagnostic techniques that are uncovering previously non-identified diseases which subsequently require treatment.
- The marketing of new medicines that offer more effective and less toxic alternatives to existing agents. Invariably these are more expensive, especially biotechnology medicines, notably monoclonal antibodies which can cost in excess of £30 000 per patient per year.
- The use of existing agents becoming more widespread as additional indications for their use are found.
- Public and patients have a higher expectation of their rights to access high-cost healthcare.

In the UK health reforms over the last decade have addressed the quality of care through promotion of clinical governance. The formation of the National Institute for Clinical Excellence (NICE) in 1998 to 'improve standards of patient care, and to reduce inequities in access to innovative treatment' has formalized this process. NICE undertakes technology appraisals of medicines and other treatments (health technologies) and addresses the clinical and cost-effectiveness of therapies and compares them with alternative uses of NHS funds. The increased use of evidence-based programmes not only concentrates on optimizing health outcomes but also utilizes health economic evaluations. Formalized health technology assessments provide an in-depth and evidence-based approach to this process. The NHS is starting to develop methods to deal with the financial implications of NICE guidance through the business planning process (Audit Commission 2005).

Terms used in health economics

Pharmacoeconomics can be defined as the measurement of both the costs and consequences of therapeutic decision making. Pharmacoeconomics provides a guide for decision makers on resource allocation but does not offer a basis on which decisions should be made. Pharmacoeconomics can assist in the planning process and help assign priorities where, for example, medicines with a worse outcome may be available at a lower cost and medicines with better outcome and higher cost can be compared. Figure 8.1 summarizes the dilemmas facing decision makers when a new medicine is introduced.

When economic evaluations are conducted it is important to categorize various costs. Costs can be direct to the organization, i.e. physicians' salaries, the acquisition costs of medicines, consumables associated with drug administration, staff time in preparation and administration of medicines, laboratory charges of monitoring for effectiveness and adverse drug reactions. Indirect costs include lost productivity from a disease which can manifest itself as a cost to the economy or taxation system as well as economic costs to the patient and the patient's family. All aspects of the use of medicines may be allocated costs, both direct, such as acquisition and administration costs, and indirect, such as the cost of a given patient's time off work because of illness, in terms of lost output and social security payments. The consequences of drug therapy include benefits for both the individual patient and society at large, which may be quantified in terms of health outcome and quality of life, in addition to purely economic impact.

It is worthwhile here to describe a number of definitions that further qualify costs in a healthcare setting. The concept of opportunity cost is at the centre of economics and identifies the value of opportunities which have been lost by utilizing resources in a particular service or health technology. This can be valued as the benefits that have been forsaken by investing the resources in the best alternative fashion. Opportunity cost recognizes that there are limited resources available for utilizing every treatment, and therefore the rationing of healthcare is implicit in such a system.

Average costs are the simplest way of valuing the consumption of healthcare resources. Quite simply, they represent the total costs (i.e. all the costs incurred in the delivery of a service) of a healthcare system divided by the units of production. For example, a hospital might treat 75 000 patients a year (defined as finished consultant episodes, FCEs) and have a total annual revenue cost of £150 million. The average cost per FCE is therefore £2000.

Fixed costs are those which are independent of the number of units of production and include heating, lighting and fixed staffing costs. Variable costs, on the other hand, are dependent on the numbers of units of productivity. The cost of the consumption of medicines is a good example of variable costs.

The inevitable increases in the medicines budget in a particular institute which is treating more patients, or treating those with a more complex pathology, have often been erroneously interpreted by financial managers as a failure to effectively manage the budget. In order to better describe the costs associated with a healthcare intervention, economists employ the term 'marginal costs' to describe the costs of producing an extra unit of a particular service. The term 'incremental cost' is employed to define the difference between the costs of alternative interventions.

Choice of comparator

Sometimes a claim is made that a treatment is cost-effective. But cost-effective against what? As in any good clinical trial, a treatment has to be compared against a reasonable comparator. The choice of comparator is crucial to this process. A comparator that is no longer in common use or in a dose that is not optimal will result in the evaluated treatment being seen as more effective than it actually is. Sadly many evaluations of medicines fall into this trap as sponsors seldom wish to undertake head-to-head studies against competitors. Again, the reader has to be careful when

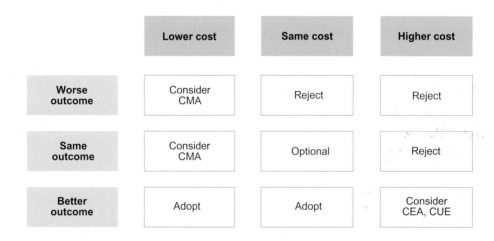

	Lower cost	Same cost	Higher cost
Worse outcome	Consider CMA	Reject	Reject
Same outcome	Consider CMA	Optional	Reject
Better outcome	Adopt	Adopt	Consider CEA, CUE

CMA: **Cost-minimization analysis**
CEA: **Cost-effective analysis**
CUA: **Cost-utility analysis**

Figure 8.1 Dilemma matrix for decision makers dealing with the economics of a new therapeutic intervention.

interpreting economic evaluations from settings which are different from those in local practice. A common error can be made when viewing international studies that have different healthcare costs and ways of treating patients and translating them directly into our own practice.

In addition, hospital charges, including those for hotel services such as heating and lighting overheads, meals and accommodation, which may constitute a major cost, should be considered. These are frequently included in an average cost per patient-day.

Types of health economic evaluations

Cost–benefit analysis (CBA)

In cost–benefit analysis consequences are measured in terms of the total cost associated with a programme where both costs and consequences are measured in monetary terms. While this type of analysis is preferred by economists, its employment in healthcare is problematical as it is frequently difficult to ascribe monetary values to clinical outcomes such as pain relief, avoidance of stroke or improvements in quality of life.

Methods are available for determining cost–benefit for individual groups of patients that centre around a concept known as contingent valuation. Specific techniques include willingness to pay, where patients are asked to state how much they would be prepared to pay to avoid a particular event or symptom, e.g. pain or nausea following day-care surgery. Willingness to pay can be fraught with difficulties of interpretation in countries with socialized healthcare systems which are invariably funded out of general taxation. Willingness to accept is a similar concept but is based on the minimum amount an individual person or population would receive in order to be prepared to lose or reduce a service.

Cost–benefit analysis can be usefully employed at a macro level for strategic decisions on healthcare programmes. For example, a countrywide immunization programme can be fully costed in terms of resource utilization consumed in running the programme. This can then be valued against the reduced mortality and morbidity that occur as a result of the programme.

Cost–benefit analysis can be useful in examining the value of services, e.g. centralized intravenous additive (CIVA) services where a comparison between a pharmacy-based intravenous additive service and ward-based preparation by doctors and nurses may demonstrate the value of the centralized pharmacy service, or a clinical pharmacokinetics service where the staffing and equipment costs can be offset against the benefits of reduced morbidity and mortality. A model for the cost–benefit analysis of the introduction of a pharmacy automated dispensing unit into a hospital setting is set out in Table 8.1.

Cost–effectiveness analysis (CEA)

Cost–effectiveness analysis can be described as an examination of the costs of two or more programmes which have the same clinical outcome as measured in physical units, e.g. lives saved or reduced morbidity. Treatments with dissimilar outcomes can also be analysed by this technique. Where two or more interventions have been shown to be or are assumed to be similar then, if all other factors are equal, e.g. convenience, side effects, availability, etc., selection can be made on the basis of cost. This type of analysis is called cost-minimization analysis (CMA). CMA is frequently employed in formulary decision making where often the available evidence for a new product appears to be no better than for existing products. This is invariably what happens in practice as clinical trials on new medicines are statistically powered for equivalence as a requirement for licensing submission.

An example of the use of cost–effectiveness analysis is shown in a study of the addition of recombinant human granulocyte-macrophage colony-stimulating factor (rhGM-CSF) after autologous bone marrow transplantation for lymphoid cancer. A randomized controlled double-blind trial was undertaken in 40 patients to ascertain the effect of rhGM-CSF with placebo. Outcomes measured included length of stay, and economic inputs included costs of medicines, total charges, departmental charges, rehospitalization and outpatient charges. In all cases except pharmacy costs, the charges were less with the rhGM-CSF treatment and indicated an overall saving to the organization and a better treatment outcome.

Table 8.1 Summary of a cost–benefit analysis for the introduction of an automated pharmacy dispensing system in a hospital setting

	Year 1	Year 2	Year 3	Year 4	Year 5
Financial costs					
Lease and maintenance	£122 000	£113 000	£113 000	£113 000	£113 000
Benefits					
Expired drugs	£42 000	£42 000	£42 000	£42 000	£42 000
Stock discrepancies	£14 400	£14 400	£14 400	£14 400	£14 400
Over-labelled drugs	£79 000	£79 000	£79 000	£79 000	£79 000
Annual stock take	£0	£5000	£5000	£5000	£5000
Difference	–£13 400	–£27 400	–£27 400	–£27 400	–£27 400

Clinical benefits:
• reduction in medication errors
• reduction in waiting times for inpatients and outpatients

As previously described, cost–effectiveness analysis examines the costs associated with achieving a defined health outcome. While these outcomes can be relief of symptoms such as nausea and vomiting avoided, pain relieved, etc., cost–effectiveness analysis frequently employs years of life gained as a measure of the success of a particular programme. This can then offer a method of incrementally comparing the costs associated with two or more interventions. For example, consider a hypothetical case of the comparison of two drug treatments for the management of malignant disease. Treatment A represents a 1-year course of treatment for a particular malignant disease. Assume that this is the current standard form of treatment and that the average total direct costs associated with this programme are £40 000 a year. This will include the costs of the medicines, antiemetics, inpatient stay, radiological and pathology costs, etc. Treatment B is a new drug treatment for the malignancy which as a result of comparative controlled clinical trials has demonstrated an improvement in the average life expectancy for this group of patients from 3.5 years for treatment A to 4.5 years for treatment B. The average annual total costs for treatment B are £55 000. A comparative table can now be constructed.

Strategy	Treatment costs	Effectiveness
Treatment A	£40 000	3.5 years
Treatment B	£55 000	4.5 years

Incremental cost–effectiveness ratio:

$$= \frac{55\ 000 - 40\ 000}{4.5 - 3.5}$$

$$= £15\ 000 \text{ per life-year gained}$$

Cost–utility analysis (CUA)

An alternative measurement for the consequences of a healthcare intervention is the concept of utility. Utility provides a method for estimating patient preference for a particular intervention in terms of the patient's state of well-being. Utility is described by an index which ranges between 0 (representing death) and 1 (perfect health). The product of utility and life years gained provides the term quality-adjusted life-year (QALY).

There are a number of methods for the calculation of utilities.

- The Rosser–Kind matrix relies on preferences from population samples from certain disease groups.
- The visual analogue scale method seeks to obtain patient preferences for their perceived disease state by scoring themselves on a line scaled between 0 and 1 as above.
- The standard gamble method requires individuals to choose between living the rest of their lives in their current state of health or making a gamble of an intervention which will restore them to perfect health. Failure of the gamble will result in instant death. The probabilities of the gamble are varied until there is indifference between the two events.
- The time trade-off method requires individuals to decide how many of their remaining years of life expectancy they would be prepared to exchange for complete health.

Using the previous model, if treatment A provides on average an increase of 3.5 years life expectancy but that this is valued at a utility of 0.9, then the health gain for this intervention is $0.9 \times 3.5 = 3.15$ QALYs. Similarly, if the increase in life expectancy with treatment B only had a utility of 0.8 (perhaps because it produces more nausea) then the health gain for this option becomes $0.8 \times 4.5 = 3.6$ QALYS. An incremental CUA can be undertaken as follows.

Strategy	Treatment costs	Effectiveness	Utility
Treatment A	£40 000	3.5 years	0.9
Treatment B	£55 000	4.5 years	0.8

Incremental cost utility ratio:

$$= \frac{55\ 000 - 40\ 000}{(4.5 \times 0.8) - (3.5 \times 0.9)}$$

$$= £33\ 333 \text{ per life QALY gained}$$

The calculation of QALYs provides a method which enables decision makers to compare different health interventions and assign priorities for decisions on resource allocation. However, the use of QALY league tables has provided much debate amongst stakeholders of healthcare as to their value and use.

Valuation of costs and consequences over time: discounting

Discounting is an economic term which is based mainly on a time preference that assumes individuals prefer to forego a part of the benefits of a programme if they can have those benefits now rather than fully in an uncertain future. The value of this preference is expressed by the discount rate. There is intense debate amongst health economists regarding the value for this annual discount level and whether both costs and consequences should be subjected to discounting. If a programme does not exceed 1 year then discounting is felt to be unnecessary.

Decision analysis techniques

Decision analysis offers a method of pictorial representation of treatment decisions. If the results from clinical trials are available, probabilities can be placed within the arms of a decision tree and outcomes can be assessed in either monetary or quality units (Fig. 8.2).

A simple decision tree might look at the three options for the management of dyspepsia in patients under 45 (see Fig. 8.3). In Option A the patient is seen by the primary care medical practitioner who undertakes testing for *Helicobacter pylori* infection and initiates eradication therapy. Option B considers symptomatic relief using proton pump inhibitors from a primary care medical practitioner and Option C involves the primary care medical practitioner referring the patient straight to a gastroenterologist for endoscopy. The quickest way to undertake decision analysis is by a computerized programme using standardized cost data to populate the decision tree. Using published information, the probabilities of complications and failures can be put into the decision tree and, from hypothetical or actual hospital cost data, the treatments can be assigned total direct costs.

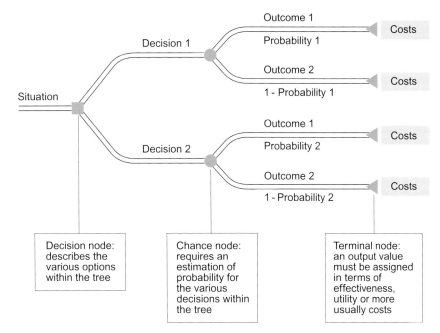

Figure 8.2 Decision tree template.

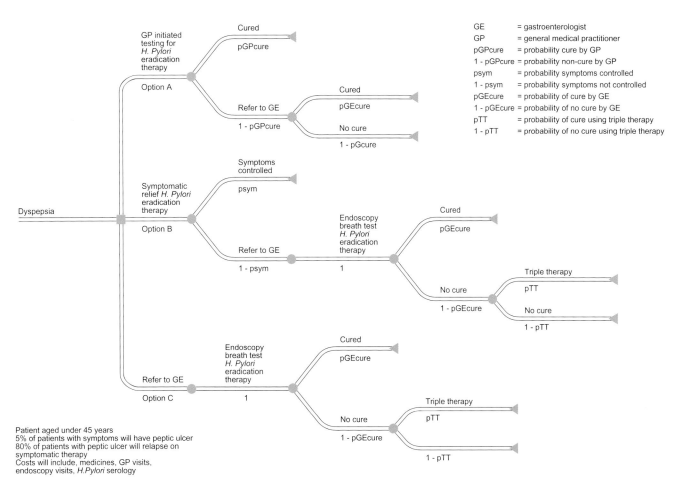

GE = gastroenterologist
GP = general medical practitioner
pGPcure = probability cure by GP
1 - pGPcure = probability non-cure by GP
psym = probability symptoms controlled
1 - psym = probability symptoms not controlled
pGEcure = probability of cure by GE
1 - pGEcure = probability of no cure by GE
pTT = probability of cure using triple therapy
1 - pTT = probability of no cure using triple therapy

Patient aged under 45 years
5% of patients with symptoms will have peptic ulcer
80% of patients with peptic ulcer will relapse on
symptomatic therapy
Costs will include, medicines, GP visits,
endoscopy visits, *H.Pylori* serology

Figure 8.3 Decision tree for the management of patients under 45 with dyspepsia.

A decision tree can then be constructed which can describe the major pathways and this is depicted in Figure 8.3. By rolling back the tree, the costs and probabilities of the model can be seen, and the tree identifies a preference for the most cost-effective option (Fig. 8.4). The model also calculates the costs of the programme at each node and, by the assignment of probabilities for each decision arm, an overall cost of the preferred option is shown to be the management of the patient by the primary care medical practitioner with *H. pylori* testing and eradication using triple therapy at an average total cost for each patient of £162.

If there is uncertainty about the robustness of the values of the variables within the tree, they can be varied within defined ranges to see if the overall direction of the tree changes. This is referred to as sensitivity analysis and is one of the most powerful tools available in an economic evaluation.

Guidelines for economic evaluations of medicines

A number of countries have introduced explicit guidelines for the conduct of economic evaluations of medicines. Others require economic evaluations before allowing a medicine onto an approved listing. Guidelines have been published which aim to provide researchers and peer reviewers with background guidance on how to conduct an economic evaluation and how to check its quality prior to appraisal (Drummond & Jefferson 1996) whilst others (NICE 2004) have set out how they incorporate health economics in the evaluation of medicines.

Risk management of unwanted drug effects

Avoiding the adverse effects of medicines has become a desirable goal of therapeutic decision makers as well as those who promote quality assurance and risk management. Not only can there be significant sequelae in terms of increased morbidity associated with adverse drug effects but the economic consequences can be considerable. For example, gentamicin is often regarded as a relatively inexpensive antibiotic but in the USA each case of nephrotoxicity has been reported to cost £1562 in terms of additional resources consumed even without any assessment of the reduction in a patient's quality of life. The increasingly

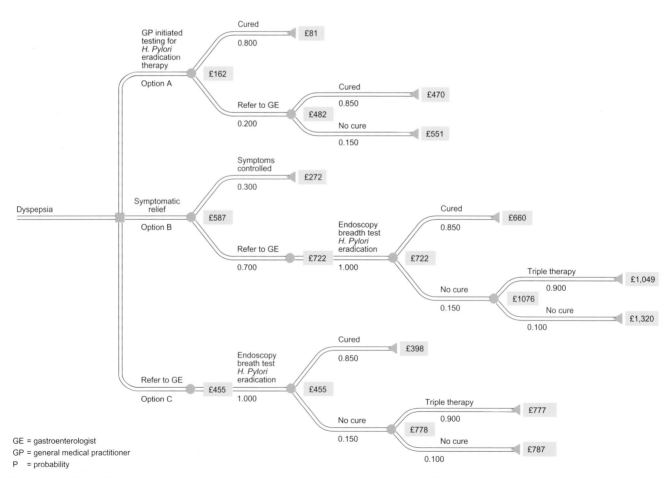

GE = gastroenterologist
GP = general medical practitioner
P = probability

Figure 8.4 Roll-out of the decision tree for the management of patients under 45 with dyspepsia. The dominant pathway is for the primary care medical practitioner to prescribe *H. pylori* eradication therapy.

litigious nature of society has resulted in economic valuation of perceived negligence, for example with irreversible vestibular toxicity associated with prolonged unmonitored aminoglycoside therapy. In England there was a target for a 40% reduction in the number of serious errors in the use of prescribed medicines by 2005 (DH 2004).

Medication non-compliance

The costs of non-compliance with medicines are considerable. In the USA it has been calculated that 11.4% of all admissions to hospital are directly associated with some form of non-compliance and at a cost of £1344 per patient. This equates to two million hospital admissions a year resulting from medication non-compliance at a total cost of £5300 million. In addition, it has been estimated that lost work productivity through non-compliance in the USA costs more than £3125 million per year.

Conclusion

A fundamental element of the use of pharmacoeconomics in practice is the viewpoint from which the analysis is conducted. Ideally this should be from a societal perspective but frequently it is from a government or Department of Health viewpoint. Purchasers of healthcare may also have a different perspective from provider units, and the viewpoint of clinicians may differ from that of patients. The pharmaceutical industry will probably have another viewpoint that will be focused on their particular products. Consequently all economic evaluations should be clear as to the perspective from which they have been analysed.

The effect of having budgets that are rigorously defended in any section of the health service, as occurs with the medicines budget, is to deny the application of economic decision making in the most efficient way for the population served. It is clear that pharmacoeconomics has an important part to play in the practice of therapeutics (Table 8.2) and needs to be an integral part of all planned therapeutic developments.

Table 8.2 Ten examples of the application of pharmacoeconomics in practice

- The value of one treatment over another in terms of the cost for each unit of health gained
- Avoidance of costs associated with the failure to use an appropriate medicine, e.g. antimicrobial surgical prophylaxis
- Avoidance of the costs of the side effects or adverse effects of a medicine
- Financial planning and horizon scanning for new medicines
- Prioritization of healthcare resources
- Health gain, quality of life issues and patient preferences
- Duration of care and balance between inpatient, day care and outpatient care
- Changes in legislative controls, e.g. reclassification of medicines from prescription only to pharmacy status
- Costs of concordance and non-concordance
- Economics of health service delivery

REFERENCES

Audit Commission 2005 Managing the financial implications of NICE guidance. Audit Commission Publications, Wetherby
Department of Health 2004 Building a safer NHS for patients: improving medication safety. Department of Health Publications, London
Drummond M F, Jefferson T O 1996 Guidelines for authors and peer reviewers of economic submissions to the BMJ. British Medical Journal 313: 275-283

National Institute for Clinical Excellence 2004 Guide to the methods of technology appraisal. National Institute for Clinical Excellence, London
Organization for Economic Co-operation and Development 2005 Health at a glance: OECD indicators. Organization for Economic Co-operation and Development, Paris

FURTHER READING

Walley T, Haycox A, Boland A (eds) 2003 Pharmacoeconomics. Elsevier, London
Bootman J L (ed) 2004 Principles of pharmacoeconomics, Harvey Whitney Books Co, Cincinnati

Rychlik R (ed) 2003 Strategies in pharmacoeconomics and outcomes research. Pharmaceutical Products Press, Binghampton

LIFE STAGES

Neonates 9

M. P. Ward Platt

The definitions of some important terms used of babies are given in Table 9.1. The earliest in pregnancy at which newborn babies can sometimes survive is 23–24 weeks' gestation, but conventionally any baby born at less than 32 weeks is regarded as being at relatively high risk of death or disability. About 7.5% of all births are technically 'premature' (<37 weeks) but only 1.4% take place before 32 weeks of gestation. Likewise, 7% of all babies are low birth weight (LBW), e.g. <2500 g, and 1.4% are very low birth weight (VLBW). However, it is the gestation at birth rather than the birth weight which is of more practical and prognostic value.

Because mothers with high-risk pregnancies will often be transferred for delivery to a hospital capable of providing neonatal intensive care, the proportion of preterm and LBW babies cared for in such units is greater than in smaller maternity units in

peripheral hospitals. In the population as a whole, between 1% and 2% of all babies will receive intensive care, and the most common reason for this among preterm babies is the need for respiratory support of some kind. Over three-quarters of babies born at 25 weeks' gestation now survive to discharge home.

Babies of less than 32 weeks' gestation invariably need some degree of special or intensive care, and generally go home when they are feeding adequately, somewhere between 35 and 40 weeks of postmenstrual age. So although in epidemiological terms the neonatal period is up to the first 28 postnatal days, babies may be 'neonatal' inpatients for as long as 3 or 4 months; during this time their weight may triple and their physiology and metabolism will change dramatically.

Drug disposition

Absorption

An important and unique source of drug absorption, available until birth, is the placenta. Maternal drugs pass to the fetus and back again during pregnancy but from delivery, any drugs present in the neonatal circulation can no longer be eliminated by that route and must be dealt with by the baby's own systems. Important examples of maternal drugs which may adversely affect the newborn baby include opiates given for pain relief during labour, β-blockers given for pregnancy-induced hypertension and benzodiazepines for seizures. In addition, a mother may be given a drug with the intention of treating not her but her fetus. An example of this is the use of corticosteroids to promote fetal lung maturation when preterm delivery is planned or expected. In this situation betamethasone is normally the drug of choice as prednisolone is metabolized in the placenta and does not reach the fetus.

Enteral drug absorption is erratic in any newborn baby, and unavailable in the ill baby because the stomach does not always empty effectively. Therefore most drugs are given intravenously to ensure maximum bioavailability. Some drugs, such as paraldehyde and diazepam (for neonatal seizures) and paracetamol (for simple analgesia), can be given rectally. The trachea may be used as the preferred route of administration when surfactant administration is required or where adrenaline (epinephrine) is given for resuscitation. The buccal route may be used to administer glucose gel in the treatment of hypoglycaemia. In the very preterm baby of 28 weeks' gestation or less, the skin is extremely thin and a poor barrier to water loss; consequently it is also permeable to substances in contact with it. This is harmful to

Table 9.1 Definitions of terms

Normal length of human pregnancy (term)	37 up to 42 completed weeks of gestation
Preterm	<37 weeks of gestation at birth
Post-term	42 completed weeks onwards
Neonatal period	Up to the 28th postnatal day
Low birth weight (LBW)	<2500 g
Very low birth weight (VLBW)	<1500 g
Extremely low birth weight (ELBW)	<1000 g

the baby if there is prolonged skin contact with alcohol, as in chlorhexidine in 70% methylated spirit, which as well as causing a severe chemical burn has resulted in systemic methyl alcohol poisoning. The intramuscular route is normally avoided in premature babies because of their small muscle bulk although the notable exceptions to this are the administration of vitamin K and naloxone.

Distribution

Drugs are distributed within a baby's body as a function of their lipid and aqueous solubility, as at any other time of life. The main difference in the neonate is that the size of the body water pool under renal control is related not to the baby's surface area but to body weight; furthermore, the absolute glomerular filtration rate increases logarithmically with postconceptional age irrespective of the length of a baby's gestation. This has implications for predicting the behaviour of water-soluble drugs such as gentamicin. The amount of adipose tissue can vary substantially between different babies. Any baby born more than 10 weeks early, and babies of any gestation who have suffered intrauterine growth restriction, may have little body fat. Conversely, the infant of a diabetic mother may have a particularly large fat layer and this affects the retention of predominantly lipid-soluble drugs. Protein binding in the plasma is influenced by the amount of albumin available and this in turn is related to gestation, with albumin values found 12 weeks prior to term being only two-thirds of adult concentrations.

Metabolism

The metabolic fate of drugs in the newborn is not qualitatively different to that in the older child, e.g. hydroxylation, oxidation and conjugation to sulphate or glucuronide. It is the efficiency with which these processes are carried out that distinguishes the baby from the older person. In addition to the immaturity of the metabolic pathways for drug disposal, drug metabolism is also affected by the physiological hyperbilirubinaemia of the newborn. The bilirubin can compete both for enzyme-binding sites and for glucuronate, and may thus affect drug metabolism for as long as unconjugated hyperbilirubinaemia persists.

Elimination

The relative immaturity of hepatic and renal function results in correspondingly slow elimination of most drugs from the neonate. This is not necessarily a disadvantage, so long as due account is taken of the slow elimination and dose intervals are modified accordingly. It may even be a useful property, as with phenobarbital, which when given as a loading dose (usually 20 mg/kg) will remain in circulation for days in useful therapeutic quantities, often avoiding the need for further doses. On the other hand, drugs such as gentamicin and vancomycin, which have a relatively narrow therapeutic index, must be given far less frequently than in children or adults and plasma drug levels must be assayed to avoid toxicity.

There has been little study of pharmacodynamics in the term or preterm neonate. Most work on the assumption that the kinetics of drug behaviour are so different in this group of patients that the pharmacodynamic properties must follow the same pattern.

In practice, the most important pharmacodynamic effect is probably that of the behaviour of opiates derived from the mother in labour. Pethidine and diamorphine are the opiates most likely to cause significant respiratory depression in the neonate. Such respiratory depression is treated with naloxone, and a special neonatal preparation (20 μg/mL) is available. However, after birth the opiates and their metabolites have a long plasma half-life in the baby whereas the naloxone is rapidly eliminated. The initial dramatic effect of naloxone can give a false sense of security, as the baby may become narcosed after a few hours following transfer to the postnatal ward. To try to prevent this late-onset narcosis, adult naloxone (400 μg/mL) may be given intramuscularly to ensure it remains active over several hours. Even when the respiratory effects have disappeared, opiates may have prolonged behavioural effects on both mother and baby.

Major clinical disorders

Respiratory distress syndrome

Among preterm babies the most commonly encountered disorder is respiratory distress syndrome (RDS; also sometimes called hyaline membrane disease (HMD) from its appearance on lung histology). The root cause of this disease is the lack of sufficient pulmonary surfactant. The condition is rare in babies born at or near term and becomes increasingly likely the more preterm a birth takes place.

Clinically, RDS is manifested by obvious difficulty with breathing, with nasal flaring, rib recession, tachypnoea and a requirement for oxygen therapy. The natural history is that RDS becomes worse over the first 2 days, reaches a plateau and then gradually improves. The use of antenatal steroid therapy to the mother, and surfactant therapy for the infant, has transformed the clinical course of this condition and greatly reduced mortality.

A relatively big baby born around 32–34 weeks of gestation may need no more treatment than extra oxygen. In contrast, smaller, more premature or more severely affected babies need some degree of mechanical assistance: either continuous positive airway pressure by nasal prongs or full artificial ventilation through an endotracheal tube. Some babies require high inspired concentrations of oxygen (up to 100%) for several days. Fortunately, pulmonary oxygen toxicity is not as much a problem to the neonate as it is to the adult, though it may have a causal role in the onset of bronchopulmonary dysplasia. The major concern is the damage that prolonged arterial hyperoxia can do to the retina, resulting in retinopathy of prematurity. The goal is to give enough inspired oxygen to keep the arterial partial pressure within a band of about 6–12 kPa.

Mechanical ventilation is not a comfortable experience, for adults or children, but it has taken a long time to appreciate that this may also be true for premature babies. Paralysing agents such as pancuronium are often given to ventilated neonates but these only prevent the baby from moving and are not sedative. Pancuronium is widely used, partly because it wears off slowly so that the baby is not suddenly destabilized. Shorter acting agents such as atracurium are often used for temporary paralysis for intubation. Whether or not the baby is paralysed, morphine is commonly given either as intermittent doses or as an infusion, to provide narcosis and analgesia to reduce the distress of neonatal intensive care.

The incidence, severity and mortality of RDS caused by surfactant deficiency may be reduced by giving corticosteroids antenatally to the mother. Antenatal steroids have been shown to reduce mortality by up to 40% among the infants of mothers so treated. Unfortunately it is not possible to identify and treat all mothers whose babies could benefit. Babies of less than 32 weeks' gestation gain most benefit because they are at greatest risk of death and disability from RDS. Optimum treatment is four oral doses of 6 mg betamethasone, each given 12-hourly, or two doses of 12 mg intramuscularly 24 hours apart (Crowley 2001).

The introduction of exogenous surfactant, derived from the pig or calf, has revolutionized the management of RDS. Natural surfactants derived from animals are currently more effective than artificial synthetic ones, but better artificial surfactants are being developed. The first dose should be given as soon as possible after birth since the earlier it is given, the greater the benefit (Yost & Soll 2001).

There are several other important ways of treating babies in respiratory failure. For some babies of at least 34 weeks of gestation and at least 2 kg birth weight, extracorporeal membrane oxygenation (ECMO), in which a baby is in effect put on partial heart–lung bypass for a few days, may be life-saving when conventional ventilation fails (ECMO Collaborative Trial Group 1996). The inhaled vasodilator nitric oxide (NO) is now widely used, and reduces the need for ECMO in some babies of 34 weeks or more, but there is little evidence that it saves lives (Van Meurs et al 2005). It may improve developmental outcome in survivors but this needs confirmation (Mestan et al 2005). Partial liquid ventilation is a technique which involves the instillation, into the trachea and bronchi, of perfluorocarbons in which oxygen is highly soluble, to abolish the water–air interface in the terminal airways (Valls-I-Soler et al 2001).

Patent ductus arteriosus

Patent ductus arteriosus (PDA) can be a problem in the recovery phase of RDS, and usually shows itself as a secondary increase in respiratory distress and/or ventilatory requirement, an increasing oxygen requirement, wide pulse pressure and a characteristic heart murmur. Physiologically, as pressure in the pulmonary artery falls because the RDS is improving, an open duct allows blood from the aorta to flow into the pulmonary artery, which engorges the lungs and reduces their compliance, while putting strain on the heart. Echocardiography is used to confirm the clinical suspicion. About one-third of all babies with birth weights less than 1000 g will develop signs of PDA, e.g. the characteristic heart murmur, but treatment is only needed when the baby is haemodynamically compromised. When treatment is needed the options are either medical treatment with indometacin or surgical ligation.

Indometacin is usually given intravenously in the UK, but can be given enterally although absorption is unpredictable. Serious potential side effects include renal impairment, gastric haemorrhage and gut perforation. These unwanted features are thought to be dose related and a low-dose, prolonged course (0.1 mg/kg daily for 6 days) has been shown to be as effective, with fewer side effects, than the same total dose given as 0.2 mg/kg, 12 hourly for three doses (Kumar & Yu 1997). Surgery is considered when one or more courses of indometacin fail to close the PDA or if indometacin is contraindicated for any reason.

The prophylactic use of indometacin in preterm babies is controversial. As well as reducing the incidence of PDA, as expected, a course of indometacin started as soon as possible after birth also has the desirable effect of reducing the incidence of cerebral haemorrhage (Fowlie 2001), but this does not appear to translate into better long-term neurodevelopment.

Bronchopulmonary dysplasia

Bronchopulmonary dysplasia (BPD) most frequently occurs in very immature babies who have undergone prolonged respiratory support. It can be defined as oxygen dependency lasting more than 28 days from birth, but this definition is not very useful in that many babies born at less than 28 weeks of gestation require oxygen for 28 days or more, but few still need it after 8 weeks. A more useful functional and epidemiological definition of established BPD is oxygen dependency at 36 weeks of postmenstrual age, in a baby born before 32 weeks. Significantly preterm babies still in oxygen at 36 weeks' postmenstrual age are likely to need oxygen at home after discharge. The factors predisposing to BPD are the degree of prematurity, the severity of RDS, infection, the occurrence of PDA, oxygen toxicity, and probably intrinsic genetic factors.

Established BPD not severe enough to need continuing mechanical ventilation is treated with oxygen, either as increased ambient oxygen delivered in the incubator or through a head box, or through nasal cannulae if the baby is in a cot. Enough oxygen must be used to maintain an oxygen saturation high enough to control pulmonary artery pressure, while avoiding chronic low-grade hyperoxia which could contribute to retinopathy of prematurity. Optimum oxygen saturations in these babies have never been rigorously defined.

Although there was enthusiasm for using dexamethasone to wean babies off ventilation and perhaps to reduce the severity of BPD, there is increasing evidence that its routine use does not improve mortality and increasing concern about steroid-related side effects, including effects on brain development. A wide variety of treatment regimens has been tested in trials and there is no standard approach. Side effects such as hypertension and glucose intolerance are common, although usually reversible, but the effects on growth and development are more serious.

BPD leads to increases in both pulmonary artery pressures and lung water content. The consequent strain on the heart can lead to heart failure, with excessive weight gain, increasing oxygen requirements and supporting clinical signs such as oedema. The treatment, as in any age group, is to give a diuretic. Thiazides improve pulmonary mechanics as well as treating heart failure (Brion et al 2001). Sometimes furosemide is used but its side effects are significant urinary loss of potassium and calcium, and renal calcification. An alternative is to combine a thiazide with spironolactone which causes less calcium and potassium loss. By reducing lung water content, diuretics can also improve lung compliance and reduce the work of breathing. However, BPD is not routinely treated with diuretics, since many babies do well without them. Systemic hypertension sometimes occurs among babies with BPD and may need treatment with antihypertensive drugs such as nifedipine or hydralazine.

Infection

Important pathogens in the first 2 or 3 days after birth are group B β-haemolytic streptococci and a variety of Gram-negative organisms, especially *Escherichia coli*. Coagulase-negative staphylococci and *Staphylococcus aureus* are more important subsequently. Superficial candida infection is common in all babies, and systemic candida infection is a risk particularly in babies receiving prolonged courses of broad-spectrum antibiotics. In general, it is wise to use narrow-spectrum agents and short courses of antibiotics whenever possible, and to discontinue blind treatment quickly, e.g. after 48 hours if confirmatory evidence of bacterial infection, such as blood culture, is negative. The most serious neonatal infections are listed in Table 9.2.

It is usual to start antibiotics prophylactically whenever preterm labour is unexplained, where there has been prolonged rupture of the fetal membranes prior to delivery, and when a baby is ventilated from birth. A standard combination for such early treatment is penicillin G and an aminoglycoside, to cover group B streptococci and Gram-negative pathogens. Treatment can be stopped after 48 hours if cultures prove negative. Blind treatment starting when a baby is more than 48 hours old has to take account of the expected local pathogens, but will always include cover for *Staphylococcus aureus*. Cephalosporins such as cefotaxime and ceftazidime have been heavily promoted for use in the blind treatment of neonatal infection on the grounds of their lower toxicity when compared to aminoglycosides, their wide therapeutic index and the absence of any need to monitor plasma concentrations. Their main disadvantage is the breadth of their spectrum which may result in fungal overgrowth or the spread of resistance, although they compare favourably with ampicillin in this regard. Since courses of blind treatment are often only for 48 hours, and the antibiotics can be stopped when cultures are negative, there is often no need to measure levels in babies receiving aminoglycosides, thereby negating much of the apparent advantage of cephalosporins. Moreover, there is now good evidence for giving gentamicin 24 hourly rather than more frequently, as it has similar efficacy and less potential for toxicity.

Methicillin-resistant *S. aureus* (MRSA) has emerged as a real problem in hospitals in recent years, but there is little evidence that neonatal units are a particularly hazardous environment.

A viral infection of increasing importance is the human immunodeficiency virus (HIV). The goal of treatment here is to prevent 'vertical' transmission from mother to baby. The main strategy to combat this is to use aggressive maternal treatment throughout pregnancy to suppress the maternal viral load. Current practice is to give the baby zidovudine, as a single agent, for 4 weeks when the maternal viral load is low, and triple therapy if the load is high.

Necrotizing enterocolitis

Necrotizing enterocolitis (NEC) is an important complication of neonatal intensive care, and can arise in any baby. However, it most commonly occurs in premature babies and those already ill. It is especially associated with being small for gestational age, birth asphyxia and the presence of a PDA. Since many sick babies have multiple problems it has been difficult to disentangle causal associations from spurious links to conditions that occur anyway in ill infants, such as the need for blood transfusion. There is general agreement that the pathophysiology is related to damage of the gut mucosa, which may occur because of hypotension or hypoxia, coupled with the presence of certain organisms in the gastrointestinal tract that invade the gut wall to give rise to the clinical condition. It almost never arises in a baby who has never been fed, whilst early 'minimal' feeding, and initiating feeding with human breast milk, appears to be protective.

A baby who becomes ill with NEC is often septicaemic and may present acutely with a major collapse, respiratory failure and shock, or more slowly with abdominal distension, intolerance of feeds with discoloured gastric aspirates and blood in the stool. The medical treatment is respiratory and circulatory support if necessary, antibiotics and switching to intravenous feeding for a period of time, usually 7–10 days. One of the most difficult surgical judgements is deciding if and when to operate to remove necrotic areas of gut or deal with a perforation.

The antibiotic strategy for NEC is to cover Gram-positive, Gram-negative and anaerobic bacteria. Metronidazole is used to cover anaerobes in the UK but clindamycin is preferred in some other countries. As with other drugs, metronidazole behaves very differently in neonates compared with older children and adults, having an elimination half-life of over 20 hours in term babies. The elimination half-life is up to 109 hours in preterm babies, partly due to poor hepatic hydroxylation in infants born before 35 weeks' gestation. There is probably a case to be made for monitoring plasma levels of this drug, but in practice this is seldom done.

Haemorrhagic disease of the newborn

Except in the very rare case of malabsorption, haemorrhagic disease of the newborn, better described as vitamin K-dependent bleeding, affects only breast-fed babies because they get very little vitamin K in maternal milk. Bottle-fed infants get sufficient vitamin K in their formula. Even without active prevention, it is a rare condition but it may cause death or disability when it presents with an intracranial bleed.

There are several possible strategies for giving vitamin K. An intramuscular injection of phytomenadione 1 mg (0.5 mL) can be given either to every newborn baby or selectively to babies who have certain risk factors such as instrumental delivery,

Table 9.2 Serious neonatal infections and pathogens

Septicaemia	*Staphylococcus epidermidis*, group B streptococci, *Escherichia coli*
Systemic candidiasis	*Candida* spp
Necrotizing enterocolitis	No single causal pathogen
Osteomyelitis	*Staphylococcus aureus*
Meningitis	Group B streptococci, *Escherichia coli*

preterm birth, etc. Vitamin K can be given orally, so long as an adequate number of doses is given, and this has been shown to be effective in preventing disease (Wariyar et al 2000). Intramuscular injections are an invasive and unpleasant intervention for the baby since muscle bulk is small in the newborn, and particularly the preterm, and other structures such as the sciatic nerve can be damaged even if the intention is to give the injection into the lateral thigh. There has also been widespread publicity about a possible link between intramuscular vitamin K and childhood malignancy which has made many parents wary of assenting to its administration. Intramuscular injections can be reserved for those babies with doubtful oral absorption, e.g. all those admitted for special care, or at high risk because of enzyme-inducing maternal drugs such as anticonvulsants.

Apnoea

Apnoea is the absence of breathing. Babies (and adults) normally have respiratory pauses, but preterm babies in particular are prone to prolonged pauses in respiration of over 20 seconds which can be associated with significant falls in arterial oxygenation. Apnoea usually has both central and obstructive components, is often accompanied by bradycardia, and requires treatment to prevent life-threatening episodes of arterial desaturation leading to convulsions and brain damage.

Apnoeic and bradycardic episodes can be treated in three ways: intubating and mechanically ventilating the baby, giving nasal continuous positive airway pressure (nCPAP) or giving respiratory stimulants such as one of the methylxanthines or doxapram. The main goal of treatment is to reduce the number and severity of the episodes without having to resort to artificial ventilation. Of the methylxanthines, caffeine appears to be as effective as theophylline or aminophylline (and both these two are partly metabolized to caffeine). Caffeine has a much wider therapeutic index than theophylline and aminophylline and there is no need to measure plasma concentrations. Doxapram is occasionally given as an adjunct to both a methylxanthine and CPAP, to avoid putting the baby on a ventilator. Most clinicians stop giving respiratory stimulants when the baby is around 34 weeks of postmenstrual age, after which time most babies will have achieved an adequate degree of cardiorespiratory stability and no longer need even the most basic forms of monitoring device.

Seizures

Seizures may arise as part of an encephalopathy, when they are accompanied by altered consciousness, or as isolated events when the baby is neurologically normal between seizure episodes. Investigations are directed to finding an underlying cause but in about half of all term babies having fits without an encephalopathy, no underlying cause can be found.

Just as with children and adults, treatment may be needed to control an acute seizure which does not terminate quickly, or given long term to prevent the occurrence of fits. In the neonate, the first-choice anticonvulsant for the acute treatment of seizures is phenobarbital because it is effective, seldom causes respiratory depression, and is active for many hours or days because of its long elimination half-life. Diazepam is sometimes used intravenously or rectally but it upsets temperature control,

causes unpredictable respiratory depression, and is very sedating compared to phenobarbital. Paraldehyde is occasionally used because it is easy to give rectally, is relatively non-sedating and short acting. It is excreted by exhalation and the smell can make the working environment quite unpleasant for staff. Phenytoin is often used when fits remain uncontrolled after two loading doses of phenobarbital (total 40 mg/kg) but is not given long term because of its narrow therapeutic index. When seizures are intractable, options include clonazepam, midazolam or lidocaine; the last two are given as infusions. There is little experience with intravenous sodium valproate in the neonate. Longer term treatment is commonly with phenobarbital but after the first few postnatal months, carbamazepine or sodium valproate is more suitable.

Hypoxic-ischaemic encephalopathy (HIE), which usually results either from intrapartum asphyxia or from an antepartum insult such as placental abruption, is an important cause of seizures. Convulsions are a marker of a more severe insult; they usually occur within 24 hours of birth and may last for several days, after which they spontaneously resolve. The less severely affected babies quickly return to neurological normality. No drug has been shown to improve outcome when given after the insult has occurred, and routine use of phenobarbital, or any other medication, before seizures occur is not recommended (Evans & Levene 2001).

The therapeutic dilemma lies in the degree of aggression with which convulsions should be treated, since no conventional anticonvulsant is very effective in reducing electrocerebral seizure activity, even when the clinical manifestations of seizures are abolished, and as stated before, convulsions tend naturally to cease after a few days. The question as to whether strenuous attempts to gain control of seizures have any effect on subsequent developmental outcome remains unanswered. However, seizures which compromise respiratory function need to be treated to prevent serious falls in arterial oxygen tension and possible secondary neurological damage. Also, babies with frequent or continuous seizure activity are difficult to nurse and cause great distress to their parents. Therefore in practice it is usual to try to suppress the clinical manifestation of seizure activity, and phenobarbital remains the most commonly used first-line treatment. Where a decision is taken to keep a baby on anticonvulsant medication, therapeutic drug monitoring can provide helpful information and may need to be repeated from time to time during follow-up.

Principles and goals of therapy

The ultimate aim of neonatal care at all levels is to maximize disability-free survival and identify treatable conditions which would otherwise compromise growth or development. It follows that potential problems should be anticipated and the complexities of intensive care avoided if at all possible.

Many of the drugs used in neonatal care are not licensed for such use, or are used off-label. There is a high potential for errors because of the small doses used, which sometimes calls for unusual levels of dilution when drawing up drugs. Constant vigilance, electronic prescribing and the use of specialized neonatal formularies are all important in preventing harm.

Rapid growth

Once the need for intensive care has passed, the growth of a premature baby can be very rapid indeed if the child is being fed with a high-calorie formula modified for use with VLBW infants. Indeed, most babies born at 27 weeks, and weighing around 1 kg, can be expected to double their birth weight by the time they are 8 weeks old. Since the dose of all medications is calculated on the basis of body weight, constant review of dose is necessary to maintain efficacy, particularly for drugs that may be given for several weeks such as respiratory stimulants, diuretics and anticonvulsants. Conversely, all that is necessary to gradually wean a baby from a medication is to hold the dose constant so that the baby gradually 'grows out' of the drug. This practice is frequently used with diuretic medication in BPD, the need for which becomes less as the baby's somatic growth reduces the proportion of damaged lung in favour of healthy tissue.

Therapeutic drug monitoring

The assay of plasma concentrations of various drugs has a place in neonatal medicine, particularly where the therapeutic index of a drug is narrow. It is routine to assay levels of antibiotics such as aminoglycosides and vancomycin, of which the trough measurement is of most value since it is accumulation of the drug which must be avoided. More rarely, it may be necessary to assay minimal inhibitory or bactericidal concentrations of antibiotics in blood or cerebrospinal fluid if serious infections are being treated, but constraints on sampling limit the frequency with which this may be undertaken. Interpretation of plasma concentrations of chloramphenicol is problematic as active metabolites do not get measured. Safer antibiotics, such as ceftazidime and cefotaxime, have mostly replaced chloramphenicol in the treatment of Gram-negative septicaemia and meningitis.

Theophylline and aminophylline are handled unpredictably and assay of plasma theophylline concentrations is a useful guide to therapy; since a baby may be on such medication for several weeks assays need to be repeated regularly (probably weekly, for convenience). The use of caffeine, which has a much wider therapeutic index, abolishes the need for routine measurement of levels, although it may occasionally be useful to measure blood levels if a normal dose appears to be ineffective. Where phenobarbital or other anticonvulsants are given long term, intermittent measurement of plasma levels can be a useful guide to increasing the dose, as with methylxanthines. Digoxin is now rarely used in this age group but regular assay of plasma concentrations is of obvious importance. All these drugs have a long half-life so it is most important that drug concentrations are not measured too early, or too frequently, to prevent inappropriate changes in dose being made before a steady state is reached.

Avoiding harm

Intramuscular injections are considered potentially harmful because of the small muscle bulk of babies. However, it is not always easy to establish venous access and occasionally it may be necessary to use the intramuscular route instead.

For sick preterm infants ventilated for respiratory failure, handling of any kind is a destabilizing influence, so the minimal necessary intervention should be the rule. Merely opening the doors of an incubator can destabilize a fragile baby. It is therefore good practice to minimize the frequency of drug administration and to try to co-ordinate the doses of different medications.

Time-scale of clinical changes

In babies, the time-scale for starting drug treatments is very short because the clinical condition of any baby can change with great rapidity. For example, where a surfactant is required it should be given as soon as possible after birth to premature babies who are intubated and ventilated. Similarly, infection can be rapidly progressive, so starting antibiotics is a priority when the index of suspicion is high or where congenital bacterial infection is likely. The same applies for antiretroviral drugs when a baby is born to a mother positive for HIV, especially if the maternal viral load is high.

For the sick preterm infant this model applies to a wide range of interventions. It is seldom possible to wait a few hours for a given drug, and this has obvious implications for the level of support required by a neonatal service.

Patient and parent care

It is all too easy to take a mechanistic approach to neonatal medicine, on the grounds that premature infants cannot communicate their needs. Such an approach to therapy is inappropriate. Even when receiving intensive care, any infant who is not either paralysed or very heavily sedated does in fact respond with a wealth of cues and non-verbal communication in relation to their needs. Monitors therefore do not replace clinical skills, but provide supplementary information and advance warning of problems. Even the most premature babies show individual characteristics, which emphasizes that individualized care is as important in this age group as in any other. In particular, neonatal pain and distress have effects on nociception and behaviour well into the childhood years.

Involvement of parents in every aspect of care is a necessary goal in neonatal clinical practice, and care is increasingly regarded as a partnership between professionals and parents rather than the province of professionals alone. Routine administration of oral medication is thus an act in which parents may be expected to participate, and for those whose baby has to be discharged home still requiring continuous oxygen, the parent will rapidly obtain complete control, with support from the hospital and the primary healthcare team. The growing number of babies who survive very premature birth but whose respiratory state requires continued support after discharge presents an increasing therapeutic challenge for the future.

CASE STUDIES

Case 9.1

A went into labour as a result of an antepartum haemorrhage at 28 weeks of gestation. There was no time to give her steroids when she arrived at the maternity unit and her son, J, was born by vaginal delivery in good condition. However, he required intubation and ventilation at the age of 10 minutes to sustain his breathing. He was not weighed at that moment but was given intramuscular vitamin K and then taken to the special care unit. On arrival in the unit, J was weighed (1270 g) and was placed in an incubator for warmth. He was connected to a ventilator. Surfactant was given, blood taken for culture and basic haematology, and he was prescribed antibiotics. A radiograph confirmed the diagnosis of RDS.

Question

1. Which antibiotic(s) would be appropriate initially for J?
Over the next 2 days J required modest ventilation and remained on antibiotics. A second dose of surfactant was given 12 hours after the first. Parenteral feeding was commenced on day 2 as per unit policy, and on day 3 very slow continuous milk feeding into his stomach was started. Blood cultures were negative at 48 hours and the antibiotics were stopped. On day 4 he was extubated into 30% oxygen.
On day 5, J looked unwell with a rising oxygen requirement, increased work of breathing and poor peripheral perfusion. Examination revealed little else except that his liver was enlarged and a little firm, his pulses rather full and easy to feel and there was a moderate systolic heart murmur. One possibility was infection.

Question

2. Which antibiotics would be appropriate for J on day 5?
Another possibility was a patent arterial duct leading to heart failure.

Question

3. How could his heart failure and PDA be treated?
After appropriate treatment he looked progressively better and when the blood culture was negative after 2 days, the antibiotics were stopped. By the age of 2 weeks, J was on full milk feeds and the duct had closed. He was in air. However, he began to have increasingly frequent episodes of spontaneous bradycardia, sometimes following apnoeic spells in excess of 20 seconds' duration. Examination between episodes showed a healthy, stable baby. Investigations such as haematocrit, serum sodium and an infection screen were normal.

Question

4. At 2 weeks, which drug of choice could be used to treat his apnoea and bradycardia? What would be the expected duration of treatment with this drug?

Answers

1. Blind antibiotic cover is usually started until negative blood cultures are received. Penicillin and gentamicin would provide good cover for streptococci and Gram-negative organisms, which are the most likely potential pathogens at this stage. A suitable dose would be 30 mg/kg of penicillin every 12 hours and 2.5 mg/kg of gentamicin every 12 hours. Alternatively, a third-generation cephalosporin such as cefotaxime could be used for initial blind treatment. If cultures were negative at 48 hours, antibiotics could be stopped provided that there were no clinical indications to continue.
2. At day 5, antibiotic treatment should take account of the likely pathogens such as *S. aureus* and others causing nosocomial infections. A suitable choice for the former would be flucloxacillin, if there was no concern about MRSA, or vancomycin if there was. The vancomycin starting dose would be 15 mg/kg every 12 hours. The addition of another agent with good Gram-negative activity such as gentamicin or a third-generation cephalosporin would provide good cover.

3. A low dose of intravenous indometacin (e.g. 100 μg/kg) would be suitable for the treatment of PDA over 6 days to reduce the incidence of adverse effects which may occur if the same total dose were to be given over 3 days. Furosemide (1 mg/kg as a single dose) is the drug of choice for acute heart failure.
4. Caffeine is as effective as and safer than theophylline to treat the apnoea of prematurity. A metabolic pathway in the immature liver, which is virtually absent in mature livers, methylates theophylline to caffeine and thus by administering the active metabolite, the complications of giving the parent drug, theophylline, are avoided. Theophylline has a narrow therapeutic range and requires plasma level monitoring. A suitable dose of caffeine for J would be a loading dose of 20 mg/kg with maintenance dose of 5 mg/kg/day, increasing to 10 mg/kg/day if necessary. The frequency of episodes of apnoea and bradycardia should decline immediately. The treatment is likely to continue until he is about 34 weeks of postmenstrual age, when his control of breathing should be mature enough to maintain good respiratory function.

Case 9.2

B was born at 25 weeks' gestation and was ventilated for 5 days before being extubated onto continuous positive airways pressure. On extubation she was initially in air, but now at the age of 4 weeks she is mostly in about 30% oxygen, fully fed on milk, and growing well. Her chest x-ray shows the pattern typical of chronic lung disease. One morning she is noticed to be in 45% oxygen, she has had a large weight gain and she looks quite oedematous all over.

Question

1. What do these symptoms suggest?
After careful evaluation, B is given an oral dose of furosemide 1 mg/kg, following which the oedema goes down, her weight falls and her oxygen requirement returns to 30%.

Question

2. What are the disadvantages of giving regular furosemide in this situation?
A thiazide diuretic and spironolactone are prescribed. Four days later, routine biochemistry tests show a sodium of 125 mmol/L.

Question

3. What is the choice the attending team has to make?

Answers

1. The symptoms suggest heart failure. Medical examination would probably have revealed an enlarged liver, and the heart might have had a 'gallop' rhythm as well. In babies, the symptoms and signs commonly suggest both left and right ventricular failure.
2. Regular treatment with furosemide causes hypercalcuria, as well as excessive loss of sodium and potassium. Chronic hypercalcuria can lead to nephrocalcinosis. For this reason, a combination of thiazides and spironolactone is commonly used.
3. The sodium is low (but the normal range in preterm babies is 130–140 mmol/L, lower than in children and adults). That it is low is probably an effect of the diuretics. The choice lies between carrying on with the diuretics and supplementing the sodium intake, or stopping the diuretics and observing the baby for any recurrence of heart failure.

REFERENCES

Brion L P, Primhak R A, Ambrosio-Perez I 2001 Diuretics acting on the distal renal tubule for preterm infants with (or developing) chronic lung disease. Cochrane Review. In: The Cochrane Library, Issue 1. Update Software, Oxford

Crowley P 2001 Prophylactic corticosteroids for preterm birth. Cochrane Review. In: The Cochrane Library, Issue 1. Update Software, Oxford

ECMO Collaborative Trial Group 1996 UK collaborative randomised trial of neonatal extracorporeal membrane oxygenation. UK Collaborative ECMO Trial Group. Lancet 348: 75-82

Evans D J, Levene M I 2001 Anticonvulsants for preventing mortality and morbidity in full term newborns with perinatal asphyxia. Cochrane Review. In: The Cochrane Library, Issue 1. Update Software, Oxford

Fowlie P W 2001 Intravenous indometacin for preventing mortality and morbidity in very low birth weight infants. Cochrane Review. In: The Cochrane Library, Issue 1. Update Software, Oxford

Kumar R K, Yu V Y H 1997 Prolonged low-dose indomethacin therapy for patent ductus arteriosus in very low birthweight infants. Journal of Paediatrics and Child Health 33: 38-41

Mestan K K, Marks J D, Hecox K et al 2005 Neurodevelopmental outcomes of premature infants treated with inhaled nitric oxide. New England Journal of Medicine 353: 23-32

Valls-I-Soler A, Alvarez F J, Gastiasoro E 2001 Liquid ventilation: from experimental use to clinical application. Biology of the Neonate 80(suppl 1): 29-33

Van Meurs K P, Wright L L, Ehrenkranz R A et al 2005 Inhaled nitric oxide for premature infants with severe respiratory failure. New England Journal of Medicine 353: 13-22

Wariyar U, Hilton S, Pagan J et al 2000 Six years' experience of prophylactic oral vitamin K. Archives of Disease in Childhood. Fetal and Neonatal Edition 82: F64-68

Yost C C, Soll R F 2001 Early versus delayed selective surfactant treatment for neonatal respiratory distress syndrome. Cochrane Review. In: The Cochrane Library, Issue 1. Update Software, Oxford

FURTHER READING

Hey E (ed) 2002 Neonatal formulary. BMJ Books, London

Klaus M H, Fanaroff A A (eds) 2001 Care of the high-risk neonate. W B Saunders, London

Rennie J M, Robertson N R C 2002 A manual of neonatal intensive care. Arnold, London

Speidel B, Fleming P, Henderson J et al (eds) 1998 A neonatal vade-mecum, 3rd edn. Arnold, London

Young T E, Magnum B 2005 Neofax 2005. Acorn Publishing, USA

Paediatrics 10

C. Barker A.J. Nunn S. Turner

KEY POINTS

- Children are not small adults.
- Patient details such as age, weight and surface area need to be accurate to ensure appropriate dosing.
- Weight and surface area may change significantly in a relatively short time period.
- Pharmacokinetic changes in childhood are important and have a significant influence on drug handling and need to be considered when choosing an appropriate dosing regimen for a child.
- The availability of a medicinal product does not mean it is appropriate for use in children.
- The use of an unlicensed medicine in children is not illegal although it must be ensured that the choice of drug and dose is appropriate.

Paediatrics is the branch of medicine dealing with the development, diseases and disorders of children. Infancy and childhood is a period of rapid growth and development. The various organs, body systems and enzymes that handle drugs develop at different rates hence drug dosage, formulation, response to drugs and adverse reactions vary throughout childhood. Compared with adult medicine, drug use in children is not extensively researched and the range of licensed drugs in appropriate dosage forms is limited.

For many purposes it has been common to subdivide childhood into the following periods:

- neonate: the first 4 weeks of life
- infant: from 4 weeks to 1 year
- child: from 1 year to 12 years.

For the purpose of drug dosing, children over 12 years of age are often classified as adults. This is inappropriate because many 12 year olds have not been through puberty and have not reached adult height and weight. The International Committee on Harmonization (2000) has suggested that childhood be divided into the following age ranges for the purposes of clinical trials and licensing of medicines:

- preterm newborn infant
- term newborn infants (0–27 days)
- infants and toddlers (28 days to 23 months)
- children (2–11 years)
- adolescents (12–16/18 years).

These age ranges are intended to reflect biological changes. The newborn (birth to 4 weeks) covers the climacteric changes after birth, 4 weeks to 2 years the early growth spurt, 2 to 11 years the gradual growth phase and 12 to 18 years puberty and the adolescent growth spurt to final adult height. Manufacturers of medicines and regulatory authorities are working towards standardizing the age groups quoted in summaries of product characteristics.

Demography

In 1992 there were 11.8 million children aged less than 16 years in the UK. The 2001 census revealed that dependent children still make up a substantial number of people, at 11.7 million, but for the first time there are more people aged 60 and over (20.9%) than there are children aged under 16 (20.2%).

Children make substantial use of hospital-based services. It has been estimated that of the 14 million attendances at hospital emergency departments reported each year in England, 3.5 million were for children. The 10 most common admission diagnoses in a specialist children's hospital over an 18-month period are shown in Table 10.1.

Congenital anomalies

Congenital anomalies remain an important cause of infant and child mortality in England and Wales, and account for an increasing proportion of infant deaths. The National Congenital Anomaly System (NCAS), established in 1964 in the wake of the thalidomide tragedy, monitors congenital anomalies nationally in England and Wales. It relies on voluntary notifications and collaborates with local registers to improve the quality and quantity of data (see Useful Paediatric Websites at end of chapter).

Between 1964 and 1975 the live-birth notification rate of one or more congenital anomalies remained steady at around 160–180 per 10 000 live births; less than 2% of live births. Notification rates for 2001 declined to 114 per 10 000 live births. A further reduction was seen in 2003, to 111.8 per 10 000 live and still births, and in 2004 to 98.9 per 10 000 live and still births. In 2004, of 6023 live-birth reports, there were 277 CNS anomalies (e.g. hydrocephalus/spina bifida), 483 cleft lip/palate, 1156 heart and circulatory, 410 hypospadias, 530 deformities of the feet, 307 polydactyly and 420 Down's syndrome.

Neural tube defects (spina bifida) are one example of devastating congenital malformations that have been influenced by dietary therapy. In 1991 the results of a long-term study (MRC Vitamin Study Research Group 1991) showed that folate supplementation prevented 72% of neural tube defects when given to women at high risk of having a child with a neural tube defect. Folate supplementation is now part of the routine advice given in antenatal clinics.

Table 10.1 Top ten diagnoses on admission to a specialist children's hospital

Ranking	Diagnosis
1	Respiratory tract infections
2	Chronic diseases of tonsils and adenoids
3	Asthma
4	Abdominal and pelvic pain
5	Viral infection (unspecified site)
6	Non-suppurative otitis media
7	Inguinal hernia
8	Unspecified head injury
9	Gastroenteritis/colitis
10	Undescended testicle

Cancer

Cancer is very rare in childhood; around 1400 new cases (0.5% of total) were diagnosed in Great Britain in 2000. About one-third of all childhood cancers are leukaemias and of these, about 80% are of the acute lymphoblastic type (ALL).

The incidence of childhood cancer has not changed very much over the past 40 years; it remains about one-fifth more common among boys than girls. However, cancer accounts for a high proportion of all childhood deaths – around 20% of all deaths among children aged 1–14 years.

As a consequence of the technical advances in treatment and the centralization of services in specialist centres, a much greater number of childhood cancer sufferers are surviving to adulthood. In 1971, there were only around 1400 such survivors, of whom about 100 were aged over 30, whilst in 2000 there were almost 15 000 adult survivors, of whom almost 7000 (over 45%) were aged over 30. Eventually, more than 1 in 1000 adults of all ages will be survivors of childhood cancer. Current indications are that the risk of developing a second primary cancer within 25 years following treatment for childhood cancer is about 4%.

Asthma, eczema and hayfever

Asthma, eczema and hayfever (allergic rhinitis) are among the most common chronic diseases of childhood but most of the affected children are managed in primary care. During the 1970s and 1980s there was considerable expansion of epidemiological research into these disorders, prompted mainly by concern about the increase in hospital admissions for childhood asthma despite the availability of effective anti-asthma medications. These studies failed to identify any demographic, perinatal or environmental factor which could explain more than a small proportion of the large changes in prevalence of asthma, hayfever or eczema.

Infections

Despite a dramatic decline in the incidence of childhood infectious diseases during the 20th century, they remain an important cause of ill health in childhood. Major advances in the prevention of infections have been achieved through the national childhood vaccination programme.

The importance of maintaining high vaccine uptake has been demonstrated by the resurgence of vaccine-preventable diseases where children have not been vaccinated. Adverse publicity surrounding the MMR vaccine, involving a possible association with Crohn's disease and autism, resulted in a loss of public confidence in the vaccine and a decrease in MMR coverage. This occurred in spite of rigorous scientific investigation and evidence refuting the claims. The annual coverage for MMR for 2 year olds declined from 92% in 1992 to 87% in 2000 and data for 2004 show that it dropped to 81.5%. Although this decline is far less than that seen for pertussis in the1970s, if MMR coverage remains at this level or declines further, resurgences of measles, mumps and rubella in primary school children will become more common.

An important gastrointestinal infection that appears to be increasing is infection with verotoxin-producing *Escherichia coli* (VTEC).This is important because it is the main cause of haemolytic uraemic syndrome, a severe condition which can lead to acute renal failure in children. VTEC is an example of an emerging infection. Before the 1980s it was unknown and during the 1990s reports of infection with VTEC in children in the UK tripled, from 172 in 1991 to 531 in 1999.

Respiratory syncytial virus (RSV) is the most important cause of lower respiratory tract infection in infants and young children in the UK, in whom it causes bronchiolitis, tracheobronchitis and pneumonia. It is responsible for seasonal outbreaks of respiratory tract infection most commonly between October and April. The main burden of disease is borne by children under 2 years and there are around 7000–10 000 confirmed laboratory reports of RSV in children in England and Wales each year. During the winter months RSV is the greatest single cause of admission to hospital in children.

Mental health disorders

Mental health disorders are another emerging concern in the child health arena. In 1999 the Office for National Statistics (ONS) carried out the first large-scale national survey of child mental health in the UK. This revealed the key public health significance of psychiatric disorders in childhood: almost 1 in 10 of 5–15 year olds were facing handicapping emotional or behavioural problems severe enough to impact on their own functioning and to place a burden on their families.

A recent study of specialist child mental health services in England and Wales found that children seen by Child and Adolescent Mental Health Services (CAMHS) typically showed a range of complex difficulties. The most common were:

- difficulties with family life and relationships
- problems involving emotional and related symptoms (including eating disorders)
- problems with peer relationships, and
- disruptive, aggressive and antisocial behaviours.

Groups at particular high risk of psychiatric disorder include children in the care system, young people who are homeless and young offenders. Longitudinal evidence has confirmed that many child psychiatric disorders persist well into adult life. Biological, psychological and social factors all seem likely to contribute to the risk of psychiatric disorders, and may often act in combination.

Drugs, smoking and alcohol

The harm that drugs, smoking and drinking can do to the health of children and young people is recognized and a number of targets have been set in an attempt to reduce prevalence.

Between 1990 and 2000, a number of surveys were carried out to determine the prevalence of drug use, smoking and drinking among children and young people. It was found that each increased with age. In 2000 14% of 11–15 year olds had used drugs in the past year; the figure rose to 27% in the 16–19 year age group. In addition, boys were more likely than girls to take drugs. Although girls were more likely than boys to smoke regularly (12% compared with 9%), the average weekly consumption of cigarettes was higher for boys.

Nutrition and exercise

Health during childhood can impact upon well-being in later life. Good nutrition and physical exercise are vital both for growth and development and for preventing health complications in later life. In addition, dietary patterns in childhood and adolescence have an influence on dietary preferences and eating patterns in adulthood.

In 2000, an international definition of overweight and obesity in childhood and adolescence was proposed to help calculate internationally comparable prevalence rates of overweight and obesity in children and adolescents. The definition interprets overweight and obesity in terms of reference points for body mass index (BMI = kg/m^2) by age and sex, and is linked to the widely used adult overweight cut-off point of 25 and adult obesity cut-off point of 30.

Between 1995 and 2000 the proportion of overweight boys (aged 2–19 years) increased by 2% and the proportion of overweight girls increased by 3%. Probable reasons for a rise in overweight and obesity in children are changes in diets and an inactive lifestyle. There is evidence that obesity at an early age tends to continue to adulthood.

Being overweight is linked to the development of type 2 diabetes, high blood pressure, heart disease, stroke, certain cancers and other types of illness. Therefore, healthy eating is not only important in relation to weight but also contributes to reducing the risk of heart disease, stroke and some cancers in later life. It is recommended that a well-balanced diet providing all the nutrients required should include at least five portions of fruit and vegetables a day. It is now practice in many areas for infant children (aged 4–7 years) to be provided with a piece of free fruit during school break time.

The normal child

Growth and development are important indicators of a child's general well-being and paediatric practitioners should be aware of the normal development milestones in childhood. In the UK development surveillance and screening of babies and children is well established through child health clinics.

Weight is one of the most widely used and obvious indicators of growth, and progress is assessed by recording weights on a percentile chart (Fig. 10.1). A weight curve for a child which deviates from the usual pattern requires further investigation. Separate recording charts are used for boys and girls and since percentile charts are usually based on observations of the white British population, adjustments may be necessary for some ethnic groups. The World Health Organization (WHO) has challenged the widely used growth charts, based on growth rates of infants fed on formula milk. In 2006 it published new growth standards based on a study of more than 8000 breast-fed babies from six countries around the world. The optimum size is now that of a breast-fed baby.

Height (or length in children less than 2 years of age) is another important tool in developmental assessment. In a similar way to weight, height or length should follow a percentile line. If this is not the case or if growth stops completely, then further investigation is required. The normal rate of growth is taken to be 5 cm or more per year and any alteration in this growth velocity should be investigated.

For infants up to 2 years of age, head circumference is also a useful parameter to monitor. In addition to the above, assessments of hearing, vision, motor development and speech are undertaken

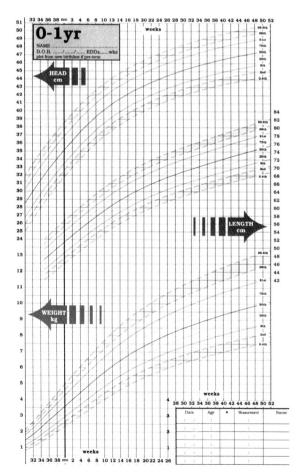

Figure 10.1 Example of a centile chart (©Child Growth Foundation).

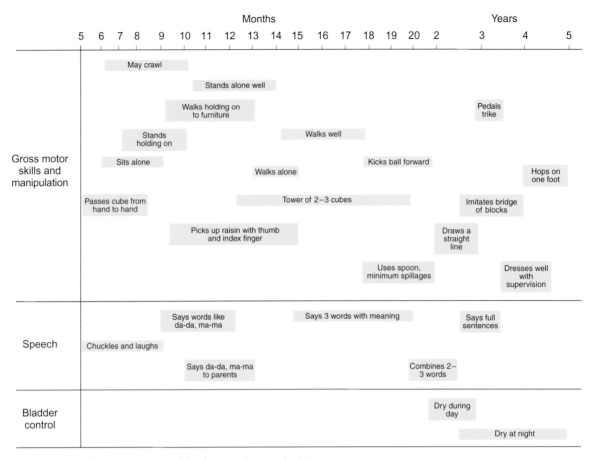

Figure 10.2 A summary of the various stages of development (Scott et al 1995).

at the child health clinics. A summary of age-related development is shown in Figure 10.2.

Child health clinics play a vital role in the national childhood immunization programme, which commences at 2 months of age. Immunization is a major success story for preventive medicine, preventing diseases that have the potential to cause serious damage to a child's health, or even death. An example of the impact that immunization can have on the profile of infectious diseases is demonstrated by the meningitis C immunization campaign, which began in November 1999. The UK was the first country to introduce the meningitis C conjugate (MenC) vaccine and uptake levels have been close to 90%. The programme was targeted at under-20 year olds and has been a huge success, with a 90% reduction in cases in that age group. Authorities are hoping to mirror the success of the meningitis C campaign with the introduction of pneumococcal vaccine into the routine UK childhood immunization schedule from April 2006.

Advice on the current immunization schedule can be found in the British National Formulary for children (BNF-C), and the Department of Health website (see Useful Paediatric Websites).

Drug disposition

Pharmacokinetic factors

An understanding of the variability in drug disposition is essential if children are to receive rational and appropriate drug therapy. For convenience, the factors that affect drug disposition will be dealt with separately. However, when treating a patient all the factors have a dynamic relationship and none should be considered in isolation.

Absorption

Oral absorption The absorption process of oral preparations may be influenced by factors such as gastric and intestinal transit time, gastric and intestinal pH and gastrointestinal contents. Posture, disease state and therapeutic interventions such as nasogastric aspiration or drug therapy can also affect the absorption process. It is not until the second year of life that gastric acid output increases and is comparable on a per kilogram basis with that observed in adults. In addition, gastric emptying time only approaches adult values at about 6 months of age.

The bioavailability of sulphonamides, digoxin and phenobarbital has been studied in infants and children of a wide age distribution. Despite the different physicochemical properties of the drugs, a similar bioavailability pattern was observed in each case. The rate of absorption was correlated with age, being much slower in neonates than in older infants and children. However, few studies have specifically reported on the absorption process in older infants or children. The available data suggest that in older infants and children orally administered drugs will be absorbed at a rate and extent similar to those in healthy adults. Changes in the absorption rate would appear to be of minor importance when compared to the age-related differences of drug distribution and excretion.

Intramuscular absorption Absorption in infants and children after intramuscular (i.m.) injection is noticeably faster than in the neonatal period, since muscle blood flow is increased. On a practical note, intramuscular administration is very painful and should, where possible, be avoided. The route should not be used for the convenience of staff if alternative routes of administration are available.

Intraosseous absorption This is a useful route of administration in patients in whom intravenous access cannot be obtained. It is especially useful in paediatric cardiorespiratory arrests where rapid access is required. A specially designed needle is usually inserted into the flat tibial shaft until the marrow space is reached. This route is considered equivalent to the intravenous route for rate of drug absorption, and most drugs can be given by this route.

Topical absorption Recent advances in transdermal drug delivery systems have led to an increased use of this route of administration. For example, patch formulations of hyoscine hydrobromide have been found to be very useful to dry up secretions in children with excess drooling; likewise fentanyl patches can be useful in pain management. Percutaneous absorption, which is inversely related to the thickness of the stratum corneum and directly related to skin hydration, is generally much greater in the newborn and young infant than in the adult. This can lead to adverse drug reactions. For example, the topical application of a preparation containing prilocaine and lidocaine (EMLA) should not be used in preterm infants because of concerns about significant absorption of prilocaine in this age group, which may lead to methaemoglobinaemia. The development of needle-free subcutaneous jet injection systems appears to bring many benefits as a method of drug administration. They have been shown to give comparable levels to standard subcutaneous injections and overcome the problems of needle phobia, with less pain on administration. This system has been used with growth hormone, insulin, sedation prior to procedures and vaccination in children.

Another route of topical absorption is ophthalmically. Significant amounts of drugs may be absorbed from ophthalmic preparations through ophthalmic or nasolacrimal duct absorption; for example, administration of phenylephrine eye drops can lead to hypertensive episodes in children.

Rectal absorption The rectal route of administration is generally less favoured in the UK than in other European countries. It can be useful in patients who are vomiting or in infants or children reluctant or unable to take oral medication. The mechanism of rectal absorption is probably similar to that of the upper part of the gastrointestinal tract, despite differences in pH, surface area and fluid content. Although some products are erratically absorbed from the rectum, the rapid onset of action can be invaluable; for example, rectal diazepam solution produces a rapid cessation of seizures in epilepsy and can be easily administered by parents in an emergency.

Buccal absorption The buccal cavity is a potentially useful route of administration in patients who cannot tolerate medications via the oral route, for example postoperative patients or those with severe nausea. Highly lipophilic drugs can rapidly cross the buccal mucosa. Fentanyl is available as a lozenge formulation (Actiq). This has been used to relax children before painful procedures and as a treatment for breakthrough pain in palliative care patients although it remains unlicensed for use in children. Midazolam has also been administered via this route for the acute treatment of seizures and is gaining favour over rectal diazepam for this purpose.

There are a number of 'melt' and 'wafer' formulations available, for example piroxicam and ondansetron. These preparations have the advantage of palatability; however, they are not absorbed via the buccal muscosa but require swallowing and enteral absorption of the active constituent. Desmopressin for buccal absorption has been introduced as an alternative to the tablet formulation; 120 µg is given buccally compared to 200 µg orally.

Intranasal absorption The intranasal route is another useful route of administration. Medicines can be administered intranasally for their local action, e.g. sympathomimetics, or for their systemic effects, e.g. desmopressin in the treatment of diabetes insipidus. Midazolam has been widely used intranasally in children for the treatment of anxiety prior to procedures and also for the treatment of childhood seizures. Highly lipophilic analgesics such as fentanyl are used via this route for the treatment of acute pain, particularly in situations where i.v. access is difficult, e.g. reduction of fractures in the emergency department. Diamorphine may be administered by nasal instillation and is preferred to intramuscular or oral morphine.

Significant systemic absorption of medicines given intranasally for their local effect can also occur; for example, corticosteroids used in the treatment of allergic rhinitis have led to cushingoid symptoms and growth suppression.

Inhalation absorption Direct delivery of drug therapies to the lungs has been the mainstay of treatment for asthma for many years. An exciting new development in this field is the administration of insulin by inhalation for the treatment of both type 1 and type 2 diabetes mellitus in adults. The first licensed product was launched in 2006 although initially it is not licensd for paediatric patients.

Systemic absorption of corticosteroids used in the treatment of asthma may produce adrenal suppression.

Distribution

A number of factors that determine drug distribution within the body are subject to change with age. These include vascular perfusion, body composition, tissue-binding characteristics and the extent of plasma protein binding.

As a percentage of total body weight, the total body water and extracellular fluid volume decrease with age (Table 10.2). Thus, for water-soluble drugs such as aminoglycosides, larger doses on a milligram per kilogram of body weight basis are required in the neonate than in the older child to achieve similar plasma concentrations.

Protein binding Despite normal blood pH, free fatty acid and bilirubin levels in infants, binding to plasma proteins is reduced as a result of low concentrations of both globulins and albumin. It has been suggested that binding values comparable with those seen in adults are reached within the third year of life for acidic drugs, whereas for basic drugs adult values are not reached until between 7 and 12 years of life. The clinical significance of this reduction in infants and older children is minimal. The influence of disease states, such as renal impairment, on plasma protein binding is more important.

Table 10.2 Extracellular fluid volume and total body water as a percentage of body weight

Age	Total body water %	Extracellular fluid %
Preterm neonate	85	50
Term neonate	75	45
3 months	75	30
1 year	60	25
Adult	60	20

Drug metabolism

At birth the majority of the enzyme systems responsible for drug metabolism are either absent or present in considerably reduced amounts compared with adult values, and evidence indicates that the various systems do not mature at the same time. This reduced capacity for metabolic degradation at birth is followed by a dramatic increase in the metabolic rate in the older infant and young child. In the 1–9 year age group in particular, metabolic clearance of drugs is shown to be greater than in adults, as exemplified by theophylline, phenytoin and carbamazepine. Thus to achieve plasma concentrations similar to those observed in adults, children in this age group may require a higher dosage than adults on a milligram per kilogram basis (Table 10.3).

Metabolic pathways that play only a minor role in adults may play a more significant role in children and compensate for any deficiencies in the normal adult metabolic pathway. For example, glucuronidation accounts for up to 70% of the metabolic pathway of paracetamol in adulthood; however, in the early newborn period glucuronidation is deficient, accounting for less than 20% of paracetamol metabolism. This is compensated for by a more pronounced sulphate conjugation and this leads to an apparently normal half-life in newborns. Paracetamol appears to be less toxic in children than in adults and this may be in part explained by the compensatory routes of metabolism.

Renal excretion

The anatomical and functional immaturity of the kidneys at birth limits renal excretory capacity. Below 3–6 months of age the glomerular filtration rate is lower than that of adults, but may be partially compensated for by a relatively greater reduction in tubular

Table 10.3 Theophylline dosage in children older than 1 year

Age	Dosage (mg/kg/day)
1–9 years	24
9–12 years	20
12–16 years	18
Adult	13

reabsorption. Tubular function matures later than the filtration process. Generally, the complete maturation of glomerular and tubular function is reached only towards 6–8 months of age. After 8 months the renal excretion of drugs is comparable with that observed in older children and adults. Changes in renal clearance of gentamicin provide a good example of the maturation of renal function (Table 10.4).

Other factors

In addition to age-related changes in drug disposition, nutritional status and disease states can influence drug handling. High plasma clearance of antibiotics such as penicillins and aminoglycosides has been demonstrated in children with cystic fibrosis; increased elimination of furosemide has been reported in children with nephrotic syndrome, while prolonged elimination of furosemide has been reported in infants with congestive cardiac failure. Altered protein binding has been demonstrated in hepatic disease, nephrotic syndrome, malnutrition and cardiac failure.

Drug therapy in children

Dosage

Doses of medicines in children should be obtained from a paediatric dosage handbook and should not be extrapolated from the adult dose. There are a number of such texts available internationally. The information within them may be based on evidence from clinical studies in children or reflect the clinical experience of the contributors. In the UK, the British National Formulary for Children (BNF-C) (see further reading section) is a national formulary which includes prescribing guidelines and drug monographs. It contains information on licensed, unlicensed and off-label use of medicines. When consulting any dosage reference resource, care should be taken to identify the dosage convention being used. Most formularies use a single dose convention and indicate the number of times the dose should be repeated in a 24-hour period. Other formularies indicate the total daily dose and the number of doses this is divided into. Some formularies combine both conventions. Confusing the total daily dose with the single dose to be repeated may have catastrophic consequences and the single dose convention has become the preferred convention.

Table 10.4 Renal clearance of gentamicin

	Plasma half-life
Small premature infants weighing less than 1.5 kg	11.5 h
Small premature infants weighing 1.5–2 kg	8 h
Term infants and large premature infants less than 1 week of age	5.5 h
Infants 1 week to 6 months	3–3.5 h
Infants more than 6 months to adulthood	2–3 h

While age, weight and height are the easiest parameters to measure, the changing requirement for drug dosage during childhood corresponds most closely with changes in body surface area (BSA). Nomograms which allow the surface area to be easily derived are available. There are practical problems in using the surface area method for prescribing; accurate height and weight may be difficult to obtain in a sick child, and manufacturers rarely provide dosage information on a surface area basis. The surface area formula for children has been used to produce the percentage method, giving the percentage of adult dose required at various ages and weights (Table 10.5).

In selecting a method of dosage calculation, the therapeutic index of the drug should be considered. For agents with a narrow therapeutic index, such as cytotoxic agents, where recommendations are quoted per square metre, dosing must be based on the calculated surface area. However, there may be exceptions, for example in children less than 1 year of age who have a proportionally larger surface area than other age groups. In children less than 1 year, dosages of chemotherapeutic agents are often based on weight rather than surface area to prevent overestimation of the dose in this age group.

For drugs with a wide therapeutic index, such as penicillin, single doses may be quoted for a wide age range. Between these two extremes, doses are quoted in milligrams per kilogram and

this is the most widely used method of calculation. Whichever method is used, the resulting dosage should be rounded sensibly to facilitate dose measurement and administration and subsequently modified according to response or adverse effects.

It is important to note that none of the available methods of dosage calculation account for the change in dosage interval that may be required because of age-related changes in drug clearance. Where possible, the use of therapeutic drug monitoring to confirm the appropriateness of a dose is recommended.

Choice of preparation

The choice of preparation and its formulation will be influenced by the intended route of administration, the age of the child, availability of preparations, other concomitant therapy and, possibly, underlying disease states. The problems of administering medicines to children have recently been reviewed by the European Medicines Evaluation Agency (EMEA 2005).

Buccal route

Drugs may be absorbed rapidly from the buccal cavity (the cheek pouch) or they may dissolve when administered and be swallowed and absorbed from the stomach. 'Melt' technology (e.g. desmopressin, piroxicam, ondansetron), in which the drug and flavourings are freeze-dried into a rapidly dissolving pellet, can be very useful. The 'melt' dissolves instantly into a very small volume which is difficult for the child to reject. Gels, sprays and liquids can also be administered into the buccal cavity, using drugs such as midazolam to treat seizures.

Oral route

The oral route is usually the most convenient but in an unco-operative child it can be the least reliable. Safe and effective drug therapy requires accurate administration, yet the 5 mL spoon is a difficult means of administering liquid medicines. Use of an oral syringe can provide controlled administration, ensure accurate measurement of the calculated dose and avoids the need for dilution of preparations with syrup. Use of oral syringes (which will not fit an intravenous Luer connector) should be mandatory in hospitals. Concentrated formulations may be administered as oral drops in a very small volume. Although convenient, there could be significant dosage errors if drops are not delivered accurately.

In general, liquid preparations are more suitable for children under 7 years of age, although some quite young children can cope with solid dose formulations. Some commercially available products contain excipients such as alcohol, propylene glycol and dyes that may cause adverse effects or be inappropriate for use in children with particular disease states. The osmolality and tonicity of preparations may be important; necrotizing enterocolitis (a disorder seen in the neonatal period) has been associated with many different factors including high-osmolality infant feeding formulae and pharmaceutical preparations, although a causal relationship has not been established. Oral liquids with high osmolality or extremes of pH may irritate the stomach and should be diluted for administration. Sugar-free preparations may be necessary in the diabetic child or be desirable in other children for the prevention of dental caries. It is, however, important to be aware of the potential problems associated with substitutes

Table 10.5 Percentage of adult dose required at various ages and body weights

	Mean weight for age lb	Mean weight for age kg	Percentage of adult dose
Newborn (full term)	7.7	3.5	12.5
2 months	10	4.5	15
4 months	14	6.5	20
1 year	22	10	25
3 years	33	15	33.3
7 years	50	23	50
10 years	66	30	60
12 years	86	39	75
14 years	110	50	80
16 years	128	58	90
Adult	150	68	100

for sucrose. The artificial sweetening agent aspartame, used in some preparations, should be used with caution in children with phenylketonuria because of its phenylalanine content. Other substitutes such as sorbitol and glycerol may not contribute to dental caries but produce diarrhoea if large doses are given. In these instances a specially formulated preparation containing a higher amount of the active drug in small volume may be preferable.

Injection solutions can sometimes be administered orally although their concentration and pH must be considered together with the presence of unsuitable excipients. Powders or small capsules may be prepared and used as an alternative. However, lactose is a common diluent in powders and caution must be exercised in children with lactose intolerance as a result of an inborn error of metabolism, or temporarily following gastrointestinal diseases or gut surgery.

Parents must be discouraged from adding the dose of medicine to an infant's feed. Quite apart from potential interactions which may arise with milk feeds, if the entire feed is not taken a proportion of the dose will be lost. It is also important to advise parents when it is not appropriate to crush solid dosage forms (e.g. sustained-release preparations).

Manufacturers are increasingly recognizing the difficulties associated with administration of medicines to children and are responding with novel formulations such as clarithromycin straws. The individual straws contain granules of medicine that are ingested when the child sips a suitable, favourite drink through the straw device. Carbonated (fizzy) drinks are preferable, as these can mask the sensation in the mouth caused by the granules.

Mini tablets of just a few millimetres diameter may be useful to ease administration and allow flexibility of dosage. They may be presented in capsules or counted from bulk and can be individually coated for positioned or sustained release. Increased surface area may present larger quantities of excipients to the child and requires careful control.

Nasogastric and gastrostomy administration

Medicines may be administered into the stomach via a nasogastric tube in the unconscious child or when swallowing is difficult. A gastrostomy tube may be placed into the stomach transcutaneously if the problem is long term, for example in some children with cerebral palsy. Enteral nutrition may also be administered through such tubes. Drugs such as phenytoin may adsorb to the plastic of the tubes and interact with enteral feeds, requiring special administration techniques to ensure bioavailability (Yeung & Ensom 2000).

Intranasal route

Several drugs, such as desmopressin, diamorphine, fentanyl and midazolam, have been shown to be absorbed from the nasal mucosa. This route may avoid the need for injections but administration may be difficult in the unco-operative child and drugs administered may irritate the mucosa or be painful.

Rectal route

Although the rectal route can be useful, it is limited by the range of products available and the dosage inflexibility associated with rectal preparations. Some oral liquid preparations such as chloral hydrate and carbamazepine can be administered rectally. The route is useful in the unconscious child in the operating theatre or intensive care unit and it is not uncommon to administer perioperative analgesics such as diclofenac and paracetamol and the antiemetic ondansetron using suppository formulations. Parents and teachers may express concerns about using this route, fearing accusations of child abuse, but it is an important route of administration for diazepam or paraldehyde in the fitting child.

When oral and rectal routes are inappropriate the parenteral route may be necessary.

Parenteral route

The problems associated with the administration of intramuscular injections in infants and children have been described earlier in this chapter. The route has a limited role in paediatric drug therapy and should not be used routinely. The intravenous route of administration is more widely used, but it is still associated with a number of potential problems that are outlined below.

Intravenous access The practical difficulties of accessing small veins in the paediatric patient do not require explanation. However, these difficulties can often explain the sites of access that are chosen. Scalp veins, commonly used in newborn infants, are often very prominent in this age group, allowing easy access. It is also more difficult for the infant to dislodge a cannula from this site than from a site on the arm or foot. Likewise the umbilical artery offers a useful route for monitoring the patient but can also be used for drug administration in some circumstances. Vasoconstrictive drugs, such as adrenaline (epinephrine), dopamine and isoprenaline, should not be given by this route.

Fluid overload In infants and children the direct administration of intravenous fluids from the main infusion container is associated with the risk of inadvertent fluid overload. This problem can be avoided by the use of a paediatric administration set and/or a volumetric infusion device to control the flow rate. A paediatric administration set incorporates a graduated volumetric chamber with a maximum capacity of 150 mL. Although this system is intended primarily as a safety device, the volume within the burette chamber can be readily adjusted, allowing its use for intermittent drug administration and avoiding the need for the 'piggy back system' commonly used in adult intravenous administration.

Dilution of parenteral preparations for infusion may also cause inadvertent fluid overload in children. In fluid-restricted or very young infants, it is possible that the volume of diluted drug can exceed the daily fluid requirement. In order to appreciate this problem, the paediatric practitioner should become familiar with the fluid volumes that children can tolerate. As a guide these volumes can be calculated using the following formula: 100 mL/kg for the first 10 kg, plus 50 mL/kg for the next 10 kg, plus 20 mL/kg thereafter. Worked examples are given in Table 10.6. It is important to remember that these volumes do not account for losses such as those caused by dehydration, diarrhoea or artificial ventilation. While the use of more concentrated infusion solutions may overcome the problem of fluid overload, stability data on concentrated solutions are often lacking. It may therefore be necessary to manipulate other therapy to accommodate the treatment or even to consider alternative treatment options.

Table 10.6   Calculation of standard daily fluid requirements in paediatric patients

15 kg patient	35 kg patient
100 mL/kg × 10 kg = 1000 mL	100 mL/kg × 10 kg = 1000 mL
Plus 50 mL/kg × 5 kg = 250 mL	Plus 50 mL/kg × 10 kg = 500 mL
Total = 1250 mL/day	Plus 20 mL/kg × 15 kg = 300 mL
	Total = 1800 mL/day

Fluid overload may also result from excessive volumes of flushing solutions. This problem is described later in this section.

Lack of suitable paediatric formulations   A large number of parenteral products are only available in adult dose sizes. The concentrations of these products can make it difficult to measure the small doses required in paediatrics and may lead to errors.

Displacement volume   Reconstitution of powder injections in accordance with manufacturers' directions usually makes no allowance for the displacement volume of the powder itself. Hence the final volume may be greater than expected and the concentration will therefore be less than expected. This can result in the paediatric patient receiving an underdose, which becomes even more significant in younger patients receiving smaller doses. Paediatric units usually make available modified reconstitution directions which take account of displacement volumes.

Rates of infusion   The slow infusion rates often necessary in paediatrics may influence drug therapy. The greater the distance between the administration port and the distal end of the delivery system, and the slower the flow rate, the longer the time required for the drug to be delivered to the patient. In very young infants and children it may take several hours for the drug to reach the patient, depending on the point of injection. This is an important consideration if dosage adjustments are being made in response to plasma level monitoring. Bolus injections should always be given as close to the patient as possible.

Dead space   Following administration via an injection port, a residual amount of drug solution can remain trapped at the port. If dose volumes are small the trapped fluid may represent a considerable proportion of the intended dose. Similarly the volume of solution required to prime the intravenous lines or the in-line filters (i.e. the dead space) can be a significant proportion of the intended dose. This problem can be minimized by ensuring that drugs are flushed into the main infusion line after administration via an injection port or through a filter, and by priming the lines initially with a compatible solution. The small volumes required to prime filters and tubing specifically designed for infants and children can be used to minimize the dead space. Modern filter materials can produce less adsorption of drugs so that more of the drug is delivered to the patient.

It is important to remember that flushing volumes can add a significant amount to the daily fluid and sodium intake, and it may be important to record the volume of flushing solutions used in patients susceptible to fluid overload.

Excipients   Analogous to oral preparations, excipients may be present in parenteral formulations and can be associated with adverse effects. Benzyl alcohol, polysorbates and propylene glycol are commonly used agents which may induce a range of adverse effects in children including metabolic acidosis, altered plasma osmolality, central nervous system depression, respiratory depression, cardiac arrhythmias and seizures. Knowledge of the products that contain these ingredients may influence drug selection.

Many hospitals have established centralized intravenous additive services (CIVAS) that prepare single intravenous doses under aseptic conditions, thus avoiding the need for preparation at ward level. Such services have not only significantly decreased the risks associated with intravenous therapy, particularly in the paediatric population, but can also produce considerable cost savings.

Pulmonary route

The use of aerosol inhalers for the prevention and treatment of asthma presents particular problems for children because of the co-ordination required. The availability of breath-activated devices and spacer devices and large-volume holding chambers has greatly improved the situation. National guidance has been published on the use of inhaler devices in children less than 5 years of age (NICE 2000) and in older children (NICE 2002). Recent experience has shown that different types of large-volume holding chambers alter drug delivery and absorption and should not be considered as interchangeable.

It must be remembered that drugs can be absorbed into the systemic circulation after pulmonary administration or may be absorbed by the enteral route when excess drug is swallowed. High-dose corticosteroid inhalation may suppress the adrenal cortical axis and growth by this mechanism.

Dose regimen selection

A summary of the factors to be considered when selecting a drug dosage regimen or route of administration for a paediatric patient is shown in Table 10.7.

Counselling adherence and concordance

Parents or carers are often responsible for the administration of medicines to their children and therefore the concordance and adherence of both parties must be considered. Literature about non-adherence and concordance in children is limited, but the problem is considered to be widespread and similar to that reported in adults.

Non-adherence may be caused by several factors such as patient resistance to taking the medicine, complicated dosage regimens, misunderstanding of instructions and apparent ineffectiveness or side effects of treatment. In older children and adolescents who may be responsible for their own medication, different factors may be responsible for non-adherence; for example, they may be unwilling to use their medication because of peer pressure.

Several general principles should be considered in an attempt to improve adherence. Adherence is usually better when fewer

Table 10.7 Factors to be considered when selecting a drug dosage regimen or route of administration for a paediatric patient

Factor	Comment
1. Age/weight/surface area	Is the weight appropriate for the stated age? If it is not, confirm the difference. Can the discrepancy be explained by the patient's underlying disease, e.g. patients with neurological disorders such as cerebral palsy may be significantly underweight for their age? Is there a need to calculate dosage based on surface area (e.g. cytotoxic therapy)? Remember heights and weights may change significantly in children in a very short space of time. It is essential to recheck the surface area at each treatment cycle using recent heights and weights
2. Assess the appropriate dose	The age/weight of the child may have a significant influence on the pharmacokinetic profile of the drug and the manner in which it is handled. In addition, the underlying disease state may influence the dosage or dosage interval
3. Assess the most appropriate interval	In addition to the influence of disease states and organ maturity on dosage interval, the significance of the child's waking day is often overlooked. A child's waking day is generally much shorter than that of an adult and may be as little as 12 hours. Instructions given to parents particularly should take account of this, e.g. the instruction 'three times a day' will bear no resemblance to 'every 8 hours' in a child's normal waking day. If a preparation must be administered at regular intervals, then the need to wake the child should be discussed with the parents or preferably an alternative formulation, such as a sustained-release preparation, should be considered
4. Assess the route of administration in the light of the disease state and the preparations and formulations available	Some preparations may require manipulation to ensure their suitability for administration by a specific route. Even preparations which appear to be available in a particular form may contain undesirable excipients that require alternatives to be found, e.g. patients with the inherited metabolic disorder phenylketonuria should avoid oral preparations containing the artificial sweetener aspartame because of its phenylalanine content
5. Consider the expected response and monitoring parameters	Is the normal pharmacokinetic profile altered in children? Are there any age-specific or long-term adverse effects, such as on growth, that should be monitored?
6. Interactions	Drug interactions remain as important in reviewing paediatric prescriptions as they are in adult practice. However, drug–food interactions may be more significant; particularly drug–milk interactions in babies having 5–6 milk feeds per day
7. Legal considerations	Is the drug licensed? If an unlicensed drug is to be used, the pharmacist should have sufficient information to support its use

medicines are prescribed. Attention should be given to the formulation, taste, appearance and ease of administration of treatment. The regimen should be simple and tailored to the child's waking day.

Many health professionals often counsel the parents/carer only, rather than involving the child in the counselling process. Where possible, treatment goals should be set in collaboration with the child. Studies have shown that parents consider the 8–10 year age group the most appropriate at which to start including the child in the counselling process. As well as verbal instruction, parents often want written information. However, current patient information leaflets must reflect the Summary of Product Characteristics (SPC) and so are often inappropriate. If a drug is used in an 'off-label' manner, statements such as 'not recommended for use in children' may cause confusion and distress. Care needs to be taken, therefore, to ensure that the information provided, whether written or spoken, is appropriate for both the parent and the child.

Medicines in schools

Children who are acutely ill will be treated with medicines at home or in hospital, although during their recovery phase it may be possible to return to school. Children with chronic illness such as asthma or epilepsy, and children recovering from acute illnesses, may require medicines to be administered whilst at school. In addition, there are some medical emergencies which may occur at school or on school trips that require prompt drug administration before the arrival of the emergency services. These emergencies include anaphylaxis (associated with food allergy or insect stings), severe asthma attacks and seizures.

Policies and guidance

There is considerable controversy over the administration of medicines in schools. There is no legal or contractual duty on school staff to administer medicine or supervise a pupil taking it. This is a voluntary role. Some support staff may have specific duties to provide medical assistance as part of their contract. Policies and procedures are required to ensure that prescribed medicines are labelled, stored and administered safely and appropriately, and that teachers and care assistants are adequately trained and understand their responsibilities.

Advice has been provided for schools and their employers on how to manage medicines in schools (Department for Education and Skills 2005). The roles and responsibilities of employers, parents and carers, governing bodies, head teachers, teachers and other staff and of local health services are all explained. The advice considers staffing issues such as employment of staff, insurance and training. Other issues covered include drawing up a healthcare plan for a pupil, confidentiality, record keeping, the storage, access and disposal of medicines, home-to-school transport, and on-site and off-site activities. It also provides general information on four common conditions that may require management at school: asthma, diabetes, epilepsy and anaphylaxis. The document also contains a set of forms which can be photocopied by users.

Responsibility for common medicines

Responsible pupils should be allowed to administer their own medication. Asthmatics should carry their 'reliever' inhaler (e.g. salbutamol or terbutaline), a spare should be available in school, and easy access before and during sports assured. There should be no need to have 'preventer' inhalers at school since two or three times daily administration schedules are appropriate and can avoid school hours. Medicines with a two or three times daily administration schedule should be supplied wherever possible so that dosing during school hours is avoided. Sustained-release preparations or drugs with intrinsically long half-lives may be more expensive but avoid the difficulties of administration at school. Sustained-release methylphenidate and atomoxetine, both used in the management of attention deficit hyperactivity disorder or ADHD, are examples. When administration at school is unavoidable, the schooltime doses can be provided in a separate, labelled container.

Special schools

Some children with severe, chronic illness will go to special rather than mainstream schools where their condition can receive attention from teachers and carers who have undergone appropriate training. Some special schools will be residential. Pupils may also attend another institution for respite care. Particular attention to communication of changes to drug treatment between parents, primary care doctors, hospital doctors and school staff is required if medication errors are to be avoided.

Monitoring parameters

Paediatric vital signs (Table 10.8) and haematological and biochemical parameters (Table 10.9) change throughout childhood and differ from those in adults. The figures presented in the tables are given as examples and may vary from hospital to hospital.

Assessment of renal function

There are a number of methods of measuring renal function in children. These include the use of ^{51}Cr-EDTA, ^{99m}Tc-DTPA and using serum and urine creatinine concentrations over a timed period. However, despite some limitations, serum creatinine and estimated creatinine clearance are the most frequently used and most practical methods for day-to-day assessment of renal function.

Table 10.8 Paediatric vital signs

	Age		
	<1 year	2–5 years	5–12 years
Heart rate (beats/min)	120–140	100–120	80–100
Blood pressure (systolic) (mmHg)	70–90	80–90	90–110
Respiratory rate (breaths/min)	25–45	25–30	16–25

Table 10.9 Biochemical and haematology reference ranges

	Neonate	Child	Adult
Albumin (g/L)	24–48	30–50	35–55
Bilirubin (µmol/L)	<200	<15	<17
Calcium (mmol/L)	1.8–2.8	2.15–2.7	2.20–2.55
Chloride (mmol/L)	95–110	95–110	95–105
Creatinine (µmol/L)	28–60	30–80	50–120
Haemoglobin (g/dL)	18–19	11–14	13.5–18.0 (males) 12–16 (females)
Haematocrit	0.55–0.65	0.36–0.42	0.4–0.45 (males) 0.36–0.44 (females)
Magnesium (mmol/L)	0.6–1.0	0.6–1.0	0.7–1.0
Phosphate (mmol/L)	1.3–3.0	1.0–1.8	0.85–1.4
Potassium (mmol/L)	4.0–7.0	3.5–5.5	3.5–5.0
Sodium (mmol/L)	130–145	132–145	135–145
Urea (mmol/L)	1.0–5.0	2.5–6.5	3.0–6.5
White cell count (× 10^9/L)	6–15	5–14	3.5–11

In adults, several formulae and nomograms are available for calculating and estimating renal function. However, these cannot be extrapolated to the paediatric population; the Cockcroft and Gault equation and the modification of diet in renal disease (eGFR) equation are validated only for patients aged 18 years and over.

A number of validated models are available for use in children. These equations use combinations of serum creatinine, height, weight, body surface area, age and sex to provide a simple estimate of creatinine clearance. A number of these equations have been further modified to better predict creatinine clearance; however, the advantage of simplicity is thereby lost. Several examples with their validated age ranges are shown below:

- Traub and Johnson (age 1–18 years)

$$\text{Creatinine clearance} \atop (\text{mL/min/1.73m}^2) = \frac{42 \times \text{height (cm)}}{\text{Serum creatinine } (\mu\text{mol/L})}$$

- Counhahan (age 2 months to 14 years)

$$\text{Creatinine clearance (mL/min/1.73m}^2) = \frac{38 \times \text{height (cm)}}{\text{Serum creatinine } (\mu\text{mol/L})}$$

- Schwarz

$$\text{Creatinine clearance (mL/min/1.73m}^2) = \frac{\kappa \times \text{height (cm)}}{\text{Serum creatinine } (\mu\text{mol/L})}$$

where κ varies dependent on the age of the patient:

low birth weight infants $= 30$
normal infants 0–18 months $= 40$
girls 2–16 years $= 49$
boys 2–13 years $= 49$
boys 13–16 years $= 60$

Whichever equation is chosen, it should be borne in mind that there are limitations to their use; for example, they should not be used in rapidly changing renal function, anorexic or obese patients, and they should not be taken as an accurate measure but as a guide to glomerular filtration rate.

Adverse drug reactions

The incidence of adverse drug reactions (ADRs) in children outside the neonatal period is thought to be less than at all other ages; however, the nature and severity of the ADRs that children experience may differ from those experienced by adults.

Studies have shown an incidence of ADRs in paediatric patients of between 0.2% and 22% of patients. The wide range reflects the limited number of formal prospective and retrospective studies examining the incidence and characteristics of ADRs in the paediatric age group and the variations in study setting, patient group and definition of adverse drug reaction used. Data can also be skewed by vaccination campaigns since adverse effects are common and reporting encouraged. One consistent finding is that the greater the number of medications the child is exposed to, the greater the risk of ADRs.

ADRs in infants and older children typically occur at lower doses than in adults, and symptoms may be atypical. Examples include:

- enamel hypoplasia and permanent discolouration of the teeth with tetracyclines
- growth suppression with long-term corticosteroids in prepubertal children
- paradoxical hyperactivity in children treated with phenobarbital
- hepatotoxicity associated with the use of sodium valproate. There are three major risk factors:
  age under 3 years
  children receiving other anticonvulsants
  developmental delay.

The mechanism is not fully understood but is thought to relate to altered metabolism and the production of a toxic metabolite.

- increased risk of Reye's syndrome with the use of salicylates in children with mild viral infection. Reye's syndrome is a life-threatening illness associated with drowsiness, coma, hypoglycaemia, seizures and liver failure. The mechanism of this toxicity remains unknown but aspirin should generally be avoided in children under 16 years.

Many adverse drug reactions occur less frequently in the paediatric population, for example gastrointestinal bleeds with NSAIDs, hepatotoxicity with flucloxacillin and severe skin reactions with trimethoprim/sulfamethoxazole.

The reporting of ADRs is particularly important because the current system of drug research and authorization not only deprives children of useful drugs because of the lack of clinical trials in children but may also exclude them from epidemiological studies of ADRs to prescribed drugs. The Commission on Human Medicines (previously the Committee on Safety of Medicines) strongly encourages the reporting of all suspected adverse drug reactions in children, including those relating to unlicensed or off-label use of medicines, even if the intensive monitoring symbol (an inverted black triangle) has been removed. The reporting scheme has been extended in recent years to allow pharmacists, nurses and patients/carers to report suspected ADRs.

Medication errors

In contrast to adverse drug reactions, medication errors occur as a result of human mistakes or system flaws. Medication errors are now recognized as an important cause of adverse drug events in paediatric practice and should always be considered as a possible causative factor in any unexplained situation. They can produce a variety of problems ranging from minor discomfort to death. In the USA it is estimated that 100–150 deaths occur annually in children in hospitals due to medication errors. The actual reported incidence of errors varies considerably between studies, ranging from 0.15% to 17% of admissions. However, different reporting systems and criteria for errors make direct comparisons between studies difficult.

The incidence of medication errors and the risk of serious errors occurring in children are significantly greater than in adults. The causes are many and include the following.

- The heterogeneous nature of the paediatric population with the corresponding lack of standard dosage.
- Calculation errors by the prescriber, dispensing pharmacist, nurse or caregiver.
- Lack of available dosage forms and concentrations appropriate for administration to children, necessitating additional calculations and manipulations of commercially available products.
- Lack of familiarity with paediatric dosing guidelines.
- Confusion between adult and paediatric preparations.
- Limited published information.
- Need for precise dose measurement and appropriate drug delivery systems leading to administration errors and the inappropriate use of measuring devices.
- Tenfold dosing errors are particularly important and potentially catastrophic; however, they appear regularly in the published literature.

The reporting and prevention of medication errors is an important aspect of the paediatric pharmacist's role. The causes of medication errors are usually multifactorial and it is essential that when investigating medication errors, particular focus should be placed on system changes.

Licensing medicines for children

Medicines licensing process

All medicines marketed in the UK must have been granted a product licence (PL) under the terms of the Medicines Act 1968, or a marketing authorization (MA) following more recent European legislation on the authorization of medicines. The aim of licensing is to ensure that medicines have been assessed for safety, quality and efficacy. In the UK, evidence submitted by a pharmaceutical company is assessed by the Medicines and Healthcare products Regulatory Agency (MHRA) with independent advice from the Commission on Human Medicines (CHM) and its paediatric expert group.

The licensed indications for a drug are published in the Summary of Product Characteristics (SPC). Many medicines granted a PL or MA for adult use have not been scrutinized by the licensing authorities for use in children. This is reflected by contraindications or cautionary wording in the SPC. There is a lack of commercial incentive to develop medicines for the relatively small paediatric market and perceived difficulties in carrying out clinical trials in this group. It is not illegal to use medicines for indications or ages not specified in the data sheet but to ensure safe and effective treatment, health professionals should have adequate supporting information about the intended use before proceeding. Failure to ensure that the use of a medicine is reasonable could result in a suit for negligence if the patient comes to harm.

Unlicensed and 'off-label' medicines

Up to 35% of drugs used in a large children's hospital and 10% of drugs used in general practice may be used outside the terms of the approved, licensed indications (McIntyre et al 2000, Turner et al 1998). In the USA the term 'off-label' is often used to describe this. Because many of these medicines will have been produced in 'adult' dose forms, such as tablets, it is often necessary to prepare extemporaneously a suitable liquid preparation for the child. This may be made from the licensed dose form, e.g. by crushing tablets and adding suitable excipients, or from chemical ingredients. An appropriate formula with a validated expiry period and ingredients to approved standards should be used. Care must be taken to ensure accurate preparation, particularly when using formulae or ingredients, such as 'old-fashioned' galenicals, which are unfamiliar.

On some occasions the drug to be used has no PL or MA, perhaps because it is only just undergoing clinical trials in adults, has been imported from another country, has been prepared under a 'specials' manufacturing licence or is being used for a rare condition for which it has not previously been employed. As with 'off-label' use, there must always be information to support the quality, efficacy and safety of the medicine as well as information on the intended use. There is always a risk in using such a medicine, which must be balanced against the seriousness of the child's illness and discussed with the parents if practicable.

Some authorities suggest that the patient should always be informed if the medicine prescribed is unlicensed or 'off label' and even that written informed consent be obtained before treatment begins. In many situations in paediatrics this would be impractical but if parents are not informed the patient information leaflet (PIL) included with many medicines may cause confusion since it may state that it is 'not for use in children'. Patient or parent information specific to the situation should be prepared and provided.

Recent legislation on medicines for children

The worldwide legislation on medicines for children is beginning to change. This is in recognition of the limited research and small number of licensed medicines brought about by a lack of incentive for commercial development. Both Europe and the USA have orphan drugs regulations designed to offer incentives for the development of medicines for rare diseases. Although not exclusively for paediatric conditions, the regulations have assisted the development of important drugs such as antiretrovirals (HIV/AIDS), alendronate (osteogenesis imperfecta), α-galactosidase (Fabry's disease), sodium phenylbutyrate (hyperammonaemia) and ibuprofen injection (closure of patent ductus arteriosus).

The USA has had regulations designed to promote the development of paediatric preparations for more than 10 years (currently Best Pharmaceuticals for Children Act 2002 and Pediatric Research Equity Act 2003). However, these regulations have resulted in few significant developments in medicines for children in other countries. In the European Union, the 'European Parliament and Council Regulation (EC) on medicinal products for paediatric use' became law in January 2007. Thereafter, pharmaceutical companies wishing to market medicines for adults must agree a Paediatric Investigation Plan with the EMEA. In return for such development the company will receive an additional 6 months market exclusivity for its product. There are also expected to be incentives for developing paediatric formulations and indications for off-patent medicines.

In preparation for the European regulations and to stimulate research, several European governments have funded paediatric clinical trials networks. In the UK, the Medicines for Children Research Network (MCRN) is part of the UK Clinical Research Network and has six local research networks in England with equivalent provision in the other UK countries. Research and development of paediatric formulations will be a part of the MCRN programme.

Service frameworks

National service frameworks (NSFs) are long-term strategies for improving specific areas of care. Two paediatric service frameworks have been published; one for paediatric intensive care (DH 2002) and another for children, young people and maternity services (DH 2004).

The service framework for paediatric intensive care defines the nature of paediatric intensive care, the elements of a high-quality paediatric intensive care service and a policy framework for the future organization of services. Standards for district general hospitals, lead centres, major acute general hospitals and specialist hospitals are set out and cover medical and nurse staffing, facilities, and clinical effectiveness and management.

Other aspects considered include retrieval services, education and training needs, and the implications for audit and research.

The NSF for children, young people and maternity services sets standards for children's health and social services, and the interface of those services with education. It establishes clear standards for promoting the health and well-being of children and young people and for providing high-quality services which meet their needs.

The recommendations that relate to the use of medicines for children and young people include the following.

- All children and young people should receive medicines that are safe and effective, in formulations that can easily be administered and are appropriate to their age, having minimum impact on their education and lifestyle.
- Medicines are prescribed, dispensed and administered by professionals who are well trained, informed and competent to work with children to improve health outcomes and minimize harm and any side effects of medicines.
- Children and young people and their parents or carers are well informed and supported to make choices about their medicines and are competent in the administration of medicines.

Markers of good practice are defined as follows.

- The use of medicines in children is based on the best available evidence of clinical and cost-effectiveness and safety, ideally derived from clinical trials but also including, where appropriate, medicines that are not licensed for their age group or for their particular health problem ('off-label') or those that do not have a licence at all ('unlicensed') in order to achieve the best possible health outcomes and minimize harm and side effects.
- In all settings and whatever the circumstances, children and young people have equitable access to safe, clinically and cost-effective medicines in age-appropriate formulations.
- Appropriate information and decision support are available for professionals who prescribe, dispense and administer medicines for children and young people.
- Children, young people and their parents/carers receive consistent, up-to-date, comprehensive, timely information on the safe and effective use of medicines.
- In all settings, professionals enable parents, young people and, where appropriate, children to be active partners in the decisions about the medicines prescribed for them.
- Primary and secondary care providers should ensure that the use of medicines in children is incorporated in their clinical governance and audit arrangements.
- The contribution of pharmacists to the effective and safe use of medicines in children is maximized.

CASE STUDIES

Case 10.1

PT
7 years old
Male
16 kg

| Presenting condition: | Presented in the emergency department with a 2-day history of worsening groin and hip pain. Could |

not weight bear. Patient was febrile with a temperature of 39.2°C, vomiting and dehydrated. There was no history of injury.

PMH:	Nil of note
Allergies:	No known drug allergies
Drug history:	Nil of note
Differential diagnosis:	Septic arthritis, osteomyelitis
Tests:	Urea and electrolytes
	Full blood count
	CRP, ESR
	Blood culture and sensitivities
	X-ray (hips and abdomen)
	Bone scan
Results:	Bone scan revealed right pubic osteomyelitis
	CRP = 56 mg/L (normal range 0–10 mg/L)
	ESR = 34 mm/h (normal range 1–10 mm/h)
	Blood culture revealed *Staphylococcus aureus* sensitive to flucloxacillin
Prescribed:	Flucloxacillin i.v. 800 mg four times a day for 2 weeks. To be followed by oral flucloxacillin 800 mg four times a day for 4 weeks
Progress:	Temperature settled and ESR/CRP decreased following initiation of antibiotic therapy

On the third day of treatment the patient developed a raised red rash which was suspected of being an allergic reaction to flucloxacillin. Treatment was changed to i.v. clindamycin 160 mg three times a day (10 mg/kg per dose) for 2 weeks followed by oral clindamycin 160 mg three times a day for a further 4 weeks.

Question

Comment on the drug therapy and any monitoring required.

Answer

There are a number of points to consider in this patient.

- Body weight appears low for age; therefore need to check the weight is correct (expected weight for a 7 year old is approx 23 kg). If incorrect, doses of medication will need to be recalculated.
- Recommended i.v. dose of flucloxacillin of 50 mg/kg/dose is correct. However, usual maximum oral dose of flucloxacillin is 25 mg/kg/dose. This is because of the increased risk of gastric side effects with high oral doses of flucloxacillin.
- There is a need to consider compliance with oral flucloxacillin therapy due to poor palatability of suspension formulation (if the child would not take capsules) and the frequent dosing regimen.
- Whilst the risk of flucloxacillin-induced hepatotoxicity is low in children, there is a need to consider measuring baseline and repeat liver function tests because of the prolonged course (more than 2 weeks) of flucloxacillin therapy.
- Clindamycin has good oral bioavailability so i.v. therapy may be unnecessary.
- The recommended dose of clindamycin by i.v. infusion is up to 10 mg/kg dose 6 hourly in severe infection. The infusion should be diluted to 6 mg/mL with sodium chloride 0.9% or dextrose 5% (or a combination) and administered over 30–60 minutes at a maximum rate of 20 mg/kg/h. Consider 160 mg in 27 mL sodium chloride 0.9% over 30 minutes.
- The recommended standard oral dose of clindamycin is 3–6 mg/kg/dose four times a day. This may contribute to problems with adherence to long-term therapy. A three times daily dosing regimen is to be preferred, particularly as this child may return to school, and four times

daily dosing would require a dose to be administered at school which may be problematic.
- Consideration should be given to how to administer clindamycin. Clindamycin palmitate suspension, which was palatable, is no longer available as a licensed preparation in the UK. Whilst extemporaneous formulations are available that use clindamycin hydrochloride capsules, the palatability of the resultant suspension is a major concern, particularly given the prolonged course of therapy. A 75 mg/5 mL suspension, licensed in Belgium, can be imported. From a safety and efficacy perspective it is preferable to use such a product, which has been through a regulatory process similar to that of the UK, than to compound an extemporaneous preparation, which has not undergone appropriate pharmaceutical/pharmacokinetic evaluation.
- Consideration could be given to decreasing the dose of clindamycin to 150 mg three times a day to accommodate capsules, although the child may have difficulty taking these.
- The most serious adverse effect of clindamycin is antibiotic-associated colitis. Therefore it is important to monitor for diarrhoea. If this arises treatment should be discontinued.

Case 10.2

CS
18 months old
Female
10 kg

Presenting condition:	Severe right-sided abdominal pain Vomiting and loss of appetite Increased temperature 38.2°C
PMH:	Nil of note
Allergies:	No known allergies
Drug history:	Nil of note
Tests:	Ultrasound
Provisional diagnosis:	Appendicitis

CS went to theatre where an appendicectomy was performed. The appendix was noted to be perforated.

Prescribed: Morphine 50 mg in 50 mL to run at 1–4 mL/h (10–40 µg/kg/h)
Paracetamol 200 mg four times a day p.r.n p.o./p.r.
Diclofenac 12.5 mg twice a day as required p.r.
or
Ibuprofen 100 mg four times a day required orally when tolerating milk

Five days of i.v. antibiotic therapy with:
- Gentamicin 70 mg daily
- Ampicillin 250 mg four times a day
- Metronidazole 75 mg three times a day

Question

Comment on the patient's drug therapy.

Answer

- The morphine dose is incorrect. If the infusion is prepared as directed, 1 mL/h will actually provide 100 µg/kg/h. This is a tenfold overdose which is a medication error frequently seen in children
- There is a need to consider how to administer the appropriate rectal dose of paracetamol to this child. Often postappendicectomy patients will need to be nil by mouth for several days. Rectal bioavailability is lower than oral bioavailability and there may be a need to consider giving a larger rather than smaller p.r. paracetamol dose, i.e. possibly 250 mg p.r. 8 hourly rather than 125 mg 6 hourly, for up to 48 hours, but not exceeding 90 mg/kg/day.
- Suggest that paracetamol and NSAID are administered regularly in addition to the morphine for at least the first few days post surgery. Multimodal analgesic therapy is recommended.
- There will be a need to monitor CS for side effects. Nausea, vomiting and pruritus all occur frequently with morphine but can be treated/prevented.
- Young children are particularly susceptible to developing myoclonic jerks with morphine. These are often worrying for parents but resolve on withdrawal of the morphine.
- NSAIDs are well tolerated by children and the risk of adverse events is much lower in children than the adult population. However, it is important to ensure adequate hydration status postoperatively, particularly when using NSAIDs. Acute renal failure has been reported in children who have been treated with NSAIDs and not adequately hydrated.
- The choice of antibiotics for CS is appropriate. High-dose (7 mg/kg) once-daily aminoglycoside (gentamicin/tobramycin) therapy is now routinely used in children. It is administered by short infusion over 20 minutes. Plasma drug levels should be monitored to achieve a 18–24 hour trough level of <1mg/L. Monitor U&E and serum creatinine. Ampicillin can be given as a bolus injection over 3–5 minutes. Metronidazole should be given as a short infusion over 20 minutes

REFERENCES

Department for Education and Skills 2005 Managing medicines in schools and early years settings. Department for Education and Skills, London. Available online at: http://publications.teachernet.gov.uk/eOrderingDownload/1448-2005DCL-ENv3final.pdf
Department of Health 2002 National service framework for paediatric intensive care. Stationery Office, London
Department of Health 2004 The national service framework for children, young people and maternity services. Stationery Office, London. Available online at: www.dh.gov.uk/ PolicyAndGuidance/HealthAndSocialCareTopics/ChildrenServices/ChildrenServicesInformation/fs/en
EMEA 2005 Reflection paper: formulations of choice for the paediatric population. European Medicines Evaluation Agency, London. Available online at: www.emea.eu.int/pdfs/human/peg/19481005en.pdf
International Committee on Harmonization 2000 Note for guidance on clinical investigation of medicinal products in the paediatric population. European Agency for the Evaluation of Medicinal Products, London
McIntyre J, Conroy S, Avery A et al 2000 Unlicensed and off label prescribing of drugs in general practice. Archives of Disease in Childhood 83: 498-501

MRC Vitamin Study Research Group 1991 Prevention of neural tube defects: results of the Medical Research Council vitamin study. Lancet 338: 131-137
National Institute for Clinical Excellence 2000 Guidance on the use of inhaler systems (devices) in children under the age of 5 years with chronic asthma. Technology Appraisal No 10. National Institute for Clinical Excellence, London
National Institute for Clinical Excellence 2002 Asthma-inhaler devices for older children. Technology Appraisal No 38. National Institute for Clinical Excellence, London
Scott E, Swanton J, McElnay J et al 1995 Pharmacists and child health. Centre for Pharmacy Postgraduate Education/HMSO, London
Turner S, Longworth A, Nunn A J et al 1998 Unlicensed and off-label drug use in paediatric wards: prospective study. British Medical Journal 316: 343-345
Yeung S C, Ensom M H 2000 Phenytoin and enteral feedings: does evidence support an interaction? Annals of Pharmacotherapy 3(7-8): 896-905

FURTHER READING

Advanced Life Support Group 2004 Emergency paediatric care. Blackwell, London

Advanced Life Support Group 2005 Pre hospital paediatric life support: the practical approach. BMJ Books, London

Behrman R E, Kliegman R M, Jenson H B (eds) 2003 Nelson textbook of pediatrics, 17th edn. W B Saunders, Philadelphia

Joint Working Party of the British Paediatric Association and the Association of the British Pharmaceutical Industry 1996 Licensing medicines for children. British Paediatric Association, London

NHS Education for Scotland (NES) 2005 An introduction to paediatric pharmaceutical care. Available online at: www.nes.scot.nhs.uk/pharmacy

Phelps S J, Hak E B 2004 Teddy bear book: pediatric injectable drugs, 7th edn. American Society of Health System Pharmacists, USA

USEFUL PAEDIATRIC DOSAGE REFERENCE SOURCES

British National Formulary for Children (BNF-C) 2006 Pharmaceutical Press, London. Available online at: www.bnfc.nhs.uk/bnfc/

Lewisham and North Southwark Health Authority 2004 Guy's, St Thomas's and Lewisham Hospitals paediatric formulary, 7th edn. Lewisham and North Southwark Health Authority, London

Royal Children's Hospital, Melbourne 2002 Paediatric pharmacopeia, 13th edn. Parville, Australia

Taketomo C, Hodding J H, Kraus D M 2006 Paediatric dosage handbook, 13th edn. Lexi-Comp, Hudson, Ohio

USEFUL PAEDIATRIC WEBSITES

- The National Congenital Anomalies System
  www.statistics.gov.uk/CCI/SearchRes.asp?term=congenital+anomalies
- Child Growth Standards
  www.who.int/childgrowth/en/
- Immunization against infectious diseases
  www.dh.gov.uk/PolicyAndGuidance/HealthAndSocialCareTopics/GreenBook/
- Royal College of Paediatrics and Child Health
  www.rcpch.ac.uk/

- Drug Information Advisory Line (Dial) – a national paediatric medicines information resource
  www.dial.org.uk
- Neonatal and Paediatric Pharmacists Group (NPPG)
  www.nppg.org.uk/
- Contact a Family (for families with disabled children)
  www.cafamily.org.uk/

Geriatrics 11

H. G. M. Shetty K. Woodhouse

KEY POINTS

- The elderly form about 18% of the population and receive about one-third of health service prescriptions in the UK.
- Ageing results in physiological changes that affect the absorption, metabolism, distribution and elimination of drugs.
- Alzheimer's disease and multi-infarct dementia are the most important diseases of cognitive dysfunction in the elderly. Donepezil, rivastigmine and galantamine are inhibitors of acetylcholinesterase and improve cognitive function in Alzheimer's disease.
- The elderly patient with Parkinson's disease is more susceptible to the adverse effects of levodopa such as postural hypotension, ventricular dysrhythmias and psychiatric effects.
- Aspirin and clopidogrel reduce the reoccurrence of non-fatal strokes in the elderly.
- Treatment of elevated systolic and diastolic blood pressure in the elderly with a low-dose thiazide diuretic, calcium antagonist or angiotensin-converting enzyme inhibitor have all been shown to be beneficial.
- Urinary incontinence can be classified as stress incontinence, overflow incontinence or due to detrusor instability. Stress incontinence is not amenable to drug therapy. The drugs most commonly used in detrusor instability are trospium and tolterodine.
- Non-steroidal anti-inflammatory drugs (NSAIDs) are more likely to cause gastroduodenal ulceration and bleeding in the elderly.

There has been a steady increase in the number of elderly people, defined as those over 65 years of age, since the beginning of the 20th century. They formed only 4.8% of the population in 1901, increasing to 15.2% in 1981 and about 18% in 2001. Between 1991 and 2031 the total population of England and Wales is expected to increase by 8%. However, the numbers of those aged between 60 and 74 years will rise by 43%, those aged between 75 and 84 by 48% and those aged over 85 years by 138%. The significant increase in the number of very elderly people will have important social, financial and healthcare planning implications.

The elderly have multiple and often chronic diseases. It is not surprising therefore that they are the major consumers of medicines. Elderly people receive about one-third of National Health Service (NHS) prescriptions in the UK. In most developed countries the elderly now account for 25–40% of drug expenditure.

A survey of drug usage in 778 elderly people in the UK showed that 70% had been on prescribed medication and 40% had taken one or more prescribed drugs within the previous 24 hours; 32% were taking cardiovascular drugs and the other therapeutic categories used in decreasing order of frequency were for disorders of the central nervous system (24%), musculoskeletal system (10%), gastrointestinal system (8%) and respiratory system (7%). The most commonly used drugs were diuretics, analgesics, hypnotics, sedatives and anxiolytics, antirheumatic drugs and β-blockers.

Institutionalized patients tend to be on larger numbers of drugs compared with patients in the community. Patients in long-term care facilities have been shown to be receiving on average eight or more drugs. Psychotropic drugs are used widely in nursing or residential homes.

For optimal drug therapy in the elderly, a knowledge of age-related physiological and pathological changes that might affect handling of, and response to, drugs is essential. This chapter discusses the age-related pharmacokinetic and pharmacodynamic changes which might affect drug therapy and the general principles of drug use in the elderly.

Pharmacokinetics

Ageing results in many physiological changes that could theoretically affect absorption, first-pass metabolism, protein binding, distribution and elimination of drugs. Age-related changes in the gastrointestinal tract, liver and kidneys include reduced:

- gastric acid secretion
- gastrointestinal motility
- total surface area of absorption
- splanchnic blood flow
- liver size
- liver blood flow
- glomerular filtration
- renal tubular filtration.

Absorption

There is a delay in gastric emptying, reduction in gastric acid output and splanchnic blood flow with ageing. These changes do not significantly affect the absorption of the majority of drugs. Although the absorption of some drugs such as digoxin may be slower, the overall absorption is similar to that in the young.

First-pass metabolism

After absorption, drugs are transported via the portal circulation to the liver, where many lipid-soluble agents are metabolized extensively (more than 90–95%). This results in a marked reduction in systemic bioavailability. Obviously, even minor reductions in first-pass metabolism can result in a significant increase in the bioavailability of such drugs.

Impaired first-pass metabolism has been demonstrated in the elderly for several drugs, including clomethiazole, labetalol, nifedipine, nitrates, propranolol and verapamil. The clinical effects of some of these, such as the hypotensive effect of nifedipine, may be significantly enhanced in the elderly. In frail hospitalized elderly patients, i.e. those with chronic debilitating disease, the reduction in presystemic elimination is even more marked.

Distribution

The age-related physiological changes which may affect drug distribution are:

- reduced lean body mass
- reduced total body water
- increased total body fat
- lower serum albumin level
- α_1-acid glycoprotein level unchanged or slightly raised.

Increased body fat in the elderly results in an increased volume of distribution for fat-soluble compounds such as clomethiazole, diazepam, desmethyl-diazepam and thiopental. On the other hand, reduction in body water results in a decrease in the distribution volume of water-soluble drugs such as cimetidine, digoxin and ethanol.

Acidic drugs tend to bind to plasma albumin, while basic drugs bind to α_1-acid glycoprotein. Plasma albumin levels decrease with age and therefore the free fraction of acidic drugs such as cimetidine, furosemide and warfarin will increase. Plasma α_1-acid glycoprotein levels may remain unchanged or may rise slightly with age, and this may result in minimal reductions in free fractions of basic drugs such as lidocaine. Disease-related changes in the level of this glycoprotein are probably more important than age per se.

The age-related changes in distribution and protein binding are probably of significance only in the acute administration of drugs because, at steady state, the plasma concentration of a drug is determined primarily by free drug clearance by the liver and kidneys rather than by distribution volume or protein binding.

Renal clearance

Although there is a considerable interindividual variability in renal function in the elderly, in general the glomerular filtration rate declines, as do the effective renal plasma flow and renal tubular function. Because of the marked variability in renal function in the elderly, the dosages of predominantly renally excreted drugs should be individualized. Reduction in dosages of drugs with a low therapeutic index, such as digoxin and aminoglycosides, may be necessary. Dosage adjustments may not be necessary for drugs with a wide therapeutic index, for example penicillins.

Hepatic clearance

Hepatic clearance (Cl_H) of a drug is dependent on hepatic blood flow (Q) and the steady-state extraction ratio (E), as can be seen in the following formula:

$$Cl_H = Q \times \frac{C_a - C_v}{C_a}$$
$$= Q \times E$$

where C_a and C_v are arterial and venous concentrations of the drug, respectively. It is obvious from the above formula that when E approaches unity, Cl_H will be proportional to and limited by Q. Drugs which are cleared by this mechanism have a rapid rate of metabolism, and the rate of extraction by the liver is very high. The rate-limiting step, as mentioned earlier, is hepatic blood flow and therefore drugs cleared by this mechanism are called 'flow limited'. On the other hand, when E is small, Cl_H will vary according to the hepatic uptake and enzyme activity, and will be relatively independent of hepatic blood flow. The drugs which are cleared by this mechanism are termed 'capacity limited'.

Hepatic extraction is dependent upon liver size, liver blood flow, uptake into hepatocytes, and the affinity and activity of hepatic enzymes. Liver size falls with ageing and there is a decrease in hepatic mass of between 20% and 40% between the third and tenth decades. Hepatic blood flow falls equally with declining liver size. Although it is recognized that the microsomal mono-oxygenase enzyme systems are significantly reduced in ageing male rodents, recent evidence suggests that this is not the case in ageing humans. Conjugation reactions have been reported to be unaffected in the elderly by some investigators, but a small decline with increasing age has been described by others.

Impaired clearance of many hepatically eliminated drugs has been demonstrated in the elderly. Morphological changes rather than impaired enzymatic activity appear to be the main cause of impaired elimination of these drugs. In frail debilitated elderly patients, however, the activities of drug-metabolizing enzymes such as plasma esterases and hepatic glucuronyltransferases may well be impaired.

Pharmacodynamics

Molecular and cellular changes that occur with ageing may alter the response to drugs in the elderly. There is, however, limited information about these alterations because of the technical difficulties and ethical problems involved in measuring them. It is not surprising therefore that there is relatively little information about the effect of age on pharmacodynamics.

Changes in pharmacodynamics in the elderly may be considered under two headings:

- those due to a reduction in homeostatic reserve
- those that are secondary to changes in specific receptor and target sites.

Reduced homeostatic reserve

Orthostatic circulatory responses

In normal elderly subjects there is blunting of the reflex tachycardia that occurs in young subjects on standing or in response to vasodilation. Structural changes in the vascular tree that occur with ageing are believed to contribute to this observation, although the exact mechanism is unclear. Antihypertensive drugs, drugs with α-receptor blocking effects (e.g. tricyclic antidepressants, phenothiazines and some butyrophenones), drugs which decrease sympathetic outflow from the central nervous system (e.g. barbiturates, benzodiazepines, antihistamines and morphine) and antiparkinsonian drugs (e.g. levodopa and bromocriptine) are therefore more likely to produce hypotension in the elderly.

Postural control

Postural stability is normally achieved by static reflexes, which involve sustained contraction of the musculature, and phasic reflexes, which are dynamic, short term and involve transient corrective movements. With ageing, the frequency and amplitude of corrective movements increase and an age-related reduction in dopamine (D_2) receptors in the striatum has been suggested as the probable cause. Drugs which increase postural sway, for example hypnotics and tranquillizers, have been shown to be associated with the occurrence of falls in the elderly.

Thermoregulation

There is an increased prevalence of impaired thermoregulatory mechanisms in the elderly, although it is not universal. Accidental hypothermia can occur in the elderly with drugs that produce sedation, impaired subjective awareness of temperature, decreased mobility and muscular activity, and vasodilation. Commonly implicated drugs include phenothiazines, benzodiazepines, tricyclic antidepressants, opioids and alcohol, either on its own or with other drugs.

Cognitive function

Ageing is associated with marked structural and neurochemical changes in the central nervous system. Cholinergic transmission is linked with normal cognitive function and in the elderly the activity of choline acetyltransferase, a marker enzyme for acetylcholine, is reduced in some areas of the cortex and limbic system. Several drugs cause confusion in the elderly: anticholinergics, hypnotics, H_2-antagonists and β-blockers are common examples.

Visceral muscle function

Constipation is a common problem in the elderly as there is a decline in gastrointestinal motility with ageing. Anticholinergic drugs, opiates, tricyclic antidepressants and antihistamines are more likely to cause constipation or ileus in the elderly. Anticholinergic drugs may cause urinary retention in elderly men, especially those who have prostatic hypertrophy. Bladder instability is common in the elderly and urethral dysfunction more prevalent in elderly women. Loop diuretics may cause incontinence in such patients.

Age-related changes in specific receptors and target sites

Many drugs exert their effect via specific receptors. Response to such drugs may be altered by the number (density) of receptors, the affinity of the receptor, postreceptor events within cells

resulting in impaired enzyme activation and signal amplification, or altered response of the target tissue itself. Ageing is associated with some of these changes.

α-Adrenoceptors

α_2-Adrenoceptor responsiveness appears to be reduced with ageing while α_1-adrenoceptor responsiveness appears to be unaffected.

β-Adrenoceptors

β-Adrenoceptor function declines with age. It is recognized that the chronotropic response to isoprenaline infusion is less marked in the elderly. Propranolol therapy in the elderly produces less β-adrenoceptor blocking effect than in the young. In isolated lymphocytes, studies of cyclic adenosine monophosphate (AMP) production have shown that on β-adrenoceptor stimulation the dose–response curve is shifted to the right, and the maximal response is blunted.

An age-related reduction in β-adrenoceptor density has been shown in animal adipocytes, erythrocytes and brain, and also in human lymphocytes in one study, although this has not been confirmed by other investigators. As maximal response occurs on stimulation of only 0.2% of β-adrenoceptors, a reduction in the number by itself is unlikely to account for age-related changes. Some studies have shown a reduction in high-affinity binding sites with ageing, in the absence of change in total receptor numbers, and others have suggested that there may be impairment of postreceptor transduction mechanisms with ageing that may account for reduced β-adrenoceptor function.

Cholinergic system

The effect of ageing on cholinergic mechanisms is less well known. Atropine produces less tachycardia in elderly humans than in the young. It has been shown in ageing rats that the hippocampal pyramidal cell sensitivity to acetylcholine is reduced. The clinical significance of this observation is unclear.

Benzodiazepines

The elderly are more sensitive to benzodiazepines than the young, and the mechanism of this increased sensitivity is not known. No difference in the affinity or number of benzodiazepine-binding sites has been observed in animal studies. Habituation to benzodiazepines occurs to the same extent in the elderly as in the young.

Warfarin

The elderly are more sensitive to warfarin. This phenomenon may be due to age-related changes in pharmacodynamic factors. The exact mechanism is unknown.

Digoxin

The elderly appear to be more sensitive to the adverse effects of digoxin, but not to the cardiac effects.

Common clinical disorders

This section deals in detail only with the most important geriatric diseases. Other conditions are mentioned primarily to highlight areas where the elderly differ from the young or where modifications of drug therapy are necessary.

Dementia

Dementia is characterized by a gradual deterioration of intellectual capacity. Alzheimer's disease (AD) and multi-infarct dementia (MID) are the most important diseases of cognitive dysfunction in the elderly. AD has a gradual onset and it progresses slowly. Forgetfulness is the major initial symptom. The patient has difficulty in dressing and other activities of daily living. They tend to get lost in their own environment. Eventually the social graces are lost. MID is the second most important cause of dementia. It usually occurs in patients in their 60s and 70s, and is more common in those with a previous history of hypertension or stroke. Abrupt onset and stepwise progression of dementia are characteristic of MID. Mood changes and emotional lability are common. There may be focal neurological deficit. A number of drugs and other conditions cause confusion in the elderly, and their effects may be mistaken for dementia. These are listed in Table 11.1.

In patients with AD, damage to the cholinergic neurones connecting subcortical nuclei to the cerebral cortex has been consistently observed. Postsynaptic muscarinic cholinergic receptors are usually not affected, but ascending noradrenergic and serotonergic pathways are damaged, especially in younger patients. Based on those abnormalities, several drugs have been investigated for the treatment of AD. Lecithin, which increases acetylcholine concentrations in the brain, 4-aminopyridine, piracetam, oxitacetam and pramiracetam, all of which stimulate acetylcholine release, have been tried but have produced no, or unimpressive, improvements in cognitive function. Anticholinesterases block the breakdown of acetylcholine and enhance cholinergic transmission. Tetrahydroaminoacridine (THA, which is a longer acting anticholinesterase) showed promise in non-blinded clinical studies. However, a controlled clinical trial did not show any benefit.

The use of donepezil, rivastigmine and galantamine for treatment of AD has received support (NICE 2001). Donepezil is a piperidine-based acetylcholinesterase inhibitor. It has been shown to improve cognitive function in patients with mild to moderately severe AD. However, it does not improve day-to-day functioning, quality of life measures or rating scores of overall dementia. It is well tolerated. Rivastigmine is a non-competitive cholinesterase inhibitor. It has been shown to slow the rate of decline in cognitive and global functioning in AD. It is associated with anorexia, nausea, vomiting and weight loss. Other adverse effects include agitation, confusion, depression and diarrhoea. Galantamine, a reversible and competitive inhibitor of acetylcholinesterase, has also been shown to improve cognitive function significantly and is well tolerated.

Deposition of amyloid (in particular the peptide β/A4) derived from the Alzheimer amyloid precursor protein (APP) is an important pathological feature of the familial form of AD that accounts for about 20% of patients. Point mutation of the gene coding for APP (located in the long arm of chromosome 21) is thought to be associated with familial AD. Future treatment strategies, therefore, might involve development of drugs which inhibit amyloidogenesis.

There have been few studies on the management of MID, although at least one report has shown that the progression of the illness may be delayed by aspirin therapy.

Parkinsonism

Parkinsonism is a relatively common disease of the elderly with a prevalence of between 50 and 150 per 100 000. It is characterized by resting tremors, muscular rigidity and bradykinesia (slowness of initiating and carrying out voluntary movements). The patient has a mask-like face, monotonous voice and walks with a stoop and a slow shuffling gait.

The elderly are more susceptible than younger patients to some of the adverse effects of antiparkinsonian drugs. Because of the age-related decline in orthostatic circulatory responses, postural hypotension is more likely to occur in elderly patients with levodopa therapy. The elderly are more likely to have severe cardiac disease, and levodopa preparations should be used with caution in such patients because of the risk of serious ventricular dysrhythmias. Psychiatric adverse effects such as confusion, depression, hallucinations and paranoia occur with dopamine agonists and levodopa preparations. These adverse effects may persist for several months after discontinuation of the offending drug and may result in misdiagnosis (e.g. of AD) in the elderly. Bromocriptine and other ergot derivatives should be avoided in elderly patients with severe peripheral arterial disease as they may cause peripheral ischaemia. Drug therapy of parkinsonism is discussed in detail in Chapter 32.

Table 11.1   Causes of confusion in the elderly

Drugs
Antiparkinsonian drugs
Barbiturates
Benzodiazepines
Cimetidine
Diuretics
Hypoglycaemic agents
Monoamine oxidase inhibitors
Opioids
Steroids
Tricyclic antidepressants

Conditions
Hypothyroidism
Vitamin B$_{12}$ deficiency
Chronic subdural haematoma
Normal pressure hydrocephalus
Alcoholism

Stroke

Stroke is the third most common cause of death and the most common cause of adult disability in UK. About 110 000 people in England and Wales have their first stroke each year and about 30 000 people go on to have further strokes. The incidence of stroke increases 100-fold from the fourth to the ninth decades (Intercollegiate Stroke Working Party 2004).

Treatment of acute stroke

About 85% of strokes are due to cerebral embolism or thrombosis resulting in ischaemia, and 15% are due to haemorrhage. A number of drugs have been investigated for treatment of ischaemic stroke (Adams et al 2005).

Thrombolytic agents The National Institute of Neurological Disorders and Stroke (1995) in the USA showed that, compared with placebo, thrombolysis with tissue plasminogen activator (rt-PA) within 3 hours of onset of ischaemic stroke improved clinical outcome at 3 months despite increased incidence (6%) of symptomatic intracranial bleeding. European co-operative acute stroke studies (ECASS I: Hacke et al 1995; ECASS II: Hacke et al 1998) of thrombolsis with rt-PA failed to show a significant benefit on an intention-to-treat primary analysis. The Canadian Alteplase for Stroke Effectiveness Study (CASES) showed excellent clinical outcome in 37% of patients treated with alteplase within 3 hours of stroke onset. Symptomatic intracranial haemorrhage occurred in 4.6% of patients in this study (Hill et al 2005). In many countries alteplase is now routinely being used to treat acute ischaemic stroke, within 3 hours of stroke onset, in appropriately selected patients.

Antiplatelet therapy Aspirin in doses of 150–300 mg commenced within 48 hours of onset of ischaemic stroke has been shown to reduce the relative risk of death or dependency by 2.7% up to 6 months after the event in two large studies, the Chinese Acute Stroke Trial (CAST) and the International Stroke Trial (IST) (Chen et al 2000).

Anticoagulation Use of intravenous unfractionated heparin and low molecular weight heparin has not been shown to be beneficial and is associated with increased risk of intracranial haemorrhage.

Neuroprotective agents A large number of neuroprotective agents have been used for treatment of acute ischaemic stroke but none has been shown to have long-term beneficial effects.

Secondary prevention

Aspirin in doses of 75–1500 mg/day has been shown to reduce the risk of non-fatal strokes. This is likely to be due to its antiplatelet effect. There is some evidence that addition of dipyridamole to aspirin may enhance the protective effect against stroke (Redman & Ryan 2001). Clopidogrel, which inhibits ADP-induced platelet aggregation, has been shown to be as effective as aspirin in secondary stroke prevention. Clopidogrel is not associated with neutropenia, unlike ticlopidine which is no longer used for stroke prevention. However, thrombotic thrombocytopenic purpura has been reported very rarely with the use of clopidogrel. Combination therapy of clopidogrel with aspirin has been shown to be associated with significant increase in the risk of life-threatening bleeding.

In patients with atrial fibrillation who have had a previous stroke or transient ischaemic attack, anticoagulation with warfarin (INR 1.5–2.7) has been shown to be significantly better than aspirin for secondary prevention. Anticoagulation has not been shown to be effective for secondary prevention in patients with sinus rhythm.

Adequate control of hypertension, diabetes and hyperlipidaemia, stopping smoking and reducing alcohol consumption are also important in secondary stroke prevention. Although there is no evidence to support the use of hypolipidaemic drugs in elderly patients aged over 75 years, the decision as to whether to treat or not should be based on appropriate risk assessment on an individual basis.

Primary prevention

A number of randomized controlled trials have shown that anticoagulation with warfarin compared with placebo reduces the risk of stroke in patients with atrial fibrillation (Benavente et al 2000). As with secondary prevention, control of risk factors such as hypertension, hyperlipidaemia, diabetes, smoking and ethanol abuse is important.

Osteoporosis

Osteoporosis is a progressive disease characterized by low bone mass and microarchitectural deterioration of bone tissue resulting in increased bone fragility and susceptibility to fracture. It is an important cause of morbidity in postmenopausal women. The most important complication of osteoporosis is fracture of the hip. Fractures of wrist, vertebrae and humerus also occur. In the UK over 200 000 fractures occur each year, costing the health service £1.5 billion per year of which 87% is spent on hip fractures.

Prevention

As complications of osteoporosis have enormous economic implications, preventive measures are extremely important (Law et al 1991). Regular exercise has been shown to halve the risk of hip fractures. Stopping smoking before the menopause reduces the risk of hip fractures by 25%.

Treatment

Vitamin D and calcium Vitamin D deficiency is common in elderly people. Treatment for 12–18 months with 800 iu of vitamin D plus 1.2 g of calcium given daily has been shown to reduce hip and non-vertebral fractures in elderly women (mean age 84 years) living in sheltered accommodation. However, recent studies indicate that vitamin D plus calcium on its own is not sufficient to protect against fractures in postmenopausal women. Except in subjects with vitamin D deficiency, supplementation of the vitamin alone has little effect on bone mineral density. Calcium supplementation on its own does not reduce fracture incidence and is no longer recommended for treatment of osteoporosis.

Calcitriol and alfacalcidol Calcitriol (1,25-dihydroxy vitamin D), the active metabolite of vitamin D, and alfacalcidol, a synthetic analogue of calcitriol, reduce bone loss and have been shown to reduce vertebral fractures, but not consistently. Serum calcium should be monitored regularly in patients receiving these drugs.

Bisphosphonates The bisphosphonates, synthetic analogues of pyrophosphate, bind strongly to the bone surface and inhibit bone resorption. The oral bisphosphonates currently used for the treatment of osteoporosis include alendronate, etidronate and risedronate. Alendronate can be given either daily (10 mg) or weekly (70 mg) with equal efficacy. It is effective in reducing vertebral, wrist and hip fractures by about 50%. Etidronate is given cyclically with calcium supplements to reduce the risk of bone mineralization defects. It reduces the risk of vertebral fractures by 50% in postmenopausal women. There is no evidence to support its effectiveness in preventing hip fractures. Risedronate reduces vertebral fractures by 41% and non-vertebral fractures by 39%. It has been shown to significantly reduce the risk of hip fractures in postmenopausal women. Ibandronate 2.5 mg daily or 150 mg monthly reduces both vertebral and non-vertebral fractures. Intravenous zoledronate, after a single dose of 4 mg, has been shown to decrease bone resorption and increase bone mineral density for up to a year.

All bisphosphonates cause gastrointestinal side effects. Alendronate and risedronate are associated with severe oesophageal reactions, including oesophageal stricture. Patients should not take these tablets at bed time and should be advised to stay upright for at least 30 minutes after taking them. They should avoid food for at least 2 hours before and after taking etidronate. Alendronate and risedronate should be taken 30 minutes before the first food or drink of the day. Bisphosphonates should be avoided in patients with renal impairment.

Hormone replacement therapy (HRT)   Oestrogens increase bone formation and reduce bone resorption. They also increase calcium absorption and decrease renal calcium loss. HRT, if started soon after the menopause, is effective in preventing vertebral fractures but has to be continued lifelong if protection against fractures is to be maintained. It is associated with increased risk of endometrial cancer, breast cancer and venous thromboembolism. One study has shown that HRT may increase the risk of deaths due to myocardial disease in elderly women with pre-existing ischaemic heart disease.

Calcitonin Calcitonin inhibits osteoclasts and decreases the rate of bone resorption, reduces bone blood flow and may have central analgesic actions. It is effective in all age groups in preventing vertebral bone loss. It is costly and has to be given parenterally or intranasally. It should not be given for more than 3–6 months at a time to avoid its inhibitory effects on bone resorption and formation, which usually disappear after 2–4 weeks. Antibodies do develop against calcitonin, but they do not affect its efficacy. Calcitonin is useful in treating acute pain associated with osteoporotic vertebral fractures.

Strontium ranelate Strontium ranelate stimulates calcium uptake in bone and inhibits bone resorption. In postmenopausal osteoporotic women it reduces vertebral fracture by 40%. It must be taken within a 4-hour fast, though this can be at bed time.

Teriparatide Teriparatide comprises the first 34 amino acids of parathyroid hormone which produce its major biological effects. It increases bone formation and bone mass without causing hypercalcaemia. Daily subcutaneous injection of teriparatide in a dose of 20 μg reduces the risk of vertebral and non-vertebral fractures. It also increases bone mineral density in vertebrae and femoral neck (Rosen 2005) but is only licensed for 18 months' use.

Arthritis

Osteoarthrosis, gout, pseudogout, rheumatoid arthritis and septic arthritis are the important joint diseases in the elderly. Treatment of these conditions is similar to that in the young. If possible, NSAIDs should be avoided in patients with osteoarthrosis. Total hip and knee replacements should be considered in patients with severe arthritis affecting these joints.

Hypertension

Hypertension is an important risk factor for cardiovascular and cerebrovascular disease in the elderly. The incidence of myocardial infarction is 2.5 times higher, and that of cerebrovascular accidents twice as high in elderly hypertensive patients compared with non-hypertensive subjects. Elevated systolic blood pressure is the single most important risk factor for cardiovascular disease and more predictive of stroke than diastolic blood pressure.

There is evidence that treatment of both systolic and diastolic blood pressure in the elderly is beneficial. One large study has shown reductions in cardiovascular events, and mortality associated with cerebrovascular accidents in treated elderly patients with hypertension (Amery et al 1986). The treatment did not reduce the total mortality significantly. Another study (SHEP 1991), which used low-dose chlortalidone to treat isolated systolic hypertension (systolic blood pressure 160 mmHg or more with diastolic blood pressure less than 95 mmHg), showed a 36% reduction in the incidence of stroke, with a 5-year benefit of 30 events per 1000 patients. It also showed a reduction in the incidence of major cardiovascular events with a 5-year absolute benefit of 55 events per 1000 patients. In addition, this study reported that antihypertensive therapy was beneficial even in patients over the age of 80 years. Subgroup meta-analysis of seven randomized controlled trials, which included 1670 patients over 80 years, showed that antihypertensive therapy for about 3.5 years reduced the risk of heart failure by 39%, strokes by 34% and major cardiovascular events by 22%.

Treatment

Non-pharmacological   In patients with asymptomatic mild hypertension, non-pharmacological treatment is the method of choice. Weight reduction to within 15% of desirable weight, restriction of salt intake to 4–6 g/day, regular aerobic exercise such as walking, restriction of ethanol consumption and stopping smoking are the recommended modes of therapy.

Pharmacological

Thiazide diuretics Thiazides lower peripheral resistance and do not significantly affect cardiac output or renal blood flow. They are effective, cheap and well tolerated and have also been shown to reduce the risk of hip fracture in elderly women by 30%. They can be used in combination with other antihypertensive drugs. Adverse effects include mild elevation of creatinine, glucose, uric acid and serum cholesterol levels as well as hypokalaemia. They should be used in low doses, as higher doses only increase the incidence of adverse effects without increasing their efficacy.

β-Blockers Although theoretically the β-blockers are expected to be less effective in the elderly, they have been shown to be as effective as diuretics in clinical studies. Water-soluble β-blockers such as atenolol may cause fewer adverse effects in the elderly.

Calcium antagonists Calcium antagonists act as vasodilators. Verapamil and, to some extent, diltiazem decrease cardiac output. These drugs do not have a significant effect on lipids or the central nervous system. They may be more effective in the elderly, particularly in the treatment of isolated systolic hypertension. Adverse effects include headache, oedema and postural hypotension. Verapamil may cause conduction disturbances and decrease cardiac output. The use of short-acting dihydropyridine calcium antagonists, such as nifedipine, is controversial. Some studies have indicated adverse outcomes with these agents, particularly in patients with angina or myocardial infarction.

Angiotensin-converting enzyme (ACE) inhibitors and angiotensin receptor blockers (ARBs) ACE inhibitors, ARBs and other vasodilators used for treatment of hypertension are discussed elsewhere. The ACE inhibitors and ARBs should be used with care in the elderly, who are more likely to have underlying atherosclerotic renovascular disease that could result in renal failure. Excessive hypotension is also more likely to occur in the elderly.

Myocardial infarction

The diagnosis of myocardial infarction in the elderly may be difficult in some patients because of an atypical presentation. In the majority of patients, chest pain and dyspnoea are the common presenting symptoms. Confusion may be a presenting factor in up to 20% of patients over 85 years of age. The diagnosis is made on the basis of history, serial electrocardiograms and cardiac enzyme estimations.

The principles of management of myocardial infarction in the elderly are similar to those in the young. Thrombolytic therapy has been shown to be safe and effective in elderly patients.

Cardiac failure

In addition to the typical features of cardiac failure, i.e. exertional dyspnoea, oedema, orthopnoea and paroxysmal nocturnal dyspnoea (PND), elderly patients may present with atypical symptoms. These include confusion due to poor cerebral circulation, vomiting and abdominal pain due to gastrointestinal and hepatic congestion, or insomnia due to PND. Dyspnoea may not be a predominant symptom in an elderly patient with arthritis and immobility. Treatment of cardiac failure depends on the underlying cause and is similar to that in the young. Diuretics, ACE inhibitors, β-blockers, nitrates and digoxin are the important drugs used in the treatment of cardiac failure in the elderly. ACE inhibitors are valuable for the treatment of cardiac failure and have been shown to reduce mortality in patients with moderate-to-severe heart failure. Treatment with β-blockers has been shown to increase left ventricular ejection fraction in patients with cardiac failure due to ischaemic or idiopathic aetiology. They do not appear to improve exercise tolerance, but some studies indicate that they may reduce mortality and the number of admissions to hospitals.

Leg ulcers

Leg ulcers are common in the elderly. They are mainly of two types: venous or ischaemic. Other causes of leg ulcers are blood diseases, trauma, malignancy and infections, but these are less common in the elderly. Venous ulcers occur in patients with varicose veins who have valvular incompetence in deep veins due to venous hypertension. They are usually located near the medial malleolus and are associated with varicose eczema and oedema. These ulcers are painless unless there is gross oedema or infection. Ischaemic ulcers, on the other hand, are due to poor peripheral circulation and occur on the toes, heels, foot and lateral aspect of the leg. They are painful and are associated with signs of lower limb ischaemia, such as absent pulse or cold lower limb. There may be a history of smoking, diabetes or hypertension.

Venous ulcers respond well to treatment and over 75% heal within 3 months. Elevation of the lower limbs, exercise, compression bandage and local antiseptic creams when there is evidence of infection, with or without steroid cream, are usually effective. Antiseptics should not be used when there is granulation tissue. Topical streptokinase may be useful to remove the slough on the ulcers. Gell colloid occlusive dressings may also be useful in treating chronic ulcers. Skin grafting may be necessary for large ulcers. Ischaemic ulcers do not respond well to medical treatment, but improving local blood flow by bypass grafting or angioplasty may help in healing (Grey et al 2006).

Urinary incontinence

Urinary incontinence in the elderly may be of three main types.

1. *Stress incontinence:* due to urethral sphincter incompetence. It occurs almost exclusively in women and is associated with weakening of pelvic musculature. Involuntary loss of small amounts of urine occurs on performing activities which increase intra-abdominal pressure, e.g. coughing, sneezing, bending, lifting, etc. It does not cause significant nocturnal symptoms.
2. *Overflow incontinence:* constant involuntary loss of urine in small amounts. Prostatic hypertrophy is a common cause and is often associated with symptoms of poor stream and incomplete emptying. Increased frequency of micturition at night is often a feature. Use of anticholinergic drugs and diabetic autonomic neuropathy are other causes.
3. *Detrusor instability:* causes urge incontinence where a strong desire to pass urine is followed by involuntary loss of large amounts of urine either during the day or night. It is often associated with neurological lesions or urinary outflow obstruction, e.g. prostatic hypertrophy, but in many cases the cause is unknown.

Stress incontinence is not amenable to drug therapy. In patients with prostatic hypertrophy α_1-blockers such as prazosin, indoramin, alfuzosin, terazosin and tamsulosin have all been shown to increase peak urine flow rate and improve symptoms in about 60% of patients. They reduce outflow obstruction by blocking α_1-receptors and thereby relaxing prostate smooth muscle.

Postural hypotension is an important adverse effect and occurs in 2–5% of patients.

5α-Reductase converts testerone to dihydrotestosterone (DHT) which plays an important role in the growth of prostate. The 5α-reductase inhibitor finasteride reduces the prostate volume by 20% and improves peak urine flow rate. The clinical effects, however, might not become apparent until after 3–6 months of treatment. Main adverse effects are reductions in libido and erectile dysfunction in 3–5% of patients.

The most commonly used drugs for detrusor instability are trospium and tolterodine, both of which are antimuscarinic. Both drugs also cause antimuscarinic side effects such as dry mouth, blurred vision and constipation.

Constipation

The age-related decline in gastrointestinal motility and treatment with drugs which decrease gastrointestinal motility predispose the elderly to constipation. Decreased mobility, wasting of pelvic muscles and a low intake of solids and liquids are other contributory factors. Faecal impaction may occur with severe constipation, which in turn may cause subacute intestinal obstruction, abdominal pain, spurious diarrhoea and faecal incontinence. Adequate intake of dietary fibre, regular bowel habit and use of bulking agents such as bran or ispaghula husk may help to prevent constipation. When constipation is associated with a loaded rectum, a stimulant laxative such as senna or bisacodyl may be given. Frail, ill elderly patients with a full rectum may have atonic bowels that will not respond to bulking agents or softening agents, and in such cases a stimulant is more effective. A stool-softening agent such as docusate sodium is effective when stools are hard and dry. For severe faecal impaction a phosphate enema may be needed. Long-term use of stimulant laxatives may lead to abuse and atonic bowel musculature.

Gastrointestinal ulceration and bleeding

Gastrointestinal bleeding associated with peptic ulcer is less well tolerated by the elderly. The clinical presentation may sometimes be atypical with, for example, patients presenting with confusion. *Heliocobacter pylori* infection is common and its treatment is similar to that in younger patients.

NSAIDs are more likely to cause gastroduodenal ulceration and bleeding in the elderly.

Principles and goals of drug therapy in the elderly

A thorough knowledge of the pharmacokinetic and pharmacodynamic factors discussed is essential for optimal drug therapy in the elderly. In addition, some general principles based on common sense, if followed, may result in even better use of drugs in the elderly.

Avoid unnecessary drug therapy

Before commencing drug therapy it is important to ask the following questions.

- Is it really necessary?
- Is there an alternative method of treatment?

In patients with mild hypertension, for example, it may be perfectly justified to try non-drug therapies which are of proven efficacy. Similarly, unnecessary use of hypnotics should be avoided. Simple measures such as emptying the bladder before going to bed to avoid having to get up, avoidance of stimulant drugs in the evenings or night or moving the patient to a dark, quiet room may be all that is needed.

Effect of treatment on quality of life

The aim of treatment in elderly patients is not just to prolong life but also to improve the quality of life. To achieve this, the correct choice of treatment is essential. In a 70-year-old lady with severe osteoarthrosis of the hip, for example, total hip replacement is the treatment of choice rather than prescribing NSAIDs with all their attendant adverse effects.

Treat the cause rather than the symptom

Symptomatic treatment without specific diagnosis is not only bad practice but can also be potentially dangerous. A patient presenting with 'indigestion' may in fact be suffering from angina and therefore treatment with H_2-blockers or antacids is clearly inappropriate. When a patient presents with a symptom every attempt should be made to establish the cause of the symptom and specific treatment, if available, should then be given.

Drug history

A drug history should be obtained in all elderly patients. This will ensure that the patient is not prescribed a drug or drugs to which they may be allergic, or the same drug or group of drugs to which they have previously not responded. It will help to avoid potentially serious drug interactions.

Concomitant medical illness

Concurrent medical disorders must always be taken into account. Cardiac failure, renal impairment and hepatic dysfunction are particularly common in the elderly, and may increase the risk of adverse effects of drugs.

Choosing the drug

Once it is decided that a patient requires drug therapy, it is important to choose the drug likely to be the most efficacious and least likely to produce adverse effects. It is also necessary to take into consideration co-existing medical conditions. For example, it is inappropriate to commence diuretic therapy to treat mild hypertension in an elderly male with prostatic hypertrophy. A calcium antagonist is more appropriate in this situation.

Dose titration

In general, elderly patients require relatively smaller doses of all drugs compared with young adults. It is recognized that the majority of adverse drug reactions in the elderly are dose related and potentially preventable. It is therefore rational to start with the smallest possible dose of a given drug in the least number of doses and then gradually increase both, if necessary. Dose titration should obviously take into consideration age-related pharmacokinetic and pharmacodynamic alterations that may affect the response to the chosen drug.

Choosing the right dosage form

Most elderly patients find it easier to swallow syrups or suspensions or effervescent tablets rather than large tablets or capsules.

Packaging and labelling

Many elderly patients with arthritis find it difficult to open child-resistant containers and blister packs. Medicines should be dispensed in easy-to-open containers that are clearly labelled using large print.

Good record keeping

Information about a patient's current and previous drug therapy, alcohol consumption, smoking and driving habits may help in choosing appropriate drug therapy when the treatment needs to be altered. It will help to reduce costly duplications and will also identify and help to avoid dangerous drug interactions.

Regular supervision and review of treatment

A UK survey showed that 59% of prescriptions to the elderly had been given for more than 2 years, 32% for more than 5 years and 16% for more than 10 years. Of all prescriptions given to the elderly, 88% were repeat prescriptions; 40% had not been discussed with the doctor for at least 6 months, especially prescriptions for hypnotics and anxiolytics. The survey also showed that 31% of prescriptions were considered pharmacologically questionable, and 4% showed duplication of drugs. It is obvious that there is a need for regular and critical review of all prescriptions, especially when long-term therapy is required.

Adverse drug reactions

It is recognized that ADRs occur more frequently in the elderly. A multicentre study in the UK in 1980 showed that ADRs were the only cause of admission in 2.8% of 1998 admissions to 42 units of geriatric medicine. It also showed that ADRs were contributory to a further 7.7% of admissions. On the basis of this study it can be estimated that up to 15 000 geriatric admissions per annum in the UK are at least partly due to an ADR. Obviously, this has enormous economic implications.

The elderly are more susceptible to ADRs for a number of reasons (Routledge et al 2003). They are usually on multiple drugs, which in itself can account for the increased incidence of ADRs. It is, however, recognized that ADRs tend to be more severe in the elderly, and gastrointestinal and haematological ADRs are more common than would be expected from prescribing

figures alone. Age-related pharmacokinetic and pharmacodynamic alterations and impaired homeostatic mechanisms are the other factors which predispose the elderly to ADRs, by making them more sensitive to the pharmacological effects of the drugs. Not surprisingly, up to 80% of ADRs in the elderly are dose dependent and therefore predictable.

Adherence

Although it is commonly believed that the elderly are poor compliers with their drug therapy, there is no clear evidence to support this. Studies in Northern Ireland and continental Europe have shown that the elderly are as adherent to their drug therapy as the young, provided that they do not have confounding disease. Cognitive impairment, which is not uncommon in old age, multiple drug therapy and complicated drug regimens may impair adherence in the elderly. Poor adherence may result in treatment failure. The degree of adherence required varies depending on the disease being treated. For treatment of a simple urinary tract infection, a single dose of an antibiotic may be all that is required and therefore compliance is not important. On the other hand, adherence of 90% or more is required for successful treatment of epilepsy or difficult hypertension. Various methods have been used to improve adherence, including prescription diaries, special packaging, training by pharmacists and counselling.

Conclusion

The number of elderly patients, especially those aged over 75 years, is steadily increasing and they are accounting for an ever-increasing proportion of healthcare expenditure in the West. Understanding age-related changes in pharmacodynamic factors, avoiding polypharmacy and regular and critical review of all drug treatment will help in the rationalization of drug prescribing, reduction in drug-related morbidity and also the cost of drug therapy for this important subgroup of patients.

CASE STUDIES

Case 11.1

An 80-year-old woman presented to an outpatient clinic with a history of severe giddiness and a few episodes of blackouts. She was being treated for angina and hypertension. She had been on bendroflumethiazide 2.5 mg once daily and slow-release isosorbide mononitrate 60 mg once daily for a few years. Her primary care doctor had recently commenced nifedipine SR 20 mg twice daily for poorly controlled hypertension. On examination her blood pressure was 120/70 mmHg while supine and 90/60 mmHg on standing up.

Question

What is the underlying problem in this patient, and could it be caused by any of the medications that she is taking?

Answer

This patient obviously has significant postural hypotension. All her drugs have the potential to produce postural hypotension and when used together, they may produce symptomatic postural hypotension.

It is important to recognize that some drugs such as nifedipine and nitrates have impaired first-pass metabolism in the elderly and that their clinical effects are enhanced. In addition, orthostatic circulatory responses are also impaired in the elderly. The need for antihypertensive drugs should be carefully assessed in all elderly patients and, if therapy is indicated, the smallest dose of drug should be commenced and increased gradually. Patients should also be told to avoid sudden changes of posture.

Case 11.2

An 85-year-old man was admitted to hospital with anorexia, nausea and vomiting. He was known to have atrial fibrillation, congestive cardiac failure and chronic renal impairment. He was on digoxin 250 µg once daily and furosemide 80 mg twice daily.

His serum biochemistry revealed the following (normal range in parentheses):

Potassium	4.5 mmol/L (3.5–5)
Urea	40 mmol/L (3.0–6.5)
Creatinine	600 µmol/L (50–120)
Digoxin	3.5 µg/L (1–2)

Question

What are the likely underlying problems in this patient and do they necessitate a change in therapy?

Answer

The patient's biochemical results confirm the presence of renal impairment and digoxin toxicity. As digoxin is predominantly excreted through the kidneys, the dose should be reduced in the presence of impaired renal function. In the presence of severe renal impairment, digitoxin, which is predominantly metabolized in the liver, can be used instead of digoxin.

Case 11.3

An 80-year-old woman with a previous history of hypothyroidism presented with a history of abdominal pain and vomiting. She had not moved her bowels for the previous 7 days. Two weeks earlier her primary care doctor had prescribed a combination of paracetamol and codeine to control pain in her osteoarthritic hips.

Question

What are the likely underlying causes of this patient's bowel dysfunction?

Answer

This patient developed severe constipation after taking an analgesic containing codeine. Ageing is associated with decreased gastrointestinal motility. Hypothyroidism, which is common in the elderly, is also associated with reduced gastrointestinal motility. Whenever possible, drugs that are known to reduce gastrointestinal motility should be avoided in the elderly.

Case 11.4

A 75-year-old lady who suffered from osteoarthritis of hip and knee joints presented with a history of passing black stools. Her drug therapy included diclofenac 50 mg three times daily and paracetamol 1 g as required.

Question

What is the likely cause of this patient's symptoms?

Answer

The likely cause is upper gastrointestinal bleeding due to the NSAID diclofenac. Elderly people are more prone to develop ulceration in stomach and duodenum with NSAIDs compared with young patients.

Case 11.5

A 70-year-old man was found to have hypertension and was commenced on lisinopril 5 mg once a day by his primary care doctor. He had a previous history of peripheral vascular disease for which he had required angioplasty. Two weeks after commencing antihypertensive treatment he presented with lack of appetite, nausea and decreased urine output.

Question

What do you think has happened? What is the most likely underlying problem?

Answer

The patient is probably developing renal failure. With a previous history of peripheral vascular disease, he is likely to have bilateral renal artery stenosis. ACE inhibitors can cause renal failure in the presence of bilateral renal stenosis by reducing blood supply to the kidneys.

REFERENCES

Adams H, Adams R, Del Zoppo G et al 2005 Guidelines for the early management of patients with ischaemic stroke: 2005 guidelines update. A scientific statement from the Stroke Council of the American Heart Association/American Stroke Association. Stroke 36: 916-923

Amery A, Birkenhager W, Brixko P et al 1986 Efficacy of antihypertensive drug treatment according to age, sex, blood pressure, and previous cardiovascular disease in patients over the age of 60. Lancet 2: 589-592

Benavente O, Hart R, Koudstaal P et al 2000 Oral anticoagulants for preventing stroke in patients with non-valvular atrial fibrillation and no previous history of stroke or transient ischaemic attacks. Cochrane Review. Cochrane Library, issue no. 3. Update Software, Oxford

Chen Z M, Sandercock P, Pan H C et al 2000 Indications for early aspirin use in acute ischaemic stroke: a combined analysis of 40,000 randomised patients from the Chinese Acute Stroke Trial and the International Stroke

Trial. On behalf of the CAST and IST collaborative groups. Stroke 31: 1240-1249

Grey J E, Enoch S, Harding K G 2006 Venous and arterial leg ulcers. British Medical Journal 332: 347-350

Hacke W, Kaste M, Fieschi C et al, for the ECASS Study Group 1995 Intravenous thrombolysis with tissue plasminogen activator for acute hemispheric stroke: the European Cooperative Acute Stroke Study (ECASS). Journal of the American Medical Association 274: 1017-1025

Hacke W, Kaste M, Fieschi C et al 1998 Randomised double-blind placebo-controlled trial of thrombolytic therapy with intravenous alteplase in acute ischaemic stroke (ECASS II). Second European–Australasian acute stroke study investigators. Lancet 352: 1245-1251

Hill M D, Buchan A M, for the CASES Investigators 2005 Thrombolysis for acute ischemic stroke: results of the Canadian Alteplase for Stroke Effectiveness Study. Canadian Medical Association Journal 172: 1307-1312

Intercollegiate Stroke Working Party 2004 National clinical guidelines for stroke, 2nd edn. Royal College of Physicians, London

Law M R, Wald N J, Mead W 1991 Strategies for prevention of osteoporosis and hip fracture. British Medical Journal 303: 453-459

National Institute for Clinical Excellence 2001 Guidance on the use of donepezil, rivastigmine and galantamine for the treatment of Alzheimer's disease. Technology appraisal guidance 19. National Institute for Clinical Excellence, London

National Institute of Neurological Disorders and Stroke rt-PA Stroke Study Group 1995 Tissue plasminogen activator for acute ischaemic stroke. New England Journal of Medicine 333: 1581-1587

Redman A R, Ryan G J 2001 Analysis of trials evaluating combinations of acetylsalicylic acid and dipyridamole in the secondary prevention of stroke. Clinical Therapeutics 23: 1391-1408

Rosen C J 2005 Postmenopausal osteoporosis. New England Journal of Medicine 353: 595-603

Routledge P A, O'Mahoney M S, Woodhouse K W 2003 Adverse drug reactions in elderly patients. British Journal of Clinical Pharmacology 57:121-126

SHEP Cooperative Research Group 1991 Prevention of stroke by antihypertensive drug treatment in older persons with isolated systolic hypertension: final results of the Systolic Hypertension in the Elderly Programme (SHEP). Journal of the American Medical Association 265: 3255-3264

FURTHER READING

Cummings J L 2004 Alzheimer's disease. New England Journal of Medicine 351: 56-67

Iqbal P, Castleden C M 1997 Management of urinary incontinence in the elderly. Gerontology 43: 151-157

Norton P, Brubaker L 2006 Urinary incontinence in women. Lancet 367: 57-67

Prisant L M, Moser M 2000 Hypertension in the elderly: can we improve results of therapy? Archives of Internal Medicine 160: 283-289

THERAPEUTICS

Peptic ulcer disease 12

S. Ghosh   M. Kinnear

KEY POINTS

- The two main types of peptic ulcer disease are those associated with *Helicobacter pylori* and those associated with non-steroidal anti-inflammatory drugs (NSAIDs).
- Ulcer-like dyspepsia does not correlate with diagnosis of peptic ulcer.
- Uninvestigated dyspepsia without alarm symptoms may be treated empirically without an endoscopic diagnosis.
- An *H. pylori* test and treat strategy means it is unknown if the patient has an ulcer.
- Triple therapy with a proton pump inhibitor (PPI), clarithromycin and amoxicillin twice daily for 7 days is currently the recommended first-line *H. pylori* eradication regimen.
- Patient compliance influences the success of *H. pylori* eradication therapy.
- *H. pylori* eradication therapy does not have a role in management of gastro-oesophageal reflux disease. Its benefit in the management of functional dyspepsia is small.
- Patients who need to continue NSAID therapy are the only patients with peptic ulcer disease in whom continued ulcer healing therapy is necessary after the ulcer has healed.
- Upper gastrointestinal symptoms in NSAID users do not correlate well with presence or absence of peptic ulcers.
- The risk of ulcers associated with NSAID use is common to all non-specific NSAIDs and is dose dependent. The risk is maintained during treatment and decreases once treatment is stopped.
- Risk factors for NSAID-induced gastrointestinal complications include age >65, previous history of peptic ulcer or gastrointestinal bleeding, concomitant use of aspirin, anticoagulants or corticosteroids.
- Adding gastroprotective agents such as a proton pump inhibitor to non-specific NSAIDs provides a similar reduction in risk of gastrointestinal toxicity to that offered by COX-2 inhibitors.
- Enteric coating or taking with food does not reduce the risk of upper gastrointestinal bleeding associated with NSAIDs and low-dose aspirin.
- Adding a gastroprotective proton pump inhibitor to aspirin is associated with lower risk of gastrointestinal bleeding than clopidogrel alone.
- Approximately one-third of deaths from gastrointestinal bleeding are due to NSAIDs, and up to one-third of NSAID/aspirin deaths are attributed to low-dose aspirin
- Criteria for stress ulcer prophylaxis are unclear but include mechanical ventilation and coagulopathy.

This definition excludes carcinoma and lymphoma, which may also cause gastric ulceration, and also excludes other rare causes of gastric and duodenal ulceration such as Crohn's disease, viral infections and amyloidosis. About 10% of the population in developed countries is likely to be affected at some time by peptic ulcer, with the prevalence for active ulcer disease being about 1% at any particular point in time.

Peptic ulcer disease often presents to clinicians as dyspepsia. However, not all patients with dyspepsia have peptic ulcer disease. Dyspepsia is defined as persistent or recurrent pain or discomfort centred in the upper abdomen. The most common causes of dyspepsia are non-ulcer or functional dyspepsia, gastro-oesophageal reflux disease (GORD) and peptic ulcer. Other causes include gastric cancer, pancreatic or biliary disease. Peptic ulcer accounts for 10–15% of dyspepsia, and oesophagitis for about 20%. However, 60–70% of patients have no obvious abnormality and have functional dyspepsia or endoscopy-negative GORD. Dyspepsia is a common symptom and affects about 40% of people annually. It is the reason for 5–10% of consultations with primary care physicians, and up to 70% of referrals to gastrointestinal units are patients with dyspepsia. However, the widely adopted test and treat recommendation for uninvestigated dyspepsia has reduced endoscopy referrals, especially if the test is negative

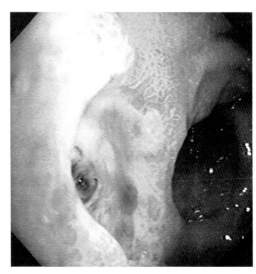

Figure 12.1 Duodenal ulcer seen at endoscopy. Note also a visible blood vessel that is a stigma of recent haemorrhage.

The term 'peptic ulcer' describes a condition in which there is a discontinuity in the entire thickness of the gastric or duodenal mucosa that persists as a result of acid and pepsin in the gastric juice (Fig. 12.1). Oesophageal ulceration due to acid reflux is generally classified under gastro-oesophageal reflux disease.

149

Epidemiology

The incidence of duodenal ulcer is now declining, which follows the decline in *Helicobacter pylori* (*H. pylori*) infection. However, hospital admission rates for gastrointestinal bleeding associated with gastric and duodenal ulcers are rising, especially in older patients. This is probably a consequence of increased prescriptions for low-dose aspirin, non-steroidal anti-inflammatory agents (NSAIDs), antiplatelets, anticoagulants and selective serotonin reuptake inhibitors (SSRI). This is despite an increase in prescriptions for ulcer-healing drugs which are also widely used for GORD and functional dyspepsia.

Infection by *H. pylori*, a spiral bacterium of the stomach, is the most important epidemiological factor in causing peptic ulcer (Fig. 12.2). Most *H. pylori* infections are acquired by oral–oral and oral–faecal transmission. The most important risk factors for *H. pylori* infection are low social class, overcrowding and home environment during childhood (e.g. bed sharing). Transmission may occur within a family, a fact demonstrated by the finding that family members, especially spouses, may have the same strain of *H. pylori*. *H. pylori* seropositivity increases with age as colonization persists for the lifetime of the host. Subjects who become infected with *H. pylori* when young are more likely to develop chronic or atrophic gastritis with reduced acid secretion that may protect them from developing duodenal ulcer. However, it may promote development of gastric ulcer as well as gastric cancer. Duodenal ulcer seems to develop in those who are infected with *H. pylori* at the end of childhood or later. However, some epidemiological data conflict with this view of pathogenesis. Basal acid output and stimulated acid output are increased in people with duodenal ulcer. The high and low rates of *H. pylori* infection in, respectively, developing and developed countries are not accurately reflected in the distribution of peptic ulcer. This indicates that other host and environmental factors besides *H. pylori* may be needed for ulcer development.

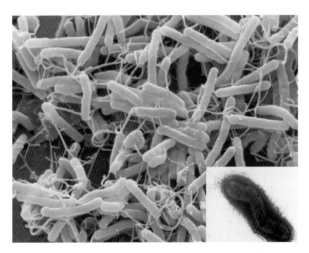

Figure 12.2 *Helicobacter pylori.* The Gram-negative spiral bacterium *Helicobacter pylori*, formerly known as *Campylobacter pylori*, was isolated serendipitously from patients with gastritis by Barry Marshall and Robin Warren in 1982. Seven years later, it was conceded that *Helicobacter pylori* is responsible for most cases of gastric and duodenal ulcer.

Pathogenesis of peptic ulcer disease

There are two common forms of peptic ulcer disease: those associated with the organism *H. pylori* and those associated with the use of aspirin and NSAIDs. Massive hypersecretion of acid occurs in the rare gastrinoma (Zollinger–Ellison) syndrome.

Helicobacter pylori

This organism is a Gram-negative microaerophilic bacterium found primarily in the gastric antrum of the human stomach (see Fig. 12.2). Ninety-five percent or more of duodenal ulcers and 80–85% of gastric ulcers are associated with *H. pylori*. The bacterium is located in the antrum and the acid-secreting microenvironment of the corpus of the stomach is less hospitable to the bacterium. In the developed world, reinfection rates are low, about 0.3–1.0% per year, whereas in the developing world reinfection rates are higher, approximately 20–30%. Ulcerogenic strains of *H. pylori*, ulcer-prone hosts, age of infection and interaction with other ulcerogenic factors such as NSAIDs determine peptic ulcer development following *H. pylori* infection. The effect of *H. pylori* in patients receiving NSAIDs is unclear.

H. pylori causing peptic ulcer disease may be more virulent than in those without ulcers. It produces cytotoxin-associated gene A (*CagA*) proteins and vacuolating cytotoxins, such as vac A, which activate the inflammatory cascade. *CagA* status and one genotype of the vac A gene are predictors of ulcerogenic capacity of a strain. *H. pylori* expresses sialic acid-specific haemagglutinins and a lipid-binding adhesion that mediate binding to the mucosal surface. A number of enzymes produced by the bacteria may be involved in causing tissue damage, such as urease, haemolysins, neuraminidase and fucosidase. Gastrin is the main hormone involved in stimulating gastric acid secretion, and gastrin homeostasis is altered in *H. pylori* infection. The hyperacidity in duodenal ulcer may result from *H. pylori*-induced hypergastrinaemia. The elevation of gastrin may be a consequence of bacterially mediated decrease of antral D cells that secrete somatostatin, thus losing the inhibitory modulation of somatostatin on gastrin, or direct stimulation of gastrin cells by certain cytokines liberated during the inflammatory process. Long-standing hypergastrinaemia leads to an increased parietal cell mass. High acid content in the proximal duodenum leads to metaplastic gastric-type mucosa, which provides a niche for *H. pylori* infection followed by inflammation and ulcer formation.

Non-steroidal anti-inflammatory drugs

Three patterns of mucosal damage are caused by NSAIDs. These include superficial erosions and haemorrhages, silent ulcers detected at endoscopy, and ulcers causing clinical symptoms and complications. Weak acid NSAIDs, such as acetylsalicylic acid, are concentrated from the acidic gastric juice into mucosal cells, and may produce acute superficial erosions via inhibition of cyclo-oxygenase (COX) and by mediating the adherence of leucocytes to mucosal endothelial cells. Enteric coating may prevent this superficial damage, but does not reduce ulcer risk. The major systemic action of NSAIDs in producing ulcers is the reduction of mucosal prostaglandin production. All NSAIDs share the ability

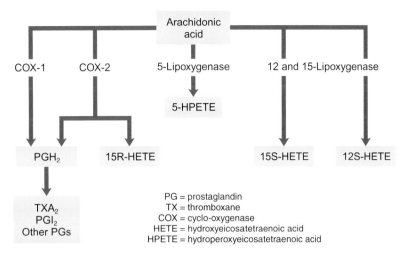

Figure 12.3 Arachidonic acid pathway.

to inhibit cyclo-oxygenase (Fig. 12.3). The presence of NSAID-induced ulcers does not correlate with abdominal pain and NSAIDs themselves often mask ulcer pain. Approximately 20% of patients taking NSAIDs experience symptoms of dyspepsia but symptoms correlate poorly with the presence of mucosal damage. Ulcers and ulcer complications occur in approximately 4% of NSAID users every year.

Each year, in the UK population over the age of 60 years, there are approximately 3500 hospitalizations and over 400 deaths associated with NSAIDs. NSAIDs increase the risk of ulcer complications (Table 12.1), and the risk is progressive depending upon the number of risk factors present (Chan & Graham 2004). NSAID-related ulcer complications increase with advancing age, particularly in those over 75 years, the risk being greatest within the first month of therapy. The risk of mucosal damage increases with even very low doses of NSAIDs, particularly aspirin. Corticosteroids alone are an insignificant ulcer risk, but potentiate the ulcer risk when added to NSAIDs, particularly in daily doses of at least 10 mg prednisolone.

Low-dose aspirin (75 mg/day) alone increases the risk of ulcer bleeding and concomitant use with NSAIDs further increases the

risk. There is no evidence that anticoagulants increase the risk of NSAID ulcers but they are associated with an increase in the risk of haemorrhage. The presence of cardiovascular disease is also considered as an independent risk factor. Enteric coating does not reduce risk (Sorensen et al 2000)

Selective cyclo-oxygenase-2 inhibitors

The gastrointestinal side effects of conventional NSAIDs are mediated through the inhibition of COX-1 (see Fig. 12.3). COX-1 stimulates synthesis of homeostatic prostaglandins while COX-2 is predominantly induced in response to inflammation. Selective COX-2 inhibitors tend not to reduce the mucosal production of protective prostaglandins to the same extent as NSAIDs. COX-2 inhibitors are therefore considered to be safer than non-selective NSAIDs in patients at high risk of developing gastrointestinal mucosal damage. Although studies have confirmed the reduction of endoscopic and symptomatic ulcers (Hooper et al 2004), an increase in cardiovascular risk, including heart attack and stroke, has resulted in the withdrawal of the COX-2 inhibitors rofecoxib and valdecoxib from the market. Additional contraindications are now in place for those COX-2 inhibitors that remain on the market. Amongst the new contraindications is the recommendation that they should not be taken by patients with established heart or cerebrovascular disease, or taken in combination with low-dose aspirin as this negates any beneficial gastrointestinal protective effects. The need for and choice of anti-inflammatory agent should therefore take into account gastrointestinal, cardiovascular and other risks such as potential cardiorenal effects. For all agents, the lowest effective dose should be used for the shortest duration.

Candidates for COX-2 inhibitors are patients at high risk of NSAID-related gastrointestinal events but who do not require low-dose aspirin therapy. The lowering of risk of gastrointestinal events is similar for COX-2 inhibitors and non-selective NSAIDs combined with a gastroprotective agent. However, dyspepsia may be more common in those receiving a COX-2 inhibitor (Lai et al 2005).

Table 12.1 Risk factors for NSAID ulcers	
Uncontroversial risk factors	Controversial risk factors
Age greater than 65 years	Smoking
Previous peptic ulceration	Alcohol
High dose of NSAID or more than one NSAID (including aspirin)	Gender of patient
Concomitant corticosteroid or anticoagulant use	H. pylori
Cardiovascular disease	

Nitric oxide-releasing NSAIDs

Nitric oxide (NO) NSAIDs are being investigated to see if the gastric mucosa protection associated with nitric oxide prevents ulceration when prostaglandins are inhibited by NSAIDs (Fiorucci et al 2001). Nitric oxide is coupled to the NSAID via an ester, resulting in prolonged release of nitric oxide. Nitric oxide itself has anti-inflammatory effects adding to the potency of the NSAID. Clinical trials are needed to assess the efficacy and safety of these agents.

Clinical manifestations

Upper abdominal pain occurring 1–3 hours after meals and relieved by food or antacids is the classic symptom of peptic ulcer disease. The relationship to meals is more marked in duodenal ulcer than in gastric ulcer. However, the symptoms of peptic ulcer disease lack specificity; they do not distinguish between duodenal ulcer, gastric ulcer and non-ulcer or functional dyspepsia. Anorexia, weight loss, nausea and vomiting, heartburn and eructation can all occur with peptic ulcer disease. Patients with predominant symptoms of heartburn are likely to have gastro-oesophageal reflux disease. Complications of peptic ulcer disease may occur with or without previous dyspeptic symptoms. These are haemorrhage, chronic iron deficiency anaemia, pyloric stenosis and perforation. In the elderly the presentation is more likely to be silent. Physical examination is either negative or may reveal epigastric tenderness. Peptic ulcers in the past tended to relapse and remit, and 70–80% of ulcers relapse within 1–2 years after being healed by medical therapy such as antisecretory therapy. This tendency to relapse is dramatically reduced by eradication of *H. pylori*.

Patient assessment

Presenting symptoms of dyspepsia require careful assessment to judge the risk of serious disease or to provide appropriate symptomatic treatment. Symptom subgroups such as ulcer, reflux and dysmotility type may be useful in identifying the predominant symptom subgroup to which a patient belongs. Many patients have symptoms which fit more than one subgroup (Table 12.2). Many patients seek reassurance, lifestyle advice and symptomatic treatment with a single consultation, others have chronic symptoms. In some cases medications may be the cause of dyspepsia and should be reviewed (Table 12.3).

Patients at any age who present with alarm features (Table 12.4) should be referred for endoscopic investigation. These groups of patients are at a higher risk of underlying serious disease such as cancer, ulcers or severe oesophagitis. Referral is also recommended for patients over the age of 55 if symptoms are unexplained or persistent despite initial management (NICE 2004, SIGN 2003).

Patients with predominant reflux-like symptoms are likely to respond to acid-suppressing therapy and one month's treatment of standard dose of proton pump inhibitor should be given in patients whose symptoms persist despite antacid and lifestyle adjustment. Eradication of *H. pylori* is not beneficial in gastro-oesophageal reflux (NICE 2004, SIGN 2003).

Table 12.2 Dyspepsia symptom subgroups

Reflux-like dyspepsia
Heartburn plus dyspepsia
Acid regurgitation plus dyspepsia

Ulcer-like dyspepsia
Localized epigastric pain
Pain when hungry
Pain relieved by food
Pain relieved by antacids or acid-reducing drugs
Pain that wakens the patient from sleep
Pain with remission and relapses

Dysmotility-like dyspepsia
Upper abdominal discomfort (pain not dominant)
Early satiety
Postprandial fullness
Nausea
Retching or vomiting
Bloating in the upper abdomen (no visible distension)
Upper abdominal discomfort often aggravated by food

Unspecified dyspepsia

Table 12.3 Drugs causing dyspepsia

NSAIDs including aspirin	Calcium channel blockers
Corticosteroids	Nitrates
Bisphosphonates	Theophylline
Potassium chloride	Drugs with antimuscarinic effects, e.g. tricyclic antidepressants
Iron	
Antibiotics	

Table 12.4 Alarm features

Dysphagia
Pain on swallowing
Unintentional weight loss
Gastrointestinal bleeding or anaemia
Persistent vomiting
On NSAIDs or warfarin

In those patients who do not have reflux-like dyspepsia, testing for the presence of *H. pylori* is recommended. Eradication treatment should be prescribed for those who test positive and empirical acid suppression for those who test negative. The small proportion of patients with ulcers should be cured. Overall, in functional dyspepsia symptom control is poor but a small but significant benefit of eradication treatment has been shown. Acid suppression is only of benefit in a small proportion of patients with functional dyspepsia. There is no evidence to support other pharmacological therapies and non-pharmacological strategies

may have a future role in functional dyspepsia. Patients should be reassured that the condition is common and not serious. National guidelines (NICE 2004) provide algorithms to guide practitioners through the management of patients presenting with dyspepsia (Fig. 12.4).

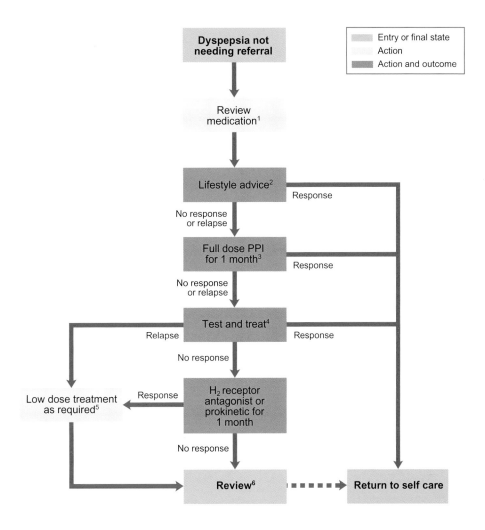

1 Review medications for possible causes of dyspepsia, for example, calcium antagonists, nitrates, theophyllines, bisphosphonates, steroids and NSAIDs.

2 Offer lifestyle advice, including advice on healthy eating, weight reduction and smoking cessation, promoting continued use of antacid/alginates.

3 There is currently inadequate evidence to guide whether full dose PPI (proton pump inhibitor) for 1 month or *H. pylori* test and treat should be offered first. Either treatment may be tried first with the other offered if symptoms persist or return.

4 Detection: use carbon-13 urea breath test, stool antigen test or, when performance has been validated, laboratory based serology.
Eradication: use PPI, amoxicillin, clarithromycin 500 mg (PAC$_{500}$) regimen or a PPI, metronidazole, clarithromycin 250 mg (PAC$_{250}$) regimen.
Do not retest even if dyspepsia remains unless there is a strong clinical need.

5 Offer low dose treatment with a limited number of repeat prescriptions. Discuss the use of treatment on an as required basis to help patients manage their own symptoms.

6 In some patients with an adequate response to therapy it may become appropriate to refer to a specialist for a second opinion. Emphasise the benign nature of dyspepsia. Review long term patient care at least annually to discuss medication and symptoms.

Figure 12.4A   Decision algorithm for management of uninvestigated dyspepsia.

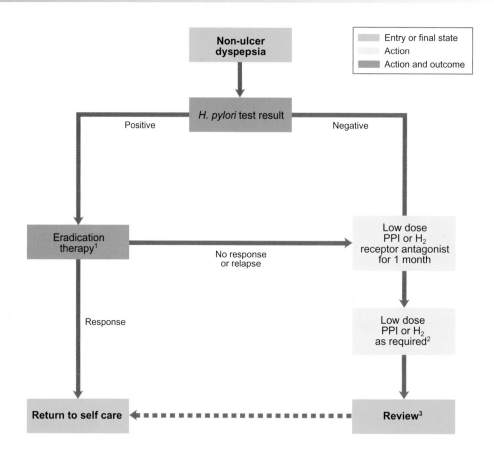

1 Use a proton pump inhibitor (PPI), amoxicillin, clarithromycin 500 mg (PAC$_{500}$) regimen or a PPI, metronidazole, clarithromycin 250 mg (PAC$_{250}$) regimen. Do not retest unless there is a strong clinical need.

2 Offer low dose treatment, possibly on an as-required basis, with a limited number of repeat prescriptions.

3 In some patients with an adequate response to therapy or new emergent symptoms it may become appropriate to refer to a specialist for a second option. Emphasise the benign nature of dyspepsia. Review long-term patient care at least annually to discuss medication and symptoms.

Figure 12.4B   Decision algorithm for management of non-ulcer dyspepsia.

Investigations

Endoscopy

Endoscopy is generally the investigation of choice for diagnosing peptic ulcer, and the procedure is sensitive, specific and safe. However, it is also invasive and expensive. Routine endoscopy in patients presenting with dyspepsia without alarm features (see Table 12.4) is not necessary. Endoscopic investigation should be undertaken in patients with alarm features and in those patients over 55 years who present with unexplained or persistent symptoms of dyspepsia. Biopsies may be taken to exclude malignancy and uncommon lesions such as Crohn's disease.

Wireless capsule endoscopy is now available to investigate NSAID-induced ulceration of the small intestine causing gastrointestinal haemorrhage and is preferable to radiological imaging.

Radiology

Double-contrast barium radiography should detect 80% of peptic ulcers. However, endoscopy is more accurate and almost always preferred. A Gastrograffin meal is used to diagnose peptic perforation in patients presenting with an acute abdomen, if a plain abdominal x-ray is not diagnostic.

Helicobacter pylori detection

There are several methods of detecting *H. pylori* infection. They include non-invasive tests such as serological tests to detect antibodies, [^{13}C] urea breath tests and stool antigen tests. Urea breath tests have a sensitivity and specificity over 90% and are accurate for both initial diagnosis and confirmation of eradication. The breath test is based on the principle that urease activity in the stomach of infected individuals hydrolyses urea to form ammonia and carbon dioxide. The test contains carbon-labelled urea which, when hydrolysed, results in production of labelled carbon dioxide which appears in the patient's breath. The stool antigen test uses an enzyme immunoassay to detect *H. pylori* antigen in stool. This test also has a sensitivity and specificity over 90% and can be used in the initial diagnosis and also to confirm eradication. However, the breath test is preferable and more convenient. Serological tests are based on the detection of anti-*H. pylori* IgG antibodies but are not able to distinguish between active or previous exposure to infection.

Invasive tests requiring gastric antral biopsies include urease tests, histology and culture. Of these, the biopsy urease test is widely used. Agar-based biopsy urease tests are designed to be read at 24 hours, whereas the strip-based biopsy urease tests can be read at 2 hours following incubation with the biopsy material. Patients on proton pump inhibitors can have false-negative results for *H. pylori* when using the urea breath test or biopsy urease test and therefore these medicines should be discontinued at least 2 weeks before testing.

The faecal occult blood test is not specific for or sensitive to detection of NSAID-induced gastric damage. A full blood count may provide evidence of blood loss from peptic ulcer.

Treatment

Complications of peptic ulcer disease

Bleeding peptic ulcer

Peptic ulcer is the most common cause of upper gastrointestinal bleeding. Most patients with bleeding peptic ulcer are clinically stable and stop bleeding without any intervention. Endoscopy allows identification of the severity of disease as well as endoscopic injection therapy which is an effective haemostatic procedure and is successful in reducing mortality. Patients who do not exhibit high-risk stigmata on endoscopy do not require endoscopic therapy. Oral proton pump inhibitors reduce the rebleeding rate and need for surgery in these patients but do not affect overall mortality (Leontiadis et al 2006).

A number of pharmacological agents have been used for endoscopic therapy such as 1:10 000 or 1:100 000 adrenaline (epinephrine), human thrombin and fibrin glue. Thermocoagulation and adrenaline (epinephrine) is routinely used in practice. Bleeding recurs in 15–20% of patients. An increase in intragastric pH is desirable for clot stabilization and haemostasis. Although acid suppression therapy does not appear to affect mortality, rebleeding rates and the need for surgery are reduced. Proton pump inhibitors are more effective than H_2-receptor antagonists and are used in practice following endoscopic injection of adrenaline (epinephrine) to reduce the risk of rebleeding. In those patients at high risk of rebleeding, a high dose infusion of omeprazole (80 mg bolus followed by 8 mg/h) for 72 hours following endoscopic haemostasis decreases the risk of rebleeding. High-dose omeprazole prior to endoscopy may also decrease the need for endoscopic injection therapy (Lau et al 2005). This may be an alternative initial management when endoscopy is unavailable or inappropriate.

After successful *H. pylori* eradication, the rate of rebleeding from peptic ulcers is markedly reduced and it is unnecessary to continue antisecretory maintenance therapy (Gisbert et al 2004). Omeprazole is superior to successful *H. pylori* eradication in preventing recurrent bleeding in patients taking non-aspirin NSAIDs, and is equivalent to successful *H. pylori* eradication in those patients taking low-dose aspirin (Chan et al 2001).

Octreotide is effective in oesophageal variceal haemorrhage and has also been used in other causes of gastrointestinal haemorrhage, especially if the source is not apparent.

Pyloric stenosis

There is limited anecdotal evidence that incomplete gastric outlet obstruction may improve within several months of successful *H. pylori* eradication. Conventional treatment with acid-suppressive therapy may also help. If medical therapy fails to relieve the obstruction, endoscopic balloon dilation or surgery may be required.

Late complications of peptic ulcer surgery

Few patients currently have peptic ulcer disease that is refractory to medical therapy. However, surgical operations were common in the 1960s and 1970s, with nearly half the patients surgically treated for peptic ulcer disease experiencing some resulting debility. Symptoms include early satiety with or without post-cibal vomiting, reactive hypoglycaemia, diarrhoea, weight loss, anaemia, bone loss and vasomotor phenomena such as flushing, palpitations, sweating, tachycardia and postural hypotension. Medical treatment of these symptoms consists of the use of pectin or guar to slow gastric emptying, metoclopramide for gastric stasis, colestyramine for postvagotomy diarrhoea, somatostatin analogues for reactive hypoglycaemia, antibiotics for bacterial colonization and antidiarrhoeal agents such as loperamide. Only a few of these treatments are supported by evidence from randomized controlled trials.

Zollinger–Ellison syndrome

This rare syndrome consists of a triad of non-β islet cell tumours of the pancreas that contain and release gastrin, gastric acid hypersecretion and severe ulcer disease. Extrapancreatic gastrinomas are also common and may be found frequently in the duodenal wall. A proportion of these patients have tumours of the pituitary gland and parathyroid gland (multiple endocrine neoplasia type I). Surgical resection of the gastrinoma may be curative. Medical management consists of greater than standard doses of proton pump inhibitors. The somatostatin analogue octreotide is also effective but has no clear advantage over proton pump inhibitors.

Stress ulcers

Severe physiological stress such as head injury, spinal cord injury, burns, multiple trauma or sepsis may induce superficial mucosal erosions or gastroduodenal ulcerations. These may lead to haemorrhage or perforation. Mechanical ventilation and the presence of coagulopathies place patients at particular risk of stress-related mucosal bleeding. Diminished blood flow to the gastric mucosa, decreased cell renewal, diminished prostaglandin production and, occasionally, acid hypersecretion are involved in causing stress ulceration. Intravenous acid suppression therapy, histamine H_2-receptor antagonists and proton pump inhibitors, and nasogastric tube administration of sucralfate (4–6 g daily in divided doses) have been used to prevent stress ulceration in the intensive care unit until the patient tolerates enteral feeding. However, the optimum strategy remains unclear (Martindale 2005). The most

commonly used regimen is intravenous ranitidine 50 mg every 8 hours reducing to 25 mg in severe renal impairment.

Uncomplicated peptic ulcer disease

Treatment of endoscopically proven uncomplicated peptic ulcer disease has changed dramatically in recent years (Fig. 12.5). Curing

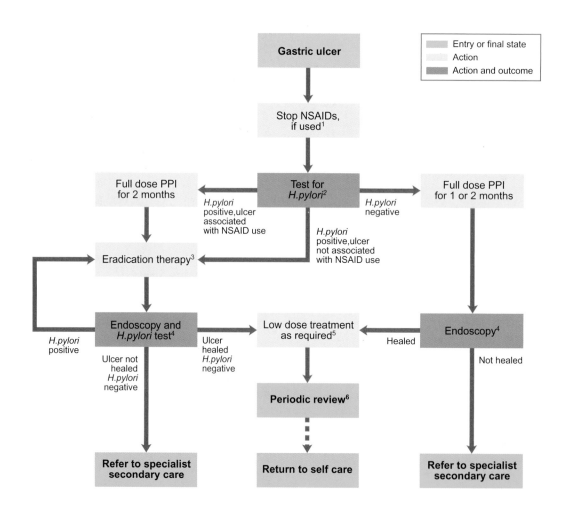

1 If NSAID continuation is necessary, after ulcer healing offer long term gastric protection or consider substitution to a newer COX-2-selective NSAID.

2 Use a carbon-13 urea breath test, stool antigen test or, when performance has been validated, laboratory based serology.

3 Use a proton pump inhibitor (PPI), amoxicillin, clarithromycin 500 mg (PAC_{500}) regimen or a PPI, metronidazole, clarithromycin 250 mg (PMC_{250}) regimen.
Follow guidance found in the *British National Formulary* for selecting second-line therapies.
After two attempts at eradication manage as *H. pylori* negative.

4 Perform endoscopy 6 to 8 weeks after treatment. If re-testing for *H.pylori* use a carbon-13 urea breath test.

5 Offer low dose treatment, possibly used on an as required basis, with a limited number of repeat prescriptions.

6 Review care annually, to discuss symptoms, promote stepwise withdrawl of therapy when appropriate and provide lifestyle advice. In some patients with an inadequate response to therapy it may become appropriate to refer to a specialist.

Figure 12.5A   Management algorithm for gastric ulcer.

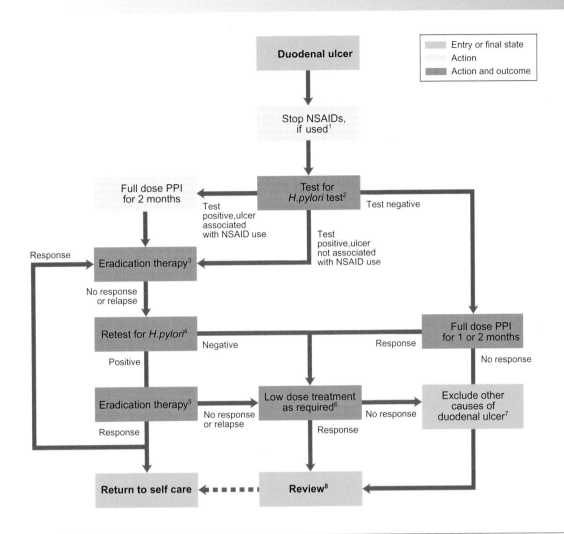

Duodenal ulcer

Entry or final state
Action
Action and outcome

Stop NSAIDs, if used[1]

Test for *H.pylori* test[2]

Full dose PPI for 2 months

Test positive, ulcer associated with NSAID use

Test negative

Test positive, ulcer not associated with NSAID use

Response

Eradication therapy[3]

No response or relapse

Retest for *H.pylori*[4]

Negative

Response

Full dose PPI for 1 or 2 months

No response

Positive

Eradication therapy[5]

No response or relapse

Low dose treatment as required[6]

No response

Exclude other causes of duodenal ulcer[7]

Response

Response

Return to self care

Review[8]

1 If NSAID continuation is necessary, after ulcer healing offer long term gastric protection or consider substitution to a newer COX-2-selective NSAID.

2 Use a carbon-13 urea breath test, stool antigen test or, when performance has been validated, laboratory based serology.

3 Use a proton pump inhibitor (PPI), amoxicillin, clarithromycin 500 mg (PAC$_{500}$) regimen or a PPI, metronidazole, clarithromycin 250 mg (PMC$_{250}$) regimen.

4 Use a carbon-13 urea breath test.

5 Follow guidance found in the *British National Formulary* for selecting second line therapies.

6 Offer low dose treatment, possibly used on an as required basis, with a limited number of repeat prescriptions.

7 Consider: non-adherence with treatment, possible malignancy, failure to detect *H. pylori* infection due to recent PPI or antibiotic ingestion, inadequate testing or simple misclassification; surreptitious or inadvertent NSAID or asprin use; ulceration due to ingestion of other drugs; Zollinger Ellison syndrome, Crohn's disease.

8 Review care annually, to discuss symptoms, promote stepwise withdrawl of therapy when appropriate and provide lifestyle advice.

Figure 12.5B *Management algorithm for duodenal ulcer.*

of *H. pylori* infection and discontinuation of NSAIDs are key elements for the successful management of peptic ulcer disease.

Helicobacter pylori eradication

It is known that *H. pylori* infection is associated with over 90% of duodenal ulcers and 80% of gastric ulcers. Cure of this infection with antibiotic therapy and simultaneous treatment with conventional ulcer-healing drugs facilitates symptom relief and healing of the ulcer and reduces the ulcer relapse rate. Antibiotics alone, or acid-suppressing agents alone, do not eradicate *H. pylori*.

Both therapies act synergistically as growth of the organism occurs at elevated pH and antibiotic efficacy is enhanced during growth. Additionally, increasing intragastric pH may enhance antibiotic absorption.

Eradication treatment regimens that consistently achieve eradication rates above 90% should be chosen. Studies have demonstrated that, currently, the highest eradication rates are achieved by 1 week of triple therapy consisting of a proton pump inhibitor and two specified antibiotics (Gisbert & Pajares 2005). The MACH-1 study (Lind et al 1996) was the first large randomized placebo-controlled trial of *H. pylori* eradication. The most effective

1- week, twice-daily regimens in this trial were the following:

- OCA: omeprazole 20 mg, clarithromycin 500 mg and amoxicillin 1 g

or

- OCM: omeprazole 20 mg, clarithromycin 250 mg and metronidazole 400 mg (Lind et al 1996).

Omeprazole may be replaced with any of the other proton pump inhibitor drugs. The MACH-1 triple therapies are consistently effective in both active gastric and duodenal ulcer disease.

In the UK, resistance to metronidazole has been reported in 11–68% of *H. pylori* isolates, and to clarithromycin in 3–10%. Resistance to amoxicillin is rare. Sensitivity testing is of little value as in vitro resistance to either drug does not preclude eradication when those drugs are used as part of a triple therapy regimen. The MACH-2 study showed that metronidazole resistance reduced the efficacy of OCM from 95% to 76%. It also showed that the potent acid suppression of a proton pump inhibitor partially overcomes metronidazole resistance (Lind et al 1999). A lower dose of clarithromycin (250 mg twice daily) is effective and recommended when combined with metronidazole (NICE 2004). However, some prescribers prefer to recommend 500 mg twice daily to achieve consistency and avoid prescribing errors. In patients with hypersensitivity to penicillin, metronidazole may be substituted for amoxicillin, but otherwise this combination should be avoided.

Ranitidine bismuth citrate (RBC) is a chemical entity which incorporates bismuth into the ranitidine molecule and which was designed for *H. pylori* eradication. There is no difference in the efficacy rate of *H. pylori* eradication between proton pump inhibitor-based and RBC-based triple therapies. Proton pump inhibitors are more effective in triple therapy regimens than H_2-receptor antagonists in similar regimens. Failure of a first-line regimen to achieve eradication will necessitate treatment with another triple therapy regimen or with a quadruple regimen. Most four-drug regimens contain bismuth subsalicylate, metronidazole, tetracycline or amoxicillin and a proton pump inhibitor and are generally not as well tolerated by patients as triple therapy regimens. In patients refractory to conventional as well as quadruple eradication therapies, the indication should be reviewed to determine the importance of eradication. This is undertaken before proceeding to endoscopic biopsies and determination of antibiotic sensitivity after culture. This strategy is rarely justified in non-ulcer dyspepsia.

Successful eradication relies upon patients adhering to their medication regimen. It is therefore important to educate patients about the principles of eradication therapy and also about coping with common adverse effects associated with their regimen. Diarrhoea is the most common adverse effect and should subside after treatment is complete. In rare cases this can be severe and continue after treatment. If this happens patients should be advised to return to their doctor as rare cases of antibiotic-associated colitis have been reported. If drugs are not taken as intended then non-adherence may result in antibiotic resistance should the antibiotic concentration at the site of infection decrease to a level where resistance may emerge.

If eradication is successful, uncomplicated active peptic ulcers heal without the need to continue ulcer-healing drugs beyond the duration of eradication therapy (Gisbert et al 2004). Patients with persistent symptoms after eradication therapy should have

their *H. pylori* status rechecked. This should be carried out no sooner than 4 weeks after discontinuation of therapy to avoid false-negative results due to suppression rather than eradication of the organism. If the patient is *H. pylori* positive, an alternative eradication regimen should be given. If eradication was successful but symptoms persist, gastro-oesophageal reflux or other causes of dyspepsia should be considered.

Patients who have had a previous gastrointestinal bleed from a gastric ulcer should continue ulcer-healing therapy until confirmation of eradication of *H. pylori*. H_2-receptor antagonists can be given after completion of the eradication regimen as they are less likely than proton pump inhibitors to result in a false-negative *H. pylori* test.

Other accepted indications for *H. pylori* eradication include mucosal-associated lymphoid tissue (MALT) lymphoma of the stomach, severe gastritis, and in patients with a high risk of gastric cancer such as those with family history of the disease.

Patients on long-term proton pump inhibitors do not warrant a test and treat strategy for *H. pylori* on grounds of long-term proton pump inhibitor treatment alone.

Treatment of NSAID-associated ulcers

NSAID-associated ulcers may be *H. pylori* positive. The effectiveness of eradicating *H. pylori* in these patients is unknown. Although the presence of *H. pylori* may enhance the efficacy of acid suppression, eradication is generally recommended in infected patients with NSAID-associated ulcers as it is difficult to determine the cause of the ulcer. One study has suggested that ulcer healing may be slower in eradicated patients compared to infected patients (Hawkey et al 1998a) but this has not been confirmed by others (Chan 2005). Two large studies compared ulcer relapse rates in patients on NSAIDs treated for 6 months with omeprazole, misoprostol or ranitidine (Hawkey et al 1998b, Yeomans et al 1998). The results supported the effect of *H. pylori* on acid suppression because the relapse rate was less in *H. pylori*-positive patients compared with *H. pylori*-negative patients.

Eradication of *H. pylori* reduces the risk of recurrent bleeding in low-dose aspirin users (Lai et al 2002). Long-term acid suppression may be required in those also taking non-aspirin NSAIDs or where eradication therapy has failed.

If NSAIDs are discontinued, most uncomplicated ulcers heal using standard doses of a proton pump inhibitor, H_2-receptor antagonist, misoprostol or sucralfate. Proton pump inhibitors are the drugs of choice for patients with large or complicated NSAID-induced ulcers because of their more rapid rate of ulcer healing. Omeprazole 20 mg or 40 mg given once daily healed ulcers within 8 weeks in 80% and 79% of patients respectively, compared with 63% of patients receiving ranitidine 150 mg twice daily (Yeomans et al 1998). Healing is impaired if NSAID use is continued and proton pump inhibitors have shown similar healing rates to misoprostol and superior healing rates to H_2-receptor antagonists in this situation. Treatment-related adverse events are more common in those treated with misoprostol.

Prophylaxis of NSAID ulceration

NSAIDs should be avoided in patients who are at risk of gastrointestinal toxicity (see Table 12.1). However, some patients with chronic rheumatological conditions may require long-term NSAID treatment, in which case the lowest effective dose should be used.

Screening and treating *H. pylori* in patients about to start NSAIDs appears to reduce ulcer risk. This effect is not apparent in low-risk long-term NSAID users (Chan 2005), perhaps explained by the fact that the ulcer risk is increased during the first few months of treatment.

Although low-dose aspirin is not as ulcerogenic as NSAIDs, its use is increasing and the place of *H. pylori* eradication in primary prevention of ulcer complications needs to be established. In some countries, e.g. Canada, *H. pylori* eradication is recommended prior to initiation of therapy with aspirin or NSAIDs.

Ulcer prophylaxis is indicated for 'at risk' patients who need to continue NSAIDs. Interpreting evidence to support gastroprotection requires outcomes to be considered and determination of whether they are symptomatic ulcers or endoscopically detected lesions. Misoprostol at a dose of 800 μg daily is effective at reducing gastrointestinal complications and symptomatic ulcers. However, adverse effects, primarily diarrhoea, abdominal pain and nausea, limit its use. Proton pump inhibitors are also effective at reducing endoscopically diagnosed ulcers but the effect on symptomatic ulcers is unclear. More people remain in remission after 6 months' treatment with omeprazole compared to misoprostol. Lansoprazole has also been shown to be as effective as misoprostol after 12 weeks' treatment at either 15 mg or 30 mg daily. Standard doses of H_2-receptor antagonists are effective at reducing the risk of endoscopic duodenal ulcers. However, reduction in the risk of gastric ulcers requires double this dose. Omeprazole 20 mg and 40 mg are more effective than ranitidine 300 mg daily but no studies have compared a proton pump inhibitor with a high-dose H_2-receptor antagonist for prevention of NSAID-induced ulcers. Gastroprotective agents licensed for prophylaxis of NSAID ulceration are listed in Table 12.5. The majority of studies on the use of these drugs with NSAIDs are based on ulcer rather than dyspepsia prophylaxis.

Gastro-oesophageal reflux disease

Gastro-oesophageal reflux disease (GORD) is the term used to describe any symptomatic clinical condition or histopathological alteration resulting from episodes of reflux of acid, pepsin and, occasionally, bile into the oesophagus from the stomach. Heartburn is the characteristic symptom, and the patient may also complain of acid regurgitation and dysphagia. Complications include oesophageal stricture, oesophageal ulceration and formation of specialized columnar-lined oesophagus at the gastro-oesophageal junction (Barrett's oesophagus). The mechanism of acid reflux is multifactorial, and involves transient lower oesophageal sphincter relaxations, reduced tone of the lower oesophageal sphincter, hiatus hernia and abnormal oesophageal acid clearance. The severity of inflammation of the oesophageal mucosa is described as categories of oesophagitis (Los Angeles A–D). However, approximately two-thirds of patients with GORD have a normal endoscopy which is called endoscopy-negative reflux disease. Hypersensitivity to normal acid exposure may be the cause of symptoms in this group of patients. Progression from endoscopy-negative reflux disease to erosive oesophagitis and Barrett's oesophagus is rare.

Management of GORD focuses on symptom control rather than endoscopic findings and therefore careful symptom evaluation is required (Table 12.6). Patients with alarm features or those who fail to respond to medical treatment should be referred for endoscopic investigation. *H. pylori* eradication plays no role in the management of GORD. However, some guidelines recommend eradication as *H. pylori* infection is associated with an increased risk of peptic ulcer and gastric cancer.

Strategies for initial treatment include lifestyle measures such as weight loss and smoking cessation in combination with antacids. These measures may be effective in patients with no significant impairment of quality of life. When quality of life is impaired, acid suppression therapy is the basis of effective treatment. A course of standard-dose proton pump inhibitor therapy is most effective for symptom relief, healing of oesophagitis and maintenance of remission in patients with GORD (Fig. 12.6). Compared with erosive oesophagitis, there is a diminished response to acid suppression in endoscopy-negative disease but proton pump inhibitors remain the most effective agents. Most patients respond after 4 weeks' treatment and after initial control of symptoms, therapy can be

Table 12.5 Drugs licensed for prophylaxis for NSAID-induced ulceration

Drug	Indication	Prophylaxis dose
Omeprazole	Prophylaxis of further DU or GU	20 mg every day
Esomeprazole	Prophylaxis of DU or GU	20 mg every day
Lansoprazole	Prophylaxis of DU or GU	15–30 mg every day
Pantoprazole	Prophylaxis of DU or GU	20 mg daily
Misoprostol	Prophylaxis of DU or GU	200 μg 2–4 times a day
Ranitidine	Prophylaxis of DU	150 mg twice a day

NSAID: non-steroidal anti-inflammatory drug; DU: duodenal ulcer; GU: gastric ulcer

Table 12.6 Symptoms associated with gastro-oesophageal reflux disease

Heartburn and regurgitation
Belching
Upper abdominal discomfort
Bloating and postprandial fullness
Chest pain
Hoarseness
Cough

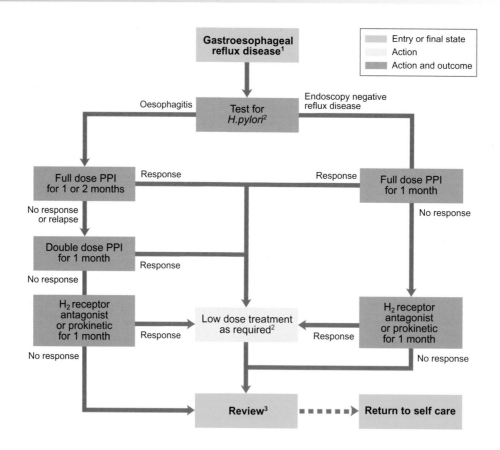

Figure 12.6   Management algorithm for gastro-oesophageal reflux disease.

1 GORD refers to endoscopically determined oesophagitis or endoscopy-negative reflux disease. Patients with uninvestigated 'reflux-like' symptoms should be managed as patients with uninvestigated dyspepsia.
There is currently no evidence that *H. pylori* should be investigated in patients with GORD.
2 Offer low dose treatment, possibly used on an as required basis, with a limited number of repeat prescriptions.
3 Review long-term patient care at least annually to discuss medication and symptoms.
In some patients with an inadequate response to therapy or new emergent symptoms it may become appropriate to refer to a specialist for a second opinion.
Review long-term patient care at least annually to discuss medication and symptoms.
A minority of patients have persistent symtoms despite proton pump inhibitor (PPI) therapy and this group remain a challenge to treat. Therapeutic options include doubling the dose of PPI therapy, adding an H_2 receptor antagonist at bedtime and extending the length of treatment.

withdrawn. If symptoms return, intermittent courses can be given or alternatively, on-demand single doses can be taken immediately as symptoms occur. Patients who relapse frequently may require continuous maintenance therapy using the lowest dose of acid suppression which provides effective symptom relief.

Escalating doses can be used in the small number of patients who do not respond to initial treatment. These patients should be investigated to confirm diagnosis. Twice-daily dosing may be required in patients with persistent symptoms. If nocturnal symptoms persist, adding an evening dose of H_2-receptor antagonist may be useful. A selected group of patients may benefit from antireflux surgery rather than the escalation of acid-suppressing treatment. Patients with endoscopically severe oesophagitis (Los Angeles class C or D) should be kept on standard-dose proton pump inhibitors long term to maintain symptom relief and prevent the development of complications such as Barrett's oesophagus or oesophageal adenocarcinoma.

Ulcer-healing drugs

Proton pump inhibitors

The proton pump inhibitors are all benzimidazole derivatives that control gastric acid secretion by inhibition of gastric H^+, K^+-ATPase, the enzyme responsible for the final step in gastric acid secretion from the parietal cell (Fig.12.7).

The proton pump inhibitors are inactive pro-drugs that are carried in the bloodstream to the parietal cells in the gastric mucosa. The pro-drugs readily cross the parietal cell membrane into the cytosol. These drugs are weak bases and therefore have a high affinity for acidic environments. They diffuse across the secretory membrane of the parietal cell into the extracellular secretory canaliculus, the site of the active proton pump (see Fig. 12.7). Under these acidic conditions the prodrugs are converted to their active form, which irreversibly binds the proton

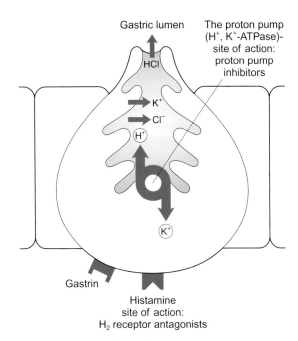

Gastric lumen

The proton pump (H⁺, K⁺-ATPase)- site of action: proton pump inhibitors

HCl

K⁺

Cl⁻

H⁺

K⁺

Gastrin

Histamine
site of action:
H_2 receptor antagonists

Figure 12.7 Receptor stimulation of acid secretion.

pump, inhibiting acid secretion. Since the 'active principle' forms at a low pH it concentrates selectively in the acidic environment of the proton pump and results in extremely effective inhibition of acid secretion. The different proton pump inhibitors (omeprazole, esomeprazole, lansoprazole, pantoprazole and rabeprazole) bind to different sites on the proton pump, which may explain their differences in potency on a milligram per milligram basis.

Proton pump inhibitors require an enteric coating to protect them from degradation in the acidic environment of the stomach. This delays absorption and a maximum plasma concentration is reached after 2–3 hours. Different formulations have been developed for patients with swallowing difficulties but these still rely upon some form of enteric coating (Table 12.7). New immediate-release formulations are under development which

may overcome problems with enteric-coated granules blocking enteral feeding tubes.

Since these drugs irreversibly bind to the proton pump they have a sustained duration of acid inhibition which does not correlate with the plasma elimination half-life of 1–2 hours. The apparent half-life is approximately 48 hours. This prolonged duration of action allows once-daily dosing of proton pump inhibitors, although twice-daily dosing is recommended in some cases of erosive oesophagitis or Barrett's oesophagus when a sustained gastric pH of greater than 4.0 is required. All proton pump inhibitors are most effective if taken about 30 minutes before a meal as they inhibit only actively secreting proton pumps. Meals are the main stimulus to proton pump activity. The optimal dosing time is 30–60 minutes before the first meal of the day.

Proton pump inhibitors are metabolized in the liver to various sulphate conjugates that are extensively eliminated by the kidneys (80%). With the exception of severe hepatic dysfunction, no dose adjustments are necessary in liver disease or in renal disease. Apart from minor differences in bioavailability in the first few days of oral dosing, pharmacokinetics are similar among all proton pump inhibitors. The antisecretory effect is also similar among all agents when administered chronically in equivalent standard doses.

Adverse drug reactions

Experience suggests that proton pump inhibitors are a remarkably safe group of drugs. The most commonly reported side effects are diarrhoea, headaches and abdominal pain which resolve on drug discontinuation (Table 12.8). Possible mechanisms for diarrhoea include bacterial overgrowth, changes in intestinal pH and bile salt abnormalities. Diarrhoea is most commonly associated with lansoprazole, particularly in the elderly. Some cases of persistent chronic watery diarrhoea associated with lansoprazole have been diagnosed as microscopic colitis. This may be explained by the unique ability of lansoprazole to inhibit colonic proton pumps which may have an effect on colonic secretion and pH. Apart from the association between lansoprazole and diarrhoea, the

Table 12.7 Available formulations of proton pump inhibitors

	Omeprazole	Lansoprazole	Pantoprazole	Rabeprazole	Esomeprazole
Capsule or tablet	√	√	√	√	√
Capsule granules can be dispersed in water or juice (pH <5) or yoghurt	√				
Capsule granules can be flushed down tube					√
Dispersible tablet	√	√			
Oral suspension		√			
Intravenous	√		√		√
Available over the counter	√				

Table 12.8 Common adverse reactions to ulcer-healing drugs

Proton pump inhibitors	H$_2$-receptor antagonists	Sucralfate
Diarrhoea	Diarrhoea	Constipation
Headache	Headache	
Abdominal pain	Abdominal pain	
Nausea/vomiting	Confusion	

incidence of adverse reactions is similar among the drugs in this group.

Loss of gastric acidity has been associated with colonization of the normally sterile upper gastrointestinal tract. Associations of long-term acid suppression with increased risk of respiratory tract infections and *Clostridium difficile*-associated disease have been reported. Further epidemiological studies are required to confirm these associations.

Drug interactions

The cytochrome P450 enzyme system is classified into a number of subgroups, several of which are involved in drug metabolism. All proton pump inhibitors are metabolized to varying degrees by the same cytochrome P450 isoenzymes, CYP2C19 and CYP3A. All except rabeprazole are metabolized primarily via the CYP2C19 isoenzyme. This suggests rabeprazole may be less influenced by other drugs metabolized through this system or by genetic changes in hepatic metabolism. The affinity of individual proton pump inhibitors for these enzymes influences the incidence of clinically relevant drug interactions.

- Pantoprazole has lower affinity for the enzyme system than the other proton pump inhibitors and is also metabolized by a sulphotransferase which is non-saturable and not part of the cytochrome P450 system. Rabeprazole is also metabolized through a non-enzymatic pathway.
- Omeprazole inhibits CYP2C9 and 2C19, the isoenzymes involved in the metabolism of, for example, phenytoin (2C9), S-warfarin (2C9), diazepam (2C19) and R-warfarin (2C19). Omeprazole 40 mg daily can decrease the clearance of phenytoin, but phenytoin levels were unchanged after a dose of 20 mg of omeprazole daily. Therefore phenytoin plasma concentrations should be monitored when omeprazole is taken concomitantly. Omeprazole may increase the coagulation time in patients receiving warfarin therapy, especially if doses higher than 20 mg daily are given. Changes in the plasma concentration of the less potent (R) enantiomer of warfarin have been observed, therefore monitoring of the international normalized ratio (INR) is recommended during concomitant therapy. The metabolism of benzodiazepines, particularly diazepam, may be decreased by omeprazole. Similar interactions are likely with esomeprazole.
- Lansoprazole is a weak inducer of CYP1A2 and concurrent administration results in increased theophylline clearance.

Other isolated interactions have been reported.

- Omeprazole can increase the concentration of ciclosporin.
- Clarithromycin increases esomeprazole concentrations; however, omeprazole has also increased clarithromycin concentration.
- Lansoprazole has reduced the efficacy of the oral contraceptive pill.
- Clarithromycin has increased plasma lansoprazole concentration.
- Lansoprazole has increased plasma concentration of tacrolimus.

Approximately 3% of the caucasian and 20% of the Asian population are poor metabolizers of proton pump inhibitors due to genetic polymorphism associated with CYP2C19. High plasma concentrations are achieved and the relative capacity for metabolism by other isoenzymes may alter and result in drug interactions. In practice, the genotype of a patient is unknown. The relative contribution of CYP2C19 to proton pump inhibitor metabolism is greatest with omeprazole and least with rabeprazole.

There have been no clinically significant interactions reported for pantoprazole or rabeprazole. The use of esomeprazole in symptom-driven, on-demand therapy may prove problematic if used concomitantly with warfarin or phenytoin. Careful monitoring should be undertaken. All acid-suppressing drugs potentially decrease the absorption of some drugs by increasing gastric pH. Reduction in absorption of ketoconazole and increased absorption of digoxin have been reported with proton pump inhibitors. The absorption of drugs formulated as pH-dependent, controlled-release products may also be altered. Very few clinically important drug interactions have been reported despite the widespread use of these agents.

Clinical use

Proton pump inhibitors relieve symptoms and heal peptic ulcers faster than H$_2$-receptor antagonists. They also heal ulcers that are refractory to H$_2$-receptor antagonists. All proton pump inhibitors provide similar eradication rates and ulcer healing when used at their recommended doses. In GORD, proton pump inhibitors heal oesophagitis and control symptoms more rapidly than H$_2$-receptor antagonists. Differences between proton pump inhibitors in terms of speed of symptom relief are observed only in the first few days of treatment. Patients with severe oesophagitis should continue long-term proton pump inhibitor therapy, whereas those with milder GORD should be stepped down in terms of acid suppression and therapy withdrawn if symptoms are controlled. Patients with non-ulcer or functional dyspepsia should not routinely be treated with proton pump inhibitors. It is recommended that the least expensive appropriate proton pump inhibitor should be used. Omeprazole 10 mg tablets can now be purchased over the counter for short-term relief of heartburn.

H$_2$-receptor antagonists

The H$_2$-antagonists are all structural analogues of histamine. They competitively block the histamine receptors in gastric parietal cells, thereby preventing acid secretion. Pepsinogen requires acid for conversion to pepsin and so when acid output is reduced, pepsin generation is, in turn, also reduced.

All the available drugs (cimetidine, ranitidine, famotidine, nizatidine) have similar properties. Maximum plasma concentration is reached within 1–3 hours after administration. First-pass hepatic metabolism varies, ranitidine being most extensively metabolized which explains the difference between the intravenous and oral dose. All H_2-antagonists are eliminated to a variable and significant extent via the kidneys, and all require dosage reduction in moderate-to-severe renal impairment. They are equally effective at suppressing daytime and nocturnal acid secretion while they do not cause total achlorhydria. The evening dose of a H_2-antagonist is particularly important because during the daytime gastric acid is buffered for long periods by food; however, during the night this does not occur and the intragastric pH may fall below 2.0 for several hours. For healing oesophagitis, intragastric pH must remain above 4.0 for 18 hours or more per day. H_2-receptor antagonists are therefore not effective in healing oesophagitis. Adding a bedtime dose of H_2-receptor antagonist to proton pump inhibitor therapy is considered to enhance nocturnal gastric pH control in patients with severe oesophagitis, in whom nocturnal gastric acid breakthrough is problematic.

The role of H_2-receptor antagonists in the management of peptic ulcer disease has diminished. H_2-receptor antagonists are less effective than proton pump inhibitors in eradication regimens, in treating ulcers when NSAIDs are continued, and in prophylaxis of NSAID-induced ulcers. H_2-receptor antagonists do effectively heal ulcers in patients who discontinue their NSAID and they also have a role in continuing acid suppression following eradication therapy. Their main role is in the empirical management of dyspepsia symptoms. If patients with mild symptoms gain adequate relief, it is not necessary to use a proton pump inhibitor. H_2-receptor antagonists are preferred over proton pump inhibitors in the second-line treatment of heartburn in pregnancy. H_2-receptor antagonists can be purchased in doses lower than those prescribed for the management of heartburn and indigestion.

Adverse drug reactions

H_2-receptor antagonists are a remarkably safe group of drugs with a lower risk of side effects than proton pump inhibitors. The risk of any adverse reaction is below 3% and serious adverse reactions account for less than 1%. Diarrhoea and headache are the most common and occasionally mental confusion and rashes have been reported (see Table 12.8). Hepatotoxicity is a rare adverse effect. Cimetidine, due to its antiandrogenic effects, has been associated with gynaecomastia and impotence when used in high doses.

Drug interactions

Although many drug interactions have been suggested with cimetidine, many have only been demonstrated in vitro and are of doubtful clinical significance. Cimetidine inhibits the activity of cytochrome P450 and consequently retards oxidative metabolism of some drugs. This interaction is potentially important for drugs with a narrow therapeutic index. The clearance of theophylline is reduced to about 40% of normal, and raised plasma levels occur as a result. Phenytoin metabolism is reduced, and toxicity is

theoretically possible. The metabolism of a number of benzodiazepines, including diazepam, flurazepam and triazolam, is impaired and levels are raised.

The interaction with warfarin has frequently been cited as justification to change to an alternative H_2-antagonist which binds less intensively to the CYP 450 system; however, careful investigation has shown that this interaction is complex. The metabolism of (R)-warfarin is affected to a greater degree than that of (S)-warfarin. As the (S) enantiomer is the more potent, the pharmacodynamic effects of the interaction may be modest although the plasma warfarin concentrations may be increased. Current opinion suggests that warfarin may safely be added with appropriate monitoring when patients are already taking cimetidine in regular daily doses. Other H_2-antagonists should be used in patients who are difficult to stabilize on warfarin or for whom frequent monitoring is not feasible.

All acid-suppressing drugs potentially decrease the absorption of drugs such as ketoconazole and other pH-dependent controlled-release products by increasing gastric pH.

Bismuth chelate

Bismuth has been included in antacid mixtures for many decades but fell from favour because of its neurotoxicity. Bismuth chelate is a relatively safe form of bismuth that has ulcer-healing properties comparable to those of H_2-antagonists. Its mode of action is not clearly understood but it is thought to have cytoprotective properties. Bismuth is toxic to *H. pylori* and was one of the first agents to be used to eradicate the organism and reduce ulcer recurrence. A combination of ranitidine and bismuth as ranitidine bismuth citrate in combination with two antibiotics results in *H. pylori* eradication rates greater than 90%. Bismuth is also included in quadruple therapy regimens used in patients resistant to triple therapy.

Adverse drug reactions

Small amounts of bismuth are absorbed from bismuth chelate, and urinary bismuth excretion may be raised for several weeks after a course of treatment. The risks of bismuth intoxication are small if these products are used at the recommended dose and for short courses of treatment. Bismuth may accumulate in patients with impaired renal function. The most commonly reported events are nausea, vomiting, blackened tongue and dark faeces.

Sucralfate

Sucralfate is the aluminium salt of sucrose octasulphate. Although it is a weak antacid, this is not its principal mode of action in peptic ulcer disease. It has mucosal protective effects including stimulation of bicarbonate and mucus secretion and stimulation of mucosal prostanoids. At pH less than 4.0 it forms a sticky viscid gel that adheres to the ulcer surface and may afford some physical protection. It is capable of adsorbing bile salts. These activities appear to reside in the entire molecular complex and are not due to the aluminium ions alone. Sucralfate has no acid-suppressing activity. At a dose of 2 g twice daily, sucralfate is effective in the treatment of NSAID-induced duodenal ulcers, if the NSAID is stopped. However, it is not effective in the treatment and prevention of NSAID-related gastric ulcers. It has also been used in the prophylaxis of stress ulceration. The liquid formulation is often used as the tablets are large and difficult to swallow.

Adverse drug reactions

Constipation appears to be the most common problem with sucralfate, and this is thought to be related to the aluminium content (see Table 12.8). About 3–5% of a dose is absorbed, and therefore there is a risk of aluminium toxicity with long-term treatment. This risk is correspondingly greater in patients with renal impairment. Caution is required to avoid oesophageal bezoar formation around a nasogastric tube in patients managed in the intensive care unit.

Drug interactions

Sucralfate may bind to other agents in the gastrointestinal tract and reduce the absorption of other drugs. Therefore it should be taken at least 2 hours following other medicines.

Antacids

Antacids have a place in symptomatic relief of dyspepsia, in particular symptoms associated with gastro-oesophageal reflux disease. They have a role in the management of symptoms which sometimes remain for a short time after *H. pylori* eradication of uncomplicated duodenal ulcer.

The choice of antacid lies between aluminium-based and magnesium-based products, although many proprietary products combine the two. Calcium-based products are unsuitable as calcium stimulates acid secretion. Antacids containing sodium bicarbonate are unsuitable for regular use because they deliver a high sodium load and generate large quantities of carbon dioxide. It should be noted that magnesium trisilicate mixtures contain a large amount of sodium bicarbonate. Some products contain other agents such as dimeticone or alginates. Products containing sodium alginate with a mixture of antacids are effective in relief of symptoms in gastro-oesophageal reflux disease but are not particularly effectual antacids.

Aluminium-based antacids cause constipation, and magnesium-based products cause diarrhoea. When combination products are used, diarrhoea tends to predominate as a side effect. Although these are termed 'non-absorbable', a proportion of aluminium and magnesium is absorbed and the potential for toxicity exists, particularly with coexistent renal failure.

Antacids provide immediate symptom relief and a more rapid response is achieved with liquid preparations. They have a limited duration of action and need to be taken several times a day, usually after meals and at bedtime. Administration should be separate from drugs with potential for chelation, such as tetracycline and ciprofloxacin, and also pH-dependent controlled-release products.

Future treatment strategies

Animal models suggest the possibility that therapeutic immunization against *H. pylori* might be a future option in the management of peptic ulcer disease. Human models are now in development. Potentially the young could be protected against the infection and existing infection could be eradicated, radically changing the epidemiology of peptic ulcer disease.

Cost of treatment

Eradication of *H. pylori* infection has revolutionized the therapeutic management of peptic ulcer disease. After successful eradication, the risk of ulcer recurrence is virtually eliminated, removing the need for maintenance therapy.

In healthcare systems where endoscopy is expensive and waiting lists are a problem, empirical therapy, either antisecretory or *H. pylori* eradication, is recommended. Prompt endoscopy is not a cost-effective strategy for the initial management of uncomplicated dyspepsia (Ford et al 2005). The economic importance of prescription of antisecretory therapy in primary care is immense. Out of 1000 patients in primary care, 15–20 will have peptic ulcer disease and 30–35 will have gastro-oesophageal reflux disease, while only one patient will have upper gastrointestinal cancer. A minority of patients with functional dyspepsia benefit from *H. pylori* eradication and many continue to use acid-suppressing therapy.

The rapidly increasing use of aspirin in prevention of cardiovascular disease and the use of non-selective NSAIDs also have economical considerations in terms of gastroprotection.

Patient care

Patient education

Patients who present with symptoms of dyspepsia should be assessed in terms of risk of serious disease. Referral for investigation is indicated if they exhibit alarm features. Patients with predominant reflux-like symptoms are likely to respond to antacid/alginate medicines. Lifestyle should be assessed as weight loss is known to improve reflux symptoms in obese patients. Smoking contributes to heartburn symptoms and delays ulcer healing. A drug history should also be undertaken to identify likely drug-induced causes of symptoms. Many drugs can give rise to symptoms of dyspepsia. Drugs that decrease lower oesophageal sphincter tone may give rise to gastro-oesophageal reflux, e.g. anticholinergics, tricyclic antidepressants and calcium channel blockers. Patients taking prescribed medication which may contribute to symptoms should be referred to the primary care doctor. If symptoms persist after 2 weeks of over-the-counter medication, the patient should also be referred to the primary care doctor. Before initiating NSAID or aspirin therapy, patients should be assessed in terms of gastrointestinal risk. Many patients present with ulcer complications and describe no prior symptoms. Benefits must outweigh risks when patients with risk factors receive NSAIDs. Appropriate prophylaxis should be prescribed. Misoprostol should not be used in pregnant women, and women of child-bearing age should be warned appropriately.

Patients should be advised to seek the pharmacist's advice when purchasing over-the-counter analgesic preparations. Preparations containing aspirin and ibuprofen should be avoided in patients

Table 12.9 Common therapeutic problems in peptic ulcer disease

	Comments
Ulcer-like symptoms of dyspepsia are not specific for peptic ulcer disease and are often present in functional (non-ulcer) dyspepsia	Predominant heartburn differentiates GORD from dyspepsia. Patients with GORD are likely to respond to antisecretory therapy
In uncomplicated patients with ulcer-like symptoms of dyspepsia, there is controversy about whether a 1-month course of acid suppression or test and for *H. pylori* should be carried out first treat	Identification and eradication of *H. pylori* will benefit those with ulcers and a small proportion of *H. pylori*-positive patients with functional dyspepsia. A course of acid suppression will have similar outcomes but ulcers may relapse. Eradication of *H. pylori* plays no role in management of GORD
A test and treat policy is cost-effective compared with initial endoscopy in patients with uncomplicated dyspepsia	There is no evidence to support widespread eradication of *H. pylori* in primary care
Patients on proton pump inhibitors can have false-negative results for *H. pylori*	Proton pump inhibitors should be withdrawn at least 2 weeks before urea breath test or biopsy urease testing (endoscopy)
Following a 7-day eradication therapy regimen, antisecretory therapy can normally be stopped	Longer courses of acid suppressive therapy should be reserved for patients with active ulcers complicated by bleeding and/or NSAID use
First-line eradication therapy comprises twice-daily proton pump inhibitor, amoxicillin 1g and clarithromycin 500mg	Metronidazole can be substituted in those patients allergic to amoxicillin and for second-line therapy. When combined with metronidazole, the dose of clarithromycin can be reduced to 250mg
In patients with NSAID-associated active peptic ulcer disease who test positive for *H. pylori*, the cause of the ulcer may not be confirmed	The ulcer should be healed with a proton pump inhibitor (PPI) for 4 weeks and *H. pylori* eradicated. Eradication of *H. pylori* may reduce the risk of recurrent bleeding
The treatment of NSAID-associated ulcers may differ depending upon whether or not the NSAID must be continued	If NSAIDs are withdrawn, healing rates are similar between H_2-receptor antagonists and PPIs after 8 weeks although PPIs heal ulcers more rapidly. Once healed, antisecretory therapy can be stopped. PPIs should be continued for prophylaxis if NSAIDs must be continued
Patients in whom low-dose aspirin is indicated but have risk factors for peptic ulcer disease	Use of aspirin should be considered carefully, especially for primary prophylaxis of cardiovascular disease. Enteric coating does not reduce this risk. A combination of aspirin and a PPI reduces the risk of gastrointestinal bleeding more than clopidogrel alone. There is no evidence to support clopidogrel in combination with a PPI
NSAID use in elderly patients	Patients over 65 years of age are at increased risk of peptic ulcer disease associated with NSAIDs and often present with 'silent ulcers'. NSAIDs (prescription and non-prescription) should be avoided in the elderly
Patients who are candidates for COX-2 inhibitors	COX-2 inhibitors are associated with less gastrointestinal toxicity than non-selective NSAIDs. Concomitant aspirin reduces any benefit of using COX-2 inhibitors. COX-2 inhibitors are associated with cardiovascular risk. The reduction in gastrointestinal risk associated with COX-2 inhibitors is similar to reduction in risk associated with non-selective NSAIDs in combination with gastroprotective agents
Criteria and regimens to administer for stress ulcer prophylaxis are unclear	Intravenous H_2-receptor antagonist therapy is given to patients at risk until enteral feeding is tolerated. Definite risk factors include mechanical ventilation, presence of coagulopathy and spinal cord injury. Controversial risks include head injury, sepsis, burns, multiple trauma, steroid therapy
Patients who require long-term proton pump inhibitor therapy	Those in whom long-term NSAIDs or low-dose aspirin are indicated and who have risk factors for associated upper gastrointestinal complications. Patients with endoscopically diagnosed GORD who either have severe erosive oesophagitis or severe symptoms which can only be controlled with maintenance therapy

with dyspepsia or in those with risk factors for peptic ulcer disease. Products containing paracetamol should be recommended.

Patients with diagnosed peptic ulcer disease need to be educated about the current principles of therapeutic management. This education should assure adherence to prescribed medication and should be directed at correcting any misunderstandings about previous ulcer healing management. In most patients a single treatment course only is required and there is no need for maintenance therapy.

Patients receiving eradication therapy for *H. pylori* should be advised of the need to treat the organism using a combination of three drugs for a short period of time. Patient adherence is necessary for successful ulcer treatment. Previous adverse reactions should be established; for example, patients who are sensitive to penicillin need an eradication regimen which does not include amoxicillin. Patients should be warned of the specific side effects to be expected from the regimen chosen for them and advised what to do should they experience any of these effects. Patients taking metronidazole must avoid alcohol as they might have a disulfiram-like reaction with sickness and headache. Patients also need to know how their therapy will be followed up.

Patient monitoring

Treatment success in peptic ulcer disease is measured by review of the patient in terms of symptom control. Patients with complicated ulcers or those who continue to have symptoms will receive a urea breath test and/or an endoscopy. Patients should be aware of what their review will entail and when their review will take place. If patients comply with their medication the review process may be kept to a minimum.

Following eradication therapy some patients continue to experience symptoms of abdominal pain. Patients should be reassured that these symptoms will resolve spontaneously, but if necessary an antacid preparation can be recommended to relieve symptoms until review. Patients receiving treatment for NSAID-induced ulceration should continue their ulcer-healing therapy until review. Only patients who continue to take an NSAID require continued prophylactic therapy.

Patients who are anaemic following a bleeding ulcer may be prescribed iron therapy. If patients suffer side effects such as constipation or diarrhoea, the dose of iron should be reduced. Treatment with iron should be for at least 3 months. Iron preparations are best absorbed from an empty stomach but if gastric discomfort is felt, the preparation should be taken with food.

Some common therapeutic problems in the treatment of peptic ulcer disease are summarized in Table 12.9.

CASE STUDIES

Case 12.1

LG, a 34-year-old woman presents in the community pharmacy with epigastric pain for which she seeks symptom relief. On enquiry, she does not have any alarm features such as weight loss, bleeding, dysphagia or persistent vomiting. The symptoms have been intermittent over the previous couple of weeks. The pain does not seem to be precipitated by food. She confirms she is not pregnant.

The symptoms are not reflux-like and do not come on with exercise or radiate to her arms or neck. Her bowel habit is not altered and she is otherwise healthy and takes no prescribed or purchased medicines.

Questions

1. Recommend a suitable initial treatment strategy.
2. LG returns a week later still complaining of discomfort. She is referred to the gastrointestinal clinic at the primary care practice for *H. pylori* testing. Which test should be used for *H. pylori* testing?
3. LG is found to be positive for *H. pylori*. She also reports an allergy to penicillin and receives a prescription for a 7-day, twice-daily course of omeprazole 20 mg, clarithromycin 250 mg and metronidazole 400 mg. What information should she receive with her prescription?

Answers

1. LG has ulcer-like epigastric pain which does not correlate with diagnosis of peptic ulcer. Functional dyspepsia is much more common than peptic ulcer and presents with similar symptoms. Relief of symptoms is the main goal of treatment together with ulcer healing if an ulcer is present. A short course of antacid therapy together with advice about healthy eating, weight reduction and smoking cessation would be appropriate initial management in line with national guidance for managing patients with uninvestigated dyspepsia. If symptoms do not respond, the next stage in management is either a trial of 1 month acid suppression therapy or *H. pylori* test and treat. Although there is inadequate evidence to guide which approach should be applied first, SIGN guidelines recommend test and treat initially to cure any unknown peptic ulcer disease. A small proportion of patients with functional dyspepsia will benefit from either of these strategies. In the absence of endoscopy, it is impossible to know if the patient has an ulcer.

2. Three non-invasive tests can be used to detect *H. pylori*: carbon-13 urea breath test, stool antigen test or laboratory-based serology. Near-patient serological tests are not recommended as they are less accurate than other available tests. Serology antibody tests cannot be used to confirm eradication of the organism as antibody concentrations remain in the plasma for a few weeks after the organism has been eradicated. The choice of test is determined by local facilities and costs.

3. Effective eradication requires combination therapy of a proton pump inhibitor (PPI) and two antibiotics, therefore the requirement to take all three medicines concomitantly should be emphasized. If the course is not completed there is a risk of eradication failure and development of antibiotic resistance. Compliance can be encouraged through provision of patient information about optimum administration of medicines and how to cope with potential adverse effects.

   The PPI is most effective if taken before meals. Clarithromycin and metronidazole may cause gastrointestinal upset and may be best taken with meals. Alcohol should be avoided with this regimen as there is a risk of metronidazole-induced inhibition of aldehyde dehydrogenase, resulting in high concentrations of acetaldehyde. 'Antabuse reactions' are uncommon but patients should be warned of the possibility of nausea, vomiting, flushing and breathlessness when alcohol is taken during and for a couple of days after a course of metronidazole. Diarrhoea is a common adverse effect associated with antibiotics. Patients should be warned of this and encouraged to cope with the inconvenience but to report to their primary care doctor if diarrhoea continues after the course of treatment is finished as there is a small risk of antibiotic-associated colitis.

   The patient should be assessed a few weeks after the 7-day course. If symptoms continue during this period, antacid should be used for relief. If symptoms persist 4 weeks after treatment, confirmation of eradication should be carried out using the urea breath test. Confirmation should not be undertaken within 2 weeks of treatment as the drugs suppress

H. pylori growth without killing the organism and false-negative results can be obtained. If eradication has failed, a further course of eradication therapy should be given using a different combination of antibiotics. If penicillin allergic, tetracycline is sometimes used.

Case 12.2

IR, a 68-year-old woman, was admitted to hospital after an episode of 'coffee ground' vomit and melaena stool. Her haemoglobin concentration was 10 g/dL with an MCV of 78 fL. Investigation revealed a gastric ulcer that stopped bleeding after endoscopic treatment with adrenaline (epinephrine). Biopsy confirmed the benign nature of the ulcer which was positive for *H. pylori*. IR was generally in good health but took ibuprofen 400 mg on an 'as required' basis for general aches and pains.

Questions

1. Were any risk factors present for NSAID-induced ulcers?
2. What treatment should she receive to heal the ulcer and prevent any recurrence?

Answers

1. IR's age places her at risk of NSAID-associated peptic ulcer disease. Risk factors include age greater than 65 years, previous history of gastrointestinal complications and concomitant use of corticosteroids, aspirin or anticoagulants. Risk is greater when multiple risk factors are present. Although the relative risk of gastrointestinal complications among non-selective NSAIDs is lowest for ibuprofen, appropriate professional advice is necessary when patients purchase this product over the counter. Patients with risk factors should be identified and preventive strategies applied such as avoidance of NSAIDs or, where benefits are clear, concomitant gastroprotection with proton pump inhibitors. NSAID ulcers are often asymptomatic and present with complications such as bleeding. It is thought that the NSAID itself may mask any pain associated with the ulcer. Many patients experience symptoms of dyspepsia with NSAID use but this is not predictive of those who develop ulcer complications. Monitoring for symptoms of dyspepsia does not safeguard against the risk of bleeding complications that often occur with no warning symptoms.

2. Endoscopic injection therapy was used to arrest the bleeding. When endoscopy services are less available, intravenous proton pump inhibitor therapy is used. Oral proton pump inhibitor therapy should be initiated to heal the ulcer and prevent re-bleeding. IR tested positive for *H. pylori*. As the cause of the ulcer is unclear and eradication also plays a role in preventing recurrent bleeding, IR should receive eradication therapy. A suitable regimen would be a 7-day course of twice-daily omeprazole 20 mg, amoxicillin 1 g and clarithromycin 500 mg. A further 3 weeks of omeprazole 20 mg may be given in patients with complicated gastric ulcers to ensure ulcer healing. A repeat endoscopy should confirm ulcer healing and successful eradication.

   As IR has no clear indication for ibuprofen, she should be educated about the risks associated with NSAIDs and advised to use simple analgesics when pain control is necessary. If the NSAID can be stopped, it is unnecessary to continue acid suppression therapy after the ulcer has healed.

Case 12.3

SB is a 43-year-old man who has been experiencing heartburn for approximately 4–6 weeks. He tends to eat his main meal in the evening and then relaxes in front of television with a glass of beer before going to bed. He is overweight but not obese and is a non-smoker. Advice was sought from the community pharmacist.

Questions

1. Is it necessary to carry out any further assessment of SB's symptoms?
2. SB returns to the pharmacy 2 weeks later. He has made an effort to modify his lifestyle but despite regular antacid/alginate use he continues to have some discomfort if he eats large meals at night. He asks if there is any other medicine he can purchase. What advice should the pharmacist give SB?
3. SB returns to the pharmacy after a further 2 weeks and reports almost complete symptom relief. He asks if he should take the medicine he purchased on a long-term basis.

Answers

1. SB's symptoms should be assessed to ensure the absence of alarm features, such as weight loss, bleeding or dysphagia, which help predict cancer. A medication history should also be taken to ensure he is not taking any prescribed or purchased medicines which are known to cause dyspepsia or heartburn. The pain of oesophageal spasm may resemble angina-like pain associated with ischaemic heart disease. However, in ischaemic heart disease the pain is usually associated with exercise and radiates to the arms and neck. A cardiovascular risk assessment may be advisable. If any of these factors are present or the symptoms are severe enough to impair quality of life, he should be referred to a primary care doctor. If there are no symptoms of concern initial management with a regular antacid/alginate regimen would be appropriate.

2. Heartburn is the characteristic symptom of gastro-oesophageal reflux disease (GORD) caused by prolonged contact of refluxed stomach contents with oesophageal mucosa. Prolonged relaxation or reduced tone of the lower oesophageal sphincter and increased gastric pressure are physiological variables which affect the period of time the oesophageal mucosa is exposed to acid and pepsin. Certain foods, posture and medicines can affect these variables and contribute to the development of GORD.

   Foods with high fat content delay gastric emptying and eating large meals at night places pressure on the lower oesophageal sphincter as well as causing postprandial fullness, discomfort, bloating and belching. Eating within a couple of hours of going to bed increases the risk of refluxing stomach contents when lying down. Wearing tight clothes and excess weight add further pressure on the stomach. Excess alcohol may cause gastritis and lower the oesophageal sphincter pressure, as does smoking. SB should be informed of the reasons why he should try eating smaller meals more often and reduce the fat content in his diet, reduce alcohol intake and try to lose some weight.

   Immediate relief from symptoms may be achieved with regular doses of an antacid/alginate preparation. These agents have a short duration of action and should be taken after meals and at bedtime. Alginates form a viscous layer on top of the gastric contents, providing a protective barrier. Domperidone may provide benefit as it increases lower oesophageal sphincter tone and accelerates gastric emptying. A record should be made of the assessment, advice and medicines provided. SB should be advised to return in 2 weeks for review of his symptoms.

   Once again, the effect of eating large meals at night should be explained and emphasized.

   Although expensive, a short course of H_2-receptor antagonist treatment or proton pump inhibitor therapy can be sold from the pharmacy. As this is the first episode of symptoms experienced by SB, and he has responded to antacid therapy, a 2-week course of H_2-receptor antagonist is appropriate although the over-the-counter dose that can be recommended is small.

3. After symptom relief is achieved, therapy should be withdrawn in all but those with endoscopically diagnosed severe oesophagitis. If symptoms return, another course of treatment is indicated. SB's records should be updated accordingly. He should be reassured and reminded about the benefits of lifestyle modification.

Case 12.4

NE, a 67-year-old woman with type 2 diabetes mellitus, presents to her primary care doctor complaining of difficulty and discomfort on swallowing. She describes regurgitation of bitter fluid into her mouth. Her diabetes and cardiovascular risk are well controlled with gliclazide, lisinopril, aspirin and simvastatin.

Questions

1. What action should be taken?
2. Investigation confirmed a diagnosis of grade C oesophagitis. Suggest a therapeutic plan for NE.

Answers

1. Endoscopic investigation is indicated in patients with alarm features such as weight loss, bleeding or dysphagia. Given her swallowing difficulties, NE should be referred urgently to a hospital specialist because of the risk of oesophageal cancer or oesophagitis.
2. Proton pump inhibitors are the most effective treatment for relief of symptoms and healing of oesophagitis. A standard dose should be given for 4–8 weeks until repeat endoscopy shows that oesophagitis has healed. If not healed, a higher dose can be given for another 4 weeks. Once healed, relapse is common in patients with severe oesophagitis, therefore maintenance treatment with a standard dose of proton pump inhibitor is indicated. The risk of gastrointestinal bleeding associated with aspirin will be reduced by concomitant proton pump inhibitor therapy. This combination is associated with lower risk than clopidogrel alone.

REFERENCES

Chan F K L 2005 NSAID-induced peptic ulcers and *Helicobacter pylori* infection. Implications for patient management. Drug Safety 28: 287-300

Chan F K L, Graham D Y 2004 Prevention of non-steroidal anti-inflammatory drug gastrointestinal complications – review and recommendations based on risk assessment. Alimentary Pharmacology and Therapeutics 19: 1051-1061

Chan F K, Chung S C, Suen B Y et al 2001 Preventing recurrent upper gastrointestinal bleeding in patients with *Helicobacter pylori* infection who are taking low dose aspirin or naproxen. New England Journal of Medicine 344: 967-973

Fiorucci S, Antonelli E, Burgaud J L et al 2001 Nitric oxide-releasing NSAIDs: a review of their current status. Drug Safety 24: 801-811

Ford A C, Qume M, Moayyedi P et al 2005. Helicobacter pylori "test and treat" or endoscopy for managing dyspepsia: an individual patient data meta-analysis. Gastroenterology 128: 1838-1844

Gisbert J P, Pajares J M 2005 Systematic review and meta-analysis: is 1-week proton pump inhibitor-based triple therapy sufficient to heal peptic ulcer? Alimentary Pharmacology and Therapeutics 21: 795-804

Gisbert J P, Khorrami S, Carballo F et al 2004 H. pylori eradication therapy vs. antisecretory non-eradication therapy (with or without long-term maintenance antisecretory therapy) for the prevention of recurrent bleeding from peptic ulcer. Cochrane Database of Systematic Reviews, issue 2. Update Software, Oxford

Hawkey C J, Tulassay Z, Szczepanski L et al 1998a Randomised controlled trial of *Helicobacter pylori* eradication in patients on non-steroidal anti-inflammatory drugs: HELP NSAIDs study. Lancet 352: 1016-1021

Hawkey C J, Karrasch J A, Szczepanski L et al 1998b Omeprazole compared with misoprostol for ulcers associated with nonsteroidal antiinflammatory drugs. The OMNIUM Study Group. New England Journal of Medicine 338: 727-734

Hooper L, Brown T J, Elliott R A et al 2004 The effectiveness of five strategies for the prevention of gastrointestinal toxicity induced by non-steroidal anti-inflammatory drugs: systematic review. British Medical Journal 329: 948-952

Lai K C, Lam S K, Chu K M et al 2002 Lansoprazole for the prevention of recurrences of ulcer complications from long-term low dose aspirin use. New England Journal of Medicine 346: 2033-2038

Lai K C, Chu K M, Hui W M et al 2005 Celecoxib compared with lansoprazole and naproxen to prevent gastrointestinal ulcer complications. American Journal of Medicine 118: 1271-1278

Lau J, Leung W K, Wu J et al 2005 Early administration of high dose intravenous omeprazole prior to endoscopy in patients with upper gastrointestinal bleeding: a double blind placebo controlled randomized trial. Gastroenterology 128: A79

Leontiadis G I, Sharma V K, Howden C W 2006 Systematic review and meta-analysis of proton pump inhibitor treatment for acute peptic ulcer bleeding. Cochrane Database of Systematic Reviews, issue 1. John Wiley, Chichester

Lind T, Veldhuyzen van Zanten S, Unge P et al 1996 Eradication of *Helicobacter pylori* using one-week triple therapies combining omeprazole with two antimicrobials: the MACH 1 study. Helicobacter 1: 138-144

Lind T, Megraud F, Unge P et al 1999 The MACH-2 study: role of omeprazole in eradication of *Helicobacter pylori* with 1-week triple therapies. Gastroenterology 116: 248-253

Martindale R G 2005 Contemporary strategies for the prevention of stress-related mucosal bleeding. American Journal of Health System Pharmacy 62(suppl 2): S11-17

National Institute for Clinical Excellence 2004 North of England Dyspepsia Guideline Development Group 2004. Dyspepsia – management of dyspepsia in adults in primary care. Clinical guideline 17. National Institute for Clinical Excellence, London

Scottish Intercollegiate Guidelines Network 2003 Dyspepsia. Guideline no. 68. Scottish Intercollegiate Guidelines Network, Edinburgh

Sorensen H T, Mellemkjaer L, Blot W J et al 2000 Risk of upper gastrointestinal bleeding associated with use of low dose aspirin. American Journal of Gastroenterology 95: 2218-2224

Yeomans N D, Tulassay Z, Juhasz L et al 1998 A comparison of omeprazole with ranitidine for ulcers associated with nonsteroidal antiinflammatory drugs. The ASTRONAUT Study Group. New England Journal of Medicine 338: 719-726

FURTHER READING

Moayyedi P, Talley N J 2006 Gastro-oesophageal reflux disease. Lancet 367: 2086-2100

Van Pinxteren B, Numans M E, Bonis P A et al 2004 Short-term treatment with proton pump inhibitors, H_2 receptor antagonists and prokinetics for gastro-oesophageal reflux disease-like symptoms and endoscopy negative reflux disease. Cochrane Database of Systematic Reviews, issue 3. John Wiley, Chichester

Inflammatory bowel disease 13

S. E. Cripps   S. Beresford

KEY POINTS

- Ulcerative colitis and Crohn's disease are the two most common inflammatory bowel disorders (IBD) of the gut. Both are chronic relapsing conditions with a high morbidity and remain largely incurable.
- Ulcerative colitis and Crohn's disease are similar but there are contrasting features which relate to the site of involvement and extent of inflammation across the bowel wall. Ulcerative colitis is limited to the large bowel and the mucosa, whereas Crohn's disease frequently involves the small intestine with inflammation extending through the bowel wall to the serosal surface.
- The aims of treatment are to control acute attacks promptly and effectively, induce remission, maintain remission and identify patients who will benefit from surgery.
- Choice and route of therapy will depend on site, extent and severity of the disease together with knowledge of current or previous treatment.
- A reduction in inflammation with corticosteroids and aminosalicylates is the mainstay of treatment, with immunosuppressants, e.g. azathioprine, methotrexate, and biologic agents, e.g. infliximab, reserved for more refractory cases.
- Although the mucosa is involved in both diseases, the single application of a drug to the inflamed mucosa might be expected to be more effective in colitis than in Crohn's disease where the systemic level of drug in blood supplying the bowel wall may be important.
- Formulations that deliver mesalazine to the colon have been used for colonic delivery of other drugs, including steroids.

Introduction

Inflammatory bowel disease (IBD) can be divided into two chronic inflammatory disorders of the gastrointestinal tract, namely Crohn's disease and ulcerative colitis. Crohn's disease affects any part of the gastrointestinal tract whereas ulcerative colitis affects the colon and rectum only. Current available treatment for IBD is not curative. IBD follows a relapsing and remitting course that is unpredictable and causes disruption to a patient's lifestyle and places a burden on the workplace and healthcare setting (NICE 2002).

Epidemiology

The incidence of IBD is more common in North America, Europe, Australia and New Zealand although the incidence in Africa, Asia and South America is rising steadily. This increase in developing countries may be due to improved sanitation and vaccination programmes along with a decreased exposure to enteric infections. Jewish and Asian people living in the USA and UK are more commonly affected by IBD than those living in Israel and Asia. There appears to be no association between IBD and social class. The peak incidence of IBD occurs between 10 and 40 years although it can occur at any age, with 15% of cases diagnosed in individuals over the age of 60 years. Up to 240 000 people are affected by IBD in the UK.

The incidence of Crohn's disease is approximately 5–10 per 100 000 population per year with a prevalence of 50–100 cases per 100 000 population. The incidence of ulcerative colitis is approximately 10–20 per 100 000 population per year with a reported prevalence of 100–200 cases per 100 000 population. The incidence of IBD is relatively stable but the prevalence is thought to be an underestimate. This underestimate arises because an average disease duration of 10 years is utilized in calculating prevalence, whereas IBD is a chronic, lifelong illness.

Aetiology

The causative agents of IBD are largely unknown although a number of factors are thought to play a role.

Environmental

Diet

Evidence that dietary intake is involved in the aetiology of IBD is inconclusive although several dietary factors have been associated with IBD, including fat intake, fast food ingestion, milk and fibre consumption, and total protein and energy intake. A large number of case–control studies have reported a causal link between the intake of refined carbohydrates and Crohn's disease (Gibson & Shepherd 2005).

During the course of the disease patients are able to identify foods which aggravate or exacerbate their symptoms, e.g. milk, spicy foods. Up to 5% of patients with ulcerative colitis improve by avoiding cow's milk whilst patients with Crohn's disease improve if they start to take elemental (amino acid based), oligomeric (peptides) and polymeric (whole protein) feeds, although symptoms may return when their normal diet is reintroduced.

Smoking

There is a higher rate of smoking amongst patients with Crohn's disease than in the general population, with up to 40% of patients with the disease being smokers. Smoking worsens the clinical course of the disease and increases the risk of relapse and the need for surgery. Fewer patients with ulcerative colitis smoke (approximately 10%). Former smokers are at the highest risk of developing ulcerative colitis, while current smokers have the least risk. This indicates that smoking may help to prevent the onset of ulcerative colitis. The explanation for this is unclear. However, it is thought that in addition to its effect on the inflammatory response, the chemicals absorbed from cigarette smoke affect the smooth muscle inside the colon, potentially altering gut motility and transit time. In some studies nicotine has been shown to be an effective treatment for ulcerative colitis.

Infection

Exposure to *Mycobacterium paratuberculosis* has been considered a causative agent of Crohn's disease although current evidence indicates it is not an aetiological factor.

Ulcerative colitis may present after an episode of infective diarrhoea, but overall there is little evidence to support the role of a single infective agent.

Enteric microflora

Enteric microflora play an important role in the pathogenesis of IBD because the gut acts as a sensitizing organ that contributes to the systemic immune response. Patients with IBD show a loss of immunological tolerance to intestinal microflora and consequently antibiotics often play a role in the treatment of IBD. More recently, manipulating the intestinal flora using probiotics, pre-biotics and synbiotics has proven to be an effective therapeutic strategy. Pro-biotics such as *Bifidobacteria* and *Lactobacilli* alter the intestinal microflora balance favourably. Pre-biotics stimulate the growth of specific, beneficial micro-organisms in the colon whilst synbiotics, a combination of both pre-biotics and pro-biotics, have been successfully used.

Drugs

Non-steroidal anti-inflammatory drugs (NSAIDs) such as diclofenac have been reported to exacerbate IBD (Felder et al 2000). It is thought this may result from direct inhibition of the synthesis of cytoprotective prostaglandins. Antibiotics may also precipitate a relapse in disease due to a change in the enteric microflora. The risk of developing Crohn's disease is thought to be increased in women taking the oral contraceptive pill, possibly caused by vascular changes.

Appendicectomy

Appendicectomy has a protective effect in both Crohn's disease and ulcerative colitis (Radford-Smith et al 2002). It is unclear whether this protective effect is immunologically based or whether individuals who develop appendicitis and consequently have an appendicectomy are physiologically, genetically or immunologically distinct from the population that is predisposed to IBD.

Stress

Some patients find that stress triggers a relapse in their IBD and this has been reproduced in animal models. It is thought that stress activates inflammatory mediators at enteric nerve endings in the gut wall. In addition to stress as a trigger factor, living with IBD can also be stressful. Its chronic nature, lack of curative treatment, distressing symptoms and impact on lifestyle make it difficult for patients to cope.

Genetic

There is mounting evidence that Crohn's disease and ulcerative colitis result from an inappropriate response of the immune system in the mucosa of the gastrointestinal tract to normal enteric flora (Ahmad et al 2004). Since the mid 1990s there has been considerable progress in understanding the contribution of genetics to IBD susceptibility and phenotype.

Ethnic and familial

Jews are more prone to IBD than non-Jews, with Ashkenazi Jews having a higher risk than Sephardic Jews. In North America IBD is more common in whites than blacks. First-degree relatives of those with IBD have a tenfold increase in risk of developing the disease. A familial link is supported from research showing a 15-fold greater concordance for IBD in monozygotic (identical) than dizygotic (non-identical) twins (Jess et al 2005).

Genetic studies

Mutations of the gene CARD15/NOD2 located on chromosome 16 have been associated with small intestinal Crohn's disease in white but not oriental populations. Two other genes have been recently linked with Crohn's disease (OCTN1 on chromosome 5 and DLG5 on chromosome 10).

Pathophysiology

In individuals with IBD, trigger factors typically cause a severe, prolonged and inappropriate inflammatory response in the gastrointestinal tract and the ongoing inflammatory reaction leads to an alteration in the normal architecture of the digestive tract. Genetically susceptible individuals seem unable to downregulate immune or antigen non-specific inflammatory responses. It is thought that chronic inflammation is characterized by increased activity of effector lymphocytes and proinflammatory cytokines that override normal control mechanisms. Others, however, have suggested that IBD may result from a primary failure of regulatory lymphocytes and cytokines, such as interleukin-10 and transforming growth factor-β, to control inflammation and effector pathways. In Crohn's disease it is also thought T-cells are resistant to apoptosis after inactivation.

The character and distribution, both macroscopic and microscopic, of chronic inflammation define and distinguish ulcerative colitis and Crohn's disease.

Crohn's disease

Crohn's disease can affect any part of the gut from the mouth to the anus. Approximately 45% of patients have ileocaecal disease, 25% colitis only, 20% terminal ileal disease, 5% small bowel disease and 5% anorectal, gastroduodenal or oral disease. Crohn's disease can involve one area of the gut or multiple areas, with unaffected areas in between being known as 'skip lesions'. The areas of the small bowel affected are typically thickened and narrow. A 'red ring' is often the first visible abnormality seen on colonoscopy. This is a lymphoid follicular enlargement with a surrounding ring of erythema, which develops into aphthoid ulceration and may progress to deep fissuring ulcers with a cobblestone appearance, fibrosis and strictures. Intestinal strictures arise from chronic and extensive inflammation and fibrosis and bowel obstruction may arise. Local gut perforation may cause abscesses which may also lead to fistulae.

Microscopically, inflammation extends through all layers of the bowel. Inflammatory cells are seen throughout, resulting in ulceration and microabscess formation. Non-caseating epithelioid cells, sometimes with Langhans' giant cells, are seen in about 25% of colonic biopsies and in 60% of surgically resected bowel. Chronic inflammation in the small intestine, colon, rectum and anus leads to an increased risk of carcinoma.

Ulcerative colitis

At first presentation ulcerative colitis is confined to the rectum (proctitis) in 40% of cases, the sigmoid and descending colon (left-sided colitis) in 40% and the whole colon (total ulcerative colitis or pancolitis) in 20% of cases. Proctitis extends to involve more of the colon in a minority, with 15–30% of patients developing more extensive disease over 10 years. The reason why some patients have extensive disease and some have limited disease is unknown. In severe total ulcerative colitis there may also be inflammation of the terminal ileum. This is known as 'backwash ileitis' but is not clinically significant. The colon appears mucopurulent, erythematous and granular with superficial ulceration that in severe cases leads to ulceration. As the colon heals by granulation, pseudopolyps may form.

Microscopically superficial inflammation is seen with inflammatory cells infiltrating the lamina propria and crypts. Crypt abscesses occur, the crypt structure is lost and goblet cell depletion arises as mucin is lost. Dysplasia, which can potentially progress to carcinoma, may be seen in biopsies taken from patients with long-standing total colitis.

Indeterminate colitis

Where chronic colitis persists, yet the pathology of the disease has not been identified as either Crohn's disease or ulcerative colitis, the term 'indeterminate colitis' is used.

Clinical manifestation

Crohn's disease

The clinical features of Crohn's disease depend largely on the site of the bowel affected, the extent, severity and the pathological process in each patient. Crohn's disease tends to be more disabling than ulcerative colitis with 25% of patients unable to work 1 year after diagnosis.

Small bowel, ileaocaecal and terminal ileal disease

Patients present with pain and/or a tender palpable mass in the right iliac fossa with weight loss and diarrhoea, which usually contains no blood. Diarrhoea is caused by mucosal inflammation, bile salt malabsorption that causes steatorrhoea or bacterial growth proximal to a stricture. Small bowel obstruction may also occur as a consequence of inflammation, fibrosis and stricture formation. Patients often describe a more generalized intermittent pain which is colicky with loud gurgling bowel sounds (borborygmi), abdominal distension, vomiting and constipation. Where inflammation or abcsesses are the predominant pathology, many patients present with constant pain, some with fever. Enteric fistulae occur and may involve the skin, bladder or vagina. Although rare, perforation of the gut may present with an acute abdomen and peritonitis. Vitamin B_{12} and folic acid deficiencies predispose patients with disease of the terminal ileum to macrocytic anaemia, while bile acid malabsorption also occurs in such patients and predisposes them to cholesterol gallstones and oxalate renal stones.

Colitis

The main symptoms are abdominal pain, profuse and frequent diarrhoea (more than six loose stools per day) with or without blood, and weight loss. Patients also complain of lassitude, anorexia and nausea and appear thin, tachycardic, anaemic, malnourished and febrile. Colitis may present insidiously with minimal discomfort. Patients with severe involvement of the colon or the terminal ileum often have electrolyte abnormalities, hypoalbuminaemia and iron deficiency anaemia. Extraintestinal complications are more common in those patients with large bowel disease.

Perianal disease

Patients may present with an anal fissure fistula or a perirectal abscess. These symptoms rarely have a significant impact on the patient's lifestyle.

Gastroduodenal and oral disease

These are both rare conditions. Gastroduodenal Crohn's disease presents as dyspepsia, pain, weight loss, anorexia, nausea and vomiting. Oral disease is very painful and may cause chronic ulceration resulting in anorexia.

Ulcerative colitis

Typical symptoms of ulcerative colitis include bloody diarrheoa with mucus, abdominal pain with fever, and weight loss in severe cases. Frank blood loss is more common in ulcerative colitis than Crohn's disease. The symptoms of ulcerative colitis are similar to Crohn's colitis with patients being tachycardic, anaemic, febrile, fatigued, dehydrated and thin. Approximately 50% of patients with ulcerative colitis have some form of relapse each year, and severe attacks can be life threatening.

Acute severe disease

In addition to the typical symptoms of ulcerative colitis, patients with acute severe disease may present with more than six bloody stools per day (10–20 liquid stools per day is not unusual), with a fever (>37.8°C), tachycardia (>90 bpm), anaemia (Hb <10.5 g/dL) or elevated inflammatory markers (ESR >30 mm/h; CRP >8).

Moderately active disease

Stool frequency is less than six motions each day with diarrhoea, mucus and rectal bleeding. Moderately active disease is more common in 'left-sided' disease. Toxic megacolon is rare in patients with rectosigmoidal involvement, and the incidence of colon cancer is much lower in these patients than those with total colitis.

Proctitis

The manifestations of active proctitis are less severe. These are tenesmus, pruritus ani, rectal bleeding and mucous discharge. Patients are often also constipated.

Extraintestinal complications and associations of IBD

Extraintestinal complications are seen more commonly in patients where IBD affects the colon. Complications affect the joints, skin, bone, eyes, liver and biliary tree and are more common in active disease.

Joints and bones

Arthropathies occur in 10% of patients with IBD, are more common in women and are a well-recognized complication of IBD. Patients with pauciarticular disease, characterized by arthritis limited to five or fewer joints, often experience a flare in the arthropathy when there is an exacerbation of the IBD symptoms. When the IBD relapse is treated, the arthropathy improves. In contrast, in polyarticular arthropathy, a chronic condition which affects more than five joints, a flare of the IBD appears not to be temporally related to the activity of the arthropathy. About 5% of patients with IBD also have ankylosing spondylitis. This is thought to be immunologically mediated and not associated with IBD activity. Osteopenia, potentially leading to osteoporosis, is often seen in patients with IBD because of chronic steroid use (particularly when the cumulative dose of prednisolone exceeds 10 g) and/or malabsorption.

Skin

Both erythema nodosum and pyoderma gangrenosum are associated with IBD. Erythema nodosum appears as tender, hot, red nodules that subside over a few days to leave a brown skin discolouration. Disease flares are normally directly related to IBD activity in the 8% of patients affected.

Pyoderma gangrenosum presents as a discrete pustule that develops into an ulcer. In the 2% of patients affected, IBD activity does not appear to be directly related to the pyoderma gangrenosum, which may begin or worsen when the IBD is quiescent.

Ocular

Less than 5% of patients with IBD develop episcleritis (intense burning and itching with localized area of blood vessels) or, more seriously, uveitis (headache, burning red eye, blurred vision). Both disorders are associated with IBD activity.

Sclerosing cholangitis

This occurs in 5% of patients with ulcerative colitis but less in those with Crohn's disease. Chronic inflammation of the biliary tree results in progressive fibrosis and biliary strictures. Patients present with obstructive jaundice, cholangitis and raised liver enzymes (alkaline phosphatase and γ-glutamyltranspeptidase). Endoscopic retrograde cholangiopancreatography (ERCP) is useful in diagnosing and aiding the stenting of strictures. There is an increased risk of cholangiocarcinoma, with a liver transplant the only cure.

Investigations

Clinical, radiological and pathological investigations help to confirm diagnosis and recurrence of disease. The key diagnostic investigation is lower gastrointestinal tract endoscopy (sigmoidoscopy and colonoscopy), which allows direct visualization of the large bowel and histopathological assessment from biopsies (Fig. 13.1). In patients with severe symptoms it is sometimes necessary to delay a full colonoscopy because of the increased risk of perforation.

Crohn's disease

Radiology

An abdominal x-ray with abdominal ultrasound is often the standard investigation in individuals with moderate-to-severe disease. To aid diagnosis contrast media are used. Upper bowel follow-through radiology tracks a barium meal through the small intestine and aids location of fistulae, fissures and strictures; a double-contrast barium enema is used where involvement of the the colon is suspected. Both contrast radiological procedures are avoided in severe active disease. Radiolabelled leucocyte scans that utilize autologous leucocytes labelled with ^{99}technetium-hexamethylenamine oxime may provide further information of disease site and severity. Computed tomography (CT scan) and magnetic resonance imagery (MRI) are also useful in locating and defining fistulae and abscesses in active disease.

Haematology, serology and biochemistry

Although not diagnostic, active disease is suggested in patients with raised inflammatory markers that include erythrocyte sedimentation rate (ESR) and C-reactive protein (CRP), in addition to a low haemoglobin and raised platelet count. Vitamin B$_{12}$ may be low in patients with chronic terminal ileal disease. Low red cell folate and serum albumin, magnesium, calcium, zinc and essential fatty acids also indicate chronic inflammation and malabsorption. Anti-*Saccharomyces cerevisiae* antibodies (ASCA)

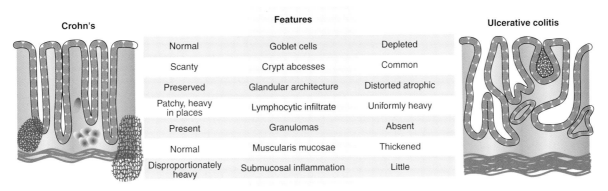

Crohn's	Features	Ulcerative colitis
Normal	Goblet cells	Depleted
Scanty	Crypt abcesses	Common
Preserved	Glandular architecture	Distorted atrophic
Patchy, heavy in places	Lymphocytic infiltrate	Uniformly heavy
Present	Granulomas	Absent
Normal	Muscularis mucosae	Thickened
Disproportionately heavy	Submucosal inflammation	Little

Figure 13.1 Histological features in the rectal biopsy that help to distinguish between ulcerative colitis and Crohn's disease (from Misiewicz et al 1994, with kind permission from Blackwell Scientific Publications, Oxford).

are more likely to be present in Crohn's disease. Serology can be used to exclude infection as a cause of diarrhoea.

Stool tests

Red and white blood cells can be seen on microscopic examination of fresh stools. Microscopic identification of infective cells such as amoeba may also be visualized. *Clostridium difficile* toxin can be assessed through culture and toxin assay. Stool tests do not diagnose IBD but contribute to excluding alternative diagnoses.

Ulcerative colitis

Radiology

The appearance of faecal residue on x-ray helps identify the extent of disease because it indicates areas of the bowel that are not inflamed. Dilated areas may also be seen. Contrast media can be used as in Crohn's disease. Ultrasound, CT scans and MRI are of less use in ulcerative colitis.

Haematology, serology and biochemistry

Malabsorption, indicated by low serum trace elements, e.g. magnesium and zinc, is not seen in ulcerative colitis. Low albumin may indicate relapse in active disease. Patients with sclerosing cholangitis often present with altered liver function tests. Perinuclear antineutrophil cytoplasmic antibodies (pANCA) are seen in ulcerative colitis.

Clinical assessment of inflammatory bowel disease

Once a diagnosis of Crohn's disease or ulcerative colitis has been made and the extent of disease determined, it is helpful to utilize a tool that can assess and monitor patient well-being, abdominal pain, diarrhoea, abdominal mass and extraintestinal symptoms when supported by laboratory tests. A number of these assessment tools are available. For Crohn's disease there is the Harvey–Bradshaw index and the Crohn's disease activity index (CDAI) (see NICE 2002 for the assessment tools) whilst for ulcerative colitis there are the criteria of Truelove and Witts.

Treatment of inflammatory bowel disease

At present there is no cure for IBD. A wide range of drugs and nutritional supplements is available to maintain the patient in long periods of remission in both Crohn's disease and ulcerative colitis. However, surgical intervention will eventually become necessary when the patient relapses and fails to respond to drug therapy.

Nutritional therapy

Nutritional therapy can be considered as an adjunctive or primary treatment. Although a potential problem for all patients with IBD, patients with Crohn's disease are at particular risk of becoming malnourished and developing a variety of nutritional deficiencies (Fig. 13.2). It is therefore important for patients to receive optimal nutrition and dietary manipulation as needed. Low-fibre diets help to reduce clinical symptoms of intestinal obstruction in Crohn's disease (Fernandes-Banares et al 1999). Functional and structural damage to the small bowel can cause malabsorption problems and occasionally patients may require a low-lactose diet.

Patients with poor oral intake and loss of appetite often respond to supplemental enteral feeds. Enteral nutrition in the form of an elemental or polymeric diet can be used as primary therapy and is widely employed in paediatrics (Heuschkel & Walker-Smith 1999).

Patients who have extensive small bowel resection may experience many nutritional deficiencies because of malabsorption. Iron depletion, hypoproteinaemia, deficiencies in water- and fat-soluble vitamins, trace elements and electrolytes may all occur and must be corrected using a suitable replacement regimen.

Where appropriate, and when enteral nutrition is not indicated or adequate, a total parenteral nutrition (TPN) regimen may be prescribed. Some patients receive concurrent enteral and parenteral feeding.

Drug treatment

The main goals of drug treatment are to induce and maintain the patient in remission, limit drug toxicity, modify the pattern of disease and avoid complications. Morbidity and mortality can

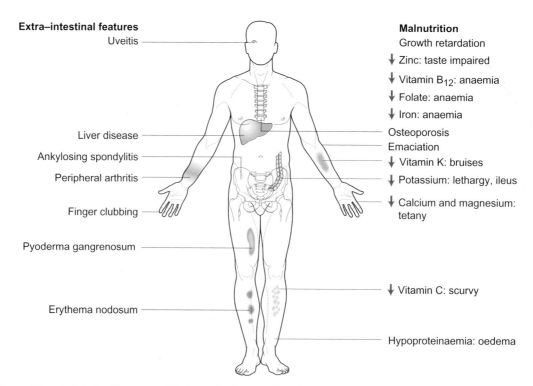

Extra–intestinal features
- Uveitis
- Liver disease
- Ankylosing spondylitis
- Peripheral arthritis
- Finger clubbing
- Pyoderma gangrenosum
- Erythema nodosum

Malnutrition
- Growth retardation
- ↓ Zinc: taste impaired
- ↓ Vitamin B$_{12}$: anaemia
- ↓ Folate: anaemia
- ↓ Iron: anaemia
- Osteoporosis
- Emaciation
- ↓ Vitamin K: bruises
- ↓ Potassium: lethargy, ileus
- ↓ Calcium and magnesium: tetany
- ↓ Vitamin C: scurvy
- Hypoproteinaemia: oedema

Figure 13.2 Some of the extraintestinal illnesses and features of malnutrition found in patients with inflammatory bowel disease (from Misiewicz et al 1994, with kind permission from Blackwell Scientific Publications, Oxford).

also be reduced by the prompt use of effective and appropriate drug therapy. The choice of drug and route of administration depends on the site, extent and severity of the disease together with the individual's treatment history. Drug therapy is often required for many years and patient preference, acceptability and possible side effects not only affect choice but will impact on medication adherence.

Corticosteroids, aminosalicylates and immunosuppressive agents such as azathioprine are the mainstays of treatment. Modern advances in treatment, such as the use of humanized monoclonal antibody preparations and other biologic agents which modify the affected biochemical inflammatory pathways, are beginning to have a significant role in treatment of the disease. These are likely to be the main area of future development.

Other drugs such as antibiotics, e.g. metronidazole, are helpful in some cases, while colestyramine, thalidomide, sodium cromoglicate, bismuth and arsenical salts, nicotine, lidocaine, sucralfate, new steroid entities, cytoprotective agents, aloe vera, probiotics and fish oils are rarely used. However, for some patients they provide alternative or supplemental therapy.

The choice of drug treatment is dependent on whether it is prescribed to induce remission or as maintenance therapy. The majority of patients are managed successfully as hospital outpatients or by their primary care doctor. Only severe extensive or fulminant disease requires hospitalization and the use of parenteral therapy and/or surgical intervention. Oral medication can be given to most patients for maintenance of moderate disease. Disease confined to the anus, rectum or left side of the colon is more appropriately treated with rectally administered topical preparations where the drug is applied directly to the site of inflammation. These topical preparations have reduced systemic absorption and fewer side effects. Rectal steroids and aminosalicylates have similar efficacy although steroids are considerably cheaper. Unfortunately, adherence to topical therapy is generally poor and good patient education is required for effective benefit. Diffuse inflammation invariably requires a combination of rectal and topical treatment. An algorithm for drug treatment in IBD is shown in Figure 13.3.

Corticosteroids

The glucocorticoid properties of hydrocortisone and prednisolone are the mainstay of treatment in active IBD. Prednisolone administered orally or rectally is the steroid of choice although in emergency situations hydrocortisone or methylprednisolone is used when the parenteral route is required. Corticosteroids have direct anti-inflammatory and immunosuppressive actions which rapidly control symptoms. They can be used either alone or in combination, with a suitable mesalazine (5-aminosalicylic acid) formulation or immunosuppressant, to induce remission.

Oral corticosteroids should not be used for maintenance treatment because of serious long-term side effects, and abrupt withdrawal should be avoided. Patients should be maintained on aminosalicylates or immunosuppressants, as appropriate, or referred for surgery.

Formulations Oral prednisolone will control mild and moderate IBD and 70% of patients improve after 2–4 weeks of 40 mg/day. This is gradually reduced over the next 4–6 weeks to prevent acute adrenal insufficiency and early relapse.

Oral corticosteroids should be taken in the morning to mimic the diurnal rhythm of the body's cortisol secretion and prevent sleep disturbance. Uncoated steroid tablets are suitable for most patients

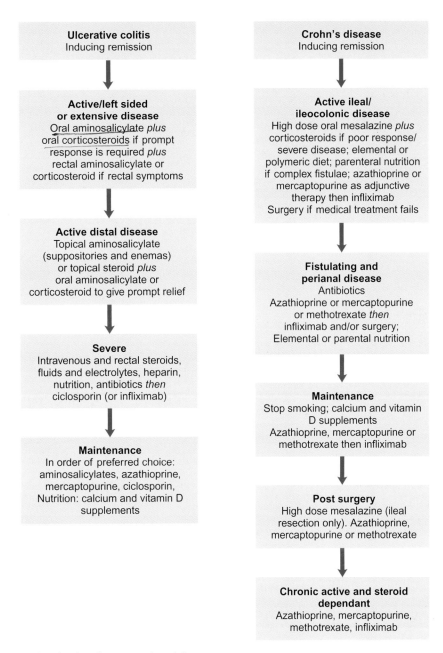

Figure 13.3 A drug treatment algorithm for inflammatory bowel disease.

while enteric-coated preparations do not offer any proven advantage and should be avoided in patients with short bowel or strictures because of poor absorption and bolus release at stricture sites.

Severe extensive or fulminant disease requires hospitalization. Patients are given either hydrocortisone sodium succinate, administered intramuscularly or intravenously at doses of 100 mg three or four times a day, or methyprednisolone 15–20 mg three or four times a day, for 5 days. No additional benefit is gained after 7–10 days. Additional therapy used in severe disease may include intravenous fluid and electrolyte replacement, blood transfusion, topical therapy for rectal and/or colonic involvement, prophylactic heparin (IBD is associated with increased coagulopathy), antibiotics and nutritional support, including possible parenteral nutrition. Oral prednisolone therapy is normally introduced as soon as possible and withdrawn over the following

6–8 weeks. Prednisolone at doses higher than 40 mg/day increases the incidence of adverse effects and has little therapeutic advantage. Short-term side effects include moon face, sleep and mood disturbance, dyspepsia and glucose intolerance. Prolonged use can cause cataracts, osteoporosis and increased risk of infection. A typical treatment algorithm for the management of an acute attack of IBD is presented in Figure 13.4.

Proctitis, left-sided disease and Crohn's disease of the anus and rectum are more appropriately treated using topical rectal preparations (Table 13.1). Rectal corticosteroid preparations are available as suppositories, foam and liquid enemas. Proctitis is best treated with suppositories. Where inflammation affects the rectum and sigmoid colon, foam enemas are preferred. In more extensive disease extending to the splenic flexure, liquid enemas are the agents of choice. However, patients often require a

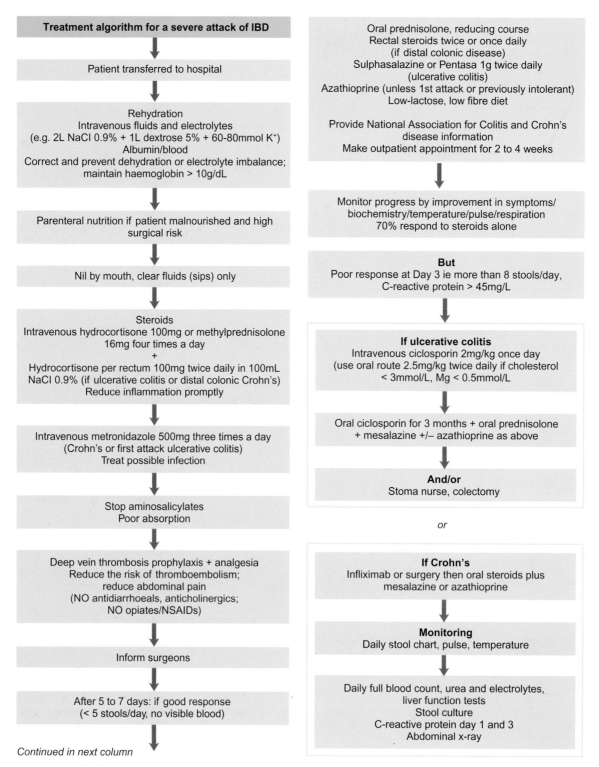

Figure 13.4 Treatment algorithm for an acute attack of IBD.

combination of different rectal preparations because, for example, over 90% of liquid enemas bypass the rectum and thereby exert no therapeutic benefit at that site. As a consequence a suppository may also be required to treat rectal inflammation. The propellant action of foam applicators also results in some preparations by-passing the rectal mucosa.

In the acute setting some hospitals make up their own liquid enemas using 100 mg hydrocortisone sodium succinate injection in 100 mL sodium chloride 0.9%. This unlicensed preparation is administered via a burette and soft catheter over 30 minutes. It is often well tolerated and gives better therapeutic results compared with commercial preparations.

Table 13.1 Comparison of commercially available preparations for rectal administration in inflammatory bowel disease

Generic name	Formulation	Site of release
Sulfasalazine	Suppositories	Rectum
	Retention enema	Transverse, descending colon and rectum
Mesalazine	Retention enema	Transverse, descending colon and rectum
	Foam enema	Rectum and rectosigmoid colon
	Suppositories	Rectum
Prednisolone sodium phosphate	Retention enema	Transverse, descending colon and rectum
	Suppositories	Rectum
Prednisolone (metasulphobenzoate or 21-phosphate)	Retention enema	Transverse and descending colon
	Foam enema	Rectum and rectosigmoid colon
Hydrocortisone (acetate)	Foam enema	Rectum and rectosigmoid colon

The choice of locally applied formulations also depends on patient acceptability and preference. Pack presentation is important to the patient because compliance will be affected by how easily the patient can open a suppository pack or insert an enema. For example, self-administration of a short-tube enema may be difficult for a patient with rheumatism but they may be able to use the long-tube version. Enema volume and viscosity may also affect ease of application and retention.

Rectal administration of prednisolone metasulphobenzoate (Predenema®) or prednisolone-21-phosphate (Predsol®) has comparable therapeutic efficacy despite the poor absorption profile of the metasulphobenzoate salt.

Other steroids

Budesonide, available orally and rectally, is currently licensed for Crohn's disease affecting the ileum and descending colon. It is less effective than conventional corticosteroids in inducing remission in active Crohn's disease, but has fewer side effects than prednisolone because of its rapid and extensive first-pass metabolism. Budesonide enemas are effective in inducing remission in distal ulcerative colitis and are comparable to conventional steroids but probably less effective than mesalazine enemas (Marshall & Irvine 1997).

Aminosalicylates

The aminosalicylates currently licensed for the treatment of IBD include sulfasalazine, mesalazine, olsalazine and balsalazide. They act on epithelial cells by a variety of mechanisms to moderate the release of lipid mediators, cytokines and reactive oxygen species. Different formulations deliver variable amounts of the active component, mesalazine (5-aminosalicylic acid, 5-ASA), to the gut lumen.

Diagnosis, disease location, activity, side effect profile, efficacy and cost all affect the choice of aminosalicylate. Available as oral or rectal preparations, aminosalicylates can be used in combination with steroids to induce and maintain remission, particularly in ulcerative colitis. Sulfasalazine is considerably cheaper but the newer aminosalicylates tend towards therapeutic benefit (Sutherland & MacDonald 2006). Aminosalicylate maintenance therapy appears to reduce the risk of colorectal cancer by up to 75% (Van Staa et al 2005).

The use of aminosalicylates in Crohn's disease is less well established (Travis et al 2006). There is evidence of patient benefit with high-dose mesalazine (over 2 g/day) in reducing relapse post small bowel resection.

Sulfasalazine consists of sulfapyridine diazotized to mesalazine. It is broken down by bacterial azoreductase in the colon to mesalazine and sulfapyridine. Sulfapyridine is absorbed in the colon, metabolized by hepatic acetylation or hydroxylation followed by glucuronidation and excreted in urine. Mesalazine is partly absorbed, metabolized by the liver and excreted via the kidneys as n-acetyl 5-aminosalicylic acid. However, the majority is acetylated as it passes through the intestinal mucosa. Sulfasalazine itself is poorly absorbed and that which is absorbed is recycled back into the gut, via the bile, either unchanged or as the n-acetyl metabolite.

Elimination of sulfapyridine depends on the patient's acetylator phenotype. Those who inherit the 'slow' acetylator phenotype experience more side effects. Mesalazine, as the active component, exerts a predominant local topical action independent of blood levels. The dissolution profile of the drug and the site of ulceration determine effectiveness (Fig. 13.5). The optimal dose of sulfasalazine to achieve and maintain remission is usually in the range of 2–4 g per day in 2–4 divided doses. Acute attacks require 4–8 g per day in divided doses until remission occurs, but at these doses associated side effects are often observed.

About 30% of patients taking sulfasalazine experience adverse effects which are either dose related and dependent on acetylate phenotype or idiosyncratic and not dose related. Dose-related side effects include nausea, vomiting, abdominal pain, diarrhoea, headache, metallic taste, haemolytic anaemia, reticulocytosis and methaemoglobinaemia. Side effects which are not dose related include rashes, aplastic anaemia, agranulocytosis, pancreatitis,

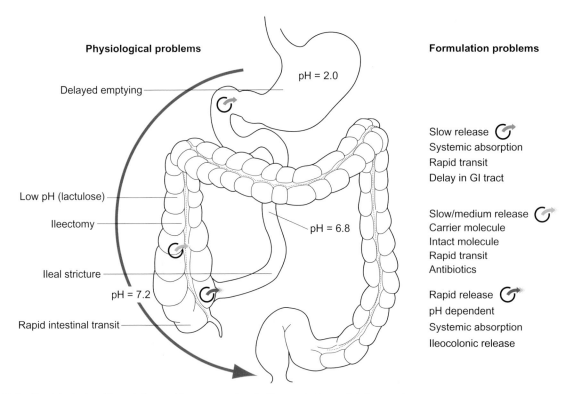

Figure 13.5 Physiological and formulation problems encountered with mesalazine oral delivery systems.

hepatic and pulmonary dysfunction, renal impairment, peripheral neuropathy and oligospermia. In 3% of patients acute intolerance may be seen. This often resembles colitis and includes bloody diarrhoea. Adverse effects usually occur during the first 2 weeks of therapy, the majority being related to plasma sulfapyridine levels. Sulfasalazine metabolites are responsible for the yellow colouration of bodily fluids and staining of soft contact lenses.

Many of the sulphonamide-related adverse effects of sulfasalazine are avoided by using one of the newer aminosalicylate formulations. However, mesalazine alone can still cause side effects, including blood disorders, pancreatitis, renal dysfunction and lupoid phenomenon. Patients should be counselled on how to recognize and report blood dyscrasias.

Formulations Mesalazine is unstable in acid medium and rapidly absorbed from the gastrointestinal tract. Therefore different approaches have been used to develop effective oral preparations (see Fig. 13.5). However, mesalazine dose is more important than the delivery system and the lowest systemic absorption preparation should be used. The different delivery systems are:

- mesalazine tablet coated with a pH-dependent acrylic resin
- ethylcellulose-coated mesalazine granules
- diazotization of mesalazine to itself or to an inert carrier.

Asacol MR tablets contain 400 mg of mesalazine coated with an acrylic resin, Eudragit-S, which dissolves at pH 7 and releases mesalazine in the terminal ileum and the colon. In vitro Mesren MR 400 mg tablets have a dissolution profile virtually identical to Asacol MR. Salofalk tablets contain 250 mg mesalazine with sodium carbonate-glycine and a cellulose ether, coated with Eudragit-L. This dissolves at pH 6 and above, releasing mesalazine in the jejunum and ileum. Similarly, Ipacol EC, containing 400 mg mesalzine, releases mesalazine at pH 6, therefore achieving a

lower ileocolonic mucosal concentration of mesalazine compared with Asacol MR or Mesren MR. Pentasa slow-release tablets 500 mg and granules 1 g comprise ethylcellulose-coated granules of mesalazine which are released in the stomach. Mesalazine is leached slowly from the granules throughout the gastrointestinal tract at all physiological pH.

It is very important to maintain patients on the same brand of mesalazine as some may relapse because of the different release profiles of the active drug. Therefore mesalazine should always be prescribed by brand. As mesalazine has a topical action on colonic epithelial cells, it depends on the release mechanism for delivery to specific sites.

Dipentum 250 mg capsules and 500 mg tablets contain olsalazine sodium, a dimer of mesalazine. Like sulfasalazine, it remains intact until it reaches the colon where it undergoes bacterial cleavage, releasing two molecules of mesalazine. Olsalazine-induced diarrhoea may help patients with distal disease and proximal constipation. Colazide 750 mg capsules contain balsalazide sodium, a pro-drug of mesalazine, which relies on bacterial cleavage in the colon, releasing mesalazine from 4-aminobenzoyl β-alanine, the inert carrier molecule. Table 13.2 compares the oral aminosalicylate preparations currently available.

An alternative to mesalazine is 4-amino salicylic acid (para-amino salicylic acid, PAS). It has been used as a 2 g enema in the treatment of distal ulcerative colitis. In the USA an oral 500 mg acrylic-coated formulation is available.

Mesalazine enemas (1 g in 100 mL), foam enemas (1 g per application) or suppositories (250 mg, 500 mg and 1 g) are effective alternatives for treating localized Crohn's disease or proctitis. The optimum rectal dose is 1 g. Rectal administrations of 5-ASA formulations are significantly better than rectal corticosteroids in inducing remission in ulcerative colitis.

Table 13.2 Comparison of available oral aminosalicylate preparations for patients with IBD

Generic (proprietary) name	Formulation	Release profile	Site of release
Sulfasalazine (Salazopyrin)	Compressed tablet, plain and film coated	Azo-linked, independent of pH	Terminal ileum and colon
Mesalazine (Asacol)	Compressed tablet, acrylic coating	Acrylic coating dissolving at pH 7	Terminal ileum and colon
Mesalazine (Mesren)	Compressed tablet, acrylic coating	Acrylic coating dissolving at pH 7	Terminal ileum and colon
Mesalazine (Salofalk)	Compressed tablet and/or capsule, acrylic coating	Acrylic coating dissolving at pH 6	Terminal ileum and colon
Mesalazine (Ipacol)	Compressed tablet and/or capsule, acrylic coating	Acrylic coating dissolving at pH 6	Mid-jejunum ileum and colon
Mesalazine (Pentasa)	Microgranules coated with ethylcellulose and compressed into tablets. Granules also available	Disintegration not dependent on pH. Slow dissolution rate	Stomach, duodenum, jejunum, ileum and colon
Olsalazine (Dipentum)	Hard gelatin capsules and tablets, uncoated	Azo-linked disintegration independent of pH	Terminal ileum and colon
Balsalazide (Colazide)	Hard gelatin capsules	Azo-linked disintegration independent of pH	Terminal ileum and colon
Polyasa	Compressed tablet and/or capsule	Azo-linked disintegration independent of pH	Terminal ileum and colon

Immunosuppressants

Azathioprine, 6-mercaptopurine, methotrexate, ciclosporin and mycophenolate are immunosuppressants used in patients unresponsive to steroids and aminosalicylates or who relapse when steroids are withdrawn. They are used to induce and maintain remission. All are unlicensed for use in IBD but are routinely used. Treatment may be for up to 5 years because earlier withdrawal increases the rate of relapse.

Azathioprine and mercaptopurine Azathioprine is metabolized to 6-mercaptopurine by the liver. Both azathioprine and 6-mercaptopurine have steroid-sparing properties. Although the action in IBD is unclear, their active metabolites inhibit purine ribonucleotide which may in turn inhibit lymphocyte function, primarily T-cells. Mercaptopurine is further metabolized to 6-thioguanine nucleotides.

Seventy percent of patients will tolerate azathioprine. Of the remaining 30%, most will tolerate mercaptopurine.

Oral maintenance doses for azathioprine are usually 2–2.5 mg/kg/day and for mercaptopurine, 1–1.5 mg/kg/day. Doses are adjusted to patient response, tolerance, white cell and platelet counts. Patients are usually prescribed a reducing dose of corticosteroid in addition because mercaptopurine and azathioprine can take several weeks to show a therapeutic benefit.

The most common side effects occur within 2–3 weeks of starting treatment and rapidly stop on withdrawal. These include flu-like symptoms (myalgia, headache), nausea and diarrhoea. Nausea is reduced by taking the medicine with food. Although rare (<3%), leucopenia can develop suddenly and unpredictably. Hepatotoxicity and pancreatitis have also been reported in less than 5% of patients.

The value of assessing thiopurine methyl transferase (TPMT) activity and genotype, especially prior to initiating treatment, is debatable. Patients who develop leucopenia and are TPMT deficient have a greater risk of myelotoxicity. However, this may not apply in IBD. Some gastroenterologists measure TPMT if a patient has relapsed on doses greater than 2 mg/kg/day to identify fast metabolizers who may respond to higher doses. Measuring TPMT activity to identify the 0.3% of non-metabolizers who are at high risk of rapid leucopenia has also been recommended (Carter et al 2004).

Methotrexate A low-dose regimen of methotrexate is effective in inducing and maintaining remission in patients with chronically active Crohn's disease. Patients receive once-weekly doses of methotrexate ranging from 15 mg to 25 mg. These can be given orally or by subcutaneous or intramuscular injection. Oral medication is more practical although parenteral administration may be more effective and better tolerated. Methotrexate is reserved for patients intolerant or unresponsive to thioguanines.

Methotrexate metabolites inhibit dihydrofolate reductase; however, inhibition of cytokine and eicosanoid may explain the drug's anti-inflammatory effect.

Adverse effects associated with methotrexate are essentially gastrointestinal (nausea, vomiting, diarrhoea and stomatitis). These may be reduced by also prescribing weekly doses of folic acid 5 mg. Folic acid should not be taken on the same day as the methotrexate. Monitoring is undertaken because of the serious side effects of hepatotoxicity, bone marrow suppression and pneumonitis.

To minimize the risk of overdose, one strength of tablet, 2.5 mg or 10 mg, should be dispensed. Methotrexate is teratogenic and all male and female patients should be counselled about using contraception while taking the medication and also for 3 months after therapy is withdrawn.

Ciclosporin Ciclosporin is a calcineurin inhibitor that acts at an early stage on precursors of helper T-cells by interfering with the release of interleukin-2. This inhibits the formation of the cytotoxic lymphocytes which cause tissue damage. Ciclosporin is reserved for the treatment of severe refractory cases of ulcerative colitis (see Fig. 13.4). Its use in Crohn's disease is unproven.

The effectiveness of ciclosporin at doses of 2–5 mg/kg/day in treating IBD has been studied in patients refractory to conventional drug therapy (Van Assche et al 2003). Patient response to this treatment has varied, with adverse effects causing withdrawal of treatment in some cases. However, some patients have stopped concurrent steroid therapy and have remained in remission for some time.

When patients with severe colitis fail to show a response to treatment with parenteral steroids then ciclosporin at an intravenous dose of 2 mg/kg/day should be considered. If patients respond to parenteral ciclosporin they can subsequently be maintained on an oral dose for 3–6 months. If the patient has a low plasma magnesium (<0.5 mmol/L) or cholesterol (<3 mmol/L) they are at an increased risk of ciclosporin-induced seizures when given intravenously. In these circumstances treatment with an oral ciclosporin preparation, e.g. Neoral, at a dose of 5 mg/kg/day is preferred. Ciclosporin therapy is used for many patients, but normally as an interim treatment prior to colectomy or starting maintenance treatment with azathioprine or mercaptopurine. Increasingly, infliximab is replacing ciclosporin use as a rescue therapy in patients with ulcerative colitis (Jarnerot et al 2005).

Forty percent of patients who receive ciclosporin develop minor side effects such as tremor, paraesthesia, headache, gum hyperplasia and hirsutism. Major complications include nephrotoxicity, neurotoxicity, hepatotoxicity and hypertension. Ciclosporin blood levels should be monitored and maintained within the range of 100–200 ng/mL. Grapefruit juice, macrolide antibiotics (mainly erythromycin and clarithromycin), ketoconazole, fluconazole, itraconazole, diltiazem, verapamil, oral contraceptives and protease inhibitors are just some of the drugs that increase ciclosporin levels and toxicity.

Mycophenolate It has been suggested that mycophenolate mofetil is effective and well tolerated in IBD. However, there is little evidence regarding its use in clinical practice.

Major concerns about the use of immunosuppressive agents are related to bone marrow suppression and hepatotoxicity. Therefore patients should be monitored regularly and have routine blood counts and liver function tests including plasma bilirubin and alkaline phosphatase. These should be undertaken every 2–3 weeks for the first 2–3 months and then bimonthly. Although often advised, there is no evidence that more frequent monitoring is more effective. Patients should be taught to recognize the signs of bone marrow suppression and educated about the need for earlier blood tests and the increased risk of infection due to immunosuppression. All patients initiated or maintained on methotrexate must carry a record card detailing current dose and blood test results. As with all patients on immunosuppressant therapy, this should be shown to their doctor and pharmacist at each visit.

The incidence of lymphomas in patients receiving immunosuppressants when compared with other treatments is of concern. It has been suggested that treatment with azathioprine or mercaptopurine should be limited to 5 years because of the risk of malignancy (McGovern & Jewell 2005). Patients should be advised to avoid live vaccines while taking immunosuppressants, including corticosteroids. Guidance on appropriate action following abnormal blood results is provided in Table 13.3.

Biologic agents

The administration of humanized monoclonal antibodies is a relatively new and highly successful development in the treatment of IBD. The first product, infliximab, a chimeric human murine monoclonal antibody, is licensed for treating severe active Crohn's

Table 13.3 Guidance on dealing with abnormal blood results for patients on immunosuppressant therapy

Baseline U&Es, LFTs and FBC should be carried out prior to initiation of therapy. These should be repeated at 2 weeks, 4 weeks then every 2–3 months.

Methotrexate should be *stopped* and the relevant expert advice obtained if any of the following occur:

WBC	<4 × 10⁹/L
Neutrophils	<2 × 10⁹/L
Platelets	<150 × 10⁹/L
AST/ALT	>3 × normal range

Unexplained respiratory symptoms, e.g. dyspnea, dry cough, especially if accompanied by fever and sweats
Renal impairment

Mouth or throat ulceration/rash/unexplained bleeding/fever/alopecia/recurrent sore throats, infections, fever or chills/nausea/vomiting/diarrhoea

Azathioprine or mercaptopurine should be *stopped* and the relevant expert advice obtained if any of the following occur:

WBC	<4 × 10⁹/L
Neutrophils	<2 × 10⁹/L
Platelets	<150 × 10⁹/L
AST/ALT	>3 × normal range

Significant reduction in renal function

Mouth or throat ulceration/rash/unexplained bleeding/fever/upper abdominal or back pain/alopecia/recurrent sore throats, infections, fever or chills/nausea/vomiting/diarrhoea

Nausea may be relieved by taking the dose with/after food or in divided doses

Ciclosporin should be *stopped* and the relevant expert advice obtained if any of the following occur:

High blood levels (will require dose adjustment)

Significant reduction in renal function

Uncontrolled hypertension

Drug blood levels should be done at similar intervals to FBC. A 12-hour trough level should be taken, i.e. before a dose. Target level within the range of 100–400 ng/mL. It takes 2–3 days to reach steady state after dose change

U&Es, urea and electrolytes; LFTs, liver function tests; FBC, full blood count; WBC, white blood cells; ALT, alanine transaminase; AST, aspartate transaminase

disease refractory or intolerant to corticosteroids or conventional immunosuppressants alone or if surgery is not appropriate. It is also licensed for fistulizing Crohn's disease provided criteria for severe active Crohn's disease are met. National guidance on the use of infliximab has been issued (NICE 2002). Clinical trials of its use in acute ulcerative colitis have also shown benefit (Rutgeerts et al 2005, Sandborn et al 2005).

Infliximab acts by inhibiting the functional activity of the pro-inflammatory cytokine tumour necrosis factor (TNF)-α, which damages cells lining the gut, causing pain, cramping and diarrhoea. Colonic biopsies post infliximab treatment show a substantial reduction in TNF-α and a reduction in the commonly elevated plasma inflammatory marker C-reactive protein.

In severe active disease infliximab is administered by intravenous infusion, at a dose of 5 mg/kg over a 2-hour period. In fistulating disease, an initial dose of 5 mg/kg is given, repeated at 2 and 6 weeks after the first infusion. Trials in inflammatory Crohn's disease have shown an 81% response rate at 4 weeks. After 12 weeks, 48% of patients still had a response. In fistulizing disease, 68% of patients experienced a 50% reduction in the number of draining fistulas at two or more consecutive visits. In those who respond to the initial induction course, maintenance therapy with infliximab infusions every 8 weeks should be considered. Fixed interval dosing may be superior to intermittent dosing because of the reduced risk of immunogenicity. Maintenance therapy is not currently recommended (NICE 2002). Unless a patient is intolerant, they should receive an immunosuppressant, e.g. azathioprine or methotrexate, because these are likely to maintain efficacy and reduce side effects.

In some patients infliximab has been associated with either infusion (during or shortly after infusion) or delayed hypersensitivity reactions. It may also affect the normal body immune responses in a significant number of patients. It is contraindicated in patients with tuberculosis and therefore all patients should have a chest x-ray prior to administration. Other contraindications include moderate-to-severe cardiac failure, malignancy and septicaemia. Intestinal stricturing is a relative contraindication (obstruction may be exacerbated through rapid healing at the stricture site). Infliximab should only be prescribed by a gastroenterologist with experience of IBD, and administered in a setting where there are adequate resuscitation facilities available and patients are closely monitored.

Adalimumab, a fully humanized anti-TNF monoclonal antibody, has shown benefit in the treatment of refractory Crohn's disease for patients who no longer respond to or are intolerant of infliximab. An effective dose is yet to be determined. Certolizumab, a new anti-TNF monoclonal antibody, has also shown efficacy in the treatment of Crohn's disease (Travis et al 2006).

Antibiotics

Metronidazole has been used in Crohn's disease associated with perianal disease, sepsis associated with fistulae, perforation and bacterial overgrowth in the small bowel. Doses of 0.6–1.5 g/day are typically used and well tolerated. Metronidazole appears to be ineffective in ulcerative colitis. The associated paraesthesia appears to be dose related, occurring frequently with treatment of greater than 3 months' duration. In such patients doses should be gradually reduced or the drug alternated with another anti-

biotic, e.g. ciprofloxacin, tetracycline or rifabutin, which have shown some limited benefit. The metabolite of metronidazole has a free nitro group and this is probably responsible for the drug's local activity. It also inhibits phospholipase A, contributing to a reduction in damage induced by polymorphonuclear leucocytes.

Other antibacterials are used if specifically indicated, especially when the causative bacterial agents have been identified.

Pseudomembranous colitis caused by *Clostridium difficile* usually occurs after prolonged or multiple antibiotics. This can be distinguished from other causes of colitis by biopsy and stool culture. If it is unclear whether a patient has pseudomembranous or acute colitis, treatment with metronidazole or vancomycin and steroids is advised. A colonoscopy can be performed once symptoms resolve.

Other treatments

Thalidomide The use of thalidomide, under specialist supervision, is restricted to refractory cases of Crohn's disease. Thalidomide acts as a TNF-α inhibitor and probably stabilizes lysosomal membranes. At therapeutic doses it also inhibits the formation of superoxide and hydroxyl radicals, both potent oxidants capable of causing tissue damage. Daily doses in the range of 50–400 mg have proved beneficial when used for periods of 1 week to several months. Side effects during treatment include sedation, dry skin and reduced libido. Thalidomide is teratogenic and should never be used in women of child-bearing age.

Antidiarrhoeals Codeine, diphenoxylate and loperamide should be used with caution to treat diarrhoea and abdominal cramping in IBD. Their use may mask inflammation, infection, obstruction or colonic dilation, thereby delaying correct diagnosis.

Colestyramine Colestyramine has been used in Crohn's disease following ileal resection to reduce diarrhoea associated with bile acid malabsorption caused by the decrease in small bowel absorptive surface area and the cathartic effect of bile salts on the colon. Doses of up to 4 g three times a day inhibit the secretion of water and electrolytes stimulated by bile acids.

Fish oils Fish liver oils containing eicosapentaenoic and docosahexaenoic acids have been used with some success in the treatment of both ulcerative colitis and Crohn's disease. These products cause unpleasant regurgitation which renders them unpalatable in long use. Enteric-coated preparations have reduced this problem. It is thought that fish oils work by diverting fatty acid metabolism from leukotriene B4 to the formation of the less inflammatory leukotriene B5.

Miscellaneous treatments There are many limited trials, studies and case series in the literature evaluating other therapies for ulcerative colitis and Crohn's disease. These include sodium cromoglicate, bismuth and arsenic salts, sucralfate, nicotine, oxygen-derived free radical scavengers, somatostatin analogues, lidocaine, chloroquine, d-penicillamine, carbomers, antituberculous agents, heparin, aloe vera and probiotics. In general these treatments are not recommended, although the variety illustrates the limitations of current therapy. When a patient is not responding to conventional agents, consideration should be given to referral to a specialist centre for a review of current therapy and a plan of future management.

Future therapy is focusing on the ability of drugs to target a specific point in the inflammatory process, such as tumour

Table 13.4 Pharmacological profile of drugs used in adults with inflammatory bowel disease

Pharmacological group	Daily dose	$t\frac{1}{2}$(h)	Metabolism
Steroids			
Hydrocortisone	125–250 mg as foam enema 100–400 mg in 0.9% w/v in sodium chloride intravenously	1.5	Hepatic metabolism 70% and 30% unchanged
Prednisolone	20–60 mg orally 20 mg as foam or liquid enema 5–10 mg as suppositories	3	Hepatic metabolism 70% and 30% unchanged
Budesonide	3–9 mg orally 2 mg as enema	2.8	90% hepatic metabolism
Aminosalicylates			
Mesalazine	500 mg–1.5 g as suppositories 1 g as enema 1.2–2.4 g orally	0.7–2.4	Local and systemic Hepatic acetylation, glucuronidation
Olsalazine	1–3 g orally	1.0	Local and systemic Hepatic acetylation, glucuronidation
Sulfasalazine	3 g as enema 1–2 g as suppositories 4–8 g orally	5–8	Colonic azo-reduction. Local and systemic acetylation Hepatic glucuronidation
4-Aminosalicylic acid	1–2 g orally 1–2 g as enema	0.75–1.0	Rapid absorption and distribution Systemic acetylation
Balsalazide	3–6.75 g orally	1.0	Local and systemic hepatic acetylation
Antibiotics			
Metronidazole	600 mg–1.2 g orally 2 g intravenously	6–24	Hepatic metabolism
Immunosuppressants			
Azathioprine	2–2.5 mg/kg orally	3	Hepatic metabolism to 6-mercaptopurine
6-Mercaptopurine	1–1.5 mg/kg orally	1.5	Hepatic metabolism to inactive metabolite
Methotrexate	15–25 mg by intramuscular or subcutaneous injection weekly 15–25 mg orally weekly	3–10	Insignificant metabolism at low doses
Ciclosporin	2 mg//kg intravenously 5 mg/kg orally	19–27	Mainly hepatic metabolism
Monoclonal antibody			
Infliximab	5 mg/kg intravenous infusion as a single dose over 2 hours	8–9 days	Unknown
Adalimumab	40 mg subcutaneous injection	10–19 days	Unknown
Miscellaneous			
Arsenic salts	250 mg–1 g rectally	72	Tissue deposition excreted unchanged
Bismuth salts	200 mg–1.2 g rectally	60–80	Tissue deposition excreted unchanged
Fish oils	3–4 g	None	Used in the arachidonic acid cycle
Sodium cromoglicate	200–800 mg orally 100–400 mg rectally	Unknown	Poorly absorbed, excreted unchanged in urine and bile
Nicotine	5–15 mg transdermally	0.5–2.0	Hepatic oxidation to cotinine 5% excreted unchanged
Lidocaine	200–800 mg rectally	1–2	Hepatic de-ethylation and hydrolysis 3% excreted unchanged Largely excreted unchanged
Human growth hormone	1.5–5 mg daily by subcutaneous injection	0.5–4	Unknown
Thalidomide	100–400 mg orally	7–16	Hydrolysis
Colestyramine	4–12 g orally		Not absorbed

necrosis factor or interleukin-10 and interleukin-11. Table 13.4 summarizes the drugs which have been used in the treatment of IBD.

Surgical treatment

In ulcerative colitis, surgical colectomy, temporary ileostomy and ileoanal pouch construction are all curative. These are the surgical interventions of choice although proctocolectomy and permanent ileostomy also have a role. Curative surgery is not possible in Crohn's disease as recurrence elsewhere in the gut is inevitable. Complications in the course of their illness result in about 70% of Crohn's patients, requiring at least one surgical procedure. If a significant length of gut is removed this can result in short gut syndrome which may require long-term parenteral nutrition and medication to control a high-output stoma if present, e.g. proton pump inhibitors, loperamide, codeine phosphate, isotonic fluids.

Patient care

Inflammatory bowel disease can result in loss of education and difficulty in gaining employment or insurance. In young patients it can cause psychological problems and growth failure or retarded sexual development. Medical treatment with corticosteroids and immunosuppressants causes secondary health problems and surgery may result in complications such as intestinal failure. The care of patients with IBD is therefore a challenge for the multidisciplinary team.

All patients should be educated about their illness and medication and reminded that even in periods of remission it is important to continue taking prescribed therapy. Certain patients such as female patients or those newly diagnosed may require more tailored information. Leaflets about IBD and insurance or employment for patients with IBD have been prepared by the National Association for Colitis and Crohn's Disease (NACC: www.nacc.org.uk).

Patients and primary care doctors may require additional reassurance as several of the treatments used, e.g. azathioprine, are unlicensed for IBD. Regular blood monitoring of aminosalicylates and immunosuppressants is essential to ensure patients avoid toxicity associated with these drugs. All patients taking steroids must be issued with a steroid card. Shared care policies between primary care doctors, gastroenterologists and patients may also be appropriate.

If relapse occurs it may be appropriate for some patients to increase the dose of their current oral therapy and/or commence rectal administration of a corticosteroid before contacting their doctor. If symptoms do not improve within 48 hours they should arrange a review with their specialist.

Effective home treatment of proctitis is important because tenesmus and occasional faecal incontinence, apart from being distressing, limit further treatment. Enemas or suppositories should be administered just before bedtime in a supine position as this allows a much longer retention time. Enemas can be warmed and should be inserted while lying in the left lateral position. Good counselling on the administration of topical therapy is important to ensure effectiveness.

IBD does not affect fertility or pregnancy. There is no evidence that the frequency of congenital abnormalities, spontaneous abortions or still births is increased. Infertility associated with sulfasalazine therapy would indicate the use of alternative aminosalicylate therapy. With the exception of methotrexate, which is contraindicated in pregnancy, most drugs used in the treatment of IBD do not present a significant hazard. However, patients are strongly advised to first discuss any plans for pregnancy with their gastroenterologist.

Encouraging patients to stop smoking, especially those with Crohn's disease, can have a significant impact on the course of the disease.

Long-term steroid use and underlying IBD both contribute to a higher risk of developing osteoporosis. This is prevalent in up to 50% of the patient population with IBD. Patients with Crohn's disease appear more susceptible to osteoporosis than those with ulcerative colitis. Regular DEXA-scanning should be considered and preventive treatment with bisphosphonate and calcium and vitamin D supplements may be necessary.

Inflammatory bowel disease patients often develop microcytic anaemia because of malabsorption and chronic blood loss. Assessment of the blood film and serum ferritin can differentiate between iron deficiency and anaemia of chronic disease. Oral iron supplements are generally poorly tolerated and parenteral iron may be required. Megaloblastic anaemias are uncommon, although vitamin B_{12} and folate deficiencies occur and may benefit from appropriate supplementation.

There is also a debate about the link between Crohn's disease and measles, measles vaccine or combined measles, mumps and rubella (MMR) immunization. However, current evidence has indicated no proven correlation.

CASE STUDIES

Case 13.1

Mr A is 40 year old with a long history of Crohn's disease. He has been admitted for reassessment of his disease with the aim of re-establishing remission following another relapse. He currently weighs 60 kg and is also planning to start a family in the next 12 months.

Current medication includes:
- Azathioprine 50 mg, daily
- Prednisolone 10 mg, daily

Questions

1. What treatment approaches would you suggest for Mr A to re-establish remission?
2. What are the problems of long-term steroid treatment in patients like Mr A?

Answers

1. The dose of azathioprine should be optimized to 2.5 mg/kg/day (up to 150 mg/day). As azathioprine is a steroid-sparing agent this should enable prednisolone to be withdrawn. If azathioprine fails or the patient is intolerant of higher doses, then methotrexate or infliximab would be alternatives. Mr A is planning a family so even in men, methotrexate should be avoided for at least 3 months prior to conception.

2. Long-term steroid use can lead to a number of problems, including osteoporosis. To prevent osteoporosis, calcium and vitamin D supplements should be considered together with a DEXA scan to assess and monitor bone density. Mr A is at increased risk of infection because of long-term immunosuppression. Diabetes, muscle wasting and reduced wound healing may also occur. The latter may be a problem if Mr A requires surgery. Mr A should always carry a steroid card.

Case 13.2

Miss B, a 30-year-old woman with a known history of ulcerative colitis, presents with bloody diarrhoea (more than 6 motions/day), pyrexia and raised inflammatory markers. She is admitted to hospital for intensive medical management with intravenous and rectal steroids, fluid and electrolyte replacement and subcutaneous heparin.

Questions

1. What is the rationale for prescribing Miss B with intravenous steroids?
2. Miss B is complaining of abdominal pain and the doctor is considering starting codeine phosphate or diclofenac. What advice would you give them?
3. By day three of intensive therapy, Miss B is still passing more than six stools a day and her C-reactive protein remains elevated. The decision is made to start ciclosporin. What dose would you recommend and what advice would you give the nursing staff about administration?

Answers

1. Intravenous administration is appropriate as absorption of oral steroids could be erratic and unpredictable in severe inflammation or in patients who are systemically unwell. A parenteral steroid also ensures rapid attainment of drug levels.
2. Regular use of opiates such as codeine phosphate should be avoided as the resulting reduction in gastrointestinal motility may precipitate a toxic megacolon and perforation. For this reason antidiarrhoeal agents such as loperamide should also be avoided. NSAIDs, by reducing cyclo-oxygenase enzyme activity, may potentially increase production of proinflammatory leukotrienes and increase bleeding. Paracetamol is safe and may be prescribed. The anti-inflammatory action of the intravenous steroids should also reduce pain. However, pain is uncommon in ulcerative colitis because the inflammation is mucosal. The patient should be reviewed to ensure perforation is not overlooked.
3. Trials have suggested an appropriate intravenous dose of ciclosporin is 2 mg/kg/day. Hypomagnesaemia should be corrected because of the risk of seizures. Likewise, cholesterol levels should be checked and if less than 3 mmol/L, an oral ciclosporin regimen, e.g. Neoral, should be used at a dose of 2.5 mg/kg twice a day since low cholesterol can also increase the risk of seizures with intravenous ciclosporin.

Intravenous ciclosporin is available as 50 mg/mL ampoules of which 1 mL should be diluted with 20 mL 5% dextrose or saline and administered over 6 hours. This is the maximum stability time, as polyethyoxylated castor oil in the injection can cause phthalate stripping from PVC tubing. It is therefore preferable that all contact with PVC is avoided. If the infusion is well tolerated, the infusion time can be reduced to 2–5 hours. Infusions should be avoided at night because of the risk of anaphylaxis. It is also recommended that infusions are given after a dose of hydrocortisone and that a blood ciclosporin level is done after 48 hours (steady state, 100–200 ng/mL).

Patients should be monitored for signs of renal and hepatic dysfunction, hypertension, hyperkalaemia, irritation at injection site, and flushing.

Case 13.3

Mr C is admitted to hospital for his first dose of infliximab to treat his severe fistulizing Crohn's disease.

Questions

1. What advice would you give Mr C about possible side effects?
2. Mr C is unsure if he will receive another dose of infliximab. What advice would you give him?

Answers

1. Rare infusion-related side effects are hypotension, shortness of breath and flushing. Blood pressure and pulse should be monitored every 30 minutes. Stopping the infusion temporarily often resolves the symptoms or they can be treated with antihistamines and paracetamol. Sometimes steroids may be required. Anaphylactic reactions are very rare but have been reported. If anaphylaxis occurs then future infusions are not advised.

A delayed reaction, joint pain and stiffness, fever, myalgia and malaise may occur if there has been an interval of more than 1 year following a previous infusion. This can be limited by pretreatment with hydrocortisone.

Infection is the main concern, especially if the patient is also prescribed an immunosuppressant. A chest x-ray should be undertaken to eliminate tuberculosis as there are reports of reactivation or development. There is also a risk of developing lymphoma although, to date, evidence from postmarketing surveillance is inconclusive.
2. Patients with fistulating disease are usually prescribed a 5 mg/kg dose at weeks 0, 2 and 6 with regular maintenance dosing at 8-weekly intervals thereafter.

Case 13.4

Mrs D is admitted to hospital for formation of an ileostomy, following unsuccessful medical management of her ulcerative colitis. Her regular drug therapy on admission includes:

- **Pentasa 1g three times a day**
- **Prednisolone 5–15 mg/day**
- **Digoxin 125 μg daily**
- **Aspirin 75 mg daily**

Question

Following her operation, Mrs D's ileostomy output is high. What treatment approaches are available for managing high-output stomas?

Answer

High-output stomas lead to dehydration and metabolic disturbance, e.g. hypokalaemia, hypernatraemia. Drinking more can make the situation worse since this flushes the small intestinal contents through and exacerbates dehydration. Food and drink can promote secretion and increase volume.

The causes of high-output stomas need to be considered and may include high lactose intake, partial obstruction, gastric hypersecretion, inappropriate diet, laxatives and diuretics. Treatment options should include high-dose omeprazole to reduce gastric acid hypersecretion and codeine phosphate (180–240 mg/day) and/or loperamide to reduce gut motility. In the absence of a colon, a dose of loperamide that exceeds 16 mg/day can be used without adverse effect. Octreotide has been used as an alternative to the antimotility drugs but would appear to offer limited benefit and is best reserved for when other measures have been tried. Intake of isotonic fluids with a sodium concentration >90 mmol/L, to allow the jejunum to absorb water, may also be of benefit.

Case 13.5

Mr E is newly diagnosed with mild ulcerative colitis. His abdominal x-ray suggests predominantly left-sided disease. His past medical history includes joint stiffness due to rheumatoid arthritis. He presents at the pharmacy with a prescription for mesalazine retention enema 1 g one at night, and mesalazine tablets, 800 mg to be taken three times a day.

Questions

1. What advice would you give Mr E about the administration of mesalazine enemas?
2. Mesalazine 400 mg tablets are available in several different brands. Does it matter which brand is supplied?

Answers

1. Rectal therapy is appropriate for mild left-sided colitis. Enemas should be administered just before bedtime when the supine position allows longer retention times. The enema can be warmed and should be inserted while lying in the left lateral position. Patients with rheumatoid arthritis may have difficulty inserting enemas and this may affect compliance and treatment success.

2. Once initiated, patients should remain on the same brand of mesalazine as different brands have different release profiles. Relapse of disease can occur if patients are inadvertently switched to another brand. Prescribers are encouraged to prescribe by brand and not by generic name.

Case 13.6

Mr F was diagnosed with Crohn's disease 4 years ago. Although relatively well, during the last year he has required two courses of prednisolone. However, when the dose has been reduced, his symptoms have flared. The decision has been made to start Mr F on azathioprine.

Question

What counselling points would you discuss with this patient?

Answer

It is important that Mr F is aware that azathioprine can take several weeks to work but that this should allow the steroid to be withdrawn.

Common side effects are nausea and flu-like symptoms with fever. The azathioprine is to be taken once a day with food as this may reduce nausea. Generalized aches and pains also affect up to 25% of patients. Some people may notice some hair loss, but this commonly reflects the severity of the inflammation rather than the medication. Inflammation of the liver or pancreas is a rare side effect.

Mr F should also be advised about the need for regular blood tests as azathioprine suppresses the bone marrow and can affect liver function. For this reason immunization with live vaccines should also be avoided.

ACKNOWLEDGEMENTS

The authors would like to thank Dr S.P.L. Travis (Consultant Gastroenterologist, John Radcliffe Hospital, Oxford) and to June Beharry (Dietitian, John Radcliffe Hospital, Oxford) for their comments on the manuscript.

REFERENCES

Ahmad T, Tamboli C P, Jewell D et al 2004 Clinical relevance of advances in genetics and pharmacogenetics of IBD. Gastroenterology 126: 1533-1549

Carter M J, Lobo A J, Travis S P L et al 2004 Guidelines for the management of inflammatory bowel disease in adults. Gut 53(suppl V): v1-v16

Felder J B, Burton I K, Rajapakse R 2000 Effects of nonsteroidal antiinflammatory drugs on inflammatory bowel disease: a case–control study. American Journal of Gastroenterology 95: 1949-1954

Fernandes-Banares F, Honojoso J, Sanchez-Lombrana J L et al 1999 Randomised clinical trial of *Plantago ovata* seeds (dietary fiber) as compared with mesalazine in maintaining remission in ulcerative colitis. American Journal of Gastroenterology 2: 427-433

Gibson P R, Shepherd S J 2005 Personal view: food for thought – western lifestyle and susceptibility to Crohn's disease. The FODMAP hypothesis. Alimentary Pharmacology and Therapeutics 21: 1399

Heuschkel R B, Walker-Smith J A 1999 Enteral nutrition in inflammatory bowel disease of childhood. Journal of Parenteral and Enteral Nutrition 23: S29-32

Jarnerot G, Hertervig E, Friis-Liby I et al 2005 Infliximab as rescue therapy in severe to moderately severe ulcerative colitis: a randomized, placebo controlled study. Gastroenterology 128: 1805-1811

Jess T, Riis L, Jespersgaard C et al 2005 Disease concordance, zygosity, and NOD2/CARD15 status: follow-up of a population-based cohort of Danish twins with inflammatory bowel disease. American Journal of Gastroenterology 100: 2486-2492

Marshall J K, Irvine E J 1997 Rectal corticosteroids versus alternative treatments in ulcerative colitis: a meta-analysis. Gut 40: 775-781

McGovern D P B, Jewell D P 2005 Risks and benefits of azathioprine therapy. Gut 54:1055

Misiewicz J J, Pounder R E, Venables C W (eds) 1994 Diseases of the gut and pancreas, 2nd edn. Blackwell Scientific Publications, Oxford

National Institute for Clinical Excellence 2002 Guidance on the use of infliximab for Crohn's disease. Technology appraisal guidance no 40. National Institute for Clinical Excellence, London

Radford-Smith G L, Edwards J E, Purdie D M 2002 Protective role of appendicectomy on onset and severity of ulcerative colitis and Crohn's disease. Gut 51: 808-813

Rutgeerts P, Feagan B G, Olson A et al 2005 A randomized placebo-controlled trial of infliximab therapy for active ulcerative colitis: Act 1 trial. Gastroenterology 128(suppl 2): A-105

Sandborn W J, Rachmilewitz D, Hanauer S B et al 2005 Infliximab induction and maintenance therapy for active ulcerative colitis: Act 2 trial. Gastroenterology 128(suppl 2): A-104

Sutherland L, MacDonald J K 2006 Oral 5-aminosalicylic acid for induction of remission in ulcerative colitis. Cochrane Database of Systematic Reviews, issue 2. John Wiley, Chichester

Travis S P L, Stange E F, Lemann M et al 2006 European evidence based consensus on the diagnosis and management of Crohn's disease: current management. Gut 55(suppl 1): i16-i35

Van Assche G, D'Haens G, Noman M et al 2003 Randomised, double blind comparison of 4 mg/kg vs. 2 mg/kg intravenous cyclosporine in severe ulcerative colitis. Gastroenterology 25: 1025-1031

Van Staa T P, Card T, Logan R F et al 2005 5-aminosalicylate use and colorectal cancer risk in inflammatory bowel disease: a large epidemiological study. Gut 54: 1573-1578

FURTHER READING

Blumberg R, Neurath M (eds) 2006 Immune mechanisms in inflammatory bowel disease. Springer-Verlag, New York

Irving P, Shanahan F, Rampton D (eds) 2006 Clinical dilemmas in inflammatory bowel disease. Blackwell, Oxford

Jewell D, Mortensen N, Steinhart A H et al (eds) 2006 Challenges in inflammatory bowel disease. Blackwell, Oxford

Kane S, Dubinsky M (eds) 2006 Pocket guide to inflammatory bowel disease. Cambridge University Press, Cambridge

Constipation and diarrhoea

14

P. Rutter

Constipation and diarrhoea are two of the most common disorders of the gastrointestinal tract. Most adults will suffer from these disorders at some time in their life and while they are often self-limiting, they can cause significant morbidity or occur as a secondary feature to a more serious disorder. For example, constipation may be secondary to hypothyroidism, hypokalaemia, diabetes, multiple sclerosis or gastrointestinal obstruction. Likewise, diarrhoea may be secondary to ulcerative colitis, Crohn's disease, malabsorption or bowel carcinoma. Both constipation and diarrhoea can also be drug induced and this should be considered when trying to identify a likely cause and determine effective management.

Constipation

In Western populations, 90% of people defaecate between three times a day and once every 3 days. It is clear, therefore, that to base a definition of constipation on frequency alone is problematic. What is perceived to be constipation by one individual may be normal to another. Most definitions of constipation include infrequent bowel action of twice a week or less that involves straining to pass hard faeces and which may be accompanied by a sensation of pain or incomplete evacuation. A pragmatic definition would simply be the passage of hard stools less frequently than the patient's own normal pattern. Standard criteria for the diagnosis of diarrhoea are available (Rome II criteria; Thompson et al 1999), although they are seldom used in practice.

Incidence

Constipation affects all age groups but is more common in the elderly: up to 20% of elderly people, compared to 8% of middle-aged and 3% of young people, seek medical advice for constipation. In the elderly, poor diet, insufficient intake of fluids, lack of exercise, concurrent disease states and use of drugs that predispose to constipation have all been identified as contributory factors.

Women are often reported to have a higher incidence of constipation than men although this probably reflects the greater likelihood that they seek medical advice. Constipation is, however, common in late pregnancy due to increased circulating oestrogens, reduced gastrointestinal motility and delayed bowel emptying caused by displacement of the uterus against the colon. It has also been reported that between 5% and 10% of children have constipation and it is more common in formula-fed babies.

Aetiology

The digestive system can be divided into the upper and lower gastrointestinal tract. The upper gastrointestinal tract starts at the mouth and includes the oesophagus and stomach and is responsible for the ingestion and digestion of food. The lower gastrointestinal tract consists of the small intestine, large intestine (colon), rectum and anus (Fig. 14.1) and is responsible for the absorption of nutrients, conserving body water and electrolytes, drying the faeces, and elimination.

The remains of undigested food are swept along the gastrointestinal tract by waves of muscular contractions called peristalsis. These peristaltic waves eventually move the faeces

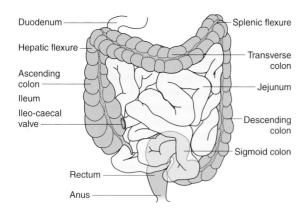

Figure 14.1 The lower gastrointestinal tract.

from the colon to the rectum and induce the urge to defaecate. By the time the stool reaches the rectum it generally has a solid consistency because most of the water has been absorbed.

Normally there is a net uptake of fluid in the intestine in response to osmotic gradients involving the absorption and secretion of ions, and the absorption of sugars and amino acids. This process is under the influence of the autonomic nervous system (sympathetic and parasympathetic). In those situations where absorption increases this will generally lead to constipation, whereas a net secretion will result in diarrhoea.

Agents that alter intestinal motility, either directly or by acting on the autonomic nervous system, affect the transit time of food along the gastrointestinal tract. Since the extent of absorption and secretion of fluid from the gastrointestinal tract generally parallels transit time, a slower transit time will lead to the formation of hard stools and constipation. Motility is largely under parasympathetic

(cholinergic) control, with stimulation bringing about an increase in motility while antagonists such as anticholinergics, or drugs with anticholinergic side effects, decrease motility and induce constipation. This mechanism is distinct from that of the other major group of drugs that induce constipation, the opioids. Opioids cause constipation by maintaining or increasing the tone of smooth muscle, suppressing forward peristalsis, raising sphincter tone at the ileocaecal valve and anal sphincter, and reducing sensitivity to rectal distension. This delays passage of faeces through the gut, with a resultant increase in absorption of electrolytes and water in the small intestine and colon.

It is normally the lower section of the gastrointestinal tract that becomes dysfunctional during constipation. For convenience, many classify constipation as originating from within the colon and rectum, or externally. Causes directly attributable to the colon or rectum include obstruction from neoplasm, Hirschsprung's disease (absence of neurones in the diseased segment of the internal anal sphincter), outlet obstruction due to rectal prolapse or damage to the pudendal nerve, typically during childbirth. Causes of constipation outside the colon include poor diet, inadequate fibre intake, inadequate water intake, excessive intake of caffeine, use of medicines with constipating side effects or systemic disorders such as hypothyroidism, diabetic autonomic neuropathy, spinal cord injury, cerebrovascular accident, multiple sclerosis or Parkinson's disease.

Differential diagnosis

Constipation is a symptom and not a disease and can be caused by many different factors (Table 14.1) but the overwhelming majority of cases in non-elderly patients will be due to lack of dietary fibre. To aid diagnosis, questions need to be asked

Table 14.1 Causes of constipation

Cause	Comment
Poor diet	Diets high in animal fats, e.g. meats, dairy products, eggs, and refined sugar, e.g. sweets, but low in fibre predispose to constipation
Irritable bowel syndrome	Spasm of colon delays transit of intestinal contents. Patients have a history of alternating constipation and diarrhoea
Poor bowel habit	Ignoring and suppressing the urge to have a bowel movement will contribute to constipation
Laxative abuse	Habitual consumption of laxatives necessitates increase in dose over time until intestine becomes atonic and unable to function without laxative stimulation
Travel	Changes in lifestyle, daily routine, diet and drinking water may all contribute to constipation
Hormone disturbances	E.g. hypothyroidism, diabetes. Other clinical signs should be more prominent, e.g. lethargy and cold intolerance in hypothyroidism and increased urination and thirst in diabetes
Pregnancy	Mechanical pressure of womb on intestine and hormonal changes, e.g. high levels of progesterone
Fissures and haemorrhoids	Painful disorders of the anus often lead patients to suppress defaecation, leading to constipation
Diseases	Many disease states may have constipation as a symptom, e.g. scleroderma, lupus, multiple sclerosis, depression, Parkinson's disease, stroke

Table 14.1 (continued)

Cause	Comment
Mechanical compression	Scarring, inflammation around diverticula and tumours can produce mechanical compression of intestine
Nerve damage	Spinal cord injuries and tumours pressing on the spinal cord affect nerves that lead to intestine
Colonic motility disorders	Peristaltic activity of intestine may be ineffective, resulting in colonic inertia
Medication	see Table 14.2
Dehydration	Insufficient fluid intake or excessive fluid loss. Water and other fluids add bulk to stools, making bowel movements soft and easier to pass
Immobility	Prolonged bedrest after an accident, during an illness or general lack of exercise
Electrolyte abnormalities	Hypercalcaemia, hypokalaemia

about the frequency and consistency of stools, nausea, vomiting, abdominal pain, distension, discomfort, mobility, diet and other concurrent symptoms or disorders the patient may be experiencing. It may also be necessary to ask about access to a toilet or commode. The individual with limited mobility may suppress the urge to defaecate because of difficulty in getting to the toilet. Likewise, lack of privacy or dependency on a nurse or carer for toileting may result in urge suppression that precipitates constipation or exacerbates an underlying predisposition. Patients with unexplained constipation of recent onset or a sudden aggravation of existing constipation associated with abdominal pain and the passage of blood or mucus, and long-standing constipation unresponsive to treatment require further investigation. Investigations include sigmoidoscopy/colonoscopy, barium enema, full blood count and biochemical monitoring including thyroid function tests (Fig. 14.2).

General management

In uncomplicated constipation, education and advice on diet and exercise are the mainstays of management and may adequately control symptoms in many individuals. Typically this advice will include reassurance that the individual does not have cancer, that the normal frequency of defaecation varies widely between individuals, and that mild constipation is not in itself harmful.

If the patient is taking medication for a concurrent disorder this must be assessed for its propensity to cause constipation. In the UK over 700 medicinal products, including ophthalmic preparations, have constipation listed as a possible side effect. Common examples of medicines involved are presented in Table 14.2.

Non-drug treatment

Non-drug treatment is advocated as first-line therapy for all patient groups, except those who are terminally ill. This often includes advising an increase in fluid intake at the same time as reducing strong or excessive intake of tea or coffee, since these act as a diuretic and serve to make constipation worse. It is generally recommended that fibre intake in the form of fruit, vegetables, cereals, grain foods, wholemeal bread, etc. be

increased to about 30 g per day. Such a diet should be tried for at least 1 month to determine if it has an effect. Most will notice an effect within 3–5 days. Unfortunately, a high-fibre diet is not without problems, with patients complaining of flatulence, bloating and distension, although these effects should diminish over a period of several months. Patients who increase their fibre intake must also be advised to drink 2 litres of water a day. Where an intake of this volume cannot be ingested it will be necessary to avoid increasing dietary fibre. An increased level of exercise should also accompany the raised fibre intake as this is thought to help relax and contract the abdominal muscles and help food move more efficiently through the gut.

A high-fibre diet is not recommended in those with megacolon or hypotonic colon/rectum because they do not respond to bulk in the colon. Similarly, a high-fibre diet may not be appropriate in those with opioid-induced constipation.

Drug treatment

Drug treatment is indicated where there is faecal impaction, constipation associated with illness, surgery, pregnancy, poor diet, where the constipation is drug induced, where bowel strain is undesirable, and as part of bowel preparation for surgery. The various laxatives available can be classified as bulk forming, stimulant, osmotic and faecal softeners. A systematic review (Tramonte et al 1997) identified 36 trials involving 1815 participants that met their inclusion criteria. Twenty of the trials compared laxative against placebo or regular diet, 13 of which demonstrated statistically significant increases in bowel movement. The remaining 16 trials compared different types of laxatives with each other. The review concluded that laxative use was superior to placebo but due to a lack of comparative data could not conclude which laxative group was most efficacious.

In general the fit, active, elderly person should be treated as a younger adult. In contrast, management of constipation in children is often complex. Early treatment is required in children to avoid developing a megarectum, faecal impaction and overflow incontinence. Encouraging the child to use the toilet after meals and increasing dietary fibre have a role alongside oral drug treatment. Depending on circumstances, behavioural therapy may be indicated.

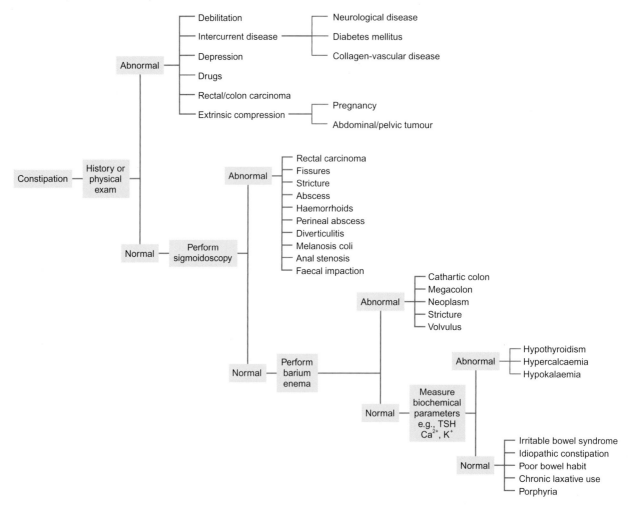

Figure 14.2 A diagnostic algorithm for constipation.

Table 14.2 Examples of medicines known to cause constipation (defined as very common [>10%] or common [1–10%])	
α-blocker	Prazosin
Antacid	Aluminium and calcium salts
Anticholinergic	Trihexyphenidyl, hyoscine, oxybutynin, procyclidine, tolterodine
Antidepressant	Tricyclics, SSRIs, reboxetine, venlafaxine, duloxetine, mirtazepine
Antiemetic	Palonosetron, dolasetron, aprepitant
Antiepileptic	Carbamazepine, oxcarbazepine
Antipsychotic	Phenothiazines, haloperidol, pimozide and atypical antipsychotics such as amisulpride, aripiprazole, olanzapine, quetiapine, risperidone, zotepine, clozapine
Antiviral	Foscarnet
β-blocker	Oxprenolol, bisoprolol, nebivolol; other β-blockers cause constipation more rarely
Bisphosphonate	Alendronic acid
CNS stimulant	Atomoxetine
Calcium channel blocker	Diltiazem, verapamil

Table 14.2 (continued)

Cytotoxic	Bortezomib, buserelin, cladribine, docetaxel, doxorubicin, exemestane, gemcitabine, irinotecan, mitozantrone, pentostatin, temozolomide, topotecan, vinblastine, vincristine, vindesine, vinorelbine
Dopaminergic	Amantadine, bromocriptine, carbegolide, entacapone, tolcapone, levodopa, pergolide, pramipexole, quinagolide
Growth hormone antagonist	Pegvisomant
Immunosuppressant	Basiliximab, mycophenolate, tacrolimus
Lipid-lowering agents	Colestyramine, colestipol, rosuvastatin, atorvastatin (other statins uncommon) gemfibrozil
Iron	Ferrous sulphate
Metabolic disorders	Miglustat
Muscle relaxant	Baclofen
NSAID	Meloxicam; other NSAIDs, e.g. aceclofenac, and COX-2 inhibitors reported as uncommon
Smoking cessation	Bupropion
Opioid analgesics	All opioid analgesics and derivatives
Ulcer healing	All proton pump inhibitors, sucralfate

Bulk-forming agents Ispaghula, methylcellulose, sterculia and bran are typical bulk-forming agents and are usually taken as granules, powders or tablets. Their use is most appropriate in situations where dietary intake of fibre cannot be increased and the patient has small hard stools, haemorrhoids or an anal fissure.

The mechanism of action for bulk-forming agents involves polysaccharide and cellulose components that are not digested and which retain fluid, increase faecal bulk and stimulate peristalsis. They may also encourage the proliferation of colonic bacteria and this helps further increase faecal bulk and stool softness. Following ingestion it usually takes 12–36 hours before any effect is seen but it may take longer. An adequate volume of fluid should also be ingested to avoid intestinal obstruction. Bulk-forming agents can be used safely long term, during pregnancy or breast feeding but many users will experience problems with flatulence and distension. The use of bulk-forming agents is not recommended in patients with colonic atony, intestinal obstruction or faecal impaction and they are less effective, or may even exacerbate constipation, in those who lack mobility.

Stimulant laxatives Drugs in this group include bisacodyl, senna and dantron. They directly stimulate colonic nerves that cause movement of the faecal mass, reduce transit time and result in the passage of stool within 8–12 hours. As a consequence of their time to onset, oral dosing at bedtime is generally recommended. For a rapid action (within 20–60 minutes) suppositories can be used. Abdominal cramps are common as an immediate side effect of stimulant laxatives, while electrolyte disturbances and an atonic colon may result from chronic use.

In the elderly, atonic colon is of less concern and prolonged use may be appropriate in a few cases. Stimulant laxatives should be avoided in patients with intestinal obstruction, and dantron alone, or in combination with a faecal softener, is restricted for use in constipation in terminally ill patients of all ages, because animal studies have demonstrated that it has carcinogenic and genotoxic properties.

Osmotic laxatives Osmotic laxatives include magnesium salts, polyethylene glycol, phosphate enemas, sodium citrate enemas, lactulose and lactitol. These agents retain fluid in the bowel by osmosis or change the water distribution in faeces to produce a softer, bulkier stool. Their ingestion should be accompanied by an appropriate fluid intake.

Rectal preparations of phosphates and sodium citrate are useful for quick relief, within 30 minutes, and bowel evacuation before abdominal radiological procedures, sigmoidoscopy and surgery. Oral magnesium salts such as the sulphate are also indicated for rapid bowel evacuation and have an effect within 2–5 hours.

Lactulose and lactitol are semisynthetic disaccharides, which are not absorbed from the gut. They increase faecal weight, volume and bowel movement and must be taken regularly. It may take 48 hours or longer for them to work. Both agents are useful in the treatment of hepatic encephalopathy since they produce an osmotic diarrhoea of low faecal pH that discourages the growth of ammonia-producing organisms.

Faecal softeners/emollient laxatives Docusate sodium is a non-ionic surfactant that has stool-softening properties. It reduces surface tension, increases the penetration of intestinal fluids into the faecal mass and has weak stimulant properties. Rectal docusate has a rapid onset of action but should not be used in individuals with haemorrhoids or anal fissure.

The classic lubricant, liquid paraffin, has no place in modern therapy. It seeps from the anus and is associated with granulomatous reactions following absorption of small quantities, lipoid pneumonia following aspiration and malabsorption of fat-soluble vitamins.

Diarrhoea

Diarrhoea is defined as the increased passage of loose or watery stools relative to the person's usual bowel habit. It may be accompanied by anorexia, nausea, vomiting, abdominal cramps or bloating. It is not a disease but a sign of an underlying problem such as an infection or gastrointestinal disorder. The most likely cause of diarrhoea in all age groups is viral or bacterial infection, therefore the following section primarily focuses on acute infective gastroenteritis but also includes reference to drug-induced diarrhoea. Diarrhoea can be associated with other conditions, e.g. irritable bowel syndrome, inflammatory bowel disease, colorectal cancer and malabsorption syndromes, but these will not be covered here.

Acute gastroenteritis is most common in children but the precise incidence is not known because many cases are self-limiting and not reported. Nevertheless, diarrhoeal illness in children leads to high consultation rates with primary care doctors and accounts for 204 consultations per 1000 consultations in the 0–4 age group. It has been estimated that children under the age of 5 years have between one and three bouts of diarrhoea per year. Children in the same age range account for over 5% of consultations to primary care doctors, with 18 000 children a year in England and Wales being admitted to hospital with rotavirus infection.

The incidence of diarrhoea in adults is, on average, just under one episode per person each year. Many of these cases are thought to be food related, with 22% of those consulting a doctor claiming to have 'food poisoning'. Traveller's diarrhoea is another common cause of diarrhoea. For high-risk travel to areas such as Africa, Asia and South America, the reported incidence is more than 20%. Over recent years *Escherichia coli* O157 has gained prominence because of a number of outbreaks in different communities associated with severe disease and even death. It is, however, an uncommon cause of diarrhoea, accounting for only 0.1% of all cases.

Aetiology

In the UK rotavirus and small round structured virus (SRSV) are the most common identified causes of gastroenteritis in children. In adults, Campylobacter followed by rotavirus are the most common causes. Other identified causes include: the bacteria *E. coli*, Salmonella, Shigella, *Clostridium perfringens* enterotoxin; viruses such as adenovirus and astrovirus; and the protozoa Cryptosporidium, Giardia and Entamoeba. These pathogens produce diarrhoea via a number of methods: for example, enterotoxigenic *E. coli* produce enterotoxins that affect gut function with secretion and loss of fluids; by interfering with normal mucosal function, for example adherent enteropathogenic *E. coli*; or by causing injury to the mucosa and deeper tissues, for example enteroinvasive *E. coli* or enterohaemorrhagic *E. coli* such as *E. coli* O157. Other organisms, for example *Staphylococcus aureus* and *Bacillus cereus*, produce preformed enterotoxins which on ingestion induce rapid-onset diarrhoea and vomiting that usually last less than 12 hours.

So-called traveller's diarrhoea frequently affects people travelling from developed to developing countries. It is caused by bacterial gastroenteritis in over 80% of cases and associated with ingestion of contaminated food or water. The organisms usually involved, in descending order, are the enterotoxigenic bacteria *E. coli*, Shigella, Salmonella, Campylobacter, Vibrio and Yersinia species. Viruses and parasites, such as Giardia, Cryptosporidium and Entamoeba, account for the remainder.

Many drugs, particularly broad-spectrum antibiotics such as ampicillin, erythromycin and neomycin, induce diarrhoea secondary to therapy (Table 14.3). With these antibiotics the mechanism involves the overgrowth of antibiotic-resistant bacteria and fungi in the large bowel after several days of therapy. The diarrhoea is generally self-limiting. However, when the overgrowth involves *Clostridium difficile* and the associated production of its bacterial toxin, life-threatening pseudomembranous colitis may be the outcome.

Table 14.3 Examples of medicines known to cause diarrhoea (defined as very common [>10%] or common [1–10%])

α-blocker	Prazosin
ACE inhibitors	Lisinopril, perindopril
Angiotensin receptor blockers	Telmisartan
Acetylcholinesterase inhibitor	Donepezil, galantamine, rivastigmine
Antacid	Magnesium salts
Antibacterial	All
Antidiabetic	Metformin, acarbose
Antidepressant	SSRIs, clomipramine, venlafaxine
Antiemetic	Aprepitant, dolasetron
Antiepileptic	Carbamazepine, oxcarbagepine, tiagabine, zonisamide, pregabalin, levtiracetam
Antifungal	Caspofungin, fluconazole, flucytosine, nystatin (in large doses), terbinafine, voriconazole

Table 14.3 (continued)

Antimalarial	Mefloquine
Antiprotozoal	Metronidazole, sodium stibogluconate
Antipsychotic	Aripiprazole
Antiviral	Abacavir, emtricitabine, stavudine, tenofovir, zalcitabine, zidovudine, amprenavir, atazanavir, indinavir, lopinavir, nelfinavir, saquinavir, efavirinez, ganciclovir, valganciclovir, adefovir, oseltamivir, ribavrin, fosamprenavir
β-blocker	Bisoprolol, carvedilol, nebivolol
Bisphosphonate	Alendronic acid, disodium etidronate, ibandronic acid, risedronate, sodium clodronate, disodium pamidronate, tiludronic acid
Cytokine inhibitor	Adalimumab, infliximab
Cytotoxics	All classes of cytotoxics
Dopaminergic	Levodopa, entacapone
Growth hormone antagonist	Pegvisomant
Immunosuppressant	Ciclosporin, mycophenolate, leflunomide
NSAIDs	All
Ulcer healing	All proton pump inhibitors
Vaccines	Pediacel (5 vaccines in 1), haemophilus, meningococcal
Miscellaneous	Calcitonin, strontium ranelate, colchicine, dantrolene, olsalazine, anagrelide, nicotinic acid, pancreatin, eplerenone, acamprosate

Signs and symptoms

Acute-onset diarrhoea is associated with loose or watery stools that will probably be accompanied by anorexia, nausea, vomiting, abdominal cramps, flatulence or bloating. When there is blood in the diarrhoea this is classed as dysentery and indicates the presence of an invasive organism such as Campylobacter, Salmonella, Shigella or *E. coli* O157.

The history of symptom onset is important. The duration of diarrhoea, whether other members of the family and contacts are ill, recent travel abroad, food eaten, antibiotic use and weight loss are all important factors to elucidate. The possibility of underlying diseases such as AIDS or infective proctitis in homosexual men must also be considered.

Dehydration is a common problem in the very young and frail elderly and the signs and symptoms must be recognized. In children, the severity of dehydration is most accurately determined in terms of weight loss as a percentage of body weight prior to the dehydrating episode. Unfortunately, in the clinical situation pre-illness weight is rarely known, therefore clinical signs of dehydration must be assessed. Symptoms that could indicate mild dehydration are vague and include tiredness, anorexia, nausea and light-headedness.

Symptoms become more prominent in moderate dehydration and include dry mucous membranes, sunken eyes, decreased skin turgor (pinch test of 1–2 seconds or longer), thirst along with tiredness, apathy, dizziness and postural hypotension. In severe dehydration the above symptoms are more marked and may also include hypovolaemic shock, oliguria or anuria, cool extremities, a rapid and weak pulse and low or undetectable blood pressure.

Investigations

Before any investigations are undertaken a medication history is required to eliminate antibiotic- and other drug-induced diarrhoeas, or the possibility of a laxative overuse-induced diarrhoea. Testing for *Clostridium difficile*-induced pseudomembranous colitis is indicated in those with severe symptoms or where hospitalization or antibiotic therapy with lincomycins, broad-spectrum β-lactams or cephalosporins has occurred within the preceding 6 weeks.

In general, stool culture is required in patients with bloody diarrhoea, severe symptoms or where there is no improvement within 48 hours. If there is a history of recent overseas travel the stool should be examined for ova, cysts and parasites. Rotavirus should be sought in those under 5 years.

Where the diarrhoea persists for more than 10 days further investigation should be undertaken to exclude parasites such as Giardia, Entamoeba and Cryptosporidium. Acute, severe or persistent diarrhoea in a homosexual male or patient with AIDS warrants referral for specialist advice.

Treatment

Acute infective diarrhoea, including traveller's diarrhoea, is usually a self-limiting disorder. However, depending on the causative agent, a number of complications may have to be dealt with. Dehydration and electrolyte disturbance can be readily treated but may, if severe, progress to acidosis and circulatory failure with hypoperfusion of vital organs, renal failure and death. Toxic megacolon due to infective colitis has been documented, associated arthritis or Reiter's syndrome may complicate the invasive diarrhoeas of Campylobacter and Yersinia, Salmonella species may infiltrate bones, joints, meninges and the gallbladder, and *E. coli* infection may, for example, be complicated by haemolytic uraemic syndrome.

General measures

Patients should be advised on handwashing and other hygiene-related issues to prevent transmission to other family members. Exclusion from work or school until the patient is free of diarrhoea is advised. In acute, self-limiting diarrhoea, healthcare workers and food handlers should be symptom free for 48 hours before returning to work. More exacting criteria for return to work, such as testing for negative stool samples, are rarely required.

In both children and adults, normal feeding should be restarted as soon as possible. In weaned and not weaned children with gastroenteritis early feeding after rehydration has been shown to result in higher weight gain, no deterioration or prolongation of the diarrhoea and no increase in vomiting or lactose intolerance (Conway & Ireson 1989, Sandhu et al 1997). Similarly, breast-feeding infants should continue to feed throughout the rehydration and maintenance phases of therapy. Avoidance of milk or other lactose-containing food is seldom justified.

Dehydration treatment

Since diarrhoea results in fluid and electrolyte loss it is important to ensure the affected individual maintains adequate fluid intake. Most patients can be advised to increase their intake of fluids, particularly fruit juices with their glucose and potassium content, and soups because of their sodium chloride content. High-carbohydrate foods such as bread and pasta can also be recommended because they promote glucose and sodium co-transport.

Young children and the frail elderly are prone to diarrhoea-induced dehydration and use of an oral rehydration solution (ORS) is recommended. The formula recommended by the World Health Organization (WHO) contains glucose, sodium, potassium, chloride and bicarbonate in an almost isotonic fluid. A number of similar preparations are available commercially in the form of sachets that require reconstitution in clean water before use (Table 14.4). Glucose concentrations between 80 and 120 mmol/L are needed to optimize sodium absorption in the small intestine. Glucose concentrations in excess of 160 mmol/L will cause an osmotic gradient that will result in increased fluid and electrolyte loss. High sodium solutions in excess of 90 mmol/L may lead to hypernatraemia, especially in children, and should be avoided. Until recently, the WHO oral rehydration solution contained 90 mmol/L sodium, as cholera is more common in developing countries and associated with rapid loss of sodium and potassium. However, a systematic review of trials using a reduced osmolarity ORS (Hahn et al 2001) concluded that solutions with a reduced osmolarity compared to the standard WHO formula were associated with fewer unscheduled intravenous infusions, a trend toward reduced stool output and less vomiting in children with mild-to-moderate diarrhoea. Based on this and other findings, the WHO oral rehydration solution now has a reduced osmolarity of 245 mOsm/L and contains 75 mmol of sodium.

Commercially available solutions in the UK contain lower sodium concentrations as diarrhoea tends to be isotonic and therefore replacement of large quantities of sodium is less important and indeed may be harmful. The presence of potassium prevents hypokalaemia occurring in the elderly, especially in those taking diuretics. Oral rehydration solutions should be routinely used in both primary and secondary care settings. There appears to be no significant difference between intravenous and oral rehydration (Gavin et al 1996).

For healthy adults an appropriate substitute for a rehydration sachet is 1 level teaspoonful of table salt plus 1 tablespoon of sugar in 1 litre of drinking water. The volume of oral rehydration solution to be taken in treating mild-to-moderate diarrhoea is dependent on age. In adults 2 litres of oral rehydration fluid should be given in the first 24 hours, followed by unrestricted

Table 14.4 Composition of oral rehydration solutions

	Osmolarity mOsm/L	Glucose mmol/L	Sodium mmol/L	Chloride mmol/L	Potassium mmol/L	Base mmol/L
Dioralyte®	240	90	60	60	20	Citrate 10
Electrolade®	251	111	50	40	20	Bicarbonate 30
Rapolyte®	250	110	60	50	20	Citrate 10
WHO ORS	245	75	75	65	20	Citrate 10

normal fluids with 200 mL of rehydration solution per loose stool or vomit. For children, 30–50 mL/kg of an oral rehydration solution should be given over 3–4 hours. This can be followed with unrestricted fluids, either with normal fluids alternating with oral rehydration solution or normal fluids with 10 mL/kg rehydration solution after each loose stool or vomit (Murphy 1998). The solution is best sipped every 5–10 minutes rather than drunk in large quantities less frequently.

Care is required in diabetic patients who may need to monitor blood glucose levels more carefully.

Drug treatment

Antimotility agents In acute diarrhoea, antimotility agents such as loperamide, diphenoxylate and codeine are occasionally useful for symptomatic control in adults who have mild-to-moderate diarrhoea and require relief from associated abdominal cramps. Antimotility agents are not generally recommended for use in children as trial results appear contradictory and any benefits are small with unacceptable levels of side effects being observed. Management should initially focus on prevention or treatment of fluid and electrolyte depletion before antimotility agents are considered.

Antimotility agents should be avoided in severe gastroenteritis or dysentery because of the possibility of precipitating ileus or toxic megacolon. All appear to have comparable efficacy but loperamide is the drug of choice given its low incidence of CNS effects.

Diphenoxylate Diphenoxylate is a synthetic opioid available as co-phenotrope in combination with a subtherapeutic dose of atropine. The atropine is present to discourage abuse but may cause atropinic effects in susceptible individuals. Administration of co-phenotrope at the recommended dosage carries minimal risk of dependence. However, prolonged use or administration of high doses may produce a morphine-type dependence. Its adverse effect profile resembles that of morphine.

In cases of suspected overdose signs may be delayed for up to 48 hours. Young children are particularly susceptible to diphenoxylate overdose where as few as 10 tablets of co-phenotrope may be fatal.

Concurrent use of diphenoxylate with monoamine oxidase inhibitors can precipitate a hypertensive crisis, while the action of CNS depressants such as barbiturates, tranquillizers and alcohol is enhanced.

Loperamide Loperamide is a synthetic opioid analogue that exerts its action by binding to opiate receptors in the gut wall, reducing propulsive peristalsis, increasing intestinal transit time, enhancing the resorption of water and electrolytes, reducing gut secretions and increasing anal sphincter tone. In uncomplicated diarrhoea it may have an effect within 1 hour of oral administration. It is relatively free of CNS effects at therapeutic doses although CNS depression may be seen in overdose, particularly in children. Because it undergoes hepatic metabolism it should be used with caution in patients with hepatic dysfunction.

Codeine and morphine The constipating side effect of the opioid analgesics codeine and morphine may be used to treat diarrhoea. Both are susceptible to misuse and, given in large doses, may induce tolerance and psychological and physical dependence. Morphine may still be obtained in combination with

agents such as the adsorbent kaolin, e.g. kaolin and morphine. However, it has no evidence of efficacy in the treatment of diarrhoea and should not be recommended.

Bismuth subsalicylate Bismuth subsalicylate is an insoluble complex of trivalent bismuth and salicylate that has been shown to be effective in reducing stool frequency. It possesses antimicrobial activity on the basis of its bismuth content while the salicylate is considered to confer antisecretory properties. At therapeutic doses it is relatively free from side effects although it may cause blackening of the tongue and stool. The relatively large quantity of the liquid preparation that has to be consumed is seen as a disadvantage.

Antimicrobials Antibiotics are generally not recommended in diarrhoea associated with acute infective gastroenteritis. Inappropriate use will only contribute further to the problem of resistant organisms. There is, however, a place for antibiotics in patients with positive stool culture where the symptoms are not receding. In patients presenting with dysentery or suspected exposure to bacterial infection, treatment with a quinolone, for example ciprofloxacin, may be appropriate. However, quinolones are not without their problems: they may cause tendon damage or induce convulsions in epileptics, in situations that predispose to seizures, and in patients taking NSAIDs. Their use in adolescents is also not recommended because of an association with arthropathy.

Where Campylobacter is the suspect causative organism, patients with severe symptoms or dysentery should receive early treatment with erythromycin or ciprofloxacin. Severe symptoms or dysentery associated with Shigella can also be treated with ciprofloxacin. Nalidixic acid can be used in children and trimethoprim may be appropriate in pregnant women where resistance is not a problem.

The use of antibiotics in patients with Salmonella is not generally recommended because of the likelihood that excretion is prolonged. Antibiotics may, however, be indicated in the very young and the immunocompromised. The benefit of antibiotic use in enterohaemorrhagic infection, for example E. coli O157, is less clear. In this situation there is evidence that antibiotics cause toxins to be released which may lead to haemolytic uraemic syndrome.

In both amoebic dysentery and giardiasis, metronidazole is the drug of choice. Diloxanide is also used in amoebic dysentery to ensure eradication of the intestinal disease. Antibiotics are not indicated in the treatment of cryptosporidiosis in immunocompromised individuals.

Probiotics Probiotics have been defined as components of microbial cells or microbial cell preparations that have a beneficial effect on health. Well-known probiotics include lactic acid bacteria and the yeast Saccharomyces. The rationale for their use in infectious diarrhoea is that they act against enteric pathogens by competing for available nutrients and binding sites, making gut contents acid and increasing immune responses. A Cochrane review (Allen et al 2003) concluded that whilst probiotics in individual studies appeared moderately effective as adjunctive therapy, there were insufficient studies of specific probiotic regimens to inform the development of evidence-based treatment guidelines.

Table 14.5 outlines some of the common therapeutic problems in constipation and diarrhoea.

Table 14.5 Common therapeutic problems in constipation and diarrhoea

Problem	Comment
Constipation	
Bulk laxative, e.g. ispaghula, taken at bedtime	Drugs such as ispaghula should not be taken before going to bed because of risk of oesophageal blockage
Urine changes colour	Anthraquinone glycosides, e.g. senna, are excreted by kidney and may colour urine yellowish-brown to red colour, depending on pH
Patient claims dietary and fluid advice ineffective in resolving constipation	May find high-fibre diet difficult to adhere to, socially unacceptable, and expect result in less than 4 weeks
Patient taking docusate complains of unpleasant aftertaste or burning sensation	Advise to take with plenty of fluid after ingestion
Sterculia as Normacol® and Normacol Plus® granules or sachets	The granules should be placed dry on the tongue and swallowed immediately with plenty of water or a cool drink. They can also be sprinkled onto and taken with soft food such as yoghurt
Methylcellulose (Celevac)	Each tablet should be taken with at least 300 mL of liquid
Diarrhoea	
Antimotility agent requested for a young child	Antimotility agents must be avoided in young children or patients with severe gastroenteritis or dysentery
Antimotility agent requested by patient with persistent diarrhoea (>10 days)	Antimotility agent inappropriate. Stool culture required to exclude parasitic infection such as Giardia, Entamoeba and Cryptosporidium
Adult with diarrhoea stops eating and drinking to allow diarrhoea to settle	Patient should eat and drink as normally as possible. Plenty of fluids required to prevent dehydration. Fruit juice (glucose and potassium), soup (salt), bread and pasta (carbohydrate) are of particular benefit
Reconstitution of oral rehydration solution	Each sachet of Diorolyte, Electrolade and Rapolyte requires 200 mL of water. They should be discarded after 1 hour after preparation unless stored in a fridge when they may be kept for 24 hours

CASE STUDIES

Case 14.1

Mr J, a man in his 30s, asks to speak with the pharmacist. He has constipation and has taken some medicine, lactulose, but he is still finding it difficult to go to the toilet. He asks for a stronger laxative.

Question

What further information do you need to be in a position to help Mr J?

Answer

Constipation is rarely a symptom of sinister pathology in someone of Mr J's age. The most likely cause is a diet low in fibre and inadequate fluid intake. Establish the duration and nature of the problem and discuss with Mr J his usual diet. Determine if there has been any change to his diet recently, which may have precipitated the constipation. Social factors also play a role in constipation so it is prudent to ask if there have been any life changes such as a loss of job or difficulties with family life. If his replies to the questions raise no suspicion of underlying medical problems then dietary advice only may be needed. However, since he has already taken lactulose it is likely he will persist in his request for a suitable laxative. Question Mr J on how he took the lactulose and for how long. Patients often have misconceptions on how quickly a medicine will work. A stimulant laxative may be a suitable alternative for Mr J as it has a quicker onset of action.

Case 14.2

Mr A's mother has recently moved in with his family following the death of his father 4 months ago. Although she was formerly a sprightly 78 year old she is now withdrawn, eats little of the meals prepared for her and no longer goes for her daily walks. Mr A knows she is taking medicine for a long-standing heart complaint and has recently started taking antidepressants. She is complaining of constipation.

Question

Mr A would like to know if there is any medicine suitable to help his mother.

Answer

Constipation is a common problem in the elderly. Activity levels often diminish and many also suffer from medicine-induced constipation exacerbated by reduced muscle tone. Pain on defaecation associated with haemorrhoids is also a common contributory factor. The elderly often have poor dental status or false teeth and consequently avoid high-fibre foods because they are more difficult to chew.

In the case of Mr A's mother, the history provides little insight into the duration of the problem although there are a number of factors that warrant further investigation. Clearly, a reduction in physical activity has occurred and her diet and fluid intake may have changed. The death of her husband and loss of independence are significant lifestyle issues for Mr A's mother that cannot readily be addressed and probably account for the recent introduction of antidepressants. The identity of her 'heart medicine' may reveal a drug-induced factor that could have been enhanced by the recent prescription for antidepressants. It is also unclear whether she has been constipated previously.

Appropriate exercise, proper diet and sufficient fluid may be the only key actions that need to be taken.

Case 14.3

Mr B is a busy 45-year-old executive who works for a large multinational company. He has noted blood in his stools over the past 2 weeks and for 3 days has had continuous abdominal discomfort. He has discussed his symptoms with his wife and they suspect haemorrhoids are the cause. Mr B is going away on business in 6 days and seeks your advice on a suitable treatment.

Question

What advice should be given to Mr B?

Answer

Blood in the stool is not necessarily serious. If the blood appears fresh and can only be seen on the surface of the stool it is likely the source is the anus or distal colon. It is probably caused by straining and bleeding from haemorrhoids or an anal fissure. Similarly if the blood appears as specks or as a smear on the toilet paper after defaecation, this is also likely to indicate haemorrhoids, particularly if such a diagnosis has been made previously following clinical examination.

If the blood is mixed with the faeces and has a dark or 'tarry' appearance then a more serious underlying cause is possible. The darker the faeces, the more suggestive they are that there has been an upper GI bleed or a substantial loss of blood from the large bowel. If this is the case the patient should have a proper clinical examination.

Iron or bismuth tablets can cause darkened stools so it is important to take a medication history from the patient.

However, given Mr B's age, recent onset of symptoms and the presence of continuous abdominal pain accompanying the constipation, a thorough clinical examination is required to eliminate sinister pathology such as bowel obstruction caused by a tumour or diverticular disease.

Case 14.4

A 7-year-old boy in previous good health was admitted to hospital with bloody diarrhoea and dehydration 4 days after attending a children's birthday party. He was treated with intravenous fluids and given nothing by mouth. The day after admission to hospital a colonoscopy revealed haemorrhagic colitis. His diarrhoea seemed to be improving up to day 5 when he experienced a generalized convulsion following which he was transferred to a children's intensive care bed. He was irritable and pale, hypertensive and an emergency laboratory report revealed thrombocytopenia, hyponatraemia and hyperkalaemia.

Questions

1. What is the likely diagnosis in this child?
2. What specific therapy is required?

Answers

1. This patient probably has haemolytic uraemic syndrome caused by *E. coli* O157. Haemolytic uraemic syndrome is the most common form

of acquired renal insufficiency in young children. It is characterized by nephropathy, thrombocytopenia and microangiopathic haemolytic anaemia. Although there are a number of potential causative factors, the most common is the toxin-producing O157 strain of *E. coli*. In 1996, 21 people died from *E. coli* O157 after eating contaminated meat from a butcher's shop in Scotland. In 2001, 13 Girl Guides and their leader contracted *E. coli* O157 after camping in a field in Inverclyde, Scotland, previously grazed by sheep and in 2005 more than 158 children from 42 schools in South Wales were affected by eating contaminated meat, one of whom died.

The syndrome typically has a pro-drome of bloody diarrhoea occurring 5–7 days before onset of renal insufficiency. Colonoscopy is usually non-specific and shows haemorrhagic colitis. At diagnosis most children are pale and very irritable. Hypertension and hyponatraemia may be associated with convulsions and are generally a consequence of a disorder of fluid and salt balance. Laboratory findings may include anaemia and thrombocytopenia, hyponatraemia, hyperkalaemia, hypocalcaemia and metabolic acidosis. The kidney typically shows signs of glomerular endothelial injury. Capillary thrombosis is quite prominent but with no evidence of immune complex deposition. Similar findings can usually be seen in all other organs including the brain, liver and intestine.

2. Treatment is usually supportive. Fluid and electrolyte balance need to be corrected and the hypertension controlled. In cases with prolonged oliguria or anuria, peritoneal dialysis may be used. Approximately 85% of patients recover normal renal function.

Case 14.5

Mr G is planning to travel to Mexico on business. He was last there 6 months ago but was incapacitated with diarrhoea for 3 of 6 days in a busy work schedule. He does not want a repeat experience on his forthcoming visit and seeks advice about taking a course of antibiotics with him to use as empirical treatment should the need arise.

Questions

1. Is there any evidence that antibiotics are of benefit in traveller's diarrhoea?
2. Are there any problems associated with empirical use of antibiotics in traveller's diarrhoea?

Answers

1. The empirical use of antibiotics has been shown to increase the cure rate in individuals suffering from traveller's diarrhoea. Studies in travellers including students, package tourists, military personnel and volunteers have compared antibiotic use against placebo (De Bruyn et al 2000). The antibiotics studied have included aztreonam, ciprofloxacin, co-trimoxazole, norfloxacin, ofloxacin and trimethoprim given for durations varying from a single dose to a 5-day treatment course. Overall, antibiotics increased the cure rate at 72 hours (defined as cessation of unformed stools or less than one unformed stool/24 hours) without additional symptoms.

2. The use of antibiotics in the treatment of traveller's diarrhoea does have problems. Adverse effects in up to 18% of recipients have been reported with gastrointestinal (cramp, nausea, anorexia), dermatological (rash) and respiratory (cough, sore throat) symptoms the most frequently reported. Antibiotic-resistant isolates have also been reported following the use of ciprofloxacin, co-trimoxazole and norfloxacin.

REFERENCES

Allen S J, Okoko B, Martinez E et al 2003 Probiotics for treating infectious diarrhoea. Cochrane Database of Systematic Reviews. Update Software, Oxford

Conway S P, Ireson A 1989 Acute gastroenteritis in well nourished infants: comparison of four feeding regimens. Archives of Disease in Childhood 64: 87-91

De Bruyn G, Hahn S, Borwick A 2000 Antibiotic treatment for travellers' diarrhoea. Cochrane Database of Systematic Reviews. Update Software, Oxford

Gavin N, Merrick N, Davidson B 1996 Efficacy of glucose-based oral rehydration therapy. Pediatrics 98(1): 45-51

Hahn S, Kim Y, Garner P 2002 Reduced osmolarity oral rehydration solution for treating dehydration due to diarrhoea in children. Cochrane Database of Systematic Reviews. Update Software, Oxford

Murphy M S 1998 Guidelines for managing acute gastroenteritis based on a systematic review of published research. Archives of Disease in Childhood 79: 279-284

Sandhu B K, Isolauri E, Walker-Smith J A et al 1997 A multicentre study on behalf of the European Society of Paediatric Gastroenterology and Nutrition Working Group on Acute Diarrhoea: early feeding in childhood gastroenteritis. Journal of Pediatric Gastroenterology and Nutrition 24: 522-527

Thompson W G, Longstreth G F, Drossman D A et al 1999 Functional bowel disorders and functional abdominal pain. Gut 45(suppl 2): 43-47

Tramonte S M, Brand M B, Mulrow C D et al 1997 The treatment of chronic constipation in adults. A systematic review. Journal of General Internal Medicine 12:15-24

FURTHER READING

Alonso-Coello P, Guyatt G, Heels-Ansdell D et al 2005 Laxatives for the treatment of hemorrhoids. Cochrane Database of Systematic Reviews. Update Software, Oxford

Anon 2000 Managing constipation in children. Drug and Therapeutics Bulletin 38: 57-60

Bartlett J G 2002 Antibiotic-associated diarrhoea. New England Journal of Medicine 346: 334-339

Borum M L 2001 Constipation: evaluation and management. Primary Care 28: 577-590

Gorelick M H, Shaw K N, Murphy K O 1997 Validity and reliability of clinical signs in the diagnosis of dehydration in children. Available online at: www.pediatrics.org/cgi/content/full/99/5/e6

Khin M U, Nyunt-Nyunt W, Khin M et al 1985 Effect on clinical outcome of breast feeding during acute diarrhoea. British Medical Journal 290: 587-589

Pappagallo M 2001 Incidence, prevalence and management of opioid bowel dysfunction. American Journal of Surgery 182(suppl 5A): 115-185

Sellin J H 2001 The pathophysiology of diarrhoea. Clinical Transplantation 15(suppl 4): 2-10

Xing J H, Soffer E E 2001 Adverse effects of laxatives. Diseases of the Colon and Rectum 44: 1201-1209

Adverse effects of drugs on the liver

15

B. E. Cadman B. Featherstone

Table 15.1 Characteristics of the different types of acute liver failure (Richardson & O'Grady 2002)

Characteristic	Hyperacute	Acute	Subacute
Transition time from jaundice to encephalopathy	0–7 days	8–28 days	29–84 days
Cerebral oedema	Common	Common	Rare
Renal failure	Early	Late	Late
Ascites	Rare	Rare	Common
Coagulation disorder	Marked	Marked	Modest
Prognosis	Moderate	Poor	Poor

An adverse drug reaction (ADR) is an effect that is unintentional, noxious and occurs at doses used for diagnosis, prophylaxis and treatment. A hepatic drug reaction is an ADR which predominantly affects the liver.

Drugs can induce almost all forms of acute or chronic liver disease, with some drugs producing more than one type of hepatic reaction. Although not a particularly common form of adverse drug reaction, drugs should always be considered as a possible cause of liver disease.

Epidemiology

The incidence of drug-induced liver disease has continued to rise steadily since the late 1960s, although the incidence of idiosyncratic reactions for most drugs remains low, occurring at therapeutic doses from 1 in every 1000 patients to 1 in every 100 000 patients. It is estimated that 15–40% of acute liver failure (ALF) cases may be attributable to drugs. Classification of ALF suggests three classes: hyperacute, acute and subacute (Table 15.1).

In the early 1990s, acute overdose with paracetamol accounted for 30–40 000 hospital admissions and over half the cases of ALF referred to liver units. It was the definite cause of at least 150 deaths a year in the UK. ALF induced by paracetamol has become an important indication for liver transplantation. Hepatotoxicity induced by such drugs as halothane, the antituberculous agents isoniazid and rifampicin, psychotropics, antibiotics and cytotoxic drugs still continues to cause concern.

Many drugs cause elevated liver enzymes with apparently no clinically significant adverse effect, although in a few patients there may be significant hepatotoxicity. For example, isoniazid causes elevated liver enzymes in 10–36% of patients taking the drug as a single agent. However, only 1% suffer significant hepatotoxicity, with the liver function tests of the majority returning to normal if therapy is discontinued. Other examples of drugs that elevate liver enzymes are shown in Table 15.2.

Although it is not possible to identify patients who will suffer adverse drug reactions manifesting in hepatic toxicity, a number of risk factors have been identified.

Risk factors

Pre-existing liver disease

Pre-existing liver disease may increase the risk of developing drug-induced hepatic injury with agents such as methotrexate, cytotoxic agents, aspirin and sodium valproate. In general, patients with liver disease are more likely to suffer ADRs.

Table 15.2 Examples of drugs that elevate liver enzymes

Drug	Percent of patients with increase in transaminases
Cefaclor	11%
Cefixime	0.7%
Ciprofloxacin	5%
Chlorpromazine	50%
Diclofenac	15%
Donepezil	MHRA reports[a]
Efavirenz	4%
Isoniazid	10–36%
Naproxen	4%
Norfloxacin	0.1%
Nevirapine	12%
Niacin	50%
Rifampicin	15–30%
Sodium valproate	11%
SSRIs	MHRA reports[a]
Statins	1–2%
Sulphonamides	10%

[a] Available at http://www.mhra.gov.uk

Age

It is generally accepted that the elderly are at an increased risk of ADRs. There are multiple reasons for this, including higher exposure rates and decreased metabolism. Drug-induced hepatic injury is more likely to occur in elderly patients than in those under 35 years of age. Similarly, halothane hepatitis and isoniazid or chlorpromazine hepatotoxicity are more likely in patients over 40 years of age. The severity of the reactions also appears to increase with age, especially in those over 60 years. Sodium valproate toxicity, on the other hand, demonstrates an increased risk of developing serious or fatal hepatotoxicity in those under 3 years, with risk decreasing as age advances. Aspirin is an example of another drug causing hepatotoxicity specifically in children. Reye's syndrome in children has been linked to the use of aspirin following a viral illness; it is life-threatening and associated with coma, seizures and liver failure.

Gender

The frequency of drug-induced hepatotoxicity is more common in females than males, particularly with halothane, isoniazid and

nitrofurantoin. There is weak evidence of a gender difference in toxicity of sodium valproate, being more common in boys before puberty and in females after puberty. Cholestatic jaundice associated with co-amoxiclav has been reported to be more common in males than females.

Genetics

Genetic differences that affect an individual's ability to metabolize certain drugs may predispose to drug-induced liver disease. For example, both fast and slow acetylators may be more susceptible to isoniazid-induced liver damage. The conventional view is that rapid acetylators are at risk of increased toxic reactions due to transformation of acetylhydrazine by cytochrome P450 into a reactive metabolite; other studies suggest slow acetylation may result in toxicity due to formation of hydrazine, which is toxic in itself. Monitoring of liver function tests (LFTs) is recommended monthly for the first 3 months, as toxicity is most likely to occur early in therapy.

Halothane-induced injury has been reported for multiple family members in one study.

It is thought that a genetic predisposition to allergic forms of drug hypersensitivity could be a factor in some types of liver disease.

Enzyme induction

Alcohol, rifampicin and other drugs that induce cytochrome P450 isoenzyme 2El potentiate the risk of hepatotoxicity with other drugs such as paracetamol, isoniazid and halothane.

Concomitant therapy with other anticonvulsants, particularly phenytoin and phenobarbital, is a risk factor for toxicity with sodium valproate, where 90% of cases of liver injury are associated with combination therapy.

Polypharmacy

A typical example of this is seen with NSAIDs. The risk of liver disease with NSAIDs is normally extremely low but is increased when NSAIDs are used with other hepatotoxic drugs.

Concurrent diseases and pregnancy

Pre-existing renal disease, diabetes, pregnancy and poor nutrition may all affect the ability of the liver to metabolize drugs effectively and may put the patient at risk of developing liver damage.

Table 15.3 summarizes the host factors that may predispose a patient to drug hepatotoxicity.

Aetiology

Drug-induced hepatotoxicity may present as an acute insult that may or may not progress to chronic disease, or it can present as an insidious development of chronic disease. The type of lesion may be cytotoxic (cellular destruction) or cholestatic (impaired bile flow). Cytotoxic damage may be further classified as necrotic (cell death) or steatic (fatty degeneration). The liver damage resulting from drug toxicity often presents as a mixed picture

Table 15.3   Examples of host factors that predispose to drug hepatotoxicity

Host factor	Drug example
Pre-existing liver disease	Methotrexate, aspirin, sodium valproate
Age	
Older	Halothane, isoniazid, chlorpromazine, co-amoxiclav
Younger	Aspirin, sodium valproate
Gender	
Female	Halothane, isoniazid, nitrofurantoin
Male	Sodium valproate (in prepubescent boys co-amoxiclav?)
Genetics	Halothane, chlorpromazine, phenytoin, carbamazepine, phenobarbital, paracetamol
Enzyme induction	Paracetamol, halothane, isoniazid, sodium valproate
Polypharmacy	NSAIDs if used with other hepatotoxic drugs
	Isoniazid with rifampicin or pyrazinamide
	Sodium valproate with phenytoin
	Paracetamol with zidovudine
Concurrent diseases	
Diabetes mellitus	Methotrexate
Renal failure	Allopurinol, i.v. tetracycline
Malnutrition	Paracetamol
HIV positive with hepatitis C or B co-infection	Antiretroviral agents

of cytotoxic and cholestatic injury. The mechanisms of drug-induced hepatic damage can be divided into intrinsic (type A) and idiosyncratic (type B) hepatotoxicity (Table 15.4). Intrinsic hepatotoxicity is predictable, dose dependent and usually has a short latency period ranging from hours to weeks. The majority of individuals who take a toxic dose are affected and exhibit the same type of injury. Examples are paracetamol, salicylates, methotrexate and tetracycline. Other examples are presented in Table 15.5. Toxicity may be avoided by ensuring the doses listed are not exceeded.

Idiosyncratic reactions occur at a low frequency, typically less than 1 in 100 individuals who are exposed to the drug. The latency period is variable, ranging from 5 to 90 days from the initial ingestion of the drug. The type of injury is less predictable and not dose related. This type of reaction may be due to either drug hypersensitivity or a metabolic abnormality. Examples of drugs that induce idiosyncratic reactions are chlorpromazine, halothane and isoniazid.

The precise mechanisms resulting in drug-induced liver disease are often not completely understood, although injury to the hepatocytes may result directly from interference with intracellular function, membrane integrity or indirectly by immune-mediated damage to cells.

Necrosis

Necrosis is characterized by cytotoxic cellular breakdown (hepatocellular destruction).

Table 15.4   Intrinsic vs idiosyncratic hepatotoxic reactions

	Intrinsic toxicity		Idiosyncratic toxicity
Mechanism	Direct toxicity	Metabolic abnormality	Hypersensitivity reaction
Dose dependent	Yes	No	No
Predictable	Yes	No	No
Latency	Hours	Weeks to months	1–5 weeks
Type of injury	Usually necrosis	Any	Any
Clinical features	Acute liver failure	Increased liver enzymes, hepatitis, jaundice	Fever, rash, eosinophilia, arthralgias, hepatitis

Table 15.5 Examples of dose-related drug-induced hepatotoxicity

Drug	Toxic dose
Paracetamol	Single dose >10 g
Tetracycline	>2 g daily (oral), increased risk of toxicity in pregnancy and renal failure
Methotrexate	Weekly dose >15 mg Cumulative dose >2 g in 3 years, increased risk of toxicity in pre-existing liver disease, alcohol abuse, diabetes
6-Mercaptopurine	>2.5 mg/kg
Vitamin A	Chronic use of 40 000 units daily
Cyclophosphamide	Daily dose >400 mg/m^2
Salicylates	Chronic use >2 g daily
Anabolic steroids	High dose >1 month
Oral contraceptive	Increased risk with higher oestrogen content, older preparations Duration of treatment
Iron	Single dose >1 g

Paracetamol causes hepatic necrosis when its normal metabolic pathway is saturated. Subsequent metabolism occurs by an alternative pathway that produces a toxic metabolite which covalently binds to liver cell proteins and causes necrosis.

Steatosis

In steatosis hepatocytes become filled with small droplets of lipid (microvesicular fatty liver) or occasionally with lipid droplets that are much larger (macrovesicular fatty liver). Tetracyclines are thought to cause steatosis by interfering with synthesis of lipoproteins that normally remove triglycerides from the liver.

Cholestasis

Some drugs injure bile ducts and cause partial or complete obstruction of the common bile duct, resulting in retention of bile acids and the condition known as cholestasis.

Cholestasis caused by anabolic and contraceptive steroids is due to inhibition of bilirubin excretion from the hepatocyte into the bile.

The penicillins, although commonly associated with allergic drug reactions, are a very rare cause of liver disease. The isoxazoyl group present in the synthetic β-lactamase resistant oxy-penicillins has been implicated as a cause of liver injury. Acute cholestatic hepatitis has increasingly been reported during treatment with flucloxacillin, and in some countries this has become the most important cause of drug-induced cholestatic hepatitis. The incidence appears to be about twice that of the related isoxazoyl penicillins cloxacillin and dicloxacillin. Moreover,

there is likely to be underreporting due to a delay in onset of up to 42 days after stopping treatment. Female sex, age over 55 years, longer courses and high daily doses also seem to be associated with a higher risk of liver reaction to flucloxacillin.

Rifampicin causes hyperbilirubinaemia by inhibiting uptake of bilirubin by the hepatocyte as well as inhibiting bilirubin excretion into bile. Other therapeutic agents affect sinusoidal or endothelial cells, which may result in veno-occlusive disease or fibrosis. Vitamin A affects the fat-storing cells, causing toxicity that leads to fibrosis.

Pathophysiology

The range of drug-induced liver diseases is illustrated in Table 15.6. Increased serum level of hepatobiliary enzymes without clinical liver disease occurs with variable frequency between drugs but for some agents it may occur in up to half the patients who receive a drug. This may reflect subclinical liver injury.

Hepatocellular necrosis

In severe cases acute hepatocellular necrosis presents with jaundice and LFT abnormalities, including a modestly raised alkaline phosphatase and a markedly elevated alanine aminotransferase level of up to 200 times the upper limit of the reference range. Prolongation of the prothrombin time occurs but depends on the severity of the injury, increasing dramatically in severe cases. Microscopy reveals necrosis of the hepatocytes in a characteristic pattern.

Steatosis

Steatosis (fatty liver) is the accumulation of fat droplets within liver cells and is associated with abnormal LFTs, although the elevation of alanine aminotransferase is not as high as that seen in acute hepatocellular necrosis. Hyperammonia, hypoglycaemia, acidosis and clotting factor deficiency may also be present. Histologically, the liver damage resembles the acute fatty liver of pregnancy. Fat distribution within the hepatocyte is either microvesicular, as occurs with tetracycline, aspirin and sodium valproate, or macrovesicular where the hepatocyte cell nucleus is displaced to the periphery by a single large fat droplet. This type of damage occurs typically with steroids, methotrexate, alcohol and amiodarone.

A less severe, more chronic form of fatty liver, steatohepatitis, also occurs. Steatohepatitis differs from diffuse fatty change. Notably the clinical symptoms and biochemistry resemble chronic parenchymal disease and the histology is similar to that seen in alcoholic hepatitis. Amiodarone is an example of a drug that can cause chronic steatohepatitis associated with phospholipidosis.

Cholestasis

Cholestasis without hepatitis is associated with a raised bilirubin and a normal or minimally raised alanine aminotransferase level. No inflammation or hepatocellular necrosis is seen. In contrast, cholestasis associated with hepatitis presents with raised bilirubin,

Table 15.6   Examples of adverse drug reactions on the liver

Adverse reaction	Drugs associated with reaction
Hepatocellular necrosis	Paracetamol Propylthiouracil Salicylates Iron salts Allopurinol Dantrolene Halothane Ketoconazole Isoniazid Mithramycin Cocaine 'Ecstasy' (methylene dioxymetamphetamine)
Fatty liver	Amiodarone Tetracyclines Steroids Sodium valproate L-Asparaginase
Cholestasis	Oral contraceptives Carbimazole Anabolic steroids Ciclosporin
Cholestasis with hepatitis	Chlorpromazine Tricyclic antidepressants Erythromycin Flucloxacillin Co-amoxiclav ACE inhibitors Sulphonamides Sulphonylureas Phenytoin NSAIDs Cimetidine Ranitidine
Granulomatous hepatitis	Phenytoin Allopurinol Carbamazepine Clofibrate Hydralazine Sulphonamides Sulphonylureas
Acute hepatitis	Dantrolene Isoniazid Phenytoin
Chronic active hepatitis	Methyldopa Nitrofurantoin Isoniazid
Fibrosis and cirrhosis	Methotrexate Methyldopa Vitamin A (dose related)
Vascular disorders	Azathioprine Dactinomycin Dacarbazine

alanine aminotransferase and alkaline phosphatase levels and a certain amount of liver damage.

Granulomatous hepatitis

Granulomatous hepatitis occurs with modestly elevated LFTs and, usually, normal synthetic liver function. Histology reveals granulomas and tissue eosinophilia.

Acute hepatitis

Acute hepatitis resembles viral hepatitis with LFTs raised in proportion to the severity of the hepatocellular damage. The best indicator of severity is the prothrombin time. Histologically, necrosis and cellular degeneration are seen in combination with an inflammatory infiltrate.

Chronic active hepatitis

Chronic active hepatitis may present as an acute injury or progress to cirrhosis. Serum transaminases are usually raised and albumin is low. The histology resembles that of autoimmune chronic active hepatitis and is associated with circulating autoantibodies. Methyldopa is an example of a drug that can cause chronic active hepatitis.

Fibrosis

In patients with fibrosis, the serum transaminase levels may be only slightly raised, and are not good predictors of hepatic damage. Microscopy shows deposition of fibrous tissues. Fibrosis may proceed to cirrhosis. Such damage may be seen with long-term methotrexate use.

Vascular disorders

A variety of drugs can cause veno-occlusive disease, which is characterized by non-thrombotic narrowing of small centrilobular veins, and is typically caused by cytotoxic agents and some herbal remedies. Use of oral contraceptives or cytotoxic agents may exacerbate an underlying thrombotic disorder and increase the risk of the Budd–Chiari syndrome (obstruction of the large veins) developing.

Tumours

Drugs have been associated with a variety of hepatic tumours. The drugs most commonly linked to malignancy are the oral contraceptives, anabolic steroids and danazol.

Clinical manifestations

The clinical features of drug-induced hepatotoxicity vary widely, depending on the type of liver damage caused.

Acute hepatocellular necrosis

In acute hepatocellular necrosis caused by paracetamol, early symptoms include anorexia, nausea and vomiting, malaise and lethargy. Abdominal pain may be the first indication of liver damage but is not usually apparent for 24–48 hours. A period of apparent recovery precedes the development of jaundice and production of dark urine. If the liver injury is severe, deterioration follows, with repeated vomiting, hypoglycaemia, metabolic acidosis, bruising and bleeding, drowsiness and hepatic encephalopathy. Oliguria (diminished urine output) and anuria (complete cessation of urine production) may result from acute tubular necrosis. Renal failure may occur even in the absence of severe liver disease. In addition to acute renal failure, myocardial injury and pancreatitis have also been reported. In fatal cases, death from acute hepatic failure occurs between 4 and 18 days after ingestion.

Steatosis

A patient presenting with steatosis generally shows fatigue, nausea, vomiting, hypoglycaemia and confusion. Jaundice is present in severe cases.

Acute hepatitis

Acute hepatitis may present with a prodromal illness with non-specific symptoms or include features of drug allergy followed by anorexia, nausea and vomiting, dark urine, pale stools and jaundice. Jaundice tends to be present in severe cases. Weight loss may also be a feature of acute hepatitis. Fatalities occur in 5–30% of jaundiced patients. Acute hepatitis is second only to paracetamol self-poisoning as a cause of drug-induced liver disease.

Chronic active hepatitis

Drug-induced chronic active hepatitis may present with tiredness, lethargy and malaise, in a manner similar to other types of chronic liver disease. The symptoms may evolve over many months. Gastrointestinal symptoms are usually present, and patients may show one or more complications of severe liver disease, including ascites, bleeding oesophageal varices or hepatic encephalopathy. If the adverse drug reaction has an allergic component, a skin rash and other extrahepatic features of a drug allergy such as lymphadenopathy, evidence of bone marrow suppression (particularly petechial haemorrhages) may be present.

Cholestasis

The main clinical feature of pure cholestasis is severe pruritus, with or without other features, according to the severity, such as dark urine, pale stools and jaundice.

Drug-induced cholestatic hepatitis usually presents with gastrointestinal symptoms following an influenza-like illness. Abdominal pain with typical features of cholestasis then occurs. The pruritus is generally less severe than with pure cholestasis.

Veno-occlusive disease

Veno-occlusive disease may present with painful hepatomegaly, ascites and jaundice along with other features of liver insufficiency. It has been reported following chemotherapy with drugs such as cyclophosphamide, doxorubicin and dacarbazine. It has also been reported as a common complication of bone marrow transplantation.

Hepatic tumours

In general patients with hepatic tumours present in a similar manner. Abdominal pain may or may not be reported, together with a feeling of fullness after eating. Weight loss, fatigue, anorexia, nausea and, occasionally, vomiting can occur, especially in advanced cases.

Investigations

Various types of investigation are used in the diagnosis of drug-induced hepatotoxicity, with the number and type of tests depending on the clinical presentation.

Biochemical tests

Routine LFTs are measured, which generally include total bilirubin, alanine transaminase and alkaline phosphatase. Impairment of the synthetic function of the liver is detected by total protein, albumin and the prothrombin time. Other biochemical tests may include measurement of γ-glutamyl transpeptidase which may be elevated in all forms of liver disease, including drug-induced disease. α-Fetoprotein may be measured to exclude malignancy. Conjugated bilirubin may be measured to establish if there is biliary obstruction.

Serological markers

Serological markers for hepatitis A, B and C and other viruses such as the Epstein–Barr virus should be determined in patients with symptoms of hepatitis with appropriate risk factors to exclude an infective cause.

Radiological investigations

Radiological investigations, such as ultrasound, computed tomography, percutaneous cholangiograms and endoscopic retrograde cholangiopancreatography, are used to look for physical obstruction of bile ducts by gallstones, masses or strictures.

Liver biopsy

Liver biopsy is seldom helpful for diagnosis but certain drugs can cause characteristic lesions, such as the distribution of microvesicular fat droplets seen with tetracyclines. Specific diagnostic tests for drug-induced disease exist for few drugs, with halothane being a notable exception.

Other causes of liver dysfunction such as autoimmune chronic active hepatitis, acute severe cholestasis, ischaemic hepatic necrosis, pregnancy-related liver disease, the Budd–Chiari syndrome, rare metabolic disorders or liver disease related to alcohol abuse must also be excluded.

Treatment

The aim of treatment for drug-induced hepatotoxicity is complete recovery. This relies on correct diagnosis, withdrawal of any and all suspected drugs, and supportive therapy, which may include liver transplantation where appropriate.

Diagnosis

Drug-induced hepatic injury should be suspected in every patient with jaundice while ruling out other causes of liver disease by the clinical history and the results of investigations. Figure 15.1 illustrates the typical process.

Drugs that are commonly prescribed, such as NSAIDs, antimicrobials and antihypertensive agents, are more likely to be implicated in drug-induced liver disease, although the frequency for the individual agents is low. Identifying the causative agent and stopping it is important in reducing the morbidity and mortality associated with drug-induced liver disease. Recovery normally follows discontinuation of a hepatotoxic drug. Serious toxicity or acute liver failure may result if the drug is continued after symptoms appear or the serum transaminases rise significantly. Failure to discontinue the drug may give grounds for claims of negligence.

A detailed and thorough drug history, including use of oral contraceptives, over-the-counter medicines, vitamins, herbal preparations and illicit drug use, should be obtained. Examples

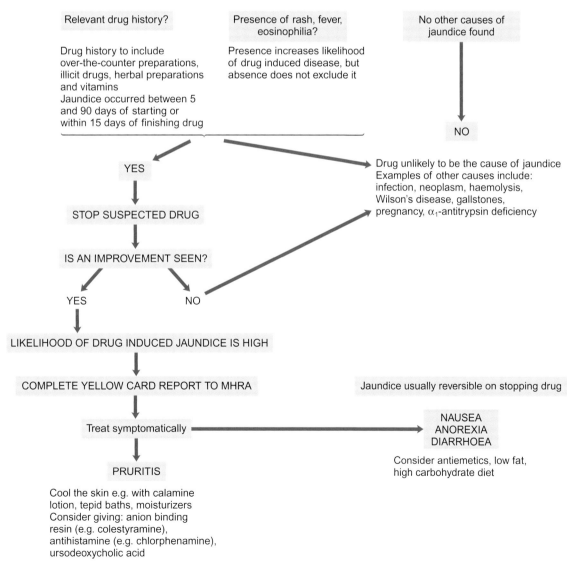

Figure 15.1 General approach to the diagnosis and management of drug-induced jaundice. (MHRA: Medicines and Healthcare Regulatory Agency)

of herbal preparations implicated in causing liver damage are listed in Table 15.7. Attention to the duration of treatment with a specific drug and the relationship to the onset of symptoms is important. The likelihood of a drug-related disease is greatest when the abnormality begins between 5 and 90 days after taking the first dose and within 15 days of taking the last dose. The latent period (the time between starting therapy and the appearance of symptoms) may vary but for many drugs is sufficiently reproducible to be of some diagnostic value.

Predisposing factors for liver toxicity should also be noted. If the liver injury is accompanied by fever, rash and eosinophilia, the likelihood of drug-induced disease increases, although lack of these features does not exclude it. Unequivocal diagnosis cannot be made in most circumstances, and improvement on withdrawal of the implicated drug may provide the strongest evidence for drug-induced disease. Time for resolution of the abnormalities is dependent on the individual drug and type of liver disease. In some cases several months may elapse.

Idiosyncratic reactions may also need to be considered and the literature consulted for previous reports. A key component of secondary prevention is the reporting of all suspected hepatic drug reactions to the appropriate monitoring agency, particularly for newer agents with fewer published cases. Many drugs are approved and licensed before the idiosyncratic reactions are identified as there is little chance of detecting the reaction in the phase III studies which typically involve 300 patients. To detect a single case of clinically significant hepatic injury due to a drug with 95% confidence, the number of patients included in the trial must be about three times the incidence of the reaction. Idiosyncratic reactions occur in about 1 in 10 000 patients so to detect the reaction, the clinical trial would have to study 30 000 patients.

Withdrawal

Once drug-induced hepatotoxicity has been recognized as a possibility, therapy should be stopped. If the patient is receiving more than one potentially hepatotoxic drug, all drugs should be stopped. Withdrawal of the agent usually results in recovery that begins within a few days. The LFTs may take many months to return to normal. Co-amoxiclav and phenytoin are examples of drugs that have been associated with a worsening of the patient's condition for several weeks after withdrawal, and a protracted recovery period of several months.

Rechallenge

When drug-induced hepatotoxicity has been confirmed by improvement on drug withdrawal, subsequent use in the patient is generally contraindicated. Rechallenge is not normally justified as this is potentially dangerous for the patient, although a positive rechallenge is the most definitive evidence of drug-induced disease. Inadvertent rechallenge may occur. If the rechallenge is negative, this is usually taken to indicate that the patient may resume using the drug. Another adverse reaction on re-exposure to the drug precludes any further use.

Management

If clinical or laboratory signs of hepatic failure appear, hospitalization is mandatory.

After withdrawal of the drug, attempts to remove it from the body are only relevant for acute hepatotoxins such as paracetamol, metals or toxic mushrooms such as *Amanita phalloides* (death cap).

If patients present a few hours post ingestion, any unabsorbed drug may best be removed by gastric lavage, rather than by use of emetics.

Antidotes

Specific antidotes are acetylcysteine and methionine for paracetamol, and desferrioxamine for iron overdose. Desferrioxamine 5–10 g in 50–100 mL of water is administered orally as soon as possible after ingestion for acute iron poisoning. Parenteral desferrioxamine is indicated in addition to oral administration, to chelate absorbed iron where the plasma levels exceed 89.5 µmol/L, where the plasma levels exceed 62.6 µmol/L and there is evidence of free iron, and in patients with signs and symptoms of acute iron poisoning.

Corticosteroids

Immunosuppression with corticosteroids has been used in the management of drug-induced hepatotoxicity, but evidence indicates their use does not affect survival of patients with acute liver failure. However, there have been anecdotal reports of impressive responses to corticosteroids that are persuasive, and it may be appropriate to conduct a short trial in rare types of drug-induced disease.

Table 15.7 Examples of herbal remedies implicated in hepatotoxicity

Borage oil
Chapparal (*Larrea tridentata*)
Chinese herbal preparations for skin disorders
Comfrey
Garcinia (*Garcinia camboge*)
Germander (*Teucrium chamaedrys*)
Kava kava (*Piper methysticum*)
Khat (*Catha edulis*)
Mistletoe (skullcap)
Passion flower (*Passiflora incarnata*)
Ubiquinone
Valerian (*Valeriana officinalis*)

Supportive treatment

For most patients there is no specific treatment available. General supportive treatment is necessary in liver failure, with appropriate attention to fluid and electrolyte balance.

Nutritional support should be along conventional medical lines. Some patients find that a low-fat, high-carbohydrate diet provides relief from the anorexia, nausea and diarrhoea that may accompany cholestasis.

Pruritus

The main symptom of drug-induced cholestasis is pruritus due to high systemic concentrations of bile acids deposited in tissues. General measures include light clothing (avoid wool) and cooling the skin with tepid baths or calamine lotion, and a general moisturizing agent such as aqueous cream. The management of liver-induced pruritus is discussed in more detail in Chapter 16.

Coagulation disorders

Coagulation disorders should be treated by correcting vitamin K deficiency with intravenous phytomenadione injection. This should correct the prothrombin time within 3–5 days. Oral phytomenadione is ineffective in cholestasis. Menadiol sodium phosphate, the water-soluble vitamin K analogue, may be effective in an oral dose of 10 mg daily. If bleeding occurs, infusion of fresh frozen plasma or clotting factor concentrates will be indicated. The administration of other fat-soluble vitamins may also be necessary. Liver transplantation is often considered the treatment of choice for patients with acute hepatic failure induced by drugs.

Long-term treatment

When the drug-induced liver disease is under control, consideration will have to be given to the treatment of the original condition for which the implicated drug was prescribed. In many cases, drug therapy will still be required and caution must therefore be exercised, as drugs with similar chemical structures may cause similar hepatotoxicity (Table 15.8).

Hepatotoxicity may occur with different derivatives of a drug. Erythromycin-induced cholestatic hepatitis has been more frequently reported with the estolate preparation than with other erythromycin esters (ethylsuccinate, stearate, propionate and

lactobionate). It is not clear which part of the drug is responsible for hypersensitivity.

Paracetamol-induced hepatotoxicity

Paracetamol causes a dose-related toxicity resulting in centrilobular necrosis. It normally undergoes the phase II reactions of glucuronidation and sulphation. However, paracetamol is metabolized by cytochrome P450 2E1 to N-acetyl-p-benzoquinoneimine (NABQI) if the capacity of the phase II reactions is exceeded or if cytochrome P450 2E1 is induced. After normal doses of paracetamol, NABQI is detoxified by conjugation with glutathione to produce mercaptopurine and cysteine conjugates. Following overdose, tissue stores of glutathione are depleted, allowing NABQI to accumulate and cause cell damage. Illness, starvation and alcohol deplete glutathione stores and increase the predisposition to paracetamol toxicity, while acetylcysteine and methionine provide a specific antidote by replenishing glutathione stores.

Ingestion of doses as low as 10–15 g of paracetamol have been reported to cause severe hepatocellular necrosis. Removal of unabsorbed paracetamol by gastric lavage may be worthwhile if more than 150 mg/kg body weight has been taken and the patient presents within 4 hours of ingestion. Activated charcoal may also be administered to reduce further absorption of paracetamol and facilitate removal of unmetabolized paracetamol from extracellular fluids. This may lessen the effect of any methionine given. A plasma paracetamol concentration should be taken as soon as possible but not within 4 hours of ingestion due to the fact that a misleading and low level may be obtained because of continuing absorption and distribution of the drug. The plasma concentration measured should be compared with a standard nomogram reference line of a plot of plasma paracetamol concentration against time in hours after ingestion. This may be a semilogarithmic (Fig. 15.2) or linear (Fig. 15.3) plot. Generally, administration of intravenous acetylcysteine is the treatment of choice for

Table 15.8 Examples of cross-sensitivity within drug groups

	Problem	Action
Phenothiazines	Cross-sensitivity	Avoid
Tricyclics	Cross-sensitivity	Avoid
NSAIDs	Cross-sensitivity	Avoid
Isoniazid, pyrazinamide	Chemically related	Avoid
Halothane	Avoid enflurane	Isoflurane appears safe

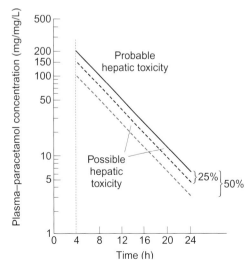

Figure 15.2 Semilogarithmic plot of plasma paracetamol concentration versus time in hours after ingestion.

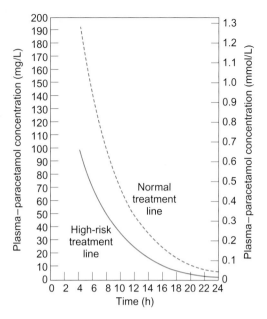

Figure 15.3 A linear plot of plasma paracetamol concentration versus time in hours after ingestion.

paracetamol overdose when the blood paracetamol level is in the range predictive of possible or probable liver injury (see Fig. 15.2). Patients allergic to acetylcysteine may receive oral methionine.

Acetylcysteine is most effective within 8 hours of overdose. However, late administration in patients who present more than 16–24 hours post ingestion may be appropriate. Acetylcysteine administered at this stage will not counteract the oxidative effects of paracetamol but it may have a cytoprotective role in hepatic failure, and has been shown to reduce morbidity and mortality in patients who have already developed acute liver failure.

Patient care

Patients may be at risk of drug-induced hepatotoxicity from prescribed drugs or from purchased drugs. Additionally, children may be at risk from medicines that are not stored properly. Parents should be reminded to store all medicines in child-resistant containers and out of reach. Deaths from liver failure have occurred in children following overdose with drugs commonly available, such as iron tablets.

Patient counselling

Patients who purchase preparations containing paracetamol should be made aware of the danger of overdosing, which may occur if other preparations containing paracetamol are taken simultaneously. Since 1994 the European guidelines on package labelling have required products containing paracetamol to warn patients of the need to avoid other products containing paracetamol. The pack size of paracetamol sold from general sales outlets has been limited to 16 tablets or capsules (32 where paracetamol is sold under the supervision of a pharmacist) with the aim of limiting availability and reducing residual stocks in the home. This appears to have reduced the incidence of ALF secondary to paracetamol overdose.

All patients should be advised of potential side effects. This information needs to be reinforced with the use of patient information leaflets.

Patients and their carers should be helped to recognize signs of liver disorder and know to report immediately symptoms such as malaise, nausea, fever and abdominal discomfort that may be significant although non-specific during the first few weeks of any change of therapy. If these are accompanied by elevated LFTs, the drug should be discontinued.

Patients who recover from drug-induced hepatotoxicity should be informed of the causative agent, warned to avoid it in the future, and advised to inform their doctor, dentist, nurse and pharmacist about the occurrence of such an event.

Parents of children commenced on sodium valproate should be warned to report side effects that may be suggestive of liver injury such as the onset of anorexia, abdominal discomfort, nausea and vomiting. Early features include drowsiness and disturbed consciousness. Fever may also be present. The time to onset is between 1 and 4 months in the majority of cases.

The challenge for all members of the healthcare team is to alert patients to the potentially toxic effects of drugs without creating so much concern that they fail to comply with vital medication. For the limited number of drugs presented in Table 15.9, careful monitoring of LFTs during the first 6 months of treatment is advisable, although not always practical. Thereafter, regular monitoring of LFTs is appropriate in patients who are at greater risk of hepatotoxicity. Such patients would include those with known liver disease, those taking other hepatotoxic drugs, those aged over 40 years, and heavy alcohol consumers. Surveillance should be particularly frequent in the first 2 months of treatment. In patients with no risk factors and normal pretreatment liver function, LFTs need only be repeated if fever, malaise, vomiting, jaundice or unexplained deterioration during treatment occurs.

Since many drugs cause elevation of LFTs there may be difficulty in assessing when to stop a drug, particularly when treating an individual for tuberculosis or epilepsy. An empirical guideline is that the drug should be stopped if the levels of alanine transaminase exceed three times the upper limit of the reference range. Any clinical features of liver disease or drug allergy would require immediate discontinuation of the drug. Conversely, a raised γ-glutamyl transpeptidase level and elevated alanine transaminase level in the absence of symptoms often reflect microsomal induction and would not indicate drug-induced injury.

It should be noted that monitoring of LFTs is not a complete safeguard against hepatotoxicity, as some drug reactions develop very quickly, and the liver enzymes are an unreliable indicator of fibrosis.

Minimizing the risk of drug-induced liver disease

Cholestatic jaundice has been reported to occur in about 1 in 6000 patients treated with co-amoxiclav. The risk of acute liver injury with co-amoxiclav is approximately six times that of amoxicillin and increases with treatment courses above 14 days (Garcia Rodriguez et al 1996). Hence the indications for co-amoxiclav

Table 15.9 Examples of drugs where regular monitoring of liver function tests is recommended

Drug	Baseline measurement*	Frequency of monitoring
Anti-TB therapy (isoniazid, rifampicin, pyrazinamide)	Yes	Patients with pre-existing chronic liver disease: check LFTs regularly, every week for the first 2 weeks, then twice a week for the first 2 months.
		Patients with normal liver function tests and no evidence of pre-existing liver disease: regular monitoring is not necessary but LFTs repeated if signs of liver dysfunction develop, e.g. fever, malaise, vomiting or jaundice.
		Patients with raised pretreatment hepatic transaminases: *two or more times normal*: check LFTs weekly for 2 weeks, then twice a week until normal. *under two times normal*: check LFTs at 2 weeks. If these transaminases have fallen, further tests are only needed if symptoms occur
Amiodarone	Yes	LFTs checked every 6 months
Cyproterone	Yes	Recheck if any symptoms
Methotrexate	Yes	LFTs checked every 2 weeks for the first 2 months, then monthly for 4 months, then every 3 months
Methyldopa	Yes	Check LFTs at intervals during the first 6–12 weeks of treatment
Sodium valproate	Yes	Check LFTs regularly during the first 6 months of therapy
Dantrolene	Yes	Repeat LFTs after first 6 weeks of therapy
Sulfasalazine	Yes	LFTs checked every 2 weeks for the first 2 months, then monthly for 4 months then every 3 months

* Baseline and subsequent LFTs difficult to interpret in critically ill patients as LFTs will be affected by multiple factors

have been restricted to cover infections caused by amoxicillin-resistant β-lactam producing infections.

Patients admitted for procedures requiring a general anaesthetic should be questioned about past exposure and any previous reactions to halothane. Halothane is well known to be associated with hepatotoxicity, particularly if patients are re-exposed. Repeated exposure to halothane within a period of less than 3 months should be avoided, while some increase in risk persists regardless of the time interval since last exposure (Ray & Drummond 1991). Unexplained jaundice or delayed-onset postoperative fever in a patient who has received halothane is an absolute contraindication to future use in that individual. Patients with a family history of halothane-related liver injury should also be treated with caution.

The individuals at greatest risk of halothane hepatitis are obese, postmenopausal women. Halothane may be present in detectable amounts even in theatres equipped with scavenging devices, and it is possible for these small concentrations to provoke a reaction in a highly sensitized individual. If electing to avoid halothane, a halothane-free circuit and operating theatre should be used. Cross-hepatotoxicity with other haloalkanes is a possibility, and enflurane should also be avoided. Isoflurane appears to be safe, as no reports of cross-sensitivity have been published. Some anaesthetists would prefer to use total intravenous anaesthesia in patients who have had a reaction to halothane.

Although hepatic adverse drug reactions are rare for most drugs, when they do occur they can cause significant morbidity and mortality. Over 600 drugs have been associated with

hepatotoxicity and any new drug released on to the market may have the potential to cause hepatotoxicity. Pemoline, troglitazone and tolcapone are examples of drugs withdrawn from the market due to reports of serious hepatic reactions. These examples help to highlight the importance of postmarketing surveillance and yellow card reporting.

Appropriate selection of drugs, an awareness of predisposing factors and avoidance of toxic dose thresholds and potentially hepatotoxic drug–drug interactions will minimize the risk to patients.

CASE STUDIES

Case 15.1

Miss RS is a 17-year-old female student who presented with jaundice and a rising bilirubin and prothrombin time. There was no previous family history of liver disease and no history of alcohol intake. She had never had an operation or received a blood transfusion and denied using illicit drugs.

She had initially developed pain in her right foot 5 weeks previously for which she was prescribed ibuprofen. Seven days before admission she started diclofenac. Two days after starting diclofenac she became increasingly tired and nauseated, and was treated with a course of ampicillin.

On examination she was jaundiced with no encephalopathy and had a blood pressure of 160/84 mmHg. There were no cardiac murmurs, hepatosplenomegaly or ascites.

	Actual value (normal range)
Albumin	24 (30–50 g/L)
Alanine transaminase	635 (0–50 units/L)
Bilirubin	331 (<17 μmol/L)
Alkaline phosphatase	213 (30–135 units/L)
Haemoglobin	12.4 (13–18 g/dL)
WBC	11.7 (4–11 × 10⁹/L)
Platelets	172 (150–450 × 10⁹/L
Prothrombin time	61 (11–14 seconds)
α_1-antitrypsin	Normal
Immunoglobulins	Normal
Creatinine clearance	127 (90–135 mL/min)
Urinary copper	1.4 μmol/24 hours (normal)
Serum copper	7 μmol/L (normal)
Caeruloplasmin	0.6 g/L (normal)
Slit-lamp examination of the eyes	No evidence of Kayser-Fleischer rings.
	No evidence of infection with cytomegalovirus or Epstein–Barr virus.

Management

Despite supportive treatment, Miss RS's prothrombin time (PT) continued to rise and she developed encephalopathy. She was listed for a liver transplant with a diagnosis of acute liver failure (ALF) possibly related to drugs. She successfully underwent orthotopic liver transplantation (OLT).

Questions

1. What is the significance of the clinical history?
2. What type of liver disease do the signs and symptoms indicate?
3. Which drug is most likely to be responsible and why?
4. What advice should the patient be given concerning medication use after a liver transplantation?

Answers

1. The patient was a student and was unlikely to be exposed to an excessive risk of infection with hepatitis A or a tropical disease as she had not travelled abroad in the recent past. The fact that Miss RS had not received a general anaesthetic recently also excludes postoperative jaundice. A negative transfusion and illicit drug use history made infections such as hepatitis B and C unlikely.

   Her alcohol consumption was minimal and this excluded alcoholic liver disease. Many possible causes of liver disease could be excluded from the clinical history alone. The results from the investigations exclude other causative factors such as cytomegalovirus or Epstein–Barr virus. α_1-Antitrypsin deficiency, an inherited disorder that may be associated with liver disease in some patients, was excluded. Wilson's disease, a disorder of copper metabolism, was excluded by the negative Kayser-Fleischer rings and measurement of serum caeruloplasmin and urinary copper excretion.

2. The patient's elevated LFTs indicate an acute hepatocellular injury. The prolonged prothrombin time also indicates a severe reaction. The fact that albumin is low is also an indicator of severity. The albumin level would also be expected to be low in chronic disease, because it reflects loss of synthetic function. In this case there is clearly no evidence to support a diagnosis of chronic disease. The rapid deterioration is not unusual in a severe drug reaction.

3. The evidence from the drug history suggests only two causative agents as the ampicillin was commenced after the initial symptoms appeared. The relationship of symptoms to the administration of drugs implicates diclofenac as the most likely cause.

   Ibuprofen is a very commonly used NSAID and is available without prescription. Hepatotoxicity with ibuprofen appears to be very rare although cases of hepatocellular injury exist and cholestasis without hepatitis has been observed. A single case of fatal liver failure associated with fatty changes has been reported. Most reported cases of hepatotoxicity have had an onset within 3 weeks of commencing ibuprofen treatment.

   There have been several reports of diclofenac-induced hepatitis published in the literature, and a considerable number reported to the regulatory authorities. A frequency of 5 cases per 100 000 patients exposed to diclofenac has been described. Females appear to be more susceptible, and there is some evidence for increased risk in patients over 65 years of age. The onset of action is usually within the first 3 months of treatment.

   Ampicillin has rarely been involved with liver injury. Reports of systemic hypersensitivity with hepatic involvement, granulomatous hepatitis and cholestasis with vanishing bile duct syndrome have been reported.

   Diclofenac appears to be the most likely candidate. All drug therapy was stopped on admission.

4. Following a liver transplant the patient will require counselling about the immunosuppressive drugs she has to take long term. Information about all aspects of drug therapy, including advice on what to do if doses are missed and advice on any potential side effects, should be covered for all drugs, which may include tacrolimus, azathioprine, prednisolone, omeprazole, antifungals, co-trimoxazole and valganciclovir.

   Over time the number of drugs and doses will be reduced. Future use of NSAIDs and diclofenac is contraindicated for this patient.

Case 15.2

Mrs X is a 79-year-old lady who presented with a 10-day history of jaundice, pale stools, dark urine, pruritus and mild abdominal discomfort. She did not have fever and had previously been fit and well. Approximately 5 weeks prior to admission she had injured her shin, a superficial ulcer had developed and she was given a course of flucloxacillin. The ulcer had not completely healed and her primary care doctor had prescribed a second course of flucloxacillin 250 mg four times a day. This second course was completed 1 week prior to admission. Mrs X did not take any other medication. There was no previous family history of liver disease. She drank approximately 2 units of alcohol per week.

On examination she was found to be jaundiced; there was no encephalopathy, ascites or hepatosplenomegaly. An ultrasound investigation showed the liver to be of normal size with no intra- or extrahepatic duct dilation. No calculi were seen in the gallbladder. Biochemical tests showed her full blood count and U&Es to be normal, other results were as follows.

	Actual value (normal range)
Albumin	35 g/dL (30–50 g/L)
Alanine transaminase	35 units/L (0–50 units/L)
Bilirubin	363 μmol/L (<17 μmol/L)
Alkaline phosphatase	476 units/L (30–135 units/L)
Prothrombin time	15.9 seconds (11–14 seconds)
Immunoglobulins	Normal
AMA, ANA, SMA, ANCA	Negative
Hepatitis serology	Negative
Liver biopsy	Hepatocellular and canalicular bile stasis with no hepatitis

Initially the bilirubin and alkaline phosphatase levels dropped. However, 3 weeks after the initial presentation Mrs X re-presented with jaundice, pruritus, weight loss, dark urine and pale stools. These symptoms gradually resolved but 6 months after initial diagnosis ultrasound showed a markedly heterogeneous nodular liver.

Questions

1. What type of liver disease do the signs and symptoms indicate?
2. What is the evidence that flucloxacillin caused the liver damage in this patient?
3. What is the significance of the nodular liver seen on ultrasound 6 months after initial diagnosis?

Answers

1. Mrs X is jaundiced and has pale stools and dark urine, indicating that she has cholestatic liver disease. This means there is an impairment of bile flow along the bile ducts. This causes a lack of bile pigment formation within the gastrointestinal tract and the formation of pale stools. Conjugated (water-soluble) bilirubin is excreted in the urine, leading to a darkening of the urine. Pruritus (intense itching) is also a sign of cholestatic liver disease due to the accumulation of bile salts in the skin. Elevations in blood levels of bilirubin and alkaline phosphatase are indicative of cholestatic liver disease.
2. Other causes for her liver disease have been excluded. Immune disease was excluded as the immunoglobulins and autoantibodies were normal. An infective cause was also excluded as her hepatitis serology was negative. The ultrasound showed no obstruction or hepatic duct dilation.

   Flucloxacillin is a well-recognized cause of drug-induced cholestatic liver disease. The risk of flucloxacillin-induced liver disease is higher in the first 45 days after exposure, with an incidence of 8.5 per 100 000 prescriptions. However, it can present weeks after the drug has been discontinued (Russman et al 2005). The risk of flucloxacillin-induced cholestasis increases in patients over 55 years old and in those receiving courses of longer than 2 weeks. Mrs X could therefore be considered to be at increased risk of flucloxacillin-induced cholestasis. Female sex is, however, not considered to be a risk factor (Fairley et al 1993).
3. The biopsy results showed hepatocellular and canalicular bile stasis with no hepatitis. This, along with ductopenia, a reduction in number or size of bile ducts, is a typical finding in flucloxacillin-induced liver disease (Eckstein et al 1993).

   The cholestasis induced by flucloxacillin typically follows a protracted course over many months. Complete remission may occur in some patients, whereas others will develop a progressive ductopenia and a secondary biliary cirrhosis. The appearance of a nodular liver on ultrasound would suggest that Mrs X's liver is still damaged. A biopsy would be needed to confirm the type of damage.

Case 15.3

Mr FD, a 45-year-old alcoholic Asian male, presented with a 2-month history of pyrexia, a mucoid, non-bloody cough, weight loss and night sweats. His CT of the chest was consistent with bronchiolitis. Cultures from early morning urine samples and bronchial alveolar lavage were positive for mycobacterium. Anti-tuberculosis therapy was started with rifampicin, isoniazid, pyrazinamide and ethambutol.

One week after initiation of therapy his bilirubin level started to rise and by 2 weeks after starting anti-TB therapy, his bilirubin level was 74 mmol/L. At this time he had no other symptoms of liver dysfunction. Initially other liver function tests remained stable but by week 9 after initiation of therapy his alanine aminotransferase had risen to 238 units/L. Clinically he was less well with malaise and vomiting.

Questions

1. What are the recommendations for monitoring liver function tests in patients on anti-TB therapy?
2. Which of the above prescribed anti-TB medications have been implicated in causing drug-induced liver damage?
3. In view of the increased bilirubin, how should this patient's anti-TB therapy be managed?
4. In view of the patient's symptoms at week 9 and his increased alanine transaminase, how should this patient's anti-TB therapy be managed?

Answers

1. Liver function tests should be checked before treatment. In patients with pre-existing chronic liver disease, liver function should be monitored regularly, weekly for the first 2 weeks and then 2-weekly for the first 2 months. In patients with normal pretreatment liver function tests and no evidence of pre-existing liver disease, regular monitoring is not necessary.

   Liver function should be repeated if signs of liver dysfunction develop, e.g. fever, malaise, vomiting or jaundice.

   In patients with pretreatment hepatic transaminases raised two or more times normal, liver function should be monitored weekly for 2 weeks, then 2-weekly until normal.

   If hepatic transaminases are under two times normal, liver function should be repeated at 2 weeks. If these transaminases have fallen, further repeat tests are only needed if symptoms occur.
2. Isoniazid (particularly in association with rifampicin), pyrazinamide and rifampicin have all been implicated in causing hepatotoxicity. Hepatic injury due to ethambutol occurs rarely, if at all.

   Minor asymptomatic rises in liver transaminases develop in 10–36% of patients receiving isoniazid. This occurs usually within the first 2 months of treatment. Approximately 1% of patients develop an acute hepatocellular necrosis resembling acute viral hepatitis. The onset of injury is usually after 6 weeks of treatment although it may occur up to a year after starting. The risk of hepatotoxicity with isoniazid increases when it is used in combination with rifampicin or pyrazinamide. Other risk factors include alcoholism, age greater than 50 years and concurrent hepatitis B infection. Injury appears to be idiosyncratic and probably involves the production of a toxic metabolite via the cytochrome P450 system.

   Rifampicin may cause transient hyperbilirubinaemia due to interference with bilirubin excretion. This is generally of little clinical consequence. Serious liver toxicity with rifampicin occurs very rarely, within the first 4 weeks of treatment and is associated with a zone three centrilobular necrosis.

   Early studies with pyrazinamide have suggested that transaminases increased in approximately 20% of patients, with overt hepatitis occurring in around 8% of patients. However, with the lower dose regimens now used, hepatotoxicity is relatively uncommon.
3. Rifampicin can cause canalicular cholestasis, resulting in transient hyperbilirubinaemia. This is due to an interference with bilirubin excretion and is generally of little clinical significance. Earlier trials of anti-TB drugs, used in short courses, noted the development of jaundice, which was not always clinically important and generally faded with continued therapy. Patients who are well, and have no symptoms of possible liver damage, should continue all anti-TB drugs and liver function tests should be monitored weekly (Campbell 1990). At this stage Mr FD showed no symptoms of liver disease and his other liver function tests were unchanged. All his therapy should be continued with weekly monitoring of liver function tests.
4. At week 9 Mr FD's alanine aminotransferase had risen to greater than five times the normal value. He also had symptoms of malaise and vomiting. At this stage his isoniazid, rifampicin and pyrazinamide should be stopped. Depending upon Mr FD's condition in relation to his tuberculosis, either no treatment is required or alternative non-hepatotoxic anti-TB therapy will be needed, e.g. ethambutol, streptomycin, moxifloxacin. Once liver function has returned to normal challenge doses of the original drugs can be reintroduced sequentially in the order isoniazid, rifampicin, pyrazinamide, with daily monitoring of the patient's condition and liver function tests.

Case 15.4

A 76-year-old man with a history of COPD was prescribed a course of co-amoxiclav 375 mg three times a day for 7 days. He presented to his primary care doctor with general malaise, vomiting and pruritus.

Questions

1. Do the clinical signs in this patient suggest liver disease?
2. Is co-amoxiclav a possible cause of liver disease? What other information is required?
3. What treatment is appropriate?

Answers

1. General malaise, tiredness and nausea and vomiting are possible signs of liver disease. Abdominal pain may also be a feature. Pruritus is associated with cholestatic jaundice as the bile salts are deposited in the skin and cause itching.

2. A full drug history, including use of over-the-counter drugs and herbal drugs, is required.

   The onset of liver disease caused by co-amoxiclav is usually within 10 days of commencing therapy but has been reported a few weeks after completing a course of treatment (Garcia Rodriguez et al 1996). Co-amoxiclav is a likely cause here, although a complete history is required to exclude other drugs or causes of illness or pre-existing liver disease.

3. Symptomatic treatment of the itch with antihistamines is appropriate. Colestyramine may be added if necessary but is poorly tolerated. Topical treatment with menthol in aqueous cream may provide relief for some patients. The reaction should be documented in the patient's medical records and an ADR report completed.

Case 15.5

A 26-year-old woman presents with increasing jaundice, nausea, vomiting and right subcostal pain and tenderness after taking 80 tablets of paracetamol 36 hours ago. The patient had vomited soon after taking the overdose and had not called the primary care doctor. Laboratory results were as follows.

	Day 1 morning	Day 1 evening	Day 2	Day 3	Day 6
Sodium (134–145 mmol/L)	144	134	135	133	134
Potassium (3.4–5.0 mmol/L)	4.1	3.1	3.6	3.8	4.4
Glucose (3.5–9.0 mmol/L)	3	4	3	3	3
Urea (<7 mmol/L)	6.7	5.4	8	11.9	33
Creatinine (35–125 µmol/L)	98	84	132	334	990
ALT (0–50 units/L)	1161	1848	Unrecordable	8435	5520
Bilirubin (<17 µmol/L)	50	42	90	80	79
Alk. phosphatase (30–135 units/L)	150	135	136	128	120
PT (11–14 seconds)	30	38	40	49	49
APPT APTT (22.5–34.5 seconds)	40	46	50	46	43
pH			7.45		
BE (±2)	−4	−3	−3	−6	−7
Lactate (<2)	3	4	4	4	4
Paracetamol (mg/L)	12	–	–	–	–
Salicylate (mg/L)	0.5	–	–	–	–
Urine output (0.5 mL/kg/h)	40–50	30	6	Anuric	Anuric

Questions

1. What treatment should be initiated for this patient?
2. What syndrome is likely to be developing?
3. Do the doses of drugs need adjusting?
4. Can the patient be prescribed paracetamol for pain?
5. What other treatment is appropriate?
6. What is the prognosis?

Answers

1. A toxic screen should always be performed to exclude other drug overdoses. A paracetamol level is required, although the prognostic value more than 15 hours after ingestion is uncertain. A plasma paracetamol concentration above the relevant treatment line should be regarded as carrying serious risk of liver disease. The extremely high ALT is characteristic of paracetamol toxicity. As the patient has overt clinical signs of liver disease, therapy with N-acetylcysteine should be commenced, as later administration has been shown to prevent or ameliorate hepatic damage and improve survival (Harrison et al 1991). Other drugs that may be used to prevent progression of the hepatorenal syndrome are dopamine, terlipressin and octreotide but further data are needed before firm treatment options can be made.

2. This patient has developing hepatorenal syndrome (HRS), the development of renal failure secondary to liver disease. Other causes of renal failure should be excluded. HRS can occur in both acute and chronic liver disease. The kidneys are likely to recover once the liver recovers. HRS is a poor prognostic sign with an associated mortality of 50–100%.

3. All drugs prescribed for the patient should be reviewed regarding potential for causing liver toxicity and enhanced side effects due to accumulation with reduced renal clearance or reduced metabolism and any necessary dose adjustments made. Any potentially nephrotoxic drugs should be stopped.

4. Ideally avoid paracetamol in the acute phase. However, if the patient needs either an analgesic or antipyretic then paracetamol in small doses may be used. No more than 2 g in 24 hours.

5. Other treatment options are shown below.

Problem	Treatment
Hypotension	Expand circulating volume Inotropes
Decreased oxygen saturation	Mechanical ventilation
Renal failure	Intermittent haemodiafiltration
Cerebral oedema	Mannitol Furosemide
Encephalopathy	Correct precipitating factors Avoid sedatives if possible Lactulose and phosphate enemas
Hypoglycaemia	Continuous glucose infusions
Bleeding	Vitamin K Fresh frozen plasma (FFP) Platelets Octreotide infusions Proton pump inhibitor (PPI)
Fluids and electrolytes	Hydration Potassium Restrict sodium to 50 mmol per day
Infection	Antifungals Broad-spectrum antibiotics

Transplantation may be considered but this patient does not meet the criteria for transplantation. The criteria for transplantation are **either** arterial pH <7.3 **or all of the following:** PT >100 seconds; encephalopathy grade 3–4; creatinine >300 µmol/L (Wendon & Williams 1995).

6. Presentation more than 36 hours following an overdose with the following criteria suggests a poor prognosis.

PT	>36 seconds
Creatinine	> 200 µmol/L
pH	<7.3
Encephalopathy	Present
Cerebral oedema	Present
Time from onset of jaundice to encephalopathy	0–7 days

A patient who develops severe liver disease and recovers does not usually suffer any long-term sequelae.

ACKNOWLEDGEMENTS

The authors would like to thank Dr Graeme Alexander for his advice in preparing this chapter and Dr Esther Unitt for her help with the flucloxacillin case.

REFERENCES

Campbell I 1990 Any questions? How should a patient be managed who is being treated for sputum positive pulmonary tuberculosis and becomes jaundiced in the third week of chemotherapy? Tubercle 71: 149

Eckstein R P, Dowsett J F, Lunzer M R 1993 Flucloxacillin induced liver disease: histopathological findings at biopsy and autopsy. Pathology 25: 223-228

Fairley C K, McNeil J J, Desmond P et al 1993 Risk factors for development of flucloxacillin associated jaundice. British Medical Journal 306: 233-235

Garcia Rodriguez L A, Stricker B H, Zimmerman H J 1996 Risk of acute liver injury associated with the combination of amoxycillin and clavulanic acid. Archives of Internal Medicine 156: 1327-1333

Harrison P M, Wendon J A, Gimson A E et al 1991 Improvement by acetylcysteine of hemodynamics and oxygen transport in fulminant liver failure. New England Journal of Medicine 324: 1852-1857

Ray D C, Drummond B G 1991 Halothane hepatitis. British Journal of Anaesthesia 67: 84-99

Richardson P, O'Grady J 2002. Acute liver disease. Hospital Pharmacist 9: 131-136

Russman S, Haye J A, Jick S S et al 2005 Risk of cholestatic liver disease associated with flucloxacillin and flucloxacillin prescribing habits in the UK: cohort study using data from the UK General Practice Research Database. British Journal of Clinical Pharmacology 60(1): 76-82

Shaw D, Leon C, Koler S et al 1997 Traditional remedies and food supplements. Drug Safety 17(5): 342-356

Wendon J, Williams R 1995 Acute liver failure. In: Williams R, Partman B, Tan K (eds) The practice of liver transplantation. Churchill Livingstone, London, 93-103

FURTHER READING

Chitturi S, George J 2002 Hepatotoxicity of commonly used drugs: nonsteroidal anti-inflammatory drugs, antihypertensives, antidiabetics, anticonvulsants, lipid-lowering agents, psychotropic drugs. Seminars in Liver Disease 22: 169-183

Farrell G C (ed) 1994 Drug-induced liver disease. Churchill Livingstone, London

Fontana R J, Shakil A O, Greenson J K et al 2005 Acute liver failure due to amoxicillin and amoxicillin/clavulanate. Digestive Diseases and Sciences 50: 1785-1790

Jaeschke H, Gores G I, Cederbaum A I et al 2002 Mechanisms of hepatotoxicity. Toxicological Science 65: 166-176

Kaplowitz N 2001 Drug-induced liver disorders: implications for drug development and regulation. Drug Safety 24: 483-490

Lee W M 1993 Acute liver failure. New England Journal of Medicine 329: 1862-1872

Lazerow S K, Abdi M S, Lewis J H 2005 Drug-induced liver disease 2004. Current Opinion in Gastroenterology 21: 283-292

Lee W M 2000 Assessing causality in drug-induced liver injury. Journal of Hepatology 33: 1003-1005

Lewis J H 2000 Drug-induced liver disease. Medical Clinics of North America 84: 1275-1311

Lewis J H 2002 The rational use of potentially hepatotoxic medications in patients with underlying liver disease. Expert Opinion on Drug Safety 1: 159-172

Lewis J H, Zimmerman H J 1999 Drug- and chemical-induced cholestasis. Clinics in Liver Disease 3: 433-464

Ryan M, Desmond P 2001 Liver toxicity: could this be a drug reaction? Australian Family Physician 30: 427-431

Thorax Editorials 1996 Hepatotoxicity of antituberculous drugs. Thorax 51: 111-113

Walgren J L, Mitchell M D, Thompson D C 2005 Role of metabolism in drug-induced idiosyncratic hepatotoxicity. Critical Reviews in Toxicology 35: 325-361

Zimmerman H J 2000 Drug-induced liver disease. Clinics in Liver Disease 4: 73-96

Liver disease 16

P. Kennedy   J. O'Grady

KEY POINTS

- The liver is a complex organ central to the maintenance of homeostasis.
- The liver is notable for its capacity to regenerate unless cirrhosis has developed.
- The spectrum of liver disease extends from mild, self-limiting conditions to serious illnesses which may carry significant morbidity and mortality.
- Liver disease is defined as acute or chronic on the basis of whether the history of disease is less than, or greater than, 6 months, respectively.
- Viral infections and paracetamol overdose are leading causes of acute liver disease but a significant number of patients have no defined aetiology.
- Alcohol abuse and chronic viral hepatitis (B and C) are the major causes of chronic liver disease.
- Cirrhosis may be asymptomatic for considerable periods of time.
- Ascites, encephalopathy, varices and hepatorenal failure are the main serious complications of cirrhosis.
- A careful assessment is required prior to the use of any drug in a patient with liver disease due to unpredictable effects on drug handling.

The liver weighs up to 1500 g in adults and as such is one of the largest organs in the body. The main functions of the liver include protein synthesis, storage and metabolism of fats and carbohydrates, detoxification of drugs and other toxins, excretion of bilirubin and metabolism of hormones, as summarized in Figure 16.1. The liver has considerable reserve capacity reflected in its ability to continue to function normally despite surgical removal of 70–80% of the organ or the presence of significant disease. It is noted for its capacity to regenerate rapidly. The distinction between acute and chronic liver disease is conventionally based on whether the history is less than, or greater than, 6 months, respectively and not on the severity of the clinical illness.

The hepatocyte is the functioning unit of the liver. Hepatocytes are arranged in lobules and within a lobule different hepatocytes perform different functions, depending on how close they are to the portal tract. The portal tract is the 'service network' of the liver and contains an artery and a portal vein delivering blood to the liver and bile duct which forms part of the biliary drainage system (Fig. 16.2). The blood supply to the liver is 30% arterial and the remainder is from the portal system which drains most of the abdominal viscera. Blood passes from the portal tract through

sinusoids that facilitate exposure to the hepatocytes before the blood is drained away by the hepatic venules and veins. There are a number of other cell populations in the liver but two of the most important are Kuppfer cells, fixed monocytes that phagocytose bacteria and particulate matter, and stellate cells responsible for the fibrotic reaction that ultimately leads to cirrhosis.

Acute liver disease

Acute liver disease is usually a self-limiting episode of hepatocyte damage which in most cases resolves spontaneously without clinical sequelae. However, in some instances which remain unclear, acute liver failure can develop. This is a rare condition in which there is a rapid deterioration in liver function with associated altered mentation (encephalopathy) and the development of a coagulopathy. Acute liver failure is a grave condition with a significant morbidity and mortality.

Chronic liver disease

Chronic liver disease occurs when permanent structural changes within the liver are present secondary to long-standing cell damage, with the consequent loss of normal liver architecture. In many cases this progresses to cirrhosis, where fibrous scars divide the liver cells into areas of regenerative tissue called nodules (Fig. 16.3). Conventional wisdom is that this process is irreversible, but there is now an increasing body of work which suggests that this is not always the case. Trials with antiviral therapies for the treatment of chronic viral hepatitis have demonstrated reversal

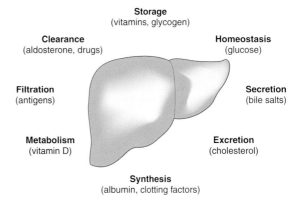

Figure 16.1   Normal physiological functions of the liver, with examples of each.

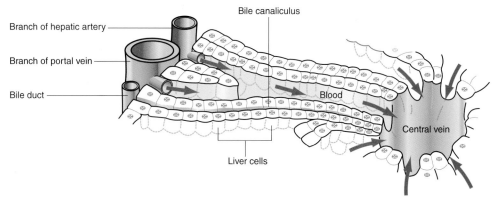

Figure 16.2 Illustration of the relationship between the three structures that comprise the portal tract, with blood from both the hepatic artery and portal vein perfusing the hepatocytes before draining away towards the hepatic veins (central veins). Each hepatocyte is also able to secrete bile via the network of bile ducts (reproduced with permission of McGraw-Hill from Vander 1980).

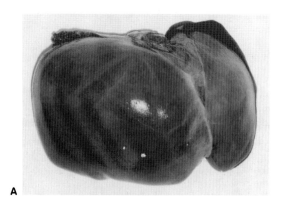

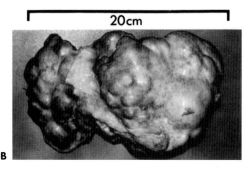

Figure 16.3 The gross post-mortem appearance of **A** a normal and **B** a cirrhotic liver demonstrating scarring and nodule formation in part B.

of cirrhotic change within the liver. Chronic liver disease with the development of cirrhosis may lead to the development of liver failure, hepatocellular carcinoma and death. Cirrhosis, which may take over 20 years to develop, is a sequel of chronic liver disease of any aetiology.

Causes of liver disease

Viral infections

Viruses commonly affect the liver, resulting in a transient and innocuous hepatitis. However, viruses which target the liver primarily are described as hepatotropic viruses, and each of these

can lead to clinically significant hepatitis and in some cases to the development of chronic viral hepatitis with viral persistence. Six human viruses have been identified, including hepatitis A (HAV), B (HBV), C (HCV), D (HDV), E (HEV) and G (HGV). Each type of viral hepatitis has a similar pathology, with the potential to cause acute inflammation of the liver, resulting in acute hepatitis. Types A and E are classically associated with an acute and sometimes severe hepatitis which is invariably self-limited, but occasionally fatal. Hepatitis B causes acute hepatitis in adults and 5% of such patients become chronic carriers, while 95% of patients infected in the neonatal period are chronically infected. Hepatitis C rarely causes an acute hepatitis but 85% of patients become chronic carriers. Both viruses cause chronic liver inflammation or hepatitis, cirrhosis and hepatocellular carcinoma.

Hepatitis A

Hepatitis A virus (HAV) is a non-enveloped RNA virus and a major cause of acute hepatitis worldwide, accounting for up to 25% of clinical hepatitis in the developed world. HAV is an enteric virus and the faecal–oral route is the main mechanism of transmission. The virus is particularly contagious and constitutes a public health problem throughout the world. The majority of attacks are mild and often pass unnoticed by the patient. Fulminant hepatitis is the most serious complication of HAV infection, which reportedly occurs in less than 1% of patients. Children in the 5–14 age group are most commonly affected, and adults are often infected by contact with their children. The virus is particularly prevalent in areas of poor sanitation, and often associated with water- and food-borne epidemics. Hepatitis A has a relatively short incubation period (2–7 weeks), during which time the virus replicates and abnormalities in liver function tests can be detected. HAV tends to run a mild subclinical course in children but a more serious disease, and even fulminant hepatitis, appears to be more frequent in adults.

Hepatitis B

Over 350 million people worldwide are chronically infected with the hepatitis B virus (HBV). Chronic HBV is defined as the presence of hepatitis B surface antigens (HBsAg) for a period of more than 6 months. In endemic areas of Africa and the Far East, up to 15–20% of the population are chronic carriers of HBV. While the majority of the population may have had a discrete acute HBV infection at some time in their life, it is thought that exposure to HBV at birth is the single most important risk factor for the development of chronic HBV infection. Carriers of HBV are at increased risk of developing cirrhosis, hepatic decompensation and hepatocellular carcinoma.

HBV can be transmitted in many ways. Vertical transmission from an HBV-infected mother to her infant during birth is a major route of infectivity in endemic areas and accounts for the high carrier rate in the Far East. However, HBV can also be transmitted parenterally, by the transfusion of blood or blood products from contaminated stocks and by intravenous drug use or needle sharing. HBV can also be transmitted sexually. There are many factors which determine the outcome of HBV infection, ranging from age and genetic factors of the host to virus characteristics. Acute HBV infection has an incubation period of 3–6 months, which is generally self-limiting and does not require antiviral therapy, with most patients recovering 1–2 months after the onset of jaundice. Chronic HBV can be associated with viraemia and hepatic inflammation; the level of viraemia is usually dependent on the presence of the hepatitis Be antigen (HBeAg), while seroconversion and HBeAg loss usually result in a reduction in HBV viraemia and a more favourable outcome. However, a significant population of patients now exists that do not express HbeAg but have elevated HBV DNA levels due to the development of what is called the 'pre-core' mutant. The majority of patients with chronic HBV will not develop hepatic complications; however, it is still estimated that 15–40% will develop serious sequelae during their lifetime. Childhood infection is associated with a different disease outcome with a higher percentage of patients developing chronic HBV infection, resulting in a higher proportion developing cirrhosis and hepatocellular carcinoma.

Hepatitis C

Over 170 million people worldwide are chronically infected with hepatitis C (HCV). HCV is a hepatotropic, non-cytopathic, predominantly blood-borne virus with greater infectivity than the human immunodeficiency virus (HIV). It is estimated that more than 2.7 million people in the USA are chronically infected with HCV, where it is the leading cause of death from liver disease. The equivalent estimate for the UK is between 200 000 and 500 000 although the vast majority have not been diagnosed. HCV is transmitted parenterally, most commonly through intravenous drug use and the sharing of contaminated needles. Prior to its identification in 1990, HCV (previously known as non-A, non-B viral hepatitis) was also contracted through contaminated blood and blood products. The introduction of widespread screening of blood donors and pooled blood products has largely consigned blood transfusion as a mode of transmission to history. There remains a small risk of HCV infection associated with tattooing, electrolysis, ear piercing, acupuncture and sexual contact. The vertical transmission rate from HCV-infected mother to child is less than 3%.

HCV infection is associated with the development of a recognized episode of acute hepatitis in only a small percentage of individuals. The majority of patients remain asymptomatic and so are often unaware of the infection or the timing at which they contracted the virus. Symptoms associated with HCV infection tend to be mild constitutional upset, with malaise, weakness and anorexia being most commonly reported. Up to 85% of subjects exposed to HCV develop chronic disease, which can lead to progressive liver damage, cirrhosis and hepatocellular carcinoma. Approximately 20–30% of patients with chronic HCV infection progress to end-stage liver disease within 20 years and a small percentage develop hepatocellular carcinoma. Patients with end-stage liver disease require a liver transplant to prevent death from the complications of cirrhosis. HCV infection is now the leading worldwide indication for liver transplantation.

Hepatitis D

Hepatitis D (HDV) is an incomplete virus that can establish infection only in patients simultaneously infected by HBV. It is estimated that 5% of HBV carriers worldwide are infected with HDV. It is endemic in the Mediterranean basin and is transmitted permucosally, percutaneously or sexually. In other geographical areas it is confined to only intravenous drug users.

Hepatitis E

Hepatitis E (HEV) is endemic in India, Asia, the Middle East and parts of Latin America. It is an RNA virus which is transmitted enterically and leads to acute hepatitis. The symptoms of HEV are no different from other causes of viral hepatitis, with an average incubation period of 42 days. In some cases, acute liver failure can result in death, particularly in pregnant women. In the majority of people there is no evidence of chronic infection and complete recovery is the outcome.

Hepatitis G

Hepatitis G virus (HGV) is a single-stranded RNA virus and a member of the Flaviviridae family. This is a relatively newly discovered virus with no definite causal relationship established between HGV and chronic hepatitis. Persistent infection with HGV is quite common; however, it is not thought to affect the clinical course of hepatitis A, B or C.

Alcohol

Alcohol is the single most significant cause of liver disease throughout the Western world, accounting for between 40% and 80% of cases of cirrhosis in different countries. In general, deaths from alcoholic liver disease in each country correlate with the consumption of alcohol per head of population, although additional factors can influence this trend. Various studies have estimated that between 20% and 30% of lifelong alcoholics will develop significant liver disease. Alcohol-induced liver disease forms a broad spectrum, from the relatively benign fatty liver disease to the development of alcoholic hepatitis. This condition may develop acutely with no preceding clinical features and in some patients progresses to death. It has an immediate mortality of between 30% and 60%. An estimated 20% of heavy drinkers develop progressive liver fibrosis, which can eventually lead to alcoholic cirrhosis, typically after a period of 10–20 years of heavy indulgence.

The central event in the development of hepatic fibrosis is the transformation of vitamin A-containing hepatic stellate cells into matrix-secreting cells, producing pericellular fibrosis. This network of collagen fibres develops around the liver cells and gradually leads to hepatocyte cell death. The extent of fibrosis progresses and micronodular fibrotic bands develop characterizing alcoholic cirrhosis. The anatomical changes within the liver hinder blood flow from the portal system, thereby causing an increase in blood pressure within this system. This results in portal hypertension, one of the major complications of cirrhosis. As the number of normally functioning liver cells reduces further, because of continued liver cell failure and death, the clinical condition deteriorates progressively. This is an unpredictable phenomenon and is reflected in the development of decompensated cirrhosis where essential synthetic, metabolic and excretory roles of the liver fail.

Immune disorders

Autoimmune disease can affect the hepatocyte or bile duct and is characterized by the presence of autoantibodies and raised immunoglobulins levels.

Autoimmune hepatitis

Autoimmune hepatitis is an unresolving inflammation of the liver of unknown cause. It is characterized by the presence of autoantibodies (anti-smooth muscle [type 1] or anti-kidney, liver microsomal [type 2]), hypergammaglobulinaemia and an interface hepatitis on liver histology. It is usually a chronic, progressive disease which can occasionally present acutely with a severe hepatitis and in some cases necessitates liver transplantation. Autoimmune hepatitis typically occurs in young women, between 20 and 40 years, often with a history or family history of autoimmune disorders.

Primary biliary cirrhosis

Primary biliary cirrhosis (PBC) is an autoimmune disease of the liver which predominantly affects middle-aged women. It is characterized by presence of antimitochondrial antibodies and a granulomatous destruction of the interlobular bile ducts leading to progressive ductopenia, fibrosis and cirrhosis. Drug regimens have had limited effect on the natural history of PBC. If the disease progresses markedly to uncontrolled pruritus, then severe jaundice or extreme lethargy, liver transplantation is often the only available treatment.

Primary sclerosing cholangitis

Primary sclerosing cholangitis (PSC) is an idiopathic chronic inflammatory disease resulting in intra- and extrahepatic biliary strictures, cholestasis and eventually cirrhosis. Often there is an association with chronic ulcerative colitis. It appears to occur predominantly in young caucasian males (mean age at presentation of 39 years). It can also occur in infancy and childhood and can affect any race. Portal hypertension and its complications are seen at the end stages of PSC, with cholangiocarcinoma developing in 10–30% of patients.

Vascular abnormalities

The Budd–Chiari syndrome (BCS) is a rare, heterogeneous and potentially fatal condition related to the obstruction of the hepatic venous outflow tract. Involvement of the portal venous system is a common sequel which adds to the gravity of the condition. The prevalence of underlying thrombophilias is markedly increased in patients with BCS. Studies have demonstrated that several thrombophilias are commonly combined in patients with BCS, and may be acquired or inherited. Affected patients are commonly women with an average age at presentation of 35. BCS can present as fulminant liver failure, but equally as an asymptomatic condition found incidentally. Early recognition and immediate use of anticoagulation have vastly improved outcome.

Metabolic and genetic disorders

There are various inherited metabolic disorders that can affect the functioning of the liver.

Haemochromatosis

Hereditary haemochromatosis (HH) is the most commonly identified genetic disorder in the caucasian population. It is associated with increased and inappropriate absorption of dietary iron resulting in deposition within the liver. This can lead to cirrhosis and hepatocellular carcinoma.

Wilson's disease

Wilson's disease is an autosomal recessive disorder of copper metabolism. The disorder leads to excessive absorption and deposition of dietary copper within the liver, brain, kidneys and other tissues. Presentation can vary widely from chronic hepatitis, asymptomatic cirrhosis and acute liver failure to neuropsychiatric symptoms with cognitive impairment.

α_1-Antitrypsin deficiency

This is an autosomal, recessively inherited disease and is the most common genetic metabolic liver disease. The disease results in a reduction in α_1-antitrypsin which is protective against a variety of proteases including trypsin, chymotrypsin, elastase and proteases present in neutrophils. The homozygous form of the disease (ZZ phenotype) is associated with the development of liver disease and cirrhosis in 15–30% of both adult and paediatric patients.

Glycogen storage disease

Glycogen storage disease is a rare condition occurring in 1 in 100 000 births. Enzymatic deficiencies at specific steps in the pathway of glycogen metabolism cause impaired glucose production and accumulation of abnormal glycogen in the liver.

Biliary tract diseases

Obstruction of bile outflow from the liver can cause inflammation, scarring and eventual cirrhosis. The obstruction may be due to gallstones or tumour, or secondary to surgical damage to the common bile duct. In developed countries primary malignant tumours of the liver and biliary tract are relatively rare. Secondary metastatic tumours are around 40 times more common than primary malignancies.

Gilbert's syndrome

Gilbert's syndrome is characterized by persistent mild unconjugated hyperbilirubinaemia. It is most frequently recognized in adolescents and young adults with an incidence of between 2% and 7% in the general population. Plasma bilirubin levels usually range between 2 and $80\,\mu mol/L$, increasing during periods of stress, sleep deprivation, prolonged fasting, menstruation and intercurrent infections. Patients usually complain of non-specific symptoms such as nausea, malaise and abdominal discomfort associated with an increase in jaundice. However, Gilbert's syndrome is otherwise a benign condition and requires no active treatment.

Clinical manifestations of liver disease

Symptoms

In patients who have liver disease, weakness, increased fatigue and general malaise are common but non-specific symptoms occurring in up to 60% of individuals. Loss of appetite and weight loss are more commonly seen in chronic liver disease. Frequently there is loss of muscle bulk from the arms and legs. Abdominal discomfort is often described by patients with an enlarged liver or spleen but this is frequently caused by distension with ascites. Abdominal pain is also common in hepatobiliary disease, frequently localized to the right upper quadrant. This is often a feature of rapid or gross enlargement of the liver. Associated tenderness is a symptom of acute hepatitis, hepatic abscess or hepatic malignancy. Jaundice is the most striking sign of liver disease. Pruritus can be a severely distressing symptom associated with jaundice. Patients usually complain that it is worse at night. Intractable jaundice related to certain conditions can be an indication for transplantation in its own right. Patients with acute and chronic liver disease can develop spontaneous bleeding. This occurs because of defective hepatic synthesis of coagulation factors and low platelet level causes abnormal blood clotting in such conditions.

Signs of liver disease

Many of the signs associated with chronic liver disease are related to the failure of the liver to carry out normal synthetic, metabolic and excretory functions. The most common signs are summarized in Table 16.1.

Cutaneous signs

Hyperpigmentation is common in chronic liver disease and results from increased deposition of melanin. It is particularly associated with primary biliary cirrhosis and haemachromatosis, often referred to as bronze diabetes. Scratch marks on the skin suggest pruritus which is a common feature of cholestatic liver disease. Vascular 'spiders', referred to as spider naevi, are small vascular malformations in the skin and are found in the drainage area of

Table 16.1 Physical signs of chronic liver disease

Common findings	End-stage findings
Jaundice	Ascites
Gynaecomastia and loss of body hair	Dilated abdominal blood vessels
Hand changes:	Fetor hepaticus
Palmar erythema	Hepatic flap
Clubbing	Neurological changes:
Dupuytren's contracture	Hepatic encephalopathy
Leuconychia	Disorientation
	Changes in consciousness
Liver mass reduced or increased	Peripheral oedema
Parotid enlargement	Pigmented skin
Scratch marks on skin	Muscle wasting
Purpura	
Spider naevi	
Splenomegaly	
Testicular atrophy	
Xanthelasma	
Hair loss	

the superior vena cava, commonly seen on the face, neck, hands and arms. Examination of the limbs can reveal several signs, none of which is specific to liver disease. Palmar erythema, a mottled reddening of the palms of the hands, can be associated with both acute and chronic liver disease. Dupuytren's contracture, thickening and shortening of the palmar fascia of the hands causing flexion deformities of the fingers, was traditionally associated with alcoholic cirrhosis. It is now considered to be multifactorial in origin and not to reflect primary liver disease. Nail changes, highly polished nails or white nails (leuconychia) can be seen in up to 80% of patients with chronic liver disease. Leuconychia is a consequence of low plasma albumin. Finger clubbing is most commonly seen in hypoxaemia related to hepatopulmonary syndrome, but is also a feature of chronic liver disease. It is reported to regress following liver transplantation.

Abdominal signs

Abdominal distension, notably of the flanks, is suggestive of ascites which can develop in both acute (less commonly) and chronic liver disease. Various other changes may be detectable on physical examination of the abdomen. An enlarged liver (hepatomegaly) is a common finding in acute liver disease. In cirrhotic patients the liver may be large but alternatively it may be small and shrunken, reflecting end-stage chronic disease. An enlarged spleen (splenomegaly) in the presence of chronic liver disease is the most important sign of portal hypertension. Dilated abdominal wall veins are a notable finding in chronic liver disease with the detection of umbilical and paraumbilical veins a feature of portal hypertension.

Jaundice

Jaundice is the physical sign regarded as synonymous with liver disease and is most easily detected in the sclerae. It reflects impaired liver cell function (hepatocellular pathology) or it can be cholestatic (biliary) in origin. Hepatocellular jaundice is commonly seen in acute liver disease, but may be absent in chronic disease until the terminal stages of cirrhosis are reached. The causes of jaundice are shown in Figure 16.4.

Portal hypertension

Increased hepatic resistance to portal flow due to cirrhosis causes portal hypertension. The increased pressure in the portal venous system leads to collateral vein formation and shunting of blood to the systemic circulation. Portal hypertension is an important contributory factor to the formation of ascites and the development of encephalopathy due to bypassing of blood from the liver to the systemic circulation. The major, potentially life-threatening complication of portal hypertension is torrential venous haemorrhage (variceal bleed) from the thin-walled veins in the oesophagus and upper stomach. Patients with portal hypertension are often asymptomatic but some may present with bleeding varices, ascites and/or encephalopathy.

Ascites

Ascites is the accumulation of fluid within the abdominal cavity. The precise mechanism by which ascites develops in chronic liver disease is unclear, but the following factors are all thought to contribute.

- Activation of the renin–angiotensin–aldosterone (RAA) axis as a consequence of central hypovolaemia, leading to a reduction in sodium excretion by the kidney and fluid retention. Reduced aldosterone metabolism due to reduced liver function may also contribute to increased fluid retention.

- A reduction in plasma albumin and reduced oncotic pressure is thought to contribute to the collection of fluid in the third space. Peripheral oedema (swollen lower limbs) occurs through this mechanism in a manner similar to the development of ascites.
- Portal hypertension and splanchnic arterial vasodilation alters intestinal capillary pressure and permeability and so facilitates the accumulation of retained fluid in the abdominal cavity.

Gynaecomastia

Endocrine changes are well documented in chronic liver disease and tend to be more common in alcoholic liver disease. Hypogonadism is common in patients with cirrhosis and in males results in testicular atrophy, female body hair distribution and gynaecomastia. This is thought in part to occur because the cirrhotic liver cannot metabolize oestrogen, leading to feminization in males. Gynaecomastia is particularly found in alcoholics but is also seen in those taking spironolactone, when there is usually associated tenderness of the nipples. In women with chronic liver disease menstrual irregularity, amenorrhoea and reduced fertility are encountered in females of reproductive age, but few detectable physical signs are seen as a result of gonadal atrophy.

Investigations

All patients with liver disease must undergo a comprehensive and thorough assessment to ascertain the underlying aetiology. Although causes of acute and chronic liver disease may differ,

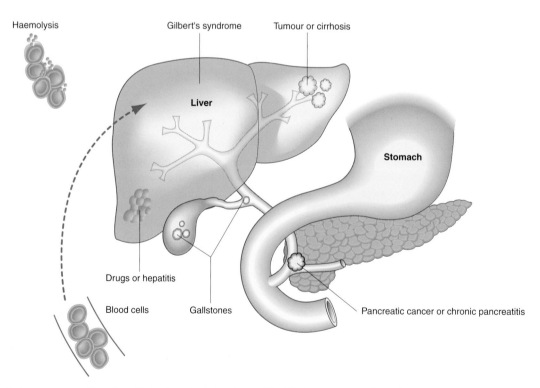

Figure 16.4 Common causes of jaundice. Obstructive: due to blockage of the bile ducts; hepatocellular: due to drugs, hepatitis, chronic liver disease or tumour formation; prehepatic: due to increased blood breakdown such as occurs in haemolysis.

a similar approach is used to investigate both patient types to ensure no primary cause or indeed co-factor is overlooked. It is not uncommon for patients to have more than one aetiology; quite often there may be a number of co-factors compounding the disease.

Imaging techniques

Ultrasonic visualization of the liver echotexture, bile duct size and patency is the modality of choice to exclude obstructive lesions contributing to impairment of liver function. Ultrasound is a non-invasive, low-risk procedure with the potential to give vital information in the detection of liver tumours, the extent of splenomegaly and the presence of ascites. Computed tomography (CT), which carries greater risk due to radiation exposure, is used to give greater detail of liver substance and the presence of varices and portal hypertension.

Liver biopsy

Liver biopsy is an invasive medical procedure with clear risks to the patient. Despite this, it remains the gold standard in establishing a diagnosis and recording the severity of chronic liver disease. In many instances liver histology will determine treatment strategies (viral hepatitis) and the presence/absence of cirrhosis will determine prognosis. In acute hepatic dysfunction, a liver biopsy is often unnecessary, especially if the condition is self-limiting. However, there are instances when a liver biopsy will be useful in confirming a diagnosis, even in acute hepatitis, and this decision will be best made by the attending physician.

Hepatitis serology

All individuals presenting with derangement of liver function should be tested for hepatitis A, B and C as part of a routine liver disease screen.

Biochemical liver function tests

Biochemical liver function tests (LFTs) are simple, inexpensive and easy to perform, but provide a relatively crude measure of liver function. These cannot be used in isolation to make a diagnosis. Biochemical parameters provide more useful information in monitoring disease progression or response to therapy. Biochemical tests can be crudely divided into the aminotransferases which reflect hepatocellular pathology and the cholestatic liver enzymes, namely bilirubin, alkaline phosphatase and γ-glutamyl transpeptidase. Bilirubin is commonly elevated in hepatocellular pathology and especially in acute hepatitis and end-stage chronic disease. Isolated elevations in one liver enzyme are unusual and abnormalities are not specific to the liver, underlining the need for a comprehensive assessment of all patients with disturbance in liver function tests.

Bilirubin

An increase in bilirubin concentration in body fluids results in jaundice and is usually clinically apparent when the plasma bilirubin level exceeds 35 μmol/L. In acute liver disease, the plasma bilirubin reflects severity of disease but is of little prognostic value. In chronic liver disease, a gradual increase for no apparent reason usually reflects serious disease progression. Hepatocellular damage, cholestasis and haemolysis can all cause elevations in the plasma bilirubin concentration.

Transaminases

Aspartate transaminase (AST) and alanine transaminase (ALT) are two intracellular enzymes present in hepatocytes which are released into the blood of patients as a consequence of hepatocyte damage or death. The aminotransferases are elevated in cases of hepatocellular diseases such as hepatitis. Extremely high values, where transaminases are recorded in the thousands, occur in acute liver disease owing to massive levels of hepatocyte killing or damage. This can be seen in viral hepatitis or acetaminophen overdose. In chronic hepatitis, plasma transaminases are rarely more than 5–8 times the normal upper limit.

Alkaline phosphatase

This enzyme is present in the canalicular and sinusoidal membranes of the liver and many other tissues, such as bone. Elevated levels of this enzyme originate predominantly from two sources: liver and bone. Concomitant elevation of the enzyme γ-glutamyl transpeptidase confirms the hepatic origin of elevated alkaline phosphatase. The plasma alkaline phosphatase activity may be raised by up to 4–6 times the normal limit in intrahepatic or extrahepatic cholestasis. It can also be raised in conditions associated with liver infiltration, such as metastases. It is frequently elevated in cirrhosis.

Albumin

Albumin is synthesized in the liver, and plasma albumin is a good marker of synthetic liver function, assuming there is no excess loss from the intestine or kidney and the patient is not in a catabolic state. It has a half-life of approximately 20 days. Changes in the plasma concentration of albumin over time can be a useful guide to the extent of chronic liver disease and its impact on liver function.

Prothrombin time

Prothrombin time (PT) is a useful short-term marker of the synthetic capacity of the liver. This is especially true in acute liver insults where it reflects the gravity of impairment of synthetic function. It is, however, also a sensitive indicator of chronic liver disease and, combined with albumin, gives an accurate picture of liver function.

Patient care

Pruritus

Pruritus is a prominent and sometimes distressing symptom of chronic liver disease. The severity of pruritus is variable and tends to be most debilitating in the context of cholestatic conditions. The pathogenesis of pruritus in liver disease is poorly understood but the deposition of bile salts within the skin is considered to be central to its development. However, the concentration of bile salts in the skin does not appear to correlate with the intensity of pruritus. Management of pruritus is variable. Relief of biliary obstruction by endoscopic, radiological or surgical means is indicated in patients with obstructed biliary systems. In other cases pharmacological agents are used initially but in some cases plasmapheresis, albumin dialysis (molecular adsorbent recycling system: MARS) or even liver transplantation may be needed.

Anion exchange resins

Colestyramine and colestipol act by binding bile acids and preventing their reabsorption. These anion exchange resins are the first line of therapy in the treatment of pruritus. Colestyramine is usually initiated at a dosage of 4 g once or twice daily, and the dose is then titrated to optimize relief without causing side effects (predominantly gastrointestinal). Such adverse effects are common and include constipation, diarrhoea, fat and vitamin malabsorption. Palatability is variable and consequently adherence is often a problem. In order to enhance compliance, patients should be advised that the benefits of therapy may take time to become apparent (often up to a week).

Anion exchange resins can reduce the absorption of concomitant therapy and such drugs should be taken 1 hour prior to or 4 hours after colestyramine or colestipol ingestion. Drugs which are susceptible to this interaction include digoxin, thyroxine, ursodeoxycholic acid (UDCA), chlorothiazide, propranolol and the antibiotics tetracycline and penicillin.

Antihistamines

Although frequently used, antihistamines are usually ineffective in the management of the pruritus caused by cholestasis and should not be considered first-line therapy. A non-sedating antihistamine such as cetirizine (10 mg once daily) or loratadine (10 mg once daily) is preferred as these avoid precipitating or masking encephalopathy. Antihistamines such as chlorphenamine or hydroxyzine provide little more than sedative properties, although they may be useful at night if the severity of pruritus is sufficient to prevent a patient from sleeping.

Ursodeoxycholic acid

The bile acid ursodeoxycholic acid (10 mg/kg daily in two divided doses) has been used frequently in cholestatic liver disease and long-term use has been shown to be effective in the treatment of pruritus. However, in some cases it has been reported to worsen pruritus.

Topical preparations

Topical therapy may benefit some patients. Calamine lotion and menthol 2% in aqueous cream are standard preparations, but improvement of pruritus with such agents is variable.

Ondansetron

The $5HT_3$ antagonist ondansetron has been reported to give a rapid reduction in pruritus after intravenous injection. The benefit is reported to last for up to 24 hours. Variable results have been reported with oral ondansetron which does not appear to have the same potency as the intravenous preparation.

Rifampicin and phenobarbital

Rifampicin and phenobarbital induce hepatic microsomal enzymes, which may benefit some patients, possibly by improving bile flow. Rifampicin administered at a dose of 600 mg per day is effective in the treatment of pruritus, albeit over a more prolonged period of time (1–3 weeks). Its use is restricted by its hepatotoxicity and drug interactions with other agents.

Opioid antagonists

A growing spectrum of opioid antagonists has been used to treat pruritus because it is believed that endogenous opioids in the central nervous system are potent mediators of itch. As a consequence the centrally acting opioid antagonists naloxone, naltrexone and nalmefene are thought to reverse the actions of these endogenous opioids. The use of such agents is limited by their route of administration. Naloxone is given by subcutaneous injection, while naltrexone and nalmefene are reported to be more substantially bioavailable after oral administration. A summary of drugs used in the management of pruritus is shown in Table 16.2.

Clotting abnormalities

The liver is the principal site for the synthesis of the clotting factors involved in coagulation, anticoagulation and fibrinolysis. Haemostatic abnormalities develop in approximately 75% of

Table 16.2 Drugs commonly used in the management of pruritus

Drug	Indication	Daily dose	Advantage	Disadvantage
Colestyramine	Cholestatic jaundice Itching (first line)	4–16 g (in two or three divided doses)	Reduce systemic bile salt levels	Poor patient compliance due to unpalatability Diarrhoea/constipation Increased flatulence Abdominal discomfort
Ursodeoxycholic acid	Cholestatic jaundice Itching	10–15 mg/kg (in two divided doses)		Variable response

Table 16.2 (continued)

Drug	Indication	Daily dose	Advantage	Disadvantage
Menthol 2% in aqueous cream	Itching	As required	Local cooling effect	Variable response
Chlorphenamine	Itching	4–16 mg (in three or four divided doses)	Sedative effects may be useful for night-time itching	May precipitate/aggravate encephalopathy
Hydroxyzine	Itching	25–100 mg (in three or four divided doses)	Sedative effects may be useful for night-time itching	May precipitate/aggravate encephalopathy
Cetirizine	Itching	10 mg (once daily)	Antihistamine with low incidence of sedation	Variable response
Naltrexone	Itching	50 mg/day	Shown to be beneficial in primary biliary cirrhosis	Opiate withdrawal symptoms, usually transient

patients with chronic liver disease, and the most frequently used indicator of defective clotting factor synthesis is the prothrombin time. The majority of clotting factors (with the exception of factor V) are dependent on vitamin K. Therefore, if following correction with vitamin K, the PT remains prolonged, severe liver disease with a poor prognosis is suggested. This is most notably in acute liver failure. For this reason the PT is used as a prognostic indicator to identify patients potentially requiring liver transplantation. The relationship of liver disease to clotting abnormalities is shown diagrammatically in Figure 16.5.

While the normal PT is between 12 and 16 seconds, prolongation of more than 3 seconds (or international normalized ratio (INR) greater than 1.2) is usually considered abnormal. Patients with liver disease who develop deranged blood clotting should receive intravenous doses of phytomenadione (vitamin K), usually 10 mg daily for 3 days. Administration of vitamin K to patients with significant liver disease does not usually improve the PT because the liver is unable to utilize the vitamin to synthesize clotting factors. Oral vitamin K is less effective than the

parenteral form and so has little or no place in the management of clotting abnormalities and bleeding secondary to liver disease.

Aspirin, non-steroidal anti-inflammatory drugs (NSAIDs) and anticoagulants should be avoided in all patients with liver disease because of the risk of altering platelet function, causing gastric ulceration and bleeding. NSAIDs have also been implicated in precipitating renal dysfunction and variceal bleeding in patients with end-stage liver disease. Although COX-2 inhibitors may cause a lower incidence of bleeding complications, currently they are avoided in patients with liver disease as their use still poses a risk.

Ascites

All patients with ascites should be evaluated for liver transplantation as the presence of ascites is associated with poor long-term survival (survival rate at 5 years is 30–40%). Conditions complicating ascites by impairing renal or circulatory function, namely refractory ascites, spontaneous bacterial peritonitis or the hepatorenal syndrome should be given priority in terms of transplantation. The aim in the treatment of ascites is to mobilize the abnormal collection of third-space fluid (intra-abdominal fluid) and this can be achieved by simple measures such as reduced sodium intake. A low-salt diet (60–90 mEq per day) may be enough to facilitate the elimination of ascites and delay reaccumulation of fluid. Salt reduction combined with fluid restriction (approximately 1–1.5 L per day) are practical measures taken to mobilize fluid and provide weight reduction and symptomatic relief.

Aggressive weight reduction in the absence of peripheral oedema should be avoided as it is likely to lead to intravascular fluid depletion and renal failure. Weight loss should not exceed 300–500 g per day in the absence of peripheral oedema and 800–1000 g per day in those with peripheral oedema to prevent renal failure. Historically, measures advocated in the management of ascites included bed rest, with reported improvement in renal perfusion, combined with strict fluid and salt restriction. However, diuretics and/or paracentesis are the cornerstone in the management of moderate-to-large volume ascites. Table 16.3 outlines a sequential approach to the management of ascites.

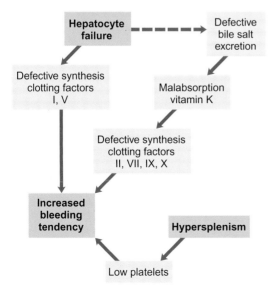

Figure 16.5 Mechanisms of deranged clotting in chronic liver disease.

Diuretics

The aldosterone antagonist spironolactone is usually used as a first-line agent in the treatment of ascites. In most instances a negative sodium balance and loss of ascitic fluid can be achieved with low doses of diuretics. Spironolactone can be used alone or in combination with a more potent loop diuretic. The specific agents and dosages used are outlined in Table 16.4. Spironolactone acts by blocking sodium reabsorption in the collecting tubules of the kidney. It is usually commenced at 100 mg/day but this varies, depending on the patient's clinical status, electrolyte levels and concomitant drug therapies. It can take many days to achieve a therapeutic effect, so dose augmentation should be conducted with caution and strict observation of the renal parameters. The addition of a loop diuretic, furosemide 40 mg/day, enhances the natriuretic activity of spironolactone, and should be used when ascites is severe or when spironolactone alone fails to produce acceptable diuresis.

The use of more potent diuretic combinations may result in excessive diuresis which can lead to renal failure of pre-renal origin. The initiation and augmentation of diuretic therapy should ideally be carried out in hospital. This allows strict urea and electrolyte monitoring to detect impending hyperkalaemia and/or hyponatraemia, which commonly occur with diuretic therapy. Aggressive and unchecked diuresis will precipitate the hepatorenal syndrome, which has a very poor prognosis. Generally, if the plasma sodium level decreases to less than 130 mmol/L or if creatinine levels rise to greater than 130 μmol/L then dose escalation of diuretics should be stopped, but this will vary from patient to patient. Diuretic therapy can be complicated by encephalopathy, hypokalaemia, hyponatraemia and azotaemia. Gynaecomastia and muscle cramps are side effects of diuretic therapy.

Refractory ascites occurs in 5–10% of patients with ascites and is associated with a 1-year survival rate of between 25% and 50%. Therapeutic strategies include repeated large-volume paracentesis with the use of plasma expanders or transjugular intrahepatic portosystemic shunts (TIPSS). In some patients liver transplantation may be indicated. Ascites is considered to be refractory or diuretic resistant if there is no response with once-daily doses of 400 mg spironolactone and 160 mg furosemide. Patients on lower doses are also considered to have refractory ascites if side effects are a problem, e.g. hepatic encephalopathy, hyperkalaemia, hyponatraemia or azotaemia.

Paracentesis

The development of severe ascites or refractory ascites is an indication for paracentesis. Repeated large-volume paracentesis in combination with albumin administration is the most widely accepted therapy for refractory ascites. Patients generally require paracentesis every 2–4 weeks and the procedure is often performed in the outpatient setting. Paracentesis, however, does not affect the mechanism responsible for ascitic fluid accumulation and so early recurrence is common. Intravenous colloid replacement or plasma expanders are used to prevent adverse effects on the renal and systemic circulation. Colloid replacement in the form of 6–8 g albumin/L of ascites removed (equivalent to 100 mL of 20% human albumin solution (HAS) (1 unit) for every 2.5 L of ascitic fluid removed) is a standard regimen.

Table 16.3 The sequential approach to the management of cirrhotic ascites

Bedrest and sodium restriction (60–90 mEq/day, equivalent to 1500–2000 mg of salt/day)

▼

Spironolactone (or other potassium-sparing diuretic)

▼

Spironolactone and loop diuretic

▼

Large-volume paracentesis and colloid replacement

Other measures

Transjugular intrahepatic portosystemic shunt (TIPSS)

Peritonovenous shunt

Consider orthotopic liver transplantation

Table 16.4 Diuretics used for ascites

Drug	Indication	Daily dose	Advantage	Disadvantage
Spironolactone	Fluid retention	50–400 mg	Aldosterone antagonist Slow diuresis	Painful gynaecomastia Variable bioavailability Hyperkalaemia
Furosemide	Fluid retention	40–160 mg	Rapid diuresis Sodium excretion	Nephrotoxic Hypovolaemia Hypokalaemia Hyponatraemia Caution in prerenal uraemia
Amiloride	Mild fluid retention	5–10 mg	As K$^+$-sparing agent or weak diuretic if spironolactone contraindicated	Lacks potency

Transjugular intrahepatic portosystemic shunting (TIPSS)

TIPSS is an invasive procedure, used to manage refractory ascites or control refractory variceal bleeding. It is carried out under radiological guidance. An expandable intrahepatic stent is placed between one hepatic vein and the portal vein by a transjugular approach (Fig. 16.6). In contrast to paracentesis, the use of TIPSS is effective in preventing recurrence in patients with refractory ascites. It reduces the activity of sodium-retaining mechanisms and improves the renal response to diuretics. However, a disadvantage of this procedure is the high rate of shunt stenosis (up to 30% after 6–12 months) which leads to recurrence of ascites. TIPSS can also induce or exacerbate hepatic encephalopathy. In addition, high cost and the limited expertise available to perform the procedure are further drawbacks.

Spontaneous bacterial peritonitis

Patients with ascites should be closely observed for spontaneous bacterial peritonitis (SBP) as it develops in 10–30% of patients and has a high mortality. Hepatorenal syndrome can complicate SBP in up to 30% of patients and also carries a high mortality. Conventional signs and symptoms of peritonitis are rarely present in such patients and if suspected, treatment with appropriate antibiotics should be started immediately after a diagnostic ascitic tap has been taken. A polymorphonuclear leucocyte count of greater than 250 cells/mm³ is diagnostic of this condition. The causative organism is of enteric origin in approximately three-quarters of infections, and originates from the skin in the remaining one-quarter. Cefotaxime 2 g, 8-hourly is effective in 85% of patients with SBP and is commonly used as first-line antimicrobial therapy. Other antibiotic regimens have been used, including co-amoxiclav, but third-generation cephalosporins are the treatment of choice. The quinolone norfloxacin (400 mg/day) has a role in the prevention of recurrence of SBP, estimated as 70% at 1 year, and is recommended for long-term antibiotic prophylaxis. However, the emergence of quinolone-resistant bacteria is a growing problem in the management of SBP.

Hepatic encephalopathy

Hepatic encephalopathy is a reversible neuropsychiatric complication that occurs with significant liver dysfunction. The precise cause of encephalopathy remains unclear, but three factors are known to be implicated, namely portosystemic shunting, metabolic dysfunction and an alteration of the blood–brain barrier. It is thought that intestinally derived neuroactive and neurotoxic substances such as ammonia pass through the diseased liver or bypass the liver through shunts and go directly to the brain. This results in cerebral dysfunction. Ammonia is thought to increase the permeability of the blood–brain barrier, enabling other neurotoxins to enter the brain and indirectly alter neurotransmission. Other substances implicated in causing hepatic encephalopathy include free fatty acids, γ-aminobutyric acid (GABA) and glutamate.

Clinical features of hepatic encephalopathy range from trivial lack of awareness, altered mental state to asterixis (liver flap) through to gross disorientation and coma. During low-grade encephalopathy, the altered mental state may present as impaired judgement, altered personality, euphoria or anxiety. Reversal of day/night sleep patterns is very typical of encephalopathy. Somnolence, semistupor, confusion and finally coma can ensue (Table 16.5).

Although hepatic encephalopathy has a wide range of presentations, it is important to differentiate between two common types which differ in progression, severity and management. Encephalopathy associated with acute liver failure is recognized by the short interval between jaundice and development of encephalopathy. In this instance, cerebral oedema is more likely and carries a high mortality in fulminant hepatic failure. In this clinical situation encephalopathy can progress from grade 1 or 2 to 4 within a matter of hours. Alternatively, encephalopathy associated with cirrhosis and portal hypertension and/or portal systemic shunts develops as a result of specific precipitating factors (Table 16.6) or an acute deterioration in liver function. This condition is usually reversible and the patient improves with correction of the precipitating cause.

Common precipitating factors include gastrointestinal bleeding, SBP, constipation, dehydration and certain drugs (including sedatives). Identification and removal of such precipitating

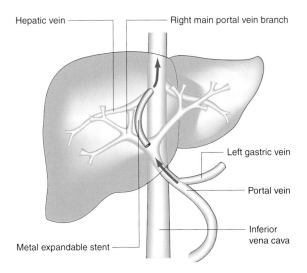

Hepatic vein — — Right main portal vein branch

Left gastric vein

Portal vein

Inferior vena cava

Metal expandable stent —

Figure 16.6 Intrahepatic stent shunt links the hepatic vein with the intrahepatic portal vein.

Table 16.5	Grading of hepatic encephalopathy
Grade 0	Normal
Subclinical	Abnormal psychometric tests for encephalopathy (e.g. number correction test)
Grade 1	Mood disturbance, abnormal sleep pattern, impaired handwriting +/− asterixis
Grade 2	Drowsiness, grossly impaired calculation ability, asterixis
Grade 3	Confusion, disorientation, somnolent but arousable, asterixis
Grade 4	Stupor to deep coma, unresponsive to painful stimuli

factors is mandatory. Therapeutic management is then aimed at reducing the amount of ammonia or nitrogenous products in the circulatory system. Treatment with laxatives increases the throughput of bowel contents, by reducing transit time, and also increases soluble nitrogen output in the faeces. Drug therapies for encephalopathy are summarized in Table 16.7.

Lactulose, a non-absorbable disaccharide, decreases ammonia production in the gut. It is widely used as it is broken down by gastrointestinal bacteria to form lactic, acetic and formic acids. The effect of lactulose is to acidify the colonic contents which leads to the ionization of nitrogenous products within the bowel, with a consequent reduction in their absorption from the gastro-intestinal tract. Lactulose is given in doses of 30–50 mL three times a day and titrated to result in 2–3 bowel motions each day. Patients unable to take oral medication or those with worsening encephalopathy are treated with phosphate enemas.

Antibiotics such as metronidazole or neomycin may also be used to reduce ammonia production from gastrointestinal bacteria. Metronidazole is the preferred option, while the use of neomycin has largely been abandoned because of associated toxicity. Other therapies investigated for the treatment of encephalopathy include L-ornithine-L-aspartate (OA), sodium benzoate, L-dopa, bromocriptine and the benzodiazepine receptor antagonist flumazenil.

Oesophageal varices

Variceal bleeding is the most feared complication of portal hypertension in patients with cirrhosis and is associated with a high mortality. A single variceal bleed carries a 6-week mortality rate of 50%. There is a 30% lifetime risk of at least one bleeding episode among patients with cirrhosis and varices. Treatment of variceal bleeding includes endoscopic banding or sclerotherapy of oesophageal varices in parallel with splanchnic vasoconstrictors and intensive medical care. Patients with variceal bleeding refractory to endoscopic intervention or patients bleeding from ectopic or gastric varices will need surgical decompressive shunts, TIPSS or in some cases even liver transplantation. Refractory variceal bleeding should therefore be managed only in centres with the appropriate expertise.

Initial treatment is aimed at stopping or reducing the immediate blood loss, treating hypovolaemic shock, if present, and subsequent prevention of recurrent bleeding. Immediate and prompt resuscitation is an essential part of treatment. Only when medical treatment has been initiated and optimized should endoscopy be performed. Endoscopy confirms the diagnosis and then allows therapeutic intervention. Fluid replacement is invariably required, and should be in the form of colloid or packed red cells and administered centrally. Saline should generally be avoided in all patients with cirrhosis. Fluid replacement must be administered with caution, as overzealous expansion of the circulating volume may precipitate further bleeding by raising portal pressure, exacerbating the clinical situation. A flowchart for the management of bleeding oesophageal varices is shown in Figure 16.7.

Endoscopic management

Endoscopic variceal sclerotherapy has been largely superseded by variceal band ligation. This technique uses prestretched rubber bands applied to the base of a varix which has been sucked into the banding chamber attached to the front of an endoscope. Variceal ligation controls bleeding in approximately 90% of cases. It is at least as effective as sclerotherapy but is associated with fewer side effects. Balloon tamponade with a Sengstaken–Blakemore balloon or Linton balloon may be used to stabilize a patient with actively bleeding varices by directly compressing the bleeding varices, until more definitive therapy can be undertaken. Balloon tamponade can control bleeding in up to 90% of cases but 50% rebleed when the balloon is deflated.

Pharmacological therapy

Several pharmacological agents are available for the emergency control of variceal bleeding (Table 16.8). Most act by lowering portal venous pressure. They are generally used to control

Table 16.6 Precipitating causes of hepatic encephalopathy
Gastrointestinal bleeding
Infection (spontaneous bacterial peritonitis, other sites of sepsis)
Hypokalaemia, metabolic alkalosis
High-protein diet
Constipation
Drugs, opioids and benzodiazepines
Deterioration of liver function
Postsurgical portosystemic shunt or TIPSS

Table 16.7 Drugs commonly used in the management of encephalopathy

Drug	Dose	Comment	Side effects
Lactulose	15–30 mL orally 2–4 times daily	Aim for 2–3 soft stools daily	Bloating, diarrhoea
Metronidazole	400–800 mg orally daily in divided doses	Metabolism impaired in liver disease	Gastrointestinal disturbance
Neomycin Used less frequently now	2–4 g orally daily in divided doses	Maximum duration of 48 h	Potential for nephro- and ototoxicity

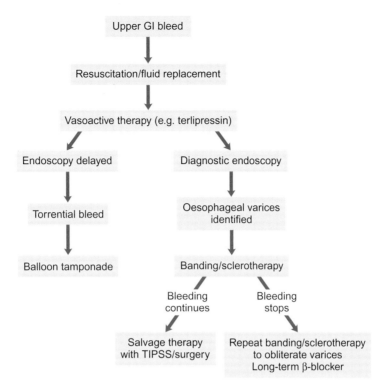

Figure 16.7 Management of oesophageal variceal haemorrhage.

Table 16.8 Drugs used in the treatment of acute bleeding varices

Drug	Dosage and administration
Terlipressin	1–2 mg bolus 4–6 hourly for 48–72 hours
Octreotide	50 µg/h i.v. infusion for 48 hours or longer if patient rebleeds

bleeding in addition to balloon tamponade and emergency endoscopic techniques. Vasopressin was the first vasoconstrictor used to reduce portal pressure in patients with actively bleeding varices. However, its associated systemic vasoconstrictive adverse effects limited its use. The synthetic vasopressin analogue terlipressin is highly effective in controlling bleeding and in reducing mortality. It can be administered in bolus doses every 4–6 hours and has a longer biological activity and a more favourable side effect profile. Somatostatin and the somatostatin analogue octreotide are reported to cause selective splanchnic vasoconstriction and reduce portal pressure. Although they are reported to cause fewer adverse effects on the systemic circulation, terlipressin remains the agent of choice.

Transjugular intrahepatic portosystemic stent shunt (TIPSS)

TIPSS is highly effective in the management of uncontrolled variceal bleeding and is the intervention of choice when endoscopic measures have failed (see Fig. 16.7).

Prevention of rebleeding

Banding (ligation) is performed at regular intervals (1–2 weeks) as part of an eradication programme to obliterate the varices. Once varices have been eradicated, endoscopic follow-up can be performed less frequently (3-monthly) for the first year, then twice yearly thereafter. If varices reappear they should be banded regularly until eradicated again.

Non-selective β-blockers, such as propranolol, are the medication of choice to prevent rebleeding and can also be used as primary prophylaxis against variceal bleeding in patients with known varices. The mechanism of action is complex, but they reduce portal hypertension by causing splanchnic vasoconstriction and reduced portal blood flow. At higher doses they can have a more marked negative effect on cardiac output and so must be titrated accordingly.

Acute liver failure

Acute liver failure (ALF) occurs when there is a sudden cessation of normal hepatic function associated with encephalopathy, development of a coagulopathy and subsequent jaundice. ALF is a rare but potentially fatal condition. It is associated with the development of cerebral oedema and renal impairment and may progress to multiorgan failure. In the past viral hepatitis was a major consideration in the aetiology of ALF. However, the development of a commercial vaccine for hepatitis B has seen a dramatic decline in the contribution of HBV to ALF. The most common cause of ALF in the USA today is drug toxicity (predominantly paracetamol toxicity). The aetiology of ALF varies according to country and so viral hepatitis has remained as the major cause of ALF in some regions. Despite the availability of a successful commercial vaccine for hepatitis A virus, worldwide only selected groups are immunized. Therefore HAV remains a significant health problem, contributing to cases of ALF.

Management of ALF is complicated, involving the central nervous system, cardiovascular and renal support. All patients with ALF are at risk of infection, and prophylactic administration of broad-spectrum antibiotics and antifungal agents is standard practice. Coagulopathy and bleeding resulting from liver failure are serious life-threatening complications which require monitoring and correction.

Liver transplantation

Liver transplantation is the established treatment for selected patients with acute liver failure, decompensated chronic liver disease, inherited metabolic disorders and primary liver cancer. However, indications for transplantation are evolving; HCV infection and alcohol-induced end-stage liver disease are the commonest indications for liver transplantation in Europe and the USA. Outcome has also improved, with 1-year post-transplant survival now exceeding 80%.

Following liver transplantation, the main problems encountered by the patient are graft rejection and opportunistic infection related to immunosuppressive therapy. An increasing number of immunosuppressive agents is now available and this has enabled clinicians to tailor immunosuppression to achieve a balance of good graft function and an acceptable side effects profile. The calcineurin inhibitors (CNIs) tacrolimus and ciclosporin are the mainstay of immunosuppressive therapy. These are most commonly used in conjunction with corticosteroids and/ or mycophenolate. Therapy is monitored closely and titrated carefully according to the needs of the patient. The emerging strategy is to withdraw corticosteroids, usually within the first year, and use mycophenolate mofetil or sirolimus to reduce reliance on CNIs.

Hepatitis A

There is still no specific therapy for HAV infection, and management of patients is generally supportive. The severity of HAV is multifactorial, with age, gender and drug toxicity all implicated. Commercial assays for the measurement of HAV RNA may prove to be a useful prognostic tool in the management of hepatitis A, as low viraemia is strongly associated with liver failure. Passive immunization with the appropriate immunoglobulin is still used in high-risk patients.

Hepatitis B

The primary goal in the management of chronic HBV infection is to prevent cirrhosis, hepatic failure and hepatocellular carcinoma. The ideal outcome is eradication of HBV before irreversible liver damage occurs. However, the presence of extrahepatic reservoirs of HBV, the integration of HBV into the host genome and the presence of an intracellular conversion pathway which replenishes the pool of transcriptional templates in the hepatocyte nucleus without the need for reinfection make the eradication of HBV impossible. Thus, therapies developed for chronic HBV

are measured in terms of HBeAg seroconversion, HBsAg loss, normalization of liver enzymes, suppression of HBV DNA and improvement in liver histopathology.

In the USA treatment strategies for chronic HBV comprise five approved therapies: interferon α-2a, lamivudine, adefovir, entecavir and pegylated interferon α-2a. In the early 1990s interferon α-2a was the only approved treatment for chronic HBV but it has now largely been superseded by pegylated interferon (peginterferon) α-2a. The approval of orally administered nucleotide or nucleoside analogues has dramatically changed the available therapies for chronic HBV, resulting in more treatment options with potentially fewer side effects and broadening the indications for treatment of HBV to include patients with decompensated cirrhosis. However, it is not yet known if oral antivirals can dramatically improve the long-term outcome of patients with HBV. One disadvantage of these new therapies is drug-resistant mutations, as data suggest that resistance rates, with extended use, may be as high as 70% for lamivudine and 15% for adefovir. Drug resistance is associated with viral breakthrough (increased HBV DNA after initial suppression), usually accompanied by deterioration in liver biochemistry and, in some rare instances, liver failure and death. The potential for resistance to one antiviral agent conferring resistance to others, thereby limiting future treatment options, is an emerging concern. This may lead to combination therapy becoming more widely used as the number of available agents increases.

A more immediate problem related to the oral antivirals is the high rate of relapse when treatment is discontinued. Studies have demonstrated a higher rate of virological relapse for lamivudine compared with peginterferon when treatment was stopped. Similar data are not available yet comparing adefovir and entecavir directly with peginterferon, but existing data suggest that relapse is more common than with interferon. The decision to treat patients with chronic HBV and, more importantly, what therapy to employ can only be taken after the advantages and limitations of each individual agent have been properly assessed and the patient fully informed.

Hepatitis C

HCV is a leading cause of chronic liver disease worldwide and liver failure secondary to HCV is the most common indication for liver transplantation. However, HCV recurrence in the graft underlines the limitations of transplantation in the management of HCV and, furthermore, emphasizes the need for more successful therapies to tackle HCV. The primary aim of treating patients with chronic HCV is viral clearance, sustained virological response (SVR), defined as the absence of viraemia 6 months after antiviral therapy has been discontinued. Viral clearance improves the patient's quality of life and reduces the risk of progression to cirrhosis and hepatocellular carcinoma.

Pegylated interferon and ribavirin combination therapy are now the standard care of chronic HCV. The SVR for treatment-naive patients is of the order of 55% for genotypes 1 and 4, and 80–85% for genotypes 2 and 3. Patients failing to achieve a significant reduction in viral load after 12 weeks of treatment are usually withdrawn from therapy. Side effects include influenza-like symptoms, decrease in haematological parameters such as haemoglobin, neutrophils, white blood cell count and platelets, gastrointestinal complaints, psychiatric disturbances (anxiety and depression), and hypo- or hyperthyrodism. These side effects may be major problems with combination antiviral therapy and may hinder compliance or necessitate significant dose reductions. Growth factors (erythropoietin, GCSF) and antidepressants may alleviate some side effects. Combination therapy is recommended for 24 weeks for the treatment of genotypes 2 and 3 and 48 weeks for the treatment of genotype 4 and the more common genotype 1.

Autoimmune hepatitis

Corticosteroids and/or azathioprine are the standard therapy for autoimmune hepatitis (AIH). Prednisone or prednisolone is usually the corticosteroid of choice, administered at doses of 40–60 mg/day alone or at lower doses when combined with azathioprine. The steroid dose is reduced over a 6-week to 3-month period to a maintenance dose of 15 mg/day or lower. The disturbance in aminotransferases usually normalizes within 6–12 weeks, but histological remission tends to lag by 6–12 months. Azathioprine at a dose of 1 mg/kg per day is used as an adjunct to corticosteroid therapy. Azathioprine used alone is ineffective in treating the acute phase of autoimmune hepatitis because it requires 3 months or more to become fully effective. In patients intolerant of azathioprine or in cases of proven treatment failure, other immunosuppressants have been used, e.g. tacrolimus and mycophenolate. Newer corticosteroids such as budesonide with fewer side effects have also been used effectively and may have a greater role in the future treatment of autoimmune hepatitis.

Primary biliary cirrhosis

Several therapies have been associated with short-term symptomatic improvements in liver function tests. Ursodeoxycholic acid (UDCA), the only medication widely used to treat primary biliary cirrhosis (PBC), reduces the retention of bile acids and increases their hepatic excretion. Therefore it is effective in protecting against the cytotoxic effects of dihydroxy bile acids which accumulate in PBC. However, UDCA does not appear to stop ongoing bile duct injury and disease progression. Therefore liver transplantation remains the only effective option in patients with end-stage disease.

Immunosuppressive agents such as ciclosporin, azathioprine and methotrexate have also been assessed for the treatment of PBC but clinically significant adverse events outweigh the benefits.

Primary sclerosing cholangitis

There is no effective treatment for this condition. UDCA can be used to manage associated cholestasis, and doses as high as 15 mg/kg/day have been advocated despite the limited evidence that they alter the natural history of the disease. Studies with various immunosuppressive agents have been disappointing and transplantation remains the only effective treatment option in patients with advanced disease.

Wilson's disease

This rare autosomal recessive condition is usually managed with chelation therapy. Penicillamine is the agent of choice in Wilson's disease as it promotes urinary copper excretion in affected patients and prevents copper accumulation in presymptomatic individuals. Initial treatment of 1.5–2 g/day is given in divided doses. Initially neurological symptoms may worsen because of deposition of mobilized copper in the basal ganglia, but symptomatic patients tend to improve over a period of several weeks. Other therapy-related adverse effects include renal dysfunction, haematological abnormalities and disseminated lupus erythematosus. Therefore, regular monitoring of full blood count and electrolytes is required as well as small doses of pyridoxine (25 mg) to counteract the antipyridoxine effect of penicillamine and the associated neurological toxicity. Patients who are unable to tolerate penicillamine may respond to trientine. This chelating agent is less potent than penicillamine but has fewer adverse effects

CASE STUDIES

Case 16.1

A 56-year-old man with alcoholic cirrhosis is admitted to hospital following a haematemesis. He has been abstinent from alcohol for 18 months and is on a waiting list for a liver transplantation because of intractable ascites. Endoscopy confirms he is bleeding from oesophageal varices which are banded. The patient is transferred 8 hours later to a specialist regional centre at their request for further management.

Laboratory data on admission are:

Na	124 (133–143 mmol/L)
K	3.0 (3.5–5.0 mmol/L)
Creatinine	131 (80–124 µmol/L)
Urea	14.3 (2.7–7.7 mmol/L)
Bilirubin	167 (3.15 µmol/L)
ALT	24 (0–35 iu/L)
PT	18.9 seconds (13 seconds)
Albumin	24 (35–50 g/dL)
Hb	8.9 (13.5–18 g/dL)

Drugs on admission:

Spironolactone 200 mg one each morning

Questions

1. What treatment would be recommended before the patient is transferred to the regional centre?
2. What options (drug and/or non-drug) are likely to be available at the regional centre for managing the patient's bleeding varices?
3. What further long-term measures are required for this patient?

Answers

1. Initial restoration of circulating blood volume with colloid, followed by cross-matched blood. Adequate fluid replacement is critical to prevent renal dysfunction. In view of the patient's ascites, saline should be avoided and dextrose 5% with added potassium (hypokalaemia present) is the crystalloid of choice. A pharmacological agent to

reduce portal pressure, such as terlipressin 1–2 mg every 4–6 hours or octreotide 50 µg/h, should be started. Current evidence supports terlipressin over octreotide. Broad-spectrum antibiotics should be started intravenously if there is suspicion of abdominal infection or sepsis, with the precise agents used being determined by local antibiotic policy. There is little evidence that gastric acid suppression is beneficial, but if the bleeding is caused by a gastric mucosal lesion, a proton pump inhibitor such as lansoprazole or omeprazole or a histamine type-2 receptor antagonist such as ranitidine can be administered.

Spironolactone is likely to be either causing or exacerbating the low sodium and should be discontinued.

Vitamin K, 10 mg intravenously once daily for 3 days, should be administered to try to correct the raised prothrombin time. As the patient has severe liver disease with varices and ascites there is a possibility he may develop encephalopathy. It would be advisable to start lactulose or, if the patient is unable to take medicines orally, administer an enema such as a phosphate enema.

2. Banding/ligation of varices is now standard therapy and injection sclerotherapy is reserved for cases where heavy blood loss impairs visualization of oesophageal varices and for bleeding gastric varices. Banding involves mechanical strangulation of variceal channels by small elastic plastic rings mounted on the tip of the endoscope.

TIPSS can be used to reduce portal pressure by creating a new passage through the liver. It is indicated mainly in patients with gastric varices and in selected cases of difficult oesophageal varices. The main problems with TIPSS are occlusion and encephalopathy, both of which occur in 20–30% of cases.

Surgery is now rarely performed but options include portal-systemic shunts and devascularization. Liver transplantation in appropriate candidates, like this patient, is a definitive treatment.

3. Banding/ligation can be performed at regular intervals of 1–2 weeks to obliterate the varices. Once varices have been eradicated, endoscopic follow-up should be undertaken every 3 months for the first year then every 6–12 months thereafter. If varices reappear they should be banded regularly until eradicated again. Non-selective β-blockers such as propranolol are used in the prophylaxis of further bleeds, with the dose adjusted until the heart rate is reduced by 25%, but to not less than 55 beats per minute.

Case 16.2

A 68-year-old woman with a long-standing history of alcoholic liver disease is admitted to hospital with a 2-week history of vomiting, confusion, increased abdominal distension and worsening jaundice. On admission laboratory data are as follows:

Na	116	(133–143 mmol/L)
K	3.8	(3.5–5 mmol/L)
Urea	8.5	(3.3–7.7 mmol/L)
Creatinine	119	(80–124 µmol/L)
Bilirubin	459	(3–17 µmol/L)
Albumin	23	(35–50 g/L)
ALT	23	(0–35 iu/L)
Alk P	524	(70–300 iu/L)
PT	18.6	(13 seconds)

Drugs on admission are as follows:

Spironolactone 300 mg each morning
Temazepam 10 mg at night
Lactulose 10 mL twice daily

Questions

Discuss the initial treatment plan for the management of:

1. Ascites
2. Nausea and vomiting
3. Confusion.

Answers

From the presenting features and LFTs on admission, it is apparent that the patient's liver disease is getting progressively worse, probably as a result of continued alcohol intake. She is confused on admission and this suggests encephalopathy, a common complication of chronic liver disease.

1. Ascites management. The patient has increased abdominal distension on admission suggestive of worsening ascites. This might be due to poor adherence with spironolactone or alternatively her ascites may have become diuretic resistant. Spironolactone therapy should be stopped in view of the low sodium and confusion, as overuse of diuretics can precipitate encephalopathy. Fluid restriction is necessary to reduce the ascites, but sufficient fluid is required to rehydrate the patient following vomiting. Paracentesis should be used to manage the ascites with every litre of ascitic fluid removed being replaced with 6–8 g of albumin. A diagnostic ascitic tap should be taken to ensure there is no infection in the ascites (spontaneous bacterial peritonitis).

2. Nausea/vomiting management. Urea is slightly raised, indicating possible dehydration as a result of vomiting. The patient should be rehydrated with dextrose 5%, not saline, as this will worsen the ascites. Additional potassium should be given to correct the low plasma potassium. Note that if the patient has been taking the spironolactone there would normally be an increase in potassium, but in this case the vomiting has probably reduced this. The patient's nausea can be managed with a suitable antiemetic such as domperidone 10 mg four times a day initially and then titrated according to the response.

3. Confusion. Confusion may be an early sign of encephalopathy in this patient. Temazepam should be stopped. The patient is on an inadequate dose of lactulose for the management of encephalopathy, so this should be increased to produce 2–3 loose motions per day. A typical dose would be 20 mL three or four times a day. In view of the patient's confusion it may be worth considering other agents in the management of the encephalopathy, such as metronidazole 400 mg twice daily.

Case 16.3

A 54-year-old woman with primary biliary cirrhosis (PBC) has been complaining of increasing backache over the last 3 months. Her general condition has deteriorated over the past year during which she has suffered from ascites and encephalopathy. Her main complaint is of continuous back pain, which disturbs her sleep.

Question

How would you manage this patient's back pain?

Answer

Back pain secondary to osteoporosis-related vertebral fractures is common in patients with chronic liver disease, and particularly in the cholestatic diseases like PBC. This is due to a marked increase in osteoclast activity. Once the diagnosis has been confirmed, the patient should be counselled that the bone pain is chronic, tends to be intermittent, and takes several months to settle after each new fracture. Bed rest is useful in the acute situation, but prolonged bed rest can accelerate bone loss.

Although there have been rapid advances in recent years in the treatment of postmenopausal osteoporosis, very few studies have addressed the problems of treating osteoporosis in patients with chronic liver disease. Calcium and vitamin D supplementation or a bisphosphonate are advised. Hormone replacement therapy is no longer advised solely for the management of osteoporosis but may be of benefit if required for other reasons.

The choice of drug is influenced by both the severity of the pain and the degree of liver impairment. For mild pain, paracetamol is the mainstay of treatment and may be used in standard doses in the majority of patients with liver dysfunction. Patients pretreated with cytochrome P450-inducing drugs or patients with a history of alcohol abuse are at increased risk of paracetamol-induced liver injury and should receive only short courses at low doses (maximum of 2 g per day for an adult).

Opioid analgesics should usually be avoided in liver disease because of their sedative properties and the risks of precipitating or masking encephalopathy. If a patient has stable mild-to-moderate liver disease then short-term use of opioids can be considered. Moderate-potency opioids, such as dihydrocodeine and codeine, are eliminated almost entirely by hepatic metabolism. Therapy should be initiated at a low dose, and the dosage interval titrated according to the response of the patient. Despite their low potency, these preparations may still precipitate encephalopathy.

In severe pain, the use of potent opioids is usually unavoidable. They undergo hepatic metabolism and are therefore likely to accumulate in liver disease. To compensate for this it is important to increase the dosage interval when using these drugs. Morphine, pethidine or diamorphine should be administered at doses at the lower end of the dosage range at intervals of 6–8 hours. The patient should be regularly observed and the dose titrated according to patient response. In any patient with liver disease receiving an opioid, it is advisable to co-prescribe a laxative as constipation can increase the possibility of developing encephalopathy.

NSAIDs should be avoided in patients with liver disease. All NSAIDs can prolong bleeding time via their effects on platelet function. Impaired liver function itself can lead to a reduced synthesis of clotting factors and an increased bleeding tendency. NSAIDs may also be dangerous due to the increased risk of gastrointestinal haemorrhage and potential to precipitate renal dysfunction.

REFERENCE

Vander A 1980 Human physiology: mechanisms of body functions, 3rd edn. McGraw-Hill Education, New Jersey

FURTHER READING

Bacon B R, O'Grady J S, DiBisceglie A M et al (eds) 2005 Comprehensive clinical hepatology. Elsevier, London

Beckingham I 2001 ABC of liver, pancreas and gall bladder. BMJ Books, London

Bosch J, Abraldes J G 2005 Variceal bleeding: pharmacological therapy. Digestive Diseases 23: 18-29

Friedman L S, Keeffe E B 2004 Handbook of liver disease. Churchill Livingstone, Edinburgh

Gines P, Cardenas A, Arroyo V et al 2004 Management of cirrhosis and ascites. New England Journal of Medicine 350: 1118-1129

Heathcote E J 2000 Management of primary biliary cirrhosis. The American Association for the Study of Liver Diseases practice guidelines. Hepatology 35: 7-13

Kjaergard L L, Liu J, Als-Nielsen B et al 2003 Artificial and bioartificial support systems for acute and acute-on-chronic liver failure: a systematic review. Journal of the American Medical Association 289: 217-222

Lai C L, Ratziu V, Yuen M F et al 2003 Viral hepatitis B. Lancet 362: 2089-2094

Leon DA, McCambridge J 2006 Liver cirrhosis mortality rates in Britain from 1950 to 2002: an analysis of routine data. Lancet 367: 52-56

Lok A S 2005 The maze of treatments for hepatitis B. New England Journal of Medicine 352: 2743-2746

Reddy K R, Faust T 2005 The clinician's guide to liver disease. Slack Inc, New Jersey

17 Chronic kidney disease and end-stage renal failure

J. Marriott   S. Smith

Chronic kidney disease is defined by reduction in the glomerular filtration rate or the presence of proteinuria. The severity of chronic kidney disease is classified from 1 to 5 depending upon the level of glomerular filtration rate (GFR) (Table 17.1). It is a common condition affecting up to 10% of the population in Western society. It is up to six times more common in some ethnic minority populations and is twice as common in females as in males. The incidence increases exponentially with age such that some degree of chronic kidney disease is almost inevitable in persons over 80 years of age. Social deprivation is also associated with higher prevalence of chronic kidney disease.

The estimated incidence of the various grades of chronic kidney disease shown in Table 17.1 has been derived from large American studies but preliminary data suggest that the rates in the UK will be similar. In the past these patients were unrecognized owing to difficulties in measuring the GFR and their health needs were largely unmet. The recent development of simple methods to estimate GFR has revealed a huge population of patients with significant kidney disease. This will pose a considerable challenge to health services in the future.

Estimation of glomerular filtration rate from the serum creatinine

The scale of the problem of chronic kidney disease has only been recognized in recent years because its detection is dependent upon making an accurate estimation of the GFR. The GFR is defined as the volume of filtrate which is produced by the glomeruli of both kidneys each minute and is a reliable indicator of renal health or disease. Unfortunately, it is impossible to measure GFR directly and therefore estimates are made by looking at the rate at which a substance, such as creatinine, is removed from the body by the kidneys. This is known as the clearance and for creatinine, the clearance is similar to the GFR, as nearly all the filtered creatinine appears in the urine. Measurements of creatinine clearance (Cl_{Cr}) require accurate collection of 24-hour urine samples with a serum creatinine sample midway through this period, which is time consuming, inconvenient and prone to inaccuracy.

The following equation may then be used:

$$Cl_{Cr} = \frac{U \times V}{S}$$

where U is the urine creatinine concentration (μmol/L), V is the urine flow rate (mL/min) and S is the serum creatinine concentration (μmol/L).

GFR can also be estimated by the clearance of infused substances such as inulin or a variety of radioisotopes but while these tests are more accurate, they are also time consuming, inconvenient and expensive.

For this reason measurement of GFR has not been routine and the serum creatinine has been used to estimate renal function. While serum creatinine concentration is related to renal function it is also dependent upon the rate of production of creatinine by the patient. This is determined by the patient's muscle mass, from where creatinine is released, which in turn is related to the patient's age, sex and weight. Creatinine is a by-product of normal muscle metabolism and is formed at a rate proportional to muscle mass. It is freely filtered by the glomerulus, with little secretion or reabsorption by the tubule. When muscle mass is stable, any change in serum creatinine levels reflects a change in its clearance by filtration. Consequently, measurement of creatinine clearance gives an estimate of the GFR.

Table 17.1 Classification of chronic kidney disease (CKD)

Stage of CKD	Glomerular filtration rate	Description	Prevalence in the USA (% of population)
1	≥90 mL/min + proteinuria	Kidney damage with normal or increased GFR	3.3
2	60–89 mL/min + proteinuria	Kidney damage with mildly decreased GFR	3.0
3	30–59 mL/min	Moderate reduction in GFR	4.3
4	13–29 mL/min	Severe reduction in GFR	0.2
5	<15 mL/min	Kidney failure	0.1

Creatinine is a useful marker of changes in GFR in an individual patient because the creatinine production rate is constant over time. However, it has been impossible to use it to define chronic kidney disease categories based on GFR because in any individual the relationship to GFR is uncertain.

It has been known for many years that the prediction of GFR from the serum creatinine would be more accurate if the creatinine generation rate for an individual patient were known. Several formulae, derived from observational studies, attempt to determine creatinine generation rate from patient parameters such as age, sex, weight, height and ethnicity. A good example is the Cockroft–Gault equation (Cockroft & Gault 1976) which uses weight, sex and age to estimate creatinine:

$$Cl_{Cr} = \frac{F\ (140\ \text{age (years)}) \times \text{weight (kg)}}{\text{serum creatinine } (\mu\text{mol/L})}$$

where F = 1.04 (females) or 1.23 (males).

Equations such as that of Cockroft & Gault (1976) are based on average population statistics and have been validated in all but the very young and the very elderly. However, they are still subject to inaccuracy owing to the influence of a number of variables upon serum creatinine. Figure 17.1 shows a range of factors, including drugs that may affect creatinine levels in serum and urine.

Although such formulae have been available for a long time they have not been widely used because they require the patient's weight or height. These are not normally recorded on laboratory request forms.

More recently a formula was derived from the Modification of Diet in Renal Disease (MDRD) study (Levey et al 1999). The MDRD formula determining GFR was developed from a multiple regression model. This used demographic and serum variables associated with low GFRs to account for inaccuracies encountered with other equations such as Cockcroft and Gault's. The independent factors associated with a lower GFR that were considered in the MDRD model included a higher serum creatinine concentration, older age, female sex, non-black ethnicity, higher serum urea levels, and lower serum albumin levels, all of which lead to inaccurate estimates of GFR using less sophisticated models.

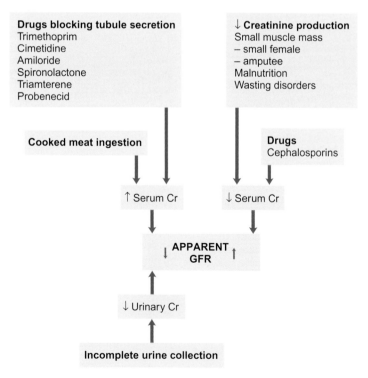

Figure 17.1 Factors that influence serum and urinary creatinine levels.

The MDRD formula:

$$eGFR = 175 \times [\text{serum creatinine} (\mu mol/L) \times 0.011312]^{-1.154} \\ \times [\text{age in years}]^{-0.203} \times [1.212 \text{ if patient is black}] \\ \times [0.742 \text{ if female}]$$

$$eGFR = \text{glomerular filtration rate} (mL/min \text{ per } 1.73\,m^2)$$

The MDRD equation to determine GFR only uses the sex and age of the patient. As it can be adjusted for ethnicity and does not require weight or height, it can be calculated by biochemistry computers from the demographic information generally available on test request forms each time a serum creatinine is measured. It is also accurate over a wide range of GFR in most ages and both sexes. Thus, for the first time there is a reliable and simple way of classifying chronic kidney disease in the general population (DH 2006).

Estimates of GFR in paediatric patients can be made using the Schwartz or Counahan formulae (see Chapter 10, Paediatrics). These both rely upon inclusion of the height of the child in estimating creatinine clearance, as height correlates with muscle mass.

It was common to assume a normal creatinine clearance of 120 mL/min and base classifications of renal impairment upon this arbitrary value. Better methods of classifying renal impairment are based upon relative changes in renal function on an individual patient basis (see Table 17.1).

Urea is also commonly used in the assessment of renal function, despite its variable production rate and diurnal fluctuation in response to the protein content of the diet. Levels of urea may also be elevated by dehydration or an increase in protein catabolism such as that accompanying gastrointestinal haemorrhage, severe infection, trauma (including surgery) and high-dose steroid therapy. Serum urea levels are therefore an unreliable measure of renal function, but can be used as an indicator of the patient's general condition and state of hydration. A rapid elevation of serum urea, before any rise in corresponding creatinine levels, is often an indication that the patient is progressing into a pre-renal state.

Significance of chronic kidney disease

Chronic kidney disease is significant as it indicates the possibility of progression to end-stage renal failure (ESRF), and the strong association with accelerated cardiovascular disease, similar in magnitude to that observed in diabetics. The cardiovascular risk increases with the severity of chronic kidney disease but is detectable at all levels. Thus, it is important to pay particular attention to other cardiovascular risk factors such as smoking, cholesterol and blood pressure in patients found to have chronic kidney disease. Progression to more severe stages and end-stage renal failure may occur, particularly if the blood pressure is inadequately controlled. However, many patients with mild chronic kidney disease remain stable for years or even decades. These patients need to be followed up to detect progression. This can usually be performed satisfactorily by their primary care clinician and long-term follow-up by a nephrologist is usually not required.

Mild levels of chronic kidney disease (grades 1–3, Table 17.1) are frequently asymptomatic. The reduction of GFR is insufficient to cause uraemic symptoms and any minor abnormalities in the urine sediment such as proteinuria or microscopic haematuria are usually unnoticed by patients. There is a frequent association with high blood pressure which may result from and cause renal damage. Recognition of chronic kidney disease classes 1–3 is important as it allows earlier treatment of cardiovascular risk factors. These patients should be investigated to determine if there is a treatable cause and followed up to identify those individuals with progressive disease.

Severe chronic kidney disease (stages 4 and 5, Table 17.1) is more frequently associated with symptoms of uraemia but these may be quite mild until the final stages of the disease when dialysis treatment is imminent. The onset of symptoms is slow and insidious so that patients get used to feeling unwell and do not realize that they are ill. It is common for patients to first present in end-stage renal failure and require immediate dialysis.

Severe chronic kidney disease is characterized by uraemia, anaemia, acidosis, osteodystrophy and neuropathy and is frequently accompanied by hypertension, fluid retention and susceptibility to infection (Fig. 17.2). It results from a significant reduction in the excretory, homeostatic, metabolic and endocrine functions of the kidney occurring over months or years.

Patients with severe chronic kidney disease often describe a long period of polyuria (excessive urine production), usually with nocturia (waking at night to pass urine). Symptoms of uraemia are usually non-specific and include lethargy, breathlessness, anorexia and nausea. When these symptoms occur they are often exacerbated by anaemia caused by a reduction in erythropoietin production. Other typical symptoms include an intractable itch, poor sleep patterns, lack of concentration and 'restless legs', that may be particularly troublesome at night. Patients may also present with muddy discolouration of the skin owing to pigment deposition.

Patients with chronic kidney disease stages 4 and 5 (see Table 17.1) should usually be followed in a hospital nephrology clinic as they require specialist management of anaemia and bone disease and, if appropriate, preparation for dialysis treatment. As they remain at high risk for vascular disease, attention to cardiovascular risk factors is very important.

Causes of chronic kidney disease

The reduction in renal function observed in chronic kidney disease results from damage to the infrastructure of the kidney. It is thought that nephrons are lost as complete units with all functions lost simultaneously. Initially the remaining nephrons cope with the increased demand. The patient remains well until so many nephrons are lost that the GFR can no longer be maintained despite activation of compensatory mechanisms. As a consequence the GFR progressively declines.

Chronic kidney disease arises from a variety of causes (Table 17.2). The difficulty in establishing a diagnosis of chronic kidney disease increases in patients aged over 65. However, establishing a cause is useful in the identification and elimination of reversible factors, in planning for likely outcomes and treatment needs, and for appropriate counselling when a genetic basis is established.

Chronic glomerulonephritis

Glomerulonephritis should not be regarded as a single disease as there are many forms, which may be either idiopathic or part

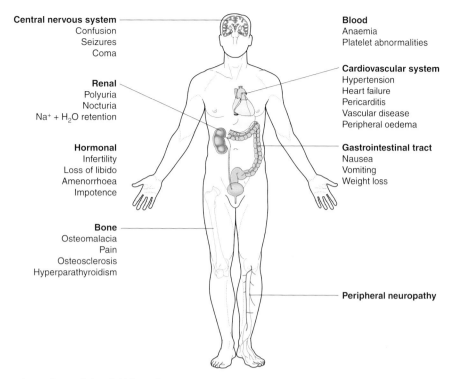

Figure 17.2 Typical signs and symptoms of chronic kidney disease.

Table 17.2 Common causes of CKD in dialysis patients in the UK (UK Renal Registry 1999)

Cause of chronic kidney disease	Percent chronic kidney disease patients
Diabetes	10
Chronic glomerulonephritis	15
Pyelonephritis and obstructive uropathy	15
Polycystic kidney disease	9
Hypertension	5
Renovascular disease	6
Other	15
Unknown	25

of systemic disease. The precise aetiology is unknown but it is thought to be mediated by deposition of immune complexes in the glomerular tuft with subsequent development of an inflammatory response. Responsible antigens include certain strains of streptococci, other infections such as malaria, endogenous antigens from, for example, neoplastic lesions, DNA, for example in systemic lupus erythematosus, and certain drugs, including non-steroidal anti-inflammatory agents, gold and penicillamine.

Hypertension

Hypertension is both a common result and a frequent cause of chronic kidney disease. It may be prevented by adequate treatment, thereby preventing a further decline in renal function.

Chronic pyelonephritis

Chronic pyelonephritis refers to chronic inflammation of the renal parenchyma with scarring of the kidney. It is generally caused by recurrent urine infection, which may be secondary to outflow obstruction or reflux nephropathy.

Metabolic diseases

Diabetes mellitus is the most common metabolic disease that may lead to chronic glomerulonephritis.

Urinary obstruction

Urinary obstruction may develop insidiously and the classic symptoms of oliguria or pain may even be absent. Causes include:

- prostate hypertrophy
- renal calculi
- congenital abnormalities
- vesicoureteric reflux.

Interstitial nephritis

Inflammation of the interstitium of the kidney with secondary involvement of the tubules is often caused by toxins. Drugs such as penicillins, analgesics and diuretics are typical toxins. Interstitial nephritis is more common in those patients aged over 65, possibly because people in this age group are prescribed greater numbers of drugs.

Congenital abnormalities

The principal congenital abnormality encountered is adult polycystic kidney disease. This is an autosomal dominant inherited condition which results in the formation of multiple cysts in both kidneys throughout life. The kidneys become enlarged and frequently fail in middle age.

Clinical manifestations

Urinary symptoms

Polyuria, where the patient frequently voids high volumes of urine, is often seen in chronic kidney disease and results from medullary damage and the osmotic effect of high plasma urea levels (greater than 40 mmol/L). The ability to concentrate urine is also lost in chronic kidney disease which, together with failure of physiological nocturnal antidiuresis, results almost invariably in nocturia, where the patient will be wakened two or three times a night with a full bladder.

Proteinuria

A degree of proteinuria invariably occurs in chronic kidney disease and can result from glomerular leaks, infection, failure of protein reabsorption in the tubules or overflow of excess plasma proteins as seen in myeloma.

Pronounced proteinuria (greater than 2 g of protein in a 24-hour collection) usually indicates a glomerular aetiology.

Fluid retention

As the GFR falls to very low levels the kidneys are unable to excrete salt and water adequately, resulting in the retention of extravascular fluid, which may manifest as both peripheral and pulmonary oedema and ascites. Oedema may be seen around the eyes on waking, the sacral region in supine patients and from the feet upwards in ambulatory patients. Volume-dependent hypertension occurs in about 80% of patients with chronic kidney disease and becomes more prevalent as the GFR falls.

Uraemia

Many substances including urea, creatinine and water are normally excreted by the kidney and accumulate as renal function decreases. Some of the substances responsible for the toxicity of uraemia are intermediate in size between small, readily dialysed molecules and large non-dialysable proteins. These are described as 'middle molecules' and include phosphate, guanidines, phenols and organic acids. Clearly, there is a wide range of uraemic toxins but it is the blood level of urea that is often used to estimate the degree of toxin accumulation in uraemia.

The symptoms of uraemia are many and various and include anorexia, nausea, vomiting, constipation, foul taste and skin discolouration, presumed to be due to pigment deposition compounded by the pallor of anaemia. The characteristic complexion is often described as 'muddy' and is frequently associated with severe pruritus without an underlying rash. In extremely severe cases crystalline urea is deposited on the skin (uraemic frost).

In uraemia there is also an increased tendency to bleed. This is further exacerbated by anaemia because of impaired platelet adhesion and modified interaction between platelets and blood vessels resulting from altered blood rheology.

Anaemia

Anaemia is an almost inevitable consequence of chronic renal failure and is generally noticeable when the GFR falls to less than 30 mL/min. The fall in haemoglobin level is a slow, insidious process accompanying the decline in renal function. A normochromic, normocytic pattern is usually seen with haemoglobin levels falling to between 6 and 8 g/dL in end-stage renal failure.

Several factors are thought to contribute to the pathogenesis of anaemia in chronic kidney disease, including shortened red cell survival, marrow suppression by uraemic toxins and iron or folate deficiency associated with poor dietary intake or increased losses, for example from gastrointestinal bleeding. However, the principal cause results from damage of peritubular cells leading to inadequate secretion of erythropoietin. This hormone, mainly but not exclusively produced in the kidney, is the main regulator of red cell proliferation and differentiation in bone marrow. Hyperparathyroidism also reduces erythropoiesis by damaging bone marrow and therefore exacerbates anaemia associated with chronic kidney disease.

Clinical findings

Anaemia is the major cause of fatigue, breathlessness at rest and on exertion, lethargy and angina often seen in patients with chronic kidney disease. These patients will also complain of feeling cold, poor concentration, reduced appetite and libido. Compensatory haemodynamic changes occur in patients with anaemia associated with chronic kidney disease. Cardiac output is increased to improve oxygen delivery to tissues although this may result in tachycardia and palpitations. As a consequence many patients cope relatively well with profoundly low haemoglobin concentrations but benefit from corrective therapy.

Electrolyte disturbances

The kidneys play a crucial role in the maintenance of volume, extracellular fluid composition and acid–base balance. Therefore it is not surprising that disturbances of electrolyte levels are seen in chronic kidney disease.

Sodium

Serum sodium levels can be relatively normal even when creatinine clearance is very low. However, patients may exhibit hypo- or hypernatraemia depending upon the condition and therapy employed (Table 17.3).

Table 17.3 Causes and mechanism of plasma sodium abnormalities in CKD

	Mechanism	Cause/effect
Hypernatraemia	Sodium overload	Drugs, e.g. antibiotic, sodium salts
	Hypotonic fluid loss	Osmotic diuresis Sweating
	↓ water intake	Unconsciousness
Hyponatraemia	Dilution by intracellular water movement	Mannitol
Hyperglycaemia	Water overload	Acute dilution by intravenous fluids, e.g. 5% dextrose infusion Excessive intake Congestive cardiac failure Nephrotic syndrome

Potassium

Potassium levels are generally elevated in chronic kidney disease. Hyperkalaemia is a potentially dangerous condition as the first indication of elevated potassium levels may be life-threatening cardiac arrest. Potassium levels of over 7.0 mmol/L are life threatening and should be treated as an emergency. Hyperkalaemia may be exacerbated in acidosis as potassium shifts from within cells.

ECG changes accompany any rise in serum potassium and become more pronounced as levels increase. T-waves peak ('tenting'), there is a reduction in the size of P-waves, an increase in the PR interval and a widening of the QRS complex. P-waves eventually disappear and the QRS complex becomes even wider. Ultimately the ECG assumes a sinusoidal appearance prior to cardiac arrest (Fig. 17.3).

Hydrogen ions

Hydrogen ions (H^+) are a common end-product of many metabolic processes and about 40–80 mmol are normally excreted via the kidney each day. In renal failure H^+ is retained, causing acidosis; the combination of H^+ with bicarbonate (HCO_3^-) results in the removal of some hydrogen as water, the elimination of carbon dioxide via the lungs, and a reduction in plasma bicarbonate level.

Hypertension and changes in chronic kidney disease

The vast majority of patients with chronic kidney disease will have hypertension. Furthermore, raised blood pressure may exacerbate renal damage and precipitate or worsen chronic kidney disease.

Severe renal impairment leads to sodium retention, which in turn produces circulatory volume expansion with consequent hypertension. This form of hypertension is often termed 'salt sensitive', as it may be exacerbated by salt intake. Lesser degrees of renal impairment reduce kidney perfusion, which activates renin production, with subsequent angiotensin-mediated

A. Normal serum potassium (3.5–5.0) mmol/L

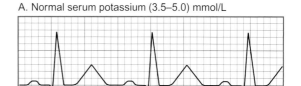

B. Serum potassium approximately 7.0 mmol/L

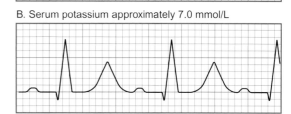

C. Serum potassium approximately 8.0–9.0 mmol/L

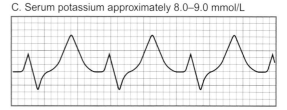

D. Serum potassium greater than 10.0 mmol/L

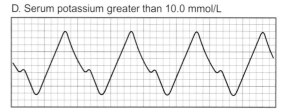

Figure 17.3 Typical ECG changes in hyperkalaemia.

vasoconstriction. Treatment of blood pressure, irrespective of choice of therapy, generally improves the course of chronic kidney disease.

Eye damage in the form of hypertensive retinopathy may be found in those patients whose blood pressure has not been adequately controlled. Appropriate and timely antihypertensive therapy can help prevent this occurring.

Renal osteodystrophy

Renal osteodystrophy describes the four types of bone disease associated with chronic kidney disease:

- secondary hyperparathyroidism
- osteomalacia (reduced mineralization)
- mixed renal osteodystrophy (both hyperparathyroidism and osteomalacia)
- adynamic bone disease (reduced bone formation and resorption).

Cholecalciferol, the precursor of active vitamin D, is both absorbed from the gastrointestinal tract and produced in the skin by the action of sunlight. Production of 1,25-dihydroxycholecalciferol (calcitriol) requires the hydroxylation of the cholecalciferol molecule at both the 1α and the 25 positions (Fig. 17.4).

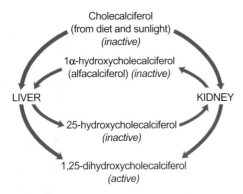

Figure 17.4 Renal and hepatic involvement in vitamin D metabolism.

Hydroxylation at the 25 position occurs in the liver, while hydroxylation of the 1α position occurs in the kidney; this latter process is impaired in renal failure. The resulting deficiency in vitamin D leads to defective mineralization of bone, and osteomalacia.

The deficiency in vitamin D with the consequent reduced calcium absorption from the gut in combination with the reduced renal tubular reabsorption results in hypocalcaemia (Fig. 17.5).

These disturbances are compounded by hyperphosphataemia caused by reduced phosphate excretion, which in turn reduces the concentration of ionized serum calcium by sequestering calcium phosphate in bone or, eventually, in soft tissue. Hypocalcaemia and a reduction in the direct suppressive action of 1,25-dihydroxycholecalciferol on the parathyroid glands results in an increased secretion of parathyroid hormone (PTH).

Since the failing kidney is unable to respond to parathyroid hormone by increasing renal calcium reabsorption, the serum PTH levels remain persistently elevated, and hyperplasia of the parathyroid glands occurs. The resulting secondary hyperparathyroidism produces a disturbance in normal architecture of bone, termed osteosclerosis (hardening of the bone). Bone pain

is the main symptom and distinctive appearances on radiography may be observed, such as 'rugger-jersey' spine, where there are alternate bands of excessive and defective mineralization in the vertebrae (Fig. 17.6).

A further possible, though by no means inevitable, consequence of the secondary hyperparathyroidism produced in response to hypocalcaemia is that sufficient bone resorption may be caused to maintain adequate calcium levels. This, in combination with the hyperphosphataemia, may result in calcium phosphate deposition and soft tissue calcification.

Neurological changes

The most common neurological changes are non-specific and include inability to concentrate, memory impairment, irritability and stupor probably caused by uraemic toxins. Fits owing to cerebral oedema or hypertension may occur. Most patients have evidence of peripheral neuropathy, although this is usually asymptomatic.

Muscle function

Muscle cramps and restless legs are common and may be major symptoms causing distress to patients, particularly at night. These conditions are probably caused by general nutritional deficiencies and electrolyte disturbances, notably of divalent cations and especially by hypocalcaemia. A proximal myopathy of shoulder and pelvic girdle muscles may rarely develop.

Diagnosis, investigations and monitoring

The diagnosis of chronic kidney disease may be suspected because of signs and symptoms of renal disease. However, more often chronic kidney disease is discovered during investigation of other medical problems or following routine screening.

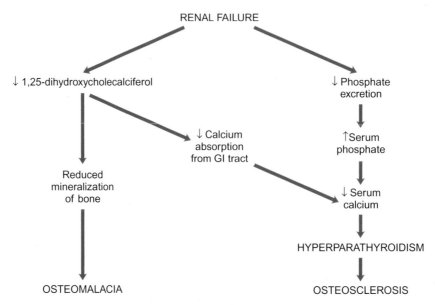

Figure 17.5 Disturbance of calcium and phosphate balance in chronic kidney disease.

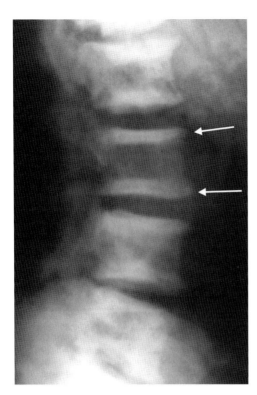

Figure 17.6 Lateral radiograph of the spine in a patient with chronic renal failure. Characteristic endplate sclerosis (arrows) are referred to as 'rugger-jersey spine' (reproduced by kind permission of Dr M. J. Kline, Department of Diagnostic Radiology, Cleveland Clinic Foundation).

Family, drug and social histories are all important in elucidating the causes of renal failure, since genetics or exposure to toxins, including prescription, over-the-counter and herbal drugs, might be implicated.

Physical examination may be very helpful. Signs of anaemia and skin pigmentation, excoriations owing to scratching and whitening of the skin with crystalline urea may indicate severe disease. Palpable or audible bruits over the femoral arteries are strongly associated with extensive arteriosclerosis and are commonly found in patients with renal vascular disease. Ankle oedema and a raised jugular venous pressure suggest fluid retention. In severe chronic kidney disease a characteristic fishy smell on the breath is observed, known as 'uraemic factor'. In some patients the kidneys may be palpable. Large irregular kidneys are indicative of polycystic disease, whereas smooth, tender, enlarged kidneys are likely to be infected or obstructed. However, in most cases of chronic kidney disease, the kidneys appear shrunken. A palpable bladder suggests outflow obstruction which in men is often due to prostatic hypertrophy.

Functional assessment of the kidney may be performed by testing serum and urine. The serum creatinine level is a more reliable indicator of renal function than the serum urea level though both are normally measured. Hyperkalaemia, acidosis with a correspondingly low serum bicarbonate level, hypocalcaemia and hyperphosphataemia are frequently present.

Urine should be examined visually and microscopically, tested with dipsticks, cultured and a 24-hour collection made for determination of GFR.

The patient may report a change in urine colour, which might result from blood staining by whole cells or haemoglobin, drugs or metabolic breakdown products. Urine may also appear milky after connection with lymphatics, cloudy following infection, contain solid material such as stones, crystals casts, or froth excessively in proteinuria.

Dipstick tests enable simple, rapid estimation of a wide range of urinary parameters including pH, specific gravity, glucose, blood and protein. Positive results should, however, be quantified by more specific methods.

Structural assessments of the kidney may be performed using a number of imaging procedures, including:

- ultrasonography
- intravenous urography (IVU)
- plain abdominal radiography
- computed tomography (CT), magnetic resonance imaging (MRI) and magnetic resonance angiography (MRA).

Ultrasonography

This method produces two-dimensional images using sound waves and is used as the first-line investigational tool in many hospitals. The technique is harmless, non-invasive, quick, inexpensive, enables measurements to be made and produces images in real time. The latter feature allows accurate and safe positioning of biopsy needles. Ultrasonography is particularly useful in the differentiation of renal tumours from cysts and in the assessment of renal tract obstruction. Doppler ultrasonography is a development that enables measurement of flow rate and direction of the intra- and extrarenal blood supply.

Intravenous urography

IVU is used less often now than in the past because it uses high doses of radiation and contrast media. Timed serial radiographs are taken of the kidneys and the full length of the urinary tract, following an intravenous injection of an iodine-based contrast medium that is filtered and excreted by the kidney. IVU will show the following:

- the presence, length and position of the kidneys; in chronic kidney disease the kidneys generally shrink in proportion to nephron loss, the exception being the enlarged kidneys seen in polycystic disease
- the presence or absence of renal scarring and the shape of the calices and renal pelvis; renal cortical scarring and caliceal distortion indicate chronic pyelonephritis
- obstruction to the ureters, for example by a stone, tumour or retroperitoneal fibrosis; these require surgical intervention
- the shape of the bladder and the presence of residual urine; enlargement and a postmicturition residue suggest urethral obstruction such as prostatic hypertrophy.

Computed tomography and magnetic resonance imaging

The similar techniques of CT and MRI provide excellent structural information about the kidneys and urinary tract. They use less radiation (none in the case of MRI) and less contrast media, although the machinery required is more expensive than needed for traditional imaging methods. MRA can also give information about renal blood supply.

Renal biopsy

If imaging techniques fail to give a cause for the reduction in renal function, a renal biopsy may be performed, although in advanced disease scarring of the renal tissue may render diagnosis difficult. Also, the small shrunken kidneys usually encountered in chronic kidney disease can be difficult to biopsy and may well subsequently bleed. In patients whose GFR is below 30 mL/min, injection of vasopressin (antidiuretic hormone, ADH) might minimize bleeding following renal biopsy.

Graphical plots of GFR

All patients with chronic kidney disease should have their serum biochemistry and haematology monitored regularly to detect any sequelae of the disease. In many forms of chronic kidney disease the decline in renal function progresses at a constant rate and may be monitored by plotting the estimated GFR against time (Fig. 17.7). The intercept with the x-axis indicates the time at which renal function will fall to zero and can be used to predict when the GFR will reach approximately 10 mL/min. This is when renal replacement therapy should be initiated (Fig. 17.7A). If an abrupt decline in the slope of a reciprocal plot is noted (Fig. 17.7B), this indicates a worsening of the condition or the presence of an additional renal insult. The cause should be detected and remedied if possible.

Prognosis

When the GFR has declined to about 20 mL/min, a continuing deterioration in renal function to end-stage renal failure is common even when the initial cause of the kidney damage has been removed and appropriate treatment instigated. The mechanism for the relentless decline in renal function is obscure but hypertension, deposition of calcium phosphate or urate crystals in the kidney and damage resulting from an increased blood flow through the remaining intact nephrons have been suggested. Serial GFR measurements should be monitored to ensure the detection of the most appropriate point at which to commence renal replacement therapy.

Treatment

The aims of the treatment of chronic kidney disease may be summarized as follows:

- reverse or arrest the process causing the renal damage, although this is usually not possible
- avoid conditions that might worsen renal failure (Table 17.4)
- relieve symptoms
- implement regular dialysis treatment and/or transplantation at the most appropriate time.

Reversal or arrest of primary disease

As indicated above, reversal or arrest of the primary cause of renal failure is unusual but sometimes possible. However, early detection of some causes may enable remedial action to be taken. A postrenal obstructive lesion such as a ureter obstructed by a stone or a ureteric tumour may be successfully treated surgically. Glomerulonephritis may respond to immunosuppressants and/or steroids. Clearly, when drug-induced renal disease is suspected the offending agent should be stopped.

Hypertension

Adequate control of blood pressure is one of the most important therapeutic measures since there is a vicious circle of events whereby hypertension causes damage to the intrarenal vasculature, resulting in thickening and hyalinization of the walls of arterioles and small vessels. This damage effectively reduces renal perfusion, leading to stimulation of the renin–angiotensin–aldosterone system. Sodium conservation and vasoconstriction result, which in turn exacerbate the degree of hypertension.

Antihypertensive therapy might produce a transient reduction in GFR over the first 3 months of treatment as the blood pressure drops. However, it is possible that control of blood pressure will ultimately lead to an improvement in renal function. This can be sufficiently dramatic that suspension of renal replacement therapy can occasionally be warranted in patients with end-stage renal failure.

The drugs used to treat hypertension in renal disease are generally the same as those used in other forms of hypertension, although allowances must be made for the effects of renal failure on drug disposition.

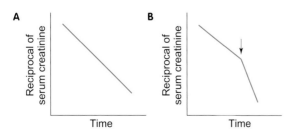

Figure 17.7 Stylized reciprocal creatinine plots. **A** Linear, uniform progression in the decline in renal function. **B** Sudden decline in renal function (arrow).

Table 17.4 Factors that might exacerbate established chronic renal failure
Reduced renal blood flow
Hypotension
Hypertension
Nephrotoxins including drugs
Renal artery disease
Obstruction, e.g. prostatic hypertrophy

Diuretics

Diuretics are of use in patients with volume overload, usually indicated by the presence of oedema. This type of hypertension may be particularly difficult to treat. The choice of agent is generally limited to a loop diuretic. Potassium-sparing diuretics are usually contraindicated owing to the risks of developing hyperkalaemia, and thiazides become ineffective as renal failure progresses.

As loop diuretics need to be filtered to exert an action, progressively higher doses are required as chronic kidney disease worsens. Doses of 500–1000 mg of furosemide or higher may be required in severe failure. Patients who do not respond to oral loop diuretic therapy alone may benefit from concomitant administration of metolazone, which acts synergistically to produce a profound diuresis. Alternatively, the loop diuretic may be given intravenously. Care must be taken to avoid hypovolaemia (monitor body weight) and electrolyte disturbances such as hypokalaemia and hyponatraemia.

Thiazide diuretics, with the notable exception of metolazone, are ineffective at a low GFR and may accumulate, causing an increased incidence of side effects.

Calcium channel blockers

These agents produce vasodilation principally by reducing Ca^{2+} influx into vascular muscle cells. They also appear to promote sodium excretion in wet hypertension. The mechanism is unclear but may revolve around the finding that high sodium levels can cause vasoconstriction by interfering with calcium transport.

Both verapamil and diltiazem block conduction across the atrioventricular node and should not be used in conjuction with β-blockers. By contrast, dihydropyridines such as nifedipine produce less cardiac depression but only dilate afferent arterioles. High systemic blood pressures can therefore cause intraglomerular hypertension and damage.

Calcium channel blockers can produce headache, facial flushing and oedema. The latter can be confused with the symptoms of volume overload but is resistant to diuretics.

Selective α₁-blockers

These vasodilators produce a variety of actions that might be of benefit in hypertension associated with chronic kidney disease. Sympathetic adrenergic activity can lead to sodium retention. These agents have also been shown to produce improvements in insulin sensitivity, adverse lipid profiles and obstruction caused by hypertrophy of the prostate, all of which might be associated with some form of chronic kidney disease.

Angiotensin-converting enzyme inhibitors and angiotensin II receptor blockers

The role of angiotensin-converting enzyme (ACE) inhibitors in hypertensive patients with renal insufficiency is complicated. ACE inhibitors reduce the amount of circulating angiotensin II, which results in vasodilation and reduced sodium retention.

They can produce a reduction in renal function by preventing the angiotensin II-mediated vasoconstriction of the efferent glomerular arteriole, which contributes to the high pressure gradient across the glomerulus. This problem is important only in patients with renal vascular disease, particularly those with bilateral renal artery stenoses. However, as ACE inhibitors preferentially dilate efferent glomerular arterioles, they lower intraglomerular pressure, thus reducing proteinuria and further development of glomerulosclerosis. Increases in GFR in hypertensive patients with renal insufficiency have been shown following ACE inhibitor therapy. Clearly, ACE inhibitors exert beneficial intrarenal haemodynamic effects in addition to actions on systemic blood pressure.

For long-term management, it is usually preferable to use an agent with a duration of action that permits once-daily dosing. There is little to choose clinically between the ACE inhibitors currently on the market; however, consideration should be given to the cost benefits of choosing an agent that does not require dose adjustment in renal failure.

It has been reported that ACE inhibitors may reduce thirst, which may be useful in those patients who have a tendency to fluid overload as a result of excessive drinking. ACE inhibitors are potassium sparing and therefore plasma potassium should be monitored carefully. A low-potassium diet may be necessary.

Angiotensin II receptor blockers have properties similar to the ACE inhibitors. Since they do not inhibit the breakdown of kinins such as bradykinin, they have the advantage that they do not cause the dry cough associated with the ACE inhibitors. The use of combined angiotensin II receptor blockers and ACE inhibitor therapy may now produce advantages in hypertension when compared with the use of either class alone.

β-blockers

β-Blockers are commonly used in the treatment of hypertension in chronic kidney disease. They exhibit a range of actions including a reduction of renin production. Consequently, they have a particular role in the rational therapy of dry hypertension. However, the β-blockers reduce cardiac output and cause peripheral vasoconstriction so they can exacerbate peripheral vascular disease.

It is advisable to use the more cardioselective β-blockers atenolol or metoprolol. As atenolol is excreted renally, dosage adjustment is required in renal failure. In practice, however, it is effective and tolerated well by renal patients at standard doses. Nevertheless, metoprolol would theoretically be a better choice since it is cleared by the liver and needs no dosage adjustment, although small initial doses are advised in renal failure since there may be increased sensitivity to its hypotensive effects.

Vasodilators

The vasodilators hydralazine and minoxidil have been used to treat hypertension in chronic kidney disease with varying degrees of success. However, they are usually only used when other measures inadequately control blood pressure. The sensitivity of patients to these drugs is often increased in renal failure so, if used, therapy should be initiated with small doses. These agents cause direct peripheral vasodilation with resultant reflex tachycardia, which may require suppression with co-prescription of a β-blocker.

Centrally acting drugs

Methyldopa and clonidine are not commonly used as antihypertensives in chronic kidney disease because of their adverse side effect profiles. If they are used in renal failure, initial doses should be small because of increased sensitivity to their effects.

Management of uraemia

Dietary modifications

Although urea is only one of the toxins encountered in uraemia, many patients experience a symptomatic improvement when dietary protein intake is reduced, presumably through a reduction in the output of nitrogenous waste. There is some evidence that, as well as reducing the symptoms of uraemia, protein restriction slows the progression of chronic kidney disease, but this remains controversial. Protein-restricted diets have been used extensively in the past but they are unpalatable and the benefits marginal so they are used infrequently in modern medical practice.

Other dietary modifications include sodium restriction to reduce the risk of fluid overload, potassium restriction to reduce the risk of hyperkalaemia, and vitamin supplementation.

Fluid retention

Oedema may occur as a result of sodium retention and the resultant associated water retention. Patients with chronic kidney disease also may have hypoalbuminaemia following renal protein loss, and this can result in an osmotic extravasation of fluid and its retention in tissues. Pulmonary and peripheral oedema is best controlled with dialysis but diuretics can be useful. The daily fluid intake should be restricted to between 1 and 3 litres, depending upon the volume of any urine produced by the patient. It is important to note that the fluid allowance must include fluids ingested in any form, including sauces, medicines and fruits in addition to drinks. The fluid restriction is very difficult to maintain. Sucking ice cubes may relieve an unpleasantly dry mouth, but the melted water must not be swallowed.

Sodium restriction Sodium intake may often be reduced to a satisfactory level of 80 mmol/day by avoiding convenience foods and snacks or the addition of salt to food at the table. This is usually tolerable to patients. It is important to be aware of the contribution of sodium-containing medications, including some antibiotics, soluble or effervescent preparations, magnesium trisilicate mixture, Gaviscon, sodium bicarbonate and the plasma expanders hetastarch and gelatin.

Potassium restriction Hyperkalaemia often occurs in chronic kidney disease and may cause life-threatening cardiac arrhythmias. If untreated, asystolic cardiac arrest and death may result. Patients are often put on a potassium-restricted diet by avoiding potassium-rich foods such as fruit and fruit drinks, vegetables, chocolate, beer, instant coffee and ice cream. Many medicines have a high potassium content, for example potassium citrate mixture, some antibiotics and ispaghula husk sachets. The use of these drugs is less of a problem in dialysed patients. Emergency treatment is necessary if the serum potassium level is above 7.0 mmol/L or if there are ECG changes. The most effective treatment is dialysis but if this is not available other measures may be tried (see Chapter 18).

The rationale and necessity for a renal diet and fluid restriction can be difficult for a patient to understand and adherence may be a problem. Consequently, involvement with a specialist renal dietician can be invaluable in optimizing dietary therapies.

Gastrointestinal symptoms

Nausea and vomiting may persist after starting a low-protein diet. In this situation, metoclopramide is useful, but sometimes accumulation of the drug and its metabolites may occur, leading to a high incidence of extrapyramidal side effects. Patients should be started on a low dose, which should then be increased slowly. Prochlorperazine or cyclizine may also be useful. The $5HT_3$-antagonists such as ondansetron have also been shown to be effective, but cost–benefit factors should be considered. The anaemic patient often becomes less nauseated when treated with epoetin.

Constipation is a common problem in patients with renal disease, partly as a result of fluid restriction and anorexia and partly as a consequence of drug therapy with agents such as aluminium supplements used as phosphate binders. It is particularly important that patients controlled by peritoneal dialysis do not become constipated, as this can reduce the efficacy of dialysis and predispose to peritonitis. Conventional laxative therapy may be used, such as bulk-forming laxatives or increased dietary fibre for less severe constipation, or a stimulant such as senna with enemas or glycerine suppositories for severe constipation. Higher doses of stimulant laxatives such as 2–4 tablets of senna at night may be required. It should be noted that certain brands of ispaghula husk preparations may contain significant quantities of potassium, and should be avoided in renal failure because of the risk of hyperkalaemia. Sterculia preparations are an effective alternative.

Pruritus

Itching associated with renal failure can be extremely severe and can often be distressing, disfiguring as a result of overenthusiastic scratching and also difficult to treat. The exact mechanism responsible is not clear and several possibilities have been suggested. Xerosis (dry skin) associated with renal failure, skin microprecipitation of divalent ions, elevated parathyroid hormone levels and increased dermal mast cell activity are all possible. Generally, however, no underlying cause is found and it is likely that a multifactorial process is responsible.

Sometimes correction of serum phosphate or calcium levels improves the condition, as does parathyroidectomy. Conventionally, oral antihistamines are used to treat pruritus; however, topical versions should not be used owing to the risks of allergy. Non-sedating antihistamines such as loratidine are generally less effective than sedating antihistamines such as chlorphenamine. Alimemazine may be useful, particularly at night. Topical crotamiton lotion and creams are also reported to be useful in some patients. Other non-drug therapies include either warming or cooling the skin using baths, three times weekly UVB phototherapy and modified electrical acupuncture.

Anaemia

The normochromic, normocytic anaemia of chronic kidney disease does not respond to iron or folic acid unless there is a co-existing deficiency. Traditionally the only treatment available was to give red blood cell transfusions. However, this is time consuming, may lead to fluid and iron overload and promotes antibody formation, which may give problems if transplantation is subsequently attempted. The introduction of recombinant human erythropoietins (epoetin-α and -β), genetically engineered forms of the hormone, has rendered treatment safer and at least as effective.

Epoetin-α and -β were thought to be indistinguishable in practical terms, and immunologically and biologically indistinguishable from physiological erythropoietin. Recently it has been recognized that the use of epoetins can be associated with the production of antierythropoietin antibodies, leading to a severe anaemia which is unresponsive to exogenous epoetin. This is known as pure red cell aplasia (PRCA) and is more commonly associated with epoetin-α when given by the subcutaneous route. Consequently although both forms of epoetin may be given by the intravenous route, only epoetin-β can be given by the subcutaneous route. The subcutaneous route is preferred by many as it provides equally effective clinical results while using similar or smaller dose (up to 30% less) when given three times a week. Most patients report a dramatically improved quality of life after starting epoetin therapy.

Novel erythropoiesis stimulating protein (NESP) is a recombinant hyperglycosylated analogue of epoetin that stimulates red blood cell production by the same mechanism as the endogenous hormone. The terminal half-life of NESP in man is three times longer than that of epoetin and consequently requires a once-weekly dosing schedule.

Iron and folate deficiencies must be corrected before therapy is initiated, while patients receiving epoetin generally require concurrent iron supplements because of increased marrow requirements. Supplemental iron is often given intravenously owing to bioavailability problems with oral forms. Maintaining iron stores ensures the effect of epoetin is optimized for minimum cost.

Epoetin therapy should aim to achieve a slow rise in the haemoglobin concentration. This is to avoid cardiovascular side effects resulting from a rapidly increasing red cell mass, such as hypertension, increased blood viscosity/volume, seizures and clotting of vascular accesses. Blood pressure should be closely monitored.

An initial subcutaneous or intravenous epoetin dose of 50 units/kg body weight is given three times weekly. This is increased, as necessary, in steps of 25 units/kg every 4 weeks, to produce a haemoglobin increase of not more than 2 g/dL per month. The target haemoglobin concentration is commonly 11–13 g/L and once this has been reached, a maintenance dose of epoetin in the region of 33–100 units/kg three times a week or 50–150 units/kg twice weekly should maintain the level.

Correcting anaemia usually helps control the symptoms of lethargy and myopathy, and often greatly reduces nausea. Improved appetite on epoetin therapy can, however, increase potassium intake and may necessitate dietary control.

Acidosis

Since the kidney is the main route for excreting H^+ ions, chronic kidney disease may result in a metabolic acidosis. This will cause a reduction in serum bicarbonate that may be treated readily with oral doses of sodium bicarbonate 1–6 g/day. As the dose of bicarbonate is not critical, it is easy to experiment with different dosage forms and strengths to suit individual patients. If acidosis is severe and persistent then dialysis may be required.

Neurological problems

Neurological changes are generally caused by uraemic toxins and improve on the treatment of uraemia by dialysis or diet. Muscle cramps are common and are often treated with quinine sulphate (see Chapter 18). Restless legs may respond to low doses of clonazepam or co-careldopa.

Osteodystrophy

The osteodystrophy of renal failure is due to three factors: hyperphosphataemia, vitamin D deficiency and hyperparathyroidism.

Hyperphosphataemia

The management of hyperphosphataemia depends initially upon restricting dietary phosphate. This can be difficult to achieve effectively, even with the aid of a specialist dietician, because phosphate is found in many palatable foods such as dairy products, eggs, chocolate and nuts. Phosphate-binding agents can be used to reduce the absorption of orally ingested phosphate in the gut, by forming insoluble, non-absorbable complexes. Phosphate binders are usually salts of a di- or trivalent metallic ion, such as aluminium, calcium or occasionally magnesium.

Aluminium hydroxide has been widely used as a phosphate binder owing to the avid binding capacity of aluminium ions. Unfortunately, a small amount of aluminium may be absorbed by patients with chronic kidney disease owing to poor clearance of this ion, which can produce toxic effects including encephalopathy, osteomalacia, proximal myopathy and anaemia. Dialysis dementia was a disease observed among haemodialysis patients. This is associated with aluminium deposition in the brain and exacerbated by aluminum in the water supply and the use of aluminium cooking pans. Desferrioxamine, 4–6 g in 500 mL of saline 0.9% per week, has been used to treat this condition by removing aluminium from tissues by chelation. The tendency of aluminium to constipate is an added disadvantage. The use of aluminium as a phosphate binder in chronic kidney disease should therefore be approached with caution.

Calcium carbonate has been used as a phosphate binder. Unfortunately, it is less effective as a phosphate binder than aluminium, and sometimes requires doses of up to 10 g daily. Calcium carbonate has advantages, as correction of concurrent hypocalcaemia can be achieved.

Calcium acetate is now also available for use as a phosphate binder. The capacity of calcium acetate and calcium carbonate to control serum phosphate appears similar. However, phosphate control is achieved using between half and a quarter of the dose of elemental calcium when calcium acetate is used. Whether this translates to a decreased likelihood of producing unwanted hypercalcaemia with calcium acetate therapy is as yet unclear.

Sevelamer, a hydrophilic but insoluble polymeric compound, is used as a phosphate binder in haemodialysis patients. Sevelamer binds phosphate with an efficacy similar to calcium acetate but with a decreased likelihood of hypercalcaemia. It does not contain either calcium or aluminium so its use is not limited by intoxication with these metals. Mean levels of total and low-density cholesterol are also reduced with sevelamer use. This compound does not appear to present any risk of toxicity but may cause bowel obstruction and is relatively expensive when compared to other phosphate binders.

Vitamin D deficiency

Vitamin D deficiency may be treated with the synthetic vitamin D analogues 1α-hydroxycolecalciferol (alfacalcidol) at 0.25–1 µg/day or 1,25-dihydroxycolecalciferol (calcitriol) at 1–2 µ/day. The serum calcium level should be monitored, and the dose of alfacalcidol or calcitriol adjusted accordingly. Hyperphosphataemia should be controlled before starting vitamin D therapy since the resulting increase in the serum calcium concentration may result in soft tissue calcification.

Hyperparathyroidism

The rise in plasma 1,25-dihydroxycolecalciferol and calcium levels that results from starting vitamin D therapy usually suppresses the production of parathyroid hormone by the parathyroids. If vitamin D therapy does not correct parathyroid hormone levels then parathyroidectomy to remove part or most of the parathyroid glands may be needed. This surgical procedure was once commonly performed on chronic kidney disease patients, but is now less frequent owing to effective vitamin D supplementation.

Cinacalcet is a calcimimetic agent which can suppress parathyroid hormone without causing hypercalcaemia. It is effective but expensive. It is particularly valuable for patients who are not fit for parathyroidectomy.

Implementation of regular dialysis treatment and/or transplantation

End-stage renal failure is the point at which, despite the conservative measures discussed above, the patient will die without the institution of renal replacement by dialysis or transplantation. This may occur very rapidly after presentation or after a period of several years.

The principle of dialysis is simple. The patient's blood and a dialysis solution are positioned on opposing sides of a semipermeable membrane across which exchange of metabolites occurs. The two main types of dialysis used in chronic kidney disease are haemodialysis and peritoneal dialysis (see Chapter 18). Neither has been shown to be superior to the other in any particular group of patients and so the personal preference of the patient is important when selecting dialysis modality.

As patients with end-stage renal failure may require dialysis treatment for many years, adaptations to the process of peritoneal dialysis have been made that enable the patient to follow as normal a lifestyle as possible. Continuous ambulatory peritoneal dialysis (CAPD) involves a flexible non-irritant silicone rubber catheter (Tenckhoff catheter) that is surgically inserted into the abdominal cavity. Dacron cuffs on the body of the catheter become infiltrated with scar tissue during the healing process, causing the catheter to

be firmly anchored in place. Such catheters may remain viable for many years. During the dialysis process thereafter, a bag typically containing 2.5 litres of warmed dialysate and a drainage bag are connected to the catheter using aseptic techniques. Used dialysate is drained from the abdomen under gravity into the drainage bag, fresh dialysate is run into the peritoneal cavity and the giving set is disconnected. The patient continues activities until the next exchange some hours later. The procedure is repeated regularly so that dialysate is kept in the abdomen 24 hours a day. This is usually achieved by repeating the process four times a day with an average dwell time of 6–8 hours.

Since CAPD is continuous and corrects fluid and electrolyte levels constantly, dietary and fluid restrictions are less stringent. Blood loss is also avoided, making the technique safer in anaemic patients.

Unfortunately, peritoneal dialysis is not an efficient process; it only just manages to facilitate excretion of the substances required and, as albumin crosses the peritoneal membrane, up to 10 g of protein a day may be lost in the dialysate. It is also uncomfortable and tiring for the patient, and is contraindicated in patients who have recently undergone abdominal surgery.

Peritonitis is the most frequently encountered complication of peritoneal dialysis. Its diagnosis usually depends on a combination of abdominal pain, cloudy dialysate or positive microbiological culture. Empirical antibiotic therapy should therefore be commenced as soon as peritonitis is clinically diagnosed. Gram-positive cocci, particularly *Staphylococcus aureus*, and Enterobacteriaceae are the causative organisms in the majority of cases, while infection with Gram-negative species and Pseudomonas species is also well recognized. Fungal infections are also seen, albeit less commonly.

Most centres have their own local protocol for antibiotic treatment of peritonitis. In one example, ceftazidime, a broad-spectrum cephalosporin with good Gram-negative activity, and vancomycin, which has excellent activity against Gram-positive bacteria, are administered in combination via the intraperitoneal route. As in all situations, the antibiotic regimen should be adjusted appropriately after the results of microbiological culture and sensitivity have been obtained.

Oral ciprofloxacin in a dose of 500 mg four times a day for 14 days has been shown to be effective, although not licensed, for the treatment of CAPD peritonitis. When this regimen is used it is important that any oral aluminium preparations are discontinued, as they reduce the absorption of ciprofloxacin by chelation.

Haemodialysis is particularly suitable for patients producing large amounts of metabolites, such as those with high nutritional demands or a large muscle mass, where these substances are produced faster than they can be removed by peritoneal dialysis. It also provides an alternative for those patients in whom peritoneal dialysis has failed.

The various techniques of haemofiltration, a technique related to haemodialysis, are also discussed in Chapter 18.

Renal transplantation

Renal transplantation remains the treatment of choice for patients with end-stage renal failure, as a relatively normal lifestyle is usually re-established. Expensive dialysis procedures are not needed, dietary restrictions are lifted and improvements are seen in anaemia and bone disease. However, there is a shortage of suitable organs for transplantation and up to 60% of patients on the dialysis programme are not physically fit enough to undergo the surgery and postoperative treatment.

Except in those rare cases where a genetically identical donor is available, the most important therapeutic aspect of transplantation is immunosuppression to prevent rejection. The major disadvantage of all immunosuppressive agents is their relative non-specificity, in that they cause a general depression of the immune system. This exposes the patient to an increased risk of malignancy and infection, which remains an important cause of morbidity and mortality.

Immunosuppressants

The major pharmacological groups of immunosuppressive agents are summarized in Table 17.5.

Most transplant centres have their own regimens involving combinations of the agents outlined in Table 17.5 for prophylaxis against rejection and for reversal of acute and chronic episodes of rejection. The regimens implemented will often depend upon the nature and source of the donor organ, e.g. cold ischaemia time, ethnic background, cadaveric or live donor, which are key factors in determining the risk of rejection. National guidance (NICE 2004) has been issued for the use of immunosuppressive therapy in kidney transplant patients.

Immunosuppression is usually commenced immediately before the grafting procedure on induction of anaesthesia (induction phase). It is continued during the perioperative period (initial therapy) and then maintained for as long as the transplanted kidney remains in situ (maintenance therapy). The induction and maintenance regimens usually differ in terms of drugs and doses used in order to achieve the best possible balance between immunosuppression and side effects.

Generally two types of induction regimen are used. Antibody-based regimens use monoclonal (e.g. muromonab-CD3), poly-clonal or anti-CD25 antibodies (e.g. basiliximab, daclizumab) for up to 8 weeks post transplant. This type of regimen prevents acute rejection effectively and enables calcineurin inhibitors to be avoided or used at reduced doses, thus minimizing nephrotoxicity.

Aggressive early immunosuppression regimens use drugs from maintenance regimens at higher doses in order to maximize immunosuppression post-transplant. These regimens carry an increased risk of nephrotoxicity.

One of the most common immunosuppressant regimens involves triple therapy with a calcineurin inhibitor, mycophenolate mofetil or azathioprine and prednisolone. Such regimens allow the dose and toxicity of individual agents to be minimized whilst maintaining adequate immunosuppression. However, the drugs and doses employed vary widely between individual transplant centres. Many tend to gradually withdraw the steroid, maintaining

Table 17.5 Mechanism of action of immunosuppressants commonly used following renal transplantation

Drug	Mechanism	Comment
Steroids	Bind to steroid receptors and inhibit gene transcription and function of T-cells, macrophages and neutrophils	Prophylaxis against and reversal of rejection
Ciclosporin	Forms complex with intracellular protein cyclophilin → inhibits calcineurin. Ultimately inhibits interleukin-2 synthesis and T-cell activation	Long-term maintenance therapy against rejection
Tacrolimus	Forms complex with an intracellular protein → inhibits calcineurin	Long-term maintenance therapy against rejection. Rescue therapy in severe or refractory rejection
Sirolimus	Inhibits interleukin-2 cell signalling → blocks T-cell cycling and inhibits B-cells	Usually used in combination with ciclosporin ± steroids
Mycophenolate	Inhibits inosine monophosphate dehydrogenase → reduces nucleic acid synthesis → inhibits T- and B-cell function	Usually used in combination with ciclosporin/tacrolimus ± steroids
Azathioprine	Incorporated as a purine in DNA → inhibits lymphocyte and neutrophil proliferation	Usually used in combination with ciclosporin/tacrolimus ± steroids
Muromonab (OKT3, mouse monoclonal anti-CD3)	Binds to CD3 complex → blocks, inactivates or kills T-cell. Short $T_{1/2}$	Prophylaxis against rejection. Reversal of severe rejection
Polyclonal horse/rabbit antithymocyte or antilymphocyte globulin (ATG, ALG)	Antibodies against lymphocyte proteins → alter T- and B-cell activity	Prophylaxis against rejection. Reversal of severe rejection
Humanized or chimaeric anti-CD25 (basiliximab and daclizumab)	Monoclonal antibodies that bind CD25 in interleukin-2 complex → prevent T-cell proliferation	Prophylaxis against acute rejection in combination with ciclosporin and steroids

patients on dual therapy, while some commonly use monotherapy for long-term treatment. In order to minimize side effects, doses of immunosuppressants are gradually reduced over a 2–6 month period to the lowest that maintain effective immunosuppression. In addition, transplants appear to become less immunogenic over a period of time (chimaerism) so lower prophylactic levels of immunosuppression are required.

Calcineurin inhibitors   The discovery and development of ciclosporin and latterly tacrolimus immunosuppression regimens have greatly increased transplant survival rates.

Calcineurin exerts phosphatase activity on the nuclear factor of activated T-cells. This factor then migrates to the nucleus, initiating IL-2 transcription. Ciclosporin and tacrolimus inhibit calcineurin through binding proteins (ciclophilin protein and tacrolimus binding protein respectively) which results in inhibition of IL-2, which is normally involved in the proliferation of T-cells.

The action of calcineurin inhibitors is partially selective in that they suppress cytotoxic T-cell production and to some extent spare B-lymphocyte activity, permitting a greater response to infection than can normally be mounted by patients using older forms of immunosuppression. Thus, there is a relatively low incidence of severe infection associated with calcineurin inhibitor therapy, although the incidence of malignancies appears to be similar to that found with other immunosuppressants.

Ciclosporin   Ciclosporin carries a high risk of side effects, including nephrotoxicity, hypertension, fine muscle tremor, gingival hyperplasia, nausea and hirsutism. Serum biochemistry can also be adversely affected, with dose-dependent increases in creatinine and urea occurring in the first few weeks of treatment. Hyperkalaemia, hyperuricaemia, hypomagnesaemia and hypercholesterolaemia may also occur. Nephrotoxicity is a particularly serious side effect and occasionally necessitates the withdrawal of ciclosporin. There is tremendous inter- and intrapatient variation in absorption of ciclosporin. Blood level monitoring is essential to achieve the maximum protection against rejection with the minimum risk of side effects. The range regarded as acceptable varies between centres, but is commonly taken as 100–200 ng/mL.

Ciclosporin is known to interact with a number of drugs. These lead to either a reduction in ciclosporin levels, causing an increased risk of rejection, or an elevation in ciclosporin levels, resulting in increased toxicity. Some drugs enhance the nephrotoxicity of ciclosporin (Table 17.6).

Ciclosporin should not be administered with grapefruit juice, which should also be avoided for at least an hour pre dose, as this can result in marked increases in blood concentrations. This effect appears to be due to inhibition of enzyme systems in the gut wall, resulting in transiently reduced ciclosporin metabolism.

Table 17.6   Examples of drug interactions involving ciclosporin

Reduce ciclosporin serum levels (hepatic enzyme inducers):
   phenytoin, phenobarbital, rifampicin, isoniazid

Increase ciclosporin serum levels (hepatic enzyme inhibitors):
   diltiazem, erythromycin, corticosteroids, ketoconazole

Enhance ciclosporin nephrotoxicity:
   aminoglycosides, amphotericin, co-trimoxazole, melphalan

Tacrolimus   Tacrolimus is chemically unrelated to ciclosporin, but acts by a similar mechanism. The side effect profile also appears to be similar to that of ciclosporin but has some subtle differences. Neurotoxicity is more common with tacrolimus, which also causes disturbances of glucose metabolism. In contrast, hirsutism is less of a problem. Tacrolimus is particularly useful when trying to reverse acute rejection episodes.

Studies have shown that ciclosporin and tacrolimus achieved similar rates of graft survival. However, several studies have showed lower rates of rejection episodes with tacrolimus.

Tacrolimus can be used in preference to ciclosporin as part of initial or maintenance immunosuppressive regimens (NICE 2004), but the choice of calcineurin inhibitor should be based upon the best likely side effect profile for the individual patient.

Steroids   Prednisolone is the oral agent commonly used for immunosuppression after renal transplantation, while methylprednisolone is used intravenously in regimens to reverse acute rejection. The maintenance dose of prednisolone is about 10–20 mg/day given as a single dose in the morning to minimize adrenal suppression. The use of steroid therapy often leads to complications, particularly if high doses are given for long periods. In addition to a cushingoid state, there may be gastrointestinal bleeding, hypertension, dyslipidaemia, diabetes, osteoporosis and mental disturbances. Patients who are temporarily unable to take oral prednisolone should be given an equivalent dose of hydrocortisone intravenously.

Azathioprine   Azathioprine is derived from 6-mercaptopurine and is therefore an antimetabolite which reduces DNA and RNA synthesis producing immunosuppression.

Azathioprine should be given in a dose of 2.5 mg/kg/day either orally or intravenously as the two routes have the same bioavailability. There is no advantage in giving it in divided doses. Since azathioprine interferes with nucleic acid synthesis, it may be mutagenic, and heathcare staff should avoid handling the tablets. The combination of azathioprine and allopurinol should be avoided because of a significant drug interaction, causing fatal marrow suppression.

Mycophenolate mofetil   Mycophenolate mofetil is a prodrug of mycophenolic acid which inhibits the enzyme inosine monophosphate dehydrogenase which is needed for guanosine synthesis. The outcome is that B- and T-cell proliferation is reduced, whereas other rapidly dividing cells are less affected, since guanosine is produced in other cells. Consequently, mycophenolate has a more selective mode of action than azathioprine.

It is licensed for prophylaxis against acute renal transplant rejection when used in combination with ciclosporin and steroids, and is given in a dose of 1 g twice daily. There is evidence that, compared to similar regimens incorporating azathioprine, it reduces the risk of acute rejection episodes. However, the risk of opportunistic infections and the occurrence of blood disorders such as leucopenia may be higher.

Using mycophenolate with azathioprine significantly increases the risks of haematological toxicity. In addition, care should be taken since blood levels are increased with concurrent administration of tacrolimus.

Mycophenolate mofetil should ideally be used only when a patient has to stop or reduce the dose of a calcineurin inhibitor. This is usually because of calcineurin inhibitor nephrotoxicity.

Sirolimus Sirolimus is a macrolide antibiotic that binds to the FKBP-25 cellular receptor. This complex initiates a sequence that produces modulation of regulatory kinases that ultimately interfere with the proliferative effects of IL-2 on lymphocytes. The progression of T-cells from the G1 to S phase is blocked, so inhibiting cell division and, therefore, cell proliferation.

Adverse effects include hyperkalaemia, hypomagnesaemia, hyperlipidaemia, hypertriglyceridaemia, leucopenia, anaemia, impaired wound healing, and joint pain. Sirolimus can be used concomitantly with tacrolimus, ciclosporin or mycophenolate mofetil. Multiple drug interactions are possible with sirolimus, especially because of its extremely long half-life. Sirolimus can be used in combination therapy, but only for those whose use of calcineurin inhibitors is limited by side effects.

Polyclonal antibodies These were the first antibodies used as immunosuppressants and polyclonal preparations contain antibodies with a number of different antigen-combining sites. Polyclonal antibodies are used perioperatively as prophylaxis against rejection and in some cases to reverse episodes of severe rejection. The main preparations are antithymocyte globulin (ATG) and antilymphocyte globulin (ALG).

Antithymocyte globulin is an antilymphocyte globulin produced from rabbit or equine serum immunized with human T-cells. It contains antibodies to human T-lymphocytes, which on injection will attach to, neutralize and eliminate most T-lymphocytes, thereby weakening the immune response. Antilymphocyte globulin is similar to antithymocyte globulin and is of equine origin. However, it is not specific to T-lymphocytes as it also acts on B-lymphocytes.

It is not certain how polyclonal antibodies act to inhibit T-cell mediated immune responses. However, depletion of circulating T-cells, modulation of cell surface receptor molecules, induction of anergy and apoptosis of activated T-cells have all been proposed.

The main drawback to the use of anti-T-cell sera is the relatively high incidence of side effects, notably anaphylactic reactions including hypotension, fever and urticaria. These reactions are more frequently observed with the first dose and may require supportive therapy with steroids and antihistamines. Severe reactions may necessitate stopping the treatment. Steroids and antihistamines may be given prophylactically to prevent or minimize allergic reactions. Pyrexia often occurs on the first day of treatment but usually subsides without requiring treatment. Tolerance testing by administration of a test dose is advisable, particularly in patients such as those with asthma who commonly experience allergic reactions. Antilymphocyte globulin and antithymocyte globulin can be substituted for each other, should adverse reactions occur.

Monoclonal antibodies Muromonab-CD3 (OKT3) is a monoclonal antibody directed against the CD3 complex associated with human T-cell receptors and has limited reactions with other tissues or cells. It blocks the function and generation of the cytotoxic T-cells responsible for kidney transplant rejection. Muromonab has a short half-life and is eventually neutralized by an antibody response. As with other anti-T-cell sera, the main drawbacks of muromonab use are its side effects. These include nausea, vomiting and diarrhoea, marked pyrexia (often over 40°C), chills, dyspnoea, chest pain and rigors. Commonly, prophylactic agents against these side effects are prescribed, especially with the initial doses of the course.

The humanized or chimaeric anti-CD25 monoclonal antibodies basiliximab and daclizumab are clinically similar and bind to CD25 in the interleukin-2 complex of activated T-lymphocytes. This renders all T-cells resistant to interleukin-2 and therefore prevents T-cell proliferation. They are used as prophylaxis against acute rejection in combination with calcineurin inhibitors and steroids. Basiliximab or daclizumab can be used for induction

Table 17.7 Common therapeutic problems in chronic kidney disease

Problem	Comment
Drug choice	Care with choice/dose of all drugs. Care to avoid renotoxic agents pre-dialysis to preserve function. Beware herbal therapies as some contain immune system boosters (reverse immunosuppressant effects) and some are nephrotoxic
Drug excretion	Chronic kidney disease will lead to accumulation of drugs and their active metabolites if they are normally excreted by the kidney
Dietary restrictions	Restrictions on patient often severe. Fluid allowance includes foods with high water content, e.g. gravy, custard and fruit
Hypertension	Frequently requires complex multiple drug regimens. Calcium channel blockers can cause oedema that might be confused with fluid overload
Analgesia	Side effects are increased. Initiate with low doses and gradually increase. Avoid pethidine as metabolites accumulate. Avoid NSAIDs unless specialist advice available
Anaemia	Epoetin requires sufficient iron stores to be effective. Absorption from oral iron supplements may be poor and i.v. iron supplementation might be required. Care required to make sure that epoetin use does not produce hypertension
Immunosuppression	Use of live vaccines should be avoided (BCG, MMR, mumps, oral polio, oral typhoid, smallpox, yellow fever)
Pruritus (itching)	Can be severe. Treat with chlorphenamine; less sedating antihistamines often less effective. Some relief with topical agents, e.g. crotamiton
Restless legs	Involuntary jerks can prevent sleep. Clonazepam 0.5–1mg at night may help

treatment in combination with other immunosuppressants, e.g a calcineurin inhibitor.

Other precautions

Transplant patients will be given prophylactic antibiotic therapy for varying periods postoperatively owing to the risks of infection associated with immunosuppression. Treatment with co-trimoxazole to prevent *Pneumocystis carinii*, isoniazid and pyridoxine to prevent tuberculosis, aciclovir or ganciclovir to prevent cytomegalovirus, and nystatin or amphotericin to prevent oral candidiasis is commonly used. Vaccination with live organisms, e.g. BCG, MMR, oral poliomyelitis, oral typhoid, must be avoided in the immunosuppressed patient.

CASE STUDIES

Case 17.1

Mr D, a 19-year-old undergraduate student, visited his university health centre complaining of a 3-month history of fatigue, weakness, nausea and vomiting that he had attributed to 'examination stress'. His previous medical history indicated an ongoing history of bed wetting from an early age. Laboratory results from a routine blood screen showed:

		Reference range
Sodium	137 mmol/L	(135–145)
Potassium	4.8 mmol/L	(3.5–5.0)
Phosphate	2.5 mmol/L	(0.9–1.5)
Calcium	1.6 mmol/L	(2.20–2.55)
Urea	52 mmol/L	(3.0–6.5)
Creatinine	620 μmol/L	(50–120)
Haemoglobin	7.5 g/dL	(13.5–18.0)

Subsequent referral to a specialist hospital centre established a diagnosis of chronic kidney disease secondary to reflux nephropathy.

Question

Explain the signs and symptoms experienced by Mr D and the likely course of his disease.

Answer

Mr D is suffering from the signs and symptoms of uraemia resulting from chronic kidney disease. Mechanical reflux damage to his kidneys has compromised renal function and resulted in an accumulation of toxins, including urea and creatinine, that in turn have contributed to his nausea, vomiting and general malaise. His biochemical results indicate other typical features of uraemic syndrome associated with chronic kidney disease. The low haemoglobin is indicative of reduced erythropoietin production following progressive kidney damage. Renal osteodystrophy is also present, as inadequate vitamin D production and the raised serum phosphate have contributed to the hypocalaemia.

This patient is likely to have remained symptom free for a period of years despite progressively worsening renal function. The kidney operates with a substantial functional reserve under normal conditions. Patients generally remain asymptomatic as their renal reserve diminishes. Eventually there is a failure in the ability of the damaged kidney to compensate and symptoms appear late in the condition.

Case 17.2

Mr K, a 43-year-old male with established chronic kidney disease, had been maintained for 3 years on continuous ambulatory peritoneal dialysis. He was admitted to hospital for cadaveric renal transplantation. On examination he was found to have slight ankle oedema. He weighed 60 kg and his blood pressure was 135/90 mmHg and pulse rate 77/min. He was administered the following immunosuppressants preoperatively: ciclosporin 150 mg i.v. (approximately 3 mg/kg), azathioprine 50 mg i.v. (approximately 1 mg/kg). Methylprednisolone 1 g was given intravenously immediately after grafting.

Question

How should the intravenous immunosuppressants be administered in this patient and how should immunosuppression be managed postoperatively?

Answer

In a patient with chronic kidney disease consideration should be given to the use of dextrose 5% as a vehicle rather than normal saline in order to reduce the sodium load and therefore minimize the risks of fluid overload. Ciclosporin should be diluted at least 1:20 and, ideally, administered over 2 hours. With cadaveric transplants, time is usually limited and the inevitable rapid administration of ciclosporin will increase the likelihood of side effects. Ciclosporin injection can precipitate severe allergic reactions and the patient should be checked regularly. Azathioprine is very irritant and the intravenous line should be flushed following administration. Intravenous triple therapy can be continued postoperatively until the patient can manage oral medication.

Typically, ciclosporin 5 mg/kg/day, azathioprine 1 mg/kg/day and methylprednisolone 300 μg/kg/day are used intravenously. However, in practice regimens vary considerably between centres.

Oral therapy should be initiated as soon as the patient can practically manage. Prednisolone should replace methylprednisolone according to the potency ratio 5:4, resulting in a daily oral dose of 22.5 mg. Azathioprine absorption can be variable; however, in most patients the oral dose is the same as that given intravenously. Ciclosporin absorption is subject to interpatient variability, although the microemulsion formulation of Neoral has led to improvements, as absorption from the gastrointestinal tract is not bile salt dependent. Generally the initial oral dose of ciclosporin should be about three times the intravenous dose, i.e. 450 mg twice daily in this patient. The dose should be individualized by measuring plasma levels after 3 days with appropriate adjustment.

Case 17.3

Mr A is a patient with chronic kidney disease secondary to chronic interstitial nephritis. He complains of chronic fatigue, lethargy and breathlessness on exertion, palpitations and poor concentration. His recent haematological results were found to be:

		Reference range
Haemoglobin	5.6 g/dL	(13.5–17.5)
Red cell count	2.92×10^9/L	(4.5–6.5×10^9/L)
Haematocrit	0.208	(0.40–0.54)
Serum ferritin	88.0 μg/L	(15–300)

Question

Explain this patient's symptoms and haematological results and outline the optimal treatment.

Answer

Mr A's symptoms are most likely to result from a normochromic, normocytic anaemia caused by renal failure. Levels of erythropoietin produced by the kidney are reduced in renal failure. Production of erythropoietin from extrarenal sites, e.g. liver, are not sufficient to maintain erythropoiesis, which is also inhibited by uraemic toxins and hyperparathyroidism. The anaemia associated with renal failure is further compounded by a reduction in red cell survival through low-grade haemolysis, bleeding from the gastrointestinal tract and blood loss through dialysis, aluminium toxicity which interferes with haem synthesis, and iron deficiency, usually through poor dietary intake.

Therapy with epoetin is the treatment of choice. However, iron and folate deficiencies should be corrected if epoetin therapy is to be successful. Iron demands are generally raised during epoetin treatment and iron status should be regularly monitored. If serum ferritin falls below 100 µg/L then iron supplementation should be started. Often intravenous iron is required to provide an adequate supply, despite the dangers associated with administration of iron by this route.

REFERENCES

Cockcroft D, Gault M 1976 Predication of creatinine clearance from serum creatinine. Nephron 16: 31-34

Department of Health 2006 Estimating glomerular filtration rate (eGFR): information for general practitioners. Available online at: www.dh.gov.uk/assetRoot/04/13/30/21/ 04133021.pdf

Levey A S, Bosch J P, Lewis J B et al 1999 A more accurate method to estimate glomerular filtration rate from serum creatinine: a new prediction equation. Modification of Diet in Renal Disease Study Group. Annals of Internal Medicine 130: 461-470

National Institute for Clinical Excellence 2004 Renal transplantation – immunosuppressive regimens (adults). The clinical effectiveness and cost effectiveness of immuno-suppressive therapy for renal transplantation. National Institute for Clinical Excellence, London

UK Renal Registry 1999 Second annual report. Renal Association, Bristol

FURTHER READING

Cassidy M J D 2003 Renal osteodystrophy. Medicine 31: 56-60

Goldsmith D J A 2003 Management of renal impairment. Medicine 31(6): 52-56

Harvey C, Hare C, Blomley M 2003 Renal imaging. Medicine 31(5): 18-28

Macdougall I C 2003 Anaemia of chronic renal failure. Medicine 31(6): 63-66

McClellan W, Schoolwerth A, Gehr T 2005 Clinical management of the chronic kidney disease. Professional Communications, USA

Mole D R, Mason P 2003 Assessment of renal function. Medicine 31(5): 5-10

O'Callaghan C A, Brenner B M 2000 The kidney at a glance. Blackwell Science, Oxford

Pereira B J G, Sayegh M, Blake PR (eds) 2004 Chronic kidney disease, dialysis, and transplantation: companion to Brenner and Rector's the kidney. WB Saunders, London

Willcocks L, Smith K 2003 Renal transplantation. Medicine 31(6): 73-77

18 Acute renal failure

J. Marriott S. Smith

KEY POINTS

- Acute renal failure (ARF) is diagnosed when the excretory function of the kidney declines rapidly over a period of hours or days and is usually associated with the accumulation of metabolic waste products and water.
- A wide range of factors can precipitate ARF, including trauma, obstruction of urine flow or any event that causes a reduction in renal blood flow, including surgery and medical conditions, e.g. sepsis, diabetes, acute liver disease.
- Drug involvement in the development of ARF is possible.
  There are no specific signs and symptoms of ARF. The condition is typically indicated by raised blood levels of urea and creatinine.
- The clinical priorities in ARF are to manage life-threatening complications, correct intravascular fluid balance and establish the cause of the renal failure, reversing factors causing damage where possible.
- The aim of medical treatment is to remove causative factors and maintain patient well-being so that the kidneys have a chance to recover.
- Creatinine clearance (Cl_{Cr}) provides a useful guide to renal function although most measures of Cl_{Cr} are inaccurate when renal function deteriorates or improves rapidly, as is usually the case in ARF.
- Treatment of ARF is essentially preventive and supportive with control of serum biochemistry, prevention of infection and early use of renal replacement therapies as support where necessary.
- ARF is a serious condition with mortality rates ranging from 5% to 90%, varying according to cause and particularly the concurrent failure of other organs; the average mortality rate is approximately 40–50% at 90 days following the event, despite improvements in management.

Definition and incidence

Acute renal failure (ARF) manifests as an abrupt decline in glomerular filtration rate occurring over a period of days or weeks. This results in an accumulation of water, nitrogenous waste products and other toxins. In patients with pre-existing renal impairment, a rapid decline in renal function is termed 'acute on chronic renal failure'.

Estimates indicate that ARF affects about 5% of hospitalized patients and up to 15% of those who are critically ill. This process may be reversed with appropriate intervention. However, severe ARF is often associated with multiple organ failures and mortality rates of up to 90% (Dishart & Kellum 2000).

Classification

ARF is not a single disease state with a uniform aetiology. Rather, it is a syndrome that results from a range of different diseases and conditions. However, it is often useful to classify ARF as a start point for the diagnostic and treatment process. The most common classification into pre-renal (functional), intrarenal (renal or intrinsic) and postrenal forms is outlined in Table 18.1.

Pre-renal ARF

The causes of pre-renal ARF are summarized in Figure 18.1. These can all produce a potentially reversible reduction in renal perfusion resulting in renal ischaemia.

Hypovolaemia

Any condition or situation that leads to hypovolaemia might result in pre-renal ARF. Examples include haemorrhage, loss of fluid associated with burns, abnormal fluid loss from the gastrointestinal tract, e.g diarrhoea, sweating and excessive renal fluid loss, for example from inappropriate use of diuretics

Hypotension

Conditions that result in hypotension will also reduce renal perfusion. Thus, hypotension associated with cardiogenic shock or sepsis can precipitate pre-renal ARF.

Renal hypoperfusion

Where a reduction in the perfusion of the kidney occurs specifically, there is a risk of developing pre-renal ARF. Examples are generally associated with renal vasoconstriction that may result from liver disease, renal vascular disease and drug use.

Table 18.1 Classification of acute renal failure (ARF)

ARF type	Typical % cases	Common aetiology
Pre-renal	40–80	Reversible ↓ renal perfusion, through hypoperfusion
Intrarenal	10–50	Renal parenchymal injury
Postrenal	<10	Urinary tract obstructions

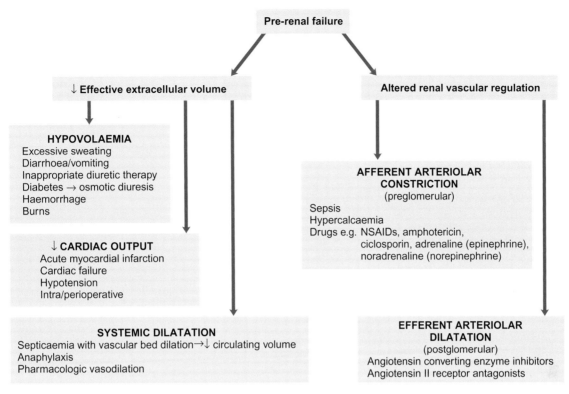

Figure 18.1 Causes of prerenal failure.

ACE inhibitor and angiotensin receptor blockers in ARF

ACE inhibitors and angiotensin receptor blockers are not nephrotoxic and there is no absolute contraindication to their use in patients with renal insufficiency. However, profound hypotension can occur if they are initiated in susceptible patients such as those on diuretics, which might result in the development of pre-renal ARF. Therefore blood pressure monitoring and careful titration of dosages should be undertaken in such patients whilst monitoring renal function. However, it is common to see increases in serum creatinine levels of up to 20% but this is not necessarily a reason to discontinue therapy with these agents.

ACE inhibitor use is absolutely contraindicated when a patient has aortic and/or bilateral renal artery stenosis (or renal artery stenosis in a patient with a single functioning kidney). If an ACE inhibitor or angiotensin receptor blocker is initiated under these circumstances then pre-renal ARF may ensue. This may occur because the renin–angiotensin system is stimulated by low renal perfusion resulting from stenotic lesions in the kidney vascular supply. Angiotensin II is produced which causes renal vasoconstriction, which amongst other things increases efferent arteriolar tone. Vasoconstriction of the efferent arterioles creates a 'back pressure' which maintains glomerular filtration pressure in an otherwise poorly perfused kidney. If angiotensin II production is inhibited by an ACE inhibitor, or binding to its receptor is blocked by an angiotensin receptor blocker, then efferent arteriole dilation will result. Since increased efferent vascular tone maintains filtration in such patients, then the overall result of such therapy will be to reduce or shut down filtration at the glomerulus, possibly leading to pre-renal ARF (Fig. 18.2).

Pre-renal failure is the most common form of renal dysfunction seen in hospitalized patients (see Table 18.1). It may progress to acute tubular necrosis (ATN), thus blurring the distinction between these conditions.

Intrarenal ARF

Any form of damage to the renal infrastructure (renal parenchyma), usually involving some form of ischaemic or nephrotoxic insult, may result in ARF. Intrarenal ARF may therefore be classified according to the renal structures principally affected.

Acute tubular necrosis

The most common form (>80% cases) of intrarenal damage encountered is acute tubular necrosis (ATN) resulting from ischaemia (e.g. from prolonged pre-renal failure) and/or direct exposure to toxins. Nephrotoxins may arise exogenously, in the form of drugs or chemical poisons, or from endogenous sources such as pigments (haemoglobin, myoglobin), crystals (uric acid, phosphate) and the toxic products from sepsis or tumours (Table 18.2). It is interesting that endogenous toxins may also be formed as a result of drug exposure. For example, myoglobin may be released (rhabdomyolysis) following muscle injury or necrosis, hypoxia, infection or drug treatment (e.g. with fibrates and statins, particularly when both are used in combination). The mechanism of the subsequent damage to renal tissue is not understood fully but probably results from a combination of factors, including hypoperfusion and ischaemia, haem catalysed

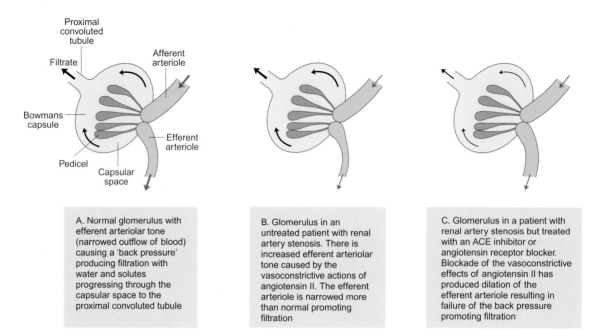

Figure 18.2 The glomerular actions of ACE inhibitors and angiotensin receptor blockers in patients with bilateral renal artery stenosis; arrow sizes indicate relative flow of blood (red) and filtrate (blue).

Table 18.2 Common clinical factors known to cause acute tubular necrosis (ATN)

Clinical factor	Mechanism
Hypoperfusion	Reduced oxygen/nutrient supply
Radiocontrast media	Medullary ischaemia may result from contrast media-induced renal vasoconstriction. The high ionic load of contrast media may produce ischaemia, particularly in diabetics and those with myeloma (who produce large quantities of light chain immunoglobulins)
Sepsis	Infection produces endotoxaemia and systemic inflammation in combination with a pre-renal state and nephrotoxins. The immunological response to sepsis involves release of vasoconstrictors and vasodilators (e.g. eicosanoids, nitric oxide) and damage to vascular endothelium with resultant thrombosis
Rhabdomyolysis	Damaged muscles release myoglobin, which can cause ATN through direct nephrotoxicity and by a reduction in blood flow in the outer medulla
Renal transplantation	The procedures and conditions encountered during renal transplantation can induce ischaemic ATN, which can be difficult to distinguish from the nephrotoxic effects of immunosuppressive drug therapy used in these circumstances
Hepatorenal syndrome	Renal vasoconstriction is frequently seen in patients with end-stage liver disease. The cause appears complex and progression to ATN common
Nephrotoxins Aminoglycosides	Aminoglycosides are transported into tubular cells where they exert a direct nephrotoxic effect. Current dosage regimens recommend once-daily doses to minimize total uptake of aminoglycoside
Amphotericin	Amphotericin appears to cause direct nephrotoxicity by disturbing the permeability of tubular cells. The nephrotoxic effect is dose dependent and minimized by limiting total dose used, rate of infusion and by volume loading. These precautions also apply to newer liposomal formulations
Immunosuppressants	Ciclosporin and tacrolimus cause intrarenal vasoconstriction that may result in ischaemic ATN. The mechanism is unclear but is enhanced by hypovolaemia and other nephrotoxic drugs
NSAIDs	Vasodilator prostaglandins, chiefly E_2, D_2 and I_2 (epoprostenol), produce an increase in blood flow to the glomerulus and medulla. In normal circumstances they play no part in the maintenance of the renal circulation. However, increased amounts of vasoconstrictor substances arise in a variety of clinical conditions such as volume depletion, chronic cardiac failure or hepatic cirrhosis associated with ascites. Maintenance of renal blood flow then becomes more reliant on the release of vasodilatory prostaglandins. Inhibition of prostaglandin synthesis by NSAIDs may cause unopposed arteriolar vasoconstriction, leading to renal hypoperfusion

Table 18.2   (continued)

Clinical factor	Mechanism
Cytotoxic chemotherapy	Cisplatin
Anaesthetic agents	Methoxyflurane, enflurane
Chemical poisons/ naturally occurring poisons	Insecticides, herbicides Alkaloids from plants and fungi, reptile venoms

free radical tubular cytotoxicity, and haem cast formation and precipitation leading to tubular necrosis and acute renal failure.

Vascular disease

The healthy kidney is a vascular organ well supplied with oxygenated blood. This renal blood flow is maintained at approximately 20% of cardiac output. However, regional blood flow within the kidney varies, resulting in relatively hypoxic regions such as the outer medulla. This area is also the site of highly metabolically active parts of the nephron. Owing to the relatively poor oxygen supply and high metabolic demands, the outer medulla is at risk of ischaemia, even under normal conditions. The regulation of regional blood flow in the kidney, and therefore oxygen supply, relies upon vasomotor mechanisms mediated in part by adenosine. Adenosine appears to exert either vasoconstrictor or dilator effects within the kidney depending upon the relative distribution of A_1 and A_2 receptors.

Clearly, any circumstance that interferes with the delicate balance of blood flow and therefore oxygen supply within the kidney can result in acute tubular necrosis because of ischaemia or through greater vulnerability to nephrotoxins. The likelihood of acute tubular necrosis is increased by underlying conditions that predispose to ischaemia such as atheroma, atheroemboli and infarction, in addition to other factors including development of a pre-renal state, sepsis and diabetes.

Common clinical precipitants of acute tubular necrosis Table 18.2 shows a summary of some of the common factors encountered clinically that may cause acute tubular necrosis.

Other renal vascular damage (intrarenal/renal artery or vein)

Occlusion of either the renal arterial or venous supply can lead to intrinsic renal damage, as can disturbances of the intrarenal vasculature, for example in vasculitis. The use of ACE inhibitors in patients with renal artery stenosis is particularly problematical.

Intrarenal obstruction

Debris, such as cholesterol, deposited within the renal vascular architecture may lead to intrinsic renal failure.

Tubulointerstitial nephritis

Interstitial damage (interstitial nephritis) is thought to be a nephrotoxin-induced hypersensitivity reaction with inflammation affecting those cells lying between the nephrons. There is usually secondary involvement of the tubules. The nephrotoxins involved are usually drugs and/or the toxic products of infection. Drugs that have been most commonly shown to be responsible include the penicillins, cephalosporins, furosemide, NSAIDs, allopurinol and azathioprine. However, many other drugs have also been implicated.

Glomerulonephritis

Glomerulonephritis is thought to be caused by the deposition of immune complexes in the glomerular tuft which elicit an inflammatory response. The antigens responsible for the immune complexes may be exogenous, and precipitate a hypersensitivity reaction, or endogenous, resulting in an autoimmune condition. Specific aetiological factors can rarely be identified, although some drugs have been implicated, including gold, penicillamine and phenytoin. Glomerulonephritis is a relatively rare cause of ARF.

Postrenal ARF

Postrenal ARF results from obstruction of the urinary tract by a variety of mechanisms. The obstruction is generally either ureteric (bilateral or affecting a solitary kidney) arising from calculi, clots, carcinoma, retroperitoneal fibrosis, stricture, surgery or in the bladder neck arising from prostatic hypertrophy/malignancy, bladder cancer, neuropathy or a blocked catheter.

It is extremely unusual for drugs to be responsible for postrenal ARF. Practolol-induced retroperitoneal fibrosis resulting in postrenal ARF is a rare example.

Differentiating pre-renal from renal ARF

It is possible to distinguish between cases of pre-renal and renal ARF through examination of biochemical markers (Table 18.3). In cases of renal ARF the patient's kidney is generally unable to retain Na^+ owing to tubular damage. This can be demonstrated by calculating the fractional excretion of sodium (FeNa).

$$FeNa = sodium\ clearance/creatinine\ clearance$$

$$FeNa = \frac{urine\ sodium \times serum\ creatinine}{plasma\ sodium \times urine\ creatinine}$$

If the FeNa is greater than 1% this indicates pre-renal ARF with preserved tubular function, whereas if the FeNa is less than 1% this is indicative of acute tubular necrosis.

This typical relationship is less likely to hold if a patient with renal ARF has glycosuria or pre-existing renal disease, has been treated with diuretics or has other drug-related alterations in renal hemodynamics, e.g. through use of ACE inhibitors or NSAIDs.

Table 18.3   Differentiating pre-renal from renal ARF

Laboratory test	Pre-renal	Renal
Urine osmolality (mOsm/kg)	>500	<400
Urine sodium (mEq/L)	<20	>40
Urine/plasma creatinine (µmol/L)	>40	<20
Urine/plasma urea (µmol/L)	>8	<3
Fractional excretion of sodium (%)	<1	>2

Clinical manifestations

The signs and symptoms of ARF are often non-specific and the diagnosis can be confounded by co-existing clinical conditions. The patient may exhibit signs and symptoms of either volume depletion or overload, depending upon the precipitating conditions, course of the disease and prior treatment.

ARF with volume depletion

In those patients with volume depletion a classic pathophysiological picture is likely to be present, with tachycardia, postural hypotension, reduced skin turgor and cold extremities (Table 18.4). The most common sign in ARF is oliguria, where the 24-hour urine production falls to between 200 and 400 mL. The oliguric kidney is unable to concentrate urine sufficiently to excrete products of metabolism. Inevitably, the serum concentration of those substances normally excreted by the kidney will rise. Diagnosis can be assisted by detecting elevated levels of creatinine, urea, potassium, hydrogen ions (acidosis) and phosphate in blood. The accumulation of urea and other waste products leads to uraemia, which describes the accumulation of excess blood metabolites together with the other signs and symptoms associated with renal failure, such as nausea, vomiting, diarrhoea, gastrointestinal haemorrhage, muscle cramps and a declining level of consciousness.

ARF with volume overload

In those patients with ARF who have maintained a normal or increased fluid intake as a result of oral or intravenous administration, it is possible to find the pulmonary and systemic signs and symptoms of fluid overload (see Table 18.4).

Diagnosis and clinical evaluation

In hospitalized patients, ARF is usually diagnosed incidentally, often by the detection of increasing serum creatinine or urea levels or by a reduction in urine output.

The assessment of renal function has been described in detail in Chapter 17. However, unless a patient is at steady state, measurement of serum creatinine does not provide a reliable guide to renal function. For example, serum creatinine levels will usually rise by only 50–100 µmol/L per day following complete loss of renal function in a previously normal patient. These changes in serum creatinine are not sufficiently responsive to serve as a practical indicator of glomerular filtration rate (GFR), particularly in ARF in critical care scenarios.

In the hospital situation, when renal impairment is detected incidentally, the cause(s) of the condition, such as fluid depletion, infection or the use of nephrotoxic drugs, are often apparent on close examination of the clinical history. In some patients, however, or in those discovered outside hospital practice, more extensive investigation is required to determine the cause. Although the majority of patients have acute tubular necrosis, other rare causes such as rapidly progressive glomerulonephritis, acute nephritis or urinary tract obstruction must be excluded. Specific longer term treatment for the underlying cause may be required.

Possible steps in the investigation of ARF are outlined in Figure 18.3.

Various other parameters should be monitored through the course of ARF. Fluid balance charts are frequently used, but are often inaccurate and should not be relied upon exclusively. Records of daily weight are more reliable, but are dependent on the mobility of the patient.

Central venous pressure (CVP) is one of a number of haemodynamic measurements that can be made following insertion of

Table 18.4   Factors associated with acute renal failure

	Volume depletion	Volume overload
History	Thirst	Weight increase
	Excessive fluid loss (sweating, diarrhoea)	Orthopnoea/nocturnal dyspnoea
	Oliguria	
Physical examination	Dry mucosae	Ankle swelling
	↓ skin elasticity	Oedema
	Tachycardia	Jugular venous distension
	↓ blood pressure	Pulmonary crackles
	↓ jugular venous pressure	Pleural effusion

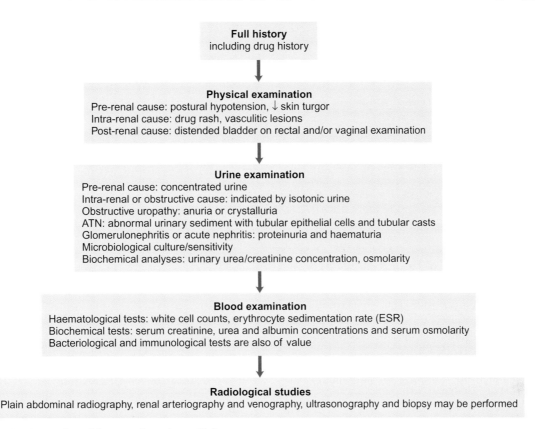

Full history
including drug history

↓

Physical examination
Pre-renal cause: postural hypotension, ↓ skin turgor
Intra-renal cause: drug rash, vasculitic lesions
Post-renal cause: distended bladder on rectal and/or vaginal examination

↓

Urine examination
Pre-renal cause: concentrated urine
Intra-renal or obstructive cause: indicated by isotonic urine
Obstructive uropathy: anuria or crystalluria
ATN: abnormal urinary sediment with tubular epithelial cells and tubular casts
Glomerulonephritis or acute nephritis: proteinuria and haematuria
Microbiological culture/sensitivity
Biochemical analyses: urinary urea/creatinine concentration, osmolarity

↓

Blood examination
Haematological tests: white cell counts, erythrocyte sedimentation rate (ESR)
Biochemical tests: serum creatinine, urea and albumin concentrations and serum osmolarity
Bacteriological and immunological tests are also of value

↓

Radiological studies
Plain abdominal radiography, renal arteriography and venography, ultrasonography and biopsy may be performed

Figure 18.3 Investigations and possible causes in acute renal failure.

a central venous catheter, and is a measure of the pressure in the large systemic veins and the right atrium produced by venous return. Although the insertion of a central catheter carries the risks of any invasive procedure, central venous pressure provides the best assessment of circulating volume and therefore the degree of fluid deficit, and reduces the risk of pulmonary oedema following over-rapid transfusion. Central venous pressure should usually be maintained within the normal range of 5–12 cmH$_2$O.

Serum electrolytes including potassium, bicarbonate, calcium, phosphate and acid–base balance should similarly be monitored.

Course and prognosis

The course of ARF caused by acute tubular necrosis may be divided into three phases. The first is the oliguric phase in which uraemia and hyperkalaemia occur unless adequate management is initiated. The oliguric phase is usually no longer than 7–14 days but may last for 6 weeks. If death does not ensue the patient with ARF will enter the diuretic phase, which is characterized by a urine output that rises over a few days to several litres per day. The diuretic phase lasts for up to 7 days and corresponds to the recommencement of tubular function. Patients who survive into this phase have a relatively good prognosis and progress to the recovery phase. Recovery of renal function where tubule cells regenerate takes place slowly over the following months, although the GFR rarely returns completely to its initial level. The elderly recover renal function more slowly and less completely.

The mortality rate of ARF varies accordingly to the cause but is typically 10–15% for an isolated episode (Dishart & Kellum 2000). Mortality rates are much higher when ARF is complicated by other factors such as multiple organ dysfunction and may be in the range 50–90%. High mortality rates are more common in patients aged over 60 years.

Death resulting from uraemia and hyperkalaemia is now less common. Consequently, the major causes of death associated with ARF are septicaemia and, to a lesser extent, gastrointestinal haemorrhage. High circulating levels of uraemic toxins that occur in ARF result in general debility. These, together with the significant number of invasive procedures such as bladder catheterization and intravascular cannulation, which are necessary in the management of ARF, render such patients prone to infection and septicaemia. Uraemic gastrointestinal haemorrhage is a recognized consequence of ARF, probably as a result of reduced mucosal cell turnover.

Management

The aim of the medical management of a patient with ARF is to prolong life in order to allow recovery of kidney function. Effective management of ARF depends upon rapid diagnosis. If the underlying acute deterioration in renal function is detected early enough, it is often possible to prevent progression. If the condition is advanced, however, management consists of mainly preventive and supportive strategies, with close monitoring and appropriate correction of metabolic, fluid and electrolyte disturbances. Specific therapies that promote recovery of ischaemic renal damage remain under investigation.

Early preventive and supportive strategies

Identification of patients at risk

Any patient who has concurrent or pre-existing conditions that increase the risk of development and progression of ARF must be identified, e.g. those with pre-existing chronic renal failure (CRF), diabetes, jaundice, myeloma and the elderly. These patients have a baseline of poor renal function and it is likely that their condition will deteriorate more quickly than others.

Withdrawal and avoidance of nephrotoxic agents

Irrespective of whether the aetiology of the ARF directly involves nephrotoxic drugs, the drug and treatment regimens (e.g. ACE inhibitors, NSAIDs, radiological contrast media, aminoglycosides) should be examined in order for potential nephrotoxins to be withdrawn and avoided in the future to prevent exacerbation of the condition. Dosages of any drugs that are renally excreted or that have active metabolites that are excreted renally should also be adjusted.

Optimization of renal perfusion

Initial treatment should include rapid correction of fluid and electrolyte balance in order to maximize renal perfusion. A central line should be inserted to facilitate ease of fluid infusion and a urinary catheter placed in order that fluid losses may be measured easily.

A diagnosis of acute deterioration of renal function caused by renal underperfusion implies that restoration of renal perfusion would reverse impairment by improving renal blood flow, reducing renal vasoconstriction and flushing nephrotoxins from the kidney. Sodium chloride 0.9% is an appropriate choice of intravenous fluid since it replaces both water and sodium ions in a concentration approximately equal to serum. The effect of fluid replacement on urine flow and, whenever possible, central venous pressure should be carefully monitored. However, fluid loading with 1–1.5 L saline at <0.5 L/h is unlikely to cause harm in most patients who do not show signs of fluid overload.

Where indicated, inotropes should be used to provide cardiac support to ensure that renal perfusion is maintained. In the past the use of subinotropic low-dose dopamine has been advocated to improve renal perfusion although there is no evidence to support this course of action.

Establishing and maintaining an adequate diuresis

If the kidneys do not respond to improving renal perfusion with fluid replacement therapy and inotropes then other measures may include:

- loop diuretics
- mannitol
- dopamine.

The conversion of oliguria or anuria to non-oliguric ARF indicates fluid overload and electrolyte disturbances are likely to be at least partially reversed. It is unclear, however, whether survival is improved.

Loop diuretics In addition to producing a substantial diuresis, loop diuretics reduce renal tubular cell metabolic demands and increase renal blood flow by stimulating the release of renal prostaglandins, a haemodynamic effect inhibited by NSAIDs. It is thought that the use of loop diuretics may thereby help salvage renal tissue. The associated increased urine flow will also reduce the likelihood of intrarenal obstruction.

Diuretic therapy should only be initiated after the circulating volume has been restored. If not, any diuresis might produce a negative fluid balance and precipitate or exacerbate a pre-renal state.

Doses up to 1–2 g of furosemide in 24 hours can be given by continuous intravenous infusion at a rate of not more than 4 mg/min. Higher infusion rates may cause transient deafness. The use of continuous infusions of loop diuretics has been shown to produce a more effective diuresis with a lower incidence of side effects than seen with bolus administration. Bolus doses of loop diuretics may induce renal vasoconstriction and be detrimental to function.

The addition of small oral doses of metolazone may also be considered. Metolazone is a weak thiazide diuretic alone but produces a synergistic action with loop diuretics.

Mannitol Mannitol has historically been recommended for the treatment of ARF. The rationale for its use in ARF arose from the concept that tubular debris may contribute to oliguria. The tubular debris causes mechanical intrarenal obstruction and the use of an osmotic diuretic will wash it out. A dose of 0.5–1.0 g/kg as a 10–20% infusion was previously recommended. However, intravenous mannitol will, before producing a diuresis, cause a considerable increase in the extracellular fluid volume by drawing water from the intracellular compartment. This expansion of the intravascular volume is potentially dangerous for patients with cardiac failure, especially if a diuresis is not produced. It is also possible that mannitol exacerbates renal medullary hypoxia (i.e. the partial pressure of oxygen (PO_2) is further reduced in the renal medulla) since increased glomerular filtration raises medullary oxygen consumption; these effects might also offset any positive benefits of mannitol in ARF. There is no evidence for mannitol producing benefit in ARF over and above aggressive hydration. Consequently, mannitol is now not recommended.

Dopamine Dopamine used to be recommended, in low dose, to improve renal blood flow and urine output. Recent research has shown it to be ineffective and it should no longer be used.

Drug therapy and renal autoregulation

Intrarenal blood flow is controlled by an autoregulatory mechanism unique to the kidney called tubuloglomerular feedback (TGF). This mechanism produces arteriolar constriction in response to an increased solute load to the distal nephrons. GFR and kidney workload are thus reduced. It has been proposed that oliguria is an adaptive response to renal ischaemia. Therefore therapy which improves GFR through increased solute load on the nephrons might increase kidney workload and worsen

ARF. Clearly, reversal of a pre-renal state with fluids is a logical therapeutic rationale. However, careful choice of therapy in intrarenal ARF is required to avoid detrimental effects on the kidney.

Non-dialysis treatment of established acute renal failure

Uraemia and intravascular volume overload

In renal failure, the symptoms of uraemia include nausea, vomiting and anorexia, and result principally from accumulation of toxic products of protein metabolism such as urea. It is often possible to reduce these symptoms by restricting protein intake to about 0.6 g/kg body weight per day. However, care should be taken to ensure the diet provides all the essential amino acids and sufficient nutrition to prevent protein catabolism. A higher intake of protein, by exceeding the body's basic requirements, permits its use as an energy source, resulting in increases in blood urea concentration; further reduction in protein intake brings about endogenous protein catabolism and again causes the blood urea concentration to increase. Fat and carbohydrate should also be given to maintain a high energy intake of about 2000–3000 kcal, or more in hypercatabolic patients, to prevent protein catabolism and promote anabolism. It should be noted, however, that excessive amounts of carbohydrate could increase production of carbon dioxide and induce respiratory acidosis in these patients.

Unfortunately, since uraemia causes anorexia, nausea and vomiting, many severely ill patients are unable to tolerate any kind of diet. In these patients and those who are catabolic, the use of enteral or parenteral nutrition should be considered at an early stage.

Intravascular fluid overload must be managed by restricting NaCl intake to about 1–2 g/day if the patient is not hyponatraemic and total fluid intake to less than 500 mL/day plus the volume of urine and/or loss from dialysis. Care should be taken with so-called 'low salt' products, as these usually contain KCl, which will exacerbate hyperkalaemia.

Hyperkalaemia

This is a particular problem in ARF, not only because urinary excretion is reduced but also because intracellular potassium may be released. Rapid rises in extracellular potassium are to be expected when there is tissue damage, as in burns, crush injuries and sepsis. Acidosis also aggravates hyperkalaemia by provoking potassium leakage from healthy cells. The condition may be life threatening by causing cardiac arrhythmias and, if untreated, can result in asystolic cardiac arrest.

Dietary potassium should be restricted to less than 40 mmol/day and potassium supplements and potassium-sparing diuretics removed from the treatment schedule. Emergency treatment is necessary if the serum potassium level reaches 7.0 mmol/L (normal range 3.5–5.0 mmol/L) or if there are the progressive changes in the electrocardiogram (ECG) associated with hyperkalaemia. These include tall, peaked T-waves, reduced P-waves with increased QRS complexes or the 'sine wave' appearance that often presages cardiac arrest (see Chapter 22, Fig. 22.3).

Emergency treatment of hyperkalaemia consists of the following.

- 10–30 mL (2.25–6.75 mmol) of calcium gluconate 10% intravenously over 5–10 minutes; this improves myocardial stability but has no effect on the serum potassium levels. The effect is short-lived, but the dose can be repeated.
- 50 mL of 50% glucose together with 10–20 units of soluble insulin. Endogenous insulin, stimulated by a glucose load or administered intravenously, stimulates intracellular potassium uptake, thus removing it from the serum. The effect lasts for 2–3 hours.
- Calcium polystyrene sulphonate (calcium resonium) 15–30 g 2–4 times a day, either orally or by enema. This ion exchange resin binds potassium in the gastrointestinal tract, releasing calcium in exchange. Rectal administration will reduce potassium over a period of 2–6 hours, while oral administration is most effective at 10–12 hours.

Ion exchange resins will not produce dramatic reductions in serum potassium alone when the starting level is dangerously high. Rather, they are used as a method of sustaining potassium reduction because the effect of glucose/insulin is only temporary. Both the oral and rectal routes of administration have disadvantages. Administration of large doses by mouth may result in faecal impaction. The oral dose can be mixed with lactulose in an attempt to prevent constipation. The manufacturers recommend that an enema should be retained for 9 hours; this is not usually a problem, rather the reverse. Constipation resulting from the use of resins may necessitate the use of laxatives.

Acidosis

The inability of the kidney to excrete hydrogen ions may result in a metabolic acidosis. This in itself is not usually a serious problem although it may contribute to hyperkalaemia. It may be treated orally with sodium bicarbonate 1–6 g/day in divided doses, or 50–100 mmol of bicarbonate ions (50–100 mL of sodium bicarbonate 8.4%) intravenously may be used. If calcium gluconate is being used to treat hyperkalaemia, care should be taken not to mix it with the sodium bicarbonate as the resulting calcium bicarbonate forms an insoluble precipitate. If elevations in serum sodium preclude the use of sodium bicarbonate, extreme acidosis (serum bicarbonate of less than 10 mmol/L) is best treated by dialysis.

Hypocalcaemia

Calcium malabsorption, probably secondary to disordered vitamin D metabolism, often occurs in ARF. Hypocalcaemia usually remains asymptomatic, as tetany of skeletal muscles or convulsions do not normally occur until serum concentrations are as low as 1.6–1.7 mmol/L (normal 2.20–2.55 mmol/L). Should it become necessary, oral calcium supplementation with calcium gluconate or lactate is usually adequate, and although vitamin D may be used to treat the hypocalcaemia of ARF, it rarely has to be added. Effervescent calcium tablets should be avoided as they contain a high sodium or potassium load.

Hyperphosphataemia

As phosphate is normally excreted by the kidney, hyperphosphataemia may occur in ARF but rarely requires treatment. Should it become necessary to treat, phosphate-binding agents may be used to retain phosphate ions in the gut. The most common agents are calcium carbonate or aluminium hydroxide in the form of mixture or capsules.

Infection

Patients with ARF are prone to infection and septicaemia, which can ultimately cause death. Bladder catheters, central catheters and even peripheral intravenous lines should be used with care to reduce the chance of bacterial invasion. Leucocytosis is sometimes seen in ARF and does not necessarily imply infection but any unexplained pyrexia must be immediately treated with appropriate antibiotic therapy, especially if accompanied by toxic symptoms such as disorientation or hypotensive episodes. Samples from blood, urine and any other material such as catheter tips should be sent for culture before antibiotics are started and therapy should cover as wide a spectrum as possible until a causative organism is identified.

Other problems

Uraemic gastrointestinal erosions

These are a recognized consequence of ARF, probably as a result of reduced mucosal cell turnover owing to high circulating levels of uraemic toxins. Proton pump inhibitors are effective and it is unlikely that any one is more advantageous than another.

Nutrition

There are two major constraints concerning the nutrition of patients with ARF:

- patients are frequently anorexic, vomiting and too ill to eat
- oliguria associated with renal failure limits the volume of enteral or parenteral nutrition that can be given safely.

The introduction of dialysis or haemofiltration allows fluid to be removed easily and therefore makes parenteral nutrition possible. Large volumes of fluid may be administered without producing fluid overload. Factors that should be considered when formulating a parenteral nutrition regimen include fluid balance, calorie/protein requirements, electrolyte balance/requirements, and vitamin and mineral requirements.

The basic calorie requirements are similar to those in a non-dialysed patient, although the need for protein may occasionally be increased in haemodialysis and haemofiltration because of amino acid loss. In all situations protein is usually supplied as 12–20 g/day of an essential amino acid formulation, although individual requirements may vary. Similarly, although lipid emulsions may theoretically reduce the efficiency of haemofiltration by blocking the filter, in practice their use does not have any noticeable effect.

Electrolyte free amino acid solutions should be used in parenteral nutrition formulations for patients with ARF as they allow the addition of electrolytes as appropriate. Potassium and sodium requirements can be calculated on an individual basis depending on serum levels. There is usually no need to try to normalize serum calcium and phosphate levels as they

will stabilize with the appropriate therapy or, if necessary, with haemofiltration or dialysis. Water-soluble vitamins are removed by dialysis and haemofiltration but these are usually replenished by the standard daily doses normally included in parenteral nutrition fluids. Magnesium and zinc supplementation may be required, not only because tissue repair often increases requirements but also because they may be lost during dialysis or haemofiltration.

It is necessary to monitor the serum urea, creatinine and electrolyte levels daily in order to make the appropriate alterations in the nutritional support. The glucose concentration should also be checked daily as patients in renal failure sometimes develop insulin resistance. The plasma pH should be checked initially to see whether the addition of amino acid solutions is causing or aggravating metabolic acidosis. It is also valuable to check calcium, phosphate and albumin levels regularly and, when practical, daily weighing gives a useful guide to fluid balance.

Renal replacement therapy

Renal replacement therapy is indicated in a patient with ARF when kidney function is so poor that life is at risk. However, it is desirable to introduce renal replacement therapy early in ARF, as complications and mortality are reduced if the serum urea level is kept below 35 mmol/L. Generally, replacement therapy is used in ARF to:

- remove toxins when severe symptoms are apparent (e.g. impaired consciousness, seizures, pericarditis)
- remove fluid resistant to diuretics (e.g. pulmonary oedema), to facilitate parenteral nutrition
- correct electrolyte and acid–base imbalances, e.g. hyperkalaemia >6.5 mmol/L or 5.5–6.5 where there are ECG changes, increasing acidosis (pH <7.1 or serum bicarbonate <10 mmol/L) despite bicarbonate therapy, or where bicarbonate is not tolerated because of fluid overload
- control the effects of sepsis (e.g. to reduce temperature).

Forms of renal replacement therapy

The common types of renal replacement therapy used in clinical practice are:

- haemodialysis
- haemofiltration
- haemodiafiltration.
- peritoneal dialysis.

Although the basic principles of these replacement therapies are similar, clearance rates, i.e. extent of solute removal, vary.

In all types of renal replacement therapy blood is presented to a dialysis solution across some form of semipermeable membrane that allows free movement of low molecular weight compounds. The processes by which movement of substances occur are as follows.

- *Diffusion.* Diffusion depends upon concentration differences between blood and dialysate and molecule size. Water and low molecular weight solutes (up to a molecular weight of about 5000) move through pores in the semipermeable membrane to establish equilibrium. Smaller molecules can be cleared from blood more effectively as they move more easily through pores in the membrane.

- *Ultrafiltration.* A pressure gradient (either +ve or −ve) across a semipermeable membrane will produce a net directional movement of fluid from relative high- to low-pressure regions. The quantity of fluid dialysed is the ultrafiltration volume.
- *Convection.* Any molecule carried by ultrafiltrate may move passively with the flow by convection. Larger molecules are cleared more effectively by convection.

Haemodialysis

In haemodialysis, blood is heparinized and diverted out of a large central venous cannula line and actively pumped through the lumen of an artificial kidney (dialyser), returning to the patient by a venous line (Fig. 18.4). In those at high risk of haemorrhage when heparinized, such as postsurgical patients, epoprostenol, a prostaglandin with a short plasma half-life of 2–3 minutes that inhibits platelet aggregation, may be used to prevent extracorporeal clotting.

The dialyser consists of a cartridge comprised of either a bundle of hollow tubes (hollow-fibre dialyser) or a series of parallel flat plates (flat-plate dialyser) made of a synthetic semipermeable membrane. Dialysis fluid is perfused around the membrane in a countercurrent to the flow of blood in order to maximize diffusion gradients. The dialysis solution is essentially a mixture of electrolytes in water with a composition approximating to extracellular fluid into which solutes diffuse. The ionic concentration of the dialysis fluid can be manipulated to control the rate and extent of electrolyte transfer. Calcium and bicarbonate concentrations can also be increased in dialysis fluid to promote diffusion into blood as replacement therapy. By manipulating the hydrostatic pressure of the dialysate and blood circuits, the extent and rate of water removal by ultrafiltration can be controlled.

Haemodialysis can be performed in either intermittent or continuous schedules. The latter regimen is preferable in the critical care situation, providing 24-hour control and minimizing swings in blood volume and electrolyte composition that are found using intermittent regimens.

The capital cost of haemodialysis is considerable, requires specially trained staff and is seldom undertaken outside a renal unit. It does, however, treat renal failure rapidly and is therefore essential in hypercatabolic renal failure where urea is produced faster than it can be removed by, for example, peritoneal dialysis. Haemodialysis can also be used in patients who have recently undergone abdominal surgery in whom peritoneal dialysis would be ill advised.

Haemofiltration

Haemofiltration is an alternative technique to dialysis whose simplicity of use, fine control of fluid balance and low cost have ensured its widespread use in the treatment of ARF.

A similar arrangement to haemodialysis is employed but dialysis fluid is not used. The hydrostatic pressure of the blood drives a filtrate similar to interstitial fluid across a high permeability dialyser (passes substances of molecular weight up to 30 000) by ultrafiltration. Solute clearance occurs by convection. Commercially prepared haemofiltration fluid may then be introduced into the filtered blood in quantities sufficient to maintain optimal fluid balance. As with haemodialysis, haemofiltration can be intermittent or continuous. In continuous arteriovenous haemofiltration (CAVH), blood is diverted, usually from the femoral artery, and returned to the femoral vein. In continuous venovenous haemofiltration (CVVH), blood is taken from a vein, usually the femoral, jugular or subclavian, and returned via a double linear catheter, the process being assisted by a blood pump. In slow continuous ultrafiltration (SCU or SCUF) the process is performed so slowly that no fluid substitution is necessary.

In addition to avoiding the expense and complexity of haemodialysis, this system enables continuous but gradual removal of fluid, thereby allowing very fine control of fluid balance in addition to electrolyte control and removal of metabolites. This control of fluid balance often facilitates the use of parenteral nutrition. Because of the advantages of haemofiltration over peritoneal dialysis and haemodialysis, continuous haemofiltration is now generally agreed to be the most appropriate form of dialysis in the majority of patients with ARF.

Haemodiafiltration

Haemodiafiltration is a technique that combines the ability to clear small molecules, as in haemodialysis, with the large molecule clearance of haemofiltration. It is, however, more expensive than traditional haemodialysis.

Peritoneal dialysis

Peritoneal dialysis is now rarely used for ARF except in circumstances where haemodialysis is unavailable.

A semirigid catheter is inserted into the abdominal cavity. Warmed sterile peritoneal dialysis fluid (typically 1–2 L) is instilled into the abdomen, left for a period of about 30 minutes (dwell time) and then drained into a collecting bag (Fig. 18.5). This procedure may be performed manually or by semiautomatic equipment. The process may be repeated up to 20 times a day, depending on the condition of the patient.

Peritoneal dialysis is relatively cheap and simple, and does not require either specially trained staff or the facilities of a renal unit. It is only used rarely in the UK because it has the disadvantages of being uncomfortable and tiring for the patient, producing a

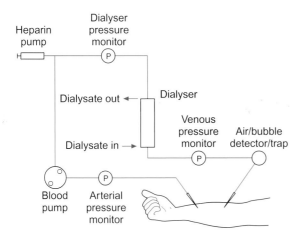

Figure 18.4 Typical haemodialysis circuit.

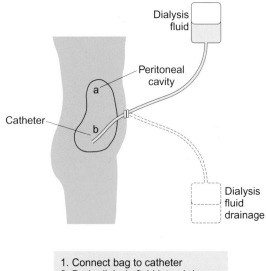

1. Connect bag to catheter
2. Drain dialysis fluid into abdomen
3. Dwell time
4. Drain fluid out
   a. perirotoneal cavity
   b. catheter

Figure 18.5 Procedure for peritoneal dialysis.

high incidence of peritonitis and also permitting protein loss, as albumin crosses the peritoneal membrane.

Drug dosage in renal replacement therapy

Whether a drug is significantly removed by dialysis or haemofiltration is an important clinical problem. Drugs that are not removed may well require dose reduction to avoid accumulation and minimize toxic effects. Alternatively, drug removal may be significant and require a dosage supplement to ensure an adequate therapeutic effect is maintained. In general, since haemodialysis, peritoneal dialysis and haemofiltration depend on filtration, the process of drug removal can be considered analoguous to glomerular filtration. Table 18.5 gives an indication of approximate clearances of common renal replacement therapies, which for continuous regimens provide an estimate for the creatinine clearance of the system.

Drug characteristics that favour clearance by the glomerulus are similar to those that favour clearance by dialysis or haemofiltration. These include:

Table 18.5 Approximate clearances of common renal replacement therapies	
Renal replacement therapy	Clearance rate (mL/min)
Intermittent haemodialysis	150–200
Intermittent haemofiltration	100–150
Acute intermittent peritoneal dialysis	10–20
Continuous haemofiltration	5–15

- low molecular weight
- high water solubility
- low protein binding
- small volume of distribution
- low metabolic clearance.

Unfortunately, a number of other factors inherent in the dialysis process affect clearance; they include:

- duration of dialysis procedure
- rate of blood flow to dialyser
- surface area and porosity of dialyser
- composition and flow rate of dialysate.

For peritoneal dialysis other factors come into play and include:

- rate of peritoneal exchange
- concentration gradient between plasma and dialysate.

In view of the above, it is usually possible to predict whether a drug will be removed by dialysis. However, it is very difficult to quantify the process except by direct measurement, which is rarely practical. Consequently, a definitive, comprehensive guide to drug dosage in dialysis does not exist. However, limited data for specific drugs are available in the literature, while many drug manufacturers have information on the dialysability of their products and some now even include dosage recommendations in their summaries of product characteristics. The most practical method for treating patients undergoing dialysis is to assemble appropriate dosage guidelines for a range of drugs likely to be used in patients with renal impairment and attempt to restrict use to these.

As drug clearance by haemofiltration is more predictable than in dialysis, it is possible that standardized guidelines on drug elimination may become available. In the interim, a set of individual drug dosage guidelines similar to those described above would be useful in practice.

Factors affecting drug use

How the drug to be used is absorbed, distributed, metabolized and excreted, and whether it is intrinsically nephrotoxic are all factors that must be considered. The pharmacokinetic behaviour of many drugs may be altered in renal failure.

Absorption

Oral absorption in ARF may be reduced by vomiting or diarrhoea, although this is frequently of limited clinical significance.

Metabolism

The main hepatic pathways of drug metabolism appear unaffected in renal impairment. The kidney is also a site of metabolism in the body, but the effect of renal impairment is clinically important in only two situations. The first involves the conversion of 25-hydroxycolecalciferol to 1,25-dihydroxycolecalciferol (the active form of vitamin D) in the kidney, a process that is impaired in renal failure. Patients in ARF occasionally require vitamin D replacement therapy, and this should be in the form of 1α-hydroxycolecalciferol (alfacalcidol) or 1,25-dihydroxycolecalciferol (calcitriol). The latter is the drug of choice in the presence of concomitant hepatic impairment. The second situation involves the metabolism of insulin. The kidney is the major site of insulin metabolism, and the insulin requirements of diabetic patients in ARF are often reduced.

Distribution

Changes in drug distribution may be altered by fluctuations in the degree of hydration or by alterations in tissue or serum protein binding. The presence of oedema or ascites increases the volume of distribution while dehydration reduces it. In practice these changes will only be significant if the volume of distribution of the drug is small, i.e. less than 50 litres. Serum protein binding may be reduced owing to either protein loss or alteration in binding caused by uraemia. For certain highly bound drugs, the net result of reduced protein binding is an increase in free drug, and care is therefore required when interpreting serum concentrations. Most analyses measure the total serum concentration, i.e. free plus bound drug. A drug level may therefore fall within the accepted concentration range but still result in toxicity because of the increased proportion of free drug. However, this is usually only a temporary effect. Since the unbound drug is now available for elimination, its concentration will eventually return to the original value, albeit with a lower total bound and unbound level. The total drug concentration may therefore fall below the therapeutic range while therapeutic effectiveness is maintained. It must be noted that the time required for the new equilibrium to be established is about four or five elimination half-lives of the drug, and this may be itself altered in renal failure. Some drugs that show reduced serum protein binding include diazepam, morphine, phenytoin, levothyroxine, theophylline and warfarin. Tissue binding may also be affected; for example, the displacement of digoxin from skeletal muscle binding sites by metabolic waste products that accumulate in renal failure results in a significant reduction in digoxin's volume of distribution.

Excretion

Alteration in renal clearance of drugs in renal impairment is the most important parameter to consider when considering dosage. Generally, a fall in renal drug clearance indicates a decline in the number of functioning nephrons. The GFR, of which creatinine clearance is an approximation, can be used as an estimate of the number of functioning nephrons. Thus, a 50% reduction in the GFR will suggest a 50% decline in renal clearance.

Renal impairment therefore often necessitates drug dosage adjustments. Loading doses of renally excreted drugs are often necessary in renal failure because of the prolonged elimination half-life leading to an increased time to reach steady state. The equation for a loading dose is the same in renal disease as in normal patients, thus:

$$\text{Loading dose (mg)} = \text{target concentration (mg/L)} \times \text{volume of distribution (L)}$$

The volume of distribution may be altered but generally remains unchanged.

It is possible to derive other formulae for dosage adjustment in renal impairment. One of the most useful is:

$$DR_{rf} = DR_n \times [(1 - F_{eu}) + (F_{eu} \times RF)]$$

where DR_{rf} is the dosing rate in renal failure, DR_n is the normal dosing rate, RF is the extent of renal impairment = patient's creatinine clearance (mL/min)/ideal creatinine clearance (120 mL/min) and F_{eu} is the fraction of drug normally excreted unchanged in the urine. For example, when RF = 0.2 and F_{eu} = 0.5, 60% of the normal dosing rate should be given.

An alteration in dosing rate can be achieved by altering either the dose itself or the dosage interval, or a combination of both as appropriate. Unfortunately, it is not always possible to obtain the fraction of drug excreted unchanged in the urine. In practice, it is simpler to use the guidelines for prescribing in renal impairment found in the British National Formularly. These are adequate for most cases, although the specialist may need to refer to other texts.

Nephrotoxicity

The list of potentially nephrotoxic drugs is long. Although the most common serious forms of renal damage are interstitial nephritis and glomerulonephritis, the majority of drugs cause damage by hypersensitivity reactions and are safe in many patients. Some drugs, however, are directly nephrotoxic and their effects on the kidney are more predictable. These include aminoglycosides, amphotericin, colistin, the polymixins and ciclosporin. The use of any drug with recognized nephrotoxic potential should be avoided where possible. This is particularly true in patients with pre-existing renal impairment or renal failure. Figure 18.6 summarizes the most important and common adverse effects of drugs on renal function, indicating the likely regions of the nephron in which damage occurs. Additional information on adverse effects can be found in Hems & Currie (2006).

Inevitably, occasions will arise when the use of potentially nephrotoxic drugs becomes necessary and on these occasions constant monitoring of renal function is essential.

In conclusion, when selecting a drug for a patient with renal failure, an agent should be chosen that approaches the ideal characteristics listed in Table 18.6.

Table 18.6 Characteristics of the ideal drug for use in a patient with renal failure

No active metabolites
Disposition unaffected by fluid balance changes
Disposition unaffected by protein-binding changes
Response unaffected by altered tissue sensitivity
Wide therapeutic margin
Not nephrotoxic

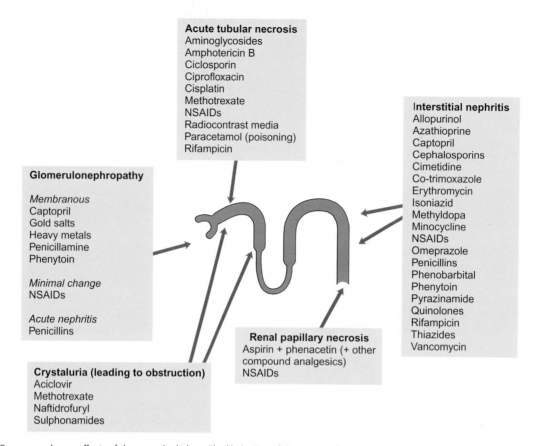

Acute tubular necrosis
Aminoglycosides
Amphotericin B
Ciclosporin
Ciprofloxacin
Cisplatin
Methotrexate
NSAIDs
Radiocontrast media
Paracetamol (poisoning)
Rifampicin

Interstitial nephritis
Allopurinol
Azathioprine
Captopril
Cephalosporins
Cimetidine
Co-trimoxazole
Erythromycin
Isoniazid
Methyldopa
Minocycline
NSAIDs
Omeprazole
Penicillins
Phenobarbital
Phenytoin
Pyrazinamide
Quinolones
Rifampicin
Thiazides
Vancomycin

Glomerulonephropathy

Membranous
Captopril
Gold salts
Heavy metals
Penicillamine
Phenytoin

Minimal change
NSAIDs

Acute nephritis
Penicillins

Renal papillary necrosis
Aspirin + phenacetin (+ other compound analgesics)
NSAIDs

Crystaluria (leading to obstruction)
Aciclovir
Methotrexate
Naftidrofuryl
Sulphonamides

Figure 18.6 Common adverse effects of drugs on the kidney. The likely sites of damage to the nephron (stylized) are indicated.

CASE STUDIES

Case 18.1

Mrs J, a 60-year-old widow, had long-standing hypertension that was unsatisfactorily controlled on a variety of agents. Her drug therapy included furosemide 40 mg once a day, verapamil SR 240 mg twice daily and a salt-restricted diet. Following a routine review of her therapy, ramipril 2.5 mg once daily was added to her treatment regimen in an attempt to improve blood pressure control.

The following day Mrs J noticed that she did not produce as much urine as usual and her ankles had started to swell. Later that evening she presented to her local hospital accident and emergency unit, where her blood pressure was found to be 100/60 mmHg and serum biochemistry revealed creatinine levels of 225 μmol/L (normal range 50–120 μmol/L), Na^+ 125 mmol/L (135–145 mmol/L) and K^+ 5.2 mmol/L (3.5–5.0 mmol/L).

Questions

1. What were the likely cause and underlying mechanism to this patient's problem?
2. What treatment should be given?

Answers

1. ACE inhibitors reduce angiotensin II production and thus attenuate angiotensin II-mediated vasoconstriction of the efferent arterioles that contributes to the high pressure gradient across the glomerulus necessary for filtration. It is not usually a problem in the majority of individuals but in patients with pre-existing compromised renal blood flow, such as renal artery stenoses, the kidney relies more heavily on angiotensin-mediated vasoconstriction of the preglomerular arterioles to maintain renal function. Hypovolaemia caused, for example, by diuretic use would tend to exacerbate this problem. Moreover, it is likely that sodium depletion would render the kidney even more dependent upon vasoconstriction of efferent arterioles through activation of the tubuloglomerular feedback system, further sensitizing the kidney to the effects of ACE inhibitors.

   Mrs J might well have been suffering from incipient renal failure, but remained asymptomatic until her renal reserve diminished.
2. The inappropriate use of an ACE inhibitor should be stopped, as should the diuretic temporarily. Mrs J should be rehydrated using sodium chloride 0.9% and kidney function markers should be monitored in the hope that recovery will occur.

Case 18.2

Mr B, a known intermittent heroin and cocaine abuser, was discovered comatose in his room early in the morning. He was admitted to hospital as an emergency. An indirect history from an acquaintance indicated that Mr B had been drinking very heavily prior to the incident (probably more than a bottle of whisky in a 24-hour period) and had smoked both heroin and cocaine of unknown source and purity.

On examination he was found to be dehydrated and serum biochemistry revealed the following.

		Reference range
Sodium	147 mmol/L	(135–145)
Potassium	6.1 mmol/L	(3.5–5.0)
Calcium	1.72 mmol/L	(2.20–2.55)
Phosphate	2.0 mmol/L	(0.9–1.5)
Creatinine	485 µmol/L	(50–120)
Creatinine kinase	120 000 iu/L	(<200 iu/L)

Urine dipstick reacted positive for blood with no signs of red blood cells on microscopy. The urine was faintly reddish-brown in colour.

Question

What is likely to have occurred and how should it be treated?

Answer

Cocaine, heroin or alcohol abuse sometimes cause muscle damage resulting in rhabdomyolysis. The mechanism is unclear but includes vasoconstriction, an increase in muscle activity, possibly because of seizures, self-injury, adulterants in the drug (e.g. arsenic, strychnine, amphetamine, phencyclidine, quinine) or compression (associated with long periods of inactivity). Acute tubular necrosis may ensue from a direct nephrotoxic effect of the myoglobin released from damaged muscle cells, microprecipitation of myoglobin in renal tubules or a reduction in medullary blood flow. The presence of myoglobin is suggested by the urine dipstick test, which reacts not only to red cells but also to free haemoglobin and myoglobin. Extremely high levels of myoglobinuria may result in urine the colour of Coca-Cola. High serum creatinine kinase levels are indicative of rhabdomyolysis together with the presence of free myoglobin in serum and urine. Serum levels of potassium and phosphate are elevated partly by the effects of incipient renal failure but also through tissue breakdown and intracellular release. Creatinine levels are often higher than expected because of muscle damage.

Treatment should involve fluid replacement with normal saline to reverse dehydration. If an adequate urine output is not achieved, the use of intravenous furosemide may be required to stimulate diuresis. In cases where urine pH is less than 6, administration of intravenous isotonic sodium bicarbonate may be of use, since acidic urine favours myoglobin nephrotoxicity. The patient's ECG should be monitored, because of the risks involved with rapid elevation in serum potassium. Timely, appropriate corrective therapy must be instigated where necessary. In 50–70% of cases with rhabdomyolysis, dialysis is required to support recovery.

Case 18.3

Mr D has been admitted to an intensive care unit with ARF, which developed following a routine cholecystectomy. His electrolyte picture shows the following.

		Reference range
Sodium	138 mmol/L	(135–145)
Potassium	7.2 mmol/L	(3.5–5.0)
Bicarbonate	19 mmol/L	(22–31)
Urea	32.1 mmol/L	(3.0–6.5)
Creatinine	572 µmol/L	(50–120)
pH	7.28	(7.36–7.44)

The patient was connected to an ECG monitor and the resultant trace indicated absent P-waves and a broad QRS complex.

Question

Explain the biochemistry and ECG abnormalities and indicate what therapeutic measures must be implemented.

Answer

Hyperkalaemia is one of the principal problems encountered in patients with renal failure. The increased levels of potassium arise from failure of the excretory pathway and also from intracellular release of potassium. Attention should also be paid to pharmacological or pharmaceutical processes that might lead to potassium elevation (e.g. inappropriate potassium supplements, ACE inhibitors, etc.). The acidosis noted in this patient, which is common in ARF, also aggravates hyperkalaemia by promoting leakage of potassium from cells. A serum potassium level greater than 7.0 mmol/L indicates that emergency treatment is required as the patient risks life-threatening ventricular arrhythmias and asystolic cardiac arrest. If ECG changes are present, as in this case, emergency treatment should be initiated when serum potassium rises above 6.5 mmol/L.

The emergency treatment should include the following.

1. Stabilization of the myocardium by intravenous administration of 10–30 mL calcium gluconate 10% over 5–10 minutes. The effect is temporary but the dose can be repeated.
2. Intravenous administration of 10–20 units of soluble insulin with 50 mL of 50% glucose to stimulate cellular potassium uptake. The dose may be repeated. The blood glucose should be monitored for at least 6 hours to avoid hypoglycaemia.
3. Intravenous salbutamol 0.5 mg in 100 mL 5% dextrose administered over 15 minutes has been used to stimulate the cellular sodium-potassium ATPase pump and thus drive potassium into cells. This may cause disturbing muscle tremors at the doses required to reduce serum potassium levels.
4. Acidosis may be corrected with an intravenous dose of 50–100 mL of sodium bicarbonate 8.4%. Correction of acidosis stimulates cellular potassium re-uptake. Hypertonic bicarbonate solutions (8.4%) can cause volume expansion and should be used with extreme caution.

REFERENCES

Dishart M K, Kellum J A 2000 An evaluation of pharmacological strategies for the prevention and treatment of acute renal failure. Drugs 59: 79-91

Hems S, Currie A 2006 Renal disorders. In: Lee A (ed) Adverse drug reactions, 2nd edn. Pharmaceutical Press, London

FURTHER READING

Aronson J K 2003 Drugs and renal insufficiency. Medicine 31: 103-109

Armitage A J, Tomson C 2003 Acute renal failure. Medicine 31: 43-48

Choi P, Brown E A 2003 Peritoneal dialysis. Medicine 31: 70-73

Gaskin G 2003 Signs and symptoms of renal disease. Medicine 31: 1-4

Glynne P, Allen A, Pusey J 2003 Acute renal failure in practice. Imperial College Press, London

Pandya P, Farrington K 2003 Haemodialysis. Medicine 31: 66-69

Short A, Cumming A 1999 ABC of intensive care: renal support. British Medical Journal 319: 41-44

Taber S S, Mueller B A 2006 Drug-associated renal dysfunction. Critical Care Clinics 22: 357-374

Hypertension 19

S. H. L. Thomas

KEY POINTS

- Hypertension can be defined as a condition in which blood pressure is elevated to an extent where benefit is obtained from blood pressure lowering. There is no clear-cut blood pressure threshold separating normal from hypertensive individuals. The risk of complications is related to the extent that blood pressure is elevated.
- The World Health Organization has identified hypertension as one of the most important preventable causes of premature morbidity and mortality in developed and developing countries.
- Hypertension should not be seen as a risk factor in isolation and decisions on management should not focus on blood pressure alone but on total cardiovascular risk
- The complications of hypertension include stroke, myocardial infarction, heart failure, renal failure and dissecting aortic aneurysm. Small reductions in blood pressure result in substantial reductions in the relative risks of these complications.
- For correct diagnosis, careful measurement of blood pressure is necessary on several occasions using well-maintained and validated equipment.
- Non-pharmacological interventions are important and include weight reduction, avoidance of excessive salt and alcohol, increased intake of fruit and vegetables and regular dynamic exercise. Other cardiovascular risk factors such as smoking, hyperlipidaemia and diabetes should be addressed.
- A large selection of antihypertensive drugs is available. It is important to use a drug that is free from adverse effects.
- The most appropriate choice of initial drug therapy depends on the age and racial origin of the patient, as well as the presence of other medical conditions. For younger white patients an ACE inhibitor is recommended as first-line treatment. For older patients and black people, a calcium channel blocker or thiazide diuretic is an appropriate initial choice.
- Many people need combinations of drugs to achieve adequate blood pressure control. Medication should be convenient to take and adverse effects should be avoided.

Hypertension (high blood pressure) is not a disease but an important risk factor for cardiovascular complications. It can be defined as a condition where blood pressure is elevated to an extent where clinical benefit is obtained from blood pressure lowering. Blood pressure measurement includes systolic and diastolic components, and both are important in determining an individual's cardiovascular risk.

Blood pressure is continuously distributed in the population and there is no clear cut-off point between hypertensive and normotensive subjects. Blood pressure values that are used as treatment thresholds or targets are therefore arbitrary. Nevertheless, there is considerable evidence from clinical trials to demonstrate that treatment of subjects with blood pressures above the thresholds currently used in clinical practice results in important clinical benefits.

The cardiovascular complications associated with hypertension are shown in Table 19.1. The most common and important of these are stroke and myocardial infarction. An increase of 5 mmHg in usual diastolic blood pressure is associated with a 35–40% increased risk of stroke. There is a similar but less steep association for coronary heart disease risk. The risk of heart failure is increased sixfold in hypertensive subjects. Meta-analysis of clinical trials has indicated that a 38% reduction in stroke and a 16% reduction in coronary events result from drug therapy which reduces blood pressure by approximately 10/6 mmHg (Collins et al 1990). A 5 mmHg reduction in blood pressure is associated with a 25% reduction in risk of renal failure.

The absolute benefits of blood pressure lowering achieved as a result of these relative risk reductions depend on the underlying level of risk in an individual subject. High-risk subjects gain more benefit in terms of events saved per year of therapy. Absolute risk is increased for those who already have evidence of cardiovascular disease, such as previous myocardial infarction, transient ischaemic attack, stroke, etc., or who have other evidence of cardiovascular dysfunction such as electrocardiogram (ECG) or echocardiographic abnormalities. Risk is also increased in the

Table 19.1 Complications of hypertension

- Myocardial infarction

- Stroke

    Cerebral/brainstem infarction
    Cerebral haemorrhage
    Lacunar syndromes
    Multi-infarct disease

- Hypertensive encephalopathy/malignant hypertension

- Dissecting aortic aneurysm

- Hypertensive nephrosclerosis

- Peripheral vascular disease

elderly and in people with diabetes or renal failure and is further enhanced by other risk factors such as smoking, hyperlipidaemia, obesity and sedentary lifestyle. In those under the age of 75, men are at greater risk than women. Cardiovascular risk in an individual who has no current cardiovascular disease can be estimated from coronary risk prediction charts (Joint British Societies 2005; see p. 353, Chapter 24).

Epidemiology

Between 10% and 25% of the population are expected to benefit from drug treatment of hypertension, the exact figure depending on the cut-off value for blood pressure and the age group considered for active treatment.

In 90–95% of cases of hypertension there is no underlying medical illness to cause high blood pressure. This is termed 'essential' hypertension. The aetiology of essential hypertension is currently unknown. Genetic factors clearly play a part and essential hypertension tends to run in families, with hypertension being twice as common in subjects who have a hypertensive parent. Genetic factors account for about one-third of the blood pressure variation between individuals although no single gene appears to be responsible except in some rare disease processes (Beevers et al 2001). The remaining 5–10% of cases are secondary to some other disease process (Table 19.2).

Blood pressure increases with age in Westernized societies and hypertension is therefore substantially more common in elderly subjects. It is also more common in black people of African Caribbean origin, who are also at particular risk of stroke and

Table 19.2 Causes of hypertension

Primary hypertension (90–95%)
• Essential hypertension

Secondary hypertension (5–10%)
• Renal diseases
• Endocrine diseases
  Steroid excess — Hyperaldosteronism (Conn's syndrome) / Hyperglucocorticoidism (Cushing's syndrome)
  Growth hormone excess — Acromegaly
  Catecholamine excess — Phaeochromocytoma
  Others — Pre-eclampsia
• Vascular causes
  Renal artery stenosis — Fibromuscular hyperplasia / Renal artery atheroma
  Coarctation of the aorta
• Drugs
  Sympathomimetic amines
  Oestrogens (e.g. combined oral contraceptive pills)
  Ciclosporin
  Erythropoietin
  NSAIDs
  Steroids

renal failure. Hypertension is exacerbated by other factors, for example high salt or alcohol intake or obesity.

Regulation of blood pressure

The mean blood pressure is the product of cardiac output and total peripheral resistance. In most hypertensive individuals cardiac output is not increased and high blood pressure arises as a result of increased total peripheral resistance caused by constriction of small arterioles.

Control of blood pressure is important in evolutionary terms and a number of homeostatic reflexes have evolved to provide blood pressure homeostasis. Minute-to-minute changes in blood pressure are regulated by the baroreceptor reflex, while the renin–angiotensin–aldosterone cascade is important for longer term salt, water and blood pressure control. Increases in blood pressure are also attenuated by local release of nitric oxide from vascular endothelium in response to increased sheer stresses in the blood vessel wall, and endothelial dysfunction is implicated in the pathogenesis of hypertension. Other mechanisms that also play a part in controlling blood pressure include secretion of atrial natriuretic peptide, endothelins, bradykinin and antidiuretic hormone (Beevers et al 2001).

Clinical presentation

Hypertension itself causes no symptoms. Although headache may be present, it is usually unclear if this is caused by hypertension or is an incidental finding. Hypertension is often an incidental finding when subjects present with unrelated conditions or may be discovered as a result of systematic population screening. In the UK, all patients under 80 years of age should have their blood pressure checked at least every 5 years, with an annual review for those with high normal values in the range 135–139 mmHg systolic or 85–89 mmHg diastolic. Hypertension may also come to light for the first time when the individual suffers a hypertension-related complication such as myocardial infarction (MI) or stroke.

Malignant (accelerated) hypertension

Malignant or accelerated hypertension is an uncommon condition characterized by greatly elevated blood pressure associated with evidence of ongoing small vessel damage. This is evident in the optic fundus, where papilloedema, haemorrhages and/or exudates may be present. Renal damage, including haematuria, proteinuria and impaired renal function, is also characteristic. The condition may be associated with hypertensive encephalopathy, which is caused by small vessel changes in the cerebral circulation associated with cerebral oedema. The clinical features are confusion, headache, visual loss and coma.

Malignant hypertension is a medical emergency that requires hospital admission and rapid control of blood pressure over 12–24 hours towards normal levels. In the absence of treatment, malignant hypertension is usually fatal, with a 1-year survival of less than 20%. Fortunately, the condition has become much less common since the advent of effective antihypertensive therapy, although there is still substantial long-term morbidity and patients require careful follow-up.

Management of hypertension

In the UK the management of hypertension is guided by consensus guidelines produced by the British Hypertension Society (BHS) (Williams et al 2004a). The guidelines are also available in summary form (Williams et al 2004b) and via the internet (www.bhsoc.org/). Guidelines for primary care management are also available from the National Institute for Health and Clinical Excellence (NICE 2004). Joint BHS/NICE guidance became available in 2006.

Diagnosis of hypertension

In the United Kingdom it is recommended that all adults have their blood pressure measured every 5 years. Those with high-normal (130–139 mmHg systolic or 85–89 mmHg diastolic) or previous high readings should have annual measurement.

Blood pressure should be measured using a well-maintained sphygmomanometer of validated accuracy. Blood pressure should initially be measured in both arms and the arm with the highest value used for subsequent readings. The subject should be relaxed and, at least at the first presentation, blood pressure should be measured in both the sitting and the standing positions. It is important to use an appropriate sized cuff since one that is too small will result in an overestimation of the patient's blood pressure. As a result a person may be falsely diagnosed as having hypertension and may receive unnecessary treatment with anti-hypertensive drugs. The arm should be supported level with the heart. It is important that the patient does not hold the arm out since isometric exercise increases blood pressure. Blood pressure is measured using the Korotkov sounds which appear (the first phase) and disappear (the fifth phase) over the brachial artery as pressure in the cuff is released. Cuff deflation should occur at approximately 2 mmHg per second to allow accurate measurement of the systolic and diastolic blood pressures. The fourth Korotkov phase (muffling of sound) has previously been used for diastolic blood pressure measurement but is not currently recommended unless Korotkov V cannot be defined.

Having established that the blood pressure is increased, the measurement should be repeated several times over several weeks, unless the initial measurement is at dangerously high levels, in which case several measurements should be made during the same clinic attendance.

Home or ambulatory blood pressure measurements

Some people develop excessive and unrepresentative blood pressure when attending the doctor's surgery, so-called 'white coat' hypertension. When the blood pressure is checked at home, it is normal. These patients can be diagnosed if they use a blood pressure machine themselves at home or by 24-hour ambulatory blood pressure monitoring. Home blood pressure measurement is inexpensive but it is important to have a machine of validated accuracy that the patient can use properly. Ambulatory blood pressure monitoring over 24 hours is also useful for patients who have unusual variability in blood pressure, resistant hypertension or symptoms suggesting hypotension. Home or ambulatory blood pressure measurements are usually lower than clinic recordings, on average by 12/7 mmHg.

Assessment of the hypertensive patient
Secondary causes

It is important to take a careful history for features that might suggest a possible secondary cause. Examples would be symptoms of renal disease, e.g. haematuria, polyuria, etc. or the paroxysmal symptoms that suggest the rare diagnosis of phaeochromocytoma. A careful physical examination should be performed for abdominal bruits (suggesting possible renal artery stenosis), radiofemoral delay (suggesting coarctation of the aorta) and palpable kidneys (suggesting renal disease). Laboratory analysis should include a full blood count, electrolytes, urea, creatinine and urinalysis. In some patients further investigations may be appropriate, for example ultrasound of the abdomen or isotope renogram where renal disease is expected, a renin–angiotensin ratio to investigate for possible hyperaldosteronism and 24-hour or overnight urinary catecholamines for phaeochromocytoma.

Contributing factors

The patient should also be assessed for possible contributory factors to hypertension such as obesity, excess alcohol or salt intake and lack of exercise. Occasionally, hypertension may be provoked by the use of drugs (see Table 19.2), including over-the-counter medicines. Other risk factors should also be documented and addressed, for example smoking, diabetes and hyperlipidaemia. It is important to establish whether there is a family history of cardiovascular disease.

Evidence of end-organ damage

The patient should also be examined carefully for evidence of end-organ damage from hypertension. This should include examination of the optic fundi to detect retinal changes. An ECG should be performed to detect left ventricular hypertrophy or subclinical ischaemic heart disease.

Determination of cardiovascular risk

An accurate assessment of cardiovascular disease risk is essential before recommending appropriate management in hypertension. Patients with documented atheromatous vascular disease, e.g. previous myocardial infarction or stroke, angina or peripheral vascular disease are at high risk of recurrent events. Those with type 2 diabetes over 40 years of age are also at high risk and can be regarded as 'coronary equivalents', i.e. with risks similar to non-diabetic patients with previous myocardial infarction. For non-diabetic patients without vascular disease it is necessary to estimate cardiovascular risk. Various methods are available based on the epidemiological data collected in Framingham, Massachusetts, including the risk prediction charts of the Joint British Societies (see p. 353 Chapter 24). A 10-year cardiovascular disease risk of 20% (equivalent to a 15% coronary heart disease risk) is regarded as an appropriate threshold for antihypertensive therapy in patients with moderate hypertension, as well as for lipid-lowering therapy (see below).

Treatment

Non-pharmacological approaches

Non-pharmacological management of hypertension is important, although the effects are often disappointing. As one element of this, general education is important to allow patients to make informed choices about management. In order to maximize potential benefit, patients should receive clear and unambiguous advice, including written information they can digest in their own time. Written advice for patients can be downloaded from the British Hypertension Society website (www.hyp.ac.uk/bhs/).

In patients who are overweight, weight loss results in reduction in blood pressure of about 2.5/1.5 mmHg per kilogram. Subjects should reduce their salt intake, for example by not adding salt to food on the plate. A daily sodium intake of <100 mmol (i.e. 6 g sodium chloride or 2.4 g elemental sodium) should be the aim. A diet high in fruit and vegetables, legumes and whole-grain cereal improves cardiovascular risk. Most subjects will need to control their intake of calories and saturated fat. Regular dynamic exercise, at a level appropriate to the individual subject, should occur on most days for at least 30 minutes for maximum benefit. This results in improved physical fitness as well as a reduction in blood pressure. Alcohol intake should be restricted to two (females) or three (males) units per day. Although smoking does not affect blood pressure, it increases cardiovascular risk and patients should quit or, if this is not possible, reduce their cigarette consumption.

Unless hypertension is severe, it is appropriate to observe the subject over several months while instituting non-pharmacological interventions. However, if there is a more urgent need for drug treatment non-pharmacological interventions should occur in parallel.

Drug treatment

Treatment thresholds

Treatment thresholds are summarized in Table 19.3. Lifestyle advice should be provided to all patients with any degree of hypertension. Patients with severe hypertension (>220/120 mmHg confirmed on several readings on the same occasion) should be treated immediately. Patients with blood pressures in the range 160–220/100–120 mmHg should be monitored over several weeks and treated if blood pressure remains in this range. The period of observation before starting treatment depends on the severity of the hypertension and the presence or absence of end-organ damage (see Table 19.3). Patients whose blood pressure is in the range 140–159/90–99 mmHg should be observed annually unless they have evidence of target organ damage, cardiovascular complications, diabetes or a calculated cardiovascular risk >15% over 10 years, in which case drug treatment should be offered. Patients with blood pressure in the range 135–139/85–89 mmHg should be reassessed annually, while those with blood pressure lower than this can be rechecked every 5 years.

Target blood pressures

Evidence from the Hypertension Optimal Treatment (HOT) study (Hansson et al 1998) suggested that the optimum target blood pressure was 139/83 for patients whose initial diastolic blood pressure was between 100 and 115. Although no harm was

Table 19.3 Threshold blood pressures for intervention

Initial blood pressure		Management
Systolic	Diastolic	
Malignant hypertension		Admit and treat immediately
>220	>120	Repeat several times at the same attendance and treat immediately if blood pressure persists in this range
180–219	110–119	Confirm over 1–2 weeks and treat if BP remains in this range
160–179	100–109	Repeat over 3–4 weeks (end-organ damage present) or 2–12 weeks (no end-organ damage), institute non-pharmacological measures and treat if blood pressure persists in this range
140–159	90–99	Repeat over several weeks. Institute non-pharmacological measures. Treat if remains in this range and patient has target organ damage, cardiovascular complications or an estimated 10-year cardiovascular risk >20%. Otherwise reassess annually
135–139	85–89	Reassess annually
<135	<85	Reassess in 5 years

demonstrated by reducing blood pressure further, patients are little disadvantaged provided their blood pressure is controlled below 150/90. This is the target blood pressure incorporated as a quality indicator for the General Medical Services Contract for primary care doctors in the UK. Diabetic patients are an exception and benefit from more aggressive blood pressure reduction. Target blood pressures for diabetic and non-diabetic subjects are summarized in Table 19.4. It should be emphasized that the audit standard will not be achieved in all patients.

Antihypertensive drug classes

Diuretics

There is substantial clinical trial evidence that benefit is obtained from the use of thiazide (e.g. bendroflumethiazide, hydrochlorothiazide) or thiazide-like (chlortalidone, indapamide) diuretics in hypertension; these drugs are both inexpensive and well tolerated by most patients. Their diuretic action is achieved by blockade of renal tubular sodium reabsorption. Initially, they reduce blood pressure by reducing circulating blood volume but in the longer term blood volume is restored towards normal and the fall in blood pressure is associated with a reduction in total peripheral resistance, suggesting a direct vasodilatory action. Thiazide-like diuretics differ in some of their ion channel-blocking properties. The clinical importance of these differences is unknown.

Although generally well tolerated, thiazide and thiazide-like diuretics may cause hypokalaemia, small increases in LDL-cholesterol and triglyceride, and gout associated with impaired urate excretion. Erectile dysfunction is also common.

Most blood pressure lowering occurs with very low doses of thiazide diuretics. Increasing the dose substantially increases the risk of metabolic disturbance without causing further blood pressure reduction. For bendroflumethiazide it is rarely (if ever) appropriate to use doses greater than 2.5 mg per day and a dose of 1.25 mg daily is often effective.

Loop diuretics are no more effective at lowering blood pressure than thiazides unless renal function is significantly impaired or the patient is receiving agents that inhibit the renin–angiotensin system. They are also a suitable choice if heart failure is present.

Spironolactone, an aldosterone antagonist, is not suitable for first-line therapy but is an increasingly important treatment option for patients with resistant hypertension. Under these circumstances high blood pressure often results from hyperaldosteronism. There is a risk of hyperkalaemia, especially if used in combination with ACE inhibitors or angiotensin receptor blockers (ARB).

Table 19.4 Target clinic blood pressures according to British Hypertension Society guidelines 2004 (Williams et al 2004a)

	Clinic blood pressure	
	No diabetes	Diabetes
Optimal treated BP	<140/85	<130/80
Audit standard	<150/90	<140/80

β-Adrenoreceptor antagonists

β-Blockers also have substantial clinical trial evidence of benefit over placebo in hypertension, and are relatively inexpensive. However, their use is likely to decline because they seem less effective at preventing stroke and they are commonly associated with adverse effects, such as lethargy, impaired concentration, aching muscles, vivid dreaming, erectile dysfunction, exacerbation of asthma, intermittent claudication or Raynaud's phenomenon. A particular concern is the effect that they have in increasing the risk of development of diabetes. They remain most suitable for younger hypertensives who have another indication for β-blockade, such as coronary heart disease.

Their mode of action in hypertension is uncertain. β-Blockade reduces cardiac output in the short term and during exercise. It also reduces renin secretion by antagonizing β-receptors in the juxtaglomerular apparatus. Central actions may also be important for some agents. Non-selective β-blockers may give rise to adverse effects as a result of antagonism of β_2-adrenoceptors, i.e. asthma and worsened intermittent claudication. However, so-called 'cardioselective' (β_1-selective) β-blockers are not free of these adverse effects. Patients who develop very marked bradycardia and tiredness may tolerate a drug with partial agonist activity such as pindolol.

Renin-angiotensin-aldosterone antagonists

ACE inhibitors block the conversion of angiotensin I to angiotensin II, while angiotensin receptor blockers block the action of angiotensin II at the angiotensin II type 2_1 receptor. Since angiotensin II is a vasoconstrictor and stimulates the release of aldosterone, antagonism results in vasodilation and potassium retention as well as inhibition of salt and water retention. ACE inhibitors also block kininase and thus prevent the breakdown of bradykinin. This appears to be important in the aetiology of cough, which is a troublesome side effect of these drugs in 10–20% of users. Angiotensin receptor blockers do not inhibit kininase and are an appropriate choice for patients who are intolerant of ACE inhibitors because of cough.

Calcium channel blockers

These agents block slow calcium channels in the peripheral blood vessels and/or the heart. The dihydropyridine group work almost exclusively on L-type calcium channels in the peripheral arterioles and reduce blood pressure by reducing total peripheral resistance. In contrast, verapamil's effects are primarily on the heart, reducing heart rate and cardiac output. Long-acting dihydropyridines are preferred because they are more convenient for patients and avoid the large fluctuations in plasma drug concentrations that may be associated with adverse effects.

Although effective for lowering blood pressure and preventing cardiovascular events, adverse effects are common, e.g. oedema and flushing. Gum hypertrophy may occur with dihydropyridines and constipation with verapamil.

Concerns have previously been raised by observational studies (Psaty et al 1995) and meta-analysis (Furberg et al 1995) that there may be an increased risk of coronary heart disease in recipients of dihydropyridine calcium channel blockers.

However, randomized clinical trials have not confirmed these observations (Gong et al 1996, Liu et al 1998, Staessen et al 1997) and have indicated that dihydropyridines are of similar efficacy to thiazide diuretics in preventing cardiovascular events (Brown et al 2000).

α-Adrenoreceptor blockers

Drugs of this class antagonize α-adrenoceptors in the blood vessel wall and thus prevent noradrenaline (norepinephrine)-induced vasoconstriction. As a result, they reduce total peripheral resistance and blood pressure. Prazosin was originally used but has the disadvantage of being short-acting and causing first-dose hypotension. Newer agents such as doxazosin and terazosin have a longer duration of action. There are concerns about the first-line use of α-blockers since the Antihypertensive and Lipid Lowering treatment to prevent Heart Attack Trial (ALLHAT) study has indicated that doxazosin is more often associated with heart failure and stroke than thiazide diuretics (ALLHAT 2000). However, they are an appropriate choice as add-in therapy for patients inadequately controlled using other agents.

Centrally acting agents

Methyldopa and moxonidine inhibit sympathetic outflow from the brain, resulting in a reduction in total peripheral resistance. Methyldopa is not widely used because it has pronounced central adverse effects, including tiredness and depression. It continues to be used in pregnancy, since it has a very good safety record. It is also sometimes needed for people with resistant hypertension. Moxonidine is a newer agent that blocks central imidazoline and α_2-adrenoceptors. It appears to have fewer central adverse effects than methyldopa. Other centrally acting agents such as clonidine and reserpine are almost never used in modern practice because of their pronounced adverse effects.

Other agents

Several other drugs are available for use for people with more resistant hypertension. Minoxidil is a powerful antihypertensive drug but its use is associated with severe peripheral oedema and reflex tachycardia. It should be restricted to patients with severe hypertension who are also taking β-blockers and diuretics. It causes pronounced hirsutism and is not a suitable treatment for women. Hydralazine can be used as add-on therapy for patients with resistant hypertension but is not well tolerated and may occasionally be associated with drug-induced systemic lupus erythematosus. Sodium nitroprusside is a direct-acting arterial and venous dilator that is administered as an intravenous infusion for treating hypertensive emergencies and for the acute control of blood pressure during anaesthesia. Hypertension has previously been treated with ganglion blockers such as guanethidine but these drugs are now of historical interest only.

Drug selection

As in other clinical situations, drugs should be chosen on the basis of efficacy, safety, convenience to the patient and cost. For assessing efficacy, it is more important to use evidence from large-scale clinical 'end-point' trials than smaller scale studies looking at the effects of drugs on blood pressure. When considering safety, it is important to recognize that these drugs will be taken in the long term and there are advantages to using drugs which have long-established safety records. It is also important to recognize the importance of symptomatic adverse effects since these may reduce compliance. Patients should feel as well during treatment of their blood pressure as they did before drug treatment was instituted. Patient convenience is another important factor and use of once-daily preparations will result in better compliance than more frequent regimens. Since the hypertensive population is very large it is necessary to be conscious of the cost of individual preparations. Combinations of low doses of antihypertensive drugs are often better tolerated than single drugs taken in high dose.

The choice of drugs available for treating hypertension is shown in Table 19.5, and common therapeutic problems are noted.

Clinical trial evidence

Initial evidence of benefit in placebo-controlled clinical trials came from studies that primarily involved thiazide diuretics or β-blockers (Table 19.6). However, there is increasing evidence of clinical benefit from newer drug classes including ACE inhibitors and calcium channel blockers.

The Blood Pressure Lowering Trialists Collaboration (2000) carried out a meta-analysis of old against new treatments. They concluded that newer treatments were no more effective than older therapies. Since this study was done several landmark comparative clinical trials have been published.

The Captopril Prevention Project (CAPPP) demonstrated that captopril was as effective as diuretics or β-blockers for preventing cardiovascular morbidity (Hansson et al 1999b). However, captopril was associated with a 25% higher stroke risk, perhaps because it did not reduce blood pressure as effectively as conventional therapy in this particular study.

The Losartan For Endpoint reduction in hypertension study (LIFE) demonstrated that losartan was more effective at preventing vascular events, especially stroke, than atenolol in just over 9000 hypertensive patients with LVH, although reductions in blood pressure were similar. Losartan was also better tolerated (Dahlöf et al 2002).

The ALLHAT study (2002) involved over 40 000 older, high-risk hypertensive patients with the aim of determining whether the occurrence of fatal coronary heart disease or non-fatal myocardial infarction was lower in those treated with newer agents (amlodipine, lisinopril or doxazosin) compared with a thiazide-like diuretic (chlortalidone). The doxazosin arm was discontinued early because of a higher rate of events, especially heart failure, compared with the diuretic. For the remaining three drugs there was no difference in occurrence of the primary end-point. Chlortalidone was more effective than amlodipine and lisinopril in lowering blood pressure and preventing heart failure and was also marginally more effective than lisinopril in preventing stroke.

The second Australian National Blood Pressure Study Group (Wing et al 2003) compared enalapril with hydrochlorthiazide in just over 6000 hypertensive subjects recruited in primary

Table 19.5 Summary of antihypertensive drugs and common therapeutic problems

Class	Examples	Major adverse effects	Notes
Diuretics	Thiazides: bendroflumethiazide	Hypokalaemia Gout Glucose intolerance Hyperlipidaemia	Cheap, effective. Efficacy proven in clinical trials Concerns about long term metabolic effects More appropriate in older patients
	Loops: furosemide K sparing: spironolactone	Impotence Uraemia Dehydration Hyperkalaemia Gynaecomastia	Especially for patients with cardiac failure Especially for resistant hypertension
β-blockers	Atenolol Propranolol Metoprolol Labetalol Celiprolol	Tiredness Reduced exercise tolerance Bradycardia Cold peripheries Claudication Wheezing Cardiac failure Impotence	Cheap Adverse effects common Possibly less effective in preventing cardiovascular events Especially for patients with ischaemic heart disease
Calcium antagonists: dihydropyridine	Nifedipine Amlodipine	Flushing Oedema Postural hypotension Headache	Not well tolerated (especially early in treatment). Recent trials confirm reductions in stroke and myocardial infarction. Similar efficacy to thiazides. Especially for elderly patients and those with ischaemic heart disease or diabetes
Calcium antagonists: rate limiting	Verapamil Diltiazem	Bradycardia/heart block Constipation (verapamil only)	Well tolerated. Suitable for patients with ischaemic heart disease who are unable to tolerate β-blockers Caution needed when used in combination with β-blockers
ACE inhibitors	Captopril Enalapril Lisinopril Perindopril Ramipril	Cough Rash, taste disturbance Renal failure Angio-oedema	More expensive. Cough very common Appropriate for use in younger patients and those with cardiac failure or diabetes
α-blockers	Prazosin Doxazosin Terazosin	Oedema Postural hypotension	More expensive. Adverse effects common. No evidence to date of long-term efficacy. Less effective than thiazides at preventing heart failure and combined cardiovascular outcomes (ALLHAT study) Second-line
Angiotensin receptor blockers	Losartan Valsartan Irbesartan	Renal failure Oedema Headache	More expensive Especially for patients in whom ACE inhibitor indicated but not tolerated due to cough More effective in preventing vascular events than atenolol in patients with LVH
Centrally acting vasodilators	Methyldopa Moxonidine	Tiredness Depression	Poorly tolerated. Only use in severe hypertension or hypertension of pregnancy Third-line
Direct-acting vasodilators	Diazoxide Minoxidil Nitroprusside	Oedema Postural hypotension Headache	Poorly tolerated. Only use in severe hypertension

Table 19.6 Placebo-controlled trials of antihypertensive drug therapy

Trial	Reference	Drugs used: first-line (second-line)
Veterans Administration Study	Veterans Administration (1970)	Thiazide (reserpine, hydralazine)
Joint National Committee on Detection, Evaluation and Treatment of High Blood Pressure	Anon (1977)	Thiazide (rauwolfia)
Australian Therapeutic Trial in Mild Hypertension	Anon (1980)	Thiazide (methyldopa, propranolol, pindolol, hydralazine, clonidine)
Medical Research Council trial of treatment of mild hypertension	MRC (1985)	Thiazide and propranolol
European Working Party on High Blood Pressure in the Elderly trial	Amery et al (1985)	Thiazide (methyldopa)
Systolic Hypertension in the Elderly Program (SHEP)	SHEP (1991)	Thiazide (atenolol)
Swedish Trial of Old Patients with hypertension (STOP – hypertension)	Dahlöf et al (1991)	Thiazide (amiloride, atenolol, metoprolol, pindolol)
Medical Research Council trial of treatment of hypertension in older adults	MRC (1992)	Thiazide and atenolol
Shanghai Trial of Nifedipine in the Elderly (STONE)	Gong et al (1996)	Nifedipine
Systolic hypertension in Europe (SYST-EUR) trial	Staessen et al (1997)	Nitrendipine (thiazide, enalapril)
Systolic hypertension in China (SYST-CHINA) trial	Liu et al (1998)	Nitrendipine (thiazide, captopril)

care. The primary end-point was any cardiovascular event or death from any cause. In this relatively small study there was a trend in favour of the ACE inhibitor which was of borderline statistical significance.

The VALUE study (Julius et al 2004) compared amlodipine and valsartan in high-risk hypertensive subjects. No differences in the primary composite cardiac end-point were observed, although non-fatal myocardial infarction was less common with amlodipine, which also lowered blood pressure to a greater extent. Conversely, onset of diabetes was less common with valsartan.

The ASCOT study (Dahlöf et al 2005) compared a modern treatment regimen based on amlodipine and perindopril with a traditional regimen based on atenolol and bendroflumethiazide. The study involved over 20 000 high-risk hypertensives. The amlodipine-based therapy was associated with better blood pressure reduction and reductions in the occurrence of cardiovascular events, total mortality and diabetes, although the primary composite end-point was not significantly affected. It is uncertain how much of the benefit can be attributed to the better blood pressure control achieved in the amlodipine-based arm and how specific these findings are to the drug doses and sequencing specified in the trial protocol for each arm of the study.

These various trials have provided results that are in part conflicting, in part because of differences in trial design and quality. However, there is increasing evidence that β-blockers may be less effective at preventing cardiovascular end-points, as suggested by LIFE and ASCOT. In a meta-analysis (Lindholm et al 2005), β-blockers were less effective than other antihypertensives at preventing stroke, although no significant differences

were observed in effects on myocardial infarction or death. There is no consistent evidence that thiazides or thiazide-like drugs are less effective than newer agents in preventing cardiovascular events.

Recommendations for drug sequencing

Current guidance on drug sequencing in hypertension in the UK has been conflicting. The British Hypertension Society advocated use of the 'AB/CD' algorithm (Williams et al 2004a). This recommends initial choice of an ACE inhibitor or angiotensin receptor blocker (A) or β-blocker (B) as first-line therapy in younger (<55 years) non-black patients. The rationale for this is that these patients often have hypertension associated with high concentrations of renin. It is therefore logical to treat these patients with drugs that antagonize the renin–angiotensin system and there is evidence that this is more effective for lowering blood pressure. Generally ACE inhibitors would be preferred because of concerns about the efficacy and safety of β-blockers. For elderly and black patients, who tend to have hypertension associated with low renin concentrations, calcium channel blockers (C) or thiazide diuretics (D) are advocated. If initial drug therapy fails to control blood pressure, A or B is combined with C or D. Subsequently a combination of A (or B) plus C plus D may be used. After this, further therapies, e.g. α-blocker, spironolactone, etc., should be added as necessary to achieve adequate control (Fig. 19.1).

National guidance was also issued on the management of adults with essential hypertension (NICE 2004). This recommended

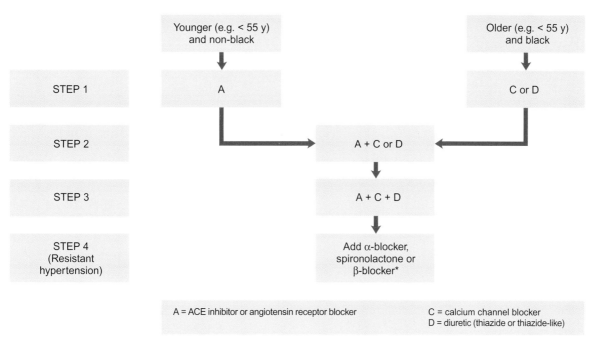

STEP 1	A		C or D
STEP 2		A + C or D	
STEP 3		A + C + D	
STEP 4 (Resistant hypertension)		Add α-blocker, spironolactone or β-blocker*	

Younger (e.g. < 55 y) and non-black

Older (e.g. < 55 y) and black

A = ACE inhibitor or angiotensin receptor blocker   C = calcium channel blocker
D = diuretic (thiazide or thiazide-like)

* As appropriate to the patient's individual circumstances

Figure 19.1 Algorithm for drug sequencing in hypertension.

use of a thiazide diuretic as first-line therapy, with the option of a β-blocker as first-line treatment for those under 55 years. Second-line therapy recommended was a β-blocker, unless the risk of developing diabetes was high, e.g. positive family history, impaired glucose tolerance, Asian or African Caribbean race, in which case an ACE inhibitor should be used. Subsequently a calcium channel blocker could be added and then other drug classes as appropriate to control blood pressure.

In 2006 the NICE (2004) guidance was revised (National Collaborating Centre for Chronic Conditions 2006). This updated guidance recommends ACE inhibitors in those under 55 years and calcium channel blockers in those over 55 years or black patients at any age, with thiazides also a first-line option for this group. β-Blockers do not feature except as add-on therapy after ACE inhibitors, calcium channel blockers and thiazide diuretics.

Special patient groups

Race

People of African Caribbean origin have an increased prevalence of hypertension and left ventricular hypertrophy and are at high risk of stroke and renal failure. They obtain particular benefit from reduced salt intake and are also sensitive to diuretic and calcium channel blockers, while β-blockers appear less effective, at least when used as monotherapy. African Caribbean people have reduced plasma renin activity and, as a result, ACE inhibitors and angiotensin receptor blockers are also less effective. This was illustrated in the ALLHAT study where stroke and coronary events were more common in black patients randomized to lisinopril compared to those receiving chlortalidone.

British Asians also have an increased prevalence of hypertension, diabetes and insulin resistance and a particularly high risk of

coronary heart disease and stroke. There is currently no evidence of a difference in drug response when compared with white Europeans. However, combinations of β-blockers and thiazides should be avoided when possible because of the higher risk of diabetes.

Elderly

The elderly have a high prevalence of hypertension, with over 70% having blood pressures greater than 140/90 mmHg. They are also at high absolute risk of cardiovascular events. Therefore the absolute benefits of blood pressure treatment are particularly large in this group. Antihypertensive therapy may also reduce the risk of heart failure and dementia (Seux et al 1999). The SCOPE study (Lithell et al 2003) was designed to investigate the effects of candesartan on the occurrence of cognitive decline or dementia but revealed no benefit, probably because of the lack of difference in blood pressure between the two arms of the study

The elderly are at particular risk of certain adverse effects of treatment such as postural hypotension and it is important that both sitting and standing blood pressure are monitored. Nevertheless, the benefits of therapy are so great that treatment should be offered at any age unless the patient is very frail or their life expectancy is very short. Isolated systolic hypertension (systolic >160, diastolic <90 mmHg) is common in the elderly and there is irrefutable evidence that drug treatment is beneficial in this group (Liu et al 1998, SHEP 1991, Staessen et al 1997). The elderly have more variable blood pressure and larger numbers of measurements may be required to confirm hypertension.

Calcium channel blockers and low-dose thiazide diuretics are safe and effective treatments for elderly hypertensive people and their use is endorsed by large-scale clinical trials. β-Blockers are less effective at reducing blood pressure and preventing clinical end-points. The Swedish Trial in Old Patients with hypertension-2

(STOP-2) compared the effects of conventional (β-blocker or thiazide) and newer drugs (ACE inhibitors or calcium channel blockers) on cardiovascular morbidity in older subjects and did not detect significant differences (Hansson et al 1999a).

Diabetes

In type 1 diabetes, the presence of hypertension often indicates the presence of diabetic nephropathy. In this group, blood pressure reduction and ACE inhibition slow the rate of decline in renal function. To achieve adequate blood pressure control combinations of drugs will be needed. Thiazides, β-blockers, calcium channel blockers and α-blockers are all suitable as add-on treatments to ACE inhibitors which should be first-line therapy. Target blood pressure should be <130/80 mmHg or <125/75 mmHg if there is diabetic nephropathy.

In type 2 (non-insulin dependent) diabetes, hypertension is particularly common, affecting 70% of people in this group. It is strongly associated with obesity and insulin resistance and control of blood pressure is more important for preventing complications than tight glycaemic control. There is particular evidence of benefit for tight blood pressure control to a target of <140/80 mmHg, and this will usually need combinations of drugs (UKPDS 1998a). It is more difficult to achieve target blood pressures in diabetics, especially those for systolic blood pressure. There is no evidence that one group of drugs is more or less effective than any other and it is not clear if ACE inhibitors have a specific renoprotective effect in this group over and above their blood pressure lowering actions. The UK Prospective Diabetes Study Group (1998b) demonstrated no difference between atenolol and captopril in terms of preventing cardiovascular complications in hypertensive patients with diabetes, although the study and its statistical power were comparatively small. In the Appropriate Blood pressure Control in Diabetes (ABCD) trial (Estacio et al 1998) and the Fosinopril versus Amlodipine Cardiovascular Events randomized Trial (FACET) (Tatti et al 1998), an ACE inhibitor was more effective than a dihydropyridine calcium channel blocker in preventing cardiovascular events. However, in both studies this was a secondary end-point. In LIFE, losartan was more effective in diabetics than atenolol, while in ALLHAT, ACE inhibitors were no better than chlortalidone in preventing cardiovascular events in diabetics.

There is now increasing evidence that angiotensin receptor blockers can delay progression of diabetic nephropathy in type 2 diabetes.

Renal disease

In patients with chronic renal impairment, good blood pressure control slows the progression of renal dysfunction. ACE inhibition reduces the incidence of end-stage renal failure but it is not clear if this is a specific effect or non-specific action as a result of blood pressure lowering. ACE inhibitors also reduce 24-hour protein loss and should be used in patients with 24-hour protein excretion of >3 g or rapidly progressive renal dysfunction. ACE inhibitors may worsen renal impairment in patients with renal vascular disease and careful monitoring of electrolytes and creatinine is mandatory. Salt restriction is particularly important in managing hypertension in renal disease. Thiazide diuretics are ineffective in patients with significant renal dysfunction and loop diuretics should be used when a diuretic is needed.

Stroke

Hypertension is the most important risk factor for stroke in patients with or without previous stroke. There is increasing evidence that in those with a previous stroke, blood pressure reduction reduces the risk of stroke recurrence as well as other cardiovascular events. The largest of these studies was PROGRESS (2001), which demonstrated that therapy based on perindopril with the addition of indapamide reduced recurrent stroke as well as other cardiovascular events and this effect could be demonstrated even in those with normal initial blood pressure.

Pregnancy

An increased blood pressure before 20 weeks gestation usually indicates pre-existing chronic hypertension that may not have been previously diagnosed. As in all younger hypertensive patients, a careful assessment is needed to exclude possible secondary causes, although radiological and radionuclide investigations should usually be deferred until after pregnancy. Hypertension diagnosed after 20 weeks gestation may also indicate chronic hypertension, which may have been masked during early pregnancy by the fall in blood pressure that occurs at that time. Patients with elevated blood pressure in pregnancy are at increased risk of pre-eclampsia and intrauterine growth retardation. They need frequent checks of their blood pressure, urinalysis and fetal growth.

Pre-eclampsia is diagnosed when the blood pressure increases by 30/15 mmHg from measurements obtained in early pregnancy or if the diastolic blood pressure exceeds 110 mmHg and proteinuria is present. There is consensus that blood pressure should be treated with drugs if it exceeds 150–160/100–110 mmHg and some clinicians use a lower threshold, for example 140/90 mmHg. Methyldopa is the most suitable drug choice for use in pregnancy because of its long-term safety record. Calcium channel blockers, hydralazine and labetalol are also used. β-Blockers, particularly atenolol, are used less often as they are associated with intrauterine growth retardation. Although diuretics reduce the incidence of pre-eclampsia they are little used in pregnancy because of concerns about decreasing maternal blood volume. ACE inhibitors and angiotensin receptor blockers are contraindicated, as they are associated with oligohydramnios, renal failure and intrauterine death.

Meta-analysis of trials suggests that antihypertensive drugs reduce risk of progression to severe hypertension and reduce hospital admissions, although excessive blood pressure reduction may reduce fetal growth.

Oral contraceptives

Use of combined oral contraceptives results, on average, in an increase of 5/3 mmHg in blood pressure. However, severe hypertension can occur in a small proportion of recipients months or years into treatment. Progesterone-only preparations do not cause hypertension so often but are less effective for contraception, especially in younger women. Combined oral contraceptives are not absolutely contraindicated in hypertension unless other risk factors for cardiovascular disease, such as smoking, are present.

Hormone replacement therapy

There is little evidence that hormone replacement therapy is associated with an increase in blood pressure and women with hypertension should not be denied access to these agents if there is an appropriate indication. However, hormone replacement therapy itself does not reduce and may increase risk of cardiovascular events. Large increases in blood pressure have occasionally been reported in individuals and it is important to monitor blood pressure during the first few weeks of therapy and 6-monthly thereafter. In women with resistant hypertension during treatment with hormone replacement therapy, the effectiveness of discontinuing hormone replacement should be assessed.

A list of the indications and contraindications to the various antihypertensive agents can be found in Table 19.7.

Table 19.7 Use of antihypertensive drugs adapted from British Hypertension Society guidelines. Strong indications and contraindications are shown, with weak/possible indications or contraindications in parentheses

Class	Indications	Contraindications
Diuretics	Elderly ISH Heart failure Secondary stroke prevention	Gout
β-blockers	Myocardial infarction Angina (Heart failure)	Asthma/chronic obstructive pulmonary disease Heart block (Heart failure) (Dyslipidaemia) (Peripheral vascular disease) (Diabetes, except with coronary heart disease)
Calcium antagonists: dihydropyridine	Elderly isolated systolic hypertension (Elderly) (Angina)	
Calcium antagonists (rate limiting)	Angina (Myocardial infarction)	Combination with β-blocker (Heart block) (Heart failure)
ACE inhibitors	Heart failure Left ventricular (LV) dysfunction Type 1 diabetic nephropathy Secondary stroke prevention (Chronic renal disease) (Type 2 diabetic nephropathy) (Proteinuric renal disease)	Pregnancy Renovascular disease (Renal impairment) (Peripheral vascular disease)
α-blockers	Benign prostatic hypertrophy (Dyslipidaemia)	Urinary incontinence (Postural hypotension) (Heart failure)
Angiotensin receptor blockers	ACE inhibitor intolerance Type 2 diabetic nephropathy Hypertension with LVH Heart failure in ACE inhibitor-intolerant subjects Post MI (LV dysfunction post MI) (Intolerance of other antihypertensive drugs) (Proteinuric renal disease) (Chronic renal failure) (Heart failure)	As ACE inhibitors
Centrally acting vasodilators	Pregnancy (methyldopa only) Resistant hypertension unresponsive to first-line therapy	
Direct-acting vasodilators	Resistant hypertension, unresponsive to first-line therapy	

Ancillary drug treatment

Aspirin

The use of aspirin reduces cardiovascular events at the expense of an increase in gastrointestinal complications. Its use should be restricted to patients who have no contraindications and either:

- have evidence of established vascular disease, or
- have no evident cardiovascular disease but who are over 50 years of age and have either evidence of target organ damage or a 10-year cardiovascular disease risk of >20%.

Blood pressure should be controlled (<150/90 mmHg) before aspirin is instituted.

Lipid-lowering therapy

There is increasing evidence from clinical trials of the benefit of lipid-lowering drug treatment in patients with hypertension. For example, in the ASCOT study lipid-lowering arm (ASCOT-LLA), treatment with atorvastatin 10 mg was associated with substantial reductions in coronary heart disease and stroke, in spite of the fact that those with total cholesterols initially higher than 6.5 mmol/L were excluded from the study (Sever et al 2003). Lipid-lowering therapy, usually with a statin, should be prescribed to patients under 80 years of age with a total cholesterol >3.5 mmol/L who either have pre-existing vascular disease or a 10-year cardiovascular risk of >20%.

CASE STUDIES

Case 19.1

A 55-year-old woman of African Caribbean origin is found to have consistently elevated blood pressure over several weeks, her lowest reading being 155/98 mmHg. She is overweight and has diabetes, and is being treated with metformin. Her renal function and urinalysis are both normal.

Questions

1. Should drug therapy be initiated for her hypertension?
2. If her hypertension was treated with drugs, which agents offer particular advantages, and which should be avoided?

Answers

1. Provided her blood pressure has been measured accurately over several weeks, it should be treated, since her diabetes is an important additional risk factor. It is important to ensure that an appropriately sized blood pressure cuff is being used, in view of her obesity. Non-pharmacological interventions should also take place in parallel. Restriction of salt intake may be particularly helpful in people of African Caribbean race and weight reduction would benefit her hypertension and her diabetes.
2. ACE inhibitors are an attractive choice for diabetic patients who have nephropathy. However, there is no evidence of nephropathy in this patient and ACE inhibitors are less effective antihypertensives in people of African Caribbean origin. β-Blockers reduce hypoglycaemic

awareness; this is not a contraindication in this case since metformin does not cause hypoglycaemia. However, β-blockers are also less effective in those of African Caribbean descent. Diuretics work well in African Caribbean hypertensives, but may worsen glucose tolerance and may not therefore be the most appropriate first choice. Calcium channel blockers do not have adverse metabolic effects and are effective in people of this origin, and would therefore be an appropriate choice. Tight blood pressure control is important and several agents may be required, including diuretics, ACE inhibitors, β-blockers and α-blockers.

Case 19.2

Mr PT, a 35-year-old man, is overweight and has a blood pressure of 178/114 mmHg. He smokes 25 cigarettes daily and drinks 28 units of alcohol per week. He has a sedentary occupation. He eats excessive quantities of saturated fat and salt.

Questions

1. How should this patient be managed?
2. What pharmacological treatment for blood pressure would be appropriate if non-pharmacological treatment was unsuccessful?

Mr PT subsequently stopped smoking and lost some weight but remained hypertensive. He was treated with atenolol 50 mg daily. His blood pressure fell to 136/84 mmHg but he developed tiredness and bradycardia and complained of erectile impotence.

Question

3. What are the treatment options for PT?

Answers

1. Since he is a young man, his absolute risk of cardiovascular events is low, at least for the time being. However, he has several additional risk factors that need to be addressed, including his sedentary lifestyle and his smoking. Non-pharmacological methods have the potential of reducing his blood pressure considerably, including reduction in weight and salt intake. Measurement of plasma cholesterol may help him modify his diet although he is unlikely to qualify for lipid-lowering therapy in view of his young age.
2. If drug treatment was appropriate, initial treatment with an ACE inhibitor would be consistent with current guidance, in view of his age. This is likely to be more effective for BP lowering than a calcium channel blocker or diuretic. β-Blockers have been recommended as an option in younger patients but are now considered less suitable as initial therapy. Other drugs could be added or substituted if he was intolerant to initial therapy or it did not reduce his blood pressure to target levels.
3. It is possible that he would feel less tired using a β-blocker with intrinsic sympathomimetic activity (e.g. pindolol) but this is by no means guaranteed. The effects on his sexual function are unpredictable. It would probably be better to change him to a drug of a different class such as an ACE inhibitor. A calcium channel blocker or thiazide diuretic (although these also commonly cause impotence) may be added if necessary.

Case 19.3

A 24-year-old woman with a family history of hypertension is prescribed an oral contraceptive. Six months after starting this, she is noted to have a blood pressure of 148/96 mmHg.

Question

How should this patient be managed?

Answer

If her blood pressure is consistently raised she may have either essential hypertension or hypertension induced by the oral contraceptive, or a combination. Her blood pressure may fall if her oral contraceptive is discontinued. She will, however, need advice on adequate contraceptive methods. A progesterone-only preparation would be one possibility. She would need careful counselling about the methods available and how successful they are. If her blood pressure remained elevated after discontinuing her oral contraceptive, she is likely to have underlying hypertension. This may be essential in nature, in view of the family history; however, because of her age she should undergo some investigations to exclude possible secondary causes of hypertension. She is at low risk of complications and there is no urgency to consider drug treatment. If there is a strong wish to use combined oral contraception, it would be important to control other risk factors as far as possible and to consider drug treatment for her hypertension.

Case 19.4

A lady of 73 has a long-standing history of hypertension and intolerance to antihypertensive drugs. Bendroflumethiazide was associated with acute attacks of gout, she developed breathlessness and wheezing while taking atenolol, nifedipine caused flushing and headache, and doxazosin was associated with intolerable postural hypotension. Four weeks earlier she had been started on enalapril but was now complaining of a dry persistent cough. Her blood chemistry has remained normal.

Questions

1. Is the patient's cough likely to be an adverse effect of enalapril?
2. What other options are available for controlling her blood pressure?

Answers

1. Yes it is. A dry cough is a common adverse effect of ACE inhibitors. It affects approximately 10–20% of recipients and is more common in women. Some patients are able to tolerate the symptom but in many the drug has to be discontinued.
2. Angiotensin receptor blockers can be used in patients intolerant of ACE inhibitors due to cough. They are unlikely to produce this symptom since they do not inhibit the metabolism of pulmonary bradykinin. Centrally acting agents such as methyldopa or moxonidine could also be considered. However, these are not well tolerated and side effects are quite likely in this patient. A non-dihydropyridine calcium channel blocker such as verapamil is another alternative. Measurement of plasma uric acid could also be considered followed by prophylactic treatment with allopurinol before introducing a diuretic. Alternatively, a trial of spironolactone could be considered.

Case 19.5

A 23-year-old woman has a normal blood pressure (118/82 mmHg) when reviewed at 8 weeks of pregnancy. In the 24th week of

pregnancy she is reviewed by her midwife and found to have a blood pressure of 148/96 mmHg. Urinalysis is normal.

Questions

1. What is the likely diagnosis?
2. What complications does the patient's high blood pressure place her at increased risk of?
3. Should she receive drug treatment? If so, with which drug? If not, how should she be managed?

Answers

1. She may have gestation-induced hypertension or chronic hypertension that had previously been masked by the fall in blood pressure that happens in early pregnancy.
2. She is at increased risk of pre-eclampsia and intrauterine growth retardation.
3. There are differences of opinion between specialists as to whether blood pressure should be treated at this level during pregnancy. In favour of treatment is the substantial rise over the earlier blood pressure recording. Some specialists would not treat unless the blood pressure was >170/110 mmHg or other complications were present. If she were treated, methyldopa would be a suitable choice. In any event, she needs close monitoring of her blood pressure, urinalysis and fetal growth.

Case 19.6

An elderly patient comes to the pharmacy with a prescription for the following medications: salbutamol inhaler 200 µg as required, beclometasone inhaler 200 µg twice daily, bendroflumethiazide 2.5 mg daily, Dilzem XL 180 mg once daily and atenolol 50 mg daily. The atenolol was being started by the patient's primary care doctor, apparently because of inadequate blood pressure control.

Question

What action should the pharmacist take?

Answer

There are two reasons to be concerned about the addition of atenolol to this patient's drug regimen. First, there is a potentially hazardous interaction with diltiazem (Dilzem XL) which may result in severe bradycardia or heart block. Second, the patient is receiving treatment for obstructive airways disease and this may be worsened by the atenolol. The prescription should be discussed with the prescriber.

Case 19.7

A patient is admitted to hospital with a stroke. A CT scan of the brain shows a cerebral infarct. The patient's blood pressure is 178/102 mmHg and remains at this level over the first 6 hours after admission to the ward.

Question

Should antihypertensive medication be prescribed?

Answer

There is no good evidence that antihypertensive drug treatment is beneficial in the early stages of acute stroke and there is a risk that lowering blood pressure may compromise cerebral perfusion further. However, in the longer term blood pressure reduction is valuable for preventing further strokes and other cardiovascular events. It would be appropriate to monitor the blood pressure and start treatment after a few days if it remains persistently elevated. A thiazide diuretic and/or ACE inhibitor are commonly used under these circumstances, following the demonstration of benefit in the PROGRESS trial.

Case 19.8

A 67-year-old man has been treated for hypertension with atenolol 50 mg daily for several years. He feels well and his blood pressure is controlled. He has read an article in the paper that suggests atenolol is not considered the most suitable drug for treating high blood pressure and enquires about changing his prescription.

Question

Should an alteration to his treatment be recommended?

Answer

There is increasing evidence that β-blockers, including atenolol, may be less effective at preventing cardiovascular events, especially stroke, than other drugs and are associated with a higher risk of development of diabetes, especially if used in combination with thiazide diuretics. They are also less effective at reducing blood pressure in older people. However, if his blood pressure is well controlled and the treatment suits him there is no strong reason to change his medication unless he is at particular risk of diabetes.

Case 19.9

A 58-year-old male patient is noted to have high blood pressure by his primary care doctor. There is no evidence of end-organ damage and he has no other cardiovascular risk factors. The blood pressure remains greater than 160/100 mmHg each time it is checked in the surgery over several weeks, in spite of salt and alcohol reduction. The patient buys a wrist blood pressure monitor in a pharmacy and takes several readings at home. These are all below 130/75 mmHg.

Question

What advice should he be given about the need for drug treatment?

Answer

He may have 'white coat' hypertension. Since this is associated with a lower risk than sustained hypertension he may not need drug treatment. However, before making this judgement it is important to check that his machine is accurate. This can be done by comparing readings with a validated machine, or by checking to see if the make of blood pressure monitor has been verified as accurate by the British Hypertension Society.

REFERENCES

ALLHAT Collaborative Research Group 2000 Major cardiovascular events in hypertensive patients randomised to doxazosin vs. chorthalidone. Antihypertensive and lipid lowering treatment to prevent heart attack trial (ALLHAT). Journal of the American Medical Association 283: 1967-1975

ALLHAT Officers and Coordinators for the ALLHAT Collaborative Research Group 2002 Major outcomes in high-risk hypertensive patients randomized to angiotensin-converting enzyme inhibitor or calcium channel blocker vs diuretic: the antihypertensive and lipid lowering treatment to prevent heart attack trial (ALLHAT). Journal of the American Medical Association 288: 2981-2997

Amery A, Birkenhäger W, Brixko P et al 1985 Mortality and morbidity results from the European working party on high blood pressure in the elderly trial. Lancet i: 1349-1354

Anon 1977 Report of the Joint National Committee on detection, evaluation, and treatment of high blood pressure: a cooperative study. Journal of the American Medical Association 237: 255-261

Anon 1980 Australian therapeutic trial in mild hypertension: report by the management committee. Lancet 1: 1261-1267

Beevers G, Lip G Y H, O'Brien E 2001 The pathophysiology of hypertension. British Medical Journal 322: 912-916

Blood Pressure Lowering Treatment Trialists Collaboration 2000 Effects of ACE inhibitors, calcium antagonists, and other blood pressure lowering drugs: results of prospectively designed overviews of randomized trials. Lancet 356: 1955-1964

Brown M J, Palmer C R, Castaigne A et al 2000 Morbidity and mortality in patients randomised to double blind treatment with a long acting calcium channel blocker or diuretic in the international nifedipine GITS study (INSIGHT). Lancet 356: 366-372

Collins R, Petro R, MacMahon S et al 1990 Blood pressure, stroke and coronary heart disease. Part 2. Short-term reductions in blood pressure: overview of randomised drugs trials in their epidemiological context. Lancet 335: 827-838

Dahlöf B, Lindholm L H, Hansson L et al 1991 Morbidity and mortality in the Swedish Trial of Old Patients with hypertension (STOP-Hypertension). Lancet 338: 1281-1285

Dahlöf B, Devereux R, Kjeldsen S E et al 2002 Cardiovascular morbidity and mortality in the Losartan For Endpoint reduction in hypertension study (LIFE): a randomised trial against atenolol. Lancet 359: 995-1003

Dahlöf B, Sever P S, Poulter N R et al, ASCOT Investigators 2005 Prevention of cardiovascular events with an antihypertensive regimen of amlodipine adding perindopril as required versus atenolol adding bendroflumethiazide as required, in the Anglo Scandinavian Cardiac Outcomes Trial – Blood Pressure Lowering Arm (ASCOT–BPLA). Lancet 366: 895-906

Estacio R O, Barrett M D, Jeffers W et al 1998 The effect of nisoldipine as compared with enalapril on cardiovascular outcomes in patients with non-insulin dependent diabetes and hypertension. New England Journal of Medicine 338: 645-681

Furberg C D, Psaty B M, Meyer J V 1995 Nifedipine: dose-related increase in mortality in patients with coronary heart disease. Circulation 92: 1326-1331

Gong L, Zhang W, Zhu Y et al 1996 Shanghai Trial Of Nifedipine in the Elderly (STONE). Journal of Hypertension 14: 1237-1245

Hansson L, Zanchetti A, Carruthers S G et al for the HOT Study Group 1998 Effects of intensive blood-pressure lowering and low-dose aspirin in patients with hypertension: principal results of the hypertension optimal treatment (HOT) randomised trial. Lancet 351: 1755-1762

Hansson L, Lindholm L H, Ekbom T et al 1999a Randomised trial of old and new antihypertensive drugs in elderly patients: cardiovascular mortality and morbidity in the Swedish Trial in Old Patients with hypertension-2 study. Lancet 354: 1751-1756

Hansson L, Lindholm L H, Niskanen L et al 1999b Effect of angiotensin-converting-enzyme inhibition compared with conventional therapy on cardiovascular morbidity and mortality in hypertension. The Captopril Prevention Project (CAPPP). Lancet 353: 611-616

Joint British Societies 2005 JBS 2: Joint British Societies' guidelines on prevention of cardiovascular disease in clinical practice. Heart 91: v1-v52

Julius S, Kjeldsen S E, Weber M et al 2004 Outcomes in hypertensive patients at high cardiovascular risk treated with regimens based on valsartan or amlodipine: the VALUE randomised trial. Lancet 363: 2022-2031

Lindholm L H, Carlberg B, Samuelsson O 2005 Should beta blockers remain first choice in the treatment of primary hypertension? A meta-analysis. Lancet 366: 1545-1553

Lithell H, Hansson L, Skoog I et al, SCOPE Study Group 2003 The Study of Cognition and Prognosis in the Elderly (SCOPE): principal results of a randomised double-blind intervention trial. Journal of Hypertension 21: 875-866

Liu L, Wang J G, Gong L et al, for the Systolic Hypertension in China (Syst-China) Collaborative Group 2003 Comparison of active treatment and placebo for older Chinese patients with isolated systolic hypertension. Journal of Hypertension 16: 1823-1829

Medical Research Council Working Party 1985 MRC trial of treatment of mild hypertension: principal results. British Medical Journal 291: 97-104

Medical Research Council Working Party 1992 MRC trial of treatment of hypertension in older adults: principal results. British Medical Journal 304: 405-412

National Collaborating Centre for Chronic Conditions 2006 Hypertension. Management of hypertension in adults in primary care: partial update. Royal College of Physicians, London. Available online at: www.nice.org.uk/page.aspx?o=CG034fullguideline

National Institute for Health and Clinical Excellence 2004 Evidence-based clinical practice guideline. Essential hypertension; managing adult patients in primary care. National Institute for Health and Clinical Excellence, London. Available online at: www.nice.org.uk/download.aspx?o=CG018fullguideline

PROGRESS Collaborative Group 2001 Randomised trial of a perindopril-based blood pressure lowering regimen amoung 6105 individuals with previous stroke or transient ischaemic attack. Lancet 358: 1033-1041

Psaty B M, Heckbert S R, Kocpsell T D et al 1995 The risk of myocardial infarction associated with antihypertensive drug therapies. Journal of the American Medical Association 274: 620-625

Seux M-L, Forette F, Staessent J A et al 1999 Treatment of isolated systolic hypertension and dementia prevention in older patients. European Society of Cardiology 1 (suppl M): M6-M12

Sever P S, Dahlof B, Poulter N R et al 2003 Prevention of coronary and stroke events with atorvastatin in patients who have average or lower-than-average cholesterol concentrations in the Anglo Scandinavian Cardiac Outcomes Trial – Lipid Lowering Arm. Lancet 361: 1149-1158

SHEP Co-operative Research Group 1991 Prevention of stroke by antihypertensive drug treatment in older persons with isolated systolic hypertension: final results of the Systolic Hypertension in the Elderly Program (SHEP). Journal of the American Medical Association 265: 3255-3264

Staessen J A, Fagard R, Thijs L et al for the Systolic Hypertension in Europe (Syst-Eur) Trial Investigators 1997 Randomised double-blind comparison of placebo and active treatment for older patients with isolated systolic hypertension. Lancet 350: 757-764

Tatti P, Pahor M, Byington R P et al 1998 Outcome results of the Fosinopril versus Amlodipine Cardiovascular Events randomised Trial (FACET) in patients with hypertension and NIDDM. Diabetes Care 21: 597-603

UK Prospective Diabetes Study Group 1998a Tight blood pressure control and risk of macrovascular and microvascular complications in type 2 diabetes: UKPDS 38. British Medical Journal 317: 703-713

UK Prospective Diabetes Study Group 1998b Efficacy of atenolol and captopril in reducing risk of macrovascular and microvascular complications in type 2 diabetes: UKPDS 39. British Medical Journal 317: 713-726

Veterans Administration Co-operative Study Group on Antihypertensive Agents 1970 Effects of treatment on morbidity in hypertension II. Results in patients with diastolic blood pressure averaging 90 through 114 mm Hg. Journal of the American Medical Association 213: 1143-1152

Williams B, Poulter N R, Brown M J et al 2004a Guidelines for the management of hypertension: report of the fourth working party of the British Hypertension Society, 2004 – BHS IV. Journal of Human Hypertension 18: 139-185

Williams B, Poulter N R, Brown M J et al 2004b The BHS Guidelines Working Party. British Hypertension Society guidelines for hypertension management, 2004 – BHS IV: Summary. British Medical Journal 328: 634-640

Wing L M H, Reid C M, Ryan P et al 2003 A comparison of outcomes with angiotensin-converting-enzyme inhibitors and diuretics for hypertension in the elderly. New England Journal of Medicine 348: 583-592

FURTHER READING

Beevers G, Lip G Y H, O'Brien E 2001 ABC of hypertension, 4th edn. BMJ Publications, London

Brown M J, Cruickshank J K, Dominiczak A F et al 2003 Better blood pressure control: how to combine drugs. Journal of Human Hypertension 17: 81-86

Grahame-Smith D G, Aronson J K 2002 The drug therapy of cardiovascular disorders: hypertension. In: Oxford textbook of clinical pharmacology and drug therapy, 3rd edn. Oxford University Press, Oxford, pp. 226-233

Hollenberg N K 2006 Atlas of hypertension, 5th edn. Current Medicine, USA

Mohler E R, Townsend R R 2005 Advanced therapy in hypertension and vascular disease. BC Decker Inc, Hamilton, Ontario

Safar M, O'Rourke M 2006 Arterial stiffness in hypertension. Elsevier, Oxford

20 Coronary heart disease

D. K. Scott   J. Dwight

Coronary heart disease (CHD), sometimes described as coronary artery disease (CAD), is a condition in which the vascular supply to the heart is impeded by atheroma, thrombosis or spasm of coronary arteries. This may impair the supply of oxygenated blood to cardiac tissue sufficiently to cause myocardial ischaemia which, if severe or prolonged, may cause the death of cardiac muscle cells, i.e. a myocardial infarction (MI). CHD kills over 6.5 million people worldwide each year. Less commonly, myocardial ischaemia can also arise if oxygen demand is abnormally increased, as may occur in severe ventricular hypertrophy due to hypertension, or where the oxygen-carrying capacity of blood is impaired, as in iron deficiency anaemia. The term ischaemic heart disease (IHD) may be used to include all causes of myocardial ischaemia.

Epidemiology

The epidemiology of CHD has been studied extensively and has led to much debate concerning the associated risk factors. Absence of established risk factors does not guarantee freedom from CHD for any individual, and some individuals with several major risk factors seem perversely healthy. Nonetheless, there is evidence that in developed countries, education and publicity about the major risk factors have led to changes in social habits, particularly with respect to a reduction in smoking and fat consumption, and this has contributed to a decrease in the incidence of CHD. The UK has had a steady decline in CHD deaths of about 4% per annum since the late 1970s. This improvement has been chiefly among those with higher incomes, however, and the less prosperous social classes continue to have almost unchanged levels of CHD. Better treatment has also contributed to a decrease in cardiac mortality although CHD still accounted for some 114 000 deaths in 2003 in the UK, including 70% of sudden natural deaths, 22% of male deaths and 16% of female deaths. In most developed countries, CHD is the leading cause of adult death but in the UK the poor outcome of lung cancer treatments makes cancer marginally the leading cause. In the UK, in comparison with caucasians, people of South Asian descent have a 45–50% higher death rate from CHD and Caribbeans and West Africans have a 35–50% lower rate.

About 3.5% of UK adults have symptomatic CHD. One-third of 50–59-year-old men have evidence of CHD, and this proportion increases with age. In the UK, there are about 1.3 million people who have survived a myocardial infarction and about 2 million who have, or have had, angina, about 5% of men and 3% of women. Approximately 260 000 experience a myocardial infarction in any year, of whom 40–50% die.

The increase in mortality with age is probably not due to a particular age-related factor but to the cumulative effect of risk factors that lead to atheroma and thrombosis and hence to coronary artery disease. In the USA, age-related death rates for CHD have fallen by 25% over a decade, but the total number of CHD deaths has fallen by only 10% because the population is ageing. Similarly, in the UK the death rates are falling but the numbers living with disease are increasing. The main risk factors are family history, hypertension, cigarette smoking and raised plasma cholesterol. Of these, the determining factor appears to be plasma cholesterol, because hypertension and smoking have little effect on the incidence of CHD in populations with low average cholesterol concentrations but a major effect in populations such as the UK with high cholesterol levels.

Other lipid-related risk factors include elevated plasma triglyceride concentrations, high saturated fat intake and a high saturated:polyunsaturated dietary fat ratio. These and other dietary factors, including energy intake and obesity, are difficult to separate out since they are all interrelated. However, it is clear that obese people have a higher risk of CHD, whatever the prime cause, and all dietary factors should be addressed simultaneously in an attempt to decrease risk. Low-fat diets are recommended whilst a number of studies have suggested a benefit from diets containing large quantities of fruit, vegetables and antioxidants (vitamins C and E and β-carotene). Unfortunately, prevention studies with pharmacological doses of these antioxidants have not shown the same benefit, and therefore dietary supplements cannot be justified although most authorities recommend at least five portions of fruit and vegetables each day. Similarly, high plasma homocysteine levels are associated with, but not proven to cause, CHD and this is of particular interest because levels may be reduced very easily by oral folic acid supplements. A study of folic acid supplementation in patients after MI successfully reduced homocysteine levels but failed to reduce the risk of a further infarction or stroke. These data reinforce the importance of not drawing oversimplified conclusions from epidemiological research.

Women appear to be less susceptible to CHD than men although they seem to lose this protection after the menopause, presumably because of hormonal changes. Race has not proved to be a clear risk factor since the prevalence of CHD seems to depend much more strongly on location and lifestyle than on ethnic origin or place of birth. It has been shown that lower social or economic class was associated with increased obesity, poor cholesterol indicators, higher blood pressure and higher C-reactive protein measurements (CRP), an indicator of inflammatory activity. It is not therefore surprising that there is increased cardiac morbidity and mortality in those classes; age-standardized CHD death rates in manual workers are 58% higher than non-manual workers.

Diabetes mellitus is a positive risk factor in developed countries with high levels of CHD but not in countries with little CHD. Insulin resistance, as defined by high fasting insulin concentrations, is an independent risk factor for CHD in men. While unusual physical exertion is associated with an increased risk of infarction, an active lifestyle that includes regular, moderate exercise is beneficial, although the optimum level has not been determined and its beneficial effect appears to be readily overwhelmed by the presence of other risk factors. A family history of CHD is a positive risk factor, independent of diet and other risk factors. Hostility, anxiety or depression are associated with increased CHD and death, especially after myocardial infarction when mortality is doubled by anxiety and quadrupled by depression. Epidemiological studies have shown associations between CHD and prior infections with several common microorganisms, including *Chlamydia pneumoniae* and *Helicobacter pylori*, but a causal connection has not been shown. The influence of fetal and infant growth conditions, and their interaction with social conditions in childhood and adult life, has been debated strongly for decades but it is clear that lower socio-economic status and thinness in very early life are linked to higher incidences of CHD (Barker et al 2001).

Aetiology

The vast majority of CHD occurs in patients with atherosclerosis of the coronary arteries (see Fig. 20.1) that starts before adulthood. The cause of spontaneous artherosclerosis is unclear, although it is thought that in the presence of hypercholesterolaemia a non-denuding form of injury occurs to the endothelial lining of coronary arteries and other vessels. This injury is followed by subendothelial migration of monocytes and the

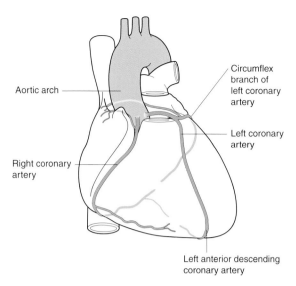

Figure 20.1 Main coronary arteries.

accumulation of fatty streaks containing lipid-rich macrophages and T-cells. Almost all adults, and 50% of children aged 11–14 years, have fatty streaks in their coronary arteries. Thereafter, there is migration and proliferation of smooth muscle cells into the intima with further lipid deposition. The smooth muscle cells, together with fibroblasts, synthesize and secrete collagen, proteoglycans, elastin and glycoproteins that make up a fibrous cap surrounding cells and necrotic tissue, together called a plaque. The presence of atherosclerotic plaques results in narrowing of vessels and a reduction in blood flow and this may become manifest as angina. Associated with the plaque is a loss of endothelium, which can serve as a stimulus for the formation of a thrombus and result in more acute manifestations of CHD, including unstable angina and myocardial infarction. Plaque rupture caused by physical stresses or plaque erosion may precipitate an acute reaction. Other pathological processes are probably involved, including endothelial dysfunction which alters the thrombosis–thrombolysis balance and the vasoconstriction–vasodilation balance. There is interest in the possible role of statins and angiotensin-converting enzyme (ACE) inhibitors in modifying endothelial function.

There is also great interest in the role of inflammation, especially in acute episodes. At postmortem, many plaques are found to contain inflammatory cells. Signs of inflammatory damage are found consistently at the sites of plaque rupture. Measures of acute phase inflammatory reactions, such as fibrinogen and CRP, have a predictive association with coronary events. High-sensitivity CRP assays have been used in populations without acute illness to stratify individuals into high-, medium- and low-risk groups. In patients with other risk factors, however, CRP adds little prognostic information. CRP is produced by atheroma, in addition to the major producer which is the liver, and is an inflammatory agent as well as a marker of inflammation. At present, although several classes of drug which are beneficial in CHD are known to reduce CRP, there is no specific therapeutic manoeuvre to reduce CRP and improve the risk level.

Oxidative stress, the uncontrolled production of reactive oxygen species (ROS) or a reduction in antioxidant species, has laboratory links to several aspects of cardiovascular pathogenesis including endothelial malfunction, lipid metabolism, atheroma formation and plaque rupture, but the clinical importance is unclear. The use of antioxidants has been disappointingly unsuccessful but there is interest in peroxisome proliferator-activated receptor (PPAR) agonists that modify ROS production; some of these are already in use for treating diabetes and are associated with favourable changes in many metabolic markers for cardiovascular disease. Other agents that reduce ROS production include statins and angiotensin antagonists.

Modification of risk factors

Common to all stages of CHD treatment is the need to reduce risk factors (Table 20.1). The patient needs to appreciate the value of the proposed strategy and to be highly committed to a plan for changing their lifestyle and habits, which may not be easy to achieve after years of smoking or of eating a particular diet. The professional carer must appreciate that preventing CHD is important but neither instant nor spectacular. It involves repeated sessions of counselling over many years to initiate and maintain healthy habits. It may also involve persuasion of patients to continue taking medication for asymptomatic disorders such as hypertension or hyperlipidaemia. The general public, with government as its agent, needs to agree that a reduction in the incidence of CHD is worth some general changes in lifestyle or liberty, such as limiting the freedom to smoke in public. National campaigns to encourage healthy eating or exercise are expensive, as is the long-term medical treatment of hypertension or hyperlipidaemia, and such strategies must have the backing of governments to succeed. It has been argued that community-wide campaigns on cholesterol reduction have had measurable benefits in Finland, the USA and elsewhere, at least in high-risk, well-educated and affluent groups. It follows that the next challenge is to extend that success to poorer, ethnically diverse groups and to those portions of the population with mild-to-moderate risk.

For every individual there is a need to act against the causative factors of CHD. Thus, attempts should be made to control or remedy hypertension, heart failure, arrhythmias, hyperlipidaemia, obesity, diabetes mellitus, thyroid disease, anaemia and cardiac valve disorders. Apart from medication, these will require careful attention to diet and exercise and will necessitate smoking cessation. Cardiac rehabilitation classes and exercise programmes improve many risk factors including obesity, lipid indices, insulin resistance, psychological state and lifestyle. They also have some measurable effects on morbidity and mortality (Lavie & Milani 2000). Similar strategies for primary prevention have not been subjected to appropriate trials.

Lipid management in coronary disease.

Lipid-related factors are of paramount importance in CHD and guidelines for patient management are being updated each year. A full treatment of this topic is given in Chapter 24. It is now clear that there is no 'safe' level of cholesterol for patients with coronary artery disease and that there is a continuum of risk down to very low cholesterol levels. A target level of low-density lipoprotein cholesterol (LDL-C) of <2 mmol/L appears to be appropriate on the basis of recent clinical trial evidence (JBS 2 2005). This is rarely achievable by diet alone which at best can achieve a 10% reduction in total cholesterol. Most protocols now recommend that all patients with coronary heart disease should be on a statin regardless of their starting cholesterol level. This is related not only to the effects of these agents on cholesterol lowering but also to other effects on the disease process (see below). Other therapeutic lipid-lowering strategies, such as fibrates and nicotinic acid therapy, may have a role in the management of these patients but in general have less trial data and are not used routinely in all patients.

Antioxidants and hormone replacement therapy

Epidemiological studies suggested that antioxidants and hormone replacement therapy may be of benefit in preventing and treating coronary disease. Unfortunately, separate randomized clinical trials of vitamin E and hormone replacement therapy suggest that

Table 20.1 Effect of interventions on risk of myocardial infarction

Intervention	Control	Benefit of intervention
Stopping smoking for ≥ 5 years	Current smokers	50–70% lower risk
Reducing plasma cholesterol plasma		2% lower risk for each 1% reduction in cholesterol
Treatment of hypertension		2–3% lower risk for each 1 mmHg decrease in diastolic pressure
Active lifestyle	Sedentary lifestyle	45% lower risk
Mild to moderate alcohol consumption (approx. 1 unit/day)	Total abstainers	25–45% lower risk
Low-dose aspirin	Non-users	33% lower risk in men
Postmenopausal oestrogen replacement	Non-users	44% lower risk

The quality of data leading to these summaries varies greatly and figures may not apply to all patient groups

these agents are not of benefit and may indeed result in higher rates of cardiovascular events.

Whilst the use of antioxidants has been disappointingly unsuccessful there is interest in PPAR agonists that modify ROS production; some of these are already in use for treating diabetes and are associated with favourable changes in many metabolic markers for cardiovascular disease. There is also evidence that brief periods of ischaemia, followed by reperfusion, confer a protective effect on myocardial tissue and reduce the extent of subsequent infarctions. This process, ischaemic pre-conditioning, may involve adenosine and potassium channel activation; the consequences for therapy are unclear but there may be a theoretical advantage from the use of potassium channel openers such as nicorandil in patients with established coronary disease.

Clinical syndromes

The primary clinical manifestation of CHD is chest pain. Chest pain arising from stable coronary atheromatous disease leads to stable angina and normally arises when narrowing of the coronary artery lumen exceeds 50% of the original luminal diameter. Stable angina is characterized by chest pain and breathlessness on exertion; symptoms are relieved promptly by rest.

A stable coronary atheromatous plaque may become unstable as a result of either plaque erosion or rupture. Exposure of the subendothelial lipid and collagen stimulates the formation of thrombus which causes sudden narrowing of the vessel. The spectrum of clinical outcomes that results is grouped together under the term acute coronary syndromes (ACS) which are characterized by chest pain of increasing severity either on minimal exertion or, more commonly, at rest. These patients are at high risk of myocardial infarction and death and require prompt hospitalization. Many aspects of the treatment of stable angina and ACS are similar but there is a much greater urgency and intensity in the management of ACS.

Stable angina

The pain of stable angina is usually described as a tightness or heaviness in the chest. This discomfort may radiate to the arms, neck, jaw or teeth. Characteristically the discomfort (it is often not described by the patient as a pain) occurs after a predictable level of exertion, classically when climbing hills or stairs, and resolves within a few minutes on resting. Unfortunately, the clinical manifestations of angina are very variable. Many patients mistake the discomfort for indigestion. Some patients, particularly diabetics and the elderly, may not experience pain at all but present with breathlessness or fatigue; this is termed silent ischaemia.

Further investigations are needed to confirm the diagnosis and assess the need for intervention. The electrocardiogram is normal in more than half of patients with angina. However, an abnormal ECG substantially increases the probability of coronary disease; in particular, it may show signs of previous myocardial infarction. Non-invasive testing is helpful. Exercise testing is useful both in confirming the diagnosis and in giving a guide to prognosis. Alternatives such as myocardial scintigraphy (isotope

scanning) and stress echocardiography (ultrasound) provide similar information. Coronary angiography is regarded as the gold standard for the assessment of coronary artery disease and involves the passage of a catheter through the arterial circulation and the injection of radio-opaque contrast media into the coronary arteries. The x-ray images obtained permit confirmation of the diagnosis, aid assessment of prognosis and guide therapy, particularly with regard to suitability for angioplasty and coronary artery bypass grafting. Non-invasive techniques, including magnetic resonance imaging (MRI) and multi-slice CT scanning, are being developed and tested as alternatives to angiography.

Treatment of stable angina is based on three principles:

- modification of risk factors
- modification of the disease process
- symptomatic treatment.

It can normally be managed by a primary care doctor or in an outpatient clinic and standard treatment should follow the ABCDE approach.

- **A**spirin and **A**ntianginals
- β-blockers and **B**lood pressure control
- **C**holesterol management and **C**igarette cessation
- **D**ietary improvements and **D**iabetes control
- **E**ducation and **E**xercise

Modification of the disease process

Aspirin and clopidogrel One of the major complications arising from atheromatous plaque is thrombus formation. This causes an increase in the plaque size and may result in myocardial infarction. Antiplatelet agents, in particular aspirin, are effective in preventing platelet activation and thus thrombus formation. Aspirin is of proven benefit in all forms of CHD.

Aspirin acts by acetylating several compounds in the thrombotic cascade, thus reducing thromboxane in platelets (see Chapter 23). This antiplatelet action is apparent within an hour of taking a dose of 300 mg. The effect on platelets lasts for the lifetime of the platelet and maintenance doses of 75–162.5 mg daily are used, depending on the tablet strength available, to deal with newly formed platelets. There is good evidence that low doses are just as effective as higher doses and have a lower risk of gastrointestinal haemorrhage. Enteric-coated preparations are no safer but it is customary to advise patients to take aspirin with food or dissolved in water and with food. Contraindications to aspirin include known allergy, including bronchospasm, and a history of gastrointestinal bleeding, while dispersible tablets should be dissolved in water before ingesting.

Clopidogrel inhibits ADP activation of platelets and is useful as an alternative to aspirin in patients who are allergic or cannot tolerate aspirin. Data from one major trial (CAPRIE Steering Committee 1996) indicate that clopidogrel is at least as effective as aspirin in patients with stable coronary disease. The usual dose is 300 mg once, then 75 mg daily. Although less likely to cause gastric erosion and ulceration, gastrointestinal bleeding is still a major complication of clopidogrel therapy and there is evidence that the combination of a proton pump inhibitor and aspirin is as effective and less costly than using clopidogrel alone in those patient with a history of upper gastrointestinal bleeding.

ACE inhibitors   ACE inhibitors have been used in the treatment of myocardial infarction for more than 10 years and in the management of heart failure for more than 20 years. ACE inhibitors have anti-inflammatory, antithrombotic and antiproliferative properties, some of which are mediated by actions on vascular endothelium; these actions might be expected to be of benefit in all patients with coronary artery disease. These agents also reduce the production of reactive oxygen species.

Their use in patients without myocardial infarction or left ventricular damage is based on two trials: the HOPE study which studied ramipril and the EUROPA study which used perindopril. These trials also identified an incidental delay in the onset of diabetes mellitus in susceptible individuals which may be of long-term benefit to them.

The HOPE study, a secondary prevention trial, investigated the effect of an ACE inhibitor on patients over 55 years old who had known atherosclerotic disease or diabetes plus one other cardiovascular risk factor. The use of ramipril decreased the combined endpoint of stroke, myocardial infarction or cardiovascular death by approximately 22%. The benefits were independent of blood pressure reduction. This has major implications for the management of CHD patients, both for the decision to treat at all and the choice of treatment. At present the use of ACE inhibitors in patients with coronary disease, but without myocardial infarction, has general acceptance.

Statins   In addition to cholesterol-lowering properties, statins also have antithrombotic, anti-inflammatory and antiproliferative properties. They are also important in restoring normal endothelial function and inhibit the production of reactive oxygen species in the vessel wall. Most stable angina patients will be on statins for cholesterol-lowering effects but it is important to recognize that these drugs may have a beneficial effect independent of cholesterol lowering which makes them valuable even in patients with 'normal' cholesterol levels.

Symptomatic therapy

Drug treatment is directed towards decreasing the workload of the heart and, to a lesser extent, improving coronary blood supply; this should provide symptomatic relief and improve prognosis. Unless otherwise contraindicated, β-blockers are first-line agents for angina although they are contraindicated in the rare Prinzmetal's angina where coronary spasm is a major factor. Patients may dislike the side effects of β-blockers but should be urged to continue wherever reasonable. Nitrates, calcium channel blockers, or both, may be added. Verapamil and diltiazem should be avoided, or used with extreme care, with β-blockers but may be used where a β-blocker is contraindicated or not tolerated. Treatment of acute attacks is by small doses of sublingual nitrates. These may also be used prior to an activity such as walking that would be expected to cause an attack.

β-blockers   β-blockers are useful for preventing angina in exercise because they suppress the rise in blood pressure, reduce the resting heart rate and decrease the force of ejection in systole. The decreased heart rate not only reduces the energy demand but also permits better perfusion of the subendocardium by the coronary circulation. A β-blocker may also reduce energy demanding supraventricular or atrial arrhythmias and counteract the cardiac effects of hyperthyroidism or phaeochromocytoma.

While β-blockers are widely used, their tendency to cause bronchospasm and peripheral vascular spasm means that they are contraindicated in patients with asthma, and used with caution in chronic obstructive airways diseases and peripheral vascular disease as well as in acute heart failure and bradycardia. They are highly beneficial but used with caution in insulin-dependent diabetics, in whom the signs of a hypoglycaemic attack may be masked, and in patients with a history of heart block. Cardioselective agents such as atenolol, bisoprolol and metoprolol are preferred because of their reduced tendency to cause bronchoconstriction but that does not override this contraindication because no agent is completely specific for the heart. Agents with low lipophilicity, e.g. atenolol, penetrate the central nervous system (CNS) to a lesser extent than others, e.g. propranolol, metoprolol, and do not so readily cause the nightmares, hallucinations and depression that are sometimes found with lipophilic agents, which should not be used in patients with psychiatric disorders. CNS-mediated fatigue or lethargy is found in some patients with all β-blockers although it must be distinguished from that of myocardial suppression. β-blockers should not be stopped abruptly for fear of precipitating angina through rebound receptor hypersensitivity.

All β-blockers tend to reduce renal blood flow, but this is only important in renal impairment. Drugs eliminated by the kidney (Table 20.2) may need to be given at lower doses in renal impairment or in the elderly, who are particularly susceptible to the CNS-mediated lassitude. Drugs eliminated by the liver have a number of theoretical interactions with other agents that affect liver blood flow or metabolic rate, but these are rarely of clinical significance since the dose should be titrated to the effect. Likewise, although there is theoretical support for the use of agents with high intrinsic sympathomimetic activity (ISA) to reduce the incidence or severity of drug-induced heart failure, there is no β-blocker that is free from that problem, and clinical trials of drugs with ISA have generally failed to show any extra benefit.

Nitrates   Organic nitrates are valuable in angina because they dilate veins and thereby decrease preload, dilate arteries to a lesser extent and thereby decrease afterload, and promote flow in collateral coronary vessels, diverting blood from the epicardium to the endocardium. They are available in many forms but all relax vascular smooth muscle by releasing nitric oxide, which was formerly known as endothelium-derived relaxing factor, which acts via cyclic GMP. The production of nitric oxide from nitrates is probably mediated by intracellular thiols, and it has been observed that when tolerance to the action of nitrates occurs, a thiol donor (such as N-acetylcysteine) may partially restore the effectiveness of the nitrate. Antioxidants such as vitamin C have also been used.

Tolerance is one of the main limitations to the use of nitrates, which remain the most useful class of agents for symptom relief in all forms of angina. While it was formerly thought that it was important to have high blood levels of nitrate at all times, it is now recognized that tolerance develops rapidly, and a 'nitrate-free' period of a few hours in each 24-hour period is beneficial in maintaining the effectiveness of treatment. The nitrate-free period should coincide with the period of lowest risk, and this is usually night time, but not early morning which is a high risk period for infarction. Many patients receiving short-acting nitrates two or

Table 20.2 β-blockers: properties and pharmacokinetics

	Blockade	Lipophilicity	ISA	Oral absorption	Elimination
Acebutolol	β_1 (some β_2)	+	+	90%[a]	Active metabolite ($t_{1/2}$ 11–13 h, renal) Gut 50% $t_{1/2}$ 3–4 h
Atenolol	β_1	–	–	50%	Renal $t_{1/2}$ 5–7 h
Betaxolol	β_1	+	–	100%	Hepatic + renal $t_{1/2}$ 15 h
Bisoprolol	β_1	+	–	90%	Hapatic + renal $t_{1/2}$ 10–12 h
Carteolol	$\beta_1\,\beta_2$	–	++	80%	Hepatic + renal $t_{1/2}$ 3–7 h
Carvedilol	$\beta_1\,\beta_2\,\alpha_1$	+	–	80%[a]	Hepatic + renal $t_{1/2}$ 4–8 h
Celiprolol	$\beta_1\,\alpha_2$	–	β_2+	30–70%	Renal + gut $t_{1/2}$ 5–6 h
Esmolol	β_1	–	–	i.v.	Blood enzymes $t_{1/2}$ 9 min
Labetalol	$\beta_1\,\beta_2\,\alpha_1$	–	–	100%[a]	Hepatic $t_{1/2}$ 6–8 h
Metoprolol	β_1	+	–	95%[a]	Hepatic $t_{1/2}$ 3–4 h
Nadolol	$\beta_1\,\beta_2$	–	–	30%	Renal $t_{1/2}$ 16–18 h
Nebivolol	β_1	+	–	12–96%[b]	Hepatic $t_{1/2}$ 8–27 h[b]
Oxprenolol	$\beta_1\,\beta_2$	+	++	90%[a]	Hepatic + $t_{1/2}$ 1–2 h
Pindolol	$\beta_1\,\beta_2$	+	+++	90%	Hepatic + renal $t_{1/2}$ 3–4 h
Propranolol	$\beta_1\,\beta_2$	+	–	90%[a]	Hepatic $t_{1/2}$ 3–6 h
Sotalol	$\beta_1\,\beta_2$	–	–	70%	Renal $t_{1/2}$ 15–17 h
Timolol	$\beta_1\,\beta_2$	+	–	90%[a]	Hepatic + renal $t_{1/2}$ 3–4 h

All figures are approximate and subject to interpatient variability. Therapeutic ranges are not well defined.
ISA, intrinsic sympathomimetic activity; $t_{1/2}$, elimination half-life.
[a] Extensive first-pass metabolism may result in a significant decrease in bioavailability.
[b] Genetically determined groups of slow and fast metabolizers have been identified.

three times a day would do well to have their doses between 7 a.m. and 6 p.m. (say, 8 a.m. and 2 p.m. for isosorbide mononitrate), but this is generally not practised in unstable angina where there is no low-risk period and where continuous dosing is used, with increasing doses if tolerance develops.

There are many nitrate preparations available, including intravenous infusions, conventional or slow-release tablets and capsules, transdermal patches and ointments, sublingual tablets and sprays and adhesive buccal tablets. The majority of stable angina patients should be controlled by conventional tablets or capsules, which are cheap, can usually be administered 2–3 times daily and which permit a nitrate-free period at night. There is no advantage in using more than one preparation. Slow-release preparations and transdermal patches are expensive, do not generally offer such flexible dosing rates and may not permit a nitrate-free period. Ointments are messy, and buccal tablets are expensive and offer no real therapeutic advantage in regular therapy. Like

sublingual sprays and tablets, however, they have a rapid onset of action and the drug bypasses the liver, which has an extensive first-pass metabolic effect on oral nitrates. The sublingual preparations, whether sprays or suckable or chewable tablets, are used for the prevention or relief of acute attacks of pain but may elicit the two principal side effects of nitrates: hypotension with dizziness and fainting, and a throbbing headache. To minimize these effects, patients should be advised to sit down, rather than lie or stand, when taking short-acting nitrates, and to spit out or swallow the tablet once the angina is relieved. Sublingual glyceryl trinitrate tablets have a very short shelf-life on exposure to air and should be stored carefully and replaced frequently. All nitrates may also induce tachycardia.

Three main nitrates are used: glyceryl trinitrate (mainly for sublingual, buccal, transdermal and intravenous routes), isosorbide dinitrate and isosorbide mononitrate. All are effective if given in appropriate doses at suitable dose intervals (Table 20.3). Since

Table 20.3 Properties of commonly used nitrates

Drug	Speed of onset	Duration of action	Notes
Glyceryl trinitrate (GTN)			
Intravenous	Immediate	Duration of infusion	
Transdermal	30 min	Designed to release drug steadily for 24 h	Tolerance develops if applied continuously
SR tablets and capsules	Slow	8–12 h	
Sublingual tablets	Rapid (1–4 min)	Less than 30 min	Inactivated if swallowed Less effective if dry mouth
Spray	Rapid (1–4 min)	Less than 30 min	
Buccal tablets	Rapid (1–4 min)	4–8 h	Nearly as rapid in onset as sublingual tablets
Isosorbide dinitrate			
SR tablets	Similar to GTN		
Intravenous			
Sublingual	Slightly slower than GTN	As for GTN	
Chewable tablets	2–5 min	2–4 h	Less prone to cause headaches than sublingual tablets
Oral tablets	30–40 min	4–8 h	
Isosorbide mononitrate			
Oral tablets	30–40 min	6–12 h	
SR tablets or capsules	Slow	12–24 h	Some brands claim a nitrate-free period if given once daily

SR sustained-release.

isosorbide dinitrate is metabolized to the mononitrate, there is a preference for using the more predictable mononitrate, but this is not a significant clinical factor. A more relevant feature may be that whereas the dinitrate is usually given three or four times a day, the mononitrate is given once or twice a day. More expensive slow-release preparations exist for both drugs.

Nicorandil Nicorandil is a compound that exhibits the properties of a nitrate but which also activates ATP-dependent potassium channels. The IONA study (2002) compared nicorandil with placebo as 'add-on' treatment in 5126 high-risk patients with stable angina. The main benefit for patients in the nicorandil group was a reduction in unplanned admission to hospital with chest pain. The study did not tell us when to add nicorandil to combinations of antianginals such as β-blockers, calcium channel blockers and long-acting nitrates. There is a theoretical benefit from these agents in their action to promote ischaemic preconditioning. This phenomenon is seen when myocardial tissue is exposed to a period of ischaemia prior to sustained coronary artery occlusion. Prior exposure to ischaemia renders the myocardial tissue more resistant to permanent damage. This mechanism is mimicked by the action of nicorandil.

Calcium channel blockers Calcium channel blockers act on a variety of smooth muscle and cardiac tissues and there are a large number of agents which have differing specificities for different body tissues. Those of importance in angina are arterial vasodilators but some also possess antiarrhythmic activity, and most are myodepressants. Nifedipine, nicardipine and other dihydropyridines have no effect on the conducting tissues and are effective arterial dilators, decreasing afterload and

improving coronary perfusion but also causing flushing, headaches and reflex tachycardia. The tachycardia is overcome by use of a β-blocker. They have a particular role in the management of Prinzmetal's (variant) angina which is thought to be due to coronary artery spasm. Nicardipine has a smaller effect on myocardial contractility but neither drug has the myodepressant effect of diltiazem or verapamil, both of which have significant effects on conducting fibres and are not suitable for use in ventricular failure. Caution should be exercised in considering their use with β-blockers because of the additive effects on bradycardia and myodepression. Verapamil and diltiazem are suitable for patients in whom β-blockers are contraindicated on grounds of respiratory or peripheral vascular disease; the most important non-cardiovascular side effect is marked constipation.

There is concern over the use of dihydropyridine compounds because rapid-onset, short-acting drugs such as nifedipine stimulate the sympathetic nervous system by reflex mechanisms, and this may exacerbate heart failure or provoke CHD and increase mortality. Use of these compounds is now rare in heart failure and subject to caution in hypertension in the absence of β-blockade. Slow-release preparations of nifedipine or slower onset compounds such as amlodipine or felodipine are more acceptable although they also stimulate reflex activity. The extensive use of nifedipine that occurred in the past was based on efficacy in trials that used surrogate markers such as blood pressure or myocardial infarction instead of mortality as their endpoint medical.

Ivabridine represents a new class of antianginal agents which block the If current. These agents act by slowing the sinus node rate but are not negatively inotropic. Ivabridine is similar in efficacy to atenolol and may be of particular use in patients in whom beta blockers are contraindicated.

Acute coronary syndromes

Definitions and causes

Acute coronary syndromes arise from an unstable atheromatous plaque. The major feature of these lesions is the presence of overlying thrombus and associated inflammation of the vessel wall. Patients with acute coronary syndromes usually present with chest pain at rest and should be admitted to hospital for evaluation and treatment. The major difference in approach to these patients arises from whether the coronary artery involved is felt to be occluded or open.

Patients with an occluded coronary artery suffer myocardial damage, the extent of which is determined by the duration and site of the occlusion. The primary strategy for these patients is the restoration of coronary flow with either thrombolysis or primary angioplasty. If the coronary artery is patent, however, then therapy with thrombolysis is unnecessary and probably harmful, although angioplasty may still be appropriate. Once the vessel is open, for both groups of patients management then focuses on the unstable coronary plaque and is therefore fundamentally similar.

The most important tool to help identify those patients in whom an artery is occluded is the ECG. The presence of ST elevation on the ECG correlates with the presence of an occluded artery and is used to determine those patients who should receive thrombolysis or primary angioplasty. The presence of characteristic ST elevation on the ECG and ischaemic chest pain is nearly always associated with myocardial damage confirmed by measurement of elevated plasma levels of troponin or cardiac enzymes. These patients have therefore had an ST elevation MI (STEMI).

Patients without ST elevation on the ECG may still have experienced myocardial damage due to temporary occlusion of the vessel or emboli from the plaque-related thrombus blocking smaller distal vessels and will have raised levels of troponin. These patients have had a non-ST elevation MI (NSTEMI). Patients without ST elevation and without a rise in troponin or cardiac enzymes are defined as having unstable angina.

An international registry of 51 000 ACS patients from a representative selection of hospitals (GRACE registry: www.outcomes-umassmed.org/GRACE/index.cfm) indicated for 2005 a roughly equal incidence of STEMI, NSTEMI and unstable angina. The definition of myocardial infarction has been refined and now includes all patients with a history of cardiac chest pain or ECG changes and elevated serum troponin. Troponins (troponin I or troponin T) are cardiac muscle proteins which are released following myocardial cell damage and are highly sensitive and specific for myocardial infarction. They are useful in diagnosing patients with ACS and for predicting response to drug therapy; they are now key to the management of these patients and have replaced cardiac enzymes such as creatinine kinase (CK), aspartate transaminase (AST) and lactate dehydrogenase (LDH).

The classification of ACS based on ECG findings and troponin measurements is shown in Figure 20.2.

The prognosis of an individual who has suffered a STEMI has improved following the widespread use of thrombolytic therapy but some 25% of individuals will die before any medical intervention occurs and some 12–15% of patients admitted to hospital will die within 6 months. The most dangerous time after a myocardial infarction is the first few hours when ventricular fibrillation (VF) is most likely to occur, Perhaps surprisingly, the long-term prognosis in NSTEMI is similar to that of STEMI. The early adverse event rate is lower but these patients are more likely to suffer death, recurrent myocardial infarction or recurrent ischaemia after hospital discharge than patients with STEMI (GRACE registry). Recently greater emphasis has been placed on the importance of improving treatment in patients with NSTEMI.

Treatment of ST elevation myocardial infarction

Treatment of STEMI may be divided into three categories:

- immediate care that is designed to remove pain, prevent deterioration and improve cardiac function
- management of complications, notably heart failure and arrhythmias
- prevention of a further infarction or death (secondary prophylaxis).

The management of heart failure and arrhythmias is covered in Chapters 21 and 22 respectively. The remaining therapeutic aims are pain relief, thrombolysis, minimization of infarct size, prophylaxis of arrhythmias and secondary prevention.

The timing of treatment is vital, since myocardial damage after onset of an acute ischaemic episode is progressive and there are pathological data to suggest that it is irreversible at 6 hours. Clinical data from large studies of thrombolysis have shown that the sooner treatment is started after the onset of pain, the better, although there is still some worthwhile benefit up to 12 hours after infarction. Sixty percent of postinfarction deaths occur within 1 hour but while treatment within 1 hour has been found to be particularly advantageous, it is extremely difficult to achieve, for logistical reasons, in anyone who has an infarct outside hospital.

Pain relief should be administered rapidly with intravenous diamorphine or morphine together with an antiemetic such as prochlorperazine or cyclizine, and oxygen. There is no benefit in leaving a patient in pain while the diagnosis is considered. The rhythm and blood pressure should be stabilized and diagnostic tests performed.

Antiplatelet agents Several large studies have shown the benefit of an aspirin tablet chewed as soon after the infarct as possible and followed by a daily enteric-coated dose for at least 1 month. Follow-up studies show additional benefit in continuing to take daily aspirin, probably for life. The reduction in mortality is additional to that obtained from thrombolytic therapy (Table 20.4). Clopidogrel, given in addition to aspirin, improved a composite endpoint that included deaths and improved coronary artery blood flow in two major trials (COMMIT/CCS-2 and CLARITY TIMI-28) but the absolute reduction in mortality was small, at approximately 0.4% (Sabatine et al 2005).

Thrombolysis In patients with STEMI early restoration of coronary artery patency results in an improved outcome;

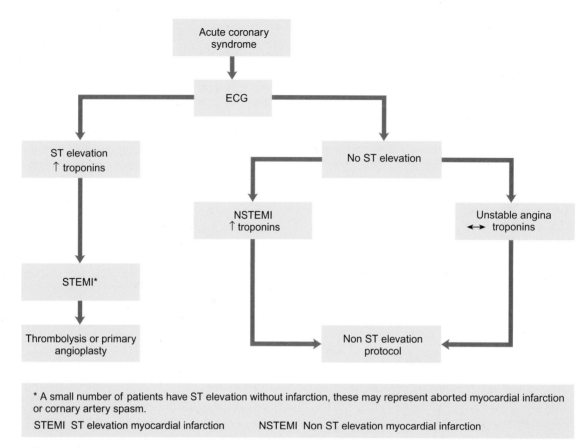

* A small number of patients have ST elevation without infarction, these may represent aborted myocardial infarction or cornary artery spasm.

STEMI ST elevation myocardial infarction   NSTEMI Non ST elevation myocardial infarction

Figure 20.2   Classification of ACS based on ECG and measurement of troponins.

this may occur spontaneously in some patients but frequently only after substantial damage has occurred. Thrombolytic agents (Table 20.5) have transformed the management of these patients by substantially improving coronary artery patency rates which has translated into a 25% relative reduction in mortality. Thrombolytic agents fall into two categories: fibrin specific (alteplase, tenecteplase and reteplase) and fibrin non-specific (streptokinase). There are theoretical advantages for the fibrin-specific agents which are superior in terms of achieving coronary artery patency in angiographic studies. Angiographic patency has been shown to correlate well with outcome in thrombolytic trials but it has been difficult to prove that this benefit translates into an improvement in mortality. Studies such as ISIS-3 and GISSI-2 demonstrated great benefit from thrombolytics given soon after the onset of pain but reveal little discernible difference between streptokinase and the more expensive tissue plasminogen

activator (rt-PA, duteplase, alteplase) in reducing mortality. The GUSTO study compared four thrombolytic regimens in a non-blinded trial and concluded that fast injection of rt-PA was better than slower infusion of streptokinase, especially in younger patients with anterior infarcts. Although the trial was large, its

Table 20.4   Vascular deaths at 35 days in the ISIS-2 study

Placebo	13.2%
Aspirin	10.7%
Streptokinase	10.4%
Aspirin + streptokinase	8.0%

Table 20.5   Fibrinolytic agents (thrombolytics)

	Fibrin specificity	Elimination	Half-life (mins)	Dosing	Antigenic	Mode of action
Streptokinase		Hepatic	18–23	1 h infusion	Yes	Activator complex
Alteplase	++	Hepatic	3–8	Bolus + 90 min infusion	No	Direct
Reteplase	+	Renal	15–18	Two boluses	No	Direct
Tenecteplase	+++	Hepatic	20–28	One bolus	No	Direct

conduct lead to controversy because of differences between results in North American centres and elsewhere.

All trials show that rapid treatment is important and that speed has a greater effect than the choice of drug; several studies indicate that giving thrombolytics an average 30–60 minutes earlier can save 15 lives per 1000 treated. Hospitals need to maintain fast-track systems to ensure maximum benefit. Further benefit is obtained if trained and appropriately equipped paramedics or primary care doctors administer thrombolytics before the patient goes to hospital, especially if the journey time is great. Tenecteplase and reteplase have been marketed with the advantage that they can be administered by bolus injection, which facilitates pre-hospital administration and reduces errors. The ASSENT 2 and GUSTO 3 studies demonstrated benefits and risks equivalent to alteplase when tenecteplase or reteplase respectively were administered with aspirin and heparin.

Patients receiving tPA also receive a 5000 unit heparin bolus followed by a 48-hour infusion adjusted to maintain the activated partial thromboplastin time (APTT) in the therapeutic range. It is not known whether low molecular weight heparin (LMWH) is superior to unfractionated heparin, although that is the inference from uncontrolled comparisons in the GRACE registry. Heparin has not been compared to placebo in trials of tenecteplase or reteplase but it is standard practice to use heparin with these agents. Heparin has no advantage with streptokinase which has a longer lasting and less specific fibrinolytic action.

Hirudin and bivalirudin are direct thrombin inhibitors, with a greater specificity for thrombus, although the increased risk of bleeding counteracts the benefits of increased vessel patency. Recent studies with newer thrombolytics and various dosing schedules, some with co-administration of glycoprotein IIb/IIIa inhibitors, have not found a regimen that increases overall survival (Menon et al 2004). All agents cause haemorrhage, which may present as a stroke or a gastrointestinal bleed, and there is an increased risk with regimens that use intravenous heparin. Recent strokes, bleeds, pregnancy and surgery are contraindications to thrombolysis. Streptokinase induces cross-reacting antibodies which reduce its potency and may cause an anaphylactoid response. Patients with exposure to streptokinase, or with a history of rheumatic fever or recent streptococcal infection, should not receive the drug. The use of hydrocortisone, to reduce allergic responses, has fallen out of favour, but patients should be carefully observed for hypotension during the administration of streptokinase.

Old age is no longer considered to be a contraindication to thrombolysis because although the risks are greater, the benefit is also greater, but the doses of alteplase and tenecteplase need to be adjusted for body weight.

All the major trials (see Table 20.6) used specific ECG criteria for entry, usually ST elevation in adjacent leads or left bundle branch block, and eliminated patients with major contraindications to thrombolysis (Table 20.7). Confusion often arises about the term 'relative contraindication'. For example, systolic hypertension is common in acute MI so most protocols recommend lowering the blood pressure with either a β-blocker or intravenous nitrates before commencing thrombolysis. Increasing numbers of patients are on warfarin and this again is regarded as a relative contraindication to thrombolysis; thresholds for the use of thrombolysis in patients on warfarin vary from an INR of 2 to 2.4. The use of thrombolytic therapy in patients with relative contraindications should take into account the site of the myocardial infarction and the likely size of the infarction. For example, in patients with a large anterior MI the benefits of thrombolysis may outweigh the risks. In patients where there is

Table 20.6 Major trials of management of acute myocardial infarction

Trial and number of patients	Intervention	Control	Main outcomes
MIAMI, 5778 (1985)	Intravenous metoprolol then oral	Placebo	↓ Mortality
ISIS-1, 16 027 (1986)	Intravenous atenolol then oral	Placebo	↓ Mortality
TIMI, 1390 (1989)	Intravenous metoprolol then oral	Later oral metoprolol	↓ Reinfarction
ISIS-2, 17 187 (1988)	Aspirin for 1 month Streptokinase	Placebo Placebo	↓ Mortality ↓ Mortality
GISSI, 11 806 (1986)	Streptokinase	Open control	↓ Mortality
GISSI-2, 12 381 (1990)	rt-PA Subcutaneous heparin	Streptokinase Placebo	No difference No benefit
ISIS-4, 41 229 (1992)	rt-PA vs. streptokinase vs. subcutaneous heparin	Anistreplase Placebo	No difference No benefit
GISSI-3, 19 394 (1994)	Glyceryl trinitrate patch Lisinopril	Placebo Placebo	No benefit ↓ mortality
ISIS-4, 58 050 (1995)	Isosorbide mononitrate Intravenous magnesium Captopril	Placebo Open control Placebo	No benefit No benefit ↓ Mortality

Table 20.6 (continued)

Trial and number of patients (date)	Intervention	Control	Main outcomes
GUSTO, 41 021 (1993)	Fast rt-PA + intravenous heparin	Slow rt-PA or streptokinase + s.c. or i.v. heparin	↓ Mortality
GUSTO IIb, 1138 (1997)	Primary angioplasty	Thrombolysis	Equivalence or small benefit
GUSTO 3, 15 059 (1997)	Two bolus reteplase	Fast rt-PA	Equivalence
ASSENT 2, 16 949 (1999)	Bolus tenecteplase	Fast rt-PA	Equivalence
OPTIMAAL, 5477 (2002)	Losartan	Captopril	Equivalence but fewer adverse effects
VALIANT, 14 703 (2003)	Valsartan / Valsartan plus captopril	Captopril / Captopril	Equivalence / Equivalence but more adverse effects

References

ASSENT 2 1999 Lancet 354: 710–722
MIAMI 1985 European Heart Journal 6: 199–226
TIMI 1989 New England Journal of Medicine 320: 618–627
GISSI 1987 Lancet 2: 871–874
GISSI-2 1990 Lancet 336: 65–71
GISSI-3 1994 Lancet 343: 1115–1122
GUSTO 1993 New England Journal of Medicine 329: 673–682
GUSTO IIb 1997 New England Journal of Medicine 336: 1621–1628

GUSTO 3 1997 New England Journal of Medicine 337: 1118–1123
ISIS-1 1986 Lancet 2: 56–66
ISIS-2 1990 Lancet 336: 71–75
ISIS-3 1992 Lancet 339: 753–770
ISIS-4 1995 Lancet 345: 669–685
OPTIMAAL 2002 Lancet 360: 752–760
VALIANT 2003 New England Journal of Medicine 349: 1893–1906

For other trials, as well as most of the above, see Fibrinolytic Therapy Trialists' Collaboration Group 1994.

Table 20.7 Contraindications to thrombolysis

Absolute contraindications

Haemorrhagic stroke of unknown origin at any time
Ischaemic stroke in preceding 6 months
Central nervous system damage or neoplasms
Recent major trauma/surgery/head injury (within preceding 3 weeks)
Known bleeding disorder
Aortic dissection

Relative contraindications

Transient ischaemic attack in preceding 6 months
Oral anticoagulant therapy
Pregnancy or within 1 week postpartum
Non-compressible punctures
Traumatic resuscitation
Refractory hypertension (systolic blood pressure >180 mmHg)

a serious concern regarding bleeding following thrombolysis, primary angioplasty should be considered.

β-blockers and calcium channel blockers β-blockers have been the subject of many studies because of their antiarrhythmic potential and because they permit increased subendocardial perfusion. In pre-thrombolysis studies, the early administration of an intravenous β-blocker was shown to limit infarct size and reduce mortality from early cardiac events. Long-term use of a β-blocker has been shown in several studies to decrease mortality in patients in whom there is no contraindication. β-blockade should be avoided in heart block, bradycardia, asthma, obstructive airways disease and peripheral vascular disease. The most convincing trial evidence concerns timolol at 5–10 mg twice a day, but other agents have been used successfully. Fears of inducing heart failure, especially in the elderly, have lead to a low usage of β-blockers or to the use of doses lower than those in the major trials. One large cohort study compared low and high doses of β-blockers with no therapy and found benefit in all treated patients with similar survival rates in the treated groups but a lower heart failure rate in the low-dose group (Rochon et al 2000).

A recent large-scale clinical trial has cast doubt on the use of intravenous β-blockade following myocardial infarction due to a reported increased incidence of cardiogenic shock (Chen et al 2005). Oral β-blockade, usually starting within 24 hours, is however regarded as standard therapy. If a β-blocker is contraindicated because of respiratory or vascular disorders, verapamil may be used, since it has been shown to reduce late mortality and reinfarction in patients without heart failure, although it showed no benefit when given immediately after an infarct. Diltiazem is less effective but may be used as an alternative. This is clearly not a class effect; other calcium channel blockers have produced different results and nifedipine increases mortality in patients following a myocardial infarction.

ACE inhibitors and angiotensin receptor blockers ACE inhibitors have been tried in various doses and durations and have proved beneficial in reducing the incidence of heart failure and mortality. In all but the earliest trials patients were given an ACE inhibitor for 4–6 weeks and treatment was continued in patients with signs or symptoms of heart failure or left ventricular dysfunction. The HOPE study (Yusuf et al 2000) found that ramipril improved survival in all groups of patients with CHD and this has lead clinicians to continue ACE inhibitors in all infarction patients over the age of 55 and in younger patients with evidence of left ventricular dysfunction. Contraindications to their use include hypotension and intractable cough.

Current research is focusing on the possible benefits of combining ACE inhibition with angiotensin II receptor blockers. Angiotensin blockade alone does not cause the accumulation of bradykinins that may be part of the benefit of ACE inhibitors, and clinical trials (OPTIMAAL Study Group 2002, VALIANT Investigators 2003) have failed to find a benefit over ACE inhibition. Nonetheless, angiotensin receptor blockers are probably suitable in patients who cannot tolerate an ACE inhibitor.

The relative benefits of ACE inhibitors and other treatments are shown in Table 20.8.

Insulin Patients with infarctions have high serum and urinary glucose levels, usually described as a stress response, while diabetics are known to do poorly after infarction. The DIGAMI trial involved patients with diabetes and showed that an intensive insulin regimen, both during admission and for 3 months afterwards, saved lives. The risk of dying was halved in patients who had not previously required insulin and who had few cardiovascular risk factors (Malmberg 1997). The promising results of this study were not, however, supported in a subsequent trial. (Malmberg et al 2005). Further work is required on defining the criteria for treatment, especially in patients who have a glucose stress response but no known diabetic history, since the presence of a stress response in a broader group of intensive care patients is itself associated with a poor outcome which is improved by intensive insulin therapy.

Table 20.8 Relative benefits of treating 1000 patients for myocardial infarction (MI)

Intervention	Events prevented
Intravenous β-adrenoceptor blocker	6 deaths
ACE inhibitor	6 deaths
Aspirin	20–25 deaths
Streptokinase (in hospital)	20–25 deaths
Alteplase (rt-PA) (in hospital)	35 deaths
Streptokinase (before hospital)	35–40 deaths
Thrombolysis 4½–1 hour earlier	15 deaths
Long-term aspirin	16 deaths/MI/strokes
Long-term β-blockade	18 deaths/MI
Long-term ACE inhibitor	21–45 deaths/MI
10% reduction in serum cholesterol	7 deaths/MI
Stopping smoking	27 deaths

Adapted from McMurray & Rankin (1994)

Antidepressants and rehabilitation A quarter of patients who have suffered a myocardial infarction subsequently experience marked depression. This is associated with poor medication compliance, a lower quality-of-life score, and a fourfold increase in mortality (Januzzi et al 2000). Antidepressant treatments have not been subjected to formal trials but it seems reasonable to try to reduce the depression. Rehabilitation programmes, which include some measure of social interaction and education, are of proven benefit. Although psychological stress clearly worsens outcomes, stress reduction interventions have not been tested and proven to work independently of other measures.

Nitrates, anticoagulation and other therapies Studies on nitrates in myocardial infarction were mostly completed before thrombolysis was widely used. Nitrates improve collateral blood flow and aid reperfusion, thus limiting infarct size and preserving functional tissue. ISIS-4 (1993) and GISSI-3 (1994) demonstrated that nitrates did not confer a survival advantage in patients receiving thrombolysis. Sublingual nitrates may be given for immediate pain relief, and the use of intravenous or buccal nitrates can be considered in patients whose infarction pain does not resolve rapidly or who develop ventricular failure.

Anticoagulation with warfarin is not generally recommended, despite promising results in trials that have practised exceptionally good anticoagulant monitoring. This is partly because of the success of aspirin therapy, which does not have the same need for expensive and time-consuming follow-up and monitoring as warfarin, and is associated with fewer drug interactions. Routine use of dipyridamole and sulfinpyrazone is not recommended after infarction. Clopidogrel has been shown to be beneficial, in addition to aspirin, in patients who have had a myorcardial infarction (COMMIT 2005).

Statins should be initiated early after an MI even though the lipid-lowering actions may not reveal themselves for some time. There is a mortality benefit to early use which presumably depends on other mechanisms. Magnesium infusions looked promising when given early after infarction in trials involving approximately 2000 patients. However, in ISIS-4, a trial involving 41000 patients, where the average delay to injection was longer, there was no reduction in mortality. Antiarrhythmics generally increase mortality and arrhythmias in postmyocardial infarction patients. They should only be used for symptomatic arrhythmias (see Chapter 22).

Early studies suggest that patients with heart failure or left ventricular dysfunction may benefit from eplerenone, an aldosterone antagonist, in addition to an ACE inhibitor and a β-blocker.

Mechanical intervention The role of early coronary artery bypass grafting and percutaneous transluminal angioplasty (PCTA), which involves the expansion of constricted vessels by a balloon device, in comparison to thrombolysis is controversial. These techniques (see Fig. 20.3) work better in well-equipped and experienced centres where both cardiac and surgical staff are available. In such circumstances PCTA is as good as thrombolysis at decreasing 30-day mortality, and better with regard to some other endpoints.

Treatment of non-ST elevation acute coronary syndromes

ACS without ST elevation is classified as either unstable angina or NSTEMI. At presentation unstable angina and NSTEMI are

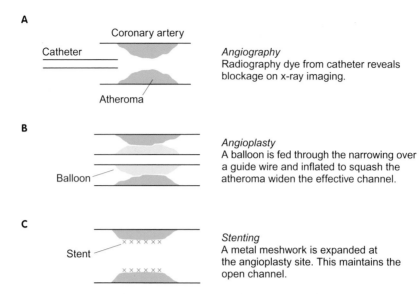

A

Coronary artery

Catheter

Atheroma

Angiography
Radiography dye from catheter reveals blockage on x-ray imaging.

B

Balloon

Angioplasty
A balloon is fed through the narrowing over a guide wire and inflated to squash the atheroma widen the effective channel.

C

Stent

Stenting
A metal meshwork is expanded at the angioplasty site. This maintains the open channel.

Figure 20.3 Procedures to overcome narrowing in atheromatous coronary vessels. The catheter is inserted from the femoral, radial or brachial arteries into the aorta and then into the coronary arteries.

indistinguishable but differ in severity of myocardial ischaemia (Table 20.9). In NSTEMI the ischaemia is severe enough to release markers of myocardial injury such as troponin I or T into the blood and these are measured 6–12 hours after the onset of pain. The death or infarction rate at 1 month is about 15–20% in some NSTEMI series compared to about 8% in unstable angina alone. One in eight NSTEMI patients will die within 6 months and one in five will have an emergency readmission to hospital. Treatment strategies differ according to the risk stratification of the patient; for example, glycoprotein IIb/IIIa antagonists appear to confer a survival advantage only in those patients who are at high risk (Fig. 20.4).

In the treatment of NSTEMI several agents are given simultaneously, rather than by stepwise addition, including oxygen, antiplatelet agents and nitrate infusions.

Aspirin has been shown to decrease the rate of myocardial infarction and death by 50% in patients with unstable angina and is recommended even in those patients where the diagnosis of coronary heart disease is uncertain.

Heparin confers additional benefit over aspirin in unstable angina (Table 20.10) but there is little evidence to support the subsequent use of oral warfarin because of the increased risk of bleeding. Comparative trials of LMWH versus unfractionated heparin indicate that LMWH is at least as effective and may be superior. Heparin therapy is usually continued for a minimum of 48 hours after presentation or until the patient has stabilized or undergone revascularization. Thrombolysis is ineffective in these patients and may be harmful.

Adding clopidogrel to aspirin is based on the CURE study where clopidogrel was given with aspirin for 3–12 months (CURE Trial Investigators 2001). Current recommendations are for 9–12 months combined therapy starting after angiography, or immediately if angiography is not expected soon, and followed by life-long aspirin (Harrington et al 2004). Clopidogrel should be stopped 5 days before CABG procedures to reduce the risk of bleeding.

Table 20.9 Examples of high-risk patients with NSTEMI
Patients with recurrent ischaemia
Recurrent chest pain
Dynamic ECG changes (ST segment depression or transient ST segment elevation)
Early postinfarction unstable angina
Extent of elevated troponin levels
Diabetes
Haemodynamic instability
Major arrhythmias (VF or VT)

Statins have also been shown to benefit patients when given early in ACS and are usually started on admission if the diagnosis of coronary artery disease is definite.

Glycoprotein IIb/IIIa inhibitors Glycoprotein IIb/IIIa inhibitors bind to the IIb/IIIa receptors on platelets (Fig. 20.5) and prevent cross-linking of platelets by fibrinogen. There are three classes of these agents: murine-human chimeric antibodies, e.g. abciximab, synthetic peptides, e.g. eptifibatide, and non-peptide synthetics, e.g. tirofiban and lamifiban. Trials of these agents in ACS (Boersma et al 2002) have yielded variable results. The synthetic peptide and non-peptide forms appear to confer advantages to patients with high-risk ACS if given intravenously soon after presentation. Oral agents are ineffective and the murine-human chimeric antibodies appear to be effective only in the context of percutaneous coronary intervention.

Interventional and adjuvant therapies in acute coronary syndromes Evidence has accumulated for the use of

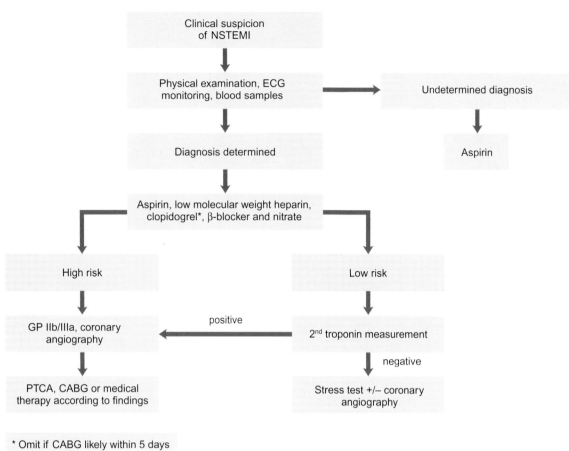

Figure 20.4 Algorithm for the management of patients with NSTEMI.

Table 20.10 Criteria that influence decision to use unfractionated heparin (UFH) or LMWH

- UFH is given intravenously or subcutaneously but, because of highly variable absorption and protein binding, has an unpredictable effect; control of therapy requires repeated measurement of APTT and this is often not done properly in real-life practice.

- LMWH are given subcutaneously once or twice daily and are much more predictable in effect; routine monitoring is not required. Different brands of LMWH vary in their composition and potency in laboratory tests but all are at least equivalent to UFH for efficacy and safety and are thus preferred because of their greater convenience and reduced monitoring. In some situations, LMWH give better outcomes and are preferred for that reason too, e.g. enoxaparin in NSTEMI.

- LMWH are not so easily reversed quickly, before an operation for example, and if an operation is anticipated UFH may be preferred.

- All heparins may cause thrombocytopenia and the immune-mediated heparin induced thrombocytopenia can be severe. Platelet counts should be monitored in anyone who is on heparin for 5 days or more.

PTCA in both STEMI and NSTEMI. Thrombolysis for STEMI has two potential drawbacks. The first is the risk of haemorrhagic stroke (around 1%) and the second a failure to adequately reperfuse the affected myocardium in approximately 50% of cases. PTCA, termed primary angioplasty when used in the context of STEMI, has the theoretical advantage of achieving adequate coronary flow in over 90% of cases and has therefore been compared to thrombolysis in a number of trials. A meta-analysis of these trials suggests that primary angioplasty was better than thrombolytic therapy at reducing overall short-term death (7% versus 9%), non-fatal reinfarction (3% versus 7%),

and stroke (1% versus 2%) (Keeley et al 2003). The success of primary angioplasty is dependent upon rapid patient transfer to a centre with skilled operators and good angiography facilities but it appears likely that primary angioplasty will supplant thrombolysis in many areas.

There is also a role for PTCA (rescue angioplasty) in the management of patients who fail to reperfuse following thrombolytic therapy. These patients continue to have ST elevation on their ECG and remain in pain. Rescue angioplasty has been studied in two trials: MERLIN (Sutton et al 2004) and REACT (Luepker et al 2000), and appears to confer some advantage.

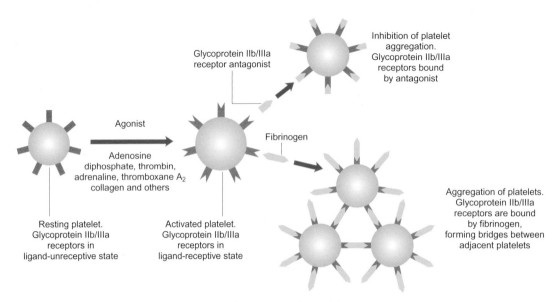

Inhibition of platelet aggregation. Glycoprotein IIb/IIIa receptors bound by antagonist

Glycoprotein IIb/IIIa receptor antagonist

Agonist

Adenosine diphosphate, thrombin, adrenaline, thromboxane A$_2$ collagen and others

Fibrinogen

Resting platelet. Glycoprotein IIb/IIIa receptors in ligand-unreceptive state

Activated platelet. Glycoprotein IIb/IIIa receptors in ligand-receptive state

Aggregation of platelets. Glycoprotein IIb/IIIa receptors are bound by fibrinogen, forming bridges between adjacent platelets

Figure 20.5 Schematic representation of mechanism of action of glycoprotein IIb/IIIa inhibitors.

It is also clear from the REACT trial that there is no role for repeat administration of the same or alternative thrombolytic in this setting. There are extensive data for angioplasty following NSTEMI where patients frequently have significant residual coronary artery narrowing despite treatment with antiplatelet agents, heparin and IIb/IIIa antagonists. These patients may either be treated with an interventional strategy, where all patients undergo angiography following admission, or conservatively where they undergo angiography and intervention only if they remain unstable or have a positive exercise test. Initial trials of early intervention did not demonstrate any benefit but with the advent of advanced angioplasty techniques using stents and adjuvant drug therapies including clopidogrel and IIb/IIIa antagonists, there appears to be a clear advantage for an interventional strategy in high-risk patients (RITA-3; Fox et al 2005).

Patients undergoing angioplasty have a significant risk of occlusion with thrombus and also of restenosis due to intimal proliferation. In addition to long-term aspirin, 3 months of oral clopidogrel is prescribed to inhibit ADP-induced platelet activation, and may be used together with an infusion of abciximab. The other intravenous IIb/IIIa antagonists, eptifibatide and tirofiban, may be marginally less effective. Although regrowth of the vessel intima to cover injured tissue is desirable, excessive intimal proliferation is a major cause of restenosis; stents that elute drugs such as sirolimus and paclitaxel to inhibit proliferation remain patent for longer but need longer courses of clopidogrel (12 months) to prevent thrombosis.

If the patient is not suitable for PTCA then coronary artery bypass grafting may be considered but with modern angioplasty techniques this is now far less common.

Patient care

Patients with CHD range from those who have investigational evidence of CHD but no symptoms to those who have major pain and exercise limitation. All need counselling on preventive measures including diet, smoking and exercise. Prophylactic medication is important and for most patients this will include aspirin and a statin. Doses of some statins are licensed to be titrated against effect, but the Heart Protection Study (2002) demonstrated that it was safe to give a 40 mg dose of simvastatin without titration or measurement of baseline lipids. Patients need advice on how to reduce the risk of gastrointestinal bleeding by taking aspirin with food and dissolved in water when the soluble preparation is prescribed. Patients should be encouraged to adopt a lifestyle that makes the most of their abilities without undue hazard to their health.

Most of the guidelines on prevention of CHD apply to all stages of the disease although the degree of exercise taken must be tailored according to the patient's threshold for angina. In general, although some patients are too cavalier, most are likely to err on the cautious side and may need to be encouraged to do more. Many centres now run cardiac rehabilitation classes to encourage patients to exercise and adopt a suitable lifestyle.

A diary of anginal attacks is very useful as a record of progress and may be used to adjust treatment. The use of sublingual glyceryl trinitrate should be recorded as well as details of the activities or circumstances that provoke angina. In view of the success of early thrombolysis in myocardial infarction, patients should be encouraged if they experience chest pain that is similar to a previous infarction, or worse than their usual angina, to call for an ambulance without summoning a primary care doctor first. There is little that general medical practitioners can do that the ambulance and casualty service cannot and any delay may worsen the patient's prognosis.

Patients should avoid over-the-counter preparations containing sympathomimetic drugs (e.g. cold cures) but the occasional aspirin for analgesia does not affect the antiplatelet action of low-dose aspirin.

Many patients will find the lifestyle changes burdensome or contrary to their wishes and it is essential they have support from their doctor, practice nurse, pharmacist or cardiology centre. This is particularly so when drugs are prescribed that may

Table 20.11   Common therapeutic problems in coronary heart disease

Problem	Comment
Used incorrectly, nitrates may cause hypotensive episodes or collapse	Advise to sit down when using nitrate sprays or sublingual tablets
A daily nitrate-free period is required to maintain efficacy of nitrates	Avoid long-acting preparations and prescribe asymmetrically (e.g. 8 a.m. and 2 p.m.)
NSAIDs are associated with renal failure when given with ACE inhibitors	Warn patients to use paracetamol as their analgesic of choice
Speed is essential when patients need fibrinolytic drugs after infarction	Arrange emergency admission to hospital where fast-track systems should exist
Aspirin may cause GI bleeding	Advise on taking with food and water. Consider use of prophylactic agents in high-risk patients
β-blockers are often considered unpleasant to take	Encourage patient to use regularly. Change the time of day. Consider a vasodilator if cold extremities are a problem. Consider verapamil or diltiazem
β-blockers are contraindicated in respiratory and peripheral vascular disease	Consider verapamil or diltiazem. Pay strict attention to other treatments and removal of precipitating factors
Patients often receive multiple drugs for prophylaxis and for treatment of co-existing disorders	Use once-daily preparations, dosing aids and intensive social and educational support. Avoid all unnecessary drugs
ACE inhibitors are contraindicated in pregnancy, especially the first trimester	Advise women of child-bearing years to avoid conception or seek specialist advice first

further diminish quality of life. Nitrates may cause headaches and hypotensive episodes and β-blockers can be associated with bad dreams, difficulty sleeping, cold extremities, fatigue, etc. Patients requiring glyceryl trinitrate should be counselled on the best way to administer sublingual doses, i.e. while sitting, not standing or lying. Nitrate tablets should be placed under the tongue only until relief is obtained, to avoid headaches, and a fresh supply should be kept in a convenient place at all times. Oral nitrates and transdermal patches should be taken or applied at the appropriate times to ensure a low nitrate period at night and a high nitrate period soon after rising.

Patients also need up-to-date advice when faced with difficult choices regarding medical treatment, angiographic procedures or surgery. Patients have good reason to be anxious at times but some patients restrict their activities unnecessarily out of fear of angina and infarction.

Common therapeutic problems in the management of coronary heart disease are described in Table 20.11.

CASE STUDIES

Case 20.1

A 55-year-old man presents to his primary care doctor complaining of tightness in his chest when he digs the garden. It eases when he has a rest. On investigation he has a raised serum glucose concentration and is considered to be a newly diagnosed non-insulin dependent type II diabetic.

Question

What cardiovascular investigations and treatments should this patient receive?

Answer

The patient's blood pressure and electrocardiogram should be checked and he should be examined for signs of hypertensive or diabetic target organ damage, including albuminuria. His serum lipid profile should be measured.

He should receive GTN spray or sublingual tablets for the chest symptoms that are almost certainly angina. He should take aspirin daily and a statin if his lipid profile is abnormal. Some prescribers would give a statin in almost all diabetic, CHD patients and likewise an ACE inhibitor. Certainly any hypertension should be treated aggressively so that the diastolic pressure is less than 80 mmHg. A β-blocker may also be useful to control blood pressure and prevent further episodes of angina, but many prescribers would wait until there was evidence of failure of the other therapies. In view of his relatively young age, a referral to a cardiologist for possible angiography would be considered. Dietary advice and help to stop smoking, if needed, would be given. Diabetic treatments should be given (see Chapter 44).

Case 20.2

The following patients are admitted for treatment of myocardial infarction:

1. **an asthmatic**
2. **a man previously treated for infarction**
3. **a patient with rheumatoid arthritis.**

Question

What contraindications, or possible contraindications, are there to standard treatments in the above people?

Answers

1. An asthmatic should not receive a β-blocker without careful consideration and supervision because of the risk of bronchoconstriction; there is also a small risk of bronchoconstriction with aspirin.
2. A previous infarct may have been treated with streptokinase and a repeat dose should be avoided. Tissue plasminogen activator should be used instead.
3. Thrombolytics are contraindicated if there is a serious risk of bleeding. A patient with rheumatoid arthritis may be receiving non-steroidal anti-inflammatory drugs (NSAIDs) or steroids and enquiries must be made into any history of gastrointestinal bleeding. NSAIDs would also not be prescribed with ACE inhibitors because of the risk of impaired renal function. Aspirin is not contraindicated with NSAIDs, and may be useful, but will increase the risk of gastrointestinal bleeding.

Case 20.3

A patient with rheumatoid disease, treated with naproxen, has coronary heart disease.

Question

Is there any benefit or harm in adding aspirin to his treatment?

Answer

Aspirin is more beneficial than any other non-steroidal anti-inflammatory agent in modifying platelet activity and reducing mortality and morbidity in coronary heart disease. There is an increased risk of gastrointestinal bleeding if two agents are given but at low doses of aspirin this should not be a major consideration. There is some evidence, however, that some NSAIDs interfere with the action of aspirin by blocking access to the active site on the COX-1 enzyme. Such agents should be avoided. Diclofenac does not block the receptor and ibuprofen has a short action and is acceptable if given 2 hours after the daily dose of aspirin.

REFERENCES

Barker D J, Forsen T, Uutela A et al 2001 Size at birth and resilience to effects of poor living conditions in adult life: longitudinal study. British Medical Journal 323: 1273

Boersma E, Harrington R A, Moliterno D J et al 2002 Platelet glycoprotein IIb/IIIa inhibitors in acute coronary syndromes: a meta-analysis of all major randomised clinical trials. Lancet 359: 189-198

CAPRIE Steering Committee 1996 A randomised, blinded, trial of clopidogrel versus aspirin in patients at risk of ischaemic events (CAPRIE). Lancet 348: 1329-1339

Chen Z M, Pan H C, Chen Y P et al 2005 Early intravenous then oral metoprolol in 45,852 patients with acute myocardial infarction: randomised placebo-controlled trial. Lancet 366: 1622-1632

COMMIT (Clopidogrel and Metoprolol in Myocardial Infarction Trial) Collaborative Group 2005 Addition of clopidogrel to aspirin in 45,852 patients with acute myocardial infarction: randomised placebo-controlled trial. Lancet 366:1607-1621

CURE (Clopidogrel in Unstable Angina to Prevent Recurrent Events) Trial Investigators 2001 Effects of clopidogrel in addition to aspirin in patients with acute coronary syndromes without ST-segment elevation. New England Journal of Medicine 345: 494-502

Fibrinolytic Therapy Trialists' Collaboration Group 1994 Indications for fibrinolytic therapy in suspected acute myocardial infarction: collaborative overview of early mortality and major morbidity results from all randomized trials of more than 1000 patients. Lancet 343: 311-322

Fox K A A, Poole-Wilson P, Clayton T et al 2005 Five-year outcome of an interventional strategy in non-ST-elevation acute coronary syndrome: the British Heart Foundation RITA 3 randomised trial. Lancet 366: 914-920

Harrington R A, Becker R C, Ezekowitz M et al 2004 Antithrombotic therapy for coronary artery disease. Chest 126: 513S-548S

Heart Protection Study Collaborative Group 2002 MRC/BHF Heart Protection Study of cholesterol lowering with simvastatin in 20,536 high-risk individuals: a randomised placebo-controlled trial. Lancet 360: 7-22

Iona Study Group 2002 Effect of nicorandil on coronary events in patients with stable angina: the Impact of Nicorandil in Angina (IONA) randomised trial. Lancet 349: 1269-1275

Januzzi J L, Stern T A, Pasternak R C et al 2000 The influence of anxiety and depression on outcomes of patients with coronary artery disease. Archives of Internal Medicine 160: 1913-1921

JBS 2 2005 Joint British Societies guidelines in prevention of cardiovascular disease in clinical practice. Heart 91: Supplement V

Keeley E C, Boura J A, Grines C L 2003 Primary angioplasty versus intravenous thrombolytic therapy for acute myocardial infarction: a quantitative review of 23 randomised trials. Lancet 361: 13-20

Lavie C J, Milani R V 2000 Benefits of cardiac rehabilitation and exercise training. Chest 117: 5-6

Luepker R V, Raczynski J M, Osganian S et al 2000 Effect of a community intervention on patient delay and emergency medical service use in acute coronary heart disease: the Rapid Early Action for Coronary Treatment (REACT) trial. Journal of the American Medical Association 284: 60-67

Malmberg K 1997 Prospective randomised study of intensive insulin treatment on long term survival after acute myocardial infarction in patients with diabetes mellitus. DIGAMI (diabetes mellitus, insulin glucose infusion in acute myocardial infarction) Study Group. British Medical Journal 314: 1512-1515

Malmberg K, Ryden L, Wedel H et al 2005 Intense metabolic control by means of insulin in patients with diabetes mellitus and acute myocardial infarction (DIGAMI 2): effects on mortality and morbidity. European Heart Journal 26: 650-661

McMurray J J V, Rankin A C 1994 Treatment of myocardial infarction, unstable angina and angina pectoris. British Medical Journal 309: 1343-1350

Menon V, Harrington R A, Hochman J S et al 2004 Thrombolysis and adjunctive therapy in acute myocardial infarction. Chest 126: 549S-575S

OPTIMAAL Study Group 2002 Effect of losartan and captopril on mortality and morbidity in high-rick patients after acute myocardial infarction: the OPTIMAAL randomized trial. Lancet 360: 752-780

Rochon P A, Tu J V, Anderson G M et al 2000 Rate of heart failure and 1-year survival for older people receiving low-dose ß-blocker therapy after myocardial infarction. Lancet 356: 639-644

Sabatine M S, Cannon C P, Gibson C M et al for the CLARITY-TIMI 28 Investigators 2005 Addition of clopidogrel to aspirin and fibrinolytic therapy for myocardial infarction with ST-segment elevation. New England Journal of Medicine 352: 1179-1189

Sutton A G, Campbell P G, Graham R et al 2004 A randomized trial of rescue angioplasty versus a conservative approach for failed fibrinolysis in ST-segment elevation myocardial infarction: the Middlesbrough Early Revascularization to Limit INfarction (MERLIN) trial. Journal of the American College of Cardiology 44: 287-296

VALIANT (VALsartan In Acute myocardial iNfarction Trial) Investigators 2003 Valsartan, captopril, or both in myocardial infarction complicated by heart failure, left ventricular dysfunction, or both. New England Journal of Medicine 349: 1893-1906

Yusuf S, Sleight P, Pogue J et al 2000 Effects of an angiotensin-converting-enzyme inhibitor, ramipril, on cardiovascular events in high-risk patients. The Heart Outcomes Prevention Evaluation (HOPE) Study Investigators. New England Journal of Medicine 342: 145-153

FURTHER READING

Abrams J 2005 Chronic stable angina. New England Journal of Medicine 352: 2524-2533

ACC/AHA/ACP-ASIM 1999 ACC/AHA/ACP-ASIM guidelines for the management of patients with chronic stable angina: executive summary and recommendations. Circulation 99: 2829-2848

Antiplatelet Trialists Collaboration 1991 Collaborative overview of randomised trials of antiplatelet therapy. British Medical Journal 308: 81-106

Antithrombotic Trialists Collaboration 2002 Collaborative meta-analysis of randomised trials of antiplatelet therapy for prevention of death, myocardial infarction and stroke in high-risk patients. British Medical Journal 324: 71-86

Braunwald E, Antman E M, Beasley J W et al 2002 ACC/AHA 2002 guideline update for the management of patients with unstable angina and non-ST-segment elevation myocardial infarction: a report of the American College of Cardiology/American Heart Association Task Force on Practice Guidelines (Committee on the Management of Patients With Unstable Angina). Available online at: www.acc.org/clinical/guidelines/unstable/unstable.pdf

Collins R, Peto R, Baigent C et al 1997 Aspirin, heparin and fibrinolytic therapy in suspected acute myocardial infarction. New England Journal of Medicine 336: 847-860

Fibrinolytic Therapy Trialists' Collaboration Group 1994 Indications for fibrinolytic therapy in suspected acute myocardial infarction: collaborative overview of early mortality and major morbidity results from all randomized trials of more than 1000 patients. Lancet 343: 311-322

Fox K A A 2004 Management of acute coronary syndromes: an update. Heart 90: 698-706

Harrington R A, Becker R C, Ezekowitz M et al 2004 Antithrombotic therapy for coronary artery disease. Chest 126: 513S-548S

Orford J L, Selwyn A P, Ganz P et al 2000 The comparative pathobiology of atherosclerosis and restenosis. American Journal of Cardiology 86(suppl): 6H-11H

Petersen S, Peto V, Scarborough P, Rayner M 2005 Coronary heart disease statistics, 2005 edition. British Heart Foundation Statistics Database. Available online at: www.heartstats.org

Snow V, Barry P, Fihn SD et al, for the American College of Physicians/American College of Cardiology Chronic Stable Angina Panel 2004 Primary care management of chronic stable angina and asymptomatic suspected or known coronary artery disease: a clinical practice guideline from the American College of Physicians. Annals of Internal Medicine 141: 562-567. Erratum in: Annals of Internal Medicine 142:79

Task Force of the European Society of Cardiology and the European Resuscitation Council 1998 The pre-hospital management of acute heart attacks. European Heart Journal 19: 1140-1164

Van de Werf F, Ardissino D, Betriu A et al 2003 Management of acute myocardial infarction in patients presenting with ST-segment elevation. The task force on the management of acute myocardial infarction of the European Society of Cardiology. European Heart Journal 24: 28-66

21 Chronic heart failure

J. McAnaw   S. A. Hudson

KEY POINTS

- Heart failure is a common condition that affects the quality of life causing fatigue, breathlessness and oedema. It also has a poor prognosis.
- The pathophysiology of heart failure is that of a maladaptive condition with haemodynamic and neurohormonal disturbances that allow a rational approach to therapeutic management.
- The aims of drug treatment are to control symptoms and improve survival.
- Diuretics are used for symptomatic treatment, especially for diastolic dysfunction. In combination with other agents, they are used to treat systolic dysfunction.
- Angiotensin-converting enzyme (ACE) inhibitors and β-blockers are first-line agents in asymptomatic and symptomatic patients with systolic dysfunction.
- Angiotensin II receptor blockers (ARBs) are the alternative of choice in patients intolerant of or resistant to ACE inhibitor therapy. Where use of an ARB is inappropriate, the combination of hydralazine and nitrate should be considered.
- Aldosterone antagonists have been shown to improve morbidity and mortality when used as adjunctive therapy in patients with heart failure due to systolic dysfunction.
- Digoxin has been shown to improve symptoms and reduce the rate of hospitalization for patients with heart failure in sinus rhythm, but has no effect on mortality.
- Multidisciplinary models of patient care improve clinical outcomes for patients and contribute to the continuity of care.

Chronic heart failure occurs when the heart's delivery of blood, and therefore oxygen and nutrients, is inadequate for the needs of the tissues. It is a complex condition associated with a number of symptoms arising from defects in left ventricular filling and/ or emptying, including shortness of breath and exertional fatigue. The symptoms of heart failure are due to inadequate tissue perfusion, venous congestion and disturbed water and electrolyte balance. In chronic heart failure, normal body compensatory mechanisms become counterproductive, and the resulting maladaptive secondary physiological effects contribute to the progressive nature of the condition.

Treatment is aimed at improving left ventricular function, controlling the secondary effects that lead to the occurrence of symptoms, and delaying progression. Drug therapy is indicated in all patients with heart failure to control symptoms, where present, improve quality of life and prolong survival. Patients with heart failure usually have their functional status assessed and categorized using the New York Heart Association (NYHA) classification system shown in Table 21.1.

Epidemiology

Chronic heart failure is a common condition with a prevalence ranging from 0.3% to 2% in the population at large, 3–5% in the population over 65 years old, and between 8% and 16% of those aged over 75 years. Heart failure accounts for 5% of adult medical admissions to hospital. There is a loss of cardiac reserve with age, and heart failure may often complicate the presence of other conditions in the elderly. More than 10% of patients with heart failure also have atrial fibrillation as a contributory factor. This combination presents a risk of thromboembolic complications, notably stroke; the risk is 2% in patients in sinus rhythm, but may exceed 10% a year in patients with atrial fibrillation who are not anticoagulated and have attendant risk factors.

Heart failure is a progressive condition with a median survival of about 5 years after diagnosis, although mortality varies according to aetiology and severity. The prognosis can be predicted according to severity of the disease. The annual mortality rate for patients with chronic heart failure is estimated at 10%. Main causes of death are progressive pump failure, sudden cardiac death and recurrent myocardial infarction.

Aetiology

Chronic heart failure is often gradual in onset, with symptoms arising insidiously and without any specific cause over a number of years. The common underlying aetiologies in patients with heart failure are coronary artery disease and hypertension. The appropriate management of these predisposing conditions

Table 21.1   New York Heart Association (NYHA) classification of functional status of the patient with heart failure

I	No symptoms with ordinary physical activity (such as walking or climbing stairs)
II	Slight limitation with dyspnoea on moderate to severe exertion (climbing stairs or walking uphill)
III	Marked limitation of activity, less than ordinary activity causes dyspnoea (restricting walking distance and limiting climbing to one flight of stairs)
IV	Severe disability, dyspnoea at rest (unable to carry on physical activity without discomfort)

is also an important consideration in controlling heart failure in the community. Identifiable causes of heart failure include aortic stenosis, cardiomyopathy, mechanical defects such as cardiac valvular dysfunction, hyperthyroidism or severe anaemia. Conditions that place increased demands on the heart can create a shortfall in cardiac output and lead to intermittent exacerbation of symptoms. Heart failure may be a consequence of hyperthyroidism, where the tissues place a greater metabolic demand, or severe anaemia, where there is an increased circulatory demand on the heart. Systolic contraction may also be compromised by bradycardia or tachycardia, or by a sustained arrhythmia such as that experienced by patients in atrial fibrillation. Atrial fibrillation often accompanies hyperthyroidism and mitral valve disease, where a rapid and irregular ventricular response may compromise cardiac efficiency. Improved management of the underlying causes, where appropriate, may alleviate the symptoms of heart failure, whereas the presence of mechanical defects may require the surgical insertion of prosthetic valve(s). However, the most common cause of heart failure is left ventricular systolic dysfunction (LVSD), and most of the available evidence from clinical trials regarding the pharmacological treatment of heart failure relates to those patients with heart failure due to left ventricular systolic dysfunction.

Pathophysiology

In health, cardiac output at rest is approximately 5 L/min with a mean heart rate of 70 beats per minute and stroke volume of 70 mL. Since the filled ventricle has a normal volume of 130 mL, the fraction ejected is over 50% of the ventricular contents, with the remaining (residual) volume being approximately 60 mL. In left ventricular systolic dysfunction the ejection fraction is reduced to below 45%, and symptoms are common when the fraction is below 35% although some patients with a low ejection fraction can remain asymptomatic. When the ejection fraction falls below 10%, patients have the added risk of thrombus formation within the left ventricle and in most cases anticoagulation with warfarin is indicated.

Left ventricular systolic dysfunction can result from cardiac injury, e.g. myocardial infarction, or by exposure of the heart muscle to mechanical stress. This may result in defects in systolic contraction, diastolic relaxation or both. Systolic dysfunction arises from impaired contractility, and is reflected in a low ejection fraction and cardiac dilation. Diastolic dysfunction arises from impairment of the filling process. Diastolic filling is affected by the rate of venous return, and normal filling requires active diastolic expansion of the ventricular volume. The tension on the ventricular wall at the end of diastole is called the preload, the volume of blood available to be pumped, which contributes to the degree of stretch on the myocardium. In diastolic dysfunction, there is impaired relaxation or reduced compliance of the left ventricle during diastole and therefore less blood is accommodated. In pure diastolic dysfunction, the ejection fraction can be normal but cardiac dilation is absent. Sustained diastolic dysfunction, which is a feature in a minority of patients with heart failure, may lead to systolic dysfunction associated with disease progression and left ventricular remodelling (structural changes and/or deterioration).

During systolic contraction, the tension on the ventricular wall is determined by the degree of resistance to outflow at the exit valve and that within the arterial tree – the systemic vascular resistance. Arterial hypertension, aortic narrowing and disorders of the aortic valve increase the afterload on the heart by increasing the resistance against which the contraction of the ventricle must work. This results in an increased residual volume and therefore leads to an increased preload as the ventricle overfills, and produces greater tension on the ventricular wall. In the normal heart, a compensatory increase in performance occurs as the stretched myocardium responds through an increased elastic recoil. In the failing heart, this property of cardiac muscle recoiling under stretch is diminished, with the consequence that the heart dilates abnormally to accommodate the increased ventricular load. With continued dilation of cardiac muscle the elastic recoil property becomes further diminished or absent. Failure of the heart to handle the increasing ventricular load leads to pulmonary and systemic venous congestion. At the same time, the increased tension on the ventricular wall in heart failure raises myocardial oxygen requirements with the risk to the patient of an episode of myocardial ischaemia or a period of arrhythmias.

The failing heart may show cardiac enlargement due to dilation, which is reversible with successful treatment. An irreversible increase in cardiac muscle mass – cardiac hypertrophy – occurs with progression of heart failure and is a consequence of longstanding hypertension. While hypertrophy may initially alleviate heart failure, the increased mass ultimately increases workload and oxygen consumption.

A reflex sympathetic discharge caused by the diminished tissue perfusion in heart failure exposes the heart to catecholamines where positive inotropic and chronotropic effects help to sustain cardiac output and produce a tachycardia. Arterial constriction diverts blood to the organs from the skin and gastrointestinal tract but overall raises systemic vascular resistance and increases the afterload on the heart.

Renin is released from the kidney in response to reduced renal perfusion due to heart failure. Circulating renin acts on blood pressure through the formation of angiotensin I and angiotensin II, a potent vasoconstrictor, and renin also prompts adrenal aldosterone release. Aldosterone retains salt and water at the distal renal tubule and so expands blood volume and increases preload. Arginine vasopressin released from the posterior pituitary in response to hypoperfusion adds to the systemic vasoconstriction and has an antidiuretic effect by retaining water at the renal collecting duct. These secondary effects become increasingly detrimental to cardiac function as heart failure progresses, since the vasoconstriction adds to the afterload and the expanded blood volume adds to the preload. The expanded blood volume promotes the release of a natural vasodilator, atrial natriuretic peptide (ANP), from the atrial myocytes to counteract the increased preload by way of attenuation.

The compensatory mechanisms for the maintenance of the circulation eventually become overwhelmed and ultimately counterproductive, leading to the emergence of clinical signs and symptoms of heart failure. The long-term consequences are that the myocardium of the failing heart undergoes biochemical and histological changes which lead to remodelling of the left ventricle, and further complicates disease progression. In those patients where the condition is severe and has progressed to an end stage, heart transplantation may be the only remaining treatment option.

Clinical manifestations

The reduced cardiac output, impaired oxygenation and diminished blood supply to muscles cause fatigue. Shortness of breath occurs on exertion (dyspnoea) or on lying (orthopnoea). When the patient lies down, the postural change causes abdominal pressure on the diaphragm which redistributes oedema to the lungs, leading to breathlessness. At night the pulmonary symptoms give rise to cough and an increase in urine production (nocturia) prompts micturition, which adds to the sleep disturbance. The patient wakens at night as gradual accumulation of fluid in the lungs provokes attacks of gasping (paroxysmal nocturnal dyspnoea, PND). Characteristically the patient describes the need to sit or stand up to seek fresh air, and usually needs to be propped up by three or more pillows to remedy the sleep disturbances due to fluid accumulation.

Patients with heart failure may appear pale and their hands cold and sweaty. Reduced blood supply to the brain and kidney can contribute to confusion and renal failure. Hepatomegaly occurs from congestion of the gastrointestinal tract, which is accompanied by abdominal distension, anorexia, nausea and abdominal pain. Oedema affects the lungs, ankles and abdomen. Signs of oedema in the lungs include crepitations heard at the lung bases. In acute heart failure, symptoms of pulmonary oedema are prominent and may be life-threatening. The sputum may be frothy and tinged red from the leakage of fluid and blood from the capillaries. Severe dyspnoea may be complicated by cyanosis and shock. Table 21.2 presents the clinical manifestations of heart failure.

Investigations

Patients with chronic heart failure are diagnosed and monitored on the basis of signs and symptoms from physical examination, history and an exercise tolerance test. On physical examination of the patient, a lateral and downward displacement of the apex beat can be identified as evidence of cardiac enlargement. Additional third and/or fourth heart sounds are typical of heart failure and arise from valvular dysfunction. Venous congestion can be demonstrated in the jugular vein of the upright reclining patient by an elevated jugular venous pressure (JVP), which reflects the central venous pressure. The jugular venous pressure is measured by noting the visible distension above the sternum and may be accentuated in heart failure by the application of abdominal compression in the reclining patient.

Echocardiography is important when investigating patients with a suspected diagnosis of heart failure. An echocardiogram allows visualization of the heart in real time and will identify whether heart failure is due to systolic dysfunction, diastolic dysfunction or heart valve defects. With the provision of direct access echocardiography services to doctors in primary care, an increasing number of patients can now be quickly referred for confirmation of suspected heart failure. However, some reports suggest that between 50% and 75% of patients referred to direct access clinics may have normal left ventricular function. This

Table 21.2 Clinical manifestations of heart failure

Venous (congestion)	Cardiac (cardiomegaly)	Arterial (peripheral hypoperfusion)
Dyspnoea	Dilation	Fatigue
Oedema	Tachycardia	Pallor
Hypoxia	Regurgitation	Renal impairment
Hepatomegaly	Cardiomyopathy	Confusion
Raised venous pressure	Ischaemia, arrhythmia	Circulatory failure

highlights the non-specific nature of heart failure symptoms and that confirming a diagnosis based solely on assessment of clinical signs and symptoms is inappropriate. Table 21.3 shows a number of investigations that are routinely performed in the diagnosis of heart failure. The use of plasma natriuretic peptide measurement in the diagnosis of patients with heart failure is currently limited by the lack of defined cut-off values, and therefore measurements are only considered in combination with ECG/chest x-ray data prior to echocardiography.

Treatment of heart failure

The goals of treatment are to relieve symptoms, delay progression, reduce hospitalization and reduce mortality. Effective therapy can considerably improve a patient's quality of life and, ultimately, improve survival.

In heart failure patients with co-morbid conditions known to contribute to heart failure, such as hyperthyroidism, anaemia, atrial fibrillation and valvular heart disease, attention must be given to ensuring these co-morbid conditions are well controlled. Patients with persistent atrial fibrillation and resultant tachycardia usually require control of their ventricular rate through suppression of atrioventricular node conduction. The use of either β-blockers or digoxin is common in such circumstances. In these patients, consideration of the use of either anticoagulant or anti-platelet agents will also be necessary. In patients diagnosed with diastolic dysfunction, there is very little evidence regarding drug treatment and therefore the use of diuretics to control symptoms is usually the chosen therapy. Figure 21.1 illustrates how therapeutic intervention affects not only cardiac function but also the complex haemodynamic and neurohormonal reflex mechanisms.

Left ventricular diastolic dysfunction

All patients with heart failure due to left ventricular systolic dysfunction should be treated with both an ACE inhibitor and a β-blocker in the absence of intolerance or contraindication. The evidence base for treatment clearly shows that use of ACE inhibitor and β-blocker therapy in patients with heart failure due to left ventricular systolic dysfunction leads to an improvement in symptoms and reduction in mortality. There is some evidence to suggest that either agent can be initiated first, as both appear

Table 21.3 Investigations performed to confirm a diagnosis of heart failure

Investigation	Comment
Blood test	The following assessments are usually performed: • Blood gas analysis to assess respiratory gas exchange • Serum creatinine and urea to assess renal function • Plasma alanine- and aspartate-aminotransferase plus other liver function tests • Full blood count to investigate possibility of anaemia • Thyroid function tests to investigate possibility of thyrotoxicosis • Plasma BNP or NT pro-BNP to indicate likelihood of a diagnosis of heart failure (screening test) • Fasting blood glucose to investigate possibility of diabetes mellitus
12-lead electrocardiogram	A normal ECG usually excludes the presence of left ventricular systolic dysfunction. An abnormal ECG will require further investigation
Chest radiograph	A chest radiograph (x-ray) is performed to look for an enlarged cardiac shadow and consolidation in the lungs
Echocardiograph	An echocardiogram is used to confirm the diagnosis of heart failure and any underlying causes, e.g. valvular heart disease

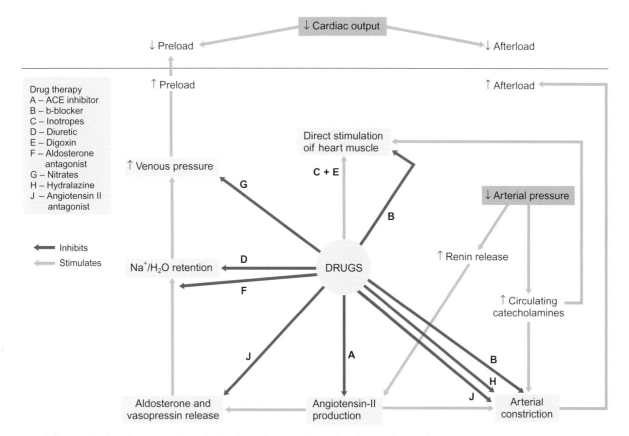

Figure 21.1   Reflex mechanisms in response to reduction in cardiac output with drug therapy intervention.

to be just as effective and well tolerated (CARMEN 2004, CIBIS III 2005). Beneficial effects on morbidity and mortality have also been shown for the use of angiotensin II receptor blockers (ARB), aldosterone antagonists, and hydralazine/nitrate combinations when used in the treatment of chronic heart failure. Digoxin has been shown to improve morbidity and reduce the number of hospital admissions in patients with heart failure, although its effect on mortality has not been demonstrated. Table 21.4 describes the treatment of acute heart failure in the hospital setting, while Figure 21.2 highlights the possible treatment options for patients with chronic heart failure due to left ventricular systolic dysfunction.

Table 21.4 Treatment of acute heart failure due to left ventricular systolic dysfunction in patients requiring hospitalization

Problem	Drug therapy indicated
Anxiety	Use of intravenous opiates to reduce anxiety and reduce preload through venodilation
Breathlessness	High-flow oxygen (60–100%) may be required in conjunction with i.v. furosemide as either direct injection or 24-hour infusion (5–10 mg/h). Venodilation with i.v. GTN is also effective at doses titrated every 10–20 min against systolic BP ≤ 110 mmHg
Arrhythmia	Digoxin useful in control of atrial fibrillation. Amiodarone is the drug of choice in ventricular arrhythmias
Expansion of blood volume blood transfusion	An elevation in preload, such as can occur acutely by expansion of blood volume after a transfusion, can exacerbate the degree of systolic dysfunction. Therefore it is necessary to continue or increase diuretic dosage during this time

The selection of adjunctive therapy beyond the use of ACE inhibitor and β-blocker therapy is largely dependent on the nature of the patient and the preference of the heart failure specialist involved in the patient's care. It is accepted that there is a limit as to how many agents any one patient can tolerate, therefore the selection of drug therapy will probably be tailored to each individual patient, meaning that treatment plans will vary.

Diuretics

In chronic heart failure, diuretics are used to relieve pulmonary and peripheral oedema by increasing sodium and chloride excretion through blockade of sodium reabsorption in the renal tubule. Normally, in the proximal tubule, about 70% of sodium is reabsorbed along with water. In mild heart failure, either a thiazide or a loop diuretic is chosen depending on the severity of the symptoms experienced by the patient and the degree of diuresis required. Thiazides are described as 'low-ceiling agents' because maximum diuresis occurs at low doses, and they act mainly on the cortical diluting segment (the point of merger of the ascending limb with the distal renal tubule) at which 5–10% of sodium is normally removed. Although thiazides have some action at this site, they fail to produce a marked diuresis since a compensatory increase in sodium reabsorption occurs in the loop of Henle, and consequently thiazides are ineffective in patients with moderate-to-severe renal impairment (creatinine clearance <25 mL/min) or persisting symptoms. Additionally, doses above the equivalent of bendroflumethiazide 5 mg have an increased risk of adverse metabolic effects with no additional symptomatic benefit. Therefore, thiazides tend to be used instead of loop diuretics where the degree of fluid retention in the patient is very mild.

Loop diuretics are indicated in the majority of symptomatic patients and most patients will be prescribed one of either furosemide, bumetanide or torasemide in preference to a thiazide.

Functional status of patient (NYHA)		Drug therapy indicated
Asymptomatic	I	In absence of contraindication or intolerance • ACE inhibitor (use Angiotensin II receptor blocker if not tolerated) • β-blocker In post-MI patient with diabetes mellitus • Eplerenone
Symptomatic	II - IV	As above, with addition of • Diuretic Where patient still symptomatic despite optimization of above therapy, consider addition of the following agents on specialist advice* • Candesartan • Digoxin (if patient in sinus rhythm) • Spironolactone (in moderate to severe heart failure) • Eplerenone (if patient post-MI or spironolactone-intolerant) • Hydralazine/ISDN (beneficial in African-American patients)

* Use of adjunctive therapy must be guided by a heart failure specialist/cardiologist, as there are certain combinations that require very close monitoring or complete avoidance according to current clinical evidence.

Figure 21.2 Outline of treatment options for patients with chronic heart failure due to left ventricular systolic dysfunction.

These agents are known as 'high-ceiling agents' because their blockade of sodium reabsorption in the loop of Henle continues with increased dose. They produce less hypokalaemia than thiazides but in high doses their intensity of action may produce hypovolaemia with risk of postural hypotension, worsening of symptoms and renal failure. However, in practice, high doses of furosemide (up to 500 mg/day) may be required to control oedema in patients with poor renal function. In the acute situation doses of loop diuretics are titrated to produce a weight loss of 0.5–1 kg per day.

Metolazone is a thiazide-like agent that is a useful adjunct to a loop diuretic in cases where the patient has severe heart failure or resistant oedema. Metolazone has a pronounced effect over 12–24 hours on the distal tubule, even at low glomerular filtration rates, and produces a synergistic effect when added to loop diuretic therapy. However, the profound diuresis poses serious risks, such as dehydration and hypotension, and patients who are prescribed metolazone in addition to an existing loop diuretic must be carefully monitored and very low doses of metolazone should be used. In practice, patients with oedema treated with loop diuretics may best be treated using a degree of self-management. Some patients are instructed to make upward adjustment of loop diuretic dose or to add metolazone therapy on particular days, for example when they self-record a gain of 2 kg or over in their ideal weight over a short period of time.

Diuretics also have a mild vasodilator effect that helps improve cardiac function and the intravenous use of loop diuretics reduces preload acutely by locally relieving pulmonary congestion before the onset of the diuretic effect. Effective diuretic therapy is indicated by normalization of filling pressure. Therefore continued elevation of the jugular venous pressure suggests a need for more diuretic unless otherwise contraindicated. Intravenous furosemide must be administered at a rate not exceeding 4 mg/min to patients with renal failure, since it can cause ototoxicity when administered more rapidly.

Table 21.5 summarizes details of diuretic therapy used in left ventricular systolic dysfunction.

ACE inhibitors

ACE inhibitors are indicated as first-line treatment for all grades of heart failure due to left ventricular systolic dysfunction, including those patients who are asymptomatic. These agents exert their effects by reducing both the preload and afterload on the heart, thereby increasing cardiac output.

ACE inhibitors act upon the renin–angiotensin–aldosterone system, and they reduce afterload by reducing the formation of angiotensin II, a potent vasoconstrictor in the arterial system. These drugs also have an indirect effect on sodium and water retention by inhibiting the release of aldosterone and vasopressin, thereby reducing venous congestion and preload. The increase in cardiac output leads to an improvement in renal perfusion, which further helps to alleviate oedema. ACE inhibitors also potentiate the vasodilator bradykinin and may intervene locally on ACE in cardiac and renal tissues.

ACE inhibitors are generally well tolerated by most patients and have been shown to improve the quality of life and survival in patients with mild-to-severe systolic dysfunction (CONSENSUS I 1987, CONSENSUS II 1992, SOLVD-P 1992,

Table 21.5 Diuretics and aldosterone antagonists used in the treatment of heart failure

Class and agent	Onset and duration of effect		Comment
Thiazide and related	**Oral**		
Bendroflumethiazide	Onset 1–2 h Duration 12–18 h		Thiazides effective in the treatment of sodium and water retention, although there is generally a loss of action in renal failure (GFR <25 mL/min). Metolazone has an intense action when added to a loop diuretic and is effective at low GFR
Metolazone	Onset 1–2 h Duration 12–24 h		
Loop	**Oral**	**Parenteral**	
Furosemide	Onset 0.5–1 h Duration 4–6 h	Onset 5 min Duration 2 h	Loop diuretics are preferred in the treatment of sodium and water retention where renal dysfunction is evident or more severe grades of heart failure present. Agents can be given orally or by infusion, and all are effective at low GFR
Bumetanide	As above	As above	
Torasemide	Onset <1 h Duration <8 h	Onset 10 min Duration <8 h	
Potassium sparing	**Oral**		
Spironolactone	Onset 7 h Duration 24 h		Can enhance diuretic effect of loop and/or thiazide. Due to slow onset of action needs 2–3 days before maximum diuretic effect reached. Spironolactone can improve survival when given as an adjunct to ACE inhibitor and diuretic therapy at a recommended dose of 25 mg daily (initial dose of 25 mg daily or on alternate days)
Aldosterone antagonist	**Oral**		
Eplerenone	Half-life 3–5 h		In post-MI patients with symptomatic heart failure (or asymptomatic patients with diabetes mellitus), eplerenone 50 mg daily improved survival when added to optimal therapy (initial dose of 25 mg daily)

SOLVD-T 1991, V-HeFT II 1991), including those patients who have experienced a myocardial infarction (AIRE 1993, SAVE 1992, TRACE 1995). When an ACE inhibitor is prescribed, it is important to ensure that the dose is increased gradually either to the target dose used in clinical trials or to the maximum dose tolerated by the patient. There is some evidence to suggest that high doses of ACE inhibitor are more effective than low doses in relation to reduction in mortality, although it is uncertain whether this is a general class effect (ATLAS 1999). In clinical practice, it is possible that some patients may be treated with ACE inhibitors at doses below those used in clinical trials. As a consequence, outcomes in heart failure treatment may not be as good as expected from the trial findings.

The introduction of an ACE inhibitor may produce hypotension, which is most pronounced after the first dose and is sometimes severe. Patients at risk include those already on high doses of loop diuretics, where the diuretics cannot be stopped or reduced beforehand, and patients who may have a low circulating fluid volume (due to dehydration) and an activated renin–angiotensin system. Hypotension can also occur where the ACE inhibitor has been initiated at too high a dose or where the dose has been increased too quickly after initiation. In the primary care setting, treatment must be started with a low dose which is usually administered at bedtime. In patients at particular risk of hypotension, a test dose of the shorter-acting agent captopril can be given to assess suitability for treatment before commencing long-term treatment with a preferred ACE inhibitor. Once it has been established that the ACE inhibitor can be initiated safely, the preferred option would be to switch to a longer-acting agent with once- or twice-daily dosing, starting with a low dose which would be gradually titrated upwards to the recommended target (Table 21.6). Monitoring of fluid balance, blood biochemistry and blood pressure are essential safety checks during initiation and titration of ACE inhibitor therapy.

One of the most common adverse effects seen with ACE inhibitors is a dry cough and this is reported in at least 10% of patients. However, since a cough can occur naturally in patients with heart failure it is sometimes difficult to determine the true cause. ACE inhibitor therapy can also compromise renal function although in patients in whom there is a reduction in renal perfusion due to worsening heart failure or hypovolaemia, renal dysfunction can also occur. Therefore, there are a number of instances where ACE inhibitor intolerance can be misdiagnosed in practice. Where ACE inhibitor intolerance is suspected, patients can usually be successfully rechallenged with an ACE inhibitor once their heart failure is more stable, although careful monitoring of the patient should be undertaken during initiation and subsequent dose titration. If the increase in the patient's serum creatinine is >100% from baseline, the ACE inhibitor should be stopped, intolerance confirmed and specialist advice sought. Where the increase from baseline is 50–100%, the ACE inhibitor dose should be halved and serum creatinine concentration rechecked after 1–2 weeks. If renal function is stable and no cough or other adverse effects are reported, therapy should be continued. Where the problem persists, an alternative treatment option might be required, e.g. angiotensin II receptor blocker (similar benefits on morbidity and mortality, but there is a possibility of similar adverse effects on blood pressure and renal function) or hydralazine-nitrate combination.

ACE inhibitors are potentially hazardous in patients with pre-existing renal disease, as blockade of the renin–angiotensin system may lead to reversible deterioration of renal function. Therefore, ACE inhibitors are contraindicated in patients with bilateral renal artery stenosis, in whom the renin–angiotensin system is activated to maintain renal perfusion. Since most ACE inhibitors or their active metabolites rely on elimination via the kidney, the risk of other forms of dose-related toxicity is also increased in the presence of renal failure. Fosinopril, which is partially excreted by metabolism, may be the preferred agent in patients with renal failure. ACE inhibitors are also contraindicated in patients with severe aortic stenosis because their use can result in a markedly reduced cardiac output due to decreased filling pressure within the left ventricle. Table 21.6 summarizes the activity and use of ACE inhibitors.

Angiotensin II receptor blockers

The use of angiotensin II receptor blockers (ARB) as an adjunct to ACE inhibitor and β-blocker therapy has been associated with significant reductions in cardiovascular events and hospitalization rate (CHARM Added 2003). Although this finding is encouraging, the impact on mortality alone has been inconsistent to date and there is no clear consensus on when to use an ARB as adjunctive therapy. In studies involving patients unable to tolerate an ACE inhibitor, ARBs have been shown to be comparable to ACE inhibitors in reducing the risk of cardiovascular death and rate of hospitalization, and in the control of symptoms in heart failure patients (CHARM Alternative 2003, Val-HeFT 2002). Therefore, ARBs are recommended for use as an alternative to ACE inhibitor therapy where intolerance has been confirmed. It is important to note that in patients who have renal failure secondary to ACE inhibitors, switching to an ARB is of no theoretical or practical benefit, as similar adverse effects are likely.

β-blockers

The use of β-blockers is recommended for all patients with heart failure, irrespective of the severity of the condition, but should only be initiated when the patient's condition is stable. A number of clinical trials provide evidence that β-blockers reduce mortality among patients with mild-to-moderate symptomatic heart failure (ANZ Carvedilol 1997, CAPRICORN 2001, CIBIS II 1999, MERIT-HF 1999, US Carvedilol 1996) and those with severe heart failure (COPERNICUS 2001). This beneficial effect also extends to the elderly heart failure population (SENIORS 2005). In heart failure due to left ventricular systolic dysfunction, β-blockers are thought to act by combating the sympathetic neurohormonal overactivity, which occurs in response to the failing heart, and minimizing the abnormal structural and physiological changes that can occur in the cardiac muscle in response to the overactivity. Carvedilol, bisoprolol, metoprolol succinate (salt not licensed for use in the UK) and nebivolol are currently recommended for use as adjunctive therapy for patients with heart failure, but require careful initiation and titration of the dose.

It is likely that patients will experience a worsening of symptoms during initiation of therapy and therefore patients are started on very low doses of β-blocker with titration occurring over a number of weeks or months with careful monitoring. Table 21.6 summarizes the activity and use of β-blockers in heart failure.

Table 21.6 Vasodilators used in the treatment of heart failure

	Dose	Frequency	Half-life (h)	Comment
ACE inhibitor				
Captopril	Target: 50–100 mg Start: 6.25 mg	Three times daily	8	First-dose hypotension may occur. May worsen renal failure. Adjust dose in renal failure. Hyperkalaemia, cough, taste disturbance and hypersensitivity may occur particularly with captopril. ACE inhibitors have been shown to improve survival, with starting and target dose for those agents used in clinical trials highlighted
Enalapril	Target: 10–20 mg Start: 2.5 mg	Twice daily	11	
Lisinopril	Target: 20–35 mg Start: 2.5–5 mg	Once daily	12	
Ramipril	Target: 10 mg Start: 2.5 mg	Once daily (or divided dose)	13–17	
Trandolapril	Target: 4 mg Start: 0.5 mg	Once daily	16–24	
Cilazapril		Once daily	9	
Fosinopril		Once daily	11–14	
Perindopril		Once daily	25	
Quinapril		Once daily	–	
β-blocker				
Carvedilol	Target: 25–50 mg Start: 3.125 mg	Twice daily	6–10	May initially exacerbate symptoms but if initiated at low dose and slowly titrated can improve long-term survival, even in elderly patients with heart failure
Bisoprolol	Target: 10 mg Start: 1.25 mg	Once daily	10–12	Metoprolol succinate is currently not licensed for use in the UK.
Metoprolol (succinate) CR/XL formulation	Target: 200 mg Start: 12.5–25 mg	Once daily	3–7	
Nebivolol	Target: 10 mg Start: 1.25 mg	Once daily	10	Half-life of nebivolol can be 3–5 times longer in slow metabolizers
Nitrates				
Glyceryl trinitrate			1–4 mins	Isosorbide dinitrate metabolized to isosorbide mononitrate. High doses needed. Tolerance can be prevented by nitrate-free period of >8 h. Protective effect against cardiac ischaemia. GTN given i.v. for sustained effect in acute/severe heart failure but limited by tolerance
Isosorbide dinitrate			1	
Isosorbide mononitrate			5	
Nitroprusside			2 mins	Light sensitive. Acts on veins and arteries. Cyanide accumulation and acidosis limit treatment duration
Angiotensin II receptor blocker				
Losartan			6–9	Comparable effectiveness to ACE inhibitor in patients with ACE inhibitor intolerance, although similar effect on renal function and blood pressure. Recent evidence suggests improved survival when ARB used as adjunctive therapy. However, increased potential for deterioration in renal function and/or hyperkalaemia
Candesartan	Target: 32 mg Start: 4–8 mg	Once daily	9	
Valsartan	Target: 160 mg Start: 40 mg	Twice daily	9	
Hydralazine			2–3	Hydralazine has a direct action on arteries. Tolerance occurs. May cause drug-induced lupus and sodium retention

Aldosterone antagonist

The use of aldosterone antagonists as an adjunct to standard treatment has been shown to have an effect on morbidity and mortality in patients with heart failure. Spironolactone has been shown to reduce mortality and hospitalization rates in patients with moderate-to-severe heart failure (RALES 1999). The use of eplerenone has also been shown to be associated with similar benefits in post-MI patients with symptomatic heart failure or post-MI diabetic patients with asymptomatic heart failure.

Aldosterone can cause sodium and water retention, sympathetic activation and parasympathetic inhibition, all of which are associated with harmful effects in the patient with heart failure. Aldosterone antagonists counteract these effects by directly antagonizing the activity of aldosterone, providing a more complete blockade of the renin–angiotensin–aldosterone system when used in conjunction with an ACE inhibitor. Although the combination of spironolactone (at a dose of 50 mg daily or more) and an ACE inhibitor is associated with an increased risk of developing hyperkalaemia, the use of a 25 mg daily dose has been shown to have little effect on plasma potassium and provides a significant reduction in mortality. The use of spironolactone is, however, contraindicated in those patients with a plasma potassium >5.5 mmol/L or serum creatinine >200 μmol/L. With eplerenone, similar contraindications exist and therefore close monitoring of blood biochemistry and renal function must be undertaken for use of either agent. The activity and use of spironolactone and eplerenone are summarized in Table 21.5.

Currently, there is no evidence available regarding the effectiveness and safety of combining an ACE inhibitor, ARB and an aldosterone antagonist, and therefore it is recommended that this combination is avoided until more information about this particular combination becomes available.

Digoxin

Although digoxin has an established role in the control of atrial fibrillation, its place in the treatment of heart failure is still the subject of debate. There is evidence to show that when digoxin has been used to treat heart failure in patients in sinus rhythm, as an adjunct to ACE inhibitor and diuretic therapy, then worsening of symptoms occurs on withdrawal of digoxin (PROVED 1993, RADIANCE 1993). While the use of digoxin in heart failure in patients in sinus rhythm has no measurable impact on mortality, it reduces the number of hospital admissions (DIG 1997). Consequently digoxin is currently recommended for use as add-on therapy at low doses in patients with moderate-to-severe heart failure who remain symptomatic despite adequate doses of ACE inhibitor, β-blocker and diuretic treatment. Due to the lack of effect on mortality, it is unlikely that digoxin would be considered before the other adjunctive therapies available.

Digoxin is a positive inotropic agent and acts by increasing the availability of calcium within the myocardial cell through an inhibition of sodium extrusion, thereby increasing sodium–calcium exchange and leading to enhanced contractility of cardiac muscle. Digoxin increases cardiac output in patients with co-existing atrial fibrillation by suppressing atrioventricular conduction and controlling the ventricular rate. In patients with atrial fibrillation, the plasma digoxin concentration usually needs to be at the higher end of the reference range (0.8–2 μg/L) or beyond to control the arrhythmia. However, a high plasma digoxin concentration is not necessarily required to achieve an inotropic effect in patients in sinus rhythm. Digoxin is also associated with both vagal stimulation and a reduction in sympathetic nerve activity, and these may play important roles in the symptomatic benefits experienced by those patients in sinus rhythm receiving lower doses. In practice, the dose prescribed will be judged appropriate by the clinical response expressed as relief of symptoms and ventricular rate. Routine monitoring of plasma digoxin concentrations in clinical decision making is not recommended, other than to confirm or exclude digoxin toxicity or investigate issues around patient compliance.

Digoxin treatment is potentially hazardous due to its low therapeutic index and so all patients receiving this drug should be regularly reviewed to exclude clinical signs or symptoms of adverse effects. Digoxin may cause bradycardia and lead to potentially fatal cardiac arrhythmias. Other symptoms associated with digoxin toxicity include nausea, vomiting, confusion and visual disturbances. Digoxin toxicity is more pronounced in the presence of metabolic or electrolyte disturbances and in patients with cardiac ischaemia. Those patients who develop hypokalaemia, hypomagnesaemia, hypercalcaemia, alkalosis, hypothyroidism or hypoxia are at particular risk of toxicity. Treatment may be required to restore plasma potassium, and in emergency situations intravenous digoxin-specific antibody fragments can be used to treat life-threatening digoxin toxicity. Table 21.7 summarizes the activity and use of digoxin.

Nitrates/hydralazine

Nitrates exert their effects in heart failure predominantly on the venous system where they cause venodilation, thereby reducing the symptoms of pulmonary congestion. The preferred use of nitrates is in combination with an arterial vasodilator such as hydralazine, which reduces the afterload, to achieve a balanced effect on the venous and arterial circulation. The combined effects of these two drugs lead to an increase in cardiac output, and there is evidence to show the combination is effective and associated with a reduction in mortality in patients with heart failure (V-HeFT I 1986). Although the combination can improve survival, the reduction in mortality is much smaller than that seen with ACE inhibitors (V-HeFT II 1991). The evidence supports the use of hydralazine 300 mg daily with isosorbide dinitrate 160 mg daily (although in practice an equivalent dose of isosorbide mononitrate is often used). Since the emergence of ACE inhibitors, with their superior effects on morbidity and mortality, the combination has mainly been reserved for those patients unable to tolerate or with contraindication to ACE inhibitor therapy. However, recent evidence suggests that using the combination of hydralazine and isosorbide dinitrate in addition to ACE inhibitor and β-blocker therapy may provide added benefits to African-American patients (A-HeFT 2004).

Organic nitrate vasodilators work by interacting with sulphydryl groups found in the vascular tissue. Nitric oxide is released from the nitrate compound and this in turn activates soluble guanylate cyclase in vascular smooth muscle, leading to the vasodilatory effect. Plasma nitric oxide concentrations are not clearly related to pharmacological effects because of their indirect action on the vasculature. Depletion of tissue sulphydryl groupings can occur during continued treatment with nitrates, and is partly responsible for the development of tolerance in patients with sustained exposure to high nitrate doses. Restoration of sulphydryl groupings occurs within hours of treatment being interrupted, therefore nitrate tolerance can be prevented by the use of an asymmetrical dosing regimen to ensure that the patient experiences a daily nitrate-free period of more than 8 hours.

In the acute setting, glyceryl trinitrate (GTN) is frequently administered intravenously, along with a loop diuretic, to patients with heart failure to relieve pulmonary congestion. When using this route of administration, it is important that a Teflon® coated catheter is used to avoid adsorption of the GTN onto the intravenous line.

Isosorbide dinitrate (ISDN) can be given orally and is completely absorbed; however, only 25% of a given dose appears as ISDN in serum with 60% of an oral dose being rapidly converted to isosorbide mononitrate. Isosorbide mononitrate (ISMN) is longer acting and therefore most of the accumulated effects of a dose of ISDN are attributable to the 5-isosorbide mononitrate metabolite. Consequently, a 20 mg dose of ISDN is approximately equivalent to a 10 mg dose of ISMN. In practice, nitrate preparations are usually given orally in the form of ISMN, and intravenously in the form of GTN.

Hydralazine has a direct action on arteriolar smooth muscle to produce arterial vasodilation. Its use is associated with the risk of causing drug-induced systemic lupus erythematosus (SLE). SLE is an uncommon multisystem connective tissue disorder that is more likely to occur in patients classified as slow acetylators of hydralazine, which accounts for almost half the UK population. The activity and use of nitrates are summarized in Table 21.6.

Inotropic agents (Table 21.7)

The use of inotropic agents (except digoxin) is almost exclusively limited to hospital practice, where acute heart failure may require the use of one or more inotropic agents, particularly the sympathomimetic agents dobutamine and dopamine, in an intravenous continuous infusion. These agents have inotrope-vasodilator effects which differ according to their action on α, β_1, β_2 and dopamine receptors (β_1 agonists increase cardiac contractility, β_2 agonists produce arterial vasodilation, dopamine agonists enhance renal perfusion). With dopamine, low doses (0–2 µg/kg/min) have a predominant effect on dopamine receptors within the kidneys to improve urine output, intermediate doses (2–5 µg/kg/min) affect β_1 receptors, producing an inotropic effect, and high doses (10 µg/kg/min) have a predominant action on α-adrenoceptors. Dobutamine has a predominantly inotropic and vasodilator action due to the action of the (+) isomer selectively on β-adrenoceptors. Tolerance to sympathomimetic inotropic agents may develop on prolonged administration, particularly in patients with underlying ischaemia, and is also associated with a risk of precipitating arrhythmias.

Noradrenaline (norepinephrine) is an α-adrenoceptor agonist whose vasoconstrictor action limits its usefulness in severely hypotensive patients such as those in septic shock. Adrenaline (epinephrine) has β_1, β_2 and α-adrenoceptor agonist effects and is used in patients with low vascular resistance. However, it is more arrhythmogenic than dobutamine and should be used with caution.

Phosphodiesterase inhibitors are rarely used in clinical practice as a consequence of trials showing an increased risk of mortality (PROMISE 1991).

Other agents

Direct-acting vasodilators such as sodium nitroprusside are rarely used, and when they are, it is in the acute setting when they are given by continuous infusion. Vasodilation occurs as a result of the catalysis of nitroprusside in vascular smooth muscle cells to produce nitric oxide. The fact that nitric oxide production in this instance is via a different route when compared to the catalysis of glyceryl trinitrate (where there is a need for sulphydryl groups) may explain why there is little tolerance seen with nitroprusside. In impaired renal function thiocyanate, a metabolic product of nitroprusside, accumulates over several days, causing nausea, anorexia, fatigue and psychosis.

Patients with coronary heart disease may be candidates for calcium-blocking antianginal vasodilators. However, some of these agents can exacerbate co-existing heart failure, since their negative inotropic effects offset the potentially beneficial arterial vasodilation. Amlodipine and felodipine have a more selective action on vascular tissue and therefore a less pronounced effect on cardiac contractility than other calcium antagonists and should be the agents of choice where appropriate.

In hospitalized patients in whom compromised respiratory function remains despite medical management of heart failure, the treatment options include mechanical ventilation, continuous positive airway pressure ventilation and the use of intra-aortic balloon pumping.

Table 21.7 Inotropic agents used in the treatment of heart failure

Class and agent	Pharmacological half-life	Comment
Cardiac glycosides		
Digoxin	39 h	In renal failure, half-life of digoxin prolonged. Dosage individualization required. Serum drug concentration monitoring used to confirm or exclude toxicity or effectiveness. Dose of digitoxin unaffected by renal failure. CNS, visual and GI symptoms linked to digoxin toxicity. No benefit in terms of mortality, but use associated with improved symptoms and reduced hospitalization for heart failure. Beneficial in AF although risk of arrhythmias with high doses. If given i.v. must be administered slowly (20 min) to avoid cardiac ischaemia
Digitoxin	5–8 days	
Phosphodiesterase inhibitors		
Enoximone	4.2 h	Used only in severe heart failure as adjunctive therapy. Associated with arrhythmias and increased mortality with chronic use
Milrinone	2.4 h	
Sympathomimetics		
Dobutamine	2 min	Continuous i.v. only. Require close monitoring in critical care setting
Dopamine	2 min	
Dopexamine	6–7 min	
Isoprenaline	>1 min	

Guidelines

Several groups have produced evidence-based consenses clinical guidelines. The focus of the various guidelines tends to be on chronic medication use (American College of Cardiology/American Heart Association 2005, European Society of Cardiology 2005, Scottish Intercollegiate Guidelines Network 2007). All guidelines confirm that ACE inhibitors and β-blockers should be given to all patients with all grades of heart failure, whether symptomatic or asymptomatic, in the absence of contraindication or intolerance.

In ACE inhibitor-intolerant patients, the preferred alternative is an ARB. However, it should be remembered that where ACE inhibitor intolerance is due to renal dysfunction, hypotension or hyperkalaemia, similar effects could be expected with an ARB. If an ARB is an unsuitable alternative, the use of hydralazine/nitrate combination or digoxin could be considered, although the latter agent has no effect on mortality. For patients with symptomatic heart failure, a loop diuretic is usually recommended to treat oedema and control symptoms. In heart failure patients who are still symptomatic despite being on optimum therapy (ACE inhibitor, β-blocker with/without a diuretic), the use of adjunctive therapies is recommended which can include ARB, aldactone antagonists, hydralazine/nitrate combination and digoxin where the patient is still in sinus rhythm.

With regard to diastolic dysfunction there is debate as to whether this is a specific diagnosis. The cause of 'apparent' heart failure symptoms can in many cases be attributed to another disease/condition such as respiratory disease, obesity or ischaemic heart disease. However, there may also be some patients in whom the cause of heart failure symptoms is uncertain. Therefore, particular recommendations for the drug treatment of diastolic heart failure are lacking.

Patient care

Heart failure remains poorly understood by the general public, amongst whom only 3% were able to identify the condition when presented with a list of typical symptoms. Patients with heart failure are often elderly with co-morbidity such as coronary heart disease and hypertension. Other complications include renal impairment, polypharmacy and variable adherence to prescribed medication regimens. Where renal function is compromised, careful attention to dosage selection is required for drugs excreted largely unchanged in the urine. Patients with heart failure are at particular risk of fluid or electrolyte imbalance, adverse effects and drug interactions. Consequently, careful monitoring is indicated to help detect problems associated with suboptimal drug therapy, unwanted drug effects and poor patient compliance.

A number of therapeutic problems may be encountered by the patient with heart failure. Notably, heart failure often complicates other serious illness, and is a common cause of hospital admission. In addition to monitoring clinical signs and symptoms in the acute setting, there should be monitoring of fluid and electrolyte balance, assessment of renal and hepatic function, and performance of chest radiograph, electrocardiograph and haemodynamic measurements where appropriate.

Patient education and self-monitoring

The patient must be in a position to understand the need for treatment and the benefits and risks offered by prescribed medication before concordance with a treatment plan can be reached. Appropriate patient education is necessary to encourage an understanding of their condition, inform them of the extent of their condition and how prescribed drug treatment will work and affect their daily lives. It is also important to encourage them to be an active participant in their care where appropriate. Specific advice should be given to reinforce the timing of doses and how each medication should be taken. Patients also need to be advised of potentially troublesome symptoms that may occur with the medication, and whether such effects are avoidable, self-limiting or a cause for concern.

Patients should be made aware that diuretics will increase urine production, and that doses are usually timed for the morning to avoid inconvenience during the rest of the day or overnight. However, there are cases where patients are reminded that they can alter the timing of the dose(s) to suit their lifestyle or commitments, with the agreement of their doctor. There are also some patients who use a flexible diuretic dosing regimen, where they take an extra dose of diuretic in response to worsening signs or symptoms as part of an agreed self-management protocol. To use such a regimen, the patient has to monitor and record their weight on a daily basis, and have clear instructions to take an extra dose of diuretic when a notable increase in weight is detected due to fluid retention, and when to seek medical attention. It is also important for patients to be aware of signs and symptoms of drug toxicity with medicines such as digoxin, e.g. anorexia, diarrhoea, nausea and vomiting, and be aware of the action to be taken should these symptoms occur.

Timing of doses is also important. If a nitrate regimen is being used, then patients must be made aware that the last dose of the nitrate should be taken mid to late afternoon to ensure that a nitrate-free period occurs overnight, thus reducing the risk of nitrate tolerance. However, patients with prominent nocturnal symptoms require separate consideration. Where β-blockers are introduced, it is important that the patient is aware of the need for gradual dose titration due to the risk of the medication aggravating heart failure symptoms. Certain medicines for the treatment of minor ailments that are available for purchase over the counter without a prescription can aggravate heart failure, such as ibuprofen, antihistamines and effervescent formulations. It is important that patients know what action to take if their symptoms become progressively worse, and whom to contact when necessary. Table 21.8 provides a general patient education and self-monitoring checklist, highlighting the typical areas where advice can be given.

Monitoring effectiveness of drug treatment

Therapeutic effectiveness is confirmed by assessing the patient for improvements in reported symptoms such as shortness of breath and oedema, and for noticeable changes in exercise tolerance. Oedema is often visible and remarked upon by patients, especially in the feet (ankles) and hands (wrists and fingers). Increased oedema may be reflected by an increase in the patient's body weight, and can be more easily assessed if the patient routinely records their weight

Table 21.8 Patient education and self-monitoring in the treatment of heart failure

Topic	Advice	Comment
Diuretics	• Will cause diuresis • Timing of dose • Flexible dosing (where indicated)	Monitor for incontinence, muscle weakness, confusion, dizziness, gout, unusual gain in weight within very short time-period (few days). Use of diary to record and monitor daily weight can help identify when to take an agreed extra dose of diuretic. Patient also able to adjust time of dose to suit lifestyle where necessary
ACE inhibitors	• Improve symptoms • Avoid standing rapidly	Monitor for hypotension, dizziness, cough, taste disturbance, sore throat, rashes, tingling in hands, joint pain
β-blockers	• Symptoms worsen initially • Gradual increase in dose	Monitor for hypotension, dizziness, headache, fatigue, gastrointestinal disturbances, bradycardia
Cardiac glycosides	• Report toxic symptoms	Monitor for signs or symptoms of toxicity, such as anorexia, nausea, visual disturbances, diarrhoea, confusion, social withdrawal
Nitrates	• Timing of dose • Postural hypotension • Avoid standing rapidly	Monitor for headache, hypotension, dizziness, flushing (face or neck), gastrointestinal upset. Ensure asymmetrical dosing pattern for nitrates to provide nitrate-free period and reduce risk of tolerance developing
Potassium salts	• Administration of dose (soluble + non-soluble)	Monitor for gastrointestinal disturbances, swallowing difficulty, diarrhoea, tiredness, limb weakness. Ensure patient knows how to take their medication safely, e.g. swallow whole immediately after food, or soluble forms to be taken with appropriate amount of water/fruit juice and allow fizzing to stop
Purchased medicines	• Choice of medicines	Ensure patient is aware of need to seek advice when purchasing medicines for minor ailments. Ask pharmacist to confirm suitability when selecting
Understanding the condition	• What heart failure is • Impact on lifestyle • Treatment goals	Ensure patient understands their condition, treatment goals and complications that may impact on their quality of life. Important to motivate the patient with respect to lifestyle modification and achievement of agreed treatment goals relative to the degree of heart failure present (asymptomatic, mild, moderate or severe)
Health issues	• Diet; sodium intake • Alcohol intake • Smoking • Exercise • Other risk factors	Issues related to diet, alcohol consumption, smoking habit, regular gentle exercise (walking). Other associated risk factors, e.g. hypertension, ischaemic heart disease, need to be addressed where appropriate

and reviews this on a daily basis. Questions about tolerance to exercise are also useful in identifying patients who may be experiencing difficulties with their condition or where the treatment plan is suboptimal. Onset or deterioration of symptoms is often slow and patients are more inclined to adapt their lifestyle gradually by moderating daily activities to compensate.

Identifying the symptoms of poor control of heart failure can be complicated by many factors, such as the presence of conditions like arthritis and parkinsonism which can also affect a patient's mobility. Poor control of respiratory disease, presenting as an increased shortness of breath or exacerbation of other respiratory symptoms, can also be mistaken for loss of control of heart failure. Therefore, consideration of these and other factors is necessary in the interpretation of presenting symptoms, as a deterioration in symptoms may not be solely due to worsening heart failure or ineffective heart failure medication.

Dietary factors can lead to loss of symptom control, where failure to restrict sodium intake may contribute to an ongoing problem of fluid retention. Simple dietary advice to avoid processed foods and not to add salt to food should be reinforced. According to some manufacturers, the absorption of ACE inhibitors, e.g. captopril, perindopril, may be slowed by food or antacids and therefore patients should be advised to take the dose before a meal in the morning to ensure maximum effect.

There are many patients with heart failure whose drug treatment is suboptimal. This is due to the fact that those agents identified as first-line therapy, i.e. ACE inhibitors and β-blockers, are either not prescribed or are given at a dosage below the recommended target dose. Those patients at risk of suboptimal treatment need to be identified, and they will require the involvement of healthcare professionals in the monitoring of symptoms and in the individualization of their therapeutic plan.

Table 21.9 provides a summary of monitoring activity required to confirm the effectiveness of drug use. Systematic patient assessment in the course of delivering care to heart failure patients can be facilitated by an audit tool designed to assess adherence to accepted evidence-based clinical guidelines. Table 21.10 shows an example of audit tool criteria based on SIGN guidelines (2007).

Table 21.9 Monitoring the effectiveness of drug treatment in patients with heart failure

Consider	Monitor for	Comment
Clinical markers	• Poor symptom control • Achievement of agreed treatment goals	Signs or symptoms of undertreatment or advancing disease need to be addressed (dyspnoea, breathlessness and/or fatigue). The aim is for good symptom control and either maintenance or improvement in quality of life. Persisting symptoms or hospitalization may indicate a revision of drug therapy or the addition of other agents where appropriate (see Fig. 21.2)
Interactions	• Drug–drug interactions	Some interactions may result in reduced effectiveness and require dosage adjustment or change in choice of drug (see Table 21.8)
Compliance	• Formulation acceptability • Dose timing and interval • Unusual time interval between requests for prescription medication	Poor compliance can result from drug being ineffective (over- or under-use), experience of side effects, a complicated drug regimen or patient behaviour (intentional non-compliance or forgetfulness). Reasons need to be identified and addressed where possible, e.g. adjusting frequency and timing of doses, review choice of formulation, education. Initiation of devices to improve compliance should be considered where appropriate
Evidence-based prescribing	• Implementation of evidence-based guidelines • Audit of prescribed treatment for heart failure	The drug of choice for a particular patient may not reflect the evidence base for treatment for patients with heart failure. It is important to ensure evidence-based treatments are considered for every patient, and choices of medication confirmed or changed where appropriate. Audit of guideline recommendations to help confirm that treatment plans are optimal can be systematically applied to help assess appropriateness of treatment
Multidisciplinary working	• Input from other healthcare professionals	It is important to be aware of what care has already been provided to minimize the risk of giving conflicting advice to the patient or duplicating work already done. It may also allow reinforcement of key information. There is an increasing evidence base for the benefits of multidisciplinary models of care for chronic heart failure patients

Monitoring safety of drug treatment

A number of issues around the safe use of medication must be considered, especially in those patients with co-morbidity where a high number of medications are prescribed. In these patients there is an increased risk of experiencing drug–drug and drug–disease interactions (Tables 21.11 and 21.12). It is important to be aware of clinically important interactions and to investigate potentially problematic combinations, as well as to regularly assess the patient for any signs or symptoms of drug therapy problems. Monitoring for problems such as negative inotropic effects, excessive blood pressure reduction, and salt and fluid retention should be undertaken and, where appropriate, laboratory measurement of plasma drug concentration (digoxin) or physiological markers (potassium, creatinine) should be performed to confirm or exclude adverse effects.

Potential problems with diuretic therapy

The use of diuretic therapy for sodium and water retention is common in the treatment of heart failure, although there can be a number of problems for the patient to contend with. Elderly patients in particular are at risk from the unwanted effects of diuretics. The increase in urine volume can worsen incontinence or precipitate urinary retention in the presence of an enlarged prostate, while overuse can lead to a loss of control of heart failure and worsening of symptoms. Rapid diuresis with a loop diuretic leading to more than a 1 kg loss in body weight per day may exacerbate heart failure due to an acute reduction in blood volume, hypotension and diminished renal perfusion, with a consequent increase in renin release. Prolonged and excessive doses of diuretics can also contribute to symptoms of fatigue as a consequence of electrolyte disturbance and dehydration. The adverse biochemical effects of excessive diuresis include uraemia, hypokalaemia and alkalosis. Diuretic-induced glucose intolerance may affect diabetic control in type 2 diabetes, but more commonly diuretics reveal glucose intolerance in patients who are not diagnosed as being diabetic. Diuretics also increase plasma urate leading to hyperuricaemia, although this may not require a change in drug therapy if symptoms of gout are absent (estimated incidence of 2%).

Hyponatraemia may occur with diuretics, and is usually due to water retention rather than sodium loss. Severe hyponatraemia (plasma sodium concentration of less than 115 mmol/L) causes confusion and drowsiness. It commonly arises when potassium-sparing agents are used in diuretic combinations.

Diuretics may also lead to hypokalaemia as a result of urinary sodium increasing the rate of K^+/Na^+ exchange in the distal tubule. Plasma potassium concentrations below 3.0 mmol/L occur in less than 5% of patients receiving diuretics. The occurrence of hypokalaemia is hazardous for patients receiving digoxin and also for those with ischaemic heart disease or conduction disorders. It is more commonly found with thiazide diuretics than loop agents, and is more likely to occur when diuretics are used for heart failure than for hypertension. This is probably due to the fact that higher doses are used and there is an associated activation of the renin–angiotensin system. Patients with a plasma potassium level of less than 3.5 mmol/L require treatment with potassium supplements or the addition of a potassium-sparing diuretic. The use of a potassium-sparing diuretic is considered to be more effective at preventing hypokalaemia than using

Table 21.10 Audit tool criteria for assessment of the drug treatment of a patient with chronic heart failure based on SIGN guideline (2007)

Treatment of heart failure	✓/✗		✓/✗

First-line therapy

1. ACE inhibitor prescribed ☐
2. Target dose for ACE inhibitor? ☐
3. Use of ARB in ACE inhibitor intolerance ☐
4. Target dose for ARB? ☐
5. Alternative used in ACE inhibitor/ARB intolerance [1] ☐
6. β-blocker prescribed ☐
7. Target dose for β-blocker? ☐

Adjunctive therapy as appropriate

8. Diuretic prescribed if sodium/water retention ☐
9. Aldosterone antagonist prescribed ☐
10. Target dose for aldosterone antagonist? ☐
11. Candesartan prescribed ☐
12. Target dose for candesartan? ☐
13. Hydralazine/nitrate prescribed ☐
14. Digoxin prescribed ☐

Treatment of co-morbidity

15. In AF, appropriate choice of antiarrhythmic agent ☐
16. History of VF, appropriate choice of antiarrhythmic agent ☐
17. In AF, warfarin prescribed ☐
18. If warfarin prescribed, INR monitored ☐
19. If calcium channel blocker required, amlodipine prescribed ☐
20. If post-MI with raised cholesterol, statin prescribed ☐
21. Pneumococcal vaccine received ☐
22. Influenza vaccine received ☐
23. Aggravating drugs avoided (see below) ☐

Lithium	Calcium channel blockers [2]
Tricyclic antidepressants	Antifungals
Erythromycin	Antiarrhythmic agents [3]
Terfenadine	NSAIDs
Other antihistamines	Carbenoxolone
Corticosteroids	High sodium-containing products
Liquorice	

[1] Refers to use of hydralazine/nitrate, or digoxin. [2] Except amlodipine/felodipine. [3] Class I + III, except amiodarone.

Table 21.11 Common drug–drug interactions with prescribed heart failure medication

Drug	Interacts with	Result of interaction
Diuretic	NSAIDs	Decreased effect of diuretic
	Carbamazepine	Increased risk of hyponatraemia
	Lithium	Excretion of lithium impaired (thiazides worse than loop diuretics)
ACE inhibitor or ARB	NSAIDs	Antagonism of hypotensive effect. Increased risk of renal impairment
	Ciclosporin	Increased risk of hyperkalaemia
	Lithium	Excretion of lithium impaired
	Diuretics	Enhanced hypotensive effect. Increased risk of hyperkalaemia with potassium-sparing drugs
Digoxin	Amiodarone	Increased digoxin level (need to halve maintenance dose of digoxin)
	Propafenone	Increased digoxin level (need to halve maintenance dose of digoxin)
	Quinidine	Increased digoxin level (need to halve maintenance dose of digoxin)
	Verapamil	Increased risk of AV block
	Diuretics	Increased risk of hypokalaemia and therefore toxicity
	Amphotericin	Increased cardiac toxicity if hypokalaemia present
Nitrates	Sildenafil	Increased hypotensive effect
	Heparin	Increased excretion of heparin
Spironolactone	Digoxin	Spironolactone may interfere with measurement of digoxin plasma levels, resulting in inaccurate interpretation
β-blocker	Amiodarone	Increased risk of bradycardia
	Diltiazem	Increased risk of AV block and bradycardia
	Verapamil	Increased risk of hypotension, heart failure and asystole

Table 21.12 Common drug–disease interactions with prescribed heart failure medication

Drug	Concurrent disease	Potential outcome
Diuretic	Prostatism	Urinary retention/incontinence
	Hyperuricaemia	Exacerbation of gout
	Liver cirrhosis	Encephalopathy
ACE inhibitor	Renal artery stenosis	Renal failure
	Severe aortic stenosis	Exacerbation of heart failure
	Renal impairment	Renal failure
	Hypotension	Hypotension and cardiogenic shock
β-blocker	Asthma	Bronchoconstriction/respiratory arrest
	Bradyarrhythmias	Exacerbation of heart failure
	Hypotension	Further hypotension and cardiogenic shock
Digoxin	Bradyarrhythmias	Exacerbation of heart failure
	Renal impairment	Exacerbation of heart failure and digoxin toxicity leading to cardiac arrhythmias

potassium supplements. Prevention of hypokalaemia requires at least 25 mmol of potassium, while treatment requires 60–120 mmol of potassium daily. Since proprietary diuretic-potassium combination products usually contain less than 12 mmol in each dose, their use is often inappropriate.

Potassium supplements are poorly tolerated at the high doses often needed to treat hypokalaemia, and a liquid formulation is more preferable to a solid form. This is mainly due to the fact that solid forms can produce local high concentrations of potassium salts in the gastrointestinal tract, with the risk of damage to the tract in patients with swallowing difficulties or delayed gastrointestinal transit. In patients with deteriorating renal function or renal failure, the use of potassium supplements or potassium-sparing diuretics might cause hyperkalaemia and therefore careful monitoring of these agents is essential.

Potential problems with ACE inhibitor and angiotensin II receptor blocker therapy

ACE inhibitors are the cornerstone of the treatment of heart failure, but there are also risks associated with their use. ARBs, which also act on the renin–angiotensin–aldosterone system, pose similar risks to those recognized for ACE inhibitors. Both agents can predispose patients to hyperkalaemia through a reduction in circulating aldosterone; therefore potassium supplements or potassium-retaining agents should be used with care when co-prescribed, and careful monitoring of plasma potassium should be mandatory. Although potassium retention can be a problem with ACE inhibitors and ARBs, it can also be an advantage by helping to counteract the potassium loss that results from the use of diuretic therapy. However, since this effect on potassium cannot be predicted, laboratory monitoring is still necessary to confirm that plasma potassium concentration remains within safe limits.

The use of an aldosterone antagonist as adjunctive therapy with an ACE inhibitor (or ARB if the patient is ACE inhibitor intolerant) can be safely undertaken with minimal effects on the plasma potassium concentration, provided that recommended target doses for the aldosterone antagonist are not exceeded (see Table 21.5). Although this is usually the case, laboratory monitoring of potassium is mandatory. Heparin therapy has also been shown to increase the risk of hyperkalaemia when used alongside ACE inhibitor or ARB therapy, and therefore a similar approach to monitoring should be taken.

When initiating ACE inhibitor or ARB therapy, volume depletion due to prior use of a diuretic increases the risk of a large drop in blood pressure occurring following the first dose. As a consequence diuretic treatment is usually withheld during the initiation phase of therapy in an effort to minimize this effect.

A dry cough, which may be accompanied by a voice change, occurs in about 10% of patients receiving an ACE inhibitor. It is more common in women and is associated with a raised level of kinins. Rashes, loss or disturbances of taste, mouth ulcers and proteinuria may also occur with ACE inhibitor therapy, particularly with captopril. These unwanted effects tend to be more common in patients with connective tissue disorders.

A number of ACE inhibitors are administered as pro-drugs so close monitoring is advised in patients with liver dysfunction, as this could reduce the benefits associated with their use. Most ACE inhibitors are dependent on the kidney for excretion, and require careful dosage titration in patients with existing renal dysfunction. Differences in the pharmacokinetic characteristics do not fully explain the differences in duration of action seen with the ACE inhibitors, as this is also related to ACE binding affinity. Throughout treatment the dose must be individualized to obtain maximum benefit in relation to symptom relief and survival, with minimum side effects. When the experience of adverse effects requires a review of therapeutic alternatives, ARBs can be considered as an alternative treatment option. Although the side effect profile of ARB therapy is very similar to that of ACE inhibitors, it is not identical.

Potential problems with digoxin therapy

Although digoxin has been shown to reduce the hospitalization of patients with heart failure, its use is associated with a range of adverse effects including non-specific signs and symptoms such as nausea, anorexia, tiredness, weakness, diarrhoea, confusion and visual disturbances. Digoxin also has the potential to cause fatal arrhythmias. It slows atrioventricular conduction and produces bradycardia, but it may also cause various ventricular and supraventricular arrhythmias. Digoxin toxicity typically causes conduction disturbances with enhanced automaticity leading to premature ventricular contractions. Patients at particular risk are those with myocardial ischaemia, hypoxia, acidosis or renal failure.

The appropriateness of digoxin dosage should be guided by assessment of the patient's renal function (from serum creatinine and creatinine clearance determinations) and from the patient's pulse rate. Renal function may also be affected by drug therapy or loss of control of heart failure, therefore any change in digoxin

Table 21.13 Monitoring the safety of drug treatment in patients with heart failure

Consider	Monitor	Comment
Clinical markers	• Side effects • Toxicity • Adverse drug reactions	There is a need to monitor for signs/symptoms of overtreatment with prescribed medication, such as diuretics (dehydration) and digoxin (nausea and vomiting). Look for signs of patient intolerance, allergy, serious adverse effects or troublesome side effects. Document unexpected adverse drug reactions if reported
Laboratory markers	• Changes in organ function • Biochemical changes • Haematological changes • Suspected digoxin toxicity	Renal function assessment and implications for drug choice and dosage individualization required, especially in the elderly and for initiation or titration of ACE inhibitor therapy (creatinine, potassium, urea). Hypokalaemia can lead to digoxin toxicity, and plasma drug concentration measurement may be performed to confirm or exclude toxicity. Haematological side effects with some drugs have been reported, e.g. ACE inhibitors, therefore laboratory checks may be required in response to clinical signs/symptoms presented
Interactions	• Drug–drug interactions • Drug–disease interactions	Some interactions may result in harm to the patient (see Table 21.8)
Co-morbidity	• Drug selection for concomitant conditions	The presence of heart failure may influence treatment choice for co-existing diseases or conditions, e.g. coronary artery disease, thyroid disease, respiratory disease. Where possible, ensure drugs known to worsen heart failure are avoided or used with caution, e.g. non-steroidal anti-inflammatory agents or corticosteroids in rheumatoid arthritis

clearance will have an impact on the plasma digoxin concentration. The possibility of a high plasma digoxin concentration should also be considered in any patient whose health deteriorates or who shows signs and symptoms of digoxin toxicity.

Potential problems with β-blocker therapy

Until recently, the use of β-blockers was contraindicated in patients with heart failure due to negative inotropic and chronotropic effects. However, β-blockers have been shown to be effective in patients with heart failure and should be used in all patients in the absence of contraindications or intolerance. Initiation of treatment and titration of dose must be under close supervision, with very small dose increments used to minimize transient worsening of heart failure symptoms. Titration of the dose to target is normally performed over a number of weeks or months, and close patient monitoring is required to ensure safety is not compromised. The maximum tolerable dose for a patient may be below the target dose and may limit further dose titration. Monitoring for excessive bradycardia or rapid deterioration of symptoms is necessary to ensure patient safety, while also monitoring the patient's prescribed dose to ensure that dosage increments are gradual and the patient is not subjected to an overall worsening of symptoms.

Potential problems with other drugs

There are a number of other cardiovascular drugs that may be prescribed for patients with diseases or conditions other than heart failure, with some agents capable of worsening or aggravating symptoms. Patients with coronary artery disease may be candidates for calcium-blocking antianginal vasodilators. However, some of these agents, for example diltiazem and verapamil, can exacerbate co-existing heart failure, since their negative inotropic effects offset the potentially beneficial arterial vasodilation. Second-generation dihydropyridines such as amlodipine and felodipine have a preferential action on the vasculature. They have less pronounced effects on cardiac contractility than other calcium antagonists, and this makes them the agents of choice where a limitation of the heart rate is not required.

Symptoms of fainting or dizziness on standing may indicate a need to review diuretic or vasodilator therapy. Patients should be reassured about mild postural effects and given advice to avoid standing from the chair too quickly. The patient and the healthcare team need to confirm the safety of the patient's treatment plan regularly, and be vigilant for any signs or symptoms suggesting otherwise.

Table 21.13 provides a summary of monitoring activity required to ensure the safety of drug use.

CASE STUDIES

Case 21.1 (part one)

Mrs EL, a 53-year-old woman weighing 60 kg, has been recently discharged from hospital and is receiving digoxin 0.375 mg, carbimazole 10 mg three times daily, furosemide 40 mg daily, and propranolol 40 mg three times daily.

Questions

1. What information is required to confirm the appropriateness of treatment for this patient? Is Mrs EL receiving a rational treatment regimen?
2. Once Mrs EL's thyroid problem has resolved, why will the medication regimen on which she was discharged need to be reviewed?

Answers

1. There is a need to obtain as much background information as possible from the patient to confirm the purpose and duration of drug

therapy and the reason for the recent hospital admission. Information relating to current symptoms, past medical and drug history, renal function, thyroid status, body weight, plasma electrolyte and digoxin determinations is required to complete the picture.

Mrs EL is receiving the antithyroid agent carbimazole to treat thyrotoxicosis, diuretic therapy possibly to treat the signs and symptoms of fluid retention associated with heart failure, and digoxin to treat atrial fibrillation (AF). Although digoxin has been used in combination with diuretics to treat heart failure, it has been largely superseded by the use of ACE inhibitors. Propranolol is probably being used to improve the symptoms of tremor and anxiety that accompany thyrotoxicosis, and is considered to be the drug of choice for this indication. Once a patient is diagnosed with thyrotoxicosis, antithyroid treatment will lead to gradual attainment of the euthyroid state over about 6 weeks (see Chapter 43). In such patients a relative resistance to the pharmacological effects of digoxin occurs, therefore the dosage requirement in thyrotoxicosis is higher than would normally be expected. High plasma digoxin concentrations are needed to suppress atrioventricular conduction in AF and to counteract the increased rate of digoxin elimination also seen in the thyrotoxic patient. Propranolol may also be beneficial in AF as it helps to control tachycardia and provide symptomatic treatment of thyrotoxicosis. Propranolol, as with all β-blockers, has a negative inotropic effect that can initially aggravate heart failure although β-blockers such as carvedilol and bisoprolol have been shown to improve symptoms and survival in such patients. However, the positive inotropic action of digoxin may afford some protection against this effect. Overall, the choice of medication for this patient would appear rational, but there are a number of issues that merit further inquiry and clarification which will include the confirmation or exclusion of heart failure due to left ventricular systolic dysfunction.

2. Once Mrs EL's thyroid status has returned to normal, inquiry into the persistence of AF and the possible existence of heart failure is required. Where heart failure is confirmed, consideration must be given to the initiation of ACE inhibitor treatment in the absence of contraindication or intolerance. The use of β-blocker treatment must also be reviewed in relation to the patient's need. Once euthyroid and hyperthyroid symptoms have resolved, consideration should be given to switching from propranolol to one of the β-blockers recommended for the treatment of heart failure. Mrs EL is also receiving furosemide and is potentially at risk of developing hypokalaemia, which is particularly hazardous in a patient receiving digoxin. Monitoring for any signs or symptoms of digoxin toxicity should be undertaken, which may include a loss of appetite, nausea, a change in bowel habit or general malaise. Visual disturbances such as haloes or yellow/green colour blindness are characteristic of digoxin toxicity but are infrequently volunteered by patients. In the case of a confirmed diagnosis of heart failure due to left ventricular systolic dysfunction, application of the audit tool to assess heart failure treatment (Table 21.10) identified the following criteria as not being met, and reasons for this should be determined or changes made to the treatment plan as appropriate.

Audit tool criteria for assessment of the drug treatment of a patient with chronic heart failure based on SIGN guideline (2006)	
ACE inhibitor prescribed?	X
In AF, warfarin prescribed?	X
Pneumococcal vaccine received	X
Influenza vaccine received	X

Case 21.1 (part two)

Two weeks after discharge Mrs EL seeks advice on what tonic preparation would be suitable for her to take with her medication. During your discussion you discover that she complains of tiredness, increased breathlessness and malaise.

Question

3. What medications/conditions might be responsible for the occurrence of these symptoms? What investigations are required?

Answer

3. There are a number of possibilities to consider when assessing the symptoms experienced by Mrs EL. Persisting hyperthyroidism or the negative inotropic effects of propranolol could be contributory factors. Alternatively, the symptoms may be due to poor control of heart failure, bradycardia or any of a variety of arrhythmias (in particular heart block and ventricular extrasystoles). The presence of anaemia may also be contributing to the symptoms reported. When considering the side effects or toxic effects of prescribed medication, it is possible that propranolol and/or digoxin may be implicated. Propranolol is associated with fatigue, while digoxin toxicity can be associated with malaise. The acute symptoms of digoxin toxicity include nausea and vomiting and are caused by an action on the chemoreceptor trigger zone. This emetic effect can occur independent of cardiotoxicity and other gastrointestinal disturbances such as anorexia, diarrhoea or constipation. The risk of digoxin toxicity is increased in patients prescribed a diuretic because of possible/concurrent hypokalaemia.

There are a number of clinical and laboratory investigations required for Mrs EL. Checking the pulse would allow an assessment of heart rate to confirm or exclude bradycardia. If necessary the propranolol should be discontinued and its place in the treatment plan re-evaluated. Laboratory tests required include the confirmation or exclusion of digoxin toxicity through measurement of the plasma digoxin concentration, and the determination of plasma potassium, urea and creatinine to investigate the possibility of hypokalaemia, dehydration or compromised renal function. If an ECG was available then the presence of bigeminy (coupling of QRS complexes) is a characteristic feature of digoxin toxicity. Where hypokalaemia is identified as a precipitant of digoxin toxicity, potassium supplementation should be administered orally, or intravenously if there is extreme hypokalaemia and life-threatening digoxin toxicity. Alternatively, high plasma digoxin (>5 µg/L) with renal impairment will require immediate treatment with intravenous digoxin antibody fragments in a single or repeated dose.

Case 21.2

Mrs FM, a 70 year old with chronic asthma and mild heart failure, has been prescribed naproxen 250 mg three times daily. On inspection of her medication record you discover that she is also receiving:

- **furosemide 40 mg each morning**
- **ramipril 5 mg in the morning**
- **prednisolone 5 mg daily**
- **salbutamol inhaler two puffs four times daily when required**
- **salmeterol 50 µg inhaler one puff twice daily**
- **beclometasone 250 µg inhaler two puffs twice daily**
- **co-magaldrox 195/220 suspension 10 mL when required.**

When you ask her about symptom control she tells you that she is still breathless at night which, in addition to her painful knee, is keeping her awake.

Questions

1. Do you think Mrs FM should be taking naproxen?
2. What other aspects of this patient's medication regimen could be improved?
3. What is the likely effect of the prescribed therapy on plasma potassium concentrations?

Answers

1. NSAIDs such as naproxen can exacerbate asthma and heart failure by inducing bronchospasm and by causing fluid retention, respectively. They can also lead to upper gastrointestinal problems, particularly when co-prescribed with oral steroids. If the painful knee is responsive to a simple analgesic such as paracetamol, this would be the preferred option. Alternatively, if a NSAID is necessary and toleralid, one such as ibuprofen in low dosage should be used as it is less likely to have an effect on respiratory and renal function although it may still aggravate symptoms of heart failure. Further investigation into the persistence of respiratory symptoms is required as it is unclear whether the patient's breathlessness is due to an exacerbation of her asthma or a worsening of her heart failure, and therefore the interpretation of this symptom is difficult.
2. It is important to establish whether the patient is receiving maximum benefit from inhaled treatment. Inhaler technique must be checked and improved if necessary and the dose of beclometasone optimized. A regular regimen of salbutamol is not advisable since it may impair control of asthma by masking the onset of exacerbations. A review of the need for an oral steroid should be undertaken, and any reduction in the use of an oral steroid must be done gradually to avoid exacerbation of the asthma and ensure that the patient does not experience adrenal insufficiency. Reduction of the oral steroid dose may benefit the heart failure and possibly reduce the need for an antacid.

    When considering the treatment of heart failure, application of the audit tool identified the following criteria which were not met.

Audit tool criteria for assessment of the drug treatment of a patient with chronic heart failure based on SIGN guideline (2006)	
Target dose for ACE inhibitor?	X
Aldosterone antagonist prescribed	X
Candesartan prescribed	X
Aggravating drugs avoided (see below) NSAID (naproxen)	X

There is scope to increase the dose of ramipril to 5 mg twice daily if tolerated, which is the target dose in heart failure patients. However, as β-blocker is contraindicated in this patient, consideration may be given to an adjunctive therapy such as spironolactone, candesartan, or an increase in the dose of furosemide provided the breathlessness is due to heart failure.

3. Mrs FM is receiving a number of medications with the potential to affect plasma potassium. Diuretics, oral and inhaled steroids (high-dose) and β-agonists can reduce potassium, while ACE inhibitors can increase potassium. It is impossible to predict the extent to which each agent will affect potassium, especially with inhaled treatments as the dose normally needs to be high before there is any significant systemic absorption. Determination of plasma potassium is necessary and if it remains low under the current treatment plan, or is at risk of being altered due to changes in drug dosage such as an increase in ramipril to 5 mg twice daily, then close observation will be required.

Case 21.3

Mr HS, 72 years old, is admitted to hospital with increasing shortness of breath at rest. He has a previous medical history of severe left ventricular systolic dysfunction (confirmed by echocardiography) and angina. Before admission he had been taking the following medication: lisinopril 10 mg daily, furosemide 80 mg each morning, digoxin 62.5 µg each morning, isosorbide mononitrate SR 60 mg daily, glyceryl trinitrate spray 1–2 doses as required, aspirin 75 mg dispersible each morning. His chest x-ray shows severe pulmonary oedema, his blood pressure is 110/70 mmHg and plasma urea and electrolytes are within normal range. During the admission, bisoprolol 5 mg daily is started.

Questions

1. What therapeutic options would you choose to treat the acute symptoms presented by Mr HS at the beginning of his admission?
2. Was the addition of bisoprolol appropriate for this patient?
3. What other drug treatment options might be considered for this patient in the longer term?

Answers

1. The administration of furosemide by the intravenous route is necessary as there is decreased absorption of oral furosemide secondary to gastrointestinal oedema in acute heart failure. Only after the oedema has resolved should the patient revert back to oral administration of diuretics. At this time, the dosage can be adjusted to maintain an appropriate fluid balance. Where diuresis is inadequate with an oral loop diuretic alone, the addition of metolazone should be considered (initially at low dose of 2.5 mg daily) to avoid rapid diuresis leading to hypotension and/or renal failure.
2. Although there is good evidence to show that β-blocker therapy is safe and effective for patients with NYHA stage IV heart failure, it is not currently recommended that it should be initiated in patients with acute symptoms of heart failure. Where β-blocker therapy is indicated, initiation should occur when the patient's heart failure has been stable for at least 2 weeks and started at a very low dose on specialist advice (i.e. bisoprolol 1.25 mg). The dose should be titrated gradually over a period of months towards the recommended target dose where appropriate, provided the patient tolerates each increment. In Mr HS's case, it is inappropriate to prescribe 5 mg bisoprolol at this time, but treatment with bisoprolol 1.25 mg daily could be considered once his heart failure has been stable for at least 2 weeks.
3. There is also scope to increase the dose of lisinopril to 20–35 mg daily provided the patient can tolerate the higher dose, as this is associated with greater benefits on morbidity and mortality. Based on his systolic blood pressure and assuming satisfactory renal function, there is no reason why this option cannot be explored and it would be reasonable to delay any titration of dosage until the symptoms become more stable. This is important since the use of large doses of loop diuretics in acutely ill patients may predispose to ACE inhibitor-induced renal impairment. Either candesartan or low-dose spironolactone could be added to Mr HS's existing drug therapy, since both would show benefits on morbidity and mortality if added to the existing treatment plan. The decision of which one to initiate first would usually lie with a heart failure specialist and would be tailored to each individual patient.

Case 21.4

Mr GF, a 57 year old, suffered a myocardial infarction 12 months ago and at the time was also found to have left ventricular systolic dysfunction on echocardiography. He is currently asymptomatic (NYHA I). At your request, he has agreed to see you for a medication review regarding his drug therapy. He has a history of type 2 diabetes mellitus (8 years) and his current prescription includes enalapril 10 mg twice daily, furosemide 40 mg daily, gliclazide 80 mg twice daily, bisoprolol 5 mg daily, aspirin 75 mg daily, and a glyceryl trinitrate spray to use when required.

Question

Is the current treatment plan for heart failure optimal?

Answer

Mr GF has echocardiographic evidence of left ventricular systolic dysfunction, but has no signs or symptoms of heart failure at present. Therefore, the absence of diuretic therapy is expected, although enquiry into the presence/absence of symptoms would form part of any review and would be included in the patient monitoring.

He is prescribed an ACE inhibitor at the recommended target dose (enalapril 10–20 mg twice daily) and treatment with this agent is optimal at present. There is scope for a further increase in dose should the need arise. When we consider β-blocker therapy, the current dose of bisoprolol (5 mg daily) is below the recommended target and should therefore be titrated to a dose of 10 mg daily or maximum tolerable dose. This titration should be implemented gradually over a period of weeks or months with close monitoring of blood pressure and heart rate. Regular assessment of the patient for side effects or signs and symptoms of heart failure should also be undertaken, as each incremental rise in β-blocker dose may be accompanied by a worsening (or in this case, appearance) of heart failure symptoms.

As Mr GF has a history of myocardial infarction and type 2 diabetes mellitus, the addition of eplerenone would be appropriate. Even though Mr GF is asymptomatic, eplerenone has been shown to improve symptoms and survival when given in addition to ACE inhibitor and β-blocker therapy. Eplerenone should be introduced at a dose of 25 mg daily and increased to a target of 50 mg daily if tolerated. Routine checks of plasma potassium and renal function should be performed before and after initiation/titration to ensure the combination of eplerenone and an ACE inhibitor is prescribed safely.

Case 21.5

Mr CH, a 78 year old, regularly visits your pharmacy for his medication and has moderately symptomatic heart failure (NYHA III). During a recent review with his doctor, Mr CH described worsening of his heart failure symptoms. His doctor has said he could take an extra dose of furosemide 40 mg if required, but Mr CH would need to be referred back to the cardiology consultant before changing any other medication. He is currently prescribed ramipril 5 mg daily, nebivolol 2.5 mg daily and furosemide 40 mg daily. His blood pressure has been measured as 103/62 mmHg (heart rate 54 bpm) and he has an estimated creatinine clearance of 20 mL/min.

Questions

1. What is the rationale behind the decision to refer Mr CH to the cardiology consultant?
2. What other drug treatment options might be considered?

Answers

1. Mr CH is prescribed both ACE inhibitor and β-blocker therapy in accordance with the evidence base for treatment. As Mr CH has symptomatic heart failure (NYHA III), he is also prescribed furosemide in response to signs and symptoms of fluid retention. When Mr CH reports deterioration in the control of his heart failure symptoms, the prescriber must consider what treatment options are available for Mr CH and make any necessary changes.

    Neither the ACE inhibitor nor β-blocker is prescribed at the recommended target dose (see Table 21.6), therefore there is scope to titrate the dose of either agent to the target dose which should result in improvement of symptoms and a reduced need for diuretic therapy. However, there may be reluctance to increase the dose of ACE inhibitor possibly due to the fact that Mr CH has a relatively low blood pressure and compromised renal function (estimated creatinine clearance 20 mL/min). Similarly, there may be reluctance to increase the dose of β-blocker due to a low blood pressure and heart rate (54 bpm). As both options may adversely affect the patient, the doctor has decided to treat the symptoms with additional diuretic when required as a short-term solution prior to Mr CH's appointment with the cardiology consultant. Advice should be sought from a heart failure specialist where a patient may be poorly tolerant of ACE inhibitor or β-blocker, or where there is a risk of hypotension or renal failure in susceptible individuals. In Mr CH's case, specialist supervision is required for optimization of therapy.
2. If there is no further scope to optimize either ACE inhibitor or β-blocker therapy due to their effects on blood pressure and/or renal function, it is also certain that other agents with similar effects (ARBs and aldosterone antagonists) might also be ruled out. Therefore, the addition of digoxin should be considered. Although digoxin has no effect on survival, it has been shown to lead to an improvement in heart failure symptoms and reduce the number of hospitalizations for heart failure. The main benefit is that improvement in symptoms will not be associated with changes in either blood pressure or renal function, and it is usually prescribed in the lower range of dosage. Caution in the use of digoxin is still required, and close attention must be paid to plasma potassium levels (hypokalaemia can cause digoxin toxicity) and heart rate (addition to a β-blocker may result in bradycardia) to ensure safety in use.

Case 21.6

Mrs JM, 66 years old, presents with a new prescription for candesartan 4 mg daily. On checking her medication record you see that she has been prescribed lisinopril 20 mg daily, bisoprolol 10 mg daily and furosemide 40 mg daily for the last 6 months to treat her heart failure. Her blood pressure was measured 2 weeks ago and was 128/78 mmHg.

Questions

1. How do you respond to the new prescription?
2. Could an aldosterone antagonist be added to Mrs JM's heart failure medication at a later date if symptoms persist?

Answers

1. It is unclear from the information given whether candesartan is prescribed as an adjunct to ACE inhibitor therapy or as an alternative to ACE inhibitor due to intolerance. Therefore, it is important to confirm the intended use of candesartan in this case through speaking to the patient and/or prescriber. If candesartan is being used as an alternative, it is important to establish the reason for intolerance. Patients are usually found to be intolerant of ACE inhibitors for

three main reasons: dry cough, hypotension or compromised renal function. As heart failure can produce symptoms of a dry cough, it can sometimes be difficult to ascertain whether the ACE inhibitor or the heart failure is responsible. Dry cough occurs secondary to the inhibition of bradykinin metabolism and is generally identified shortly after initiation of an ACE inhibitor; therefore inquiry into the timing of symptoms attributed to ACE inhibitor intolerance is important. If the reason is due to persistent dry cough, an ARB would be a suitable alternative. However, if the ACE inhibitor intolerance is related to hypotension or renal dysfunction, it is likely an ARB would induce similar adverse effects and therefore another alternative agent may have to be selected, e.g. hydralazine-nitrate combination.

If candesartan is being used as adjunctive therapy, which is supported by the current evidence base for treatment, careful introduction and titration of dose must be undertaken due to the increased risk of hypotension, renal dysfunction and hyperkalaemia (ACE inhibitors and ARBs are both potassium conserving). The addition of candesartan would normally be under the guidance of a heart failure specialist, and should be initiated at a low dose and gradually titrated up to the target (32 mg daily) or maximum tolerable dose. It is important to note that dose increases during the titration period should be at least 2 weeks apart. Although Mrs JM has a normal blood pressure measurement at present, it is unclear whether renal function or blood biochemistry has previously been checked and it is important that this is confirmed prior to starting candesartan. The monitoring plan for Mrs JM should include regular checks of blood pressure, plasma creatinine (and estimation of renal function), plasma potassium and clinical assessment for any signs/symptoms of adverse effects/intolerance. This should be done 7–14 days after initiation and final dose titration. As the addition of candesartan should improve heart failure symptom control, regular patient monitoring will allow an assessment of the effectiveness of therapy.

2. At present, Mrs JM is prescribed an ACE inhibitor, diuretic and β-blocker and is starting treatment with an ARB. From the available evidence, it is difficult to confirm whether the addition of an aldosterone antagonist to ACE inhibitor and ARB therapy will produce additional benefit, but the additional risk of the patient developing hyperkalaemia and renal dysfunction from combining these three agents is much greater. Therefore, the combination of an ACE inhibitor, ARB and aldosterone antagonist is not recommended at this time.

REFERENCES

A-HeFT (Taylor A L, Ziesche S, Yancy C et al) 2004 Combination of isosorbide dinitrate and hydralazine in blacks with heart failure. New England Journal of Medicine 351: 2049-2057

AIRE (Acute Infarction Ramipril Efficacy (AIRE) Study Investigators) 1993 Effect of ramipril on mortality and morbidity of survivors of acute myocardial infarction with clinical evidence of heart failure. Lancet 342: 821-828

American College of Cardiology/American Heart Association Task Force on Practice Guidelines 2005 Guideline update for the diagnosis and management of chronic heart failure in the adult – summary article. Circulation 112: e154-235

ANZ Carvedilol 1997 Australia/New Zealand Heart Failure Research Collaborative Group. Randomised, placebo-controlled trial of carvedilol in patients with congestive heart failure due to ischaemic heart disease. Lancet 349: 375-380

ATLAS (Packer M, Poole-Wilson P A, Armstrong P W et al) 1999 Comparative effects of low and high doses of the angiotensin-converting enzyme inhibitor, lisinopril, on morbidity and mortality in chronic heart failure. ATLAS Study Group. Circulation 100: 2312-2318

CAPRICORN Investigators 2001 Effect of carvedilol on outcome after myocardial infarction in patients with left-ventricular dysfunction: the CAPRICORN randomised trial. Lancet 357: 1385-1390

CARMEN (Komajda M, Lutiger B, Madeira H et al) 2004 Tolerability of carvedilol and ACE-inhibition in mild heart failure. Results of CARMEN (Carvedilol ACE-Inhibitor Remodelling Mild CHF EvaluatioN). European Journal of Heart Failure 6: 467-475

CHARM Added (McMurray J J, Ostergren J, Swedberg K et al) 2003 Effects of candesartan in patients with CHF and reduced left-ventricular systolic dysfunction taking angiotensin-converting-enzyme inhibitors: the CHARM Added trial. Lancet 362: 767-771

CHARM Alternative (Granger C B, McMurray J J, Yusuf S et al) 2003 Effects of candesartan in patients with CHF and reduced left-ventricular systolic function intolerant to angiotensin-converting-enzyme inhibitors: the CHARM Alternative trial. Lancet 362: 772-776

CIBIS II Investigators Committees 1999 The cardiac insufficiency bisoprolol study II (CIBIS II): a randomised trial. Lancet 353: 9-13

CIBIS III (Willenheimer R, van Veldhuisen D J, Silke B et al) 2005 Effect on survival and hospitalization of initiating treatment for chronic heart failure with bisoprolol followed by enalapril, as compared with the opposite sequence: results of the randomized Cardiac Insufficiency Bisoprolol Study (CIBIS) III. Circulation 112: 2426-2435

CONSENSUS I (CONSENSUS Trial Study Group) 1987 Effects of enalapril on mortality in severe congestive heart failure. New England Journal of Medicine 316: 1429-1435

CONSENSUS II (Swedberg K, Held P, Kjekshus J et al) 1992 Effects of the early administration of enalapril on the mortality in patients with acute myocardial infarction. Results from the co-operative new Scandinavian enalapril survival study II. New England Journal of Medicine 327: 678-684

COPERNICUS (Packer M, Coats A J, Fowler M B et al for the Carvedilol prospective randomized cumulative survival study group) 2001 Effect of carvedilol on survival in severe chronic heart failure. New England Journal of Medicine 334: 1651-1658

DIG (Digitalis Investigation Group) 1997 The effect of digoxin on mortality and morbidity in patients with heart failure. New England Journal of Medicine 336: 525-533

European Society of Cardiology 2005 The Task Force for the Diagnosis and Treatment of CHF of the European Society of Cardiology. Guidelines for the diagnosis and treatment of chronic heart failure: full text (update 2005). European Heart Journal 26: 1115-1140

MERIT-HF Study Group 1999 Effect of metoprolol CR/XL in chronic heart failure: metoprolol CR/XL randomised intervention trial in congestive heart failure (MERIT-HF). Lancet 353: 2001-2007

PROMISE (Packer M, Carver J R, Rodeheffer R J et al for the PROMISE Study Research Group) 1991 Effect of oral milrinone on mortality in severe chronic heart failure. New England Journal of Medicine 325: 1468-1475

PROVED (Uretsky B F, Young J B, Shahidi F E et al for the PROVED Investigative Group) 1993 Randomized study assessing the effect of digoxin withdrawal in patients with mild to moderate chronic congestive heart failure: results of the PROVED trial. Journal of the American College of Cardiology 22: 955-962

RADIANCE (Packer M, Gheorghiade M, Young J B et al) 1993 Withdrawal of digoxin from patients with chronic heart failure treated with angiotensin-converting-enzyme inhibitors. RADIANCE study. New England Journal of Medicine 329: 1-7

RALES (Pitt B, Zannad F, Remme W J et al for the Randomized Aldactone Evaluation Study Investigators) 1999 The effect of spironolactone on morbidity and mortality in patients with severe heart failure. New England Journal of Medicine 341: 709-717

SAVE (Pfeffer M A, Braunwald E, Moye L A et al) 1992 Effect of captopril on mortality and morbidity in patients with left ventricular dysfunction after myocardial infarction. Results of the survival and ventricular enlargement trial (SAVE). New England Journal of Medicine 327: 669-677

Scottish Intercollegiate Guidelines Network (SIGN) 2007 Management of chronic heart failure (Guideline 95). Scottish Intercollegiate Guidelines Network, Edinburgh. Available online at: www.sign.ac.uk

SENIORS (Flather M D, Shibata M C, Coats A J et al) 2005 Randomized trial to determine the effect of nebivolol on mortality and cardiovascular hospital admission in elderly patients with heart failure (SENIORS). European Heart Journal 26: 215-225

SOLVD-P (SOLVD Investigators) 1992 Effect of enalapril on mortality and the development of heart failure in asymptomatic patients with reduced left ventricular ejection fractions. New England Journal of Medicine 327: 685-691

SOLVD-T (SOLVD Investigators) 1991 Effect of enalapril on survival in patients with reduced left ventricular ejection fractions and congestive heart failure. New England Journal of Medicine 325: 293-302

TRACE (Trandolapril Cardiac Evaluation Study Group) 1995 A clinical trial of the angiotensin-enzyme inhibitor trandolapril in patients with left ventricular dysfunction after myocardial infarction. New England Journal of Medicine 333: 1670-1676

US Carvedilol (Packer M, Bristow M R, Cohn J N et al) 1996 The effect of carvedilol on morbidity and mortality in patients with chronic heart failure. US Carvedilol Heart Failure Study Group. New England Journal of Medicine 334: 1349-1355

Val-HeFT (Maggioni A P, Anand I, Gottlieb S O et al) 2002 Effects of valsartan on morbidity and mortality in patients with heart failure not receiving angiotensin-converting enzyme inhibitors. Journal of the American College of Cardiology 40: 1422-1424

V-HeFT I (Cohn J, Archibald D, Ziesche S et al) 1986 Effect of vasodilator therapy on mortality in chronic congestive heart failure. Results of a Veterans Administration cooperative study. New England Journal of Medicine 314: 1547-1552

V-HeFT II (Cohn J N, Johnson G, Ziesche S et al for the V-HeFT II study) 1991 A comparison of enalapril with hydralazine-isosorbide dinitrate in the treatment of chronic congestive heart failure. New England Journal of Medicine 325: 303-310

FURTHER READING

McMurray J, Cohen-Solal A, Dietz R et al 2005 Practical recommendations for the use of ACE inhibitors, β-blockers, aldosterone antagonists and angiotensin receptor blockers in heart failure: putting guidelines into practice. European Journal of Heart Failure 7: 710-721

Cardiac arrhythmias 22

D. K. Scott

An arrhythmia is an abnormal cardiac rhythm, usually involving a change in rate or regularity, and is monitored by an electrocardiograph. The term dysrhythmia is probably better since arrhythmia implies 'without rhythm'.

Physiology

The heart contains many different types of cell, including muscle cells and some specialized cells that generate or conduct electrical stimuli and cause the muscles to contract. Several types of cardiac cell are capable of automaticity-generating impulses, with the overall heart rhythm determined by the cells that do so most rapidly. When a cell is stimulated it passes on the impulse to adjacent cells and then enters a latent phase (refractory period) during which it cannot be restimulated. Cells that possess automaticity depolarize steadily until they reach a threshold potential at which they depolarize rapidly and generate an impulse (Fig. 22.1). In the normal heart (Fig. 22.2), sinoatrial (SA) node cells depolarize quickest and thus control the heart rhythm. The impulses are conducted from the SA node across the atria to the atrioventricular (AV) node and then down the bundle of His to the Purkinje fibres and the ventricles. This is termed sinus rhythm.

The activity of the heart is controlled by the sympathetic nervous system, which stimulates the SA node and penetrates most cardiac tissue, and the parasympathetic vagus nerve, which reduces conduction through the AV node and slows the SA node. When functioning normally, the AV node prevents the conduction of excess atrial beats, such as those which occur in atrial

fibrillation, to the ventricles but permits the passage of beats from a normal sinus rhythm. Excessive vagal stimulation results in bradycardia. This may occur in abdominal surgery, following oesophageal intubation or even in some very fit athletes when they stop exercise. Anticholinergic drugs such as tricyclic antidepressants or atropine may remove vagal control and cause tachycardia.

If the SA node is prevented from operating normally, the AV node will usually take over as pacemaker or, if both are disabled, the ventricular conducting tissues will serve as pacemaker. Whenever the SA node is not the controlling pacemaker the heart beat is less well co-ordinated. This may result in inefficient pumping, with an increase in energy expenditure to maintain an adequate circulation, or ineffective pumping with an inadequate circulation.

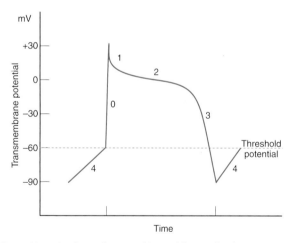

Figure 22.1 Cardiac cell potential (see Table 22.9 for dominant ion movement in each phase 0-4).

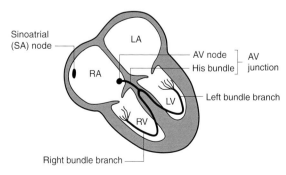

Figure 22.2 Heart conduction system.

Aetiology and epidemiology

It is estimated that 3.9 million people in USA have a cardiac rhythm disturbance and that this results in 730 000 hospital admissions each year. About 45 000 death certificates cite an arrhythmia as the main cause of death each year but about 500 000, a quarter of all deaths, mention arrhythmias. The most common clinically significant arrhythmia is atrial fibrillation and in the UK each year about 46 000 new cases are diagnosed. Over the age of 50 the prevalence of atrial fibrillation doubles with each decade and it is associated with many cardiac and non-cardiac illnesses. Arrhythmias result from abnormal impulse formation or abnormal impulse conduction and these changes may be brought about in several ways.

1. An infarction may cause the death of pacemaker cells or conducting tissue.
2. A cardiac tissue disorder, e.g. fibrosis or rheumatic fever, or a multisystem connective tissue disorder, e.g. sarcoidosis, disrupts the conduction network.
3. Sympathetic or parasympathetic control changes, e.g. stress, anxiety, exercise or smoking.
4. Circulating drugs, e.g. antiarrhythmics or inotropes, or other substances, e.g. caffeine, alcohol or bile salts, affect the heart directly or via the nervous system.
5. Hypothyroidism, hyperthyroidism, hypoadrenalism, hyperkalaemia and hypokalaemia or other electrolyte disturbances may predispose the heart to arrhythmias.

Patients who have pre-existing cardiac disorders including heart failure, hypertension or a recent infarction are at greater risk of arrhythmias. Older age is an independent risk factor and arrhythmias are also more common in pregnancy and following surgery. Some patients have occasional arrhythmias that may be attributed to the temporary ischaemia of angina, physical activity or stress but others have paroxysmal arrhythmias for no discernible reason. Most apparently normal adults have occasional ectopic beats, while in some studies up to 20% have brief periods of atrial fibrillation, and nearly half have both ventricular and supraventricular arrhythmias. In general, these arrhythmias are asymptomatic and treatment is not recommended. Many young adults have resting sinus rhythms of as little as 40 beats per minute, which would be defined as bradycardia in an older or active patient.

Atrial arrhythmias are more common than ventricular arrhythmias and atrial fibrillation (AF) is the commonest chronic arrhythmia. The 2-year incidence of AF increases with age from less than 0.1% in the 30–39 year age group to above 1% in 70–79-year-old men. The prevalence in men aged over 70 years is about 10% and the hospital stay required for treating AF exceeds the total for all ventricular and junctional rhythms. Among emergency medical admissions to UK general hospitals, 7% of patients have AF. Eighty-five percent of the patients with chronic AF and 40% of patients with paroxysmal AF have an identifiable cause, mostly valve disease, hypertension or ischaemic heart disease. Women have a lower risk of AF but respond less well to treatment and have a higher risk of dying. Women also have a lower risk of sudden cardiac death, defined as death within 1 hour of symptom onset in the absence of another probable cause and presumed to be due to arrhythmia, but have a higher risk of drug-induced arrhythmias.

Description of arrhythmias

All cardiac rhythms can be described by a phrase which includes terms that relate to rate, origin and pattern. Table 22.1 lists terms that may be combined into a single phrase. For example, 'atrial flutter' denotes a fast, regular rhythm originating in the atria. The term 'flutter' includes both rate and pattern. Even complex phrases can be broken down into the same three elements; for example, 'paroxysmal atrial tachycardia with block' denotes a fast rhythm that originates from a single atrial focus and which occurs in bursts with some other rhythm in between. There is also a delay in conducting the beat from the atria to the ventricles.

Terms denoting how long the arrhythmia has been present may be used, with varying definitions. Guidelines standardizing the phrases in relation to atrial fibrillation recommend that *paroxysmal* refers to self-terminating episodes of up to 7 days, although in

Table 22.1 Nomenclature for describing arrhythmias

Term	Notes
Rate	
Tachycardia	Both terms imply an SA node rhythm unless otherwise stated
Bradycardia	Often a regular rhythm Normal limits for rate vary according to the age and activity of the patient Bradycardia is slow, tachycardia is fast
Origin	
Sinus	SA node
Atrial	From the atria but not the SA node
Nodal	Atrioventricular node
Supraventricular	Usually, but not necessarily, from the AV node
Re-entrant	A circuit involving retrograde (backward) conduction and an accessory pathway whereby impulses travel in a loop, e.g. the Wolff–Parkinson–White syndrome
Ventricular	From the ventricular tissue
Pattern	
Ectopic	From a focus other than the SA node
Premature contraction	May be isolated or repeated
Paroxysmal	Occurs in bursts
Flutter	A fast, regular rhythm from a single ectopic focus
Fibrillation	A fast, chaotic rhythm from multiple foci
Block	A delay in, or absence of, conduction through the AV node
Mobitz	Terms used to describe particular
Wenckebach	varieties of second-degree block
Torsades de pointes	A form of ventricular tachycardia with complexes of varying amplitude
Electromechanical dissociation	Electrical impulses (as recorded on an ECG) do not lead to mechanical activity (as detected by pulse)

practice they are usually less than 1 day in duration; *persistent* refers to non-self terminating rhythms over periods longer than 7 days; *permanent* refers to rhythms that have not responded to cardioversion attempts. *Recurrent* refers to paroxysmal or persistent rhythms that return after having stopped or having been stopped.

Traditional names are still used for a few arrhythmias, such as torsades de pointes, a fast ventricular rhythm with polymorphic QRS complexes and a characteristic electrocardiogram (ECG) pattern. Some terms, for example supraventricular, have a general meaning such as originating above the ventricles, but can commonly denote something more specific, such as from the AV node. This terminology arises partly because all descriptions depend on an indirect measure of the function of the heart, namely the ECG recording. The ECG records patterns of electrical activity in the heart; it does not refer to how well the heart is functioning as a pump or to the physical state of heart tissues. The pumping ability of the heart may be measured by pulse and blood pressure, and it is important that patients are treated on the basis of their heart function and not just on the basis of an electrical recording.

The ECG is useful, however, in providing clues to the nature and cause of an arrhythmia (Fig. 22.3). The P-wave represents atrial depolarization and the QRS complex represents ventricular depolarization. The interval between the two, the PR interval, is the time taken to conduct the beat through the AV node, and is lengthened in AV block. The QRS complex is generally narrow when the ventricles are controlled from above and wide when they are not. The T-wave denotes ventricular repolarization and the QT interval the time between depolarization and polarization of the ventricles. The QT interval may be altered by drugs such as tricyclic antidepressants, antiarrhythmics and antihistamines (Table 22.2). Some of these drugs, such as the antihistamines, are more likely to cause changes if given together with drugs that inhibit their metabolism, including erythromycin and

Table 22.2 Drugs associated with prolonged QT intervals
Astemizole
Clarithromycin
Erythromycin
Halofantrine
Haloperidol
Lithium
Mizolastine
Phenothiazines
Pimozide
Sertindole
Terfenadine
Tizanidine
Tricyclic antidepressants
Class IA or III antiarrhythmics

the antifungal drugs fluconazole, itraconazole, ketoconazole and miconazole (Moss 1999). The QT interval varies with heart rate and a corrected figure (QTc) is used. A prolonged QTc predisposes to torsades de pointes and may be drug induced or, more rarely, an inherited characteristic.

Signs and consequences of arrhythmias

Arrhythmias are associated with increased morbidity and mortality but good data are available only for common varieties. AF roughly doubles the risk of a person having a stroke, triples the risk of heart failure and doubles mortality risk. Signs and symptoms of arrhythmias may include: dizziness or collapse because of a poor blood supply to the brain; shortness of breath because of poor oxygenation; angina associated with a poor coronary circulation and/or increased cardiac workload arising from a tachycardia; and weakness (Table 22.3). Palpitations are the

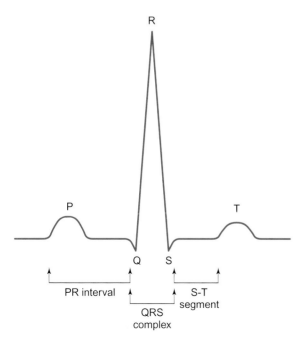

Figure 22.3 The electrocardiogram (ECG).

Table 22.3 Symptoms present at the emergency presentation of atrial fibrillation	
Shortness of breath	52%
Pain (including angina)	34%
Palpitations	22%
Collapse or dizziness	19%

awareness of one's heart beat and may be due to extra beats or the absence of a beat; they may range from a minor sensation to a distressing problem. Since these signs are not unique to arrhythmias, intermittent arrhythmias are not always easy to diagnose and 24-hour recordings of the ECG, or implantable recording devices activated when the patient has symptoms, may be used.

It is estimated that 80% of an individual's cardiac output comes from ventricular action, even when this is not co-ordinated with the atria. Thus, many patients with an abnormal rhythm but a regular ventricular rate experience little difficulty in normal daily living; indeed, only one in 12 patients with paroxysmal AF has symptoms. AF is sometimes described as slow or fast depending on the ventricular rate, which can vary between 50 and 200 beats per minute, depending on the degree of AV conduction. A patient with slow AF, in which an effective AV node block permits only a small proportion of impulses to pass from the atria to the ventricles, may not need treatment. In contrast, fast AF, which occurs in patients with an ineffective AV node block, features rapid and irregular ventricular beats and consequent inefficient filling of the ventricles and inefficient circulation.

Treatment

Treatment of arrhythmias involves consideration of five 'Cs'; causes, coagulation, control, conversion, and cure. In all cases, physicians will need to look for causes that can be removed and consider protecting the patient against stroke with anticoagulant therapy; this is particularly important in atrial fibrillation. Control of ventricular rate, to ensure good cardiac output despite an abnormal atrial rhythm, is an alternative to converting the heart to a normal rhythm by means of electricity or drugs. Cure of the patient means that the arrhythmia does not return.

Criteria for treatment

Treatment of arrhythmias is often disappointing with significant adverse effects and therefore guidelines for treatment often emphasize safety above efficacy or ' first, do no harm'. Care must be taken not to overtreat patients.

Suitable criteria for treatment of an arrhythmia include:

- the arrhythmia causes haemodynamic failure (poor circulation)
- haemodynamic failure has not occurred but the present arrhythmia is known to be a predictor of a more serious arrhythmia. For example, patients who experience an episode of ventricular tachycardia following myocardial infarction have a 30% risk of dying within 1 year, probably from ventricular fibrillation
- the patient is distressed by an awareness of extra or missed beats (palpitations).

Tachycardias are known to lead to an increased risk of the development, over months or years, of cardiomyopathy (heart muscle damage) and therefore prolonged tachycardias may be an indication for treatment in their own right.

The aim of treatment is to restore a satisfactory circulation and to prevent further episodes of poor circulation or distress.

While it is thought that arrhythmias are implicated in many cases of sudden death, the main evidence comes from patients who died while having their ECG recorded continuously on a tape (Holter monitoring). Such patients may not represent the general population but confirm a general impression that ventricular tachyarrhythmias are a more common cause of death than bradyarrhythmias (Table 22.4). Patients who have heart failure, or who have already been admitted to hospital for another reason, have a greater risk of dying from asystole or a muscle rupture.

Hazards of treatment

Since arrhythmias can occur without apparent ill effect, it follows that their presence does not automatically mandate treatment; indeed, the use of an antiarrhythmic agent may generate a worse arrhythmia. Such proarrhythmic effects are common to all antiarrhythmics but are probably less common in class II and class IV. The arrhythmias generated are many and varied and range from a rate change to a life-threatening pattern such as torsades de pointes. Table 22.5 lists some of the more common features of drug-induced arrhythmias.

Ten percent of patients with postinfarction ventricular ectopics deteriorate if treated. The cardiac arrhythmia suppression trials (CAST) in the USA (CAST Investigators 1989, 1992) showed that the use of class IC drugs in such patients increased the risk of sudden death, and a meta-analysis of the use of lidocaine in myocardial infarction (Hine et al 1989) and a study of d-sotalol (Sanderson 1996) also demonstrated increased mortality when these drugs were used prophylactically, despite a reduction in arrhythmias. Table 22.6 shows estimates for the number of Americans who may have died as a result of misguided therapy with class I agents, in comparison to other causes.

Atrial and supraventricular arrhythmias are common in pregnancy; if treatment is required, then amiodarone should be avoided because of its effects on the fetus but β-blockers and adenosine are

Table 22.4 Analysis of fatal arrhythmias in monitored patients

Ventricular tachycardia leading to fibrillation	50%
Ventricular fibrillation	11%
Torsades de pointes	18%
Bradycardia	21%

Table 22.5 Common features of drug-induced arrhythmias

Incessant tachyarrhythmias
Bizarre arrhythmias
Cardiac arrest
New VT in a patient with SVT
Torsades de pointes
Acceleration of original rhythm

Table 22.6 Deaths in US citizens, 1965–75	
Vietnam war	55 000
Road accidents	100 000
Homicide	200 000
Class I antiarrhythmics	1 000 000

thought to be safer options. Long-established drugs such as digoxin and quinidine are probably safe but may not be effective.

Role of drugs

In recent years, drugs have decreased in importance and electrical interventions have increased. Electrical mapping of arrhythmias, to identify the origin and exact nature of the disturbance, is now available in a number of UK centres. Electrodes are inserted through catheters into the chambers of the heart and internal cardiograms are used to create a detailed map of the heart surface; this can take several hours and may be performed under anaesthesia. Once the origin and nature of the rhythm have been characterized, electrodes are used to burn out aberrant pathways or ectopic foci. This has been done most successfully in the case of atrial flutter where the origin is usually close to the pulmonary veins in the left atrium; a circle of tissue may be destroyed around the veins and usually prevents the flutter. This process of pulmonary vein isolation may also be used for atrial fibrillation where it reduces the recurrence of arrhythmias, improves quality of life scores and reduces hospital admissions, when compared to drug therapy. There are considerable hazards associated with the procedure, including oesophageal perforation, stroke and pulmonary vein stenosis, but these risks are limited in experienced centres. Electrical therapy is also favoured for AV nodal disease where drugs are often unsuccessful.

Pacemakers

The role of pacemakers to stimulate the heart to contract and implantable defibrillators to stop the heart and allow the underlying natural rhythm to pick up is also increasing as the technology and battery life improve. These devices are inserted under the skin, usually on the chest wall, and wires are inserted through a vein into the heart chambers. The most common varieties sense the heart's rhythm and have an algorithm that determines whether or not the device should issue a pacing stimulus or even a cardioverting shock. Most are programmable from outside the body by an electromagnetic probe and most record their own activity and any unusual rhythms detected. Some work only in the right ventricle but others have dual-chamber sensing and stimulating modes, usually in the right atrium and ventricle. A pacemaker is often less than $5 \times 5 \times 1$cm in size, costs some £12 000 and has batteries that last several years; implantable defibrillators are a little larger, cost more and do not last as long. Defibrillators were formerly unsuitable for atrial arrhythmias because they did not distinguish the rhythms sufficiently accurately and might shock a well patient, but are now improving.

Pacemakers may be used with drugs, where the drug is used to control a fast rhythm and the pacemaker prevents adverse consequences from drug-induced bradycardia, or where the patient has both fast and slow rhythms on different occasions.

Bradyarrhythmias

Bradyarrhythmias are generally caused by tissue damage, a decrease in sympathetic autonomic tone or an increase in parasympathetic tone mediated by the vagus nerve. Such changes in autonomic function may be caused or mimicked by drugs such as hyoscine, β-blockers, digoxin and verapamil or by deficiencies in thyroid or corticosteroid hormones. Increased vagal tone causes AV block of varying degree which reduces the rate of impulses reaching the ventricles. A ventricular escape rhythm involving ectopics, an idioventricular rhythm or even a tachycardia may then result, which should be recognized as secondary to the fault at the AV node and not treated as a primary disorder.

AV block may be classified into three types.

- First-degree block describes instances where all beats are conducted through the AV node, but with some delay. This does not require treatment but may be a warning to avoid drugs that would worsen the block, such as β-blockers and class IV agents.
- Second-degree block implies that some, but not all, beats are conducted through the AV node, and there are further subdivisions of this class, e.g. Mobitz and Wenckebach. The need for treatment depends upon whether a satisfactory ventricular rate and output can be maintained.
- Third-degree block implies that there is no conduction of sinus or atrial beats through the AV node, and treatment is usually required.

The treatment of bradycardia should include identification and treatment of the cause, such as treatment of jaundice or hypothyroidism, and removal of causative drugs. Immediate treatment is normally to decrease vagal tone with intravenous atropine, which will decrease AV block and increase the SA rate. It is important to note that it will take a minute or longer to see initial signs of benefit and at least 5 minutes to observe maximum effect. Doses of 300–600 µg of atropine may be given up to six times at 1-minute intervals until benefit is observed. If atropine is ineffective, intravenous adrenaline (epinephrine) or isoprenaline may be used.

Ultimately a pacemaker may be required to pace the heart from the right ventricle or from both the right atrium and ventricle. This approach may also be used where the patient has bouts of tachycardia and bradycardia, as seen in the sick sinus syndrome. In such cases the tachycardia may be controlled by β-blockers, amiodarone or class IV drugs, but an undesirable consequence may be the worsening of the bradycardia for which the only suitable treatment is a pacemaker.

2 Tachyarrhythmias

The primary treatment of any tachyarrhythmia is to remove the cause. Removal of arrhythmogenic drugs or stimulants such as caffeine, alcohol and smoking may solve the problem, and investigation of other medical causes, including abnormal thyroid function and abnormal serum electrolyte concentrations, is essential. Behavioural modifications to avoid stress and anxiety may help, and physical procedures such as the Valsalva manoeuvre have been useful in terminating re-entrant tachycardias.

Acute tachyarrhythmias

Tachyarrhythmias that compromise cardiac output will require rapid control by external electric shock, antiarrhythmic drugs or radiofrequency electric currents that destroy the aberrant conducting tissue. This last method is applied by a catheter passed through the great veins until the tip is close to the conducting pathways. It is of greatest value in junctional arrhythmias, where drug therapy is generally much less successful. External electric shocks, formerly direct current shocks but now often a less damaging biphasic waveform, can be delivered from semi-automated apparatus, as in hospitals, or from fully automated machines sometimes available in public places such as airports or train stations for lay personnel to use. The automated devices will only generate a shock if the rhythm they detect is suitable.

Drugs may be used to convert an abnormal rhythm to sinus rhythm (cardioversion), to control the ventricular rate, e.g. digoxin or β-blockers, or as prophylaxis of further arrhythmias after electrical cardioversion. Cardioversion with drugs is more likely to be successful soon after the arrhythmia starts and is unlikely to work in the presence of structural abnormalities or after 3 months, due to remodelling of the atria. In some cases, where there is no immediate danger to the patient, drugs may be used to prepare a patient for electrical cardioversion, e.g. amiodarone for AF. Paroxysmal supraventricular tachyarrhythmias are usually easily converted to sinus rhythm by adenosine, flecainide or verapamil with success rates of between 70% and 100%. Flecainide also works well for atrial fibrillation, better than class IA drugs, which in turn are better than class III drugs. Atrial flutter responds less well, and generally only to class III drugs; class IC may convert the flutter to a worse rhythm by removing the AV block that protects the ventricles.

Ventricular tachyarrhythmias are harder to terminate with drugs. Despite years of use, lidocaine is effective in less than a quarter of patients, whereas sotalol and amiodarone have higher success rates.

Chronic tachyarrhythmias

In chronic tachyarrhythmias, the class of drug to be used, based on the Vaughan-Williams system (see below), must be selected. That choice is based upon the origin of the arrhythmia, regardless of its pattern. Table 22.7 lists the classes of drug considered useful for arrhythmias of various origin. Whatever the origin, the preference of one class over another may vary, depending on a clinician's experience with particular drugs, on the presentation of the arrhythmia and on patient characteristics. Such factors also govern the choice of drug within a class. The drug chosen should have the dosing schedule and adverse effect profile that best suit the patient or inconvenience them least (see Tables 22.11 and 22.14). Thus, for example, a patient with glaucoma or prostatism should not be given disopyramide which possesses marked anticholinergic properties, and a patient with obstructive airways disease should preferably not have a β-blocker (class II), though if considered essential they could have a cardioselective agent.

Table 22.8 illustrates some of the factors affecting the choice of drug to treat atrial fibrillation.

It should be noted that it is not necessary to cure all arrhythmias to satisfy the criteria for treatment. Atrial arrhythmias may be well tolerated provided the ventricular rate is controlled and the patient is not distressed. Thus, digoxin may provide satisfactory control of the number of impulses that pass through the AV node to the ventricles without converting the patient to sinus rhythm. It used to be thought that this kind of rate-control strategy was inferior to attempts to induce sinus rhythm or rhythm control. This has now been disproved in several good clinical studies and, on average, patients receiving rate-control therapies, e.g. digoxin or β-blockers, have fewer hospital admissions and fewer adverse effects.

It is also important to consider all measures of treatment success when selecting a drug. For example, in a comparison of sotalol and amiodarone in persistent atrial fibrillation (Singh et al 2005) conversion rate, time to recurrence and the influence of coronary

---

Table 22.7 Drug classes used in chronic tachyarrhythmias

	SA node	Atria	AV node	Accessory pathway*	Ventricles
Commonly used	II	II	IV (for urgent cardioversion)	IC	II
		IV	II		III
Also used		Digoxin	Digoxin	II	I
		III	IC	IA	
		IC			
		IA			

Class I drugs are not generally used in the context of acute illness (e.g. acute myocardial infarction, sepsis, etc.) or heart failure because of myodepression and increased proarrhythmic properties. Digoxin is most often used to control ventricular rate. *AV-nodal and accessory pathway arrhythmias respond poorly to drugs in the long term but respond well to radiofrequency catheter ablation in which the aberrant pathway is destroyed. See Blomström-Lundqvist et al (2003) for details of drug usage and alternatives.

Table 22.8 Drug choice in treating chronic or persistent atrial fibrillation

Associated factors	First choice	Second choice	Avoid
Acute systemic illness	Nothing or II	IV, III	I
Paroxysmal			
Exercise induced	II	Sotalol, IC	Digoxin
Vagal origin	Disopyramide	Sotalol, IC	
Elderly	Sotalol/Amiodarone		
Sustained AF			
Ventricular rate control	II	Digoxin, IV	
Cardioversion	IC	IA, III	II, IV, digoxin
Respiratory disorders			II, sotalol
Ischaemic heart disease	Sotalol	Amiodarone	I
Heart failure	Amiodarone	Digoxin	I
Hypertension	Sotalol	Amiodarone	

heart disease were considered. Both drugs converted similar numbers of patients at 1 month (24% and 27% respectively) and direct current (DC) shock failed in similar proportions (28% and 25%) but the median time to recurrence of AF varied markedly (487 and 74 days respectively compared to 6 days for placebo). In patients with ischaemic heart disease, the differences were not statistically significant (569 and 428 days). Adverse events were similar in the two groups.

Adjunctive therapy, such as ACE inhibitors or angiotensin blockers, to counteract atrial remodelling and make arrhythmias more susceptible to treatment is showing considerable promise.

Chronic ventricular tachycardias

Most patients who have episodes of ventricular tachycardia (VT) have coronary artery disease or cardiomyopathy, are at high risk of recurrence of VT and require secondary prophylaxis. Those who have non-sustained VT or ventricular ectopics, without overt heart disease, have a prognosis no different from the normal population, and they should not automatically have treatment (Landers & Reiter 1997). Prophylaxis against ventricular tachyarrhythmias is difficult and patients at high risk may have a DC defibrillator implanted in the same way as a pacemaker. The device monitors the ECG and is programmed to recognize ventricular fibrillation or ventricular tachycardia and deliver an electric shock through electrodes sewn into the heart. A β-blocker is often given at the same time to reduce the risk of sympathetically driven arrhythmias and decrease the number of shocks delivered. Defibrillators have proved to be more successful than class I drugs but only a little better than amiodarone. Combinations of amiodarone and β-blockers are showing promise in trials. The cardioverting shock, while life-saving, is unpleasant for the patient and there are often complications that necessitate hospital admission. Similar devices for atrial fibrillation have not been

as successful because of difficulty in detecting fibrillation and patients' objections to repeated shocks.

Antithrombotic therapy

Atrial fibrillation is associated with a high incidence of stroke, about 5% per year or 2–7 times that of matched populations without AF, regardless of its impact on circulation. This is thought to be related to thrombus formation in the disorganized blood flow in the atrium. Nearly all patients with AF should be given oral anticoagulants or, if that is contraindicated, aspirin. The exceptions are young patients with no co-existent cardiovascular disease or lone AF, who should be treated with aspirin 300 mg daily, and patients whose risk of stroke is low and who are judged to have a high risk of bleeding on warfarin.

Older patients were formerly excluded from warfarin therapy because of increased bleeding, but it is now recognized that old age, diabetes, hypertension, heart failure, thyrotoxicosis, prosthetic heart valves and previous strokes or transient ischaemic attacks (TIAs) are strong independent risk factors for stroke in AF; some groups have an annual incidence of 15%. Warfarin, adjusted to give an international normalized ratio (INR) in the range 2.0–3.0, reduces stroke rate by two-thirds in all patient groups, with little risk of excess bleeding. Patients with valvular disorders may require a higher INR but this carries a greater risk of bleeding. In comparison, aspirin reduces stroke risk by one-fifth (Atrial Fibrillation Investigators 1994, Benavente et al 2000). There is a small amount of evidence for adding dipyridamole to aspirin in patients who have already had a TIA or stroke (Diener et al 1996), but the role of newer agents such as clopidogrel and ximelagatran is unclear.

DC cardioversion may lead to strokes, especially in patients with an established arrhythmia, and so elective cardioversion for AF that has lasted more than 48 hours is usually preceded by

3 weeks of anticoagulation and followed by 4 weeks of further treatment.

Emergency treatment of arrhythmias in adults

Acute life-threatening arrhythmias may result in haemodynamic failure, the so-called cardiac arrest. Fast but careful management is required to prevent permanent damage or death. The emergency treatment options are set out in Figure 22.4 which is simplified from guidelines issued by the European Resuscitation Council.

Adrenaline (epinephrine), atropine and lidocaine can be administered by endotracheal tube at double the intravenous dose in 10 mL of isotonic saline. The use of lidocaine or bretylium as an adjunct to electrical defibrillation is controversial but common.

Acidosis may cause widespread problems, including serious arrhythmias, and sodium bicarbonate (50 mmol) may be given to counteract acidosis after prolonged resuscitation. Overdose is hazardous, however, and arterial blood gas measurements should be made where possible, before giving repeat doses.

Severe bradycardia should be managed with atropine first and adrenaline (epinephrine) second.

Fast rhythms in which the origin is unclear, and may be ventricular, atrial or nodal, can be analysed by giving adenosine very rapidly to produce a temporary AV block. The underlying rhythm may then be apparent and can be treated. Adenosine (see Class IV, below) is given in a series of escalating doses until an effect is evident. It is one of the few drugs that has to be given very rapidly, at less than 3 seconds per injection, to work.

A more general approach to the management of an arrhythmia is presented in Figure 22.5.

Treatment of arrhythmias after myocardial infarction

Despite the increased risk of death from arrhythmias post infarction, trials of antiarrhythmics have generally demonstrated that they increase the death rate still further. Presumably this arises because of their proarrhythmic properties although many drugs are known to act differently in normal compared to ischaemic tissue. Trials have shown increased risks from class I drugs and from d-sotalol (class III) but marginal benefit from amiodarone. β-Blockers are useful in most patients, not only because they are antiarrhythmics but also because of their hypotensive and sympatholytic properties (Hjalmarson & Olsson 1991; see also Chapter 20). Approximately one-third of patients have non-sustained ventricular tachycardia that lasts less than 30 seconds in the acute postinfarction phase and the appropriate treatment is either reassurance or a β-blocker. Some will die early due to left ventricular failure but those who survive to leave hospital have the same prognosis as patients who did not have VT.

Classification of antiarrhythmic drugs

The most widely accepted classification is the Vaughan–Williams system based on electrophysiological data, illustrated in Tables 22.9 and 22.10 and Figure 22.1. It is not only physiologically acceptable but it provides a good basis for clinical choices since drugs in the same class have similar therapeutic effects. Table 22.9 and Figure 22.1 relate to His–Purkinje fibres or fast fibres, which have a sodium-dependent phase 0. Other fibres have different characteristics, notably the slow fibres in

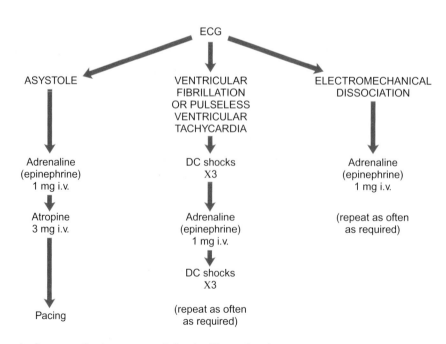

In all cases cardiopulmonary resuscitation should be continued throughout and any specific cause removed or countered.

Figure 22.4 Emergency treatment options for arrhythmias in adults.

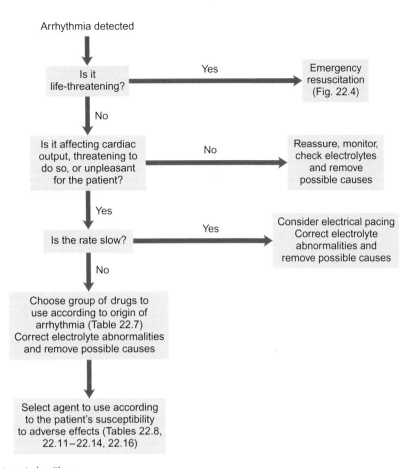

Figure 22.5 Arrhythmia treatment algorithm.

the SA node and upper AV node, where phase 0 is calcium dependent and overlaps phase 1 and 2. The clinical consequences are that class I drugs, and especially IB, have less effect on SA or AV nodal arrhythmias than those which originate from ventricular cells, while class IV drugs have major effects on the SA and AV nodes.

Most drugs have several modes of action and their effectiveness as antiarrhythmic agents depends upon the summation of

Table 22.9 Effect of different drug classes on phases of action potential in His–Purkinje fibres

Phase	Dominant ion movement	Drug class	Effect
0	Sodium inward	IA	Block ++
		IB	Block +
		IC	Block +++
2	Calcium inward	IV	Block
3	Potassium outward	III	Marked slowing
4	Sodium inward, potassium outward	I, II, IV	Slows

Table 22.10 Electrophysiological effects of some antiarrhythmics

Class	Antiarrhythmic agents	Effects on duration of QRS	Effects on duration of QT	Sinus rate
IA	Quinidine, procainamide, disopyramide	+	+	+
IB	Lidocaine (lignocaine), mexiletine, tocainide, phenytoin, aprindine	0/–	0	0
IC	Flecainide, encainide, lorcainide, propafenone, moracizine	++	+	0
II	Atenolol, metoprolol, sotalol, esmolol	0	++	– –
III	Amiodarone, bretylium, sotalol	0	+++	–
IV	Verapamil, diltiazem, adenosine	0	0	– –

+, increased; –, decreased; 0, no change

these effects. For example, class IB agents shorten the duration of the action potential, thereby decreasing the refractory period and increasing the risk of sustaining a tachyarrhythmia. In contrast, they also slow phase 4, which increases the overall refractory period. The net result is a decrease in the risk of sustaining a tachyarrhythmia.

It is important to note that all antiarrhythmics are also proarrhythmic.

Class I

All class I agents slow down sodium currents in phases 0 and 4 of the action potential but vary in their effects on phases 2 and 3. All may be used in ventricular tachyarrhythmias but class IB are of no value in atrial disorders and are more effective in ischaemic tissue than in normal tissue. The use of class I agents is diminishing in favour of classes II and III. Lidocaine may be used for prophylaxis of ventricular tachycardia or ventricular fibrillation and for management of ventricular ectopics and ventricular tachycardia, although it should be reserved for symptomatic patients. While it is also indicated in the management of VF, it is only an adjunct to DC electric shock. Lidocaine is not available orally and is usually administered by an intravenous infusion regimen in which the dose is decreased with time, for example:

- 4 mg/min for 30 minutes then
- 2 mg/min for 2 hours then
- 1 mg/min to continue.

It is unusual to continue for longer than 24–48 hours, after which an oral agent should be used if required.

Class IA agents are all potentially toxic but have a role as reserve agents in patients who have no contraindication to their use (Table 22.11). They may be used on their own or combined cautiously with digoxin for atrial arrhythmias. Quinidine and disopyramide are particularly prone to cause torsades de pointes but disopyramide is valuable in treating the Wolff–Parkinson–White syndrome, in which it inhibits both anterograde and retrograde conduction. All three class IA agents may be used in VT but individual variation in response to these agents is probably greater than in any other class. It may be useful, therefore, to try a second class IA agent if the first is not successful.

Class IC agents are effective in atrial and ventricular tachyarrhythmias but they also cause arrhythmias in a significant number of patients. The CAST (1989, 1992) studies demonstrated that flecainide, moracizine and encainide increased mortality when used in the management of ventricular ectopics after myocardial infarction. These agents are usually restricted to the management of ventricular arrhythmias resistant to other drugs although single-dose intravenous flecainide may be used to terminate atrial or supraventricular tachycardias. Longer-term use in AF is more common in the USA but is usually accompanied by a β-blocker to minimize the risk of proarrhythmia.

Class II

β-Blockers are useful for treating arrhythmias that are provoked or exacerbated by sympathetic autonomic nervous stimulation or by circulating catecholamines. They are valuable in arrhythmias originating from the SA or AV nodes that are provoked by anxiety, stress or exercise. They are also useful, along with α-receptor blockers, in the arrhythmias of phaeochromocytoma. β-Blockers are contraindicated in patients with extensive infarcts because of their myodepressant actions, but have a cardioprotective effect in uncomplicated acute myocardial infarction (see Chapter 20) and in heart failure (see Chapter 21).

Table 22.11 Adverse effects of antiarrhythmic drugs (class I)

Drug	Cardiac	Non-cardiac	Caution or avoid in
Disopyramide	Torsades de pointes Myodepressant	Anticholinergic (urinary retention, constipation, dry mouth, blurred vision)	Glaucoma, prostatism, hypotension
Procainamide		Lupus, nausea, diarrhoea	Myasthenia gravis, slow acetylators (increased risk of lupus)
Quinidine	Torsades de pointes Vasodilation (i.v.)	Diarrhoea, nausea, tinnitus, headache, deafness, confusion, visual disturbances, blood dyscrasias	Myasthenia gravis
Lidocaine (lignocaine)		Convulsions in overdose, paraesthesiae	Liver failure (reduce dose)
Mexiletine		Nausea, paraesthesiae	2nd- or 3rd-degree heart block
Tocainide		Thrombocytopenia, nausea, pulmonary fibrosis, paraesthesiae	Use only if other agents have failed
Flecainide	Proarrhythmic Myodepressant	Paraesthesiae, tremor	Use only if other agents have failed
Propafenone	Proarrhythmic Myodepressant	Gastrointestinal disturbances	Use only if other agents have failed

β-Blockers are contraindicated in patients with asthma or chronic obstructive airway disease. However, if other agents have been tried and failed, a cardioselective β-blocker may be used at low doses. It should be noted that cardioselectivity is a relative term and no agent is free from respiratory effects. Membrane-stabilizing activity and intrinsic sympathomimetic activity have no impact upon the choice of drug for arrhythmias. The risk of bradycardia is a threat with all β-blockers, especially in patients with myocardial disease, heart block or a mixed tachycardia-bradycardia (sick sinus syndrome). β-Blockers with partial agonist activity have not proved useful in such cases despite theoretical promise. In general, β-blockers may also exacerbate peripheral vascular disease and cause nightmares or depression. There is little value in changing to a second β-blocker if the first agent has not been successful.

Atenolol, metoprolol and esmolol are available for intravenous use, and esmolol, with its short duration of action, is the most appropriate β-blocker for urgent use in SA, atrial or atrioventricular arrhythmias. Verapamil and adenosine (class IV) are also suitable. Care must be taken if both class II and IV agents are to be used since they have additive effects in suppressing the AV node and in depressing contractility. The combination is most dangerous if intravenous verapamil follows intravenous or oral β-blockers that have a prolonged action.

Sotalol has some class III activity as well as class II effects and bretylium is considered to have class II activity in addition to class III.

Class III

Class III drugs (amiodarone, bretylium, sotalol) prolong the action potential and bring greater uniformity among different cell types, thus reducing the means for generation of arrhythmias. Although they are all powerful antiarrhythmics, there the similarities end. Each drug has a different side effect profile (Table 22.12) and other electrophysiological properties. Amiodarone can cause sodium channel blockade and has powerful class I activity and ancillary class II activity, bretylium is an adrenergic neurone blocking agent, while sotalol is a β-blocker. Sotalol is a racemic mixture of which the d-isomer has class III activity and the l-isomer is a β-blocker. This combination is more successful than either element alone and d-sotalol alone has increased mortality in postinfarction patients. Amiodarone has an extensive range of side effects, both trivial and fatal, that prevent its wider use. It is commonly restricted to serious ventricular arrhythmias that have proved resistant to other therapy, although it is increasingly being used in atrial arrhythmias and has a role in re-entrant rhythms such as the Wolff–Parkinson–White syndrome. A significant disadvantage to its use is its long half-life (about 1 month), which necessitates intensive oral loading, for example 200 mg three times daily for a week, then 200 mg twice daily for a week followed by 200 mg daily. The long half-life results in a slow onset of action and very prolonged effects after discontinuing therapy. Intravenous doses are effective immediately but there are hazards associated with rapid intravenous doses and incompatibility problems with common infusion fluids.

In contrast to amiodarone, bretylium has a rapid onset of action and short half-life, is only available parenterally and is not effective in atrial arrhythmias. It has been used mostly in emergency resuscitation for ventricular tachycardia or fibrillation, either to aid electric defibrillation or to cardiovert patients on its own. The major problem has been severe hypotension although, paradoxically, there may be an initial sympathetic stimulation that precedes the sympathetic block and causes hypertension and arrhythmias. Whereas amiodarone and bretylium have minimal

Table 22.12   Adverse effects of antiarrhythmic drugs (classes II–IV)

Drug	Cardiac	Non-cardiac	Caution or avoid in
β-blockers (general)	Myodepressant Heart block	Bronchoconstriction (β_2) Vasoconstriction Hallucinations/vivid dreams (lipophilic compounds) Decreased renal blood flow Changes in serum lipid profile Drowsiness, fatigue	Asthma, COAD, Raynaud's disease, gangrene, diabetes mellitus, depression
Azimilide Dofetilide Ibutilide Sotalol	Torsades de pointes		Combination with disopyramide or amiodarone or drugs in Table 22.2
Amiodarone	Torsades de pointes	Hyper-/hypothyroidism, pneumonitis, myopathy, neuropathy, hepatitis, corneal deposits, photosensitivity	Thyroid disease
Bretylium	Hypotension	Initial sympathomimetic response, nausea	
Verapamil	Heart block	Constipation, headaches, flushing, ankle oedema, light-headedness	
Adenosine	Heart block	Bronchoconstriction, flushing, chest pain	Asthma, COAD, combination with dipyridamole

myodepressant activity, sotalol is a significant myodepressant and also has the standard side effect profile of a β-blocker. It is less effective than amiodarone but, despite its problems, a lot safer; it is available orally and it may be of particular benefit in treating arrhythmias in hypertension, in angina and after acute myocardial infarction. It is rarely used for non-antiarrhythmic purposes.

All three agents, by virtue of their class III activity, prolong the QT interval and increase the risk of torsades de pointes, especially in hypokalaemia or when combined with a bradycardic drug such as a class IA agent. Newer agents with a more pure class III action include ibutilide, dofetilide and azimilide; they have been used in trials for several years but have not been licensed in Europe.

Class IV

Verapamil and diltiazem inhibit slow channel conduction through the AV node and are referred to by a number of terms, including the general name calcium antagonists or calcium channel blockers. Other calcium antagonists such as nifedipine and other 4,5-dihydropyridines have no antiarrhythmic effect. The potassium channel opener adenosine and its pro-drug ATP act as indirect calcium antagonists and resemble verapamil in their antiarrhythmic scope. The ultra-short duration of action of intravenous adenosine makes it very suitable as a diagnostic aid and for interrupting supraventricular arrhythmias without the myosuppressant effects of verapamil. Adenosine is, however, a bronchoconstrictor and causes dyspnoea, flushing, chest pain and further transient arrhythmias in a high proportion of patients, and its metabolism is inhibited by dipyridamole (see Table 22.12). All class IV agents should be avoided in second- or third-degree heart block and sick sinus syndrome, unless the patient has a pacemaker to overcome bradycardia. Likewise, combined therapy with a β-blocker is hazardous because of the risk of excessive AV block, although in some cases it may be useful to treat chronic atrial fibrillation or flutter with digoxin and a calcium antagonist where either agent alone has failed. Calcium antagonists may cause conversion to sinus rhythm but are used chiefly to control ventricular rate. Verapamil has a greater dilatory effect on systemic arteries than diltiazem and may be especially useful in patients with hypertension or angina.

Both agents cause myocardial suppression and are thus contraindicated in heart failure although their depressant actions on the SA node are usually offset by the reflex response to arterial vasodilation. Side effects are mostly predictable and include ankle oedema, flushing, dizziness, light-headedness and headache. Constipation is common in patients receiving verapamil.

Digoxin

Digoxin is one of a group of cardiac (digitalis) glycosides with a well-defined role in the management of atrial tachyarrhythmias, in the presence of congestive heart failure. Digoxin inhibits conduction through the AV node and thus protects the ventricles from rapid atrial rhythms. In addition, some patients with established atrial fibrillation may convert to sinus rhythm although this is unusual in atrial flutter and in atrial fibrillation of recent origin (less than 1 week). Digoxin is ineffective in the presence of high sympathetic nervous activity, such as in exercise, and its use is diminishing as the use of amiodarone, sotalol and class II

drugs increases. Digoxin also causes both atrial and ventricular ectopic beats and is a potent cause of arrhythmias (Table 22.13). Both beneficial and toxic effects are enhanced by hypokalaemia and hypercalcaemia, and the AV block is enhanced by β-blockers and calcium antagonists. There are numerous other drug interactions (Table 22.14), some of which are pharmacokinetic and some of which are pharmacological. Digoxin is the only antiarrhythmic for which therapeutic drug monitoring is widely used. It has a narrow therapeutic range of 1–2 ng/mL. This range is modified by serum electrolyte concentrations and by the concurrent use of other drugs, but the extent of the modification is not defined. Since digoxin is excreted by the liver and the kidney (70% renal elimination in normal renal function), reduced renal function increases digoxin levels and necessitates reduced doses, notably in the elderly.

Table 22.15 summarizes the pharmacokinetics of antiarrhythmics, Table 22.16 lists some common interactions, and Table 22.17 lists common therapeutic problems in the management of arrhythmias.

Table 22.13 Adverse effects of digoxin

Cardiac
- Ventricular ectopics including bigeminy
- Ventricular tachycardia
- AV junctional beats or tachycardia
- 2nd- or 3rd-degree heart block
- Atrial tachycardia (often paroxysmal) with block
- SA node arrest

Non-cardiac
- Anorexia, nausea, vomiting
- Diarrhoea (less common)
- Fatigue, confusion
- Abnormal colour vision (excess yellow/green)

Table 22.14 Interactions involving digoxin

Serum levels increased by:	Amiodarone, verapamil, diltiazem, quinidine, propafenone, clarithromycin, broad-spectrum antibiotics (erythromycin, tetracyclines), decreased renal blood flow (β-blockers, NSAIDs), renal failure, heart failure
Serum levels decreased by:	Colestyramine, sulfasalazine, neomycin, rifampicin, antacids, improved renal blood flow (vasodilators), levothyroxine (thyroxine)
Effects of digoxin increased by:	Hypokalaemia, hypercalcaemia, hypomagnesaemia Antiarrhythmic classes IA, II, IV Diuretics that cause hypokalaemia, corticosteroids Myxoedema, hypoxia (acute or chronic), acute myocardial ischaemia or myocarditis
Effects of digoxin decreased by:	Hyperkalaemia, hypocalcaemia, thyrotoxicosis

Patient care

Patients with arrhythmias may experience considerable anxiety about the possibility that they will have a serious arrhythmia at any moment and may therefore need considerable reassurance. This anxiety will not be helped by the fact that most antiarrhythmic drug treatments work in only a proportion of patients and several treatment options may be tried before the most appropriate is identified. Encouragement and realistic reassurance are required, with regular follow-up. The patient's family and friends may need to be advised on what to do in the event of an acute arrhythmia.

Stressful situations, smoking, cocaine and amphetamine use, alcohol binges and excessive caffeine intake should all be avoided.

Patients should give informed consent for all interventions, but their response to treatment options may not be the same as

Table 22.15	Pharmacokinetics of antiarrhythmics			
	Oral absorption	% protein-binding	Approx. therapeutic range	Elimination, metabolism, half-life
Amiodarone	Slow, variable	>95	0.5–2.5 mg/L	Extensive metabolism, very variable rate, $t_{1/2}$ 2 days initially increasing to 40–60 days
Bretylium	Intravenous/intramuscular only	Unbound	1–3 mg/L	Renal, $t_{1/2}$ 5–10 h
Digoxin	Variable, 70%	25	0.8–2 ng/mL	70% renal, variable, $t_{1/2}$ 36 h
Diltiazem	40% absorbed	80	0.05–0.3 mg/L	Hepatic, $t_{1/2}$ 3 h
Disopyramide	Rapid, >80%	30–90	2–4 mg/L (depends on extent of binding)	50% renal, 15% bile, active metabolite, $t_{1/2}$ 4–10 h
Flecainide	Complete, slow	40	0.2–1 mg/L	30% renal, $t_{1/2}$ 20 h
Lidocaine	Intravenous/intramuscular only	60–80	1.5–5 mg/L	10% renal, rapid hepatic metabolism to CNS-toxic products, $t_{1/2}$ 8–100 min increases with duration of dosing
Mexiletine	> 90%	60–70	0.5–2 mg/L	10% renal, $t_{1/2}$ 10–12 h, hepatic metabolites mostly inactive
Moracizine	Rapid	95	0.2–3.6 mg/L	Hepatic metabolism to active metabolites, $t_{1/2}$ 2–6 h, metabolite >80 h
Phenytoin	Variable rate and extent	>90	10–20 mg/L	Capacity-limited hepatic metabolism, $t_{1/2}$ 10–60 h but variable because of non-first order elimination
Procainamide	Rapid, > 75%	15–20	3–10 mg/L	50% renal, 25–40% converted to N-acetylprocainamide (active, $t_{1/2}$ 6 h), procainamide $t_{1/2}$ 2.5–4.5 h
Propafenone	Complete, rapid	>95	0.06–1 mg/L	Extensive first-pass metabolism, capacity-limited, $t_{1/2}$ 2–12 h
Quinidine	Rapid, >80%	80–90	2–6 mg/L	Mixed renal and hepatic, $t_{1/2}$ 6 h
Tocainide	Complete, rapid	>10	4–10 mg/L	40% renal, 60% hepatic, $t_{1/2}$ 15 h
Verapamil	Rapid, >90%	90	0.1–0.4 mg/L	Hepatic, $t_{1/2}$ 4–12 h, marked first-pass effect
Dofetilide	Rapid, >92%		Not determined	60% renal, 40% oxidation, $t_{1/2}$ 7.1–9.7 h
Azimilide	Complete	94	Not determined	>90% hepatic, $t_{1/2}$ 4–5 d
Ibutilide	Extensive first-pass metabolism, not used directly	40	Not determined	95% hepatic, $t_{1/2}$ 5.7–8.8 h

All values quoted are subject to marked interindividual variability. Most therapeutic ranges are poorly defined. Oral absorption does not account for drug lost by first-pass hepatic metabolism. Rapid absorption indicates a peak plasma concentration in less than 2 hours.
$t_{1/2}$ elimination half-life at normal renal function.
For the pharmacokinetics of β-blockers and other calcium channel blockers see Chapter 20.

Table 22.16   Common interactions involving antiarrhythmic agents (excluding digoxin)

Antiarrhythmic	Other drug	Effect
Disopyramide	Anticholinergics	Increased anticholinergic effects
	Pyridostigmine	Decreased anticholinergic effects of disopyramide
		Decreased cholinergic effects of pyridostigmine
	Class II, IV	Increased hypotension
	Class III	Torsades de pointes
Procainamide	Class III	Torsades de pointes
	Cimetidine	Decreased renal clearance
Quinidine	Class II, IV	Increased hypotension
	Class III	Torsades de pointes
	Warfarin	Increased anticoagulation
	Enzyme inducers	Decreased serum levels
	Enzyme inhibitors	Increased serum levels
Lidocaine (lignocaine)	β-blockers, cimetidine	Decreased elimination of lidocaine
	Enzyme inducers	Increased elimination of lidocaine
Mexiletine	Theophylline	Increased theophylline levels
Propafenone	Warfarin	Enhanced anticoagulation
Amiodarone	Warfarin	Enhanced anticoagulation

Additive antiarrhythmic or myosuppressant effects are not included.
Interactions between antiarrhythmics are listed under the first named drug only.
Enzyme inducers include barbiturates, rifampicin, smoking.
Enzyme inhibitors include cimetidine

Table 22.17   Common therapeutic problems in the management of arrhythmias

Problem	Comment
Narrow therapeutic range of digoxin	Encourage compliance and check serum electrolytes regularly
β-Blockers are generally contraindicated in bronchial and peripheral vascular disease	Consider verapamil or diltiazem
Verapamil-induced constipation	If it occurs, give regular osmotic laxatives
All antiarrhythmics are proarrhythmic	Prevention is better than cure. Minimize the requirement for drugs by careful attention to precipitating factors. Consider use of pacemakers or electrical therapies if appropriate
Amiodarone is commonly associated with an increased tendency to sunburn	Warn all patients to stay covered up when outdoors, use sun block or stay indoors
Diagnosis of paroxysmal arrhythmias is difficult	Use continuous monitoring by tapes or implantable event recorders
Torsades de pointes may be precipitated by taking other medication with amiodarone or disopyramide	Patients should remind members of healthcare team that they are taking antiarrhythmic drugs

that of prescribers. A study of patients' and prescribers' attitudes to the use of aspirin and warfarin for stroke prevention in atrial fibrillation (Devereaux et al 2001) demonstrated not only that prescribers differ markedly on the balance of risks between stroke prevention and bleeding caused by treatment but also that patients feared stroke more than doctors did. This affected their decisions about taking warfarin or aspirin. Prescribers should seek and respect patients' views on such treatment choices, rather than assume all patients are the same or that they will agree with the prescriber's own views.

CASE STUDIES

Case 22.1

A middle-aged man with a medical history of stable angina treated with GTN spray when necessary and verapamil 80 mg three times daily presents to his primary care doctor with complaints of a fluttering sensation in his chest from time to time. It is a bit disconcerting but not painful. It occurs mainly in the morning after coffee. It does not limit him in his activities.

Question

What should the primary care doctor do?

Answer

This sounds like typical atrial fibrillation but needs an ECG investigation and a careful history. Caffeine in the coffee may be a precipitant and if so, should be avoided, but if the verapamil is a recent prescription then that too should be withdrawn. Dependent upon the nature of the angina and any risk of bronchoconstriction or peripheral vascular disease, the verapamil could be replaced by sotalol or another β-blocker, even if the prescription is long term. If the palpitations are only short-lived and do not trouble the patient unduly, he may be reassured and no treatment offered, but a thorough review of the management of his angina and fibrillation is probably indicated.

Case 22.2

A patient who is in intensive care with septicaemia following a bacterial chest infection is on permanent bedside ECG monitoring. She is febrile, has tachycardia and is observed to have ventricular ectopic beats occasionally. She then develops atrial ectopics and short runs of atrial fibrillation. Her cardiac output decreases by about 10% during the fibrillatory episodes.

Question

How should this patient be managed?

Answer

Acutely ill patients often develop arrhythmias, especially atrial ectopics and fibrillation. These are usually not a significant problem and do not merit treatment unless the cardiac output is seriously compromised. Ventricular ectopics are also normal in all adults and only if they occur frequently or occur in runs of three or more consecutive beats are they an indicator of a possible poor outcome. In an intensive care unit patient, a 10% decrease in cardiac output, which is reversed when the rhythm is back to normal, is not a serious problem. If it becomes worse, the normal treatment would be a β-blocker but this lady has a respiratory problem and amiodarone or verapamil may be preferred. Since she is in intensive care, however, there is some protection against the risk of bronchoconstriction because intravenous access is probably in place and ventilators should be readily available. Other causes of arrhythmias should be sought, especially amongst her other prescribed medication (see Table 22.2).

REFERENCE

Atrial Fibrillation Investigators 1994 Risk factors for stroke and efficacy of antithrombotic therapy in atrial fibrillation: analysis of pooled data from five randomised controlled trials. Archives of Internal Medicine 154: 1449-1457

Benavente O, Hart K, Koudstaal P et al 2000 Antiplatelet therapy for preventing stroke in patients with non-valvular atrial fibrillation and no previous history of stroke or transient ischaemic attacks. Cochrane Review. Cochrane Library, issue 4. Update Software, Oxford

Blomström-Lundqvist C, Scheinman M M, Aliot E M et al 2003 ACC/AHA/ESC guidelines for the management of patients with supraventricular arrhythmias. American College of Cardiology. Available online at: www.acc.org/clinical/guidelines/arrhythmias/sva_index.pdf

Cardiac Arrhythmia Suppression Trial (CAST) Investigators 1989 Preliminary report: effect of encainide and flecainide on mortality in a randomised trial of arrhythmia suppression after myocardial infarction. New England Journal of Medicine 321: 406-412

Cardiac Arrhythmia Suppression Trial II Investigators 1992 Effect of the antiarrhythmic agent moracizine on survival after myocardial infarction. New England Journal of Medicine 327: 227-233

Devereaux P J, Anderson D R, Gardner M J et al 2001 Differences between perspectives of physicians and patients on anticoagulation in patients with atrial fibrillation: observational study. British Medical Journal 323: 1218

Diener H C, Cunha L, Forbes C et al 1996 European stroke prevention study, 2: Dipyridamole and acetylsalicylic acid in the secondary prevention of stroke. Journal of the Neurological Sciences 143: 1-13

Hine L K, Laird N, Hewitt P et al 1989 Meta-analytic evidence against prophylactic use of lidocaine in acute myocardial infarction. Archives of Internal Medicine 149: 2694-2698

Hjalmarson A, Olsson G 1991 Myocardial infarction: effects of beta-blockade. Circulation 84: VI101-VI107

Landers M D, Reiter M J 1997 General principles of antiarrhythmic therapy for ventricular tachyarrhythmias. American Journal of Cardiology 80: 31G-44G

Moss A J 1999 The QT interval and torsades de pointes. Drug Safety 21: 5-10

Sanderson J 1996 The SWORD of Damocles. Lancet 348: 2-3

Singh B N, Singh S N, Reda D J et al 2005 Amiodarone versus sotalol for atrial fibrillation. New England Journal of Medicine 352: 1861-1872

FURTHER READING

Brugada R, Hong K, Cordeiro J M et al 2005 Short QT syndrome. Canadian Medical Association Journal 173: 1349-1354

Fuster V, Rydén LE, Asinger R et al 2001 ACC/AHA/ESC guidelines for the management of patients with atrial fibrillation: executive summary. Circulation 104: 2118-2150

Goldstein R N, Stambler B S 2005 New antiarrhythmic drugs for prevention of atrial fibrillation. Progress in Cardiovascular Disease 48: 193-208

Iqbal M B, Taneja A K, Lip G Y H et al 2005 Recent developments in atrial fibrillation. British Medical Journal 330: 238-243

Joglar J A, Page R L 1999 Treatment of arrhythmias during pregnancy: safety considerations. Drug Safety 20: 85-94

Lévy S, Breithardt G, Campbell R W F et al 1998 Atrial fibrillation: current knowledge and recommendations for management. European Heart Journal 19:1294-1320

Nattel S, Opie L H 2006 Controversies in atrial fibrillation. Lancet 367: 262-272

Roberts R 2006 Genomics and cardiac arrhythmias. Journal of the American College of Cardiology 47: 9-21

23 Thrombosis

P. A. Routledge   H. G. M. Shetty

Venous thromboembolism

- Venous thromboembolism has an incidence of 2–5%.
- Combinations of sluggish blood flow and hypercoagulability are the commonest causes of venous thromboembolism. Vascular injury is also a recognized causative factor.
- Treatment of venous thromboembolism involves the use of anticoagulants and, in severe cases, thrombolytic drugs.
- Anticoagulant therapy usually involves an immediate-acting agent such as heparin followed by maintenance treatment with warfarin.
- Unfractionated heparins increase the rate of interaction of thrombin with antithrombin III 1000-fold and prevent the production of fibrin from fibrinogen.
- Low molecular weight heparins inactivate factor Xa, have a longer half-life and produce a more predictable response than unfractionated heparins.
- Warfarin is the most widely used coumarin because of potency, reliable bioavailability and an intermediate half-life of elimination (36 h).
- Warfarin consists of an equal mixture of two enantiomers, (R)- and (S)-warfarin, that have different anticoagulant potencies and routes of metabolism.

Arterial thromboembolism

- Arterial thromboembolism is normally associated with vascular injury and hypercoagulability.
- Acute myocardial infarction is the commonest form of arterial thrombosis.
- Arterial thromboembolism affecting the cerebral circulation results in either transient ischaemic attacks (TIAs) or, in severe cases, cerebral infarction (stroke).
- Investigation of TIAs is necessary and prophylaxis using aspirin (or another antiplatelet agent) or warfarin is often beneficial, depending on the pathophysiology.
- If the source of embolism is from the heart, prophylaxis with oral anticoagulants is the treatment of choice.

Thrombosis is the development of a 'thrombus' consisting of platelets, fibrin, red cells and white cells in the arterial or venous circulation. If part of this thrombus in the venous circulation breaks off and enters the right heart, it may be lodged in the pulmonary arterial circulation, causing pulmonary embolism (PE). In the left-sided circulation, an embolus may result in peripheral arterial occlusion, either in the lower limbs or in the cerebral circulation (where it may cause thromboembolic stroke). Since the pathophysiology of each of these conditions differs, they will be discussed separately under the headings venous thromboembolism and arterial thromboembolism.

Venous thromboembolism

Epidemiology

Venous thromboembolism is common, with an incidence of 2–5%. Pulmonary embolism is now the commonest cause of maternal death and deep vein thrombosis may result in not only pulmonary embolism but also subsequent morbidity as a result of the postphlebitic limb. Thromboembolism appears to increase in prevalence over the age of 50 years, and the diagnosis is more often missed in this age group.

Aetiology

Venous thromboembolism occurs primarily due to a combination of stagnation of blood flow and hypercoagulability. Vascular injury is also a recognized causative factor but is not necessary for the development of venous thrombosis. In venous thromboembolism, the structure of the thrombus is different from that in arterial thromboembolism. In the former, platelets seem to be uniformly distributed through a mesh of fibrin and other blood cell components, whereas in arterial thromboembolism the white platelet 'head' is more prominent and it appears to play a much more important initiatory role in thrombus.

Sluggishness of blood flow may be related to bedrest, surgery or reduced cardiac output, e.g. in heart failure. Factors increasing the risk of hypercoagulability include surgery, pregnancy, oestrogen administration, malignancy, myocardial infarction and several acquired or inherited disorders of coagulation, e.g. antithrombin III deficiency, protein C deficiency, resistance to activated protein C, or primary antiphospholipid syndrome.

Protein C

Protein C deficiency is inherited by an autosomal dominant transmission. Such patients are at increased risk not only of venous thromboembolism but also of warfarin skin necrosis. This occurs because protein C (and its closely related co-factor, protein S) is a vitamin K-dependent antithrombotic factor that can be further suppressed by the administration of warfarin. Thrombosis in the small vessels of the skin may occur if large loading (induction) doses of warfarin are given to such patients when the suppression of the antithrombotic effects of these factors occurs before the antithrombotic effects of blockade of vitamin K-dependent clotting factor (II, VII, IX and X) production has occurred. Although the prevalence of protein C deficiency is 0.2%, only one subject in 70 (i.e. 0.0003%) will be symptomatic, and the condition accounts for around 4% of patients presenting with thromboembolic disease before the age of 45 years.

Protein S deficiency

Protein S deficiency is probably even rarer than protein C deficiency but the familial form, inherited in an autosomal dominant fashion, is a high-risk state, accounting for possibly 5–8% of cases of the thromboembolism in patients less than 45 years old.

Factor V Leiden

The presence of another, additional clotting defect may be a trigger factor for problems in patients with deficiency of one of these factors. One of these conditions is activated protein C deficiency. This results from the presence of factor V Leiden, a point mutation in the factor V gene, which causes the activated factor V molecule to be resistant to deactivation by activated protein C (APC). This defect may have a prevalence of 9% in the general population, and higher in patients with thromboembolic disease, and may in itself be of little consequence until there is another risk factor, such as immobility or use of the contraceptive pill. In these circumstances, the combination of risks may be responsible for the increased predisposition to thromboembolism in a high proportion of affected individuals.

Antithrombin III deficiency

Antithrombin III deficiency is a rare autosomal dominantly inherited abnormality associated with a reduced plasma concentration of this protein. The defect may not result in clinical problems until pregnancy or until patients enter their fourth decade, when venous and (to a lesser extent) arterial thrombosis becomes more common. Nevertheless, it has been estimated to be responsible for between 2% and 5% of thromboembolism occurring before age 45.

Lupus anticoagulant

Lupus anticoagulant, an antibody against phospholipid, is so named because it increases the clotting time in blood when measured by some standard coagulation tests. Patients affected are more prone to thromboembolism. This factor is found in 10% of patients with systemic lupus erythematosus (SLE) where it is associated with a threefold increase in thromboembolic risk; it is also found in the primary antiphospholipid syndrome (PAPS), where it may signify an increased risk of venous and arterial thrombosis and of recurrent miscarriage.

Oestrogens

Oestrogens increase the circulating concentrations of clotting factors I, II, VII, VIII, IX and X and reduce fibrinolytic activity. They also depress the concentrations of antithrombin III, which is protective against thrombosis. This effect is dose related, and venous thrombosis was more often seen with the high (50 μg) oestrogen-containing contraceptive pill than with the present lower-dose preparations.

Malignancy

Venous thromboembolism is also commoner in malignancy (the risk may be up to fivefold greater). Although first described in association with carcinoma of the pancreas, all solid tumours seem to be associated with this problem. This may be related to the expression of tissue factor or factor X activators, but several other mechanisms may also be responsible.

Surgery

The increased risk of venous thromboembolism in surgery is related in part to stagnation of venous blood in the calves during the operation but also to tissue trauma, since it appears to be more common in operations that involve marked tissue damage, such as orthopaedic surgery. This may in turn be related to release of tissue thromboplastin and to reduced fibrinolytic activity. The most important risk factors associated with clinical thromboembolism after surgery are age and obesity.

Clinical manifestations

In 90% of patients, deep vein thrombosis occurs in the veins of the lower limbs and pelvis. In up to half of cases this may not result in local symptoms or signs, and the onset of pulmonary embolism may be the first evidence of the presence of venous thromboembolism. In other cases patients classically present with pain involving the calf or thigh associated with swelling, redness of the overlying skin and increased warmth. In a large deep venous thrombosis that prevents venous return, the leg may become discolored and oedematous. Massive venous thrombus can occasionally result in gangrene, although this occurs very rarely now that effective drug therapies are available.

Pulmonary embolism may occur in the absence of clinical signs of venous thrombosis. It may be very difficult to diagnose because of the non-specificity of symptoms and signs. Clinical diagnosis is often made because of the presence of associated risk factors. Obstruction with a large embolus of a major pulmonary artery may result in acute massive pulmonary embolism, presenting with sudden shortness of breath and dull central chest pain, together with marked haemodynamic disturbance, e.g. severe hypotension and right ventricular failure, sometimes resulting in death due to acute circulatory failure unless rapidly treated.

Acute submassive pulmonary embolus occurs when less than 50% of the pulmonary circulation is occluded by embolus, and the embolus normally lodges in a more distal branch of the pulmonary artery. It may result in some shortness of breath but if the lung normally supplied by that branch of the pulmonary artery becomes necrotic, pulmonary infarction results with pleuritic pain and haemoptysis (coughing up blood), and there may be a pleural 'rub' (a sound like Velcro being torn apart when the patient breathes in) as a result of inflammation of the lung. Patients may, rarely, develop recurrent thromboembolism. This may not result in immediate symptoms or signs but the patient may present with increasing breathlessness and signs of pulmonary hypertension (right ventricular hypertrophy) and, if untreated, progressive respiratory failure.

Investigations

Deep vein thrombosis

Although several conditions may mimic deep vein thrombus, such as a Baker's cyst, which involves rupture of the posterior aspect of the synovial capsule of the knee, deep vein thrombosis is the commonest cause of pain, swelling and tenderness of the leg. The clinical diagnosis of venous thrombosis is relatively unreliable, and venography is the most specific diagnostic test.

Venography Venography involves injection of radio-opaque contrast medium, normally into a vein on the top of the foot, and subsequent radiography of the venous system.

Ultrasound Ultrasound is a non-invasive alternative to venography that does not involve exposure to ionizing radiation or potentially allergenic contrast media. It is now the initial investigation of choice in clinically suspected deep vein thrombosis, although it is less sensitive for below-knee and isolated pelvic deep vein thrombosis.

Magnetic resonance imaging Magnetic resonance imaging (MRI) is also non-invasive and avoids radiation exposure. When used with direct thrombus imaging (DTI), which detects methaemoglobin in the clot, MRI DTI is sensitive and specific, even with below-knee and isolated pelvic deep vein thrombosis. However, it is not widely clinically available and ultrasound remains the primary initial investigation.

Pulmonary embolism

Pulmonary arteriography The diagnosis of pulmonary embolism is most often made using one of two techniques: pulmonary arteriography or ventilation–perfusion scanning. Pulmonary arteriography is the most specific test. This requires catheterization of the right side of the heart and an injection of contrast medium into the pulmonary artery. Adequate facilities and experienced personnel are therefore required and it is now generally reserved for those situations where massive or submassive pulmonary embolism is suspected but non-invasive tests have given indeterminate results.

Ventilation–perfusion scanning Ventilation–perfusion scanning involves the injection of a radiolabelled substance into the vein and measurement of the perfusion via the pulmonary circulation, using a scintillation counter. This is often combined with a ventilation scan in which radiolabelled gas, normally xenon, is inhaled by the patient. Pulmonary embolism classically results in an area of under- or non-perfusion of a part of the lung that, nevertheless, because the airways are patent, ventilates normally. This pattern is called ventilation–perfusion mismatch and is a specific sign of pulmonary embolism.

Spiral computed tomography Computed tomography angiography (CT angiography) using helical or spiral CT (sCT) is now being increasingly used in some centres, and has a high accuracy rate. Although subsegmental emboli can be missed, visualization of smaller arterial branches, and therefore detection of small emboli, may improve with the availability of multidetector scanners. Not only does sCT enable direct visualization of emboli, but visualization of the lung parenchyma and mediastinum may help in the differential diagnosis in non-embolic cases. Magnetic resonance imaging is also being developed for the diagnosis of pulmonary embolism and early results are promising.

Other findings Other findings occur in pulmonary embolism, such as changes in the chest radiograph, e.g. a raised right hemidiaphragm as a result of loss of lung volume (pulmonary embolism more commonly affects the right than the left lung). Hypoxia is also seen, and this is worse the larger the pulmonary embolus. The electrocardiogram may show signs of right ventricular strain. The echocardiogram may show right ventricular overload and dysfunction in massive pulmonary embolism. However, all these changes are relatively non-specific and do not obviate the need for the specific tests mentioned above.

Treatment

The aim of treatment of venous thrombosis is to allow normal circulation in the limbs and, wherever possible, to prevent damage to the valves of the veins, thus reducing the risk of the swollen postphlebitic limb. Second, it is important to try to prevent associated pulmonary embolism and also recurrence of either venous thrombosis or pulmonary embolism in the risk period after the initial episode.

In acute massive pulmonary embolism the initial priority is to correct the circulatory defect that has caused haemodynamic upset and, in these circumstances, rapid removal of the obstruction using thrombolytic drugs or surgical removal of the embolus may be necessary. In acute submassive pulmonary embolism, the goal of treatment is to prevent further episodes, particularly of the more serious acute massive pulmonary embolism. In both deep vein thrombosis and pulmonary embolism, a search must be made for underlying risk factors, such as carcinoma, which may occur in up to 10% of patients, and particularly in those with repeated episodes of venous thromboembolism.

The treatment of venous thromboembolism consists of the use of anticoagulants and, in severe cases, thrombolytic drugs. Anticoagulant therapy involves the use of immediate-acting agents (particularly heparin) and oral anticoagulants, the commonest of which is warfarin. Not only do these treat the acute event, but they also prevent recurrence and may be necessary for some time after the initial event, depending on the persistence of risk factors for recurrent thromboembolism.

Heparins

Conventional or unfractionated heparin (UFH) is a heterogeneous mixture of large mucopolysaccharide molecules ranging widely in molecular weight between 3000 and 30000, with immediate anticoagulant properties. It acts by increasing the rate of the interaction of thrombin with antithrombin III by a factor of 1000. It thus prevents the production of fibrin (factor I) from fibrinogen. Heparin also has effects on the inhibition of production of activated clotting factors IX, X, XI and XII, and these effects occur at concentrations lower than its effects on thrombin.

Unlike UFH, low molecular weight heparins (LMWHs) contain polysaccharide chains ranging in molecular weight between 4000 and 6000. Whereas UFH produces its anticoagulant effect by inhibiting both thrombin and factor Xa, LMWHs predominantly inactivate only factor Xa. In addition, unlike UFH, they inactivate platelet-bound factor Xa and resist inhibition by platelet factor 4, which is released during coagulation. Bemiparin, dalteparin, enoxaparin, reviparin and tinzaparin are LMWHs with similar efficacy and adverse effects.

Because unfractionated and LMWHs all consist of high molecular weight molecules that are highly ionized (heparin is the strongest organic acid found naturally in the body) they are not absorbed via the gastrointestinal tract and must be given by intravenous infusion or deep subcutaneous (never intramuscular) injection. Unfractionated heparin is highly protein bound and it appears to be restricted to the intravascular space, with a consequently low volume of distribution. It does not cross the placenta and does not appear in breast milk. Its pharmacokinetics are complex but it appears to have a dose-dependent increase in half-life. The half-life is normally about 60 minutes, but is shorter in patients with pulmonary embolism. It is removed from the body by metabolism, possibly in the reticuloendothelial cells of the liver, and by renal excretion. The latter seems to be more important after high doses of the compound.

LMWHs have a number of potentially desirable pharmacokinetics features compared with UFH. They are predominantly excreted renally and have longer and more predictable half-lives than UFH and so have a more predictable dose response than UFH. They can therefore be given once or, at the most, twice daily in a fixed dose, sometimes based on the patient's body weight, without the need for laboratory monitoring (except for patients given treatment doses and at high risk of bleeding).

The major adverse effect of all heparins is haemorrhage, which is commoner in patients with severe heart or liver disease, renal disease, general debility and in women aged over 60 years. The risk of haemorrhage is increased in those with prolonged clotting times and in those given heparin by intermittent intravenous bolus rather than by continuous intravenous administration. UFH is monitored by derivatives of the activated partial thromboplastin time, for example the kaolin–cephalin clotting time (KCCT); in those patients with a KCCT three times greater than control, there is an eightfold increase in the risk of haemorrhage. The therapeutic range for the KCCT during UFH therapy therefore appears to be between 1.5 and 2.5 times the control values. Rapid reversal of the effect of heparin can be achieved using protamine sulphate, but this is rarely necessary because of the short duration of action of heparin. LMWHs may produce fewer haemorrhagic complications, and monitoring of effect is not routinely required. At doses normally used for treatment, they do not significantly affect coagulation tests and routine monitoring is not necessary (British Committee for Standards in Haematology 2006b).

Heparins, particularly UFH, may also cause thrombocytopenia (low platelet count). This may occur in two forms. The first occurs 3–5 days after treatment and does not normally result in complications. The second type of thrombocytopenia occurs after about 6 days of treatment and often results in much more profound decreases in platelet count and an increased risk of thromboembolism. LMWHs are thought to be less likely to cause thrombocytopenia but this complication has been reported, including in individuals who had previously developed thrombocytopenia after UFH. For these reasons, patients should have a platelet count on the day of starting UFH and the alternate-day platelet counts should be performed from days 4 to 14 thereafter. For patients on LMWH, the platelet counts should be performed at 2–4 day intervals from day 4 to 14 (British Committee for Standards in Haematology 2006c). If the platelet count falls by 50% and/or the patient develops new thrombosis or skin allergy during this period, heparin-induced thrombocytopenia (HIT) should be considered and, if strongly suspected or confirmed, heparin should be stopped and an alternative agent such as a heparinoid or hirudin commenced.

Heparin-induced osteoporosis is rare but may occur when the drug is used during pregnancy, and may be dose related. The exact mechanism is unknown. Other adverse effects of heparin are alopecia, urticaria and anaphylaxis, but these are also rare.

It has been shown that there is a non-linear relationship between the dose of UFH infused and the KCCT. This means that disproportionate adjustments in dose are required depending on the KCCT if under- or overdosing is to be avoided (Table 23.1). Since the half-life of UFH is 1 h, it would take 5 h (five half-lives of the drug) to reach a steady state. A loading dose is therefore administered to reduce the time to achieve adequate anticoagulation. UFH in full dose can also be given by repeated subcutaneous injection, and in these circumstances the calcium salt appears to be less painful than the sodium salt. Opinions differ as to whether the subcutaneous or intravenous route is preferable. The subcutaneous route may take longer to reach effective plasma heparin concentrations but avoids the need for infusion devices.

Heparin is normally used in the immediate stages of venous thrombosis and pulmonary embolism until the effects of warfarin become apparent. In the past it has been continued for 7–10 days, but recent evidence indicates that 3–5 days of therapy may be sufficient in many instances. This shorter treatment may also reduce the risk of the rare but potentially very serious complications of severe heparin-induced thrombocytopenia, which

---

Table 23.1 Guidelines to control unfractionated heparin (UFH) treatment

Loading dose

5000 iu over 5 minutes

Infusion

Start at 1400 iu/h (e.g. 8400 iu in 100 mL of normal saline over 6 h). Check after 6 h. Adjust dose according to ratio of the KCCT to the control value using the values below

KCCT ratio	Infusion rate change
>7.0	Discontinue for 30 min to 1 h and reduce by >500 iu/h
>5.0	Reduce by 500 iu/h
4.1–5.0	Reduce by 300 iu/h
3.1–4.0	Reduce by 100 iu/h
2.6–3.0	Reduce by 50 iu/h
1.5–2.5	No change
1.2–1.4	Increase by 200 iu/h
<1.2	Increase by 400 iu/h

After each dose change, wait 10 h before next KCCT estimation unless KCCT >5, when more frequent (e.g. 4-hourly) estimation is advisable. Developed using Diogen (Bell and Alton); local validation may be necessary.
KCCT, Kaolin–cephalin clotting time.
Modified from Fennerty et al 1986 and reproduced in British Committee for Standards in Haematology 1998

normally occurs after the 6th day. LMWHs are used for similar lengths of time, but are normally given subcutaneously without a loading dose, and without routine monitoring. They are more expensive than UFH but the increased efficacy and convenience of administration may well make them cost-effective in treatment and prevention in certain situations, for example outpatient treatment.

Heparinoids

Danaparoid is a heparinoid that is licensed for prophylaxis of deep vein thrombosis in patients undergoing general or orthopaedic surgery. It is a mixture of the low molecular weight sulphated glycosaminoglycuronans: heparin sulphate, dermatan sulphate and a small amount of chondroitin sulphate. It acts by inhibiting factor Xa and, like LMWHs, is given by subcutaneous injection. It normally has a low cross-reactivity rate with heparin-associated antiplatelet antibodies and can be used in the treatment of individuals who develop HIT but still need ongoing anticoagulation. It is administered intravenously, with monitoring of anti-Xa activity only required in those at high risk of bleeding, e.g. renal insufficiency.

Hirudins

Lepirudin, a recombinant hirudin, is licensed for anticoagulation in patients with type II (immune) heparin-induced thrombocytopenia who require parenteral antithrombotic treatment. The dose of lepirudin is adjusted according to the activated partial thromboplastin time (APTT), and it is given intravenously by infusion. Haemorrhage is greater in those with poor renal function. Severe anaphylaxis occurs rarely in association with lepirudin treatment and is more common in previously exposed patients (British Committee for Standards in Haematology 2006c). Bivaluridin is a direct thrombin inhibitor. It is licensed for anticoagulation in patients undergoing percutaneous coronary intervention (PCI) and the activated clotting time (ACT) is used to assess its activity. Haemorrhage is an important adverse effect of this agent also.

Fondaparinux

Fondiparinux sodium is a synthetic pentasaccharide that binds to antithrombin III, thus inhibiting factor Xa but without effect on factor IIa. Therefore at doses normally used for treatment, it does not significantly affect coagulation tests and routine monitoring of these is not necessary.

It is licensed for prophylaxis of venous thromboembolism in high-risk situations and for treatment of acute deep vein thrombosis and treatment of acute pulmonary embolism, except in haemodynamically unstable patients or patients who require thrombolysis or pulmonary embolectomy. It is given subcutaneously and haemorrhage is the most important adverse effect.

Oral anticoagulants

Although not the only coumarin anticoagulant available, warfarin is by far the most widely used drug in this group because of its potency, duration of action and more reliable bioavailability. Acenocoumarol (nicoumalone) has a much shorter duration of action and phenindione may be associated with a higher incidence of non-haemorrhagic adverse effects. When given by mouth, warfarin is completely and rapidly absorbed, although food decreases the rate (but not the extent) of absorption. It is extremely highly plasma protein bound (99%) and therefore has a small volume of distribution (7–14 L). It consists of an equal mixture of two enantiomers, (R)- and (S)-warfarin. They have different anticoagulant potencies and routes of metabolism.

Both enantiomers of warfarin act by inducing a functional deficiency of vitamin K and thereby prevent the normal carboxylation of the glutamic acid residues of the amino-terminal ends of clotting factors II, VII, IX and X. This renders the clotting factors unable to cross-link with calcium and thereby bind to phospholipid-containing membranes. Warfarin prevents the reduction of vitamin K epoxide to vitamin K by epoxide reductase. (S)-warfarin appears to be at least five times more potent in this regard than (R)-warfarin. Since warfarin does not have any effect on already carboxylated clotting factors, the delay in onset of the anticoagulant effect of warfarin is dependent on the rate of clearance of the fully carboxylated factors already synthesized. In this regard the half-life of removal of factor VII is approximately 6 h, that of factor IX 24 h, factor X 36 h and factor II 50 h. Some of the variability in response to warfarin may be related to genetic variations in the gene encoding the vitamin K epoxide reductase multiprotein complex (VKORC1 gene).

The effect of warfarin is monitored using the one-stage prothrombin time, for example the international normalized ratio (INR). This test is sensitive chiefly to factors VII, II and X (and to a lesser extent factor V, which is not a vitamin K-dependent clotting factor). However, factor VII, to which the INR is sensitive, is the most important factor in the extrinsic pathway of clotting. The optimum therapeutic range for the INR differs for different clinical indications since the lowest INR consistent with therapeutic efficacy is the best in reducing the risk of haemorrhage. Examples of therapeutic ranges recommended for certain indications are given in Table 23.2 (British Committee for Standards in Haematology 1998, 2006a).

Warfarin is metabolized by the liver via the cytochrome P450 system. Only very small amounts of the drug appear unchanged in the urine. The average clearance is 4.5 L/day and the half-life ranges from 20 to 60 h (mean 40 h). It thus takes approximately 1 week (around five half-lives) for the steady state to be reached after warfarin has been administered. The enantiomers of warfarin are metabolized stereo-specifically, (R)-warfarin being mainly reduced at the acetyl side-chain into secondary warfarin alcohols while (S)-warfarin is predominantly metabolized at the coumarin ring to hydroxywarfarin. The clearance of warfarin may be reduced in liver disease as well as during administration of a variety of drugs known to inhibit either the (S) or (R), or both, enantiomers. These are shown in Table 23.3 which is not exhaustive. The number of possible interactions and the potential severity of their outcome mean that it is essential not to prescribe any medicine concomitantly with warfarin until a thorough check on all possible interactions has been undertaken. The British National Formulary contains comprehensive tables listing possible interactions between warfarin and other medicines.

Table 23.2 Recommended target INRs for different conditions and grade of recommendation

Indication	Target INR	Grade of recommendation
Pulmonary embolus	2.5	A
Proximal deep vein thrombosis	2.5	A
Calf vein thrombus	2.5	A
Recurrence of venous thromboembolism when no longer on warfarin therapy	2.5	A
Recurrence of venous thromboembolism while on warfarin therapy	3.5	C
Symptomatic inherited thrombophilia	2.5	A
Antiphospholipid syndrome	3.5	A
Non-rheumatic atrial fibrillation	2.5	A
Atrial fibrillation due to rheumatic heart disease, congenital heart disease, thyrotoxicosis	2.5	C
Cardioversion	2.5	B
Mural thrombus	2.5	B
Cardiomyopathy	2.5	C
Mechanical prosthetic heart valve (caged ball or caged disk), aortic or mitral*	3.5	B
Mechanical prosthetic heart valve (tilting disc or bileaflet), mitral*	3.0	B
Mechanical prosthetic heart valve (tilting disc), aortic*	3.0	B
Mechanical prosthetic heart valve (bileaflet), aortic*	2.0	B
Bioprosthetic valve	20. (if anticoagulated)	A
Ischaemic stroke without atrial fibrillation	Not indicated	C
Retinal vessel occlusion	Not indicated	C
Peripheral arterial thrombosis and grafts	Not indicated	A
Arterial grafts	2.5 (if anticoagulated)	
Coronary artery thrombosis	2.5 (if anticoagulated)	
Coronary artery graft	Not indicated	A
Coronary angioplasty and stents	Not indicated	A

INR, international normalized ratio.
A, at least one randomized controlled trial (RCT); B, well-conducted clinical trials but no RCT; C, expert opinion but no studies.
* If the valve type is not known, a target INR of 3.0 is recommended for valves in the aortic position and 3.5 in the mitral position.
British Committee for Standards in Haematology 1998, 2006a.

Renal function is thought to have little effect on the pharmacokinetics of, or anticoagulant response to, warfarin. Some of the variability in warfarin dose requirement is related to genetic polymorphisms of the cytochrome (CYP2C9) mediating the rate of hepatic metabolism of (S)-warfarin. Individuals with the variant isoform (either heterozygotes or in particular homozygotes) metabolize this more active enantiomer more slowly and so require lower doses.

The major adverse effect of warfarin is haemorrhage, which often occurs at a predisposing abnormality such as an ulcer or tumour. The risk of bleeding is increased by excessive anticoagulation, although this may not need to be present for severe

Table 23.3 Some clinically important drug interactions with warfarin

Interacting drug	Effect of interaction on anticoagulant effect	Probable mechanism(s)
Colestyramine Colestipol	Reduced anticoagulant effect	Impaired absorption and increased elimination of warfarin. N.B. Long-term treatment may cause impaired vitamin K absorption and enhance anticoagulant effect
Barbiturates Carbamazepine Griseofulvin Phenytoin (see also below) Primidone Rifampicin Rifabutin St John's wort	Reduced anticoagulant effect	Induction of warfarin metabolism
Amiodarone Azapropazone Chloramphenicol Cimetidine Ciprofloxacin Clarithromycin Dextropopoxyphene Erythromycin Fluconazole Fluvastatin Itraconazole Ketoconazole Mefenamic acid Metronidazole Miconazole Nalidixic acid Norfloxacin Ofloxacin Phenylbutazone Sulfinpyrazone Sulphonamides (e.g. in co-trimoxazole) Voriconazole Zafirlukast	Increased anticoagulant effect	Inhibition of warfarin metabolism
Anabolic steroids Bezafibrate Danazol Gemfibrozil Levothyroxine Phenytoin (see also above) Salicylates/aspirin (high-dose) Stanozolol Tamoxifen Testosterone	Increased anticoagulant effect	Pharmacodynamic potentiation of anticoagulant effect
Cranberry juice	Increased anticoagulant effect	Mechanism unknown
NSAIDs (including aspirin at all doses) Clopidogrel	Increased risk of bleeding	Additive effects on coagulation and haemostasis
Oral contraceptives, oestrogens and progestogens Vitamin K (e.g. in some enteral feeds)	Reduced anticoagulant effect	Pharmacodynamic antagonism of anticoagulant effect

haemorrhage to occur. Close monitoring of the degree of anticoagulation of warfarin is therefore important, and guidelines for reversal of excessive anticoagulation are shown in Table 23.4. It is also important to reduce the duration of therapy of the drug to the minimum effective period in order to reduce the period of risk.

Skin reactions to warfarin may also occur but are rare. The most serious skin reaction is warfarin-induced skin necrosis, which may occur over areas of adipose tissue such as the breasts, buttocks or thighs, especially in women, and which is related to relative deficiency of protein C or S. This is important because these deficiencies result in an increased risk of thrombosis and therefore warfarin may more often be used in such subjects. Preventing excessive anticoagulation in the initial stages of induction of therapy may reduce the severity of the reaction. A dosing schedule which helps to achieve this is shown in Table 23.5.

Warfarin may also be teratogenic, producing in some instances a condition called chondrodysplasia punctata. This is associated with 'punched-out' lesions at sites of ossification, particularly of the long bones but also of the facial bones, and may be associated with absence of the spleen. Although it has been associated predominantly with warfarin anticoagulation during the first trimester of pregnancy, other abnormalities, including cranial nerve palsies, hydrocephalus and microcephaly, have been reported at later stages of pregnancy if the child is exposed.

Although other oral anticoagulants are available, in the vast majority of cases these have not been shown to have any clear benefits over warfarin. They may be used occasionally where a patient does not tolerate warfarin. The necessary duration of anticoagulation in venous thrombosis and pulmonary embolus is still uncertain. On the basis of the available evidence, therapy may be required for approximately 6 months after the first deep vein thrombosis or pulmonary embolus. It may be possible to reduce the duration of therapy in patients who have had a postoperative episode since it is likely that the risk factor has been reversed (unless immobility continues). In patients with a second episode, therapy may be required for even longer and in patients with more than two episodes, life-long treatment may be necessary in order to reduce the risk of recurrence (British Committee for Standards in Haematology 1998).

Fibrinolytic drugs

Thrombolytic therapy is used in life-threatening acute massive pulmonary embolus. It has been used in deep vein thrombosis, particularly in those patients where a large amount of clot exists and venous valvular damage is likely. However, fibrinolytic drugs are potentially more dangerous than anticoagulant drugs, and evidence is not available in situations other than acute massive embolism to show a sustained benefit from their use.

Streptokinase was the first agent available in this class. It was produced from streptococci and is a large protein that binds to and activates plasminogen, thus encouraging the breakdown of formed fibrin to fibrinogen degradation products. It also acts

Table 23.4 Recommendations for management of bleeding and excessive anticoagulation in patients receiving warfarin

Cause	Recommendation
3.0<INR<6.0 (target INR 2.5) 4.0<INR<6.0 (target INR 3.5)	1. Reduce warfarin dose or stop 2. Restart warfarin when INR <5.0
6.0<INR<8.0, no bleeding or minor bleeding	1. Stop warfarin 2. Restart when INR <5.0
INR>8.0, no bleeding or minor bleeding	1. Stop warfarin 2. Restart warfarin when INR <5.0 3. If other risk factors for bleeding give 0.5–2.5 mg of vitamin K (oral)
Major bleeding	1. Stop warfarin 2. Give prothrombin complex concentrate 50 units/kg or FFP 15 mL/kg 3. Give 5 mg of vitamin (oral or i.v.)

INR, international normalized ratio; FFP, fresh frozen plasma.
British Committee on Standards in Haematology 1998.

Table 23.5 Suggested warfarin induction schedule

Day	INR	Warfarin dose (mg)
First	<1.4	10
Second	<1.8	10
	1.8	1
	>1.8	0.5
Third	<2.0	10
	2.0–2.1	5
	2.2–2.3	4.5
	2.4–2.5	4
	2.6–2.7	3.5
	2.8–2.9	3
	3.0–3.1	2.5
	3.2–3.3	2
	3.4	1.5
	3.5	1
	3.6–4.0	0.5
	>4.0	0 (Predicted maintenance dose)
Fourth	<1.4	>8
	1.4	8
	1.5	7.5
	1.6–1.7	7
	1.8	6.5
	1.9	6
	2.0–2.1	5.5
	2.2–2.3	5
	2.4–2.6	4.5
	2.7–3.0	4
	3.1–3.5	3.5
	3.6–4.0	3
	4.1–4.5	Miss out next day's dose then give 2 mg
	>4.5	Miss out 2 days' doses then give 1 mg

INR, international normalized ratio.
Modified from Fennerty et al 1984.

on the circulating fibrinogen to produce a degree of systemic anticoagulation. Since it is a large protein molecule, it cannot be administered orally and has to be given by intravenous infusion. The half-life of removal from the body is 30 minutes. It is cleared chiefly by the reticuloendothelial system in the liver.

Its major adverse effect is to increase the risk of haemorrhage but it may also be antigenic and produce an anaphylactic reaction. It may also cause hypotension during infusion and in some patients, particularly those who have been administered the drug within the previous 12 months, a relative resistance to the drug may occur. Thrombolytic therapy is contraindicated in patients who have had major surgery or with active bleeding sites in the gastrointestinal or genitourinary tract, those who have a history of stroke, renal or liver disease, and those with hypertension. It should also be avoided during pregnancy and the postpartum period.

Tissue plasminogen activator (rt-PA) or alteplase was developed using recombinant DNA technology. Although this agent is much more expensive than streptokinase, it can be used in those situations where streptokinase may be less effective because of development of antibodies, for example within 1 year of previous streptokinase use or where allergy to streptokinase has previously occurred. Because it produces a lesser degree of systemic anticoagulation (it is more active against plasminogen associated with the clot), immediate use of heparin subsequently is necessary to prevent recurrence of thrombosis.

Reteplase, and more recently tenecteplase, are also fibrin-specific agents and so heparin is required to prevent rebound thrombosis. They have a similar efficacy to alteplase and are also more expensive than streptokinase. They are presently only licensed for acute myocardial infarction (see section on arterial thromboembolism, below). In this clinical situation, reteplase is administered as an intravenous bolus, followed by a second bolus 30 minutes later (double bolus), and tenecteplase is given as a single intravenous bolus. They therefore have the advantage of convenience of administration compared with alteplase, and are the preferred option in pre-hospital settings, particularly when administerd by paramedics (NICE 2002a).

Patient care

The patient on oral anticoagulants should be given full information on what to do in case of problems and what circumstances and drugs to avoid. An anticoagulant card with previous INR values and doses should also be provided. The patient should be told of the colour code for the different strengths of warfarin tablet and advised to carry their treatment card at all times. The likely duration of anticoagulant therapy should be made clear to the patient to avoid unnecessary and potentially dangerous prolongations of treatment. Patients who have received a fibrinolytic agent should also carry a card identifying the drug given and the date of administration.

Arterial thromboembolism

Epidemiology

Acute myocardial infarction is the commonest clinical presentation of acute arterial thrombosis. Stroke is commonly caused by atherothromboembolism from the great vessels or embolism arising from the heart (approximately 80% of strokes). The annual incidence of stroke in the developed world is approximately 1 per 2000 of the population, and the incidence is likely to increase as the population ages. Peripheral arterial occlusive thrombosis is normally associated with atherothromboembolism but is rare, even in patients with increased risk of thromboembolism, e.g. atrial fibrillation.

Aetiology

Arterial thromboembolism is normally associated with vascular injury and hypercoagulability. Vascular injury is most often due to atheroma, itself aggravated by smoking, hypertension, hyperlipidaemia or diabetes mellitus. Although the exact mechanism is not clear, it is thought that platelet aggregation may be induced by the sheer stresses caused by stenosis of an atherosclerotic vessel. This thrombotic material may embolize to cause occlusion further downstream. Hypercoagulability is also a risk factor. It may be associated with increased plasma fibrinogen levels and an increase in circulating cellular components, e.g. polycythaemia or thrombocythaemia. As mentioned earlier, the thrombus formed in the artery contains a much larger proportion of platelets, possibly reflecting the fact that other blood components that are not as readily adherent may be dissipated by the higher flow rates in the arterial circulation.

Oestrogens, by the mechanisms described earlier, are likely to increase the risk of arterial as well as venous thrombosis. Hyperlipidaemia may also increase the risk of hypercoagulability as well as enhancing thrombotic risk through its role in the progression of atheroma and vascular injury.

Clinical manifestations

Arterial thromboembolism affecting the cerebral circulation results in either transient ischaemic attacks (TIAs) or, in severe cases, cerebral infarction (one form of stroke). A transient ischaemic attack is defined as symptoms of acute ischaemia of the brain lasting for less than 24 h with complete recovery. The distinction between a transient ischaemic attack and a stroke is therefore one of degree. It may involve weakness of the limbs or cause disturbance of vision. If the vertebrobasilar territory is affected, nausea, vomiting and dizziness may be the most prominent features. In stroke, features are similar but persist for longer than 24 h. Clinical findings, however, vary markedly and it may be difficult on clinical grounds to separate cerebral infarction from the even more serious cause of stroke, cerebral haemorrhage. Patients with cerebral haemorrhage, however, more often have severe headache and coma, and less often have a preceding history of transient ischaemic attacks.

Arterial thromboembolism affecting a limb (normally a lower limb) most often presents as a sudden onset of pain in the limb associated with loss of peripheral pulses and coldness of the affected limb.

Investigations

The diagnosis of a transient ischaemic attack is a clinical one since, by definition, no permanent damage to the brain substance is caused by these episodes. The investigations therefore help to identify risk factors for transient ischaemia and will include investigations of factors known to increase blood viscosity or hypercoagulability, estimation of plasma glucose and lipid levels. Other investigations include CT head scan, imaging of the carotid vessels (normally by Doppler ultrasound) and a search for any cardiac sources of emboli (echocardiography). Evidence of arterial disease elsewhere increases the suspicion of transient ischaemic episodes.

The diagnosis of cerebral infarction includes the investigations previously mentioned for transient ischaemic attacks and computed axial tomography (CT scanning) is the initial investigation of choice. In cerebral infarction, areas of low density occur within a day or two of the episode. In cerebral haemorrhage, an area of high density occurs, often immediately after the episode. MRI and magnetic resonance angiography (MRA) may help to further localize the thrombus and to assess the severity of damage when required, but these investigations are not routinely available at present

Thromboembolism in a peripheral artery may be detected by Doppler ultrasound, but angiography is the definitive modality for investigation of the site and extent of blockage and the response to treatment.

Treatment and prevention

Transient ischaemic attacks resolve spontaneously and major aspects of their management include risk factor modification and prophylaxis (see aspirin, below). In patients with cerebral infarction, aspirin in a dose of 300 mg should be administered as soon as possible after the diagnosis is established. Intravenous alteplase, if administered within 3 h of onset of ischaemic stroke, has been shown to be beneficial but is associated with increased risk of intracerebral bleeding. Several neuroprotective agents have been investigated for treatment of ischaemic stroke but none has been shown to be effective. Anticoagulants may increase the risk of conversion of infarction of brain substance to haemorrhage and are contraindicated. Maintenance of adequate nutrition and the prevention and treatment of aspiration pneumonia, deep vein thrombosis, pressure sores and constipation are important. Risk factors for recurrent cerebral infarction such as hypertension, diabetes and hyperlipidaemia should be treated. Stopping smoking, avoiding excessive alcohol consumption and exercise are also important.

Anticoagulant therapy is effective in prophylaxis against cardiothromboembolic TIA or stroke (e.g. in patients with atrial fibrillation) but is not normally instituted until at least 2 weeks after the event. UK guidelines for the management of atrial fibrillation and the choice of thromboprophylaxis (aspirin or warfarin) are available (NICE 2006). If the source of emboli is from the great vessels, then prophylaxis with aspirin or other antiplatelet agent is more likely to be of benefit and is also likely to be safer than warfarin therapy (see below).

Aspirin

Aspirin is a potent inhibitor of the enzyme cyclo-oxygenase, which catalyses the production of prostaglandins. It reduces the production of thromboxane A_2 in the platelet, an effect that lasts for the life of the platelet. It also prevents the production of the antiaggregatory prostaglandin epoprostenol (prostacyclin) in the endothelial lining of the blood vessel, but there is still debate as to the optimal dose for aspirin to achieve the maximum ratio of inhibition of thromboxane versus epoprostenol production.

Aspirin is well absorbed after oral administration. It is rapidly metabolized by esterases in the blood and liver to salicylic acid and other metabolites that are excreted in the urine. In the doses used in prophylaxis against thromboembolism, aspirin is largely metabolized by the liver but in overdose, urinary excretion of salicylate becomes a limiting factor in drug elimination.

The major adverse effect of aspirin is gastrointestinal irritation and bleeding. This problem is much more common with higher doses of aspirin (600 mg or more) that were once used in the prevention of arterial thromboembolism but are less common with the doses (150–300 mg) now recommended. There is evidence that concomitant use of ulcer-healing drugs, e.g. misoprostol, H_2-receptor antagonists or omeprazole, can reduce the risk of non-steroidal anti-inflammatory drug (NSAID)-induced peptic ulceration in patients susceptible to the problem, but haemorrhagic risk may not be significantly reduced. There is also little evidence that buffered or enteric-coated preparations of aspirin are safer in this respect. However, the vast majority of patients tolerate low-dose aspirin well, and it is normally given as a single oral dose of soluble aspirin. Aspirin may also, rarely, induce asthma, particularly in patients with co-existing reversible airways obstruction. Other patients have a form of aspirin hypersensitivity that may result in urticaria and/or angiooedema. In this situation there may be cross-reactivity with other NSAIDs.

Clopidogrel

Clopidogrel is a pro-drug that is metabolized in part to an active thiol derivative. The latter inhibits platelet aggregation by rapidly and irreversibly inhibiting the binding of adenosine diphosphate (ADP) to its platelet receptor, thus preventing the ADP-mediated activation of the glycoprotein IIb/IIIa receptor for the life of the platelet. It is orally active and is given once daily for the reduction of atherosclerotic events in those with pre-existing atherosclerotic disease. In this respect, it may be a useful alternative to aspirin in aspirin-allergic subjects but haemorrhage occurs with the same frequency as aspirin, and thrombocytopenia (sometimes severe) may be commoner than with aspirin therapy. Clopidogrel is also licensed for combination use with low-dose aspirin in the management of acute coronary syndrome without ST segment elevation, when it is given for up to 12 months after the initial event (NICE 2004, 2005). The combination of these agents is associated with a greater risk of haemorrhage than warfarin in patients with atrial fibrillation, despite being significantly less effective than warfarin treatment in stroke prevention in this situation.

Dipyridamole

Dipyridamole is used by mouth as an adjunct to oral anticoagulation for prophylaxis of thromboembolism associated with prosthetic heart valves. Modified-release preparations are licensed (alone or in combination with low-dose aspirin) for secondary prevention of ischaemic stroke and transient ischaemic attacks (see treatment of stroke). It is a phosphodiesterase inhibitor and thus elevates concentrations of cyclic AMP. It may also block the uptake of adenosine by erythrocytes and other cells. Adverse effects include headache (to which tolerance may gradually develop) gastrointestinal problems, flushing and hypotension.

Glycoprotein IIb/IIIa inhibitors

Glycoprotein IIb/IIIa inhibitors prevent platelet aggregation by blocking the binding of fibrinogen to receptors on platelets. Abciximab is a monoclonal antibody which binds to coronary glycoprotein IIb/IIIa receptors and to other related sites; it is licensed as an adjunct to heparin and aspirin for the prevention of ischaemic complications in high-risk patients undergoing percutaneous transluminal coronary intervention. Abciximab should be used once only to avoid any further risk of thrombocytopenia.

Eptifibatide and tirofiban also inhibit glycoprotein IIb/IIIa receptors; they are licensed for use with heparin and aspirin to prevent early myocardial infarction in patients with unstable angina or non-ST segment elevation myocardial infarction. Abciximab, eptifibatide and tirofiban should be used by specialists only (NICE 2002b).

Patient care

Aspirin is normally well tolerated at the doses used for stroke prevention (150–300 mg). However, it should not be given to patients with a history of gastrointestinal ulceration. Since it may induce bronchospasm in susceptible individuals, it should be used cautiously in such circumstances. It is best tolerated if taken once daily as soluble aspirin after food.

CASE STUDIES

Case 23.1

A 75-year-old patient receiving warfarin to prevent deep vein thrombosis and previously well controlled comes to the clinic with an INR of 12, despite having the same dose of drug. There is no evidence of bleeding.

Question

What should be done?

Answer

Since the patient has a risk factor for haemorrhage (>70 years old), he/she should be given vitamin phytomenadione (vitamin K) 500 μg by slow intravenous injection to reduce the INR to around 2 within 24 h. For partial reversal of anticoagulation by the oral route, it is possible to give smaller oral doses of phytomenadione, e.g. 0.5–2.5 mg using the intravenous preparation orally. After either oral or intravenous therapy, a further dose of phytomenadione can be given if the INR is still too high after 24 h. However, a single dose often helps the INR to return to close to the target level at 24 h without causing warfarin resistance subsequently. A search for clinical conditions or drugs which might cause warfarin sensitivity should also be made. Measurement of plasma warfarin concentration may help in difficult cases

Case 23.2

A patient receiving heparin for 7 days for extensive venous thromboembolism develops arterial thrombosis.

Question

What would you suspect in this situation and what should be done?

Answer

The rare but serious heparin-induced thrombocytopenia (HIT) may be responsible. The platelet count should be measured urgently and if HIT is strongly suspected or confirmed, the heparin should be discontinued immediately. An alternative anticoagulant should be started in full dosage whilst specific confirmatory tests are being performed unless there are significant contraindications. Danaparoid and lepirudin may be considered as alternative anticoagulants in these circumstances.

Case 23.3

A patient admitted to an acute hospital with suspected myocardial infarction says that he had a myocardial infarction 4 years ago and was treated with a drug to 'dissolve the clot in the coronary artery'. The chest pain started 4 h earlier and his electrocardiogram shows ST segment elevation in the anterior leads.

Question

What relevance may his previous treatment and present history and findings have to his management on this occasion?

Answer

Thrombolytic drugs are indicated for any patient with acute myocardial infarction, provided the likely benefits outweigh the possible risks. Trials have shown that the benefit is greatest in those with ECG changes that include ST segment elevation (especially in those with anterior infarction) and in patients with bundle branch block. The patient has received a thrombolytic, possibly streptokinase. He should be asked if he was given a card with the identity of the therapy to carry with him. If the prior treatment was with streptokinase or anistreplase (no longer available), prolonged persistence of antibodies to streptokinase may reduce the effectiveness of subsequent treatment. Therefore, streptokinase should not be used again beyond 4 days of first administration of streptokinase (or anistreplase) and urgent consideration should be given to the use of an alternative thrombolytic agent such as alteplase, reteplase or tenecteplase.

Case 23.4

A 64-year-old male patient is to be prescribed aspirin therapy following an acute myocardial infarction.

Question

What questions should you ask the patient before starting treatment with aspirin?

Answer

The patient should be asked if he has had aspirin before and, if so, whether he tolerated it. Caution is necessary in patients with a history previous gastrointestinal ulceration and those with uncontrolled hypertension, and active peptic ulceration is a contraindication. Other contraindications include severe hepatic impairment and severe renal failure. It may induce bronchospasm or angio-oedema in susceptible individuals, e.g. in asthmatics, and caution should be exercised in these circumstances.

Case 23.5

A 56-year-old woman on warfarin therapy for atrial fibrillation with mitral stenosis appears to become resistant to warfarin after previously good control on 5 mg daily. Her INR does not rise above 1.4 even when her warfarin dose is increased to 20 mg daily.

Question

What can be done to find the cause of the resistance?

Answer

The patient should be asked about any new medications which might have been introduced recently, including over-the-counter and herbal preparations. Some proprietary medicines may contain vitamin K which could cause resistance. Other medicines, including the herbal medicine St John's wort, might induce warfarin metabolism and result in resistance (see Table 23.3). One cause of apparent resistance to warfarin is poor compliance and this should therefore be considered. Supervised administration of the dose and/or measurement of plasma warfarin concentration may be of value if the latter is suspected.

REFERENCES

British Committee for Standards in Haematology 1998 Guidelines on oral anticoagulation (warfarin): third edition. British Journal of Haematology 132: 277-285. Available online at: www.bcshguidelines. com/publishedHO.asp?tf=Haemostasis%20and%20Thrombosis&status

British Committee for Standards in Haematology 2006a Guidelines on oral anticoagulation (warfarin): third edition, 2005 update. British Journal of Haematology 132: 277-285. Available online at: www.bcshguidelines. com/publishedHO.asp?tf=Haemostasis%20and%20Thrombosis&status

British Committee for Standards in Haematology 2006b Guidelines on the use and monitoring of heparin. British Journal of Haematology 133: 19-34. Available online at: www.bcshguidelines.com/publishedHO. asp?tf=Haemostasis%20and%20Thrombosis&status

British Committee for Standards in Haematology 2006c The management of heparin induced thrombocytopenia. British Journal of Haematology 133: 259-269. Available online at: www.bcshguidelines.com/ publishedHO.asp?tf=Haemostasis%20and%20Thrombosis&status

Fennerty A, Dolben J, Thomas P et al 1984 Flexible induction dose regimen for warfarin and prediction of maintenance dose. British Medical Journal 288: 1268-1270

Fennerty A G, Renowden S, Scolding N et al 1986 Guidelines for the control of heparin treatment. British Medical Journal 292: 579-580

National Institute for Clinical Excellence 2002a The clinical effectiveness and cost effectiveness of early thrombolysis for treatment of myocardial infarction. Technology appraisal 52. National Institute for Clinical Excellence, London. Available online at: www.nice.org.uk/page.aspx?o=t a052&c=cardiovascular

National Institute for Clinical Excellence 2002b Acute coronary syndromes – glycoprotein IIb/IIIa inhibitors (review). Technology appraisal 47. National Institute for Clinical Excellence, London. Available online at: www.nice.org.uk/page.aspx?o=TA047&c=cardiovascular

National Institute for Clinical Excellence 2004 Clopidogrel in the treatment of non-ST-segment-elevation acute coronary syndrome. Technology appraisal 80. National Institute for Clinical Excellence, London. Available online at: www.nice.org.uk/page.aspx?o=TA080&c=cardiovascular

National Institute for Clinical Excellence 2005 Clopidogrel and dipyridamole for the prevention of atherosclerotic events. Technology appraisal 90. National Institute for Clinical Excellence, London. Available online at: www.nice.org.uk/page.aspx? o=TA090&c=cardiovascular

National Institute for Clinical Excellence 2006 Atrial fibrillation. Clinical guideline 36. National Institute for Clinical Excellence, London. Available online at: www.nice.org.uk/page.aspx?o= 336576

24 Dyslipidaemia

R. Walker

- Elevated concentrations of total cholesterol (TC) and low-density lipoprotein (LDL-C) increase the risk of coronary heart disease (CHD), while high-density lipoprotein (HDL-C) confers protection.
- Two-thirds of the UK population have a plasma total cholesterol above 5 mmol/L.
- Dyslipidaemia may be secondary to disorders such as diabetes mellitus, hypothyroidism, chronic renal failure, nephrotic syndrome, obesity, high alcohol intake and some drugs.
- Androgens, β-blockers, ciclosporin, oral contraceptives, diuretics, glucocorticoids and vitamin A derivatives can have an adverse effect on the lipid profile.
- There are five main classes of lipid-lowering agents: statins, fibrates, resins, nicotinic acid derivatives and absorption blockers.
- Statins are generally the drugs of choice in the treatment of primary prevention and secondary prevention of coronary heart disease.
- The aim of treatment in primary prevention (>20% risk of cardiovascular disease over 10 years) and secondary prevention includes the lowering of total cholesterol to either less than 4 mmol/L or a reduction by 25%, whichever results in the lowest level. The equivalent target for LDL-C is 2 mmol/L or a reduction of 30%, whichever results in the lowest level.

Disorders of lipoprotein metabolism together with high fat diets, obesity and physical inactivity have all contributed to the current epidemic of atherosclerotic disease seen in developed countries. Disorders of lipoprotein metabolism that result in elevated plasma concentrations of total cholesterol (TC) and low-density lipoprotein cholesterol (LDL-C) increase the risk of an individual developing coronary heart disease (CHD). In contrast, high-density lipoprotein cholesterol (HDL-C) confers protection against coronary heart disease, with the risk reducing as HDL-C increases. It is therefore clear that the term hyperlipidaemia, which was formerly used to describe disorders of lipoprotein metabolism, is inappropriate. It is more appropriate to use the term dyslipidaemia, which encompasses both abnormally high levels of specific lipoproteins, e.g. LDL-C, and abnormally low levels of other lipoproteins, e.g. HDL-C, as well as disorders in the composition of the various lipoprotein particles. It is particularly appropriate when considering the individual at risk of coronary heart disease with a normal or high total cholesterol and low HDL-C (total cholesterol:HDL-C ratio).

Epidemiology

Lipid and lipoprotein concentrations vary among different populations, with countries consuming a Western type of diet generally having higher total cholesterol and LDL-C levels than those where regular consumption of saturated fat is low.

The ideal plasma lipid profile is unknown and varies between different populations, even across Europe, and also within a given population. For practical purposes the values presented in Table 24.1 represent the target levels for total cholesterol and LDL-C in the UK for individuals receiving treatment for primary prevention (>20% risk of cardiovascular disease over 10 years) or secondary prevention. For completeness, the values for triglycerides and HDL-C are also presented although the benefit of achieving the stated targets is less clear.

A relationship between total cholesterol and the development of coronary heart disease is recognized, as is its contribution to the 1 in 4 deaths from coronary heart disease that occurs each year in the UK. A reduction in the mean level of total cholesterol in the population will reduce the development of coronary atherosclerosis and the prevalence of coronary heart disease. In the individual there is little evidence of a level below which a further reduction of total cholesterol or LDL-C is not associated with a lower risk of coronary heart disease.

A population approach to screening for raised total cholesterol and LDL-C would be expensive to implement and must run in parallel with programmes that identify individuals with dyslipidaemia and/or other risk factors for coronary heart disease. Some believe only individuals under the age of 20 years

Table 24.1 Optimal plasma lipid profile

[a]Total cholesterol (TC)	<4.0 mmol/L
[a]LDL cholesterol (LDL-C)	<2.0 mmol/L
[b]Triglycerides	<1.7 mmol/L
HDL cholesterol (HDL-C)	>1.0 mmol/L in men
	>1.2 mmol/L in women

[a]Target levels in individuals with established atherosclerotic disease, coronary heart disease, stroke, peripheral arterial disease, diabetes mellitus or where there is a cardiovascular disease risk >20% over 10 years. In these identified individuals the aim is to achieve the value stated in the table or a 25% reduction in total cholesterol and a 30% reduction in LDL-C from their baseline levels should these set target levels lower than those stated in the table.
[b] Fasting levels

should be screened to detect those with a familial disorder who will develop premature atherosclerosis and therefore benefit from lifelong management; whilst opportunistic screening is appropriate for the rest. Current guidance (Joint British Societies 2005) recommends all adults from the age of 40 years should have their total cholesterol and LDL-C measured once every 5 years as part of an opportunistic cardiovascular disease (CVD) risk assessment in primary care.

Lipid transport and lipoprotein metabolism

The clinically important lipids in the blood (unesterified and esterified cholesterol, and triglycerides) are not readily soluble in plasma and are rendered miscible by incorporation into lipoproteins. There are six main classes of lipoproteins: chylomicrons, chylomicron remnants, very low-density lipoproteins (VLDL-C), intermediate-density lipoproteins (IDL-C), low-density lipoproteins (LDL-C) and high-density lipoproteins (HDL-C).

The protein components of lipoproteins are known as apoproteins (apo), of which apoproteins A-I, E, C and B are perhaps the most important. Apoprotein B exists in two forms: B-48, which is present in chylomicrons and associated with the transport of ingested lipids, and B-100, which is found in endogenously secreted VLDL-C and associated with the transport of lipids from the liver (Fig. 24.1).

When dietary cholesterol and triglycerides are absorbed from the intestine they are transported in the intestinal lymphatics as chylomicrons, the largest of the lipoprotein particles and of which approximately 80% of the lipid core are triglycerides. The chylomicrons pass through blood capillaries in adipose tissue and skeletal muscle where the enzyme lipoprotein lipase is located, bound to the endothelium. Lipoprotein lipase is activated by apoprotein C-II on the surface of the chylomicron. The lipase catalyses the breakdown of the triglyceride in the chylomicron to free fatty acid and glycerol, which then enter adipose tissue and muscle. The cholesterol-rich chylomicron remnant is taken up by receptors on hepatocyte membranes, and in this way dietary cholesterol is delivered to the liver and cleared from the circulation.

VLDL-C is formed in the liver and transports triglycerides, which again make up approximately 80% of its lipid core, to the periphery. The triglyceride content of VLDL-C is removed by lipoprotein lipase in a similar manner to that described for chylomicrons above, and forms IDL-C particles. The core of IDL-C particles is roughly 50% triglyceride and 50% cholesterol esters, acquired from HDL-C under the influence of the enzyme lecithin-cholesterol acyltransferase (LCAT). Approximately 50% of the body's IDL particles are cleared from plasma by the liver.

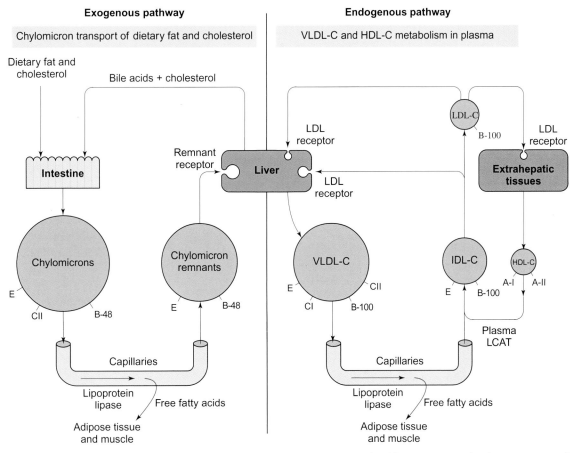

Figure 24.1 Schematic representation of lipoprotein metabolism in plasma. Dietary cholesterol and fat are transported in the exogenous pathway. Cholesterol produced in the liver is transported in the endogenous pathway.

The other 50% of IDL-C are further hydrolysed and modified to lose triglyceride and apoprotein E1 and become LDL-C particles. LDL-C is the major cholesterol-carrying particle in plasma.

LDL-C provides cholesterol, an essential component of cell membranes, bile acid and a precursor of steroid hormones to those cells that require it. LDL-C is also the main lipoprotein involved in atherogenesis, although it only appears to take on this role after it has been modified by oxidation. For reasons that are not totally clear, the arterial endothelium becomes permeable to the lipoprotein. Monocytes migrate through the permeable endothelium and engulf the lipoprotein, resulting in the formation of lipid-laden macrophages that have a key role in the subsequent development of atherosclerosis. The aim of treatment in dyslipidaemia is normally to reduce concentrations of LDL-C (and consequently atherogenesis) and thus reduce total cholesterol at the same time.

While VLDL-C and LDL-C are considered the 'bad' lipoproteins, HDL-C is often considered to be the 'good' antiatherogenic lipoprotein. In general, about 65% of total cholesterol is carried in LDL-C and about 25% in HDL.

High-density lipoprotein

HDL-C is formed from the unesterified cholesterol and phospholipid removed from peripheral tissues and the surface of triglyceride-rich proteins. The major structural protein is apoA-I. HDL-C mediates the return of lipoprotein and cholesterol from peripheral tissues to the liver for excretion in a process known as reverse cholesterol transport.

Reverse cholesterol transport pathway

The reverse cholesterol transport pathway (Fig. 24.2) controls the formation, conversion, transformation and degradation of HDL-C and is the site of action for a number of new, novel drugs. Newly created (nascent) HDL particles are formed primarily in the liver. These particles (lipid-poor apoA-I particles) are secreted into the plasma and are involved in the removal of cholesterol and phospholipids from peripheral tissues (Von Eckardstein et al 2001). This transfer of lipid from the plasma membrane of cells to apoA-I results in the formation of discoidal pre-β HDL, and is mediated by the membrane transporter ATP-binding cassette transporter 1 (ABCA1). The free cholesterol on the surface of the pre-β HDL is esterified by LCAT and changes from a disc-like appearance to a spherical shape. The spherical HDL (namely HDL$_3$) continues to accept more free cholesterol from cells and becomes larger HDL$_2$ particles. The HDL$_2$ particles exchange cholesterol and triglycerides with LDL-C and VLDL-C under the influence of cholesterol ester transfer protein (CETP). The degradation of HDL$_2$ takes place in the liver following selective uptake by scavenger receptor class B type 1 (SR-B1) and the apoA-I from the degradation is recycled to create new HDL particles. To illustrate the importance of the reverse cholesterol transport pathway, inhibition of CETP by drugs such as torcetrapib have been developed

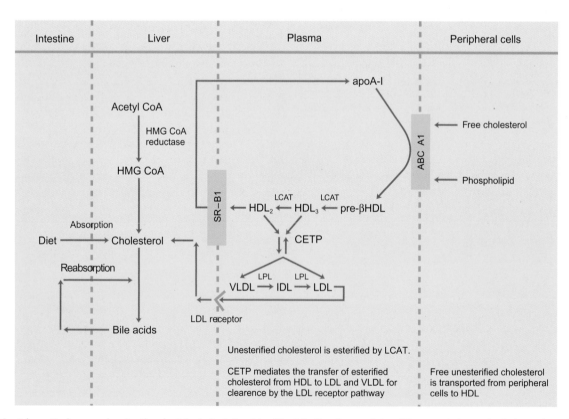

Figure 24.2 Schematic diagram showing the physiological relationship of the intestine, liver, peripheral tissue and plasma in cholesterol metabolism and reverse cholesterol transport. Key enzymes, receptor transfer proteins and lipoproteins involved in cholesterol synthesis, transport and metabolism are also shown. SR-B1, scavenger receptor class B type 1; LCAT, lecithin cholesterol acyltransferase; ABC A1, ATP binding cassette transporter A1; CETP, cholesterol ester transfer protein; LPL, lipoprotein lipase; apoA-I, apolipoprotein A-I.

and shown to increase levels of HDL-C by 16–91%. Unfortunately the side effect profile of these agents have, to date, prevented any of them reaching the market.

From the above it is evident that HDL-C plays a major role in maintaining cholesterol homeostasis in the body. As a consequence it is considered desirable to maintain both levels of the protective HDL-C and the integrity of the reverse cholesterol transport pathway. Low levels of HDL-C are found in 17% of men and 5% of women and may be a risk factor for atherogenesis that is comparable in importance to elevated levels of LDL-C. Drugs that reduce HDL-C levels are considered to have an undesirable effect on lipid metabolism and increase the risk of developing cardiovascular disease.

Triglycerides

The role of hypertriglyceridaemia as an independent risk factor for coronary heart disease is unclear because triglyceride levels are confounded by an association with low HDL-C, hypertension, diabetes and obesity, and a synergistic effect with LDL-C and/ or low HDL-C. An isolated elevation of triglyceride may be the consequence of a primary disorder of lipid metabolism, it may be secondary to the use of medicines or it may be a component of the metabolic syndrome or type 2 diabetes mellitus. Many individuals will be found to have a mixed dyslipidaemia that includes elevated levels of triglycerides, but reduction of LDL-C remains the primary focus.

Aetiology

Primary dyslipidaemia

Up to 60% of the variability in cholesterol fasting lipids may be genetically determined although expression is often influenced by interaction with environmental factors. The common familial (genetic) disorders can be classified as:

- the primary hypercholesterolaemias such as familial hypercholesterolaemia in which LDL-C is raised
- the primary mixed (combined) hyperlipidaemias in which both LDL-C and triglycerides are raised
- the primary hypertriglyceridaemias such as type III hyperlipoproteinaemia, familial lipoprotein lipase deficiency and familial apoC-II deficiency.

Familial hypercholesterolaemia

Heterozygous familial hypercholesterolaemia (often referred to as FH) is a common inherited metabolic disease and affects approximately 1 in 500 of the population. Familial hypercholesterolaemia is caused by a range of mutations in the LDL receptor gene that varies from family to family. Given the key role of LDL receptors in the catabolism of LDL-C, patients with familial hypercholesterolaemia may have plasma levels of LDL-C 2–3 times higher than the general population from birth. It is important to identify and treat these individuals from birth, otherwise they will be exposed to high concentrations of LDL-C and will suffer the consequences.

In patients with heterozygous familial hypercholesterolaemia it has been estimated that coronary heart disease occurs about 20 years earlier than in the general population, with some individuals, particularly men, dying from atherosclerotic heart disease often before the age of 40 years. The adult heterozygote typically exhibits the signs of cholesterol deposition such as corneal arcus (crescentic deposition of lipids in the cornea), tendon xanthomas (yellow papules or nodules of lipids deposited in tendons) and xanthelasma (yellow plaques or nodules of lipids deposited on eyelids) in their third decade.

In contrast to the heterozygous form, homozygous familial hypercholesterolaemia is extremely rare (1 per million) and associated with an absence of LDL receptors and almost absolute inability to clear LDL-C. In these individuals involvement of the aorta is evident by puberty and usually accompanied by cutaneous and tendon xanthomas. Myocardial infarction has been reported in homozygous children as early as 1.5–3 years of age. Up to the 1980s, sudden death from acute coronary insufficiency before the age of 20 years was normal.

Familial combined hyperlipidaemia

Familial combined hyperlipidaemia has an incidence of 1 in 200 and is associated with excessive synthesis of VLDL-C. In addition to increases in triglyceride and LDL-C levels, patients also typically have raised levels of apoB and elevated levels of small, dense LDL particles. It is associated with an increased risk of atherosclerosis and occurs in approximately 15% of patients who present with coronary heart disease before the age of 60 years.

Familial type III hyperlipoproteinaemia

Familial type III hyperlipoproteinaemia has an incidence of 1 in 5000. It is characterized by the accumulation of chylomicron and VLDL remnants that fail to get cleared at a normal rate by hepatic receptors due to the presence of less active polymorphic forms of apoE. Triglycerides and total cholesterol are both elevated and accompanied by corneal arcus, xanthelasma, tuberoeruptive xanthomas (groups of flat or yellowish raised nodules on the skin over joints, especially the elbows and knees) and palmar striae (yellow raised streaks across the palms of the hand). The disorder predisposes to premature atherosclerosis.

Familial lipoprotein lipase deficiency

Familial lipoprotein lipase deficiency is characterized by marked hypertriglyceridaemia and chylomicronaemia, and usually presents in childhood. It has an incidence of 1 per million and is due to a deficiency of the extrahepatic enzyme lipoprotein lipase, which results in a failure of lipolysis and the accumulation of chylomicrons in plasma. The affected patient presents with recurrent episodes of abdominal pain, eruptive xanthomas, lipaemia retinalis (retinal deposition of lipid) and enlarged spleen. This disorder is not associated with an increased susceptibility to atherosclerosis; the major complication is acute pancreatitis.

Familial apolipoprotein C-II deficiency

In the heterozygous state, familial apoC-II deficiency is associated with reduced levels of apoC-II, the activator of lipoprotein lipase. Typically, levels of apoC-II are 50–80% of normal. This level of activity can maintain normal lipid levels. In the rare homozygous state there is an absence of apolipoprotein C-II and despite normal levels of lipoprotein lipase, it cannot be activated. Consequently, homozygotes have triglyceride levels from 15 to above 100 mmol/L (normal range <1.7 mmol/L) and may develop acute pancreatitis. Premature atherosclerosis is unusual but has been described.

Lipoprotein(a)

There are many other familial disorders of lipid metabolism in addition to those mentioned above but most are very rare. However, a raised level of lipoprotein(a), otherwise known as Lp(a), is emerging as a major genetically inherited determinant of coronary heart disease. Lp(a) was first described more than 40 years ago. It is found in the plasma of virtually everyone in a wide concentration range (0.01–2 g/L) with up to 70% of the variation in plasma concentration being genetically determined. The concentration of Lp(a) is not normally distributed and the contribution of inheritance to circulating Lp(a) levels is more pronounced than for any other lipoprotein or apoprotein. A parental history of early-onset coronary heart disease is associated with raised concentrations of Lp(a), and these appear to play a role in both atherogenesis and thrombosis. An important component of Lp(a) is apo(a), which is structurally and functionally similar to plasminogen and may competitively bind to fibrin and impair fibrinolysis.

Concentrations of Lp(a) above 0.3 g/L occur in about 20% of caucasians and increase the risk of coronary atherosclerosis twofold, and this may increase to fivefold if LDL-C concentrations are also raised. However, the role of Lp(a) plasma levels in the clinical assessment of coronary heart disease risk remains to be resolved.

Secondary dyslipidaemia

Dyslipidaemias that occur secondary to a number of disorders (Table 24.2), dietary indiscretion or as a side effect of drug therapy (Table 24.3) account for up to 40% of all dyslipidaemias. Fortunately, the lipid abnormalities in secondary dyslipidaemia can often be corrected if the underlying disorder is treated, effective dietary advice implemented or the offending drug withdrawn.

On occasion, a disorder may be associated with dyslipidaemia but not the cause of it. For example, hyperuricaemia (gout) and hypertriglyceridaemia co-exist in approximately 50% of men. In this particular example, neither is the cause of the other and treatment of one does not resolve the other. There are, however, two notable exceptions to the rule with this example: nicotinic acid and fenofibrate. Both drugs reduce triglyceride levels but nicotinic acid increases urate levels while fenofibrate reduces them by an independent uricosuric effect.

Many of the disease states associated with secondary dyslipidaemia are listed in Table 24.2. The impact and severity of the lipid disorder will depend on the individual's genetic or nutritional predisposition to hyperlipidaemia. Some of the more common disorders that cause secondary dyslipidaemia include the following:

Table 24.2 Examples of disorders known to adversely affect the lipid profile

Anorexia nervosa
Bulimia
Type 1 diabetes
Type 2 diabetes
Hypothyroidism
Pregnancy
Inappropriate diet
Alcohol abuse
Chronic renal failure
Nephrotic syndrome
Renal transplantation
Cardiac transplantation
Hepatocellular disease
Cholestasis
Myeloma

Diabetes mellitus

Premature atherosclerotic disease is the main cause of reduced life expectancy in patients with diabetes. The atherosclerotic disease is often widespread and complications such as plaque rupture and thrombotic occlusion occur more often and at a younger age. The incidence of coronary heart disease is up to four times higher among diabetic patients.

Type 1 diabetes In patients with type 1 diabetes HDL-C may appear high but for reasons which are unclear, it does not impart the same degree of protection against coronary heart disease as in those without diabetes. It is therefore not appropriate to use coronary risk prediction charts that utilize the TC:HDL-C ratio in patients with type 1 diabetes. Those with type 1 diabetes are often, but not exclusively, children or young adults and they carry a 2–3-fold increased risk of developing coronary heart disease or having a stroke in later life.

Type 2 diabetes Patients with type 2 diabetes typically have increased triglycerides and decreased HDL-C. Levels of total cholesterol may be similar to those found in non-diabetic individuals but the patient with type 2 diabetes often has increased levels of highly atherogenic small dense LDL particles.

Individuals with type 1 or type 2 diabetes and aged over 40 years, but without coronary heart disease, are often considered to have the same coronary heart disease risk as patients without diabetes who have survived a myocardial infarction. This assumption is generally appropriate but is clearly influenced by the age of the patient, duration of diabetes and whether there

Table 24.3 Typical effects of selected drugs on lipoprotein levels

Drug	VLDL-C	LDL-C	HDL-C
Alcohol	↑	0	↑
Androgens, testosterone	↑	↑	↓
ACE-inhibitors	0	0	0
β-Blockers	↑	0	↓
Calcium channel blockers	0	0	0
Ciclosporin	↑	↑	↑
Oestrogens, oestradiol	↑	↓	↑
Glucocorticoids	↑	0	↑
Isotretinoin	↑	0	↓
Progestins	↓	↑	↓
Protease inhibitors	↑	0	0
Sertraline	↑	↑	0
Tacrolimus	↑	↑	↑
Thiazide diuretics	↑	↑	↓
Valproate	↑	0	↓

Effect seen may vary depending on dose and duration of exposure.
↓, reduction; ↑, increase; 0, no change.

are any complications and other patient-related risk factors. Where the individual fulfils the above criteria treatment with a statin is normally recommended even where there is a low HDL-C and elevated triglycerides. The role of fibrates (see below) and nicotinates remains unclear.

Individuals aged 18–39 with type 1 or type 2 diabetes are candidates for treatment with a statin where there is evidence of:

• retinopathy
• nephropathy
• poor glycaemic control
• elevated blood pressure
• metabolic syndrome (central obesity, raised triglycerides and/or reduced HDL-C)
• history of first-degree relative with premature CVD.

Hypothyroidism

Abnormalities of plasma lipid and lipoprotein levels are common in patients with untreated hypothyroidism. Hypothyroidism may elevate LDL-C because of reduced LDL receptor activity and it frequently causes hypertriglyceridaemia and an associated reduction in HDL-C as a result of reduced lipoprotein lipase activity. Remnants of chylomicrons and VLDL-C may also

accumulate. However, once adequate thyroid replacement has been instituted the dyslipidaemia should resolve.

Chronic renal failure

Dyslipidaemia is frequently seen in patients with renal failure in the predialysis phase, during haemodialysis or when undergoing chronic ambulatory peritoneal dialysis. The hypertriglyceridaemia that most commonly occurs is associated with reduced lipoprotein lipase activity and often persists despite starting chronic maintenance renal dialysis.

Nephrotic syndrome

In patients with the nephrotic syndrome, dyslipidaemia appears to be caused by an increased production of apoB-100 and associated VLDL-C along with increased hepatic synthesis of LDL-C and a reduction in HDL-C. The necessary use of glucocorticoids in patients with the nephrotic syndrome may exacerbate underlying lipoprotein abnormality.

Obesity

Chronic, excessive intake of calories leads to increased concentrations of triglycerides and reduced HDL-C. Obesity per se can exacerbate any underlying primary dyslipidaemia. Individuals with central obesity appear to be at particular risk of what has become known as the metabolic or DROP (**d**yslipidaemia, insulin **r**esistance, **o**besity and high blood **p**ressure) syndrome which represents a cluster of risk factors. Obesity and sedentary lifestyle coupled with diet and genetic factors interact to produce the syndrome (Kolovou et al 2005).

Alcohol

In the heavy drinker the high calorie content of beer and wine may be a cause of obesity with its associated adverse effect on the lipid profile. In addition, alcohol increases hepatic triglyceride synthesis, which in turn produces hypertriglyceridaemia.

Light to moderate drinkers (1–3 units/day) have a lower incidence of coronary heart disease and associated mortality than those who do not drink. This protective effect is probably due to an increase in HDL-C, and appears independent of the type of alcohol. The optimum consumption for men (21 units/week) is higher than that recommended for women (14 units/week).

Drugs

A number of drugs can adversely affect plasma lipid and lipoprotein concentrations (see Table 24.3).

Antihypertensive agents Hypertension is a major risk factor for atherosclerosis, and the beneficial effects of lowering blood pressure are well recognized. It is, however, a concern that treatment of patients with some antihypertensives has reduced the incidence of cerebrovascular accidents and renal failure but had no major impact in reducing the incidence of coronary heart disease. It has been suggested that some of these antihypertensive agents have an adverse effect on lipids and lipoproteins that override any beneficial reduction of blood pressure.

Diuretics Thiazide and loop diuretics increase VLDL-C and LDL-C by mechanisms that are not completely understood. Whether these adverse effects are dose dependent is also unclear. Use of a thiazide for less than 1 year has been reported to increase total cholesterol by up to 7% with no change in HDL-C. However, there is evidence that the short-term changes in lipids do not occur with the low doses in current use. Studies of 3–5 years' duration have found no effect on total cholesterol.

β-Blockers The effects of β-blockers on lipoprotein metabolism are reflected in an increase in plasma triglyceride concentrations, a decrease in HDL-C, but with no discernible effect on LDL-C. β-Blockers with intrinsic sympathomimetic activity appear to have little or no effect on VLDL-C or HDL-C. Pindolol has intrinsic sympathomimetic activity but is rarely used as an antihypertensive agent since it may exacerbate angina. Acebutolol and oxprenolol have half the intrinsic sypathomimetic activity of pindolol and may be useful if a β-blocker has to be used in a patient susceptible to altered lipoprotein metabolism. Alternatively, the combined α- and β-blocking effect of labetalol may be of use since it would appear to have a negligible effect on the lipid profile.

Overall, the need to use a diuretic or a β-blocker must be balanced against patient considerations. A patient in heart failure should receive a diuretic if indicated regardless of the lipid profile. Likewise, the patient with heart failure may also benefit from a β-blocker such as bisoprolol or carvedilol. Patients who have had a myocardial infarction should be considered for the protective effect of a β-blocker and again the benefits of use will normally override any adverse effects on the lipid profile.

If an antihypertensive agent is required that is without adverse effects on lipoproteins, many studies would suggest that angiotensin converting enzyme (ACE) inhibitors, angiotensin II receptor antagonists, α-adrenoceptor blockers or calcium channel blockers could be used.

Oral contraceptives Oral contraceptives containing an oestrogen and a progestogen provide the most effective contraceptive preparations for general use and have been well studied with respect to their harmful effects.

Oestrogens and progestogens both possess mineralocorticoid and glucocorticoid properties that predispose to hypertension and diabetes mellitus, respectively. However, the effects of the two hormones on lipoproteins are different. Oestrogens cause a slight increase in hepatic production of VLDL-C and HDL-C, and reduce plasma LDL-C levels. In contrast, progestogens increase LDL-C and reduce plasma HDL-C and VLDL-C.

The specific effect of the oestrogen or progestogen varies with the actual dose and chemical entity used. Ethinyloestradiol at a dose of 30–35 μg or less would appear to create few problems with lipid metabolism, while norethisterone is one of the more favourable progestogens even though it may cause a pronounced decrease in HDL-C.

Corticosteroids The effect of glucocorticoid administration on lipid levels has been studied in patients treated with steroids for asthma, rheumatoid arthritis and connective tissue disorders. Administration of a glucocorticoid such as prednisolone has been shown to increase total cholesterol and triglycerides by elevating LDL-C and, less consistently, VLDL-C. The changes are generally more pronounced in women.

Alternate-day therapy with glucocorticoids has been suggested to reduce the adverse effect on lipoprotein levels in some patients.

Ciclosporin Ciclosporin is primarily used to prevent tissue rejection in recipients of renal, hepatic and cardiac transplants. Its use has been associated with increased LDL-C levels, hypertension and glucose intolerance. These adverse effects are often exacerbated by the concurrent administration of glucocorticoids. Without doubt the combined use of ciclosporin and glucocorticoid contributes to the adverse lipid profile seen in transplant patients. Unfortunately, the administration of a lipid-lowering drug to patients treated with ciclosporin increases the incidence of myositis and rhabdomyolysis (dissolution of muscle associated with excretion of myoglobin in the urine) and its use is therefore contraindicated in such patients.

Hepatic microsomal enzyme inducers Drugs such as carbamazepine, phenytoin, phenobarbital, rifampicin and griseofulvin increase hepatic microsomal enzyme activity and can also increase plasma HDL-C. The administration of these drugs may also give rise to a slight increase in LDL-C and VLDL-C. The overall effect is one of a favourable increase in the TC:HDL-C ratio. It is interesting to note that patients treated for epilepsy have been reported to have a decreased incidence of coronary heart disease.

Risk assessment

Primary prevention

In patients with no evidence of coronary heart disease, the Joint British Societies (2005) have developed cardiovascular disease risk prediction charts for males (Fig. 24.3) and females (Fig. 24.4) that offer a pragmatic way forward. They recommend that all adults from the age of 40 years, with no history of cardiovascular disease or diabetes, and not receiving treatment for raised blood pressure or dyslipidaemia, should receive opportunistic screening every 5 years in primary care. Factors that need to be taken into account at screening include the following.

- *Age*: in individuals <40 years and >70 years the appropriate risk chart plus clinical judgement should be used to determine if there is a need for treatment.
- *Gender*: there are separate charts for men and women.
- *Ethnicity*: the risk prediction charts have only been validated in white caucasians and will underestimate risk in Asians by a factor of 1.4, although whether this holds true after adjusting for diabetes is unclear (Bhopal 2000).
- *Smoking history*: an estimate of lifetime exposure to tobacco is required.
- *Family history*: risk increases when coronary heart disease has occurred in a first-degree relative (parent, offspring, sibling), when a number of family members have developed coronary heart disease, and the younger the age of those affected (see Table 24.4). The risk prediction charts are of little value for those with familial dyslipidaemia as they are at high risk and require treatment.
- *Body weight and height*: body mass index (BMI) should be calculated. A BMI >25 kg/m^2 indicates overweight and >30 kg/m^2 obesity.

NON-DIABETIC MEN

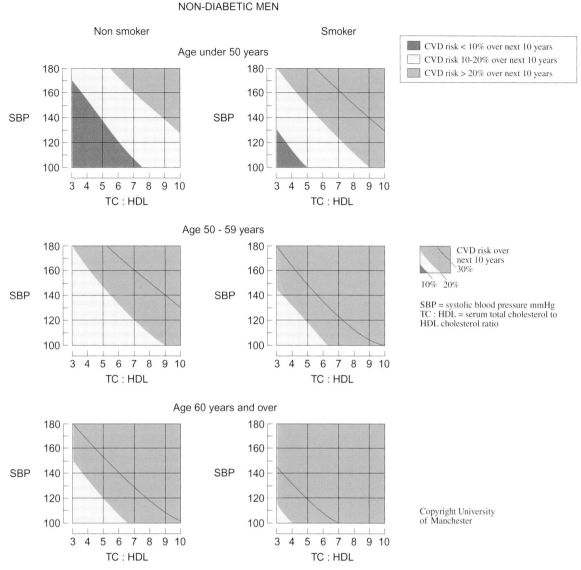

Figure 24.3 Joint British Societies' cardiovascular disease risk prediction chart for non-diabetic men. Reproduced with permission of the BMJ Publishing Group from Heart 2005; suppl 5:v1-v52

- *Waist circumference*: central obesity is present where the waist circumference >102 cm in men or >80 cm in women.
- *Blood pressure*: target blood pressure in a non-diabetic individual should be <140/90 mmHg.
- *Non-fasting lipids*: total cholesterol <4 mmol/L and LDL-C <2 mmol/L.
- Non-fasting blood glucose: if non-fasting glucose >6.1 mmol/L, the individual should be assessed for impaired glucose regulation or diabetes.

The risk prediction charts can be used for estimating the total risk of developing cardiovascular disease (coronary heart disease + stroke) over 10 years. If diabetes is diagnosed during the screening process there is no need to estimate risk as these individuals are considered to be at high risk and require therapy. Individuals with established cardiovascular disease or diabetes do not require formal assessment as they will be well above the threshold for treatment.

To use the charts to predict the risk of developing cardiovascular disease over the next 10 years, knowledge of age, gender, smoking history, systolic blood pressure and the ratio of non-fasting total cholesterol to HDL-C is all that is required. No single factor should be taken in isolation, unless exceptionally abnormal, as this will give an inadequate guide to the predicted risk for that individual. For example, there may be two individuals with the same total cholesterol of 5.4 mmol/L but only one may require treatment because of the contribution of other risk factors.

The risk factor calculated using the charts is based on the number of cardiovascular events expected over the next 10 years in 100 women or men with the same risk factor as the individual being assessed. Those with a cardiovascular risk >20% over 10 years are deemed to require treatment although individuals with a risk as low as 8% over 10 years will gain some benefit, but this will be small.

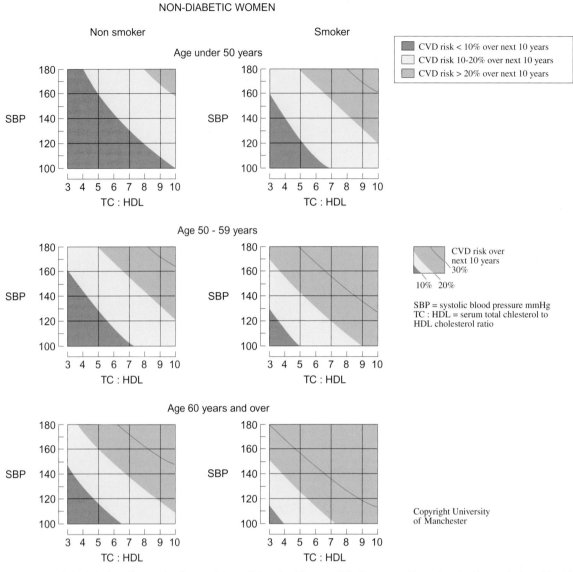

Figure 24.4   Joint British Societies' cardiovascular disease risk prediction chart for non-diabetic women. Reproduced with permission of the BMJ Publishing Group from Heart 2005; suppl 5:v1-v52.

Table 24.4   Criteria that indicate familial hypercholesterolaemia

Family history of dyslipidaemia, or cardiovascular disease:

• in first-degree female relative less than 65 years old
• in first-degree male relative less than 55 years old

Xanthelasma or corneal arcus under the age of 45

ᵃTendon xanthomata + total cholesterol >7.5 mmol/L at any age
ᵃTendon xanthomata + LDL-C > 4.9 mmol/L

ᵃTendon xanthomata may not be readily apparent in younger people.

Secondary prevention

Patients with coronary heart disease and levels of total cholesterol >4 mmol/L and LDL-C >2 mmol/L are the ones most likely to benefit from treatment with lipid-lowering agents. Typical of individuals who fall into this category are patients with a history of angina, myocardial infarction, coronary artery bypass graft, coronary angioplasty or cardiac transplantation.

As in the situation with primary prevention outlined above, if an individual is to receive a lipid-lowering agent as part of a secondary prevention strategy, the possibility of a familial dyslipidaemia and the need to assess other family members must not be overlooked.

Treatment

Lipid profile

When a decision has been made to determine an individual's lipid profile a random plasma total cholesterol and HDL-C will often suffice. If a subsequent decision is made to commence treatment and monitor outcome, a more detailed profile that includes triglycerides is required.

Plasma concentrations of triglycerides increase after the ingestion of a meal, and therefore patients must fast for 12–15 hours before they can be measured. Patients must also be seated for at least 5 minutes prior to drawing a blood sample. Cholesterol levels are little affected by food intake, and this is therefore not a consideration if only total cholesterol is to be measured. However, it is important that whatever is being measured reflects a steady-state value. For example, during periods of weight loss, lipid concentrations decline as they do following a myocardial infarction. In the case of the latter, samples drawn within 24 hours of infarct onset will reflect the preinfarction state. In general, measurement should be deferred for 2 weeks after a minor illness and for 3 months after a myocardial infarction, serious illness or pregnancy.

Once the total cholesterol, HDL-C and triglyceride values are known it is usual to calculate the value for LDL-C using the Friedewald equation:

$$LDL\text{-}C = (Total\ cholesterol - HDL\text{-}C) - (0.45 \times triglyceride)\ mmol/L$$

The Friedewald formula should not be used in non-fasting individuals, it is less reliable in individuals with diabetes and is not valid if the plasma triglyceride concentration >4 mmol/L.

Although lipid target levels are normally only defined for total cholesterol and LDL-C, increasingly non-HDL-C is measured. The value for non-HDL-C is obtained by subtracting the value for HDL-C from total cholesterol. Non-HDL-C consequently represents the total of cholesterol circulating on apoprotein B particles, i.e. both LDL and triglyceride-rich lipoproteins, and represents the main atherogenic particles. A desirable value is <3 mmol/L.

Lifestyle

Before a decision is made to start treatment with a lipid-lowering agent, other risk factors must also be tackled as appropriate, such as smoking, obesity, high alcohol intake and lack of exercise (Table 24.5). Underlying disorders such as diabetes mellitus and hypertension should be treated as appropriate. Issues around body weight, diet and exercise will be briefly covered below.

Body weight and waist measurement

The overweight patient is at increased risk of atherosclerotic disease and typically has elevated levels of plasma triglycerides, raised LDL-C and a low HDL-C. This adverse lipid profile is often compounded by the presence of hypertension and raised blood glucose i.e. the metabolic syndrome. A reduction in body weight will generally improve the lipid profile and reduce overall cardiovascular risk.

It is useful to classify the extent to which an individual is overweight by calculating their body mass index (BMI). The BMI in all but the most muscular individual gives a clinical measure of adiposity.

- BMI 18.5 – underweight
- BMI 18.6 to 24.9 – ideal
- BMI 25 to 29.9 – overweight (low health risk)
- BMI 30 to 40 – obese (moderate health risk)
- BMI >40 – obese (high health risk)

The distribution of body fat is increasingly being recognized as a factor that influences cardiovascular disease risk. Measurement of waist circumference is perhaps the easiest and most practical indicator of central obesity. Target waist circumference should be <102 cm in white caucasian men, <88 cm in white caucasian females and, in Asians, <90 cm in men and <80 cm in females.

Diet

Diet modification should always be encouraged in a patient with dyslipidaemia but is rarely successful alone in bringing about a significant improvement in the lipid profile. Randomized controlled trials of dietary fat reduction or modification have shown

Table 24.5 Lifestyle targets (adapted from Joint British Societies 2005)

Do not smoke
Maintain ideal body weight (body mass index 20–25 kg/m²). Avoid central obesity
Reduce total dietary intake of fat to ≤30% of total energy intake
Reduce intake of saturated fats to ≤10% of total fat intake
Reduce intake of dietary cholesterol to <300 mg/day
Replace saturated fats by an increased intake of monounsaturated fats
Increase intake of fresh fruit and vegetables to at least five portions per day
Regularly eat fish and other sources of ω3 fatty acids (at least two portions of fish each week)
Limit alcohol intake to <21 units/week for men and <14 units/week for women
Restrict intake of salt to <100 mmol day (<6 g of sodium chloride or <2.4 g sodium per day)
Undertake regular aerobic exercise of at least 30 mins per day, most days of the week

variable results on cardiovascular morbidity and mortality (Hooper et al 2001). In pragmatic, community-based studies, reductions in total cholesterol of only 3–6% have been achieved. The overall picture is that patients with dyslipidaemia should receive dietary advice and a small number of those who adhere to the advice will experience a substantial fall in total cholesterol.

There is a common misconception that a healthy diet is one that is low in cholesterol. However, generally it is the saturated fat content that is important, although many components of a healthy diet are not related to fat content. For example, the low incidence of coronary heart disease in those who consume a Mediterranean diet suggests an increased intake of fruit and vegetables is also important. The typical Mediterranean diet has an abundance of plant food (fruit, vegetables, breads, cereals, potatoes, beans, nuts and seeds) minimally processed, seasonally fresh, and locally grown; fresh fruit as the typical daily dessert, with sweets containing concentrated sugars or honey consumed a few times per week; olive oil as the principal source of fat; dairy products (principally cheese and yoghurt) consumed daily in low to moderate amounts; 0–4 eggs consumed weekly; and red meat consumed in low to moderate amounts. This diet is low in saturated fat (<8% of energy) and varies in total fat content from <25% to >35% of energy.

Fish Regular consumption of the long chain ω3 fatty acids, principally ecosapentaenoic acid and docosahexaenoic acid, typically found in fatty fish and fish oils, has been linked to the low levels of coronary heart disease seen in Inuits (Eskimos). A meta-analysis (Bucher et al 2002) showed the risk of fatal myocardial infarction in those with cardiovascular disease was reduced by 30% when consuming ω3 fatty acids. Consumption of ω3 fatty acids decreased triglyceride levels but had little effect on LDL-C or HDL-C. The proposed mechanisms is thought to involve the ω3 fatty acids and their antiarrhythmic properties, ability to reduce blood pressure and heart rate, lower triglyceride levels, stimulate endothelial-derived nitric oxide, increase insulin sensitivity, decrease platelet aggregation and decrease proinflammatory eicosanoids. Although there would appear to be clear benefits in consuming oily fish (approximately 100 g daily) in those who have had a myocardial infarction, the evidence for their consumption in other individuals is equivocal (Hooper et al 2006).

Trans fats Trans fats are unsaturated fatty acids with at least one double bond in the trans configuration. They are formed when vegetable oils are hydrogenated to convert them into semisolid fats that can be incorporated into margarines or used in commercial manufacturing processes. Trans fats are typically found in deep fried fast foods, bakery products, packaged snack foods, margarines and crackers. When the calorific equivalent of saturated fats, cis unsaturated fats and trans fats are consumed, trans fats raise LDL-C, reduce HDL-C and increase the ratio of total cholesterol:HDL-C. In addition to these harmful effects, trans fats also increase the blood levels of triglycerides, increase levels of Lp(a) and reduce the particle size of LDL-C, all of which further increase the risk of coronary heart disease. It is therefore necessary to reduce the dietary intake of trans fatty acids to less than 0.5% of total energy intake (Mozaffarian et al 2006). This may be difficult for many individuals because of poor food labelling, or lack of labelling in the case of bakeries, restaurants and other food outlets.

Stanol esters and plant sterols The availability of margarines and other foods enriched with plant sterols or stanol esters increases the likelihood that LDL-C can be reduced by dietary change. Both stanol esters and plant sterols at a maximum effective dose of 2 g/day inhibit cholesterol absorption from the gastrointestinal tract and reduce LDL-C by an average of 10%. They compete with cholesterol for incorporation into mixed micelles, thereby impairing its absorption from the intestine. However, as with other dietary changes the reduction seen varies between individuals and is probably dependent on the intial cholesterol level. Single meal studies show that phytosterols are bioactive at doses as low as 150 mg and the small amounts that naturally occur in foods are also probably important in the management of total cholesterol.

Antioxidants Antioxidants occur naturally in fruit and vegetables and are important components of a healthy diet. Their consumption is thought to be beneficial in reducing the formation of atherogenic, oxidized LDL-C. Primary and secondary prevention trials with antioxidant vitamin supplements, however, have not been encouraging. Neither vitamin E nor β-carotene supplements would appear to reduce the risk of coronary heart disease but likewise have not been shown to be harmful.

Salt Dietary salt (sodium) has an adverse effect on blood pressure and therefore a potential impact on coronary heart disease and stroke. As part of dietary advice the average adult intake of sodium should be reduced from approximately 150 mmol (9 g) to 100 mmol (6 g) of salt. This intake can be reduced by consuming fewer processed foods, avoiding many ready meals and not adding salt to food at the table.

Exercise Moderate amounts of aerobic exercise (brisk walking, jogging, swimming, cycling) on a regular basis have a desirable effect on the lipid profile of an individual. These beneficial effects have been demonstrated within 2 months in middle-aged men exercising for 30 minutes, three times a week. Current advice for adults who are not routinely active is to undertake 30 minutes of moderate-intensity activity on at least 5 days of the week. For active individuals, additional aerobic exercise of vigorous intensity is recommended for 20–30 minutes three times a week. Exercise per se probably has little effect on total cholesterol levels in the absence of a reduction in body weight, body fat or dietary fat. Perhaps the most important effect of regular exercise is to raise levels of HDL-C in a dose-dependent manner according to energy expenditure (Durstine et al 2002).

Overall, comprehensive dietary and lifestyle changes (stopping smoking, stress management training and moderate exercise) can bring about regression of coronary atherosclerosis. Unfortunately many find it difficult to attain or sustain the necessary changes. In others, dietary and lifestyle changes alone will never be adequate or will not bring about the necessary improvement in lipid profile quickly enough. As a consequence, the use of lipid-lowering drugs is widespread.

Drugs

Before starting lipid-lowering therapy, dietary and lifestyle changes should ideally be tried for 3–6 months. If this does not achieve the required beneficial effect on the lipid profile then drug therapy can be started but involves a long-term commitment to treatment and appropriate dietary and lifestyle adjustments. In an individual requiring treatment for secondary prevention a delay of up to 6 months in starting treatment may not be appropriate.

Primary prevention

It cannot be overemphasized that dyslipidaemia should not be treated in isolation and must be embarked upon with clear goals. Appropriate management, in addition to lifestyle advice, will not only address management of dyslipidaemia but will also seek to optimize use of antihypertensive agents, other cardiovascular protective therapies and achieve tight blood glucose control. In patients without evidence of arterial disease, treatment must be considered if the risk of cardiovascular disease is >20% or more over 10 years (Joint British Societies 2005). Treatment will normally include:

- a lipid-lowering agent to lower total cholesterol to less than 4 mmol/L or reduce total cholesterol by 25%, whichever results in the lowest level (equivalent figures for LDL-C are 2 mmol/L or a reduction of 30%, whichever results in the lowest level)
- personalized information on modifiable risk factors including physical activity, diet, alcohol intake, weight and tight control of diabetes
- advice to stop smoking
- advice and treatment to achieve blood pressure below 140 mmHg systolic and 85 mmHg diastolic.

Secondary prevention

In individuals with diagnosed cardiovascular disease or other occlusive arterial disease, treatment should include:

- a lipid-lowering agent to lower total cholesterol to less than 4 mmol/L or reduce total cholesterol by 25%, whichever results in the lowest level (equivalent figures for LDC-C are

2 mmol/L or a reduction of 30%, whichever results in the lowest level)
- advice to stop smoking
- personalized information on modifiable risk factors including physical activity, diet, alcohol intake, weight and diabetes
- advice and treatment to achieve blood pressure below 130 mmHg systolic and 80 mmHg diastolic
- tight control of blood pressure and glucose in those with diabetes
- low-dose aspirin (75 mg daily)
- ACE inhibitors for those with left ventricular dysfunction
- β-blocker for those who have had a myocardial infarction
- warfarin or aspirin for those over 60 years who have atrial fibrillation.

Lipid-lowering therapy

There are five main classes of lipid-lowering agents available:

- statins
- fibrates
- bile acid binding agents
- cholesterol absorption inhibitors
- nicotinic acid and derivatives.

Agents such as soluble fibre and fish oils have also been used to reduce lipid levels. A number of new agents are also under investigation for their novel effect on different parts of the cholesterol biosynthesis pathway (Table 24.6).

The choice of lipid-lowering agent depends on the underlying dyslipidaemia, the response required and patient acceptability. The various groups of drugs available have different mechanisms of action and variable efficacy depending on the lipid profile of an individual. Table 24.7 demonstrates the comparable effectiveness of the different groups in improving the lipid profile.

Table 24.6 Mechanism of action of lipid-lowering agents under investigation

Drug group	Mechanism
Acyl-coenzyme A: cholesterol acyltransferase (ACAT) inhibitors	ACAT esterifies excess intracellular cholesterol. Inhibition of ACAT prevents transport of cholesterol into the arterial wall and thereby prevents atheroma developing. Lowers VLDL-C and triglycerides
Bile acid sequestrants	Related to first-generation resins but improved patient tolerance. Sequester bile acids and prevent reabsorption. Reduce LDL-C while HDL-C and triglycerides increase or remain unchanged
Cholesteryl ester transfer protein (CETP) inhibitors	CETP is responsible for the transfer of cholesteryl ester from HDL-C to the atherogenic LDL-C and VLDL-C
Lipoprotein lipase (LPL) activity enhancers	LPL is responsible for VLDL-C catabolism with subsequent loss of triglycerides and increase in HDL-C. Protects against atherosclerosis
Microsomal triglyceride transfer protein (MTP) inhibitors	Inhibit absorption of lipid and reduce hepatic secretion of lipoproteins, thereby reducing atherosclerotic plaque formation
Peroxisome proliferator-activated receptor (PPAR) activators	PPAR-α and -γ regulate the expression of genes involved in lipid metabolism and inhibit atherosclerotic plaque rupture. They reduce entry of cholesterol into cells, lower LDL-C and triglycerides, and increase HDL-C
Squalene synthase inhibitors	Inhibit squalene synthase, upregulate LDL receptor activity and enhance removal of LDL-C

Table 24.7 Comparison of reported change in lipid profile at optimal dose of single drug

Drug group	TC (%)	Triglycerides (%)	LDL-C	HDL-C
Bile acid binding agents	↓15–30%	↑5–30%	↓15–30%	↑3–8%
Fibrates	↓10–20%	↓30–50%	↓20–25%	↑10–25%
Statins	↓20–45%	↓10–45%	↓25–60%	↑2–15%
Nicotinic acid and derivatives	↓15–30%	↓20–60%	↑15–40%	↑10–20%
Fish oils	↑or↓	↓10–60%	↑or↓	↑5–10%
Absorption blockers	↓10–20%	↓5–10%	↑15–30%	↑2–5%

However, this table must be interpreted with caution as not all members of each group will bring about the changes quoted. The statins are currently the drugs of choice in the majority of patients with dyslipidaemia.

Statins

The discovery of a class of drugs, the statins, that selectively inhibit 3-hydroxy-3-methylglutaryl-CoA reductase (HMG-CoA reductase) was a significant advance in the treatment of dyslipidaemia. Their primary site of action is the inhibition of HMG-CoA reductase in the liver and the subsequent inhibition of the formation of mevalonic acid, the rate-limiting step in the biosynthesis of cholesterol. This results in a reduction in intracellular levels of cholesterol, an increase in expression of hepatic LDL receptor, and enhanced receptor-mediated catabolism and clearance of LDL-C from plasma. Production of VLDL-C, the precursor of LDL-C, is also reduced. The overall effect is a reduction in total cholesterol, LDL-C, VLDL-C and triglycerides with an increase in HDL-C. The reduction in LDL-C occurs in a dose-dependent manner, with a lesser and dose-independent effect on VLDL-C and triglycerides.

Simvastatin was the first member of the group to be marketed in the UK and it was followed by pravastatin, fluvastatin, atorvastatin, cerivastatin and rosuvastatin. Cerivastatin was withdrawn from the market in 2001 because of fatal rhabdomyolysis whilst rosuvastatin, the newest member of the group, was launched in March 2003. Although lovastatin has been available in the USA for many years there have been no attempts to market it in Europe until recently.

The efficacy of statins has been demonstrated in a number of landmark, randomized placebo-controlled trials (Table 24.8). A greater absolute benefit is seen in those trials that involved established cardiovascular disease, i.e. secondary prevention studies, compared to those that involved individuals without established cardiovascular disease, i.e. primary prevention studies. Statins are currently the lipid-lowering agents of choice in both primary and secondary prevention of coronary heart disease.

Table 24.8 Summary of key statin trials

Abbreviated trial name	Trial name	Study details
4S	Scandanavian Simvastatin Survival Study (4S) Group	First of the large clinical trials that enrolled 4444 patients and demonstrated the efficacy of simvastatin as secondary prevention against a mortality endpoint and other CHD events. Mean duration 5.4 years. Scandinavian Simvastatin Survival Study Group 1994 Randomised trial of cholesterol lowering in 4444 patients with coronary heart disease. The Scandinavian Simvastatin Survival Study (4S). Lancet 344: 1383-1389.
WOSCOPS	West of Scotland Coronary Prevention Study	Over 6000 men enrolled with moderately elevated cholesterol (LDL-C ≥ 4 mmol/L) and no previous MI. The efficacy of pravastatin against placebo was demonstrated in primary prevention for reducing MI and CHD death. Mean duration 4.9 years Shepherd J, Cobbe SM, Ford J et al 1995 Prevention of coronary heart disease with pravastatin in men with hypercholesterolaemia. New England Journal of Medicine 333: 1301-1307.
CARE	Cholesterol And Recurrent Events trial	4159 patients enrolled with previous MIs but average cholesterol levels. Efficacy of pravastatin compared to placebo demonstrated for secondary prevention of recurrent cardiac events. Median duration 5 years. Sacks FM, Pfeffer MA, Moye LA et al 1996 The effect of pravastatin on coronary events after myocardial infarction in patients with average cholesterol levels. New England Journal of Medicine 335: 1001-1009

Table 24.8 (continued)

Abbreviated trial name	Trial name	Study details
AFCAPS/ TexCAPS	Airforce/Texas Coronary Atherosclerosis Prevention Study.	The efficacy of lovastatin v placebo was demonstrated in 5608 men and 997 women for primary prevention of a first acute major coronary event in individuals without clinically evident atherosclerotic cardiovascular disease. Mean duration 5.2 years. Downs JR, Clearfield M, Weis S et al 1998 Primary prevention of acute coronary events with lovastatin in men and women with average cholesterol levels: results of AFCAPS/TexCAPS. Journal of the American Medical Association 279: 1615-1622.
LIPID	Long-term Intervention with Pravastatin in Ischaemic Disease	The efficacy of pravastatin v placebo as secondary prevention against mortality from CHD was demonstrated in over 9000 patients with a history of CHD and a wide range of initial cholesterol levels. Mean duration 6.1 years. The Long-Term Intervention with Pravastatin in Ischaemic Disease (LIPID) Study Group 1998 Prevention of cardiovascular events and death with pravastatin in patients with coronary heart disease and a broad range of initial cholesterol levels. New England Journal of Medicine 339: 1349-1357.
MIRACL	Myocardial Ischemia Reduction with Aggressive Cholesterol Lowering	The benefit of early initiation of atorvastatin within 24–96 h after an acute coronary syndrome event was demonstrated. Atorvastatin successfully reduced recurrent ischemic events in the following 16 weeks. Schwartz GG, Olsson Ag, Ezekowitz ME et al 2001 Effects of atorvastatin on early recurrent ischemic events in acute coronary syndromes: the MIRACL study: a randomised controlled trial. Journal of the American Medical Association 285: 1711-1718.
PROSPER	PROspective Study of Pravastatin in the Elderly at Risk	5804 patients aged 70–82 years were randomized to 40 mg pravastatin or placebo. Pravastatin improved all elements of the lipid profile and reduced primary and secondary endpoints. Mean duration 3.2 years. Shepherd J, Blauw GJ, Murphy MB et al 2002 Pravastatin in elderly individuals at risk of vascular disease (PROSPER): a randomised controlled trial. Lancet 360: 1623-1630.
LIPS	Lescol Intervention Prevention Study	This was the first randomized trial involving 1677 patients to show a significant reduction in the risk of cardiac events in patients started on fluvastatin immediately following a successful percutaneous coronary intervention independent of baseline cholesterol. Median duration 3.9 years. Serruys PW, de Feyter P, Macaya C et al 2002 Fluvastatin for prevention of cardiac events following successful first percutaneous coronary intervention: a randomised controlled trial. Journal of the American Medical Association 287: 3215-3222.
HPS	Heart Protection Study	20 536 high-risk individuals recruited into a placebo-controlled trial of simvastatin. The addition of simvastatin to existing best medicine produced additional benefits irrespective of initial cholesterol level. Mean duration of trial 5 years. Heart Protection Study Collaborative Group 2004 MRC/BHF Heart Protection Study of cholesterol lowering with simvastatin in 25,536 high risk individuals: a randomised placebo controlled trial. Lancet 360: 7-22.
ASCOTT-LLA	Anglo-Scandinavian Cardiac Outcomes Trial-Lipid Lowering Arm	Over 10 000 patients were recruited to the lipid-lowering arm of this trial designed primarily to assess different antihypertensive strategies in patients with hypertension and ≥3 other cardiovascular risk factors. The trial was terminated early due to the efficacy of atorvastatin and the confounding effect of open-label statin as add-on therapy, making continuation of the off-atorvastatin arm unethical. Median trial duration 3.3 years. Sever PS, Dahlö FB, Poulter NR et al 2003 Prevention of coronary and stroke events with atorvastatin in hypertensive patients who have average or lower-than-average cholesterol concentrations, in the Anglo-Scandinavian Cardiac Outcomes Trial – Lipid Lowering Arm (ASCOT-LLA): a multicentre randomised controlled trial. Lancet 261: 1149-1158.
ALERT	Assessment of LEscoll in Renal Transplantation	A study in 2012 high-risk renal transplant patients. The efficacy of fluvastatin was demonstrated against major cardiac events. Mean trial duration 5.1 years. Holdaas H, Fellström B, Jardine AG et al 2003 Effect of fluvastatin on cardiac outcomes in renal transplant recipients: a multicentre, randomised, placebo controlled trial. Lancet 361: 2024-2031.

continued

Table 24.8 (continued)

Abbreviated trial name	Trial name	Study details
REVERSAL	Reversal of Atherosclerosis with Aggressive Lipid Lowering	A trial of 654 patients that used intravascular ultrasound to demonstrate 40 mg of pravastatin was associated with progression of atherosclerotic disease but 80 mg atorvastatin halted, or even regressed, progression. Trial duration 18 months. Nissen SE, Tuzcu EM, Schoenhagen P et al 2004 Effect of intensive compared with moderate lipid-lowering therapy on progression of coronary atherosclerosis: a randomised controlled trial. Journal of the American Medical Association 291: 1071-1080.
PROVE IT – TIMI 22	Pravastatin or Atorvastatin Evaluation and Infection Therapy – Thrombolysis in Myocardial Infarction 22	Standard therapy with 40 mg pravastatin v intensive therapy with 80 mg atorvastatin in 4162 patients hospitalized for an acute coronary syndrome event. Intensive therapy with atorvastatin achieved a greater reduction in LDL-C and improved outcome against death or major cardiovascular event. Mean trial duration 24 months. Cannon CP, Braunwald E, McCabe CF et al 2004 Intensive versus moderate lipid lowering with statins after acute coronary syndromes. New England Journal of Medicine 350: 1495-1504.
CARDS	Collaborative Atorvastatin Diabetes Study	A placebo-controlled trial in 2828 patients with type 2 diabetes. Atorvastatin 10 mg demonstrated efficacy as primary prevention for lowering the risk of cardiovascular disease. Median trial duration 3.9 years. Colhoun HM, Betteridge DJ, Durrington PM et al 2004 Primary prevention of cardiovascular disease with atorvastatin in type 2 diabetes in the Collaborative Atorvastatin Diabetes Study (CARDS): multicentre randomised placebo-controlled trial. Lancet 264: 685-696.
A to Z	Aggrastat to Zocor	A two-part trial of simvastatin 40 mg for 1 month followed by 80 mg thereafter or placebo for 4 months followed by simvastatin 20 mg in 4497 patients following an acute coronary syndrome. Early initiation of the aggressive simvastatin regimen resulted in a trend to reduction of major cardiovascular events. Trial duration from 6 to 24 months. Lemos JA, Blazing MA, Wiviott SD et al 2004 Early intensive vs a delayed conservative simvastatin strategy in patients with acute coronary syndromes: phase Z of the A to Z trial. Journal of the American Medical Association 292: 1307-1316.
TNT	Treating to New Targets	A randomized double-blind study to assess whether lowering LDL-C below recommended levels (<2.6 mmol/L) was beneficial in patients with stable coronary heart disease. 10 001 patients received either 10 mg or 80 mg atorvastatin. Atorvastatin 80 mg provided significant clinical benefit above that of the 10 mg dose. Median trial duration 4.9 years. LaRosa JC, Grundy SM, Waters DD 2005 Intensive lipid lowering with atorvastatin in patients with stable coronary disease. New England Journal of Medicine 352: 1425-1435.
ASTEROID	A Study to Evaluate the effect of Rosuvastatin On Intravascular ultrasound-Derived coronary atheroma burden	Open-label, prospective cohort study of 507 patients who had a coronary angiography and received rosuvastatin 40 mg. Trial outcome revealed significant atheroma reduction in 349 evaluable patients. Trial duration 2 years. Nissen SE, Nicholls SJ, Sipahi I et al 2006 Effect of very high intensity statin therapy on regression of coronary atherosclerosis. The ASTEROID trial. Journal of the American Medical Association 295: 1556-1565.

There is much debate around which should be the statin of choice. Perhaps more important is the need to identify patients who need treatment and ensure they receive an appropriate, effective dose of a statin. Rosuvastatin is the most potent of the statins but there is limited evidence from clinical trials regarding its impact on morbidity and mortality to support routine use. It would appear best reserved for those individuals that have an inadequate response to other statins. There are also concerns about its safety profile, and rhabdomyolysis in particular, when used at the higher dose of 40 mg/day. It is recommended that this dose should only be used under specialist supervision, whilst the maximum dose for Asian patients should not exceed 20 mg/day.

All the statins require the presence of LDL receptors for their optimum clinical effect, and consequently they are less effective in patients with heterozygous familial hypercholesterolaemia because of the reduced number of LDL receptors. However, even in the homozygous patient with no LDL receptors they can bring about some reduction of plasma cholesterol although the mechanism is unclear.

Adverse effects

Many side effects appear mild and transient. The commonest include gastrointestinal symptoms, altered liver function tests and muscle aches. Less common are elevation of transaminase levels in excess of three times the upper limit of normal, hepatitis, rash, headache, insomnia, nightmares, vivid dreams and difficulty concentrating.

Myopathy (unexplained muscle soreness or weakness) leading to myoglobulinuria secondary to rhabdomyolysis is also a rare but serious potential adverse effect of all the statins. Guidelines have been issued (CSM 2002) which indicate the risk of myopathy is increased:

- when there are underlying muscle disorders, renal impairment, untreated hypothyroidism, alcohol abuse, or the recipient is aged over 70 years
- where statins are co-prescribed with other lipid-lowering drugs, e.g. fibrates, nicotinic acid
- when there is a past history of myopathy with another lipid-lowering drug
- where there is co-prescription of simvastatin or atorvastatin with drugs that inhibit CYP3A4,

The statins are a heterogeneous group metabolized by different CYP450 isoenzymes. Simvastatin, atorvastatin and lovastatin are metabolized by CYP3A4, fluvastatin is metabolized by CYP 2C9, and pravastatin and rosuvastatin are eliminated by other metabolic routes and less subject to interactions with CYP450 isoenzymes than other members of the family. Nevertheless, caution is still required as a 5–23-fold increase in pravastatin bioavailability has been reported with ciclosporin. Simvastatin and atorvastatin do not alter the activity of CYP3A4 themselves, but their plasma levels are increased by known inhibitors of CYP3A4 (Table 24.9). Advice has been published for the prescribing of simvastatin and atorvastatin with inhibitors of CYP3A4 (Table 24.10).

Pleiotropic properties

While the effect of statins on the lipid profile contributes to their beneficial outcome in reducing morbidity and mortality from coronary heart disease, other mechanisms, known as pleiotropic effects, may also play a part (Werner et al 2002). These mechanisms include plaque stabilization, inhibition of thrombus formation, reduced plasma viscosity and anti-inflammatory and antioxidant activity. These pleiotropic properties, i.e. cholesterol-independent effects, are far reaching and reveal a clinical impact beyond a process of reducing total cholesterol. For example, lowering total cholesterol produces only modest reductions of a fixed, atherosclerotic, luminal stenosis but results in a qualitative change of the plaque and helps stabilize it. This protects the plaque from rupturing and triggering further coronary events.

Inflammation is thought to play a prominent part in the development of atherosclerosis and increased levels of C-reactive protein have been used to identify individuals at risk of plaque rupture and consequent myocardial infarction and stroke. Statins have been shown to reduce the levels of C-reactive protein in several trials. The mechanism is unclear but probably involves a direct effect on macrophages within the atherosclerotic plaque, suppression of macrophage growth and their expression of metalloproteinases and tissue factor.

An important aspect of vascular endothelium dysfunction is the impaired synthesis, release and activity of endothelial-derived

Table 24.9 Examples of drug interactions involving statins and the cytochrome P450 enzyme pathway

CYP 450 isoenzyme	Inducers	Inhibitors
CYP3A4		
Atorvastin, lovastatin, simvastatin	Phenytoin Barbiturate Rifampicin Dexamethasone Cyclophosphamide Carbamazepine Omeprazole	Ketoconazole Itraconazole Fluconazole Erythromycin Clarithromycin Tricyclic antidepressants Nefazodone Venlafaxine Fluoxetine Sertraline Ciclosporin Tacrolimus Diltiazem Verapamil Protease inhibitors Mldazolam Corticosteroids Grapefruit juice Tamoxifen Amiodarone
CYP2C9		
Fluvastin	Rifampicin Phenobarbitone Phenytoin	Ketoconazole Fluconazole Sulfaphenazole

Table 24.10 Advice for prescribing simvastatin or atorvastatin with inhibitors of CYP3A4 (CSM 2004)

Avoid simvastatin with potent inhibitors of CYP3A4:	HIV protease inhibitors, azole antifungals, erythromycin, clarithromycin, telithromycin
Do not exceed the following doses:	Simvastatin 10 mg daily with ciclosporin, gemfibrozil or niacin (>1 g/day) Simvastatin 20 mg daily with verapamil or amiodarone Simvastatin 40 mg daily with diltiazem
Avoid grapefruit juice when taking simvastatin	
Atorvastatin to be used cautiously with CYP3A4 inhibitors:	Additional care required at high doses of atorvastatin avoid drinking large quantities of grapefruit juice

nitric oxide, an important and early marker of atherosclerosis. After the administration of a statin one of the earliest effects observed (within 3 days) is an increased endothelial nitric oxide release, thereby mediating an improvement in vasodilation of the endothelium.

For some while it has been thought that part of the beneficial effect of statins on cardiovascular disease could be attributed to an effect on blood coagulation. It is now evident that statins, amongst their many actions, decrease platelet activation and activity, decrease prothrombin activation, factor Va generation, fibrinogen cleavage and factor XIII activation, and increase factor Va inactivation.

Over-the-counter sale

Low-dose (10 mg) simvastatin can be purchased from community pharmacies in the UK to treat individuals at moderate cardiovascular risk. Men aged 55–70 years with or without risk factors and men aged 45–54 years or women aged 55–70 years with at least one risk factor (smoker, obese, family history of premature coronary heart disease or of South Asian origin) are eligible for treatment. Simvastatin cannot be sold to individuals who have cardiovascular disease, diabetes or familial dyslipidaemia or are taking lipid-lowering agents or medication that may interact with simvastatin. The rationale for over-the-counter sale is to reduce the risk of a first major coronary event in adults at moderate risk. Unfortunately, the evidence base to support the use of 10 mg simvastatin and achieve long-term cardiovacular benefit is limited.

Fibrates

Members of this group include bezafibrate, ciprofibrate, fenofibrate and gemfibrozil. They are thought to act by binding to peroxisome proliferator-activated receptor α (PPAR-α) on hepatocytes. This then leads to changes in the expression of genes involved in lipoprotein metabolism. Consequently, fibrates reduce triglyceride and, to a lesser extent, LDL-C levels while increasing HDL-C. Fibrates take 2–5 days to have a measurable effect on VLDL-C, with their optimum effect present after 4 weeks. In addition to their effects on plasma lipids and lipoproteins, the fibrates may also have a beneficial effect on the fibrinolytic and clotting mechanisms. The fibrates also produce an improvement in glucose tolerance, although bezafibrate probably has the most marked effect. In the patient with elevated triglycerides and gout only fenofibrate has been reported to have a sustained uricosuric effect on chronic administration. Overall there appears little to differentiate members of the group with regard to their effect on the lipid profile, with fenofibrate and ciprofibrate being the most potent members of the group.

In patients with diabetes the typical picture of dyslipidaemia is one of raised triglycerides, reduced HDL-C and near normal LDL-C. Despite the effect of fibrates to reduce triglycerides and increase HDL-C, statins remain the first-line lipid-lowering agent in most guidelines because of a lack of clear evidence that fibrates prevent cardiovascular disease in diabetes. It was hoped that a 5-year study of fenofibrate in individuals with type 2 diabetes (FIELD Investigators 2005) would clarify the issue. However, in the final analysis the results provided little convincing evidence to change from recommending a statin.

Adverse effects

Overall, the side effects of fibrates are mild and vary between members of the group. Their apparent propensity to increase the cholesterol saturation index of bile renders them unsuitable for patients with gallbladder disease. Gastrointestinal symptoms such as nausea, diarrhoea and abdominal pain are common but transient, and often resolve after a few days of treatment. Myositis has been described, and is associated with muscle pain, unusual tiredness or weakness. The mechanism is unclear but it is thought fibrates may have a direct toxic action on muscle cells in susceptible individuals.

Fibrates have been implicated in a number of drug interactions (Table 24.11), of which two in particular are potentially serious. Fibrates are known to significantly increase the effect of anticoagulants, while concurrent use with a statin is associated with an increased risk of myositis and, rarely, rhabdomyolysis. Concurrent use of cerivastatin and gemfibrozil was noted to

Table 24.11 Typical drug interactions involving bile acid binding agents and fibrates

Drug group	Interacting drug	Comment
Bile acid binding agents (colestyramine/colestipol)		All medication should be taken 1 h before or 4–6 h after colestyramine/colestipol to avoid reduced absorption caused by binding in the gut
	Acarbose	Hypoglycaemia enhanced by colestyramine
	Digoxin	Absorption reduced
	Diuretics	Absorption reduced
	Levothyroxine	Absorption reduced
	Mycophenolate mofetil	Absorption reduced
	Paracetamol	Absorption reduced
	Raloxifene	Absorption reduced
	Valproate	Absorption reduced
	Statins	Absorption reduced by up to 50%
	Vancomycin	Effect of oral vancomycin antagonized by colestyramine
	Warfarin	Increased anticoagulant effect due to depletion of vitamin K or reduced anticoagulant effect due to binding or warfarin in gut

Table 24.11 (continued)

Drug group	Interacting drug	Comment
Fibrates	Antidiabetic agents	Improvement in glucose tolerance
	Ciclosporin	Increased risk of renal impairment
	Bile acid binding agent	Reduced bioavailability of fibrate if taken concomitantly
	Statin	Increased risk of myopathy
	Warfarin	Increased anticoagulant effect

cause rhabdomyolysis and this contributed to the withdrawal of cerivastatin from clinical use in 2001.

Bile acid binding agents

The two members of this group in current use are colestyramine and colestipol. Both were formerly considered first-line agents in the management of patients with hypercholesterolaemia but now have limited use. They reduce total cholesterol but either have no effect on, or show a slight increase in, triglyceride levels. As a consequence they are unsuitable for use in patients with elevated triglyceride levels.

Following oral administration, neither colestyramine nor colestipol is absorbed from the gut. They bind bile acids in the intestine, prevent their reabsorption and produce an insoluble complex that is excreted in the faeces. The depletion of bile acids results in an increase in hepatic synthesis of bile acids from cholesterol. The depletion of hepatic cholesterol increases LDL receptor activity in the liver and this removes LDL-C from the blood. Both colestyramine and colestipol also increase hepatic VLDL-C synthesis and thereby increase plasma triglycerides in some patients.

Colestyramine and colestipol can reduce total cholesterol levels within 24–48 hours, and thereafter continue to gradually reduce levels for up to 1 year. The starting dose of colestyramine is one 4 g sachet twice a day. Over a 3–4 week period the dose should normally be built up to 12–24 g daily taken in water or a suitable liquid as a single dose, or up to four divided doses each day. Occasionally 36 g a day may be required although the benefits of increasing the dose above 16 g a day are offset by gastrointestinal disturbances and poor patient adherence. Colestipol is also available in granular form and mixed with an appropriate liquid at a dose of 5 g once or twice daily. This dose can be increased every 1–2 months to a maximum of 30 g in a single or twice-daily regimen.

Although licensed and marketed in countries other than the UK, colesevelam is a new member of this class. It is a non-absorbed water-insoluble polymer that sequesters bile and is up to six times as potent as traditional bile acid binding agents, probably because of a greater binding to glycocholic acid. Colesevelam is administered as a tablet and appears to achieve a far higher compliance than colestyramine or colestipol.

Adverse effects

Side effects are more likely to occur with high doses and in patients aged over 60 years. Bloating, flatulence, heartburn and constipation are common complaints. Constipation is the major subjective side effect, and although usually mild and transient, it may be severe.

Colestyramine and colestipol are known to interact with many drugs (see Table 24.11), primarily by interfering with absorption. Consequently, medication should be taken 1–2 hours before or 4–6 hours after these agents. Although the data are limited, studies with colesevelam have not revealed clinically significant effects on absorption of other drugs. For patients on multiple drug therapy, colestyramine and colestipol are clearly not the best choice.

Cholesterol absorption inhibitors

Ezetimibe is a 2-azetidinone derivative that interacts with a putative cholesterol transporter in the intestinal brush border membrane and thereby blocks cholesterol absorption from the gastrointestinal tract. It can reduce LDL-C by 15–20% when added to diet, or by 20–25% when added to diet with a statin. Ezetimibe also brings about a small increase in HDL-C and a reduction in triglycerides. It should be used either with a statin, a fibrate or a nicotinic acid derivative or by itself in statin-intolerant individuals. Although apparently well tolerated, there are no long-term randomized controlled trials that demonstrate reduced cardiovascular morbidity or mortality

Cholesterol ester transfer protein inhibitors

Low levels of cholesterol ester transfer protein (CETP) are associated with increased levels of HDL-C and reduced cardiovascular risk. In the body CETP transfers cholesterol from HDL-C to LDL-C and VLDL-C, thereby altering the HDL-C:LDL-C ratio in a potentially unfavourable manner. As a consequence of this, inhibitors of CETP are expected to have a beneficial cardiovascular effect. Torcetrapib is a potent inhibitor of CETP and in trials has demonstrated a dose-dependent ability to increase HDL-C, with little effect on LDL-C or triglycerides. Increases in plasma HDL-C of more than 100% have been reported but whether this will transfer to reduced cardiovascular morbidity and mortality is unclear.

Nicotinic acid and derivatives

Nicotinic acid in pharmacological doses (1.5–6 g) lowers both plasma LDL-C and VLDL-C levels and increases HDL-C.

The major mechanism of action for nicotinic acid appears to be the ability to reduce the release of VLDL-C which in turn leads to decreased levels of IDL-C and LDL-C. In addition, it reduces the release of free fatty acids from adipose tissue into the general circulation and consequently reduces the available substrate for triglyceride synthesis. The mechanism by which nicotinic acid increases HDL-C is not known although a decrease in HDL-C catabolism has been reported. Nicotinic acid has also been shown to reduce levels of Lp(a).

Acipimox is structurally related to nicotinic acid, has similar beneficial effects on the lipid profile and a better side effect profile but appears to be less potent. An extended-release preparation of nicotinic acid has also been marketed to reduce the incidence of the troublesome side effects, but up to 30% of users still report problems.

Adverse effects

Despite the established long-term safety of nicotinic acid it is of limited use in practice because of its side effects. These are very common and unpleasant and include troublesome flushing of the skin, headache, postural hypotension, diarrhoea, exacerbation of peptic ulcers, hepatic dysfunction, gout and increased blood glucose levels. While acipimox shares many of these side effects, though to a lesser extent, it does not have an adverse effect on blood glucose nor does it share the property of exacerbating peptic ulcers.

Fish oils

Fish oil preparations rich in ω3 fatty acids have been shown to markedly reduce plasma triglyceride levels by decreasing VLDL-C synthesis although little change has been observed in LDL-C or HDL-C levels. However, the effect is inconsistent and significant increases in LDL-C have also been reported to accompany the use of fish oils. Data from several studies suggest that ω3 fatty acids protect against coronary heart disease mortality, particularly sudden death, rather than non-fatal events. The protective effects in secondary prevention are achieved by consumption of 1 g daily, equivalent to 100 g of oily fish.

Soluble fibre

Preparations containing soluble fibre, such as ispaghula husk, have been shown to reduce lipid levels. The fibre is thought to bind bile acids in the gut and increase the conversion of cholesterol to bile acids in the liver. However, its role in the management of dyslipidaemia is unclear and it is much less effective than statins in reducing total cholesterol and LDL-C.

Patient care

Diet

The management of dyslipidaemia should always include lifestyle changes once underlying causes have been eliminated. Dietary advice is the cornerstone of management and should be supported by advice to stop smoking, undertake regular exercise and moderate alcohol intake. Patients should be encouraged to increase their intake of complex carbohydrates, fruit and vegetables, and oily fish. Soluble fibre found in lentils, beans, peas and oats may also have some beneficial effect in reducing cholesterol as may the dietary intake of stanol esters and plant sterols.

Drugs

Statins

In patients receiving an HMG-CoA reductase inhibitor, a once-daily regimen involving an evening dose is often preferred. Several of the HMG-CoA reductase inhibitors are claimed to be more effective when given as a single dose in the evening compared to a similar dose administered in the morning. This has been attributed to the fact that cholesterol biosynthesis reaches peak activity at night. However, atorvastatin may be taken in the morning or evening with similar efficacy. A reduction in TC and LDL-C is usually seen with all HMG-CoA reductase inhibitors within 2 weeks, with a maximum response occurring by week 4 and maintained thereafter during continued therapy.

Bile acid binding agents

Palatability is often a major problem, with patients needing to be well motivated and prepared for the problems they may encounter.

Both colestyramine and colestipol are available in an orange flavour and/or as a low sugar (aspartame-containing) powder. Colestipol is without taste and is odourless. Each sachet of colestyramine or colestipol should be added to at least 120 mL of liquid and stirred vigorously to avoid the powder clumping. The powder does not dissolve but disperses in the chosen liquid, which may be water, fruit juice, skimmed milk or non-carbonated beverage. Both may also be taken in soups, with cereals, and with pulpy fruits with high moisture content, such as apple sauce.

All patients receiving colestipol or colestyramine must be aware that any concurrent medication must be taken 1–2 hours before or 4–6 hours after the bile acid binding agent. Gemfibrozil can be administered with colestipol if the two drugs are taken 2 hours apart.

Other lipid-lowering agents

To achieve optimum effect, patients taking a fibrate should be advised to take their medication 30 minutes before a meal.

The adverse effect profile of nicotinic acid has been discussed above. For those patients who find the flushing particularly troublesome, a single dose of aspirin 75 mg, taken some 30 minutes before the nicotinic acid, has been shown to give relief from the prostaglandin-mediated flushing. Extended-release dosage forms of nicotinic acid have also been shown to reduce the incidence of flushing and pruritus.

CASE STUDIES

Case 24.1

Mr DF is a 43-year-old man who has been relatively fit and well for the past 20 years during which he has rarely visited his primary care doctor. Two weeks ago he was admitted to hospital having suffered a

myocardial infarction. On questioning it was revealed that his brother had died in a road traffic accident at the age of 19 and his father had died from coronary heart disease aged 54 years.

Examination of Mr DF revealed a corneal arcus and tendon xanthomas. Blood drawn within 2 h of the onset of the myocardial infarction revealed total cholesterol 7.8 mmol/L, HDL-C 0.9 mmol/L and triglycerides 2.3 mmol/L.

Questions

1. Calculate the concentration of Mr DF's LDL-C and comment on the findings.
2. What is the likely diagnosis and treatment for Mr DF on discharge?
3. Mr DF wants to know why he was not identified as being at high risk of coronary heart disease before he suffered his myocardial infarction.

Answers

1. The value for LDL-C can be calculated from the Friedewald formula where:

$$\text{LDL-C} = (\text{Total cholesterol} \times \text{HDL-C}) - (0.45 \times \text{triglycerides}) \text{ mmol/L}$$
$$= (7.8 - 0.9) - (0.45 \times 2.3)$$
$$= 5.9 \text{ mmol/L}$$

The ideal value of LDL-C is <2 mmol/L.

2. Mr DF has the signs and family history of classic heterozygous familial hypercholesterolaemia, most likely due to a genetic defect in the LDL receptor on hepatocytes. His level of LDL-C is high and action is required to reduce it. Appropriate lifestyle advice is necessary but a statin will be required to achieve the desired outcome. Typically a high dose of simvastatin (80 mg day) will have to be used.

3. Unfortunately Mr DF's father probably died of heart disease at a time when the practice of detecting affected families and screening first-degree relatives was not widespread. The early, unrelated death of his brother and Mr DF's previous good health would not have given an opportunity to identify any underlying familial disorder.

From population data it is known that the prevalence of heterozygous familial hypercholesterolaemia is about 1 in 500. Consequently 120 000 cases would be expected in the UK. However, far fewer cases are known and screening programmes to track cases in affected families are now in place. A family history of elevated total cholesterol or death from coronary heart disease before the age of 55 in a first-degree male relative, as in the case of Mr DF, is an important sign that should highlight the potential risk to other family members.

Case 24.2

Mr PT is a 52-year-old active school teacher. Four years ago he was found to have a raised total cholesterol and elevated blood pressure for which he was started on 10 mg simvastatin and 2.5 mg bendroflumethiazide. Over the years his dose of simvastatin has been gradually increased to 40 mg a day, but apart from this his medication has remained unchanged. He presents at the clinical complaining of aches and pains in his legs over the past 10 days. On questioning he reveals that over recent months he has been eating fresh grapefruit and consuming the occasional glass of grapefruit juice. A tentative diagnosis of myopathy is initially made.

Questions

1. What is the likelihood that grapefruit juice has contributed to Mr PT's problem?
2. Would atorvastatin, rosuvastatin or pravastatin be a more appropriate statin to prescribe if Mr PT wanted to continue with the occasional glass of grapefruit juice?

Answers

1. Grapefruit juice is known to interact with statins through its inhibition of the cytochrome P450 CYP3A4 enzyme. It has been suggested that it is the furanocoumarin in the grapefruit juice which binds to CYP3A4 and inactivates it in both the liver and the gastrointestinal tract. As little as 200 mL of grapefruit juice may inhibit CYP3A4, thereby prolonging the half-life of the statin and increasing plasma levels. When taken on a regular basis this can increase the risk of dose-related side effects such as rhabdomyolysis and increase the risk of myopathy. Current advice is that grapefruit juice should be avoided altogether when taking simvastatin, regardless of whether it is fresh grapefruit or grapefruit juice, grapefruit juice diluted from concentrate or frozen grapefruit juice.

2. Atorvastatin is also metabolized by CYP3A4. Although the effect is less dramatic than with simvastatin, the concurrent intake of large quantities of grapefruit juice with atorvastatin is not recommended. Neither pravastatin nor rosuvastatin is substantially metabolized by P450 and may be better alternatives. However, when there is a past history of myopathy the need for caution remains as the risk of recurrence is enhanced whatever lipid-lowering agent is prescribed. It should also be noted that rosuvastatin, unlike pravastatin, has no clinical outcome data and would not be appropriate for use in this patient. There are also separate concerns regarding the muscle toxicity of rosuvastatin, especially when used at the higher dose of 40 mg. This again would indicate that rosuvastatin is not the best option for Mr PT.

Case 24.3

Mrs MC is a very active, 51-year-old caucasian lady who for the past 6 months has been suffering from the classic symptoms of the menopause. Six months ago on a routine visit to her doctor she had her lipid profile measured and this revealed an HDL-C of 0.8 mmol/L and total cholesterol of 5 mmol/L. Her blood pressure was 140/80 mmHg. She is currently prescribed no medication but is receiving intensive lifestyle support to lower her cholesterol. She has no other medical history of note other than a record that her mother died at the age of 66 years from a heart attack.

Mrs MC would like to be prescribed hormone replacement therapy to control her menopausal symptoms and reduce her risk of cardiovascular disease.

Questions

1. Is it appropriate to prescribe hormone replacement therapy to reduce Mrs MC's cardiovascular risk?
2. What is the value of measuring HDL-C?
3. Does Mrs MC have a risk of cardiovascular disease that requires treatment with a lipid-lowering agent?

Answers

1. Most epidemiological studies have demonstrated a beneficial effect of hormone replacement therapy on the development of coronary heart disease in postmenopausal women. However, randomized controlled trials with defined clinical endpoints have failed to demonstrate a reduction in cardiovascular events. Whether this has arisen because of how the body responds to hormone replacement therapy, the age of the women studied or the influence of the type of hormone replacement therapy, the dose, route of administration and duration of treatment is unclear. At present there are no compelling data to justify the use of hormone replacement therapy for the prevention or treatment of cardiovascular disease in postmenopausal women. The fact that Mrs MC's menopausal symptoms may benefit from treatment with hormone replacement therapy and the likely duration of this

therapy are additional issues that must be taken into account in the decision of whether or not to prescribe hormone replacement therapy.

2. HDL-C is a major fraction of cholesterol in plasma and an important determinant of cardiovascular risk in men and women, even when the level of total cholesterol appears to be within the normal range. The incidence of myocardial infarction is positively correlated with the cholesterol concentration and inversely related to the concentration of HDL-C. The TC:HDL-C ratio is another way to represent this risk and has been shown to have good predictive capabilities in women.

3. With reference to the Joint British Societies risk prediction charts, it can be determined that with a TC:HDL-C ratio of 6.25 (5/0.8) and a systolic blood pressure of 140 mmHg, Mrs MC has a 10–20% risk of developing cardiovascular disease over the next 10 years. This would not automatically make her a candidate for treatment with a lipid-lowering agent as her 10-year cardiovascular risk is not >20%. Knowledge of Mrs MC's body mass index and blood glucose level would be useful additional information, as would a more detailed insight into her family history of cardiovascular disease. It is only when all the relevant information has been gathered that a final decision on the use of a lipid-lowering agent can be made. It would also be of interest to determine whether the lifestyle support has brought about any improvement in Mrs MC's lipid profile or blood pressure.

Case 24.4

Mr EC is a 48-year-old executive for a large multinational company who works long hours and frequently has to travel abroad. He has a family history of coronary heart disease and 9 months ago he attended a coronary screening clinic for a health check. At the clinic he was found to have a normal blood pressure but a blood screen revealed a total cholesterol of 6.7 mmol/L and triglycerides of 11.8 mmol/L. When he revisited the clinic 4 weeks later after trying to follow dietary advice, a fasting blood sample revealed a total cholesterol of 5 mmol/L and triglycerides of 2.7 mmol/L. Liver function tests were normal. He is a non-smoker and claims never to drink more than 10 units of alcohol per week.

After repeated requests to revisit the clinic he eventually turned up stating he had been away from home for 6 months on a series of business trips. He was trying to keep to a low-fat diet and his blood profile revealed total cholesterol 5.7 mmol/L, triglycerides 4.3 mmol/L, HDL-C 0.8 mmol/L and LDL-C 3 mmol/L.

Questions

1. Is Mr EC at high risk of coronary heart disease?
2. Is Mr EC a candidate for lipid-lowering therapy?
3. Should the children of Mr EC be screened for dyslipidaemia?

Answers

1. Mr EC has a TC:HDL-C ratio of 7.1 (5.7/0.8). If the Joint British Societies risk charts were used they would indicate he has a 10-year risk of coronary heart disease of 10–20% and does not require lipid-lowering treatment. However, the tables underestimate the risk of coronary heart disease in those with familial hyperlipidaemia or a history of premature coronary heart disease.

   Mr EC would appear to have a mixed lipaemia although it is difficult to interpret non-fasting triglycerides because of the influence of food intake. The low HDL-C suggests he is overweight and/or has a non-ideal lifestyle. Exclusion of diabetes, high alcohol intake, liver and renal impairment is necessary. The possibility of impaired glucose tolerance should not be overlooked and a glucose tolerance test should be performed.

2. Given the elevated triglycerides and total cholesterol, Mr EC is certainly a candidate for lifestyle advice. The use of a statin may be considered if the lifestyle changes do not bring about the necessary improvements in the lipid profile. However, the dyslipidaemia may be secondary to obesity, alcoholism, diabetes or hypothyroidism. If any of these disorders are present the appropriate treatment may correct the underlying dyslipidaemia.

3. The family history of coronary heart disease is important but is only significant if the age of onset in a parent or sibling was under 55 years of age for an affected male or under 65 years for an affected female. A rare familial disorder, e.g. familial dysbetalipoproteinaemia, may be the causative factor. If this was confirmed his children should be screened after puberty as the offending gene may not express itself in the younger child.

   Mr EC was subsequently found to have diabetes for which he initially received metformin together with a statin. In this scenario where a patient is diagnosed with type 2 diabetes, it is also important to consider advising children about lifestyle issues and the need to control weight throughout life.

REFERENCE

Bhopal R 2000 What is the risk of coronary heart disease in South Asians? A review of UK research. Journal of Public Health Medicine 22: 375-385

Bucher H C, Hengstle P, Schindler C et al 2002 n-3 polyunsaturated fatty acids in coronary heart disease: a meta-analysis of randomized controlled trials. American Journal of Medicine 112: 298-304

CSM 2002 HMG CoA reductase inhibitors (statins) and myopathy. Current Problems in Pharmacovigilance 28: 2

CSM 2004 Statins and cytochrome P450 interactions. Current Problems in Pharmacovigilance 30: 1-2

Durstine J L, Grandjean P W, Cox C A et al 2002 Lipids, lipoproteins and exercise. Journal of Cardiopulmonary Rehabilitation 22: 385-398

FIELD Investigators 2005 Effects of long-term fenofibrate therapy on cardiovascular events in 9795 people with type 2 diabetes mellitus (the FIELD study): randomised controlled trial. Lancet 366: 1849-1861

Hooper L, Summerbell C D, Higgins P T et al 2001 Dietary fat intake and prevention of cardiovascular disease: systematic review. British Medical Journal 322: 757-763

Hooper L, Thompson R L, Harrison R A 2006 Risks and benefits of omega 3 fats for mortality, cardiovascular disease, and cancer: systematic review. British Medical Journal 332: 752-760

Joint British Societies 2005 JBS 2: Joint British Societies' guidelines on prevention of cardiovascular disease in clinical practice. Heart 91: v1-v52

Kolovou G D, Anagnostopoulou K K, Cokkinos D V 2005 Pathophysiology of dyslipidaemia in the metabolic syndrome. Postgraduate Medical Journal 81: 358-366

Mozaffarian D, Katan M B, Ascherio A et al 2006 Medical progress: trans fatty acids and cardiovascular disease. New England Journal of Medicine 354: 1601-1613

Von Eckardstein A, Nofer J R, Assmann G 2001 High density lipoproteins and arteriosclerosis. Role of cholesterol efflux and reverse cholesterol transport. Arteriosclerosis, Thrombosis and Vascular Biology 21: 13-27

Werner N, Nickenig G, Laufs U 2002 Pleiotropic effects of HMG-CoA reductase inhibitors. Basic Research in Cardiology 97: 105-116

Asthma 25

K. P. Gibbs   D. Cripps

KEY POINTS

- Asthma is a common and chronic inflammatory condition of the airways whose cause is not completely understood.
- Common symptoms are caused by hyperresponsive airways and include coughing, wheezing, chest tightness and shortness of breath.
- The only reliable, simple and objective way to diagnose asthma is to demonstrate reversible airflow limitation.
- Asthma mortality is about 1500 per year in the UK with annual NHS costs of around £850 million.
- Asthma is still a poorly controlled disease despite effective treatments.
- Asthma triggers should be avoided or controlled.
- Pharmacological therapy should involve early anti-inflammatory treatment in all but the mildest asthmatics and follow national, evidence-based guidance.
- Optimum treatment involves the lowest doses of therapy that provide good symptom control with minimal or no side effects, and the best drug delivery device is one that the patient can use correctly.
- Patients should be educated to take an active role in their disease management, be given individualized self-management plans and be regularly supervised by the healthcare team.

Asthma literally means 'panting'. It is a broad term used to refer to a disorder of the respiratory system that leads to episodic difficulty in breathing. The national UK guidelines (BTS/SIGN 2005) define asthma as 'a chronic inflammatory disorder of the airways…in susceptible individuals, inflammatory symptoms are usually associated with widespread but variable airflow obstruction and an increase in airway response to a variety of stimuli. Obstruction is often reversible either spontaneously or with treatment'.

Epidemiology

The exact prevalence of asthma remains uncertain because of the differing ways in which airway restriction is reported, diagnostic uncertainty (especially for children under 2 years) and the overlap with other conditions such as chronic obstructive pulmonary disease. It has been estimated that about 4% of the British and American populations have asthma. with over 5.1 million people being treated for asthma in the UK (National Asthma Campaign 2001). Mortality from asthma is estimated at approximately 0.4 per 100 000 and about 1500 deaths per annum in the UK. Most deaths occur outside hospital and the most common reasons for death are thought to be inadequate assessment of the severity of airway obstruction by the patient and/or clinician, and inadequate therapy of an acute attack.

The probability of children having asthma-like symptoms is estimated to be between 5% and 12%, with a higher occurrence in boys than girls and in children whose parents have an allergic disorder. Between 30% and 70% of children will become symptom free by adulthood. However, individuals who develop asthma at an early age do have a poorer prognosis.

The prevalence of asthma actually appears to be rising despite advances in therapy. However, there is some doubt about this due to the differing criteria for the diagnosis of asthma used in different studies. Asthma is considered to be one of the consequences of Western civilization, and appears to be related to a number of environmental factors. Air pollution resulting from industrial sources and transport may be interacting with smoking, dietary and other factors to increase the incidence of this debilitating problem.

Aetiology

The specific abnormality underlying asthma is hyperreactivity of the lungs to one or more stimuli. This can also occur in certain patients with chronic bronchitis and allergic rhinitis but usually to a lesser extent. There are a number of possible trigger factors (Table 25.1).

One of the most common trigger factors is the allergen found in the faeces of the house dust mite, which is almost universally present in bedding, carpets and soft furnishing. Pollen from grass (prevalent in June and July) can lead to seasonal asthma. The role of occupation in the development of asthma has become apparent with increased industrialization. There are many causes of occupational asthma and bronchial reactivity may persist for years after exposure to the trigger factor. Food allergy usually results in gastrointestinal disturbances and eczema rather than asthma. Drug-induced asthma can be severe and the most common causes are β-blocker drugs and prostaglandin synthetase inhibitors. The administration of β-adrenoceptor blockers to a patient, even in the form of eye drops, can cause β_2-receptor blockade and consequent bronchoconstriction. Selective β-adrenoceptor blockers are thought to pose slightly less risk but as these lose their selectivity at higher doses, it is generally recommended that this group of drugs is avoided altogether in asthma patients. Aspirin and related non-steroidal anti-inflammatory drugs can cause severe bronchoconstriction in susceptible individuals. Aspirin inhibits the enzyme cyclo-oxygenase, which normally converts

Table 25.1 Examples of trigger factors that may cause asthma

Trigger	Examples
Allergens	Pollens, moulds, house dust mite, animals (dander, saliva and urine)
Industrial chemicals	Manufacture of, for example, isocyanate-containing paints, epoxy resins, aluminium, hair sprays, penicillins and cimetidine
Drugs	Aspirin, ibuprofen and other prostaglandin synthetase inhibitors, β-adrenoceptor blockers
Foods	A rare cause but examples include nuts, fish, seafood, dairy products, food colouring, especially tartrazine, benzoic acid and sodium metabisulfite
Other industrial triggers	Wood or grain dust, colophony in solder, cotton dust, grain weevils and mites; also environmental pollutants such as cigarette smoke and sulphur dioxide
Miscellaneous	Cold air, exercise, hyperventilation, viral respiratory tract infections, emotion or stress

arachidonic acid to prostaglandins. When this pathway is blocked an alternative reaction predominates, leading to an increase in production of bronchoconstrictor leukotrienes. Figures from differing studies vary, but between 5% and 20% of the adult asthma population are thought to be sensitive to aspirin.

Pathophysiology

The discovery of the antibody IgE led to the description of extrinsic or allergic asthma ('eosinophilic' asthma, IgE-mediated sensitization to common allergens) and non-IgE-mediated intrinsic asthma ('non-eosinophilic' asthma). Extrinsic asthma is common in children, associated with a genetic predisposition, and is precipitated by known allergens. Intrinsic asthma develops in adulthood, with symptoms triggered by non-allergenic factors such as a viral infection, irritants which cause epithelial damage and mucosal inflammation, emotional upset which mediates excess parasympathetic input or exercise which causes water and heat loss from the airways, triggering mediator release from mast cells. Mast cells, eosinophils, epithelial cells, macrophages and activated T-lymphocytes are all key features of the inflammatory process of asthma. These cells act on the airways to cause inflammation, either directly or through neural mechanisms. Their exact roles and interrelationships with each other and with the causative allergenic or non-allergenic mechanisms have, however, yet to be fully determined (Douwes et al 2002, Holgate 2002). Figure 25.1 outlines the theoretical cellular mechanisms involved.

These cell-derived mediators play a role in causing the main features of asthma: marked hypertrophy and hyperplasia of bronchial smooth muscle, mucus gland hypertrophy leading to excessive mucus production and airway plugging, airway oedema, acute bronchoconstriction and impaired mucociliary clearance. Mast cell components are released as a result of an IgE antibody-mediated reaction on the surface of the cell. Histamine and other mediators of inflammation are released from mast

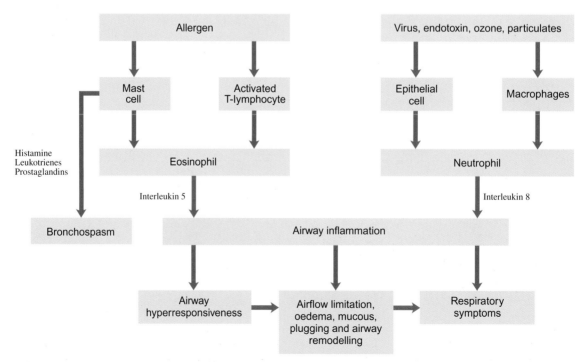

Figure 25.1 Postulated cellular mechanisms involved in airway inflammation (adapted from Douwes et al 2002).

cells, for example leukotrienes, prostaglandins, bradykinin, adenosine, prostaglandin-generating factor of anaphylaxis, as well as various chemotactic agents that attract eosinophils and neutrophils. Macrophages release prostaglandins, thromboxane and platelet-activating factor (PAF). PAF appears to sustain bronchial hyperreactivity and cause respiratory capillaries to leak plasma, which increases mucosal oedema. It also facilitates the accumulation of eosinophils within the airways, a characteristic pathological feature of asthma. Eosinophils release various inflammatory mediators such as leukotriene C_4 (LTC_4) and PAF. Epithelial damage results and thick viscous mucus is produced that causes further deterioration in lung function.

Mucus production is normally a defence mechanism but in asthma patients there is an increase in the size of bronchial glands and goblet cells that produce mucus. Mucus transport is dependent on its viscosity. If it is very thick it plugs the airways, which also become blocked with epithelial and inflammatory cell debris. Mucociliary clearance is also decreased due to inflammation of epithelial cells.

Clinical manifestations

Asthma can present in a number of ways. It may manifest as a persistent cough. Most commonly, it is described as recurrent episodes of difficulty in breathing (dyspnoea) associated with wheezing (a high-pitched noise due to turbulent airflow through a narrowed airway). Diagnosis is usually made from the clinical history from the patient or patient's representative confirmed by demonstration of reversible airflow obstruction, with repeated measures of lung function. The history of an asthma patient often includes the presence of atopy and allergic rhinitis in the close family. Symptoms of asthma are often intermittent, and the frequency and severity of an episode can vary from individual to individual. Between periods of wheezing and breathlessness patients may feel quite well. However, the absence of an improvement in ventilation cannot rule out asthma, and in younger children it is sometimes very difficult to perform lung function tests; in this case, diagnosis relies on subjective symptomatic improvement in response to bronchodilator therapy.

Acute severe asthma is a dangerous condition that requires hospitalization and immediate emergency treatment. It occurs when bronchospasm has progressed to a state where the patient is breathless at rest and has a degree of cardiac stress. This is usually progressive and can build up over a number of hours or even days. The breathlessness, with a peak flow rate <100 litre per minute, is so severe that the patient cannot talk or lie down. Expiration is particularly difficult and prolonged as air is trapped beneath mucosal inflammation. The pulse rate can give an indication of severity; severe acute asthma can increase the pulse rate to more than 110 beats per minute. It is common to see hyperexpansion of the thoracic cavity and lowering of the diaphragm, which means that accessory respiratory muscles are required to try to inflate the chest. Breathing can become rapid (>30 breaths/min) and shallow, leading to low arterial oxygen tension (PaO_2) with the patient becoming fatigued, cyanosed, confused and lethargic. The arterial carbon dioxide tension ($PaCO_2$) is usually low in acute asthma. If it is high it should respond quickly to emergency therapy. Hypercapnia (high $PaCO_2$ level) that does not diminish

is a more severe problem, and indicates progression towards respiratory failure.

Investigations

The function of the lungs can be measured to help diagnose and monitor various respiratory diseases. A series of routine tests has been developed to assess asthma as well as other respiratory disease such as chronic obstructive pulmonary disease (COPD).

The most useful test for abnormalities in airway function is the forced expiratory volume (FEV). This is measured by means of lung function assessment apparatus such as a spirometer. The patient inhales as deeply as possible and then exhales forcefully and completely into a mouthpiece connected to a spirometer. The FEV_1 is a measure of the forced expiratory volume in the first second of exhalation. Another volume that is commonly measured is the forced vital capacity (FVC), an assessment of the maximum volume of air exhaled with maximum effort after maximum inspiration. The FEV_1 is usually expressed as a percentage of the total volume of air exhaled, and is reported as the FEV_1/FVC ratio. This ratio is a useful and highly reproducible measure of the capabilities of the lungs. Normal individuals can exhale at least 75% of their total capacity in 1 second. Any reduction indicates a deterioration in lung performance (Fig. 25.2).

The peak flow meter is a useful means of self-assessment for the patient. It gives slightly less reproducible results than the spirometer but has the advantage that the patient can do regular tests at home with the hand-held meter. The peak flow meter measures peak expiratory flow rate (PEFR), the maximum flow rate that can be forced during expiration. The PEFR can be used to assess the improvement or deterioration in the disease as well as the effectiveness of treatment. For all three measurements (FEV_1, FVC and PEFR) there are normal values with which the patient's results can be compared. However, these normal values vary with age, race, gender, height and weight. The measurement of FEV_1, FVC or PEFR does not detect early deterioration of lung function such as bronchospasm and mucus plugging in the smaller airways.

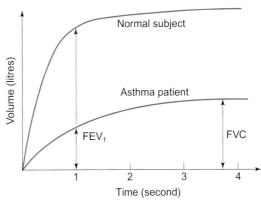

Figure 25.2 Typical lung spirometry in normal subjects and asthma patients. FEV_1/FVC is an index of airways obstruction. A decrease in FEV_1/FVC indicates obstruction.

The diagnosis of asthma can be confirmed by measuring the response to a bronchodilator or by examining a patient's day-to-day variation in PEFR readings. A variability in reading of more than 20% (and of at least 60 mL) for 3 days in a week is highly suggestive of asthma. However, individuals may not have airflow obstruction at the time of the test so the absence of an improvement does not rule out asthma. In this situation peak flow readings can be done at home with repeated pre- and post-bronchodilator readings taken at various times of the day.

Treatment

Since asthma involves inflammation and bronchoconstriction, treatment should be directed towards reducing inflammation and increasing bronchodilation. Restoration of normal airways function and prevention of severe acute attacks are the main goals of treatment. Anti-inflammatory drugs should be given to all but those with the mildest of symptoms. Other measures, such as avoidance of recognized trigger factors, may also contribute to the control of this disease. The lowest effective dose of drugs should be given to minimize short-term and long-term side effects. It should, however, always be remembered that asthma is a potentially life-threatening illness and is often undertreated. Common therapeutic problems encountered in the management of asthma are outlined in Table 25.2.

Chronic asthma

The pharmacological management of asthma depends upon the frequency and severity of a patient's symptoms. Infrequent attacks can be managed by treating each attack when it occurs, but with more frequent attacks preventive therapy needs to be used.

The preferred route of administration of the agents used in the management of asthma is by inhalation. This allows the drugs to be delivered directly to the airways in smaller doses and with fewer side effects than if systemic routes were used.

Table 25.2 Common therapeutic problems in asthma

- Asthma is underdiagnosed, especially in the elderly

- Failing to avoid or reduce the effect of allergens

- Lack of patient knowledge about the condition and its management

- Knowing when to start anti-inflammatory therapy

- Taking anti-inflammatory therapy on an 'as required' basis rather than regularly as no short-term benefit is felt by the patient

- Patients or health professionals missing the signs of rapidly deteriorating asthma control

- Incorrect technique in the use of inhalers and drug delivery devices

- Little published evidence to guide the best management of asthma in children under 12 years, particularly the under-2 year old age group

---

Inhaled bronchodilators also have a faster onset of action than when administered systemically and give better protection from bronchoconstriction.

Treatment of chronic asthma is usually given in a stepwise progression, as outlined in Figure 25.3, according to the severity of the patient's asthma symptoms and response to current treatment. At each stage the patient's inhaler technique should be assessed. If necessary, the type of inhalation device used should be changed to improve patient compliance.

To help in patient education, the terms used to describe the effects of asthma medication are similar across all manufacturers and sources of education. 'Reliever' is used for agents that give immediate relief of symptoms. Agents that act to reduce inflammation or give long-term bronchodilation are referred to as 'controllers', 'protectors' or 'preventers'.

Reliever medication

β-Adrenoceptor agonist bronchodilators β-Adrenoceptor agonists are the mainstay of asthma management. Salbutamol and terbutaline are selective β_2-agonists and have few β_1-mediated side effects, particularly cardiotoxicity. β_2-Receptors are, however, also present in myocardial tissue; cardiovascular stimulation resulting in tachycardia and palpitations is still the main dose-limiting toxicity with these agents when used in high dosage.

An inhaled β_2-agonist is the first-line agent in the management of asthma. This is used as required by the patient for the symptomatic relief of breathlessness and wheezing, for example salbutamol 200 µg when required. This may be the only treatment necessary for those with infrequent symptoms. There is no advantage to regular administration.

Additional bronchodilators Additional bronchodilators may be required if the above therapy does not adequately control symptoms (Tables 25.3 and 25.4).

Inhaled anticholinergic agents These block muscarinic receptors in bronchial smooth muscle and can be added to the treatment regimen, for example as an alternative at step 3 of Figure 25.3. They have a slower onset of action than β_2-agonists but a longer duration of action. The anticholinergics may be especially helpful in the elderly in whom asthma may be complicated by a degree of obstructive airways disease.

Oral bronchodilators Oral bronchodilators can also be added, for example theophylline at step 3 or β_2-agonists at step 4 for additional symptom control. Slow-release forms should be used; these are especially useful in a single night-time dose if nocturnal symptoms are troublesome although twice-daily dosing is more usual. Oral bronchodilators may also become necessary in patients who are unable to use inhaler therapy effectively. Side effects are more pronounced with oral therapy.

Theophylline should be started at a dose of 400–500 mg/day in adults and, if required, increased after 7 days to 800–1000 mg/day. In children higher doses may be required but this will be determined by the age of the child (see Chapter 10, Paediatrics, for explanation).

Theophylline has a narrow therapeutic index and its hepatic metabolism varies greatly between individuals. Theophylline clearance is affected by a variety of factors, including disease states and concurrent drug therapy. The dose used should

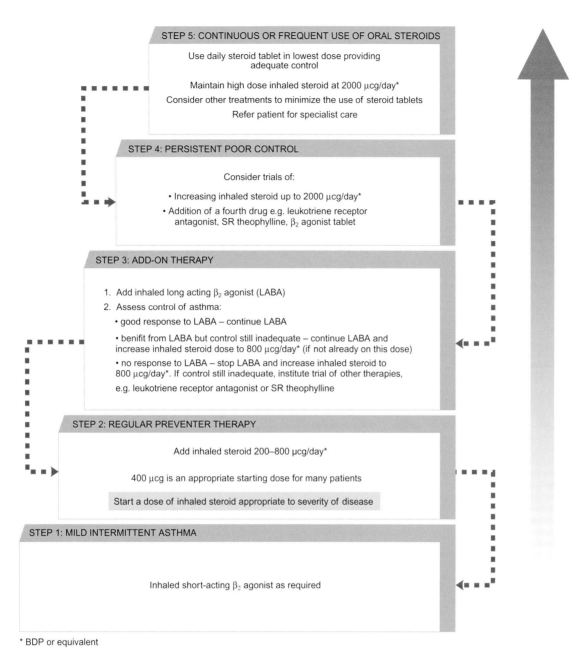

STEP 5: CONTINUOUS OR FREQUENT USE OF ORAL STEROIDS

Use daily steroid tablet in lowest dose providing
adequate control

Maintain high dose inhaled steroid at 2000 μcg/day*

Consider other treatments to minimize the use of steroid tablets

Refer patient for specialist care

STEP 4: PERSISTENT POOR CONTROL

Consider trials of:

• Increasing inhaled steroid up to 2000 μcg/day*

• Addition of a fourth drug e.g. leukotriene receptor
antagonist, SR theophylline, β₂ agonist tablet

STEP 3: ADD-ON THERAPY

1. Add inhaled long acting β₂ agonist (LABA)

2. Assess control of asthma:

• good response to LABA – continue LABA

• benifit from LABA but control still inadequate – continue LABA and
increase inhaled steroid dose to 800 μcg/day* (if not already on this dose)

• no response to LABA – stop LABA and increase inhaled steroid to
800 μcg/day*. If control still inadequate, institute trial of other therapies,

e.g. leukotriene receptor antagonist or SR theophylline

STEP 2: REGULAR PREVENTER THERAPY

Add inhaled steroid 200–800 μcg/day*

400 μcg is an appropriate starting dose for many patients

Start a dose of inhaled steroid appropriate to severity of disease

STEP 1: MILD INTERMITTENT ASTHMA

Inhaled short-acting β₂ agonist as required

* BDP or equivalent

Figure 25.3 Stepwise management of asthma in adults (reproduced by permission of the BMJ Publishing Group, from BTS/SIGN 2005).

therefore take into account these factors, which are listed in Table 25.5. Plasma levels may be taken after 3–4 days at the higher dose and it has been normal practice to adjust the dose to keep the plasma level within a therapeutic window of 10–20 mg/L although improvements in respiratory function are seen at levels as low as 5 mg/L in some patients. Because the bronchodilating effects of theophylline are proportional to the log of the plasma concentrations, there is proportionally less bronchodilation as the plasma level increases. The mild side effects such as nausea and vomiting are seen at concentrations as low as 13 mg/L but are more common over 20 mg/L. Significant cardiac symptoms, tachycardia and persistent vomiting are usually seen at concentrations of 40 mg/L while severe CNS effects, such as

seizures, have been seen at 30 mg/L but are more common above 50 mg/L.

Only modified-release preparations should be used and once stabilized on a particular product, the patient should not be changed to another theophylline preparation, as there are large differences in plasma profiles with the different preparations. Normal-release theophylline preparations should not be used because of their rapid absorption and highly variable clearance, giving short and unpredictable durations of action.

High-dose β₂-agonists High-dose β₂-agonists are only considered if conventional doses do not achieve adequate symptom control. Nebulized drugs such as salbutamol 2.5–5 mg per dose are given.

Table 25.3 Comparison of inhaled bronchodilators

Drug	Onset of action (min)	Peak action (min)	Duration of action (h)
Ipratropium	3–10	60–120	4–6
Oxitropium	5–10	60–120	7.5–12
Salbutamol	5–15	60[a]	4–6
Salmeterol	14[a]	150[a]	12[a]
Terbutaline	5–30	60–120	3–6

[a] Approximate or median value

Terbutaline has been given by continuous subcutaneous infusion in the treatment of 'brittle' asthma, where there is an unpredictable and rapid development of airway narrowing, causing sudden onset of acute, severe life-threatening asthma.

Controller medication

Inhaled anti-inflammatory agents   Regular anti-inflammatory treatment should be used for patients with recent exacerbations, nocturnal asthma, impaired lung function or if using their inhaled bronchodilator more than once a day (BTS/SIGN 2005). Corticosteroids are the most commonly used anti-inflammatory agents but others such as the cromones are available (Table 25.6). The molecular mechanism of action of corticosteroids has still to be fully elucidated (Barnes 2003).

Table 25.4 Daily dose range for selected bronchodilators

Drug and route	Age and total daily dosage range			
Aminophylline				
Intravenous injection	Adult 5 mg/kg (single dose)	1 month–18 years 5 mg/kg (single dose) up to 500 mg maximum		
Intravenous infusion	16 years–adult 500 µg/kg/h	9–16 years 800 µg/kg/h	1 month–9 years 1 mg/kg/h	
Oral	12 years–adult 225–450 mg m/r twice a day	3–12 years 6–20 mg/kg m/r twice a day		
Formoterol				
Inhaled	6 years–adult 4.5–24 µg twice a day			
Ipratropium bromide				
Inhaled	6 years–adult 20–40 µg 3–4 times daily	1 month–6 years 20 µg 3–4 times daily		
Nebulized for acute bronchospasm	Adult 500 µg repeated as necessary	6–12 years 250–500 µg repeated as necessary (max. 1 mg daily)	Under 6 years 125–250 µg repeated as necessary (max. 1 mg daily)	
Salbutamol				
Inhaled	Adult 200 µg when required, up to four times a day	Child 100 µg when required, up to four times a day		
Nebulized for acute severe bronchospasm	Adult 2.5–5 mg repeated as necessary	6–18 years 2.5–5 mg repeated every 20–30 min if necessary	2–5 years 2.5 mg repeated every 20–30 min if necessary	Under 2 years 2.5 mg repeated every 20–30 min if necessary
Salmeterol				
Inhaled	12 years–adult 50–100 µg twice a day	4–12 years 50 µg twice a day	2–4 years 25 µg twice a day	
Terbutaline				
Inhaled	Adult 250–500 µg when required, up to four times a day	1 month–18 years 250–500 µg when required, up to four times a day		
Nebulized for acute severe bronchospasm	Adult 5–10 mg repeated as necessary	6–18 years 5–10 mg repeated every 20–30 min if necessary	2–5 years 5 mg repeated every 20–30 min if necessary	Under 2 years 5 mg repeated every 20–30 min if necessary
Theophylline Oral	12 years–adult 175–500 mg (m/r) twice a day	6–12 years 175–250 mg (m/r) twice a day		

Table 25.5 Factors affecting theophylline clearance

Decreased clearance	Increased clearance
Congestive cardiac failure	Cigarette smoking
Cor pulmonale	Children 1–12 years
Chronic obstructive pulmonary disease	High-protein, low-carbohydrate diet
Viral pneumonia	Barbecued meat
Acute pulmonary oedema	Carbamazepine
Cirrhosis	Phenobarbital
Premature and term babies	Phenytoin
Elderly	Sulfinpyrazone
Obesity	
High-carbohydrate, low-protein diet	
Cimetidine	
Erythromycin	
Oral contraceptives	
Ciprofloxacin	
Propranolol	

Corticosteroids   Corticosteroids suppress the chronic airway inflammation associated with asthma. At present, inhaled corticosteroids are the initial drugs of choice, with a starting dose for an adult of beclometasone or budesonide 400 μg per day (or an equivalent) given in divided doses.

The threshold frequency of β_2-agonist use which prompts the start of corticosteroid therapy has not been fully established but national guidance (BTS/SIGN 2005) recommends considering steroids for patients with any of the following.

- Exacerbations of asthma in the last 2 years.
- Using inhaled β_2-agonists three times a week or more.
- Symptoms three times a week or more, or waking one night a week.

If symptoms persist the steroid dose is increased stepwise accordingly. The dose of inhaled corticosteroid should be reduced, if possible, once symptoms and peak expiratory flow rates have improved and stabilized.

If a patient's asthma cannot be controlled by the above dose of inhaled corticosteroid and the inhaler technique and compliance are adequate, the dose can be increased to a maximum of 1.5–2 mg a day. Adrenal suppression may occur at these maximal doses so patients should carry a steroid warning card. Oropharyngeal side effects such as candidiasis are also more common at the higher doses of steroids, e.g. 500 μg a day or more of fluticasone (Table 25.7). Measures to minimize this can be tried, such as using a large-volume spacer device and rinsing the mouth with water or brushing teeth after inhalation, but there is little evidence to confirm how effective these are.

Cromones   Inhaled sodium cromoglicate and nedocromil sodium are less effective than cortocosteroids in asthma. Although rarely used, they may be possible alternatives if corticosteroids cannot be tolerated.

Long acting β-adrenoreceptor agonist bronchodilators (LABA)   When low-dose inhaled steroids fail to control asthma symptoms adequately at step 3, long-acting β_2-agonists should be added instead of increasing the steroid dose. Symptom relief after a trial period, e.g. 4–6 weeks, must then be assessed to see if the LABA has been effective and whether treatment needs to

Table 25.6 Drugs used for the prophylaxis of asthma

Drug and age range	Total daily dosage range	
	Standard dose	High dose
Beclometasone diproprionate or budesonide		
Adult	100–400 μg twice a day	400–1000 μg twice a day
12–18 years	100–400 μg twice a day	400–1000 μg twice a day
5–12 years	100–200 μg twice a day	Up to 400 μg twice a day
2–5 years	100–200 μg twice a day	Up to 400 μg twice a day
Under 2 years	50–100 μg twice a day	Up to 200 μg twice a day
Beclometasone diproprionate CFC-free (Qvar® brand)[a]		
Adult	50–200 μg twice a day	200–500 μg twice a day
Ciclesonide		
Adult	80 μg once daily	160 μg once daily
Fluticasone		
Adult	50–200 μg twice a day	400–1000 μg twice a day
12–18 years	50–200 μg twice a day	400–1000 μg twice a day
5–12 years	50–100 μg twice a day	100–200 μg twice a day
Under 5 years	50–100 μg twice a day	100–200 μg twice a day
Mometasone		
Adult	200–400 μg once daily	400 μg twice a day

[a] Owing to the bioavailability differences in non-CFC steroid inhalers, dosing is quoted for the individual brand.

Table 25.7 Adverse reactions associated with drugs used in the management of asthma

β_2-agonists
- By inhalation: adverse drug reactions are uncommon
- Nebulization, orally or parenterally: fine tremor (usually the hands), nervous tension, headache, peripheral vasodilation, tachycardia. The adverse reactions often diminish as tolerance develops with continued administration
- High doses: hypokalaemia, aggravation of angina

Inhaled corticosteroids
- Hoarseness, oral or pharyngeal candidiasis
- Adrenal suppression may occur with high doses, e.g. beclometasone diproprionate above 1500 μg daily

Oral corticosteroids
- Prolonged use of these results in exaggeration of some of the normal physiological effects of steroids
- Mineralocorticoid effects include: hypertension, potassium loss, muscle weakness, and sodium and water retention. These effects are most notable with fludrocortisone, are significant with hydrocortisone, occur only slightly with prednisolone and methylprednisolone and are negligible with dexametasone and betametasone
- Glucocorticoid effects include: precipitation of diabetes, osteoporosis, development of a paranoic state, depression, euphoria, peptic ulceration, immunosuppression, Cushing's syndrome (moon face, striae and acne), growth suppression in children, worsening of infection: skin thinning, striae atrophicae, increased hair growth, perioral dermatitis and acne
- Adrenal suppression occurs with high doses and/or prolonged treatment. Steroid therapy must be gradually withdrawn in these patients to avoid precipitating an adrenal crisis of hypotension, weight loss, arthralgia and, sometimes, death

Ipratropium bromide
- Occasionally: dry mouth
- Precipitation of acute glaucoma with nebulized therapy, possibly worsened by co-administration of salbutamol. A mouthpiece should be used to minimize the exposure of the eyes to the nebulized drug
- Rarely: systemic anticholinergic effects such as urinary retention and constipation

Methotrexate
- Myelosuppression, mucositis and, rarely, pneumonitis

Nedocromil sodium
- Mild and transient nausea, coughing, transient bronchospasm, throat irritation, headache and a bitter taste

Sodium cromoglicate
- Coughing, transient bronchospasm and throat irritation due to inhalation of the powder

Theophylline
- Although about 5% of the population experience minor adverse effects (nausea, diarrhoea, nervousness and headache), increasing the plasma concentration results in more serious effects. The following is a guide to the plasma levels at which the adverse reactions usually occur:
  - Above 20 mg/L: persistent vomiting, insomnia, gastrointestinal bleeding, cardiac arrhythmias
  - Above 35 mg/L: hyperglycaemia, hypotension, more serious cardiac arrhythmias, convulsions, permanent brain damage and death
- Individual patients may suffer these effects at plasma levels other than those quoted, for example convulsions have occurred in patients at 25 mg/L

Leukotriene receptor antagonists
- Abdominal pain, headache, diarrhoea, dizziness, upper respiratory tract infections
- Rarely: acute hepatitis (associated with zafirlukast), Churg–Strauss syndrome

be added to or changed. Patients should be reminded that these agents are an addition to their short-acting agents, not a replacement, and are unsuitable for acute symptom relief due to their slower onset of action.

Leukotriene antagonists Drugs are being developed with the goal of attenuating the effects of leukotrienes in asthma. Two leukotriene receptor antagonists, montelukast and zafirlukast, are currently licensed in the UK. They are less effective than corticosteroids in controlling asthma but are effective in combination with steroids and are included in step 4 as add-on therapy for adult patients. Although available only in oral formulations, they are generally well tolerated. If these agents are initiated then a 4–6 week trial should be undertaken; if there is no improvement in control, the drug should be stopped. They seem to be of particular value in aspirin-induced asthma, possibly due to the role of leukotrienes in this form of asthma.

Anti-IgE monoclonal antibodies The first of these agents to reach the market was omalizumab. Although its role in the stepwise management of asthma has yet to be determined, it may be of benefit to patients with severe persistent allergic asthma. The high cost of these agents may influence their cost-effectiveness and ultimate place in therapy.

Oral corticosteroids Oral corticosteroids should only be used, at step 5, if symptom control cannot be achieved with maximum doses of inhaled bronchodilators and steroids. They should be given as a single morning dose to minimize adrenal suppression. Alternate-day dosing produces fewer side effects but is less effective in controlling asthma.

Short courses (of up to 3 weeks) of high-dose oral steroids, 30–60 mg daily, can be safely used during exacerbations of asthma.

Steroid-sparing agents Some agents are being investigated in patients who are dependent on systemic steroids in an attempt to reduce the steroid dose. Methotrexate, ciclosporin and gold have been tried with varying success. All have potentially toxic side effects and need to be closely monitored.

Acute severe asthma

The management of acute asthma depends on the severity of the attack and its response to treatment, as well as an appreciation of the patient's past history and present treatment. If an acute attack becomes persistent and difficult to treat, it is known as acute severe asthma.

The aims of treatment are to prevent any deterioration in the patient's condition and hasten recovery.

Prevention of an acute attack

The ideal way of treating an acute attack is to educate patients to recognize when their condition is deteriorating so that they can initiate treatment to prevent the attack becoming severe. This can be achieved with an individualized self-management plan

The dose of inhaled β_2-agonist should be increased, and a short course of oral steroids commenced, e.g. prednisolone at a dose of 40–60 mg every morning for 1 week. The dose of inhaled corticosteroid is often also increased but there is limited evidence to support this.

If the condition deteriorates further, hospital admission may become necessary. This could be a self-referral from the patient, responding to criteria drawn up by the doctor, such as their PEFR falling below 50% of their usual best. The education of patients and their relatives in the management of acute attacks should always stress the prompt initiation of further treatment and early referral.

Immediate management of acute severe asthma

The immediate treatment of acute severe asthma should take place in the patient's home, during the ambulance journey or immediately on admission to hospital. One suggested treatment protocol for management in the emergency department is outlined in Figure 25.4.

Oxygen is administered in a high concentration, at high flow rates, particularly for severe and life-threatening exacerbations. A β_2-agonist is administered, which should give prompt bronchodilation lasting 4–6 hours.

In mild-to-moderate exacerbations the β_2-agonist can be administered by metered dose inhaler with a spacer attachment (4–6 puffs) as there is no demonstrable difference between this and using a nebulizer. With severe symptoms, nebulizers are used in preference to conventional inhalers because they permit a high dose (10–20 times the dose of a metered dose inhaler)

and they require no co-ordination on the part of the patient between inspiration and actuation, which is helpful in those distressed or for those who panic. Some devices also allow the co-administration of oxygen. Patients undergoing an acute attack often have an inspiratory rate that is too low to use a metered dose inhaler effectively. If a nebulizer is not immediately available, multiple actuations of a metered dose inhaler into a large-volume spacer device is an acceptable alternative. Salbutamol at doses of 2–5 mg (20–50 puffs, given five puffs at a time into the spacer) has been used.

Corticosteroids are also given in the acute attack. If PEFR is below 50%, oral prednisolone (40–50 mg, for 5 days) is given. Intravenous hydrocortisone (100 mg) should only be used if the patient cannot take oral medication. This reduces and prevents the inflammation that causes oedema and hypersecretion of mucus and hence helps to relieve the resultant smooth muscle spasm. The clinical response to both oral and parenteral steroids has an onset at 1–2 hours with a peak effect at 6–8 hours.

If life-threatening features are present, such as cyanosis, bradycardia, confusion, exhaustion or unconsciousness, higher dose bronchodilators are used: salbutamol 5 mg with ipratropium bromide 500 μg, repeated after 15 minutes and regularly if required. The addition of the anticholinergic often gives a response that is greater than that of the two agents used alone. Intravenous aminophylline can be given with a bolus dose of 250 mg over 30 minutes, followed by a continuous infusion of 500 μg/kg/h. The bolus should be omitted if the patient is known to take oral theophylline or aminophylline. The choice between intravenous aminophylline and β_2-agonist depends on concurrent therapy and side effect profiles. The dose of intravenous aminophylline used must also take into account recent theophylline therapy in addition to other factors (Table 25.8). Serious toxicity can occur with parenteral aminophylline and patients must be carefully monitored for nausea and vomiting, the most common early signs of toxicity. If the aminophylline infusion is continued for more than 24 hours, the plasma theophylline concentration may be measured to guide any necessary alteration in infusion rate in order to maintain the level in the optimum range of 10–20 mg/L.

Intravenous magnesium sulphate, 1.2–2 g as a 20-minute infusion, has been shown to help in some patients who have not had a good response to initial treatment. There is, however, no evidence to support repeated dosing regardless of therapeutic outcome.

Further deterioration in condition may require assisted mechanical ventilation on an intensive care unit. Regular monitoring of arterial blood gases and oxygen saturation is performed to help detect any deterioration in condition.

Antibiotics are only indicated where there is evidence of a bacterial infection.

Subsequent management of acute severe asthma

The subsequent management of acute severe asthma depends on the patient's clinical response. All patients should be monitored throughout their treatment with objective measures of their PEFRs before and after bronchodilator treatment and with continual monitoring of their arterial blood gas concentrations to ensure adequate oxygen is being given.

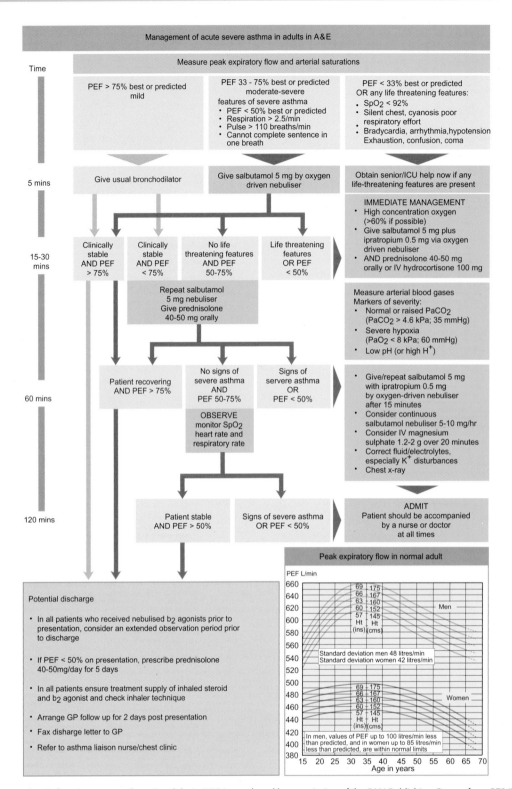

Figure 25.4 Management of acute severe asthma in adults in A&E (reproduced by permission of the BMJ Publishing Group, from BTS/SIGN 2005).

As the patient responds to treatment, infusions can be stopped and other treatment changed or tailed off as described above. As improvement continues, an inhaled β2-agonist is substituted for the nebulized form and the oral corticosteroids stopped or reduced to a maintenance dose if clinically necessary. Throughout the treatment programme, potential drug interactions should be anticipated and managed appropriately (Table 25.9).

All patients should have their inhaler technique checked, and any observed problems should be corrected before discharge. If necessary, alternative devices may be tried. A self-management

Table 25.8 Intravenous aminophylline dosing in acute severe asthma

	Aminophylline dose	Patient characteristics
Loading dose	5 mg/kg over 20–30 min	Adults and children
	3 mg/kg over 10–15 min	Previous theophylline therapy (although some authorities do not use a loading dose in these patients)
Maintenance dose	500 µg/kg/h	Non-smoking adults
	700 µg/kg/h	Children under 12 or smokers
	200 µg/kg/h	Cardiac failure, liver impairment, pneumonia

plan should be drawn up and discussed with each patient. Early primary care follow-up and referral to a hospital specialist are recommended.

Patient care

The correct use of drugs and the education of patients are the cornerstones of asthma management. There are three main steps in the education of the asthmatic patient.

1. The patient should have an understanding of the action of each of the medicines they use.
2. The appropriate choice of inhalation device(s) should be made and the patient educated to use them correctly.
3. An individualized action (self-management) plan should be developed for each patient.

All members of the healthcare team should provide education and support for the asthmatic patient at regular intervals. The need for each patient to understand their asthma and its management must be balanced against the dangers of overwhelming the patient with information, particularly when the asthma has been newly diagnosed. To try to overcome this, a 'ladder of asthma knowledge' has been proposed. Patients are counselled in a gradual manner, each session adding to the previous one in content and reinforcing existing knowledge (Table 25.10).

Patient knowledge of asthma treatment

Increasing patients' knowledge about their asthma therapy is a necessary component of asthma management. However, education alone has not been shown to have a beneficial effect on morbidity. Education programmes must, therefore, also look at modifying a patient's behaviour and attitude to asthma. Counselling should lead to increased patient confidence in the ability to self-manage asthma, decrease hospital admission rates and emergency visits by primary care doctors, increase compliance and improve quality of life.

Table 25.9 Common clinically significant interactions with drugs used in the management of asthma

Drug	Interacting drug	Probable mechanism and clinical result
β₂-agonists	β-Adrenoreceptor antagonists	Antagonism of bronchodilator effect. More marked with non–selective antagonists
	Corticosteroids	Increased risk of hypokalaemia with high-dose β₂-agonists
	Diuretics	Increased risk of hypokalaemia with high-dose β₂-agonists
	Methyldopa	Acute hypotension possible with β₂-agonist infusions
Corticosteroids	Anticoagulants	High-dose steroids enhance anticoagulant effect of coumarins
	β₂-agonists	Increased risk of hypokalaemia with high doses
	Antifungals	Metabolism of steroids possibly affected by antifungal agents
	Carbamazepine	Reduced steroid effect due to increased metabolism
	Barbiturates	Accelerates steroid metabolism
	Ciclosporin	Increases plasma concentration of prednisolone
	Methotrexate	Increased risk of haematological toxicity
Theophylline	Azithromycin	May increase theophylline plasma levels
	β₂-agonists (high dose)	Increased risk of hypokalaemia
	Carbamazepine	Induction of theophylline metabolism resulting in decreased plasma levels
	Clarithromycin	Inhibition of theophylline metabolism resulting in increased plasma levels
	Cimetidine	Inhibition of theophylline metabolism resulting in increased plasma levels
	Ciprofloxacin	Increased plasma concentration. Possible risk of convulsions
	Diltiazem	Increased theophylline plasma levels
	Erythromycin (oral)	Inhibition of theophylline metabolism resulting in increased plasma levels

continued

Table 25.9 (continued)

Drug	Interacting drug	Probable mechanism and clinical result
Theophylline (continued)	Fluconazole	Possible increase in theophylline plasma level
	Fluvoxamine	Increased theophylline plasma levels, halve theophylline dose
	Isoniazid	May increase theophylline plasma levels
	Ketoconazole	Possible increase in theophylline plasma level
	Lithium carbonate	Reducing plasma lithium concentrations as theophylline enhances lithium renal clearance
	Norfloxacin	Increased plasma concentration. Possible risk of convulsions
	Phenytoin	Plasma concentrations of theophylline and phenytoin both reduced
	Primidone	Induction of theophylline metabolism resulting in decreased plasma levels
	Rifampicin	Induction of theophylline metabolism resulting in decreased plasma levels
	Smoking (tobacco)	Induction of theophylline metabolism resulting in decreased plasma levels
	St John's wort	Reduced theophylline plasma levels
	Verapamil	Increased theophylline plasma levels

Table 25.10 Ladder of asthma knowledge for patients

Step 1	Patient/carer understands what relief medication does, side effects which may occur, aims of treatment, what is happening to them and their chest. Education material is made available
Step 2	Patient/carer accepts and agrees about use of medication, importance of preventers and recognition of symptoms
Step 3	Patient/carer knows how to monitor peak expiratory flow (PEF) and symptoms, when to increase dose of inhaled steroids and contact their medical practice
Step 4	Patient/carer confident to manage own medication, increasing and decreasing dose using PEF or symptom monitoring, start oral steroids and attend their medical practice

Specific counselling on drug therapy should concentrate on three areas: drugs used to relieve symptoms, drugs used to prevent asthma attacks and those drugs which are given only as reserve treatment for severe attacks.

Choice of inhalation device

The choice of a suitable inhalation device is vital in asthma management. The incorrect use of inhalers will lead to suboptimal treatment. This has been demonstrated to occur in up to 75% of patients using metered dose inhalers. There is no demonstrable difference in efficacy between the various devices available. Other factors, therefore, need to be considered when choosing the appropriate device, including the patient's age, severity of disease, manual dexterity, co-ordination and personal preference. The range of different devices available for the drugs commonly used in asthma is shown in Table 25.11.

Metered dose aerosol inhalers The pressurized, metered dose inhaler (MDI), illustrated in Figure 25.5, is the most widely prescribed inhalation device in the UK. It usually contains a suspension of active drug, with a typical particle size of 2–5 μm, in a liquefied propellant. Operation of the device releases a metered dose of the drug with a droplet size of 35–45 μm. The increased droplet size is due to the propellant, which evaporates when expelled from the inhaler. A transition from the older chlorofluorocarbon (CFC) propellants to newer hydrofluoroalkanes, which do not damage the ozone layer, has taken place. Care must be taken when converting a patient from CFC to non-CFC propellant inhalers as with some formulations the dosage is not equivalent. Changes in response and symptom control should be monitored. Patients should be advised that the taste and 'plume', i.e. the spread and velocity of the actuation, may also change.

MDIs have the advantage of being multidose, small and widely available for most of the drugs used for asthma management. Their main disadvantage is that correct use requires a good technique. A particular problem for many patients is co-ordinating the beginning of inspiration with the actuation of the inhaler. Even when this is done correctly, MDIs only deliver about 10% of drug to the airways, with 80% deposited in the oropharynx. Other disadvantages include irritation in the pharynx and bronchi, which inhibits further inspiration, caused by the cold propellant. Corticosteroids administered by MDIs can cause dysphonia and oral candidiasis. The candidiasis can be minimized either by advising patients to gargle with water after using the inhaler and to expel the water from the mouth afterwards, or by using a spacer device.

Younger children in particular find MDIs difficult to use and the addition of a spacer device can make this easier, allowing inhalation over several ambient breaths.

The correct technique for using metered dose inhalers is as follows.

1. MDIs have a mouthpiece dustcap which has to be removed before use (often patients do not remove this). The cap must be replaced after use to prevent subsequent inhalation of foreign bodies.
2. The MDI must be vigorously shaken. This distributes the drug particles uniformly throughout the propellant (newer CFC-free inhalers may be solutions and not require shaking – see manufacturer's literature). The MDI must be held upright.

Table 25.11 Inhalation devices and spacer devices available

Drug	Type of inhaler device						
	Metered dose inhaler	Breath-actuated metered dose inhaler	Single-dose dry powder	Multiple-dose dry powder	Nebulizer	Large-volume spacer for MDI	Small-volume spacer for MDI
Salbutamol	✓	✓	✓	✓	✓	✓	✓
Ipratropium	✓		✓		✓		✓
Terbutaline				✓	✓		
Salmeterol	✓	✓		✓		✓	✓
Formoterol			✓	✓			
Tiotropium[a]			✓				
Beclometasone	✓	✓	✓	✓		✓	✓
Budesonide	✓			✓	✓	✓	✓
Ciclesonide	✓						✓
Fluticasone	✓			✓	✓	✓	✓
Mometasone				✓			
Cromoglicate	✓	✓	✓		✓	✓	✓
Nedocromil	✓					✓	✓

[a] Only licensed for use in COPD

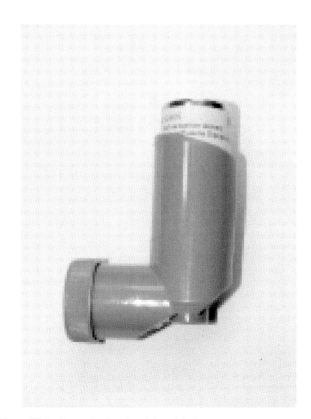

Figure 25.5 Pressurized metered dose inhaler.

3. The patient should breathe out gently, but not fully.
4. The tongue should be placed on the floor of the mouth and the inhaler placed between the lips, which are then closed round the mouthpiece.
5. The patient should now start to breathe in slowly and deeply through the mouth.
6. The canister is pressed to release the dose while the patient continues to breathe in. This synchronization of inspiration and actuation, so that there is a supporting stream of air to carry the drug to the lungs, is probably the most common point of failure in those with bad inhalation technique. Patients who are very short of breath, for example during a severe asthma attack, find this particularly difficult.
7. The breath is held for at least 10 seconds. This allows the drug particles reaching the periphery of the lung to settle under gravity. Using this technique, about 15% of a dose may reach the lungs. Exhalation should be through the nose.
8. If a second dose is called for, at least 1 minute should elapse before repeating the inhalation procedure. During actuation, the temperature of the MDI actuator stem and valve drops, and should theoretically be allowed to warm up. In practice, however, this may not be very important.

Studies indicate that personal tuition improves inhaler technique, particularly if regularly repeated. Other methods of instruction include videos (see http://medguides.medicines.org. uk/demonstrations.aspx), package inserts and information leaflets or booklets provided by Asthma UK and the pharmaceutical industry.

The scoring of inhalation technique using checklists (Table 25.12) has been advocated, which can be kept as a permanent record by any of the healthcare professionals.

Metered dose inhaler with a spacer extension Extension devices allow greater evaporation of the propellant, so reducing particle size and velocity. This also reduces oropharyngeal deposition and potentially increases lung deposition. Oral candidiasis and dysphonia (impaired voice) from inhaled corticosteroids may be reduced by using these devices. Spacers are useful for people who have poor co-ordination between inspiration and actuation. Several types are available. In younger children these offer advantages over MDIs alone with respect to compliance. Recommendations have been published regarding device choice (NICE 2000, 2002) (see Table 25.13).

Large-volume (750 mL) spacers are available and include the Volumatic (Fig. 25.6) and the Nebuhaler; these are manufacturer specific and have not been fully assessed with devices of other companies. These spacers have one-way inhalation valves that allow several inhalations of one dose from the spacer's chamber.

No co-ordination is required between actuation of the MDI and inhalation. A large-volume spacer has been used instead of a nebulizer to deliver high doses of a β_2-agonist in acute severe asthma attacks. Disadvantages of these spacers include their large size, which renders them less portable, and their proven efficacy only with inhalers from the same manufacturer. Spacers should be washed regularly in warm, soapy water and left to drip dry without rinsing. Cloths should not be used for drying as this affects the antistatic coating of plastic spacers; a metal one is available without this problem. All spacers should be replaced every 6–12 months. Facemasks are available for young children.

Small- and medium-volume spacer devices are also available, either as an integral part of the design of some MDIs or as a separate device (Fig. 25.7). These spacers have also been used to compensate for poor inhalation technique in adults and reduce oropharyngeal deposition of steroid. These are more convenient to carry around than the larger spacers and often will fit devices from several manufacturers. The published evidence of additional benefit from these devices in either increasing efficacy or decreasing adverse effects is limited.

Breath-actuated metered dose inhalers These MDIs are actuated automatically by inspiratory flow rates of about 22–36 L/min. One type is illustrated in Figure 25.8. These eliminate the need for the correct co-ordination of inspiration and actuation but require priming before each actuation.

Dry powder inhalers Several types of dry powder inhalers (DPI) are available. These are propellant free and are designed to be easier to use than conventional MDIs. They are useful for those who have difficulty co-ordinating an MDI and can be used by children as young as 4 years old. Table 25.13 gives the current recommendations for device choice in children (NICE 2000, 2002).

Dry powder inhalers are available as either single-dose or multiple-dose devices (Fig. 25.9). Single-dose devices pierce or break a gelatin capsule to release the contents and must be regularly cleaned to avoid powder clogging the device. Multiple-dose devices are preferred by many patients since they avoid having to reload for each dose. Care must be taken to hold these devices in the correct orientation to avoid the powder falling out of the device before inhalation.

Nebulizers A nebulizer produces an aerosol by blowing air or oxygen through a solution to produce droplets of 5 μm or less in size. Nebulizers require little co-ordination from the patient as any drug is inhaled through a facemask or mouthpiece using

Table 25.12 MDI technique score chart
1. Shake vigorously
2. Remove cap
3. Hold upright
4. Breathe out gently, not fully
5. Start breathing in slowly and deeply
6. Actuate during inspiration
7. Continue slow inhalation
8. No aerosol loss is visible
9. Hold breath 10 seconds
10. Next dose after 1 minute

Score 1 for each correct step undertaken. This gives a score out of 10 that can be used to monitor a patient's performance and highlight any problem areas.

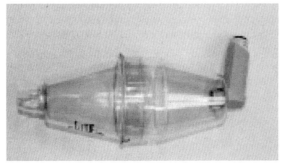

Figure 25.6 Large-volume spacer (Volumatic®).

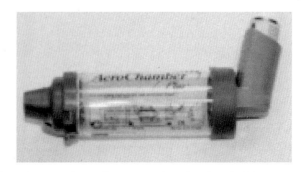

Figure 25.7 Medium-volume spacer (Aerochamber Plus®).

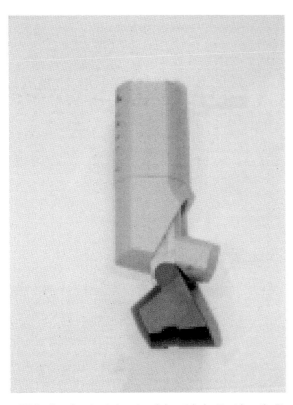

Figure 25.8   Breath-actuated metered dose inhaler (Easi-breathe®).

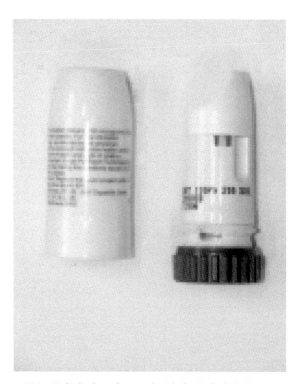

Figure 25.9   Multiple-dose dry powder inhaler (Turbohaler®).

Table 25.13   Inhaler device choice for children

Age group	Drug group	1st choice device	2nd choice device
0–2 years	All	MDI + spacer + facemask	Nebulizer
3–4 years	All	MDI + spacer	Nebulizer or dry powder
5–15 years	Bronchodilators	MDI or dry powder or breath-actuated MDI	
5–15 years	Corticosteroids	MDI + spacer	Dry powder or breath-actuated MDI

normal tidal breathing. Only about 13% of the dose used is deposited in the lungs, but because the doses used are higher than those used in other aerosol devices, patients will generally receive a higher dose than from an MDI. In clinical practice, however, for example in mild and moderate asthma exacerbations, no benefit has been shown over using 4–6 puffs of a MDI.

Nebulizers are useful in patients who are unable to use conventional inhalers, for example children under 2 years old, patients with severe attacks of asthma unable to produce sufficient inspiratory effort and those lacking the co-ordination to use other inhalers. Nebulized bronchodilators can be used in acute severe asthma attacks, often avoiding the need for intravenous drugs,

and in conjunction with prophylactic agents in the treatment of chronic asthma unresponsive to or poorly controlled by conventional treatment.

Most of the short-acting β_2-agonists, as well as ipratropium bromide, fluticasone, budesonide and sodium cromoglicate, are available for nebulization. The majority of these preparations are made up in isotonic 0.9% sodium chloride and are available in preservative-free, unit dose presentations. The use of solutions that are either hypertonic or hypotonic, particularly after dilution with water, or that contain a preservative such as benzalkonium chloride or EDTA, has been associated with bronchoconstriction.

The safe and correct use of nebulizers requires careful counselling, especially if they are to be used in the home. The following points are critical for the correct use of a nebulizer.

1. Nebulizers should only be driven by compressed air or by oxygen at flow rates of at least 5–6 L/min to ensure that droplets of the correct size are produced.
2. To maximize nebulized drug, a minimum volume of 3–4 mL should ideally be nebulized. This volume is required to reduce the amount of drug that is unavoidably left in a 'dead-space' fluid volume of about 1 mL at the end of nebulization, although this is less with newer nebulizers and no further dilution of commercial nebulizer solutions is used. Sodium chloride 0.9% must be used if solutions are diluted.
3. Most nebulizer chambers are disposable but will last 3–4 months when used by a patient at home. The chamber must be emptied after use and each day the chamber should be rinsed in hot water and dried by blowing air through the device. Several centres advocate that once a week the chamber should be sterilized using 0.02% hypochlorite to prevent

Table 25.14 Example of a self-management plan setting out the action required in response to a given peak flow reading and/or symptoms

Peak flow	Symptoms	Action
>85% of normal best value	Intermittent or few symptoms	When required, β$_2$-agonist for symptom relief
		Continue regular inhaler corticosteroid, consider reducing the dosage every 3 months if stable
70–85% of best	Waking at night Symptoms of a cold	Double dose of inhaled corticosteroid
50–70% of best	Increasing breathlessness or using a β$_2$-agonist every 2–3 hours	Start oral corticosteroid course Contact a doctor
<50% of best	Severe attack Poor response to β$_2$-agonist	Call emergency doctor or ambulance urgently

bacterial contamination. The chamber is thoroughly rinsed to remove all traces of hypochlorite and then dried.

4. The nebulizer should be serviced at least once a year.

There are disadvantages with the use of nebulizers. There may be overreliance on the nebulizer by the patient which can result in a delay in seeking medical advice, while the high doses of bronchodilators used increase the incidence of side effects.

Self-management plans

Every asthmatic should be considered for an individualized action plan (often referred to as a 'self-management plan'). These plans are a means of giving patients more confidence by involving them in the management of their own asthma. The patient should then be able to deal with any fluctuation in their condition and know when to seek medical advice. Personalized action plans have been shown to improve health outcomes in asthma patients when written down as part of self-management education (Gibson et al 2002).

Key elements of an action plan include being able to monitor symptoms, peak flow measurements, drug usage and knowing how to deal with fluctuations in severity of asthma according to written guidance. Symptom diaries, management guidance cards and peak flow reading diary cards are available from Asthma UK and from some of the pharmaceutical companies who manufacture asthma products.

An action plan would also include details of when to increase the dose of an inhaled steroid, when to take a short course of oral corticosteroids and when to self-refer to a general medical practitioner or local hospital (Table 25.14).

CASE STUDIES

Case 25.1

Miss RP, a 21-year-old asthmatic, diagnosed in her early teens, has a normal best peak expiratory peak flow reading of 450 L/min. She weighs 55 kg. Her normal medication is:

- **Salbutamol MDI** — **Two puffs when required**
- **Symbicort® 200/6 Turbohaler®** — **One actuation twice a day.**

Over the past few days she developed a cold and was becoming more breathless with falling peak flow readings. Her Symbicort had run out 10 days before and she had not had time to renew the prescription.

Her clinician admits Miss RP to hospital. On arrival she was slightly confused, talking in broken sentences, with a blood pressure of 110/44 mmHg and a respiratory rate of 110 breaths per minute. Her PEF on admission was 220 L/min. She was given 60% oxygen and prescribed:

- **50 mg oral prednisolone daily**
- **salbutamol 5 mg via a nebulizer, 4-hourly**
- **ipratropium bromide 500 μg via a nebulizer, 4-hourly**
- **amoxicillin 500 mg three times s day**
- **erythromycin 500 mg four times a day.**

After one hour she was still hypoxic with blood gas measurements of:

- **pCO$_2$** **30 mmHg (normal range: 35–45)**
  (–7.5 mmHg = approx. 1 kPa)
- **pO$_2$** **59.1 mmHg (normal range: 75–100)**
  (–7.5 mmHg = approx. 1 kPa)
- **HCO$_3^-$** **18.9 mmol/L**
- **base excess** **–6.7 mmol/L.**

She was prescribed intravenous hydrocortisone 200 mg, magnesium sulphate 2 g and aminophylline 250 mg as single doses, followed by an aminophylline infusion.

Questions

1. What dose of intravenous aminophylline should Miss RP be given and how should it be monitored?
2. What counselling should Miss RP receive at her follow-up at the medication review clinic?
3. On further review 4 months later she has had no recurrence of symptoms. Should her medication be altered?

Answers

1. With no previous theophylline therapy, the aminophylline infusion requires a loading dose of 5 mg/kg body weight, administered over 20–30 minutes in order to rapidly obtain therapeutic plasma levels. With a weight of 55 kg this dose should be 275 mg but a single ampoule contains 250 mg so this was chosen for convenience.

   Miss RP does not smoke so the subsequent infusion rate should be 500 μg per kg per hour, commonly administered as a 1 mg per mL solution in 0.9% sodium chloride, giving an infusion rate of 27.5 mL per hour.

Erythromycin inhibits theophylline's metabolism and causes a rise in plasma theophylline levels in 2–7 days. This rise may not be clinically significant for all patients but switching to the newer macrolides, azithromycin or clarithromycin, which interact less significantly, would be sensible. Whichever macrolide is used, theophylline plasma levels should be monitored to watch for any effects, particularly if the level is near the top of the therapeutic range.

Plasma theophylline concentrations should be measured 4–6 hours after starting an intravenous infusion; the aim is to achieve target plasma levels between 10 and 20 mg/L. Some patients exhibit improvement in respiratory function below these levels, so a target of 10 mg/L is often used in asthma. Monitoring thereafter should be every 2–3 days or daily with interacting drugs.

2. It is likely that the acute attack suffered by Miss RP was due to a combination of a bacterial infection precipitating an attack in combination with not taking her corticosteroid and LABA bronchodilator for 10 days. No change to her normal therapy was made on hospital discharge, only a finish of her 5-day course of prednisolone and antibiotics.

In general, asthma consultations often underestimate persisting morbidity from the disease both by the patient and the health professional. The Royal College of Physicians recommends that three questions should always be asked to avoid this and to help structure a consultation.

- Have you had difficulty sleeping because of your asthma symptoms (including cough)?
- Have you had your usual asthma symptoms during the day (cough, wheeze, chest tightness or breathlessness)?
- Has your asthma interfered with your usual activities (e.g. housework, work/school, etc.)?

Discussion with Miss RP should also cover:

- the importance of regular preventer therapy and always keeping a spare inhaler at home to avoid running out
- inhaler technique. It has been estimated that up to 75% of patients using a pressurized MDI have suboptimal inhaler technique. Miss RP is using two different inhaler devices. The choice of device should be carefully tailored to a patient's manual dexterity, co-ordination, age, disease severity and personal preference. Miss RP could switch both devices to a Turbohaler (changing salbutamol to terbutaline) or a pressurized MDI, depending on her technique and preferences
- how to identify trigger factors and reduce their effect, although the evidence for successful allergen avoidance is limited
- how to recognize deteriorating asthma symptoms. A peak flow of less than 70–80% of 'best' or symptoms at night are indicative of deteriorating asthma
- the point at which to start an emergency course of steroids
- when to call for help.

3. In stable disease a step down in therapy should be considered. Which element of treatment to step down will depend on (BTS/SIGN 2005):

- the severity of the asthma
- the side effects of the treatment
- the beneficial effects achieved
- the patient's preference.

In Miss RP's case it would seem reasonable to attempt a 25–50% reduction in corticosteroid dose, ask her to keep twice-daily PEF readings and a symptom diary for a few weeks and review in 3 months unless symptoms deteriorate before then. Reducing her steroid dose by 50% whilst keeping her LABA dose the same is achieved by prescribing a Symbicort® 100/6 Turbohaler at 2 puffs twice a day.

Case 25.2

Mr PG is a 42-year-old recently diagnosed asthmatic. He is a non-smoker. He has been measuring his PEF regularly since diagnosis and has a morning-to-night diurnal variation of between 380 and 500 L/min (his best value). His current medication is:

- **beclometasone pressurized MDI 200 μg twice a day**
- **salbutamol pressurized MDI 200 μg when required.**

He comes to you for his next review. During your discussion, Mr PG tells you that he has noticed that he is wheezing more at night than previously and wakes up two or three times a night. He is also affected by the cold air whilst walking to work, necessitating the use of his salbutamol most mornings.

Questions

1. How has monitoring peak flows changed since 2004?
2. What could be done to reduce his diurnal PEF variation and reduce his current symptoms?
3. The beclometasone inhaler that Mr PG is using contains CFCs. He would like a non-CFC containing inhaler. What could this be changed to?
4. What would you include in an action plan for Mr PG?

Answers

1. The portable peak flow meters which are used by patients in the UK and Europe were altered in 2004 to a new European standard. These 'EU-scale' meters have a more accurate scale than the older 'Wright-scale' meters. Although most patients should have changed there may still be some with the older version (these have a scale with a black background and white text). These should be changed to the newer one (this has a yellow background and blue text). More information and an on-line calculator to convert old readings to new is available at: www.peakflow.com.

2. There are two main choices at this stage in management. Either the beclometasone dose could be increased to 800 μg a day or a long-acting β_2-agonist could be added. There is no evidence that either route is more effective so the decision should be discussed with Mr PG on the basis of preference, possible side effects and suitability. The opportunity to assess Mr PG's inhaler technique must be taken at this point. If he is still able to use a pressurized MDI effectively then a suitable LABA may be a salmeterol pressurized MDI at a dose of 50 μg twice daily.

3. An example of a suitable CFC-free beclometasone inhaler is Qvar®. This inhaler has a hydrofluoroalkane propellant that does not contain CFCs. The bioavailability of the particles delivered by this device means that the Qvar dose must be reduced by 50% from the CFC-containing inhaler dose to maintain equivalence. Mr PG must also be warned that the taste of the inhaler will change.

4. An action plan should contain elements from the following.

- Advice about recognizing loss of asthma control, as assessed by symptoms and PEF readings.
- The action to take if asthma deteriorates, including how to seek emergency help and when to commence a course of emergency oral steroids, which should be prescribed in advance.
- Some clinicians double the dose of inhaled steroids when symptoms deteriorate (e.g. PEF less than 70% of best or waking at night). There is little published evidence to support this as a short-term measure although it is widely practised.

Further information and help for both patients and health professionals is available from Asthma UK at: www.asthma.org.uk

Case 25.3

Mrs JS is attending the hospital respiratory outpatient clinic, 3 weeks after her fourth hospital admission for exacerbation of her asthma in a year. She is 44 and has been diagnosed with asthma since the age of 4.

Her current medication is:

- **salbutamol pressurized MDI 2 puffs when required**
- **Seretide-250 pressurized MDI 2 puffs twice daily**
- **prednisolone tablets 8 mg once daily**
- **theophylline M/R 500 mg twice daily**
- **methotrexate tablets 10 mg once a week.**

She has required oral steroids in addition to her Seretide for 3 years; she started at 15 mg daily and is now reduced to 8 mg. She has been taking the methotrexate for 3 months but has not managed to reduce her oral steroid dose. She has also tried oral ciclosporin in the past year to try and help reduce this, with no effect.

Questions

1. What step of the BTS/SIGN (2005) management ladder is Mrs JS currently on?
2. What monitoring should be performed in order to prevent or minimize the long-term side effects of steroids?
3. What treatment options are available to reduce Mrs JS's dependence on oral steroids?
4. A trial of continuous subcutaneous terbutaline was decided upon. What dose should be used and what monitoring and patient counselling should be performed?

Answers

1. Mrs JS is currently at step 5 of the BTS/SIGN stepwise management guidelines – continuous or frequent use of oral steroids. She belongs to a subgroup of around 5–10% of asthma patients who remain symptomatic despite high-dose treatment. These patients are at risk of dying from their asthma and have continued morbidity from both the disease and the oral steroids. These patients are often described as having 'difficult' asthma which includes the clinical subgroups of brittle asthma and corticosteroid-dependent asthma. It is important that a full review is undertaken in order to look for any fixed airflow obstruction indicative of COPD or for evidence of bronchiectasis in order to confirm the current diagnosis. There is also a co-existent

psychiatric illness in a proportion of these patients (Robinson et al 2003).

2. Mrs JS is at risk of the long-term side effects of steroids such as hypertension or the onset of diabetes mellitus, requiring frequent monitoring of blood pressure and for the signs of diabetes. Steroid-induced osteoporosis is also of concern if continuous corticosteroid is used or if patients have to take frequent short courses (e.g. 3–4 a year). There appears to be a threshold dose at which osteoporosis can occur, of over 7.5 mg per day of prednisolone. Guidance is available from the National Osteoporosis Society at: www.nos.org.uk. Mrs JS should be investigated with bone densitometry because of the length of time she has been receiving oral steroids. General measures are also suggested.

   - General lifestyle measures; not smoking or drinking alcohol to excess, taking regular exercise, taking measures to avoid falls.
   - Calcium and vitamin D supplementation if the diet is not adequate or in at-risk groups such as the elderly or housebound.
   - Hormone replacement therapy may be considered for postmenopausal women.

3. Inhaled steroids are the treatment of choice, with up to 2000 μg per day of beclometasone (or equivalent) if necessary. Mrs JS is currently taking 1000 μg of fluticasone which is equivalent to 2000 μg of beclometasone. Although increasing this dose would be an option, there is little evidence to support this. Additional agents such as a leukotriene antagonist could be added for a 6-week trial. Oral gold could be substituted for methotrexate as an immunosuppressant; the main limitation to this is the side effect of persistent diarrhoea. Continuous subcutaneous β_2-agonists, such as terbutaline, have also been tried. Although some patients do benefit from this therapy there is no evidence available from randomized controlled trials to back up this treatment. Omalizumab may be of benefit but only in patients who have confirmed IgE-mediated allergic asthma.

4. The usual starting dose is 6 mg over 24 hours, which can be increased to 8 or even 12 mg over 24 hours if necessary. A portable syringe driver is required to administer this so the patient will need instruction in how to set this up, or a district nurse visit arranged in order to help. Terbutaline prescribed as a continuous subcutaneous infusion over 24 hours is an unlicensed use and the doses often exceed those stated in the Summary of Product Characteristics; the prescriber, therefore, takes full legal responsibility for its use. Monitoring and counselling include the following.

   - Plasma potassium, owing to the risk of hypokalaemia. This risk is greater in severe asthma due to hypoxia and the concomitant use of theophylline and corticosteroids.
   - Mrs JS may experience a fine tremor, usually of the hands, while receiving terbutaline infusion.
   - The cannula site should be routinely checked for any signs of irritation during the infusion.

REFERENCES

Barnes P J 2003 How do corticosteroids work in asthma? Archives of Internal Medicine 139: 359-370

British Thoracic Society/Scottish Intercollegiate Guidelines Network (BTS/SIGN) 2005 Update: British guideline on the management of asthma. Thorax 58 (suppl 1): i1-i94. Available online at: www.brit-thoracic.org.uk

Douwes J, Gibson P, Pekkanen J et al 2002 Non-eosiniphilic asthma: importance and possible mechanisms. Thorax 57: 643-648

Gibson P G, Powell H, Coughlan J et al 2002 Self-management education and regular practitioner review for adults with asthma (Cochrane review). In: The Cochrane Library, Issue 1. Update Software, Oxford

Holgate S 2002 Asthma: more than an inflammatory disease. Current Opinion in Allergy and Clinical Immunology 2: 27-29

National Asthma Campaign 2001 Out in the open. A true picture of asthma in the United Kingdom today. National Asthma Campaign Asthma Audit 2001. Asthma Journal 6 (3): 1-14

National Institute for Clinical Excellence 2000 Guidance on the use of inhaler systems (devices) in children under 5 years with chronic asthma. Technology Appraisal Guidance 20. National Institute for Clinical Excellence, London

National Institute for Clinical Excellence 2002 Inhaler devices for routine treatment of chronic asthma in older children (aged 5–15 years). Technology Appraisal Guidance 38. National Institute for Clinical Excellence, London

Robinson D S, Campbell D A, Durham S R et al 2003 Systematic assessment of difficult-to-treat asthma. European Respiratory Journal 22: 476-483

FURTHER READING

Currie G P, Devereux G S, Lee D K C, Ayres J G 2005 Recent developments in asthma management. British Medical Journal 330: 585-589

Dolovici M B, Ahrens R C, Hess D R et al 2005 Device selection and outcomes of aerosol therapy: evidence-based guidelines. Chest 127: 335-371

Gibson P G, Powell H, Coughlan J et al 2002 Self-management education and regular practitioner review for adults with asthma. Cochrane Database of Systematic Reviews, Issue 3. Update Software, Oxford

GINA Global Initiative for Asthma 2004 Global strategy for asthma management and prevention.
Available online at: www.ginasthma.com/

Winzel S 2003 Severe asthma: epidemiology, pathophysiology and treatment. Mount Sinai Journal of Medicine 70 (3): 185-190

26 Chronic obstructive pulmonary disease

K. P. Gibbs D. Cripps

KEY POINTS

- Chronic obstructive pulmonary disease (COPD) is a leading cause of morbidity and mortality worldwide, and results in an economic and social burden that is both substantial and increasing.
- COPD is the most prevalent manifestation of obstructive lung disease and mainly comprises chronic bronchitis and emphysema.
- The reduction of overall personal exposure to tobacco smoke, occupational dusts, chemicals and pollutants is an important goal to prevent the onset and progression of COPD.
- Risk factors for COPD include host factors (α_1-antitrypsin deficiency and airway hyperresponsiveness) and exposures (tobacco smoke, occupational dusts and chemicals, indoor and outdoor pollutants, infections) and socio-economic status.
- Smoking cessation is the single most effective intervention to reduce the risk of developing COPD and slow disease progression. This should be the primary focus of management.
- The management of COPD should follow guidance set out both nationally and internationally
- COPD care should be delivered by a multidisciplinary team; assessing and managing patients, advising patients on self-management strategies and exercise, identifying and monitoring patients at high risk of exacerbations and educating patients and other health professionals.
- Patients should undergo non-pharmacological pulmonary rehabilitation, such as breathing exercises.

Chronic obstructive pulmonary disease (COPD) is a disease state characterized by airflow limitation that is not fully reversible. The airflow limitation is usually both progressive and associated with an abnormal inflammatory response of the lungs to noxious particles or gases (GOLD 2005).

COPD is a general term that covers a variety of other disease labels, including chronic obstructive airways disease (COAD), chronic obstructive lung disease (COLD), chronic bronchitis and emphysema.

Epidemiology

COPD is the fourth leading cause of death in the world and expected to rise to the third by 2020. COPD causes about 30 000 deaths each year in the UK, is the largest single cause of lost working days in the UK, is accountable for more than 10% of all hospital admissions and directly costs the NHS around £491m per year. The burden of COPD on the UK healthcare system exceeds that of asthma and is outlined in Table 26.1.

Respiratory diseases including chronic bronchitis are more common in areas of high atmospheric pollution and in people with dusty occupations such as foundry workers and coal miners. Areas that are highly industrialized generally have the highest incidence of COPD.

Pathology

The major pathological changes in COPD affect four different compartments of the lung and all are affected in most individuals in varying degrees (ATS/ERS 2004).

Central airways (<2 mm diameter, cartilaginous)

The bronchial glands hypertrophy and goblet cell proliferation occurs. This results in excessive mucus production (chronic bronchitis). Epidemiologically chronic bronchitis is defined as a chronic or recurrent cough with sputum production on most days for at least 3 months of the year during at least 2 consecutive years, in the absence of other diseases recognized to cause sputum production. There is a loss of ciliary function with increase in inflammatory cells, notably lymphocytes, macrophages and, later in disease, neutrophils.

Peripheral airways (<2 mm diameter, non-cartilaginous)

Bronchiolitis is present from early disease with a pathological increase in goblet cells and in inflammatory cells in the airway walls. With disease progression, fibrosis develops along with increased deposition of collagen in the airway walls.

Lung parenchyma (respiratory bronchioles, alveoli and capillaries)

In emphysema elastases destroy elastin, thus resulting in dilation and destruction of the respiratory bronchioles and alveolar sacs

Table 26.1   Annual morbidity from COPD (NICE 2004)

	Hospital admissions	Consultant episodes	GP consultations
England and Wales	109 243	161 965	20 patients suspected of COPD per GP per year.

and ducts. Because of this there is a loss of the alveolar wall attachments and peripheral airway collapse.

Emphysema is defined as an abnormal enlargement of the air spaces distal to the terminal bronchioles. There are two main forms: (1) centrilobular emphysema which involves dilation and destruction of respiratory bronchioles, alveolar ducts and alveoli; and (2) panacinar emphysema which involves destruction of the whole acinus. The former predominates in COPD, the latter in patients with α_1-antitrypsin deficiency.

Pulmonary vasculature

Vessel walls thicken early in the course of the disease along with endothelial dysfunction. The vessel walls become infiltrated by inflammatory cells, including macrophages and lymphocytes, and there is increased vascular smooth muscle. In advanced disease there is emphysematous destruction of the vascular bed and collagen deposition.

Aetiology

Tobacco smoking is the most important and dominant risk factor in the development of COPD but other noxious particles also contribute, such as occupational exposure to chemical fumes, irritants, dust and gases. A person's exposure can be thought of in terms of the total burden of inhaled particles. These cause a (normal) inflammatory response in the lungs; smokers, however, seem to have an exaggerated response which eventually causes tissue destruction and impaired repair mechanisms. As well as inflammation, the other main processes involved in the

pathogenesis of COPD are an imbalance of proteinases and antiproteinases in the lungs, and oxidative stress.

Not all smokers go on to develop clinically significant COPD; genetic factors seem to modify each individual's risk. The age when starting to smoke, total pack-years smoked, and current smoking status are predictive of COPD mortality. Passive exposure to cigarette smoke may also contribute to respiratory symptoms and COPD by increasing the lungs' total burden of inhaled particles and gases (GOLD 2005). Tobacco exposure is quantified in 'pack-years':

$$\text{Total pack year} = \frac{(\text{number of cigarettes smoked per day})}{20} \times \frac{\text{number of years}}{\text{of smoking}}$$

Additional risk factors include the natural ageing process of the lungs. Males are currently more at risk of developing chronic bronchitis, but as the number of women who smoke increases, the incidence of chronic bronchitis in females will also rise. The major risk factors are summarized in Table 26.2.

Inflammation

COPD is characterized by chronic inflammation throughout the airways, parenchyma and pulmonary vasculature. This is a different pattern of inflammation from that of asthma, with an increase in neutrophils, macrophages and T-lymphocytes (particularly CD8[+]); increased eosinophils occur in some patients during exacerbations. These inflammatory cells cause the release of inflammatory mediators and cytokines such as leukotriene B4, interleukin-8 and tumour necrosis factor-α. Over

Table 26.2 Risk factors for the development of COPD

Risk factor	Comment
Smoking	Risk increases with increasing consumption but there is also large inter- individual variation in susceptibility
Age	Increasing age results in ventilatory impairment; most frequently related to cumulative smoking
Gender	Male gender was previously thought to be a risk factor but this may be due to a higher incidence of tobacco smoking in men. Women have greater airway reactivity and experience faster declines in FEV_1 so may be at more risk than men
Occupation	The development of COPD has been implicated with occupations such as coal and gold mining, farming, grain handling and the cement and cotton industries
Genetic factors	α1-Antitrypsin deficiency is the strongest single genetic risk factor, accounting for 1–2% of COPD. Other genetic disorders involving tissue necrosis factor and epoxide hydrolase may also be risk factors
Air pollution	Death rates are higher in urban areas than in rural areas. Indoor air pollution from burning biomass fuel is also implicated as a risk factor, particularly in underdeveloped areas of the world
Socio-economic status	More common in individuals of low socio-economic status
Airway hyper-responsiveness and allergy	Smokers show increased levels of IgE, eosinophils and airway hyper-responsiveness but how these influence the development of COPD is unknown

time the actions of these mediators damages the lungs and leads to the characteristic pathological changes observed.

Proteinase and antiproteinase imbalance

The observation that α_1-antitrypsin deficient individuals are at increased risk of developing emphysema has led to the theory that an imbalance between proteinases and antiproteinases leads to lung destruction. In COPD there is either an increased production/activity of proteinases or a decreased production/activity of antiproteinases. The main proteinases, proteolytic enzymes such as neutrophil elastin, are released by macrophages or neutrophils. The antiproteinases inhibit the damage caused by the proteolytic enzymes. The main antiproteinase is α_1-antitrypsin, also known as α_1-proteinase inhibitor. Cigarette smoke has been shown to inactivate this protein. Oxidative stress also decreases the activity of antiproteinases.

Oxidative stress

An imbalance of oxidants and antioxidants exists in COPD with the balance in favour of the oxidants. This state of oxidative stress contributes to the development of the disease by damaging the intracellular matrix, oxidizing biological molecules which cause cell destruction and promoting histone acetylation. There also seems to be a link between oxidative stress and the poor response to corticosteroids seen in COPD. To work, corticosteroids must recruit histone deacetylase (HDAC) to switch off the transcription of inflammatory genes. In COPD, the activity of HDAC is impaired by the oxidative stress, thereby reducing the responsiveness to corticosteroids Cigarette smoke also impairs the function of HDAC.

Pathophysiology

The pathogenic mechanisms and pathological changes described above lead to the physiological abnormalities of COPD: mucus hypersecretion, ciliary dysfunction, airflow limitation and hyperinflation, gas exchange abnormalities, pulmonary hypertension and systemic effects (ARS/ERS 2004).

Mucus hypersecretion, ciliary dysfunction and complications

Enlarged mucus glands cause hypersecretion of mucus and the squamous metaplasia of epithelial cells results in ciliary dysfunction. These are typically the first physiological abnormalities in COPD.

Normally cilia and mucus in the bronchi protect against inhaled irritants, which are trapped and expectorated. The persistent irritation caused by cigarette and other smoke causes an exaggeration in the response of these protective mechanisms and leads to inflammation of the small bronchioles (bronchiolitis) and alveoli (alveolitis). Cigarette smoke also inhibits mucociliary clearance, which causes a further build-up of mucus in the lungs. As a result, macrophages and neutrophils infiltrate the epithelium and trigger a degree of epithelial destruction. This, together with a proliferation of mucus-producing cells, leads

to plugging of smaller bronchioles and alveoli with mucus and particulate matter.

This excessive mucus production causes distension of the alveoli and loss of their gas exchange function. Pus and infected mucus accumulate, leading to recurrent or chronic viral and bacterial infections. The primary pathogen is usually viral but bacterial infection often follows. Common bacterial pathogens include *Streptococcus pneumoniae*, *Moraxella catarrhalis* and *Haemophilus influenzae*.

Bronchiectasis is a pathological change in the lungs where the bronchi become permanently dilated. It is common after early attacks of acute bronchitis during which mucus both plugs and stretches the bronchial walls. In severe infections the bronchioles and alveoli can become permanently damaged and do not return to their normal size and shape. The loss of muscle tone and loss of cilia can contribute to COPD because mucus has a tendency to accumulate in the dilated bronchi.

Airflow limitation and hyperinflation

Fibrosis and narrowing (airway remodelling) of the smaller conducting airways (<2 mm diameter) is the main site of expiratory airflow limitation in COPD. This is compounded by the loss of elastic recoil (destruction of alveolar walls), destruction of alveolar support/attachments and the accumulation of inflammatory cells mucus and plasma exudates during exercise. The degree of airflow limitation is measured by spirometry.

This progressive destructive enlargement of the respiratory bronchioles, alveolar ducts and alveolar sacs is referred to as emphysema. Adjacent alveoli can become indistinguishable from each other, with two main consequences. The first is loss of available gas exchange surfaces, which leads to an increase in dead space and impaired gas exchange. The second consequence is the loss of elastic recoil in the small airways, vital for maintaining the force of expiration, which leads to a tendency for them to collapse, particularly during expiration. Increased thoracic gas volume and hyperinflation of the lungs result. The causes of airflow limitation in COPD are summarized in Table 26.3.

Table 26.3 Causes of airflow limitation in COPD

Irreversible	Fibrosis and narrowing of the airways
	Loss of elastic recoil due to alveolar destruction
	Destruction of alveolar support that maintains patency of small airways
Reversible	Accumulation of inflammatory cells, mucus and plasma exudates in the bronchi
	Smooth muscle contraction in peripheral and central airways
	Dynamic hyperinflation during exercise

From GOLD 2005

Gas exchange abnormalities

This occurs in advanced disease and is characterized by arterial hypoxaemia with or without hypercarbia. The anatomical changes during COPD result in an abnormal distribution of ventilation and perfusion within the lungs and creates the abnormal gaseous exchange.

Pulmonary hypertension and cor pulmonale

Pulmonary hypertension develops late in COPD after gas exchange abnormalities have developed. The thickening of the bronchiole and alveolar walls resulting from chronic inflammation and oedema leads to blockage and obstruction of the airways. Alveolar distension and destruction result in distortion of the blood vessels that are closely associated with the alveoli. This causes a rise in the blood pressure in the pulmonary circulation. Reduction in gas diffusion across the alveolar epithelium leads to a low partial pressure of oxygen in the blood vessels (hypoxaemia) due to an imbalance between ventilation and perfusion. By a mechanism that is not clearly established, chronic vasoconstriction results and causes a further increase in blood pressure and further compromises gas diffusion from air spaces into the bloodstream. The chronic low oxygen levels lead to polycythaemia (increase in number of erythrocytes), which makes the blood more viscous. In advanced disease, this persistent hypoxaemia develops along with pathological changes in the pulmonary circulation. Sustained pulmonary hypertension results in a thickening of the walls of the pulmonary arterioles, with associated pulmonary remodelling and an increase in right ventricular pressure within the heart.

The consequence of continued high right ventricular pressure is eventual right ventricular hypertrophy, dilation and progressive right ventricular failure (cor pulmonale). Pulmonary oedema develops as a result of physiological changes subsequent to the hypoxaemia and hypercapnia, such as activation of the renin–angiotensin system, salt and water retention and a reduction in renal blood flow.

Systemic effects

Systemic inflammation and skeletal muscle wasting can also occur in COPD which limit exercise capacity and worsen prognosis.

Clinical manifestations

Diagnosis

A diagnosis of COPD is usually considered in any patient who has symptoms of cough, sputum production or dyspnoea and/or a history of exposure to COPD risk factors (see Table 26.2). Spirometry is then used to confirm the diagnosis.

COPD is a progressive disorder, which passes through a potentially asymptomatic mild phase, before the moderate phase and then severe disease.

Clinical features

The traditional description of COPD symptoms, particularly in severe disease, depends on whether bronchitis or emphysema predominates. Chronic bronchitic patients exhibit excess mucus production and a degree of bronchospasm, resulting in wheeze and dyspnoea. Hypoxia and hypercapnia (high levels of carbon dioxide in the tissues) are common. This type of patient has a productive cough, is often overweight and finds physical exertion difficult due to dyspnoea. The bronchitic patient is sometimes referred to as a 'blue bloater'. This term is used because of the tendency of the patient to retain carbon dioxide caused by a decreased responsiveness of the respiratory centre to prolonged hypoxaemia that leads to cyanosis, and also the tendency for peripheral oedema to occur. Bronchitic patients lose the ability to increase the rate and depth of ventilation in response to persistent hypoxaemia. The reason for this is not clear, but decreased ventilatory drive may result from abnormal peripheral or central respiratory receptors. In severe disease the chest diameter is often increased, giving the classic barrel chest. As obstruction worsens, hypoxaemia increases, leading to pulmonary hypertension. Right ventricular strain leads to right ventricular failure, which is characterized by jugular venous distension, hepatomegaly and peripheral oedema, all of which are consequences of an increase in systemic venous blood pressure. Recurrent lower respiratory tract infections can be severe and debilitating. Signs of infection include an increase in the volume of thick and viscous sputum, which is yellow or green in colour and may contain bacterial pathogens, squamous epithelial cells, alveolar macrophages and saliva, but pyrexia may not be present.

The clinical features of emphysema are different from those of bronchitis. A patient with emphysema will experience increasing dyspnoea even at rest, but often there is minimal cough and the sputum produced is scanty and mucoid. Cough is usually more of a problem after dyspnoea is apparent. The patient will breathe rapidly (tachypnoea), because the respiratory centres are responsive to mild hypoxaemia, and will have a flushed appearance. Typically a patient with emphysema will be thin and have pursed lips in an effort to compensate for a lack of elastic recoil and exhale a larger volume of air. Such a patient will tend to use the accessory muscles of the chest and neck to assist in the work of breathing. Hypoxaemia is not a problem until the disease has progressed. Pulmonary hypertension is usually mild and cor pulmonale is uncommon until the terminal stages of the disease. Generally, bronchial infections tend to be less common in emphysema. The patient with emphysema is sometimes referred to as a 'pink puffer' because he or she hyperventilates to compensate for hypoxia by breathing in short puffs. As a result, the patient appears pink with little carbon dioxide retention and little evidence of oedema. Eventually the patient is unable to obtain enough oxygen in spite of rapid breathing.

The bronchitic 'blue bloater' and emphysemic 'pink puffer' represent two ends of the COPD spectrum. In reality the underlying pathophysiology may well be a mixture, and the resulting signs and symptoms somewhere between the two extremes described.

Additional specific problems are also common in patients with COPD:

- obstructive sleep apnoea hypopnoea syndrome (OSAHS)
- acute respiratory failure.

The sleep apnoea syndrome is a respiratory disorder characterized by frequent or prolonged pauses in breathing during sleep. It leads to a deterioration in arterial blood gases and a decrease in the saturation of haemoglobin with oxygen. Hypoxaemia is often accompanied by pulmonary hypertension and cardiac arrhythmias, which may lead to premature cardiac failure.

Acute respiratory failure is said to have occurred if the PaO_2 suddenly drops and there is an increase in $PaCO_2$ that decreases the pH to 7.3 or less. The most common cause is an acute exacerbation of chronic bronchitis with an increase in volume and viscosity of sputum. This further impairs ventilation and causes more severe hypoxaemia and hypercapnia. The clinical signs and symptoms of acute respiratory failure include restlessness, confusion, tachycardia, cyanosis, sweating, hypotension and eventual unconsciousness.

Investigations

Lung function tests are used to assist in diagnosis. A spirometer is used to measure lung volumes and flow rates. The main measurement made is the forced expiratory volume in the first second of exhalation (FEV_1). Other tests can be performed, such as:

- vital capacity (VC): the volume of air inhaled and exhaled during maximal ventilation
- forced vital capacity (FVC): the volume of air inhaled and exhaled during a forced maximal expiration after full inspiration
- residual volume (RV): the volume of air left in the lungs after maximal exhalation.

Airflow obstruction is defined as:

- FEV_1 less than 80% of that predicted for the patient
- and FEV_1/FVC less than 0.7.

Vital capacity decreases in bronchitis and emphysema. Residual volume increases in both cases but tends to be higher in patients with emphysema due to air being trapped distal to the terminal bronchioles. Total lung capacity is often normal in patients with bronchitis but is usually increased in emphysema, again due to

air being trapped. Smoking increases the normal deterioration in FEV_1 over time, from about 30 mL per year to about 45 mL per year. The major criticism of measuring FEV_1 and FVC is that they detect changes only in airways greater than 2 mm in diameter. As airways less than 2 mm in diameter contribute only 10–20% of normal resistance to airflow, there is usually severe obstruction and extensive damage to the lungs by the time the lung function tests (FEV_1 and FVC) detect abnormalities.

Both UK and international COPD guidelines use spirometry to categorize the severity of COPD. These are summarized in Table 26.4.

At diagnosis and evaluation, patients may receive other investigations as outlined in Table 26.5.

Chest radiographs reveal differences between the two disease states. A patient with emphysema will have a flattened diaphragm with loss of peripheral vascular markings and the appearance of bullae. These are indicative of extensive trapping of air. A bronchitic patient will have increased bronchovascular markings and may also have cardiomegaly (increased cardiac size due to right ventricular failure) with prominent pulmonary arteries.

Table 26.4 Assessment of severity of airflow obstruction

FEV_1	Severity (NICE)	Severity (GOLD)
Normal spirometry with chronic symptoms (cough, sputum production)		Stage 0: At risk
Greater than 80% predicted		Stage I: Mild
50–80% predicted	Mild	Stage II: Moderate
30–49% predicted	Moderate	Stage III: Severe
Less than 30% predicted	Severe	Stage IV: Very severe

Adapted from NICE 2004 and GOLD 2005

Table 26.5 Additional investigations at the diagnosis of COPD

Investigation	Note
Chest x-ray	To exclude other pathologies
Full blood count	To identify anaemia or polycythaemia
Serial domiciliary peak flow measurements	To exclude asthma if there is a doubt about diagnosis
α_1-Antitrypsin	Particularly with early-onset disease or a minimal smoking/family history
Transfer factor for carbon monoxide (TLCO)	To investigate symptoms that seem disproportionate to the spirometric impairment
CT scan of the thorax	To investigate symptoms that seem disproportionate to the spirometric impairment To investigate abnormalities seen on the chest x-ray To assess suitability for surgery
ECG	To assess cardiac status if features of cor pulmonale

Table 26.5 (continued)

Echocardiogram	To assess cardiac status if features of cor pulmonale
Pulse oximetry	To assess need for oxygen therapy. If cyanosis or cor pulmonale is present or if FEV_1 <50% of predicted value
Sputum culture	To identify organisms if sputum is persistently present and purulent

Treatment

Stable COPD

The clinical progress of COPD depends on whether bronchitis or emphysema predominates. Bronchitic patients will experience an increasing frequency of exacerbations of acute dyspnoea triggered by excess mucus production and obstruction. There is a progressive decline in lung function with complications such as cor pulmonale, hypercapnia and polycythaemia. Eventually cardiorespiratory failure with hypercapnia will occur, which may be severe, unresponsive to treatment and result in death. Emphysema patients will become progressively dyspnoeic without exacerbations triggered by increased sputum production. Eventually cor pulmonale will develop very rapidly, usually in the late stages of the disease, and lead to intractable hypercapnia and respiratory arrest.

Drug treatment together with other measures such as physiotherapy and artificial ventilation have not been shown to improve the natural progression of COPD. Quality of life and symptoms will, however, improve with suitable treatment and it is likely that the correct management of the patient will lead to a reduction in hospital admissions and may prevent premature death. In patients with severe COPD and hypoxaemia, long-term oxygen therapy is the only treatment known to improve the prognosis.

The aims of treatment for patients with COPD are shown in Table 26.6 and the common therapeutic problems associated with COPD in Table 26.7. Drug treatment itself can only relieve symptoms; it does not modify the underlying pathology. Most patients with COPD are considered to have irreversible obstruction, in contrast to asthmatics, but a significant number do seem to respond to bronchodilators. Treatment options at each stage of COPD are outlined in Figure 26.1.

Smoking

Smoking is the most important factor in the development of obstructive airways disease. Every smoker with chronic airflow obstruction must be advised to stop. Individually targeted advice may prove to be more successful in persuading individuals to give up, especially in those motivated to do so.

Smokers who have a strong physical type of dependence will benefit from agents such as nicotine replacement therapy. The nicotine absorbed reduces the effects associated with reducing cigarette smoking such as irritability, sleep disturbances, fatigue, headache and increased appetite.

Table 26.6 Treatment aims for patients with COPD

Prevent disease progression
Relieve symptoms
Improve exercise tolerance
Improve health status
Prevent and treat complications such as hypoxaemia and infections
Prevent and treat exacerbations
Reduce mortality

Table 26.7 Common therapeutic problems associated with COPD

- Failure of patient to stop smoking
- Inadequate inhaler technique leading to subtherapeutic dosing
- Poor concordance with treatment regimen
- Failure to assess corticosteroid reversibility before prescribing inhaled corticosteroids
- Inappropriate prescribing of antibiotics in an acute exacerbation of COPD
- Failure to properly assess a patient for home nebulizer therapy
- Failure to ensure compliance with 15 hours a day of home oxygen therapy

Antibiotics and vaccines

Prophylactic antibiotics have no place in the management of COPD. Antibiotic therapy is, however, vital if a patient develops purulent sputum. If patients frequently develop acute infective exacerbations of bronchitis they should be given a supply of antibiotics to keep at home and start on the first sign of an exacerbation.

Initial routine sputum cultures are unhelpful in these patients as they are unreliable in identifying the pathogenic organisms.

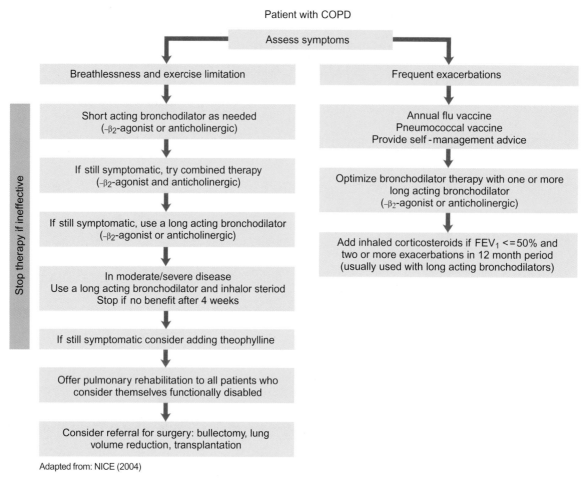

Patient with COPD

Assess symptoms

Breathlessness and exercise limitation

Frequent exacerbations

Short acting bronchodilator as needed
($-\beta_2$-agonist or anticholinergic)

If still symptomatic, try combined therapy
($-\beta_2$-agonist and anticholinergic)

If still symptomatic, use a long acting bronchodilator
($-\beta_2$-agonist or anticholinergic)

In moderate/severe disease
Use a long acting bronchodilator and inhalor steriod
Stop if no benefit after 4 weeks

If still symptomatic consider adding theophylline

Offer pulmonary rehabilitation to all patients who
consider themselves functionally disabled

Consider referral for surgery: bullectomy, lung
volume reduction, transplantation

Stop therapy if ineffective

Annual flu vaccine
Pneumococcal vaccine
Provide self-management advice

Optimize bronchodilator therapy with one or more
long acting bronchodilator
($-\beta_2$-agonist or anticholinergic)

Add inhaled corticosteroids if $FEV_1 <= 50\%$ and
two or more exacerbations in 12 month period
(usually used with long acting bronchodilators)

Adapted from: NICE (2004)

Fig 26.1 Stepwise approach to the pharmacological management of chronic COPD.

The normal pathogens involved are *Streptococcus pneumoniae*, *Haemophilus influenzae* or *Moraxella catarrhalis*. The usual antibiotics of choice are co-amoxiclav, amoxicillin, erythromycin or doxycycline. If the infection follows influenza, *Staphylococcus aureus* may be present and an anti-staphylococcal agent such as flucloxacillin should be added to the regimen. If the infection is considered atypical in presentation or if the purulent sputum is still present after 1 week of treatment, then sputum cultures should be taken to try to identify the pathogenic organisms.

Prophylactic immunization

A single dose of pneumococcal vaccine and annual influenza vaccinations have been shown to reduce hospitalizations and the risk of death in the elderly with chronic lung disease, and should be offered to those with chronic airflow obstruction. The prevalent strains of influenza change so the vaccine composition is, correspondingly, altered annually.

Bronchodilators

Bronchodilators in COPD are used to reverse airflow limitation. As the degree of limitation varies widely, their effectiveness should be assessed in each patient using respiratory function tests and by assessing any subjective improvement reported by

the patient. Patients may experience improvements in exercise tolerance or relief of symptoms such as wheeze and cough.

Inhaled β_2-adrenoceptor agonists Selective β_2-agonists should be tried initially since they provide rapid relief and have a low incidence of side effects. Inhaled treatment is as efficacious as oral agents and is therefore preferred, having fewer side effects. The dose–response curve for β_2-agonists in COPD is almost flat and there is little benefit in giving more than 1 mg. The effects of short-acting β_2-agonists last for 4 hours and they can be used either regularly or 'as required' for symptom relief. Used before exercise, they can improve exercise tolerance. Poor patient response to bronchodilators may be due to poor inhalation technique so this should be checked as often as possible and the inhaler device changed if necessary. Regular four times a day therapy can result in poor patient compliance.

If patients remain symptomatic despite a short-acting β_2-agonist, then a long-acting agent can be added. The national guidance recommends that long-acting agents are used if a patient has two or more exacerbations in a year (BTS 2005).

Anticholinergic drugs In COPD patients, parasympathetic (vagal) airway muscle tone is the major reversible component. Inhaled anticholinergic drugs reverse this vagal tone and have a significant bronchodilator effect, especially in the elderly. Only one short-acting agent, ipratropium bromide, and one long-acting agent, tiotropium, are currently available in the UK.

The national guidance allows the use of either β_2-agonists or ipratropium for the management of mild disease. Higher doses of ipratropium bromide may be required than are used in patients with asthma, for example 80 µg used 6-hourly. If symptoms do not respond to a single agent then combination therapy may produce additive bronchodilation.

Tiotropium has a 24-hour duration of action and trial results indicate that it can reduce exacerbation rates, exercise tolerance and rates of hospital admissions. As with long-acting β_2-agonists, tiotropium can be used when short-acting agents fail to control symptoms, patients have two or more exacerbations in the last year or as an adjunct to corticosteroid therapy in more severe disease. Combining tiotropium with a long-acting β_2-agonist can also be tried but should be assessed for benefit (in activities of daily living, exercise capacity or lung function) after a 4-week trial. As more evidence emerges about the benefits of tiotropium it may become first-line treatment after short-acting agents (Vincken 2005).

Theophyllines Theophyllines are weak bronchodilators but seem to have useful additional physiological effects in COPD such as increased respiratory drive, improved diaphragmatic function and improved cardiac output, but the exact clinical benefits of these have not been established. The use of theophylline should only be considered after a trial of short-acting with long-acting bronchodilators. Whenever theophylline is tried in the management of COPD, an initial therapeutic trial of several weeks should be carried out. If subjective and objective measures of lung function show an improvement, then theophylline can be continued as maintenance therapy. Persistent nocturnal symptoms such as cough or wheeze may be helped by the night-time use of long-acting theophylline.

Care must be taken when prescribing theophylline. Its clearance is affected by many factors, including cigarette smoking, viral pneumonia, heart failure and concurrent drug treatment, such as macrolide antibiotics used during exacerbations (see Chapter 25).

Theophylline is being investigated in low concentrations for its ability to reverse the decrease in histone deacetylase activity associated with oxidative stress. This may prove to be of benefit in reversing corticosteroid resistance.

High-dose and nebulized bronchodilators Although most patients will benefit from standard-dose bronchodilators, some with severe disease will benefit from higher doses. European guidelines (Boe et al 2001) recommend that hand-held inhalers are still used for doses of bronchodilators up to 1 mg of salbutamol or 160 µg of ipratropium bromide. Doses above this may be more conveniently given using a nebulizer. These patients should have their inhaled therapy optimized, possibly using a protocol as outlined in Table 26.8, and assessed as detailed in the guidelines.

Corticosteroids

Patients with COPD show a poor response to corticosteroids and have a largely steroid-resistant pattern of inflammation (Barnes 2004). It is postulated that the oxidative stress of COPD inhibits the mechanism by which corticosteroids, acting through histone deacetylase (HDAC), switch off activated inflammatory genes.

The long-term benefits of inhaled corticosteroids in COPD have only been shown in patients with moderate-to-severe disease, with an FEV_1 less than 50% of predicted value. A reduction in the number of exacerbations and a slowing of the decline

---

Table 26.8 Optimization of inhaled therapy for patients with severe COPD

1. Check diagnosis and confirm severity. Ensure optimal inhaler technique

2. Ensure all other therapies have been tried: long-acting bronchodilator, theophylline, corticosteroid, LTOT and pulmonary rehabilitation

3. Optimize hand-held inhaler dosing, for example:
   - ESalbutamol 200–400 µg four times a day
   - Ipratropium bromide 40–80 µg four times a day
     Or a combination of these agents

4. Try further increasing the dose of the hand-held inhaler to:
   - Salbutamol up to 1 mg four times a day, and/or
   - Ipratropium bromide up to 160–240 µg four times a day (although the effect of alternative use of tiotropium at this stage is unknown)

5. If a poor response at step 4 consider a period of home nebulizer therapy with careful examination of patient response, over at least 2 weeks

6. Initial therapy: try nebulized salbutamol 2.5 mg or terbutaline 5 mg four times a day and assess response at 2 weeks

7. If the response to monotherapy is poor, consider one or more of the following:
   - Salbutamol 5 mg or terbutaline 10 mg four times a day, or
   - Iptratropium bromide 250–500 µg four times a day, or the combination
   - Salbutamol 2.5–5 mg and ipratropium 500 µg four times a day

8. Decide which treatment in step 7 was the most beneficial

in health status have been shown, but no effect on improving lung function.

Inhaled corticosteroids should be used although there is no consensus over the minimum effective dose. No inhaled steroid is licensed for sole use in COPD in the UK.

There is little place for oral steroids in stable COPD. Some patients with advanced disease may require maintenance oral therapy if this cannot be withdrawn after a short course for an exacerbation. In this instance the lowest dose possible should be used and the patient regularly assessed for the development of osteoporosis and need for osteoporosis prevention; patients over 65 years and receiving maintenance therapy should automatically have prophylactic treatment for osteoporosis.

Mucolytics

Mucolytics may be of benefit in stable COPD if there is a chronic cough that is productive of sputum. Benefit must be assessed, for example with a reduction in the frequency of cough and/or sputum production.

Acute exacerbations of COPD

Patients with COPD suffer acute worsenings of the disease, referred to as acute exacerbations. These exacerbations can be spontaneous but are often precipitated by infection and lead to respiratory failure with hypoxaemia and retention of carbon dioxide. Many patients can be managed at home (see NICE 2004) but some will require admission to hospital.

Bronchodilators

Bronchodilators are used to treat the increased breathlessness that is associated with exacerbations. These can be given by MDI or nebulizer although, practically, breathless patients are often unable to use MDIs effectively. A β_2-agonist can be given with or without an anticholinergic agent, depending on the benefits obtained.

Antibiotics

Bacteria can be isolated from the sputum of patients with stable COPD but antibiotics can be used to treat exacerbations of COPD associated with a history of more purulent sputum. The choice of antibiotic should be dependent on local policy, sensitivity patterns and any previous treatments. An aminopenicillin or a macrolide with increased activity against *H. influenzae* or oxytetracycline is generally suitable as a first-line agent. Sputum should be sent for culture in order to check the appropriateness of initial therapy, and the antibiotic changed if necessary.

Corticosteroids

A short course of oral steroids has been shown to benefit FEV_1 and reduce the duration of hospitalization. Patients managed at home who have increased breathlessness which interferes with daily activities and all those admitted to hospital should be treated. A suitable course is prednisolone 30 mg every morning, given for 7–14 days.

Other treatment

Intravenous aminophylline can be considered, if there is an inadequate response to bronchodilators. The loading dose and maintenance dose required should be carefully chosen as these depend on various factors (see Chapter 25).

Oxygen therapy is necessary to improve hypoxia. In patients with a hypoxic drive, the administration of high concentration oxygen will cause a fall in ventilation, carbon dioxide retention and respiratory acidosis. To avoid this but administer enough to overcome potentially life-threatening hypoxia, the goal is an oxygen saturation of between 90% and 93%. The initial concentration used should be 40% and then titrated to oxygen saturation. Arterial blood gases should be monitored regularly.

During an acute attack, pyrexia, hyperventilation and the excessive work of breathing can result in an inability to eat or drink and thus lead to dehydration; intravenous hydration is given to correct this.

Chest physiotherapy is employed to mobilize secretions, promote expectoration and expand collapsed lung segments. Nebulized 0.9% sodium chloride has been used to help in this.

Although largely superseded by non-invasive ventilatory support, doxapram (as a continuous infusion at a rate of 1–4 mg per minute) can be tried in patients with acute respiratory failure, carbon dioxide retention and depressed ventilation. Doxapram stimulates the respiratory and vasomotor centres in the medulla, increases the depth of breathing and may slightly increase the rate of breathing. Arterial oxygenation is usually not improved because of the increased work of breathing induced by doxapram. This agent has a narrow therapeutic index with side effects such as arrhythmias, vasoconstriction, dizziness and convulsions and may be harmful if used when the $PaCO_2$ is normal or low.

Treatment of cor pulmonale

COPD is responsible for over 90% of cases of cor pulmonale. Treatment is symptomatic and involves managing the underlying airways obstruction, hypoxaemia and any pulmonary oedema that develops. Peripheral oedema is managed by using thiazide or loop diuretics although there are concerns over their metabolic effects reducing respiratory drive. Oxygen is used to treat hypoxaemia, and this should also promote a diuresis. All patients should be assessed for the need for long-term oxygen therapy.

Domiciliary oxygen therapy

The aim of therapy is to improve oxygen delivery to the cells, increase alveolar oxygen tension and decrease the work of breathing to maintain a given PaO_2. Domiciliary oxygen therapy can be given in two ways.

Intermittent administration Intermittent administration is used to increase mobility and capacity for exercise and to ease discomfort. Intermittent administration is of most benefit in patients with emphysema.

Continuous long-term oxygen therapy (LTOT) LTOT for at least 15 hours per day has been shown to improve survival in patients with severe, irreversible airflow obstruction, hypoxaemia and peripheral oedema (MRC Working Party 1981). LTOT can only be prescribed if specific conditions are met, as described in Table 26.9. The main aim of treatment is to achieve a PaO_2 of at least 8 kPa without causing a rise in $PaCO_2$ of more than 1 kPa, achieved by adjusting the oxygen flow rate. Before LTOT can be prescribed each individual must be assessed accordingly (see Table 26.9).

Oxygen can be prescribed as oxygen cylinders but 15 hours per day at 2 L/min requires 10×1340 L cylinders a week. A more convenient system is to use a concentrator, which converts ambient air to 90% oxygen using a molecular sieve. The concentrator is sited in a well-ventilated area in the home with plastic tubing to terminals in rooms such as the living room and bedroom. Tubing from the terminals delivers oxygen to the patient, who wears a mask or uses the more convenient nasal prongs. This tubing should be long enough to allow some mobility.

Patient care

Pulmonary rehabilitation

Patients should participate in a co-ordinated programme of non-pharmacological treatment which includes:

- advice and support on stopping smoking
- nutritional assessment
- aerobic exercise training to increase capacity and endurance for exercise
- strength training for upper and lower limbs
- relaxation techniques
- breathing retraining, for example diaphragmatic and pursed lips breathing to improve the ventilatory pattern and improve gas exchange
- education about their medicines, nutrition, self-management of their disease and lifestyle issues
- psychological support because COPD patients often have decreased capacity to participate in social and recreational activities and can become anxious, depressed or fatigued.

A multidisciplinary team should deliver these programmes. This care should be individually tailored to optimize each patient's physical and social performance and autonomy and last for a minimum of 6 weeks and a maximum of 12 weeks of exercise (NICE 2004).

Table 26.9 Guidelines for prescribing long-term oxygen therapy (LTOT)

A   Chronic hypoxaemia. When PaO_2 is consistently below 7.3 kPa whilst the patient is clinically stable.

The PaO_2 can be between 7.3 and 8 kPa if either secondary polycythaemia or pulmonary hypertension is present

B   Nocturnal hypoventilation

C   For palliative use to relieve dyspnoea in pulmonary malignancy and other causes of disabling dyspnoea due to terminal disease

From British Thoracic Society 2005

Pulmonary rehabilitation programmes that include at least 4 weeks exercise training have been shown to improve dyspnoea and the patient's COPD control. These benefits were greater than those seen with bronchodilators. However, the long-term effect of these programmes has yet to be established although personalized education to COPD patients about their condition has been shown to reduce their need for health services.

Stopping smoking

The health hazards associated with smoking are well known and publicized. To give up smoking, which has been described as a form of drug addiction, requires self-motivation. Stopping smoking does not, however, have an immediate effect: a reduction in COPD mortality is not seen until about 10 years or more after cessation of smoking. Members of the healthcare team can educate smokers about the dangers and actively encourage and motivate those who want to give up. Brief chats between individuals and health professionals about stopping smoking are both effective and cost-effective in encouraging individuals to quit (NICE 2006).

Once a decision to quit has been made, it is the degree of dependence rather than the level of motivation that will influence the success rate. Smokers need both initial advice from all healthcare professionals and follow-up support. For example, especially in the early stages, symptoms such as coughing increase after the cigarettes are stopped. The patient must be closely supported to avoid a return to the habit. Most professional organizations have issued advice on helping patients stop smoking (see Department of Health website at www.givingupsmoking.co.uk/CNI/).

There are a number of therapeutic options to help an individual stop smoking and these include nicotine replacement therapy (NRT), bupropion and varenicline.

Nicotine replacement

The major mode of action of NRT is thought to be the stimulation of nicotine receptors in the brain and the subsequent release of dopamine. This, together with the peripheral effects of nicotine, leads to a reduction in nicotine withdrawal symptoms. NRT may also act as a coping mechanism, making cigarette smoking less rewarding. NRT does not, however, completely eliminate the effects of withdrawal as none of the available products reproduces the rapid and high levels of nicotine obtained from cigarettes.

There is little research comparing the relative effectiveness of NRT products, but all seem to have similar success rates. Choice of product should be made on the number of cigarettes smoked (irrespective of the nicotine content), the smoker's personal preference and tolerance to side effects. An individual is more likely to stick to the cessation programme if using a product which suits him or her. The types of NRT available are summarized in Table 26.10.

NRT approximately doubles smoking cessation rates compared with controls (either placebo or no NRT), irrespective of the intensity of adjunctive therapy. The strongest clinical trial evidence is with patches and gum; trials with other forms of NRT were generally smaller. The choice of product and initial dose is also influenced by the degree of tobacco dependence; heavy smokers (15–20+ cigarettes a day and/or smoking within

Table 26.10 Comparison of selected nicotine replacement products

Formulation	Use and comments	Specific side effects
Patch 24 hour: 7, 14 and 21mg 16 hour: 5, 10 and 15mg	One daily on clean, non-hairy, unbroken skin. Remove before morning (16 h) or next morning (24 h). Apply to fresh site or non-hairy skin, usually at the hip, trunk or upper arm. Should not be applied to broken skin	Local skin irritation and rashes, insomnia. Do not use with generalized skin disease
Gum 2 and 4mg	Chew until taste is strong then rest gum between gum and cheek; chew again when taste has faded. Repeat this for 30 minutes or until taste dissipates. Avoid acidic drinks for 15 min before and during chewing the gum	Jaw ache, headache and dyspnoea. Mild burning sensation in the mouth and throat
Sublingual tablet 2 or 4mg each	Rest under tongue until dissolved	
Lozenge 1, 2 or 4mg each	Place between gum and cheek and allow to dissolve. Delivers slightly more nicotine than the equivalent gum	Nasal irritation, rhinorrhoea, sneezing, throat irritation and cough. This usually dissipates with continued use
Inhalator 10mg per cartridge	Inhale as required. Helps to satisfy the hand-to-mouth ritual of using a cigarette which may help some people. The nicotine is absorbed through the mouth rather than the lungs. Use with caution in asthmatics	Nasal irritation, rhinorrhoea, sneezing, throat irritation and cough. This usually dissipates with continued use
Nasal spray 0.5mg per spray	One spray into each nostril as needed. More rapidly absorbed than other forms of NRT so often used for acute relief of cravings. Not recommended for people with nasal or sinus conditions, allergies or asthma	

30 minutes of waking) will require higher NRT doses. The available types of NRT product are as follows.

Long acting Transdermal patches are considered to be most suitable for people who smoke regularly through the day. The 24-hour patch, worn overnight, is better for people who crave nicotine first thing in the morning. This can cause insomnia or vivid dreams, so the patch can either be removed before bedtime or a 16-hour patch used. Heavy smokers should be started on the high-dose patches.

Short acting There are several short-acting products available:

- *Gum.* It is important to chew correctly when using nicotine gum. It is advised that the gum should be chewed slowly until the taste becomes strong and then allowed to rest between the cheek and teeth to allow absorption. When the taste has faded the gum should be chewed again. Nicotine gum is therefore not a good choice for people with dentures or other vulnerable dental work. Most gum users do not consume enough in a day to match the nicotine levels from smoking. Patients should be encouraged to use the 10–15 pieces of gum a day, for example as one piece an hour.
- *Lozenge.* These are allowed to dissolve in the mouth and periodically moved around, until completely gone. One lozenge per hour is recommended during the initial period of use to provide adequate nicotine absorption.
- *Inhalator.* This method of NRT may be particularly useful for people who miss the physical act of smoking. Nicotine is absorbed via the buccal mucosa with this device, peaking in 20–30 minutes. To achieve sufficient blood levels, the user should puff on the inhalator for 2 minutes each hour, changing the cartridge after three 20-minute sessions.
- *Nasal spray.* This is most useful for people who smoke 20 or more cigarettes per day. The side effects of sneezing and burning sensation in the nose usually wear off after a day or two so patients should be encouraged to persevere.
- *Sublingual tablets.* These tablets dissolve under the tongue and so may be useful for people with dentures who have difficulty using nicotine gum. Hourly use should be recommended.

Bupropion amfebutamone

Originally used as an antidepressant, this drug has been licensed for use in smoking cessation. Bupropion inhibits neuronal noradrenaline and dopamine uptake, reducing tobacco withdrawal symptoms by increasing CNS dopamine levels. Treatment should be started while the patient is still smoking and a target stop date set during the second week. Treatment should then be continued for 7–9 weeks, initially at a dose of 150mg daily for 6 days, increasing to 150mg twice a day thereafter (with at least 8 hours between doses). Trial evidence shows that it is as effective as NRT, alongside intensive behavioural support. There is no clear evidence of benefit over NRT but there is some evidence of better results if combined with NRT.

Bupropion should not be used in patients with a current or previous seizure disorder or in patients with bulimia, anorexia nervosa, bipolar disorder, severe hepatic cirrhosis or those taking monoamine oxidase inhibitors. Bupropion inhibits cytochrome P450 enzymes and so may inhibit the metabolism of other drugs.

The main side effects experienced include dry mouth, insomnia (avoid bedtime dosing), headache, dizziness, allergic reactions, taste disorder and seizures.

Varenicline

Varenicline is a new oral selective partial nicotinic agonist. Trial evidence suggests use may result in a higher abstinence rate than bupropion but its exact place in therapy has yet to be established. The main side effects are nausea, abnormal dreams and insomnia.

Use of inhaled therapy

For those patients with obstructive airways disease with a degree of reversibility, the correct use of inhaled therapy is a vital part of overall management.

Medication counselling needs to highlight the modes of action of the bronchodilators, particularly the more rapid onset of the β_2-agonists to relieve breathlessness rather than the slower-acting anticholinergics. If inhaled steroids are prescribed, the importance of regular administration must be stressed. The incorrect use of any inhaler will lead to subtherapeutic dosing. The correct use of inhalers is, therefore, as vital in the management of COPD patients as it is for patients with asthma (see Chapter 25). The

advantages and disadvantages of each type of inhaler device are summarized in Table 26.11.

Domiciliary oxygen therapy

Studies have shown that only about 50% of patients on LTOT comply with the requirement for 15 hours of treatment a day. Counselling will be required to persuade the patient to comply with this minimum figure. Emphasis must be given to the improvement in quality of life gained from treatment rather than the idea of being continually 'tied' to the oxygen supply. If an oxygen concentrator is used, limited mobility can be gained by installing at least two terminals for the unit (usually in the living room and bedroom) with long tubing between the terminal and nasal prongs.

Patients should be actively encouraged to stop smoking if they still do; they are a fire risk if they use LTOT. Moreover, the carbon monoxide present in tobacco smoke binds to haemoglobin and forms carboxy-haemoglobin, which decreases the amount of oxygen that can be transported by the blood and will partially or completely negate the beneficial effects of LTOT.

The long-term, chronic nature of COPD may leave a patient with a fear of exercise as this will cause dyspnoea (breathlessness). Thus the patient with COPD may decide not to undertake any exercise. Ambulatory oxygen cylinders can be used to encourage

Table 26.11   Comparison of inhaler devices

Inhaler type	Compact	Hand–lung co-ordination required	Easy to use	Reduces oropharynx deposition
MDI	+	+	−	−
MDI + small spacer	+	±	±	+
MDI + large spacer	−	−	±	+
Breath-actuated MDI	+	−	+	−
Dry powder	+	−	±	−
Breath-actuated dry powder	+	−	+	−
Nebulizer	−	−	±	−

MDI, metered dose inhaler; +, feature present; ±, feature present for some patients; −, feature absent.

Table 26.12   Oxygen delivery for ambulatory oxygen therapy

How long is the oxygen used by the patient?	Best type of delivery device
Less than 90 minutes	Small cylinder
90 minutes to 4 hours	Small cylinder with oxygen-conserving device
More than 4 hours	Liquid oxygen
More than 30 minutes, with flow rates greater than 2 L/min	Liquid oxygen

From NICE 2004

Table 26.13   Practice points

- The impact of COPD on an individual patient will depend not only on the degree of airflow limitation but also on the severity of their other symptoms such as exercise capacity and breathlessness.

- COPD can be classified according to FEV_1 measurements but there is not a predictable relationship between the presence of symptoms and the degree of airflow limitation.

- Pharmacological therapy is used to:
  - prevent and control the symptoms of COPD
  - reduce the frequency and severity of exacerbations
  - improve health status
  - improve exercise tolerance.

- All COPD patients still smoking should be encouraged to stop, and offered help to do so, at every opportunity.

- The choice of drug used should take into account the patient's response to a trial of the drug, the drug's side effects, patient preference, ease of use and cost.

- Drug administration via a nebulizer should be carefully and systematically considered for patients with distressing or disabling breathlessness despite maximal therapy with inhalers.

- Cor pulmonale can develop. The use of domiciliary oxygen therapy for 15 hours a day reduces the associated mortality.

- Pneumococcal vaccination and yearly influenza vaccination should be given to patients with COPD.

mobility and increase exercise tolerance during travel outside the home.

Patients using domiciliary oxygen are followed up to provide education and support, to assess the oxygen's effect on the oxygen saturation of the patient and to assess the suitability of the delivery device for ambulatory oxygen if provided. Suitable devices have been suggested by NICE (2004) depending on the amount of time required for use (Table 26.12).

CASE STUDIES

Case 26.1

Mrs CB is a 68-year-old retired farmer's wife who lives alone. She has been diagnosed with COPD for 18 months which is managed by a salbutamol MDI taken as required. Her FEV_1 readings are mildly reduced at 77% of the predicted value. She presents with a 2-day history of coughing and increasing shortness of breath and today started to expectorate yellow-coloured sputum. She stopped smoking 4 months ago and has remained abstinent.

Amoxicillin 500 mg 8-hourly and a 10-day course of prednisolone 30 mg every morning are prescribed by her primary care doctor and she is asked to take her salbutamol regularly, four puffs four times a day.

Three days later she can no longer go out of her house because of worsening shortness of breath and can no longer cope with her daily tasks. A pulse oximetry reading shows an oxygen saturation of 88% whilst breathing air. Her pulse rate is 93 beats per minute and she has a blood pressure of 177/90 mmHg.

Questions

1. Is the choice of antibiotic appropriate?
2. Does this patient need to be admitted to hospital?

Answers

1. The most likely bacterial causes of this acute exacerbation are *Haemophilus influenzae, Streptococcus pneumoniae* or *Moraxella catarrhalis*. Sometimes infection can be caused by *Chlamydia pneumoniae*. Acute bronchitis may also be caused by a viral infection, which would not be treated with antibiotics.

   Amoxicillin does not cover all *H. influenzae* infections. A suitable alternative would be co-amoxiclav as this gives better cover against *H. influenzae*. Other alternative agents would be doxycycline, clarithromycin or azithromycin, although there is increasing resistance to the macrolides in some areas. Local antibiotic policies should always be followed.

   Another factor to be considered is the extent to which the antibiotic penetrates the sputum. Commonly the amount of penetration reduces as COAD tissue damage progresses. β-Lactam antibiotics such as amoxicillin only reach sputum concentrations of approximately 5–20% of those in plasma. In order to obtain sufficient concentrations of antibiotics in the sputum, intravenous therapy may be required in patients with severe exacerbations or those unable to take medication orally.

2. Although COPD exacerbations should be managed at home wherever possible, worsening symptoms require hospital admission and management. The national guidelines (NICE 2004) give advice on when patients should be referred. Mrs CB's condition is deteriorating, she can no longer cope at home and has an oxygen saturation of below 90%. For these reasons she needs to be admitted to hospital.

Case 26.2

Mr NR is a 61-year-old retired dock worker whose medical history is COPD and chronic heart failure. He has recently started a pulmonary rehabilitation programme and asks you for advice on the best way to give up smoking. He currently smokes around 25 cigarettes a day and has been smoking since he was 20.

Questions

1. Why is it important for Mr NR to give up smoking?
2. What should be discussed when helping someone stop smoking?
3. What non-pharmacological support will help Mr NR in giving up?
4. Which smoking cessation product should be chosen?
5. Is this choice safe in someone with cardiac disease?

Answers

1. Stopping smoking is the single most important way of affecting a patient's outcome at all stages of COPD. Giving up smoking will slow down the gradual decline in FEV_1 that is seen in smokers. Mr NR should be told that stopping smoking will not prevent the onset of heart disease but that it will 'reduce the odds' for him personally.
2. There are five key steps in helping a smoker to stop smoking: the 'five As'.

   - **Ask** about tobacco use. This should include an assessment of the degree of addiction
   - **Advise** to quit
   - **Assess** willingness to make an attempt
   - **Assist** in quit attempt
   - **Arrange** follow-up

   Motivation from the patient is the key to giving up smoking but is related to the degree of dependence on tobacco. Heavy smokers may exhibit low motivation to quit as they lack confidence in their ability to do so.
3. It is thought that around 3% of smokers quit every year on their own but that percentage increases when given simple advice whilst encouraging the quit attempt. Several non-pharmacological strategies exist to help.

   - Written self-help material.
   - Counselling and behavioural therapy. These aim to motivate the smoker and help with the skills and strategies to cope with nicotine withdrawal, psychological pressures to smoke and coping with situations of temptation to smoke.

   In all cases pharmacological therapy should also be offered as appropriate.
4. Mr NR can be classed as a heavy smoker; smoking 25 cigarettes a day means that he is absorbing approximately 30–40 mg of nicotine each day. The patches are considered to be most suitable for people who smoke regularly through the day and so a high-dose 21 mg a day patch would seem a suitable first choice for Mr NR, particularly if he craves nicotine first thing in the morning. If he suffers from insomnia or vivid dreams, the patch can either be removed before bedtime or a 16-hour patch used. A suitable alternative would be the short-acting gum, lozenge or nasal spray. Mr NR would require the 4 mg gum and should be encouraged to use the 8–12 pieces of gum a day to provide approximately 20 mg of absorbed nicotine per day. As the nasal spray is most useful for people who smoke 20 or more cigarettes per day this may be the preferred formulation.

   Mr NR may benefit from a combination of products. Although this practice is not recommended by product manufacturers, this restriction is arbitrary and not evidence based (NICE 2004) and may be appropriate for some patients. If breakthrough cravings are felt despite a background patch then the addition of the other acute dosing forms may be used as 'rescue' medication.

   A date on which to quit smoking should be set. NRT should be prescribed in blocks of 2 weeks. Mr NR should be seen and helped regularly throughout this process, before and after his quit date. The NRT can be discontinued if Mr NR remains abstinent for 6–8 weeks.
5. NRT is safe in a patient with stable cardiac disease. In acute cardiovascular conditions such as acute myocardial infarction, unstable angina or stroke, NRT will act as a potent vasoconstrictor and should

be used with caution. Continued smoking is, however, likely to cause more harm than NRT even in these patients, so a balanced decision has to be made with the patient. If NRT is used then rapidly reversible products should be chosen such as gum, lozenges, nasal spray or the inhalator, as nicotine absorption ceases when the product is withdrawn.

Case 26.3

Mr MM is a 65-year-old male, 5'9" tall, who was diagnosed with COPD over 3 years ago. His condition was stable until about 18 months ago when he began to deteriorate slightly. His current medication is:

- salbutamol breath-actuated MDI (Easi-breathe) 2 puffs four times a day
- ipratropium dry powder inhaler (Aerocaps) 80 µg three times a day
- tiotropium 18 µg once a day.

His inhaler technique is poor with a standard MDI, despite repeated counselling.

In the last 6 months, he has had three exacerbations of his disease, the last one requiring hospitalization 2 weeks ago. Tiotropium was started during his hospital admission. His current FEV_1 is 254 L/min, with a predicted value of 565 L/min.

Questions

1. Can his inhalers be rationalized?
2. COPD guidance (NICE 2004) does not differentiate between long-acting anticholinergics or β_2-agonists if symptoms persist using short-acting bronchodilators alone. Are there any advantages of tiotropium?
3. As Mr MM is experiencing frequent exacerbations what are the possible treatment options at this stage?
4. What other measures can be taken to help prevent further exacerbations?

Answers

1. Mr MM should not be taking two anticholinergic agents; the ipratropium should have been discontinued when the tiotropium was started.

   He is using two inhaler devices but that is unavoidable with these drugs as there is no common device. His inhaler technique should be assessed; if he is having difficulty with the breath-actuated inhaler then a dry powder device may be more appropriate.
2. There is little published evidence to allow a clinically meaningful comparison between a long-acting anticholinergic and a long-acting β_2-agonist. A study is under way to investigate this question. Tiotropium does have noted advantages over ipratropium; it is given once a day and has more M_1 and M_3 selectivity. Comparisons between tiotropium and ipratropium or placebo show that tiotropium may reduce the number of exacerbations and improve exercise capacity, dyspnoea and health-related quality of life. As with other medication currently available for COPD, tiotropium has not demonstrated any effect on mortality or decline in lung function over time.

   In patients with severe symptoms it seems reasonable to combine both a long-acting anticholinergic and a long-acting β_2-agonist as additional benefits, similar to combining the short-acting agents, should be observed.
3. Mr MM's current FEV_1 is 48% of his predicted value. The addition of an inhaled steroid at this point would be appropriate as his current FEV_1 is less than 50% predicted. This should help to reduce the frequency of his exacerbations although there will be no effect on disease progression. There is no evidence or consensus regarding the minimum dose of steroid required for this indication. Doses which

have been used in trials include budesonide 800–1600 μg per day and fluticasone 1000 μg per day. No inhaled steroid is licensed in the UK for sole use, only combinations with long-acting β₂-agonists are licensed (Seretide, Symbicort). The choice, therefore, is to use an unlicensed product or add a long-acting β₂-agonist at the same time. Pragmatically a steroid alone should be added first. Mr MM can then be reviewed after a suitable period and if still symptomatic then the long-acting β₂-agonist can be added. When stable, a combination inhaler can be substituted for the individual inhalers if the doses are appropriate.

4. Mr MM should be encouraged to join a local pulmonary rehabilitation programme. These have been shown to lead to significant improvements in exercise capacity, quality of life and health status (Man et al 2004, NICE 2004).

   Mr MM should also be offered pneumococcal vaccination and yearly influenza vaccinations; these may help to prevent further exacerbations, particularly in the elderly. Even though there is no specific evidence that pneumococcal vaccine is helpful in COPD, its use is routinely recommended (NICE 2004).

   Self-management of exacerbations could be discussed. This would include:

- when to take maximal bronchodilator therapy
- when to start a course of oral steroids, e.g. if symptoms persist despite maximal bronchodilator dose, use 30 mg prednisolone for up to 14 days, stopping 2 days after symptoms resolve
- when to start antibiotics, e.g. when the sputum turns yellow or green
- when to call for an ambulance, e.g. if very short of breath or chest pain or feeling drowsy, agitated or confused.

REFERENCES

American Thoracic Society/European Thoracic Society (ATS/ERS) 2004 Standards for the diagnosis and management of patients with COPD. American Thoracic Society/European Thoracic Society. Available online at: www.ersnet.org/lrPresentations/copd/files/main/index.html

Barnes P J 2004 Corticosteroid resistance in airway disease. Proceedings of the American Thoracic Society 1: 264-268

Boe J, Dennis J H, O'Driscoll B R 2001 European Respiratory Society guidelines on the use of nebulizers. European Respiratory Journal 18: 228-242

British Thoracic Society (BTS) 2005 Clinical component for the home oxygen service in England and Wales. Available online at: www.brit-thoracic.org.uk/

GOLD 2005 Global strategy for the diagnosis, management, and prevention of chronic obstructive pulmonary disease. Global Initiative for chronic Obstructive Lung Disease. National Heart, Lung, and Blood Institute. Available online at: www.nhlbi.nih.gov/health/prof/lung/copd/copd_wksp.pdf

Man W D, Polkey M I, Donaldson N et al 2004 Community pulmonary rehabilitation after hospitalisation for acute exacerbations of chronic obstructive pulmonary disease: randomised controlled study. British Medical Journal 329: 1209

MRC Working Party 1981 Long-term domiciliary oxygen therapy in chronic hypoxic cor pulmonale complicating chronic bronchitis and emphysema. Lancet 1(8222): 681-686

National Institute for Clinical Excellence 2004 Chronic obstructive pulmonary disease. Clinical Guideline 12. National Institute for Clinical Excellence, London

National Institute for Clinical Excellence 2006 Brief interventions and referral for smoking cessation in primary care and other settings. Public Health Intervention Guidance 1. National Institute for Clinical Excellence, London

Vincken W 2005 Bronchodilator treatment of COPD: long acting anticholinergics. European Respiratory Review 14 (94): 23-31

FURTHER READING

Barnes P 2000 Chronic obstructive pulmonary disease. New England Journal of Medicine 343 (4): 269

Barnes P, Shapiro S D, Pauwels R A 2003 Chronic obstructive pulmonary disease: molecular and cellular mechanisms. European Respiratory Journal 22: 672-688

Braman S 2006 Chronic cough due to acute bronchitis: ACCP evidence-based clinical practice guidelines. Chest 129(1 suppl): 95S-103S

Britton J (ed) 2002 ABC of smoking cessation. BMJ Publishing, London. Also available online at: www.bmj.bmjjournals.com

Henningfield J E, Fant R V, Buchalter A R et al 2005 Pharmacotherapy for nicotine dependence. CA Cancer Journal for Clinicians 55: 281-299

MacNee W, Calverley P M A 2003 Chronic obstructive pulmonary disease 7: management of COPD. Thorax 58: 261-265

Morgan M D, Britton J R 2003 Chronic obstructive pulmonary disease 8: non-pharmacological management of COPD. Thorax 58: 453-457

National Collaborating Centre for Chronic Conditions 2004 Chronic obstructive pulmonary disease. Thorax 59 (suppl 1): 1-232

Drug-induced lung disease 27

N. P. Keaney

An adverse drug reaction (ADR) can involve the lung in a variety of ways and the clinical presentation is mainly determined by the site of the damage. Thus the airways may be principally affected, as in an allergic reaction to penicillin, or the parenchyma of the lung may be the sole site of involvement in various chronic fibrotic reactions. The symptoms and signs of an ADR may not, therefore, be easily distinguished from those of a naturally occurring illness. Likewise, the changes in pulmonary function, as measured by spirometry or by the carbon monoxide transfer factor, and the radiological abnormalities seen on a chest x-ray are usually non-specific.

A high index of suspicion is therefore required if an ADR is to be diagnosed and it can be very difficult to establish a cause-and-effect relationship without re-exposing the patient to one or more suspected drugs. Because of many uncertainties this is not a technique that is regularly used to confirm a suspected pulmonary ADR, e.g. a chronic reaction may have so disabled a patient that the risk:benefit ratio is unfavourable or provocation of an asthma attack may cause a life-threatening situation. Other dilemmas of drug rechallenge relate to the size and duration of dosage which must be chosen to ensure, on one hand, that an ADR is identifiable and, on the other, that only a safe reaction

occurs. In some circumstances rechallenge may not be necessary, because the ADR is merely an aspect of the therapeutic effect of a suspected drug, because an alternative is readily available or because of previous reports of a similar ADR to the drug.

ADRs are typically classified into those which are predictable on the basis of the known pharmacological action of the drug (Type A) and those that are of an idiosyncratic nature (Type B). Allergic (anaphylactic) reactions are defined as Type B, although in the airways, some apparently allergic reactions, i.e. asthmatic reactions, may be due to a recognized non-allergic mechanism. For most ADRs, however, the underlying mechanism is ill understood and the classification into Type A and B reactions cannot be easily applied. For example, some pulmonary reactions to cytotoxic drugs, although unpredictable in any particular patient, in essence may be a direct consequence of some, as yet unidentified, action of the drug or be exacerbated by environmental factors (see Case 27.1).

A range of drug-induced pulmonary syndromes can be identified (Table 27.1) It is convenient, therefore, to discuss induced lung disease on the basis of the respiratory structure principally affected and giving rise to the clinical syndrome characteristic for that site. Thus the bronchi and small airways, the parenchyma of the lung, the pulmonary circulation and the pleural space will be treated separately as much as is possible. All the ADRs described below are infrequent or rare phenomena and the descriptions of incidence, whether explicit or implied, should be read with that in mind.

Table 27.1 Syndromes typical of drug-induced pulmonary disease

Asthma
Bronchiolitis obliterans
Hypersensitivity infiltrate
Interstitial pneumonitis
Interstitial fibrosis
Non-cardiogenic pulmonary oedema
Pleural effusions
Pulmonary infiltrates with eosinophilia
Pulmonary vascular disease

Bronchi and small airways

Airflow obstruction

Local anaphylaxis in airways causes asthma due to release of preformed and newly synthesized mediators, involves IgE and mast cells in immediate reactions, and polymorph neutrophils, eosinophils, lymphocytes and platelets in late and sustained reactions. It is helpful to consider the various ways in which drugs may interact with the above processes as they modify the physiological control of the calibre of the airways (Table 27.2).

Drugs as antigens

Antibiotics are the drugs most often responsible for allergic reactions. These vary in severity, and acute asthma can accompany such local or systemic anaphylaxis. With penicillins, the group most commonly involved, there is almost always a history of uneventful exposure to a previous course of treatment. Fatal reactions seem to occur in patients with a recognized allergic predisposition such as asthma or a previous ADR to a penicillin. Historically sensitivity to penicillins has been due to persisting impurities such as a polyvalent penicilloyl antigen and sometimes to the β-lactam itself. Identification of penicillin sensitivity by patch or prick skin testing is not reliable and intradermal testing has been associated with fatality. As penicillin allergy may not be attributable to the β-lactam ring, it can be appreciated that cross-reactivity with another group of β-lactam antibiotics, the cephalosporins, is not an inevitable consequence of allergy to penicillin. Patients who report an allergy to penicillin should be assessed to determine whether it is likely that the reaction was immunologically mediated. Skin testing is only predictive for reactions mediated by IgE, such as anaphylaxis, angio-oedema, urticaria and asthma. Desensitization should be carried out in a hospital by a person with appropriate training.

Direct release of mediators

Histamine can be released from mast cells by a number of drugs and this phenomenon is readily demonstrated by intradermal injection of morphine or quaternary ammonium compounds such as tubocurarine; also in the clinical context marked bronchoconstriction has been reported after intravenous injection of muscle relaxants. This latter group of drugs is used in conjunction with intravenous anaesthetic agents which themselves can cause anaphylaxis. The combination of thiopentone and suxamethonium has been most often implicated in anaesthetic ADRs affecting the airways. When individual patients cross-react with other induction agents and/or relaxants an allergic process is unlikely. Direct release of mediators is probable with this combination of drugs and is clearly the mechanism for the high incidence of anaphylactoid reactions with the former anaesthetic agent Althesin. Althesin was a combination of two steroids solubilized with polyoxyethylated castor oil (Cremophor EL). This surface-active agent effected disruption of the membrane of mast cells, with ensuing release of granules and mediators. The cytotoxic agents, the taxols, are also formulated with Cremophor EL, but a slower rate of infusion has still been associated with anaphylactoid reactions.

Iodinated intravenous radiological contrast media have been systematically studied and in one survey the incidence of anaphylaxis was 1 in 14 000, accompanied in 12% of cases by severe bronchospasm. Individuals who are thought to be sensitive to contrast media can be tested with small intravenous doses. Pretreatment with an H_1-antagonist such as chlorphenamine may only be prophylactic in two-thirds of susceptible patients. Other drugs for which direct mediator release has been invoked include hydrocortisone sodium succinate, methylprednisolone and N-acetylcysteine. Using the phosphate salt of hydrocortisone, however, avoids this problem. Benzalkonium, which acts as a preservative and is incorporated in a number of preparations, probably acts in the same way and has been removed from solutions intended to be administered by nebulization (e.g. ipratropium).

Altered mediator synthesis

Aspirin and other non-steroidal anti-inflammatory drugs (NSAIDs) can precipitate asthma in sensitive individuals. These attacks develop about half an hour after ingestion and are frequently accompanied by flushing and rhinorrhoea. Random population surveys have found that 4–9% of asthmatics were affected.

Table 27.2 Various mechanisms whereby bronchospasm may be drug induced

Site of reaction	Mechanism	Typical drug
Interaction with IgE	Drug as antigen	Penicillin, dextrans
Direct release of mediators	Displacement of histamine	Iodinated contrast media, quaternary amines
Altered mediator synthesis	Cyclo-oxygenase inhibition	Aspirin, NSAIDs
Reflex bronchoconstriction	Non-specific irritation	Dry powder (lactose), metabisulfite,
Direct effect on smooth muscle	Agonist	Pilocarpine
Inhibit hydrolysis of mediator	Inhibition of enzyme	Neostigmine, captopril
Antagonism at β-receptors	Mast cell sensitization	Timolol, propafenone
Agonists at β-receptors	Tolerance (genetic poly-morphism)	Isoprenaline, fenoterol, salmeterol

Cross-sensitivity between aspirin and the many differently structured NSAID molecules argues against an allergic mechanism. One theory suggests that their common action as inhibitors of cyclo-oxygenase decreases prostaglandin E_2 (PGE_2) synthesis and creates an imbalance between bronchodilator and broncho-constrictor prostanoids and leukotrienes respectively. PGE_2 is thought to act as a brake on cys-leukotriene synthesis and on the release of other mediators from mast cells. Some individuals with this type of sensitivity to aspirin cross-react to the food colourant tartrazine (E102). A syndrome of late-onset asthma, nasal poly-posis and intermittent attacks of rhinorrhoea, angio-oedema or urticaria has been reported. Extrinsic asthmatics are also susceptible. The severity of an attack is variable but even mild asthmatics have been known to suffer a fatal reaction. A genetic predisposition may be relevant to familial clustering of cases but the expression of the abnormality is variable, with challenge results positive in those unaware of any history and negative in a significant proportion of those reporting previous aspirin sensitivity. Interestingly, a refractory period occurs for 2–5 days after a reaction to aspirin or a NSAID during which rechallenge does not precipitate asthma. This phenomenon has been used to desensitize patients who must take the drug regularly, thus maintaining the refractory state. Analgesia in this group of patients can be safely provided by the use of codeine or dihydrocodeine; paracetamol is without hazard for all but a few.

Reflex bronchoconstriction

The modern management of bronchial asthma utilizes the inhaled route of administration. In view of the hyperreactivity of the airways in asthmatics it should not be surprising that with a number of inhaled drugs bronchoconstriction may be brought about by a vagal reflex due to a non-specific stimulation of bronchial mucosal irritant receptors. This is especially problematic with dry powders. As an example of the need to overcome this side effect, the dry powder sodium cromoglicate administered via a Spinhaler (Fisons) was formerly available as a combination formulation with isoprenaline, a bronchodilator with a rapid onset of action.

Wheeze following inhalation of beclometasone dipropionate is well recognized and may be of some concern if an allergic reaction is responsible. In one study the abnormal reaction could be prevented by prior inhalation of cromoglicate, suggesting that an allergic basis was possible. However, the patients had a similar response to a placebo inhaler containing propellant alone. This suggested that a non-specific irritant action was the cause. There are now a number of alternative inhaled corticosteroid molecules presented in dry powder format. For instance, the multi-dose Pulmicort Turbohaler delivers budesonide, has no filler and should be without ill effect. The prior use of a bronchodilator would, of course, prevent this particular ADR.

Paradoxical bronchoconstrictor reactions to inhaled ipratropium have been reported with the nebulizer solution and, as mentioned above, the preservative benzalkonium was implicated. However, the major factor in this adverse response was undoubtedly the hypotonicity of the solution. Unit-dose vials with an isotonic preservative-free sterile formulation have more or less eliminated this ADR. Sporadic reports are now likely to be due to non-specific irritation and to involve metered dose inhalers.

Direct effect on smooth muscle

Cholinoceptor agonists such as carbachol, pilocarpine (eye drops) and methacholine (bronchial challenge testing) have all been identified as causative agents that can aggravate asthma or produce unexpectedly severe bronchoconstriction.

Inhibition of mediator hydrolysis

Anticholinesterases such as neostigmine are used after general anaesthesia to reverse the effects of competitive muscle antagonists and may also be used in patients with spinal cord injury to promote colonic emptying. Because of the risks of bronchospasm caused by excess acetylcholine, a muscarinic antagonist may be given simultaneously.

Angiotensin converting enzyme (ACE) inhibitors also inhibit other proteases such as those that inactivate bradykinin and other vasoactive peptides. The incidence of cough with this group of drugs has been reported to vary from 0.2% to 3%. This adverse effect has been ascribed to sensitization of non-myelinated nerve fibres in the airways by excess kinins. There is conflicting evidence as to whether ACE inhibitors affect bronchial hyper-reactivity. It is clear, however, that asthma is a much less likely side effect than cough with these agents.

Antagonism at β-adrenoreceptors

Non-selective β-receptor antagonists given orally block the β-receptors in the heart, peripheral vasculature, bronchi, pancreas and liver, etc. There may be some argument for using a selective β-agonist such as atenolol, metoprolol or bisoprolol in a patient with reversible airflow obstruction due to chronic bronchitis and without asthma. In this situation one might expect the inhaled $β_2$-agonist would need to be administered in a large dose to overcome the bronchial $β_2$-blockade which occurs to some extent even with 'selective' $β_1$-blockers. The issue is not simply one of agonist/antagonist interaction as pharmacokinetic considerations must be borne in mind. The inhaled route of administration results in selective distribution of supramaximal doses of bronchodilator to the airways. The effect is most likely to be inhibited by a competitive β-receptor antagonist towards the end of the expected duration of action, when the concentration of agonist will have declined substantially, i.e. after 3–4 hours. Whilst it would appear appropriate to use a β-agonist more frequently or to change to the anticholinergic agent ipratropium, the solution is really to avoid the use of β-adrenoreceptor blockers if inhaled bronchodilator therapy is required. Nowadays there are many alternatives to β-receptor blockers which can be used in the treatment of disorders such as hypertension and angina.

In asthmatic subjects there is an added risk to the use of a β-receptor blocker, namely that acute severe bronchospasm may be precipitated. This can occur even with the low systemic concentrations achieved following topical application of timolol eye drops. The mechanism of this ADR is uncertain. It is unlikely to be due to simple antagonism of circulating adrenaline or neurally released noradrenaline. It may possibly relate to an effect on mast cells which are stabilized by β-agonists at therapeutic concentrations; pretreatment of asthmatic subjects with cromoglicate will stabilize mast cells and protect from bronchoconstriction induced by propranolol. One must be aware that some drugs may have β-receptor blocking properties and can exacerbate asthma even though this may not be obvious at first sight. Examples of such agents include xamoterol, which has been marketed for use in mild cardiac failure, and propafenone, a class Ic antiarrhythmic drug.

Agonists at β-adrenoreceptors

The suggestion has been made in the past, and resurrected recently, that regular use of bronchodilators may result in a deterioration in the control of asthma. High doses of isoprenaline were implicated as the principal factor in the epidemic of sudden death from asthma which was recorded in a number of countries in the 1960s. This concern has been made all the more relevant by more recent epidemiological findings from New Zealand which attributed an increase in asthmatic mortality to self-treatment with nebulized fenoterol. With isoprenaline it seemed likely that inadequate education of patients about the use of prophylactic and emergency steroid therapy was combined with an overreliance on high doses of a non-selective β-agonist bronchodilator. Similar arguments have been presented for the data from New Zealand, where fenoterol was the standard nebulized bronchodilator therapy for severe asthma. Tolerance is thought to have developed in a proportion of patients who abused high-dose inhaled isoprenaline. The indirect evidence for this is based on an increase in the duration of action seen in those who reverted to using the drug appropriately.

Experiments designed to test tolerance to high-dose salbutamol by establishing successive dose–response curves before, during and after chronic dosing with oral or inhaled β-agonist have not consistently demonstrated tolerance in either asthmatic patients or volunteers. The probable explanation for the variation in these experiments is genetic polymorphism of β-receptors. One phenotype demonstrates a propensity to develop functional tolerance associated with downregulation of pulmonary β-receptors.

The discussion about the safety of β-receptor agonists has been further developed with sporadic reports that regular bronchodilator therapy might itself result in a deterioration of asthma control even when prophylactic inhaled steroid therapy is constant. The long-acting β-agonists (LABA) salmeterol and formoterol, with a duration of bronchodilator action of up to 12 hours, have also been the subject of reports of deterioration of asthma. A recent meta-analysis (Salpeter et al 2006) concluded that long-acting β-agonists increased severe and life-threatening exacerbations of asthma as well as asthma-related deaths. Whether this was due to β-adrenoreceptor desensitization and downregulation or increased bronchial hyperreactivity with regular β-agonist use is unclear, In children and adolescents tolerance to the protective effect of salmeterol on exercise-induced bronchconstriction in asthmatics has been shown after 1 week of treatment. Inhaled corticosteroid therapy has a protective effect. A similar pattern of results has been shown with allergen challenge in mild asthmatics. In practice this degree of tolerance found in the laboratory does not translate into significant problems for the majority of patients treated with a long-acting β-agonist.

Another concern relates to the rate of onset of bronchoconstriction during an acute asthmatic attack, especially in the presence of a long-acting bronchodilator. In this circumstance the functional antagonism between the bronchodilator and endogenous spasmogens means that dilated airways require a higher concentration of mediators to achieve a given degree of bronchoconstriction. It has been shown for the bronchoconstrictors histamine and methacholine that, following pre-treatment with salbutamol, the rate of decline of FEV_1, once it begins, is more rapid with the higher concentrations required to overcome the pre-existing salbutamol-induced bronchodilation. This evidence has been extrapolated to justify inclusion in guidelines which recommend that in an informed, motivated, self-monitoring patient bronchodilators should be used on an intermittent basis, as required for symptomatic relief, provided that there is an additional therapeutic background of anti-inflammatory prophylaxis. More symptomatic patients, particularly those with nocturnal wheezing, have reported significant improvements in their quality of life when they use a long-acting bronchodilator and, despite the concerns outlined above, large and prolonged clinical trials have not shown an increase in the rate of exacerbations with salmeterol.

Lung parenchyma

ADRs affecting the lung parenchyma can be broadly classified into acute and chronic reactions, reflecting hypersensitivity and fibrosis as the predominant mechanisms of toxic response respectively. Subacute reactions, intermediate between acute and chronic in their onset, also occur. Although there is little understanding of the processes underlying the aetiology and pathogenesis of these ADRs, certain clinical patterns are identifiable.

Hypersensitivity pneumonitis

In general, these acute reactions are of an allergic nature, have a dramatic clinical presentation, and demand urgent diagnosis and withdrawal of the offending agent. With early treatment the affected individual has an excellent chance of a complete recovery (Lacasse & Cormier 2006). When a patient develops a cough with breathlessness and wheezing many probable causes are considered before this symptom complex is attributed to an ADR. However, in the context of a patient receiving a disease-modifying antirheumatic drug (DMARD) a heightened awareness of the importance of such symptoms is required. A patchy bilateral infiltrate distributed peripherally on the chest radiograph and eosinophilia on a blood count should lead to review of recent drug therapy. Such a presentation in an individual whose lungs have previously been normal and in whom infection has been excluded will be more confidently identified as an ADR if the history reveals ingestion of a candidate drug. A diagnosis will usually be made on the grounds of high clinical suspicion but further investigations will include pulmonary function testing with spirometry and measurement of the transfer factor for carbon monoxide. However, these results will merely characterize the type of defect.

In recent years the technique of bronchoscopic bronchoalveolar lavage has been applied to these cases. It has proved possible to identify an increase in the cellular yield (pleocytosis) in hypersensitivity pneumonitis with eosinophilia and/or lymphocytosis in the fluid obtained at bronchoalveolar lavage. With more sophisticated facilities the pattern of various lymphocytic subtypes can be assessed. Alternatively an in vitro analysis of the transformation of lavaged lymphocytes can be performed and the effects of challenge with the suspected drug studied. Pleural effusions sometimes are a feature and eosinophilia may be found in the pleural fluid or on pleural biopsy. The rapid onset of the symptoms will usually ensure the speedy withdrawal of the offending drug (usually by the patient) and it seems likely that many minor reactions are never reported. The probability of complete recovery is excellent and the rate of improvement may be accelerated by systemic corticosteroid therapy.

Drug-induced hypersensitivity pneumonitis is not a sufficiently frequent occurrence for trials of treatment to be compared. It seems logical to use a corticosteroid with a view to suppressing the inflammatory reaction and so prevent a subacute illness or chronic inflammation which could progress to pulmonary fibrosis and permanent impairment of pulmonary function.

Non-steroidal anti-inflammatory drugs

Among the drugs which are recognized to cause hypersensitivity pneumonitis, NSAIDs such as indomethacin, azapropazone, diclofenac, piroxicam and ibuprofen have all been identified.

Gold

Parenteral gold (aurothiomalate) when used in the treatment of rheumatoid arthritis has also been found to cause acute breathlessness with bilateral 'alveolar' infiltrates on the chest x-ray. The symptoms can follow the second to the fifth or sixth injection. There is approximately a 50% chance of complete resolution if the gold treatment is discontinued. A genetic predisposition to this ADR is probable.

Salazopyrin

Salazopyrin is widely used in the management of patients with rheumatoid arthritis. It too has been implicated as a cause of pulmonary eosinophilia although the majority of reports have related to its use in inflammatory bowel disease. The reaction is mostly related to the sulphonamide rather than the 5-aminosalicylate moiety (mesalazine). A typical presentation is detailed in Case 27.2.

Other drugs

Many other drugs have featured in sporadic reports of drug-induced pulmonary eosinophilia, especially antibiotics. Nitrofurantoin causes both acute pneumonitis (90% of cases) and, rarely, chronic pulmonary fibrosis. It is of particular interest as it resembles paraquat in its capacity to undergo cyclical reduction and oxidation. The reoxidation liberates a free electron and generates toxic O_2^- radicals and a reactive nitrofurantoin molecule which may act as a hapten. The acute reaction usually occurs after 4 weeks or so of continuous treatment although even more rapid reactions have been observed. In the 10 years from 1995 the Australian ADR Advisory Committee received reports of 46 pulmonary reactions to nitrofurantoin, most often in elderly females, this gender bias reflecting usage.

With cytotoxic immunosupressent drugs acute reactions are uncommon. Methotrexate is implicated most often but this reflects its higher usage compared with procarbazine, mitomycin, bleomycin or azathioprine, all of which have been associated with the development of eosinophilic pneumonitis. Corticosteroid therapy will hasten clinical improvement of these ADRs and re-exposure to the offending drug is not recommended.

Pulmonary fibrosis

Drug-induced pulmonary fibrosis is an ADR which is somewhat more reliably diagnosed than other parenchymal reactions, particularly with cytotoxic drugs. For such drugs the cumulative dose, the patient's age, renal dysfunction, previous radiotherapy, oxygen administration and concurrent cytotoxic therapy have been implicated as predisposing factors (Dimopoulou et al 2006). The antiarrhythmic agent amiodarone has also been implicated as a cause of pulmonary fibrosis.

Bleomycin

Bleomycin was found to cause pulmonary damage during early animal experiments but nevertheless it was introduced into clinical practice and the predictability of this reaction led to its experimental use and research into mechanisms of toxicity. The high ambient oxygen tension in the lung facilitates the generation of superoxide radicals by bleomycin and this effect also accounts for the risks of oxygen therapy mentioned above. A relationship between the dose of bleomycin and its toxicity becomes evident when more than 450 mg has been administered; below this dose toxicity occurs in 3–5% of patients, whereas at 450–550 mg and over 550 mg, incidences of 13% and 17% respectively have been observed.

The clinical onset of the chronic pneumonitis/pulmonary fibrosis syndrome is usually insidious with symptoms of malaise, dry cough, fever and breathlessness developing and progressing over a period of several weeks or months. The chest x-ray is usually abnormal with basal infiltrates initially and widespread infiltrates in more severely affected patients. CT scanning is a more sensitive method of detecting pulmonary abnormalities. (Nodules resembling metastatic deposits from the primary tumour have also been seen on CT scanning.) Pulmonary function testing has shown abnormalities in asymptomatic individuals with no radiological changes, yielding presumed prevalences of toxicity of 33% and 71% in two surveys. However, some of the effects attributed to bleomycin were minor and unlikely to be clinically deleterious, e.g. a 10% reduction in gas transfer occurred after the first dose of bleomycin in one study but did not decrease further.

The course of the pulmonary damage caused by bleomycin is variable. With mild disease the radiological changes may resolve over a period of 6–12 months if the drug is withdrawn and symptoms may disappear. High-dose corticosteroid therapy in more severely affected patients has led to improvement. Mortality from bleomycin-induced pulmonary fibrosis ranges from 1 to 2% in large series to 10% in patients receiving 550 mg. Despite this profile of toxicity bleomycin is used in a variety of malignant tumours as it is often curative.

Busulphan

Pulmonary parenchymal damage caused by other cytotoxic drugs is regularly observed and reported in the literature. The alkylating agent busulphan has a low risk estimated at 4% but autopsy studies have found a much higher incidence of abnormalities (46%) that had not been clinically evident during life. Chlorambucil, cyclophosphamide and melphalan are the subjects of sporadic reports of fibrotic ADRs involving the lung. In one bizarre incident, a pharmacist treated himself with melphalan because myelomatosis had been mentioned in a differential diagnosis. He died from progressive pulmonary fibrosis and did not have any disorder requiring cytotoxic therapy.

Carmustine

The nitrosoureas, especially carmustine, seem to be capable of causing a syndrome of delayed pulmonary fibrosis. Carmustine is usually used alone in primary cerebral malignant tumours which rarely involve the lung. The attribution of a pulmonary ADR to this drug can be made much more clearly and confidently in this circumstance than, for example, when multiple cytotoxic drugs are used for an intrathoracic tumour which is subsequently irradiated. For carmustine high dosage is correlated with the early development of pulmonary fibrosis but the incidence of this ADR increases as survivors are followed up. In one series of 31 children treated with carmustine, only 17 were cured of their tumour. Of these survivors, six died from pulmonary fibrosis (two within 3 years of treatment) and six of the remaining eight patients, who could be traced, were found to have evidence of severe fibrotic damage to the lungs with an active fibrotic process recognized up to 17 years after treatment.

Amiodarone

The antiarrhythmic drug amiodarone has an unusual pharmacokinetic profile due to its high lipid solubility. The parent drug and its principal desethyl metabolite have exceptionally low rates of elimination ($t_{1/2}$ 45–60 days) from huge volumes of distribution (5000 litres) resulting in concentrations in the lung 1000 times greater than in plasma. This accumulation favours a direct toxic effect and daily doses in excess of 400 mg for more than 2 months result in pulmonary toxicity in 6% of patients. A mortality rate of 10–20% is expected. Chronic pneumonitis with fibrosis is the usual toxic manifestation and this can be readily diagnosed on transbronchial biopsy performed via a bronchoscope. Foamy alveolar macrophages seen on light microscopy contain dense lamellar cytoplasmic inclusions on electron microscopy which are a consequence of pulmonary accumulation of phospholipid with amiodarone and desethylamiodarone and are seen even in the absence of clinical evidence of pneumonitis or fibrosis.

Up to 25% of patients with amiodarone-induced pulmonary damage may have 'organizing pneumonia', a steroid-responsive condition with characteristic histological features. This type of reaction is thought to have an immunological basis and treatment with prednisolone is recommended for all patients in case some areas of pneumonitis are of this nature. This treatment should be continued for some months after withdrawal of amiodarone, because of its prolonged elimination half-life.

Amiodarone is heavily iodinated and increases the density of tissues, e.g. pulmonary opacities seen on CT scans can be ascribed to this drug's toxicity from the radiological appearances. Oxygen therapy, e.g. during general anaesthesia, may aggravate pulmonary toxicity and in some instances precipitate respiratory failure in patients with subclinical amiodarone toxicity.

Pulmonary vasculature

Pulmonary embolism

In the early 1960s there were many reports of venous thrombosis in association with the use of oral contraceptive agents. The sporadic reports were followed by many systematic surveys, both retrospective and prospective, that established a risk of thromboembolism 5–6 times greater in women on the contraceptive pill. Further studies related the risk to the dose of oestrogen and, despite a general dose reduction, a small risk persists. In a prospective study of 17 000 married women aged 25–39 years, 105 episodes of venous thromboembolism occurred, the incidence (events per thousand woman-years) being 0.43 in users and 0.06 in non-users of oral contraceptives. Seventy-one of the certain or probable diagnoses were in postoperative patients and confined to current users of oral contraceptives. Further evidence suggests that the risk of pregnancy, and associated incidence of thromboembolic disease, is such that a combined oral contraceptive should not be discontinued preoperatively. The use of a progestogen-only pill would undoubtedly carry less risk.

The implications of oestrogen in hormone replacement therapy (HRT) have been extensively studied and a twofold to fourfold risk of thromboembolism reported with both oestrogen alone and oestrogen/progestogen combinations. Hormone replacement therapy is a purely preventive therapy and so the risk/benefit relationships should be assessed, bearing in mind that in an older population of women, factors such as gross obesity, previous venous thrombosis and/or a family history of venous thrombosis must be taken into account.

Pulmonary hypertension

About 30 years ago a small epidemic of pulmonary hypertension was identified, particularly in Switzerland. The problem seemed to be confined to countries where the appetite suppressant aminorex fumarate was marketed. The evidence for this ADR was circumstantial as no animal model was found that reproduced the syndrome. Withdrawal of the drug brought the epidemic to an end. Now sporadic cases associated with other anorectic drugs such as amphetamines, fenfluramine and most recently dexfenfluramine have been reported.

Pulmonary hypertension, once initiated, usually progresses to a clinical syndrome characterized by increasing breathlessness, right-sided cardiac failure and sudden death. Pulmonary hypertension also follows severe or recurrent pulmonary thromboembolism and is therefore linked with oestrogen therapy and the oral contraceptive. Intravenous drug abusers inject particulate matter, e.g. from crushed tablets, impaction of which in pulmonary arterioles may give rise to a clinical presentation typical of pulmonary embolism. Progression to severe pulmonary hypertension does occur and corn starch, talc and microcrystalline cellulose have each been found in the lung on histological examination.

Eosinophilia/myalgia with L-tryptophan

In 1989 a new syndrome occurred typified by pain in muscles and a rash, with cough and breathlessness being common. There was marked eosinophilia of peripheral blood but even in the most breathless patients the chest x-ray looked surprisingly normal. Pulmonary hypertension was often found and was the cause of the respiratory distress. Treatment with an anti-inflammatory high-dose corticosteroid was rapidly beneficial.

The majority of patients were taking L-tryptophan as a 'health food' supplement but subsequently cases were described from psychiatric clinics where L-tryptophan was prescribed for a depressive illness. The causative factor of this eosinophilia/myalgia syndrome is obscure. It is intriguing to consider how such an adverse reaction could be due to a naturally occurring amino acid. An individual producer of L-tryptophan was linked epidemiologically to many cases in the USA and it has been suggested that an impurity, identified as 1,1'ethylene (bis)tryptophan, arising from the manufacturing process, was the cause.

Pulmonary vasculitis

Drug-induced pulmonary vasculitis is caused by an immune mechanism, e.g. due to the presence of intravascular immune complexes formed when excess antigen (drug or metabolite) and antibody combine and are deposited on the vascular endothelium. The complement system is then activated and the sequential changes set up an inflammatory reaction. The result is a vasculitis which produces different clinical manifestations, the pattern of which depends on the size and site of the blood vessels targeted by the immune complexes and on the persistence of the cellular response. Our understanding of these and other parenchymal reactions is limited by the absence of suitable animal models and the paucity of adequate histological evidence in most patients, so that many cases of pulmonary vasculitis will be overlooked.

Pulmonary vasculitis is frequently a capillaritis and the conventional diagnostic appearances associated with an arteritis will be absent. The involvement of capillaries weakens them and, as they are largely unsupported by connective tissue, bleeding into the alveolar walls and alveoli occurs. If this diffuse intrapulmonary haemorrhage is associated with glomerulonephritis and is of idiopathic aetiology, it is called Goodpasture's syndrome. The diagnostic marker is a circulating antibody against the glomerular basement membrane (anti-GBM). This anti-GBM is not detected in cases of drug-induced diffuse intrapulmonary haemorrhage (with or without glomerulonephritis), typically due to penicillamine, but also described with aminoglutethimide, nitrofurantoin, amphotericin and cocaine smoking.

Pulmonary oedema

Non-cardiogenic pulmonary oedema or adult respiratory distress syndrome (ARDS) occurs as a consequence of increased pulmonary alveolar capillary permeability. Classically the air spaces in the lung become filled with a proteinaceous fluid. This ADR can be mistaken for left ventricular failure from which it differs by having a normal pulmonary venous 'wedge' pressure. Breathlessness and hypoxaemia may progress to respiratory failure. In 1880 Osler described pulmonary oedema as a complication of heroin abuse and it still occurs in addicts. This particular ADR occurs with both intravenously and orally administered opiates. It has been reported after overdose of dextropropoxyphene and codeine and even with naloxone (although this drug is only likely to be given to patients who have already taken an opiate). Other drugs known to cause non-cardiogenic pulmonary oedema are listed in Table 27.3.

Pleural reactions

Pleural reactions, either effusions or fibrosis, may be associated with various parenchymal ADRs or may be an isolated finding. Bromocriptine, like methysergide, is an ergot derivative and while both have been found to cause pulmonary fibrosis, an unusual feature of this ADR has been the presence of pleural effusions and/or pleural thickening. It is tempting to relate the reaction to an effect involving 5HT receptors but which cell type is involved is unclear. Other drugs associated with pleural effusion are listed in Table 27.4 and at least six subgroups can be identified.

Table 27.3 Drugs causing non-cardiogenic pulmonary oedema

Adrenaline
Amitriptyline*
Antilymphocytic globulin
Aspirin
Codeine*
Dextropropoxyphene*
Diamorphine (heroin)
Hydrochlorothiazide
Indometacin
Interleukin-2
Methadone
Mono-octanoin
Ritodrine
Salbutamol
Terbutaline

*ADR occurs with overdose

Table 27.4 Examples of drugs associated with pleural effusion and/or thickening

Drug	Association
Amiodarone	Parenchymal reaction
Cytotoxics	
Methotrexate	Pleuritic pain
Dantrolene	
Nitrofurantoin	Eosinophilia
L-tryptophan	
Interleukin-2	
Bromocriptine	
Methysergide	5HT receptors
Pergolide	
Oesophageal sclerosants	Direct toxicity
Procainamide	Drug-induced systemic lupus erythematosus

CASE STUDIES

Case 27.1

A 51-year-old man receiving chemotherapy in January collapsed on leaving hospital. His breathing was distressed and noisy. He was thought to be fitting and was taken to the hospital accident and emergency department. An initial assessment suggested asthma but nebulized salbutamol was not helpful. Stridor was then recognized as he improved in the warmer temperature.

Comment

Reflex laryngeal spasm is part of the recognized neurotoxicity of oxaloplatin and the cold air probably triggered sensitized sensory neurones in his larynx, resulting in vocal cord adduction (laryngospasm), stridor and collapse. Avoidance of cold air is the best policy in this case as the reaction is likely only in the immediate aftermath of oxaloplatin administration.

Case 27.2

Shortly after knee joint replacement, a 75-year-old ex-miner developed classic rheumatoid arthritis. Diclofenac, a parenteral steroid, and salazopyrin (as a DMARD) were introduced with significant early relief from the steroid and continued improvement with the salazopyrin. After 3 months he mentioned a cough with purulent sputum and an antibiotic was prescribed. A year later he was admitted to hospital where he was treated for community-acquired pneumonia. Response to antibiotic therapy was poor and the chest x-ray showed persistent shadowing. A CT scan demonstrated pulmonary fibrosis and features of pneumonitis.

Comment

An ADR to salazopyrin was considered the likely causative agent. This drug was discontinued and prednisolone given with subsequent clinical and radiological improvement. The rheumatoid arthritis was eventually satisfactorily controlled with leflunomide.

REFERENCES

Dimopoulou I, Bamias A, Lyberopoulos P et al 2006 Pulmonary toxicity from novel antineoplastic agents. Annals of Oncology 17: 372-379

Lacasse Y, Cormier Y 2006 Hypersensitivity pneumonitis. Orphanet Journal of Rare Diseases 1:25. Available online at: www.ojrd.com/content/1/1/25

Salpeter S R, Buckley N S, Ormiston T M, Salpeter E E 2006 Meta-analysis: effect of long-acting β agonists on severe asthma exacerbations and asthma-related deaths. Annals of Internal Medicine 144: 904-912

FURTHER READING

Camus P, Gibson G J 2003 Adverse pulmonary effects of drugs and radiation. In: Gibson G J, Geddes D M et al (eds) Respiratory medicine. W B London

Camus P, Foucher P, Bonniaud P et al 2001 Drug-induced infiltrative lung disease. European Respiratory Journal 18: 93s-100s

Gruchalla R S, Pirmohamed M 2006 Antibiotic allergy. New England Journal of Medicine 354: 601-609

Keaney N P 2003 Respiratory disorders. In: Davies D M, Ferner R E, de Glanville H (eds) Textbook of adverse drug reactions. Oxford University Press, Oxford

Talbot J, Waller P (eds) 2004 Stephens' detection of new adverse drug reactions. John Wiley, Chichester

Useful website: Pneumotox online. Available online at: www.pneumotox. com/lungdrug

Insomnia and anxiety 28

C. H. Ashton

Definitions and epidemiology

Insomnia and anxiety are among the commonest symptoms seen in general practice. Each can arise from a number of causes and often, though not always, they occur together. Insomnia refers to difficulty in falling asleep or staying asleep, or to lack of refreshment from sleep. Complaints of poor sleep increase with increasing age and are twice as common in women as in men (Sateia & Nowell 2004). Thus by the age of 50, a quarter of the population are dissatisfied with their sleep, the proportion rising to 30–40% (two-thirds of them women) among individuals over 65 years.

Anxiety, a feeling of apprehension or fear, combined with symptoms of increased sympathetic activity, is a normal response to stress. A clinical problem may arise if the anxiety becomes severe or persistent and interferes with everyday performance. Clinical subtypes of anxiety include panic disorder, agoraphobia, other phobias and generalized anxiety but these subtypes may merge into a 'general neurotic' syndrome (Tyrer 1989). The prevalence of such syndromes in the general population is about 10–20% and there is a high rate of co-morbidity with depressive disorders. The overall female-to-male ratio is nearly 2:1. The age of onset of most anxiety disorders is in young adulthood (twenties and thirties), although the maximum prevalence of generalized anxiety and agoraphobia-panic in the general population is in the 50–64 year age group.

Pathophysiology

Anxiety and insomnia reflect disturbances of arousal and/or sleep systems in the brain. These systems are functionally interrelated and their activity determines the degree and type of alertness during wakefulness and the depth and quality of sleep.

Arousal systems

Arousal is maintained by at least three interconnected systems: a general arousal system, an 'emotional' arousal system and an endocrine/autonomic arousal system (Fig. 28.1). The general arousal system, mediated by the brainstem reticular formation, thalamic nuclei and basal forebrain bundle, serves to link the cerebral cortex with incoming sensory stimuli and provides a tonic influence on cortical reactivity or alertness. Excessive activity in this system, due to internal or external stresses, can lead to a state of hyperarousal as seen in anxiety and insomnia. Emotional aspects of arousal, such as fear and anxiety, are contributed by the limbic system which also serves to focus attention on selected aspects of the environment. There is evidence that increased activity in certain limbic pathways is associated with anxiety and panic attacks.

These arousal systems activate somatic responses to arousal, such as increased muscle tone, increased sympathetic activity and increased output of anterior and posterior pituitary hormones. Inappropriate increases in autonomic activity are often associated with anxiety states; the resulting symptoms (palpitations, sweating, tremor, etc.) may initiate a vicious circle which increases the anxiety.

Several neurotransmitters have been particularly implicated in arousal systems. Acetylcholine is the main transmitter maintaining general arousal but there is evidence that heightened emotional arousal is particularly associated with increased noradrenergic and serotonergic activity. Drugs which antagonize such activity have anxiolytic effects. In addition, the inhibitory neurotransmitter γ-aminobutyric acid (GABA) exerts an inhibitory control on other transmitter pathways and increased GABA activity may have a protective effect against excessive stress reactions. Many drugs which increase GABA activity are potent anxiolytics.

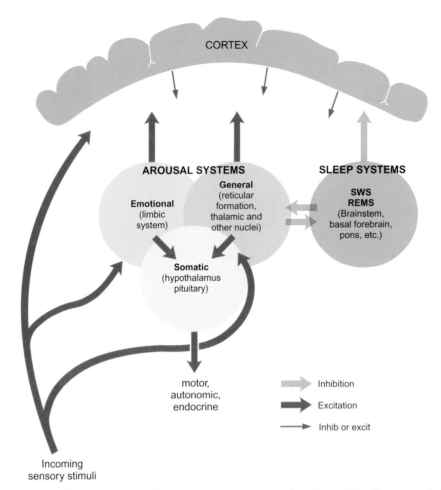

Figure 28.1 Diagram of arousal and sleep systems. Arousal systems receive environmental and internal stimuli, cause cortical activation and mediate motor, autonomic and endocrine responses to arousal. Reciprocally connected sleep systems generate slow-wave sleep (SWS) and rapid eye movement sleep (REMS). Either system can be excited or inhibited by cognitive activity generated in the cortex.

Sleep systems

At the other end of the arousal spectrum, the phenomenon of sleep is actively induced and maintained by neural mechanisms in several brain areas, including the lower brainstem, pons and parts of the limbic system. These mechanisms have reciprocal inhibitory connections with arousal systems, so that activation of sleep systems at the same time inhibits waking and vice versa (see Fig. 28.1). Normal sleep includes two distinct levels of consciousness, orthodox sleep and paradoxical sleep, which are promoted from separate neural centres.

Orthodox sleep normally takes up about 75% of sleeping time. It is somewhat arbitrarily divided into four stages (1–4) which merge into each other, forming a continuum of decreasing cortical and behavioural arousal. Stages 3 and 4 are associated with increasing amounts of high-voltage δ slow waves (1–3 Hz) shown on the electroencephalograph (EEG). These latter stages represent the deepest level of sleep and are also termed slow-wave sleep (SWS).

Paradoxical sleep (rapid eye movement sleep, REMS) normally takes up about 25% of sleeping time and has quite different characteristics. The EEG shows unsynchronized fast activity similar to that found in the alert conscious state and the eyes show rapid jerky movements. Peripheral autonomic activity is increased during REMS and there is an increased output of catecholamines and free fatty acids. Vivid dreams and nightmares most often occur in REMS, although brief frightening dreams (hypnagogic hallucinations) can occur in orthodox sleep, especially at the transition between sleeping and waking. Normally stage 4 sleep occurs mostly in the first few hours of the night, while REMS is most prominent towards the morning. Brief awakenings during the night are normal. Both SWS and REMS are thought to be essential for brain function and both show a rebound after a period of deprivation, usually at the expense of lighter (stage 1 and 2) sleep which appears to be expendable.

Aetiology and clinical manifestations

Insomnia

Insomnia may be caused by any factor which increases activity in arousal systems or decreases activity in sleep systems. Many causes act on both systems (Morin 2003). Increased sensory stimulation activates arousal systems, resulting in difficulty in falling asleep. Common causes include pain or discomfort and external stimuli such as noise, bright lights and extremes of temperature. Anxiety may also delay sleep onset as a result of increased emotional arousal.

Drugs are an important cause of insomnia. Difficulty in falling asleep may result directly from the action of stimulants, including caffeine, theophylline, sympathomimetic amines and some antidepressants. Drug withdrawal after chronic use of central nervous system depressants, including hypnotics, anxiolytics and alcohol, commonly causes rebound insomnia with delayed or interrupted sleep, increased REMS and nightmares. With rapidly metabolized drugs, such as alcohol or short-acting benzodiazepines, this rebound may occur in the latter part of the night, resulting in early waking. Certain drugs, including neuroleptics, tricyclic antidepressants and propranolol, may occasionally cause nightmares.

Difficulty in staying asleep is characteristic of depression. Patients typically complain of early waking but sleep records show frequent awakenings, early onset of REMS and reduced SWS. Alteration of sleep stages, increased dreaming and nightmares may also occur in schizophrenia, while recurring nightmares are a feature of post-traumatic stress disorder. Interference with circadian rhythms, as in shift work or rapid travel across time zones, can cause difficulty in falling asleep or early waking.

Frequent arousals from sleep are associated with myoclonus, 'restless legs syndrome', muscle cramps, bruxism (tooth grinding), head banging and sleep apnoea syndromes. Reversal of the sleep pattern, with a tendency to poor nocturnal sleep but a need for daytime naps, is common in the elderly, in whom it may be associated with cerebrovascular disease or dementia.

Anxiety

Anxiety is commonly precipitated by stress but vulnerability to stress appears to be linked to genetic factors such as trait anxiety and many patients presenting for the first time with anxiety symptoms have a long history of high anxiety levels going back to childhood. Anxiety may also be induced by central stimulant drugs (caffeine, amphetamines), withdrawal from chronic use of central nervous system depressant drugs (alcohol, hypnotics, anxiolytics) and metabolic disturbances (hyperventilation, hypoglycaemia, thyrotoxicosis). It may form part of a depressive disorder and may occur in temporal lobe lesions and in rare hormone-secreting tumours such as phaeochromocytoma or carcinoid.

Apart from the psychological symptoms of apprehension and fear, somatic symptoms may be prominent in anxiety and include palpitations, chest pain, shortness of breath, dizziness, dysphagia, gastrointestinal disturbances, loss of libido, headaches and tremor. Panic attacks are experienced as storms of increased autonomic activity combined with a fear of imminent death or loss of control. If panics become associated with a particular environment, commonly a crowded place with no easy escape route, the patient may actively avoid similar situations and eventually become agoraphobic.

Investigations and differential diagnosis

Many patients complaining of insomnia overestimate their sleep requirements. Although most people sleep for 7–8 hours daily, some healthy subjects require as little as 3 hours of sleep and sleep requirements decline with age. Such 'physiological insomnia' does not usually cause daytime fatigue, although the elderly may take daytime naps. If insomnia is causing distress, primary causes such as pain, drugs which disturb sleep, psychiatric disturbance including anxiety and depression and organic causes such as sleep apnoea should be identified and treated before hypnotic therapy is prescribed. There is growing concern that daytime sleepiness resulting from insomnia increases the risk of industrial, traffic and other accidents.

In patients presenting with symptoms and clinical signs of anxiety, it is important to exclude organic causes such as thyrotoxicosis, excessive use of stimulant drugs such as caffeine and the possibility of alcoholism or withdrawal effects from benzodiazepines. However, unnecessary investigations should be avoided if possible. Extensive gastroenterological, cardiological and neurological tests may increase anxiety by reinforcing the patient's fear of serious underlying physical disease.

Treatment

Hypnotic drugs

Hypnotic drugs provide only symptomatic treatment for insomnia. Although often efficacious in the short term, they do little to alter the underlying cause which should be sought and treated where possible. Simple explanation of sleep requirements, attention to sleep hygiene, reduction in caffeine or alcohol intake and the use of analgesics where indicated may obviate the need for hypnotics (Drug & Therapeutics Bulletin 2004, Morin 2003, Sateia & Nowell 2004). Behavioural techniques are sometimes helpful. Nevertheless, about 20 million prescriptions for hypnotics are issued each year in the UK and these drugs can improve the quality of life if used rationally.

The ideal hypnotic would gently suppress brain arousal systems while activating systems that promote deep and satisfying sleep, allowing a return to normal sleep patterns. It should have a rapid onset of action with a duration of less than 8 hours without hangover effects the next day and should not induce tolerance or dependence if used long term or cause withdrawal effects when stopped. It should not depress respiration and should be safe for use in the elderly patient. Unfortunately, no such hypnotic exists; all presently available hypnotics are general central nervous system depressants which inhibit both arousal and sleep mechanisms. Thus they do not induce normal sleep and often have adverse effects, including daytime sedation ('hangover') and rebound insomnia on withdrawal. They are unsuitable for long-term use because of the development of tolerance and dependence.

Benzodiazepines

By far the most commonly prescribed hypnotics are the benzodiazepines. A number of different benzodiazepines are available (Table 28.1). These drugs differ considerably in potency (equivalent dosage) and in rate of elimination but only slightly in clinical effects. All benzodiazepines have sedative/hypnotic, anxiolytic, amnesic, muscular relaxant and anticonvulsant actions with minor differences in the relative potency of these effects.

Pharmacokinetics   Most benzodiazepines marketed as hypnotics are well absorbed and rapidly penetrate the brain, produc-

Table 28.1 Profile of selected hypnotic drugs

Drug	Site of action	Elimination half-life (h)	Recommended hypnotic dose (mg)[a]
Benzodiazepines	GABA/benzodiazepine receptor		
Diazepam[b]		20–100 (36–200)[c]	5–15
Loprazolam		6–12	1
Lormetazepam		10–12	0.5–1.5
Nitrazepam		15–38	5–10
Temazepam		8–15	10–20
Non-benzodiazepines	GABA/benzodiazepine receptor		
Zaleplon		1	10
Zolpidem		2	10
Zopiclone		5–6	7.5
Antihistamines	Histamine (H₁) receptor		
Promethazine			25–50

[a] Recommended adult doses, approximately equivalent in hypnotic potency. Dosage should be halved in the elderly.
[b] Diazepam, though classed as an anxiolytic drug, has useful hypnotic properties when administered as a single dose.
[c] Half-life of pharmacologically active metabolite shown in parentheses.

ing hypnotic effects within half an hour after oral administration. Rates of elimination vary, however, with elimination half-lives of from 6 to 100 hours (see Table 28.1). The drugs undergo hepatic metabolism via oxidation or conjugation and some form pharmacologically active metabolites with even longer elimination half-lives. Oxidation of benzodiazepines is decreased in the elderly, in patients with hepatic impairment and in the presence of some drugs, including alcohol.

Pharmacokinetic characteristics are important in selecting a hypnotic drug. A rapid onset of action combined with a medium duration of action (elimination half-life about 6–8 hours) is usually desirable. Too short a duration of action may lead to, or fail to control, early morning waking, while a long duration of action (nitrazepam) may produce residual effects the next day and may lead to cumulation if the drug is used regularly. However, frequency of use and dosage are important. For example, diazepam (5–10 mg) produces few residual effects when used occasionally, despite its slow elimination, although chronic use impairs daytime performance. Large doses of short-acting drugs may produce hangover effects, while small doses of longer acting drugs may cause little or no hangover.

Effects on sleep A major site of the hypnotic action of benzodiazepines is the brainstem reticular formation which, as mentioned above, is of central importance in arousal. The reticular formation is extremely sensitive to depression by benzodiazepines which decrease both spontaneous activity and responses to afferent stimuli. Similar depression of limbic arousal systems adds to hypnotic efficacy in patients with insomnia due to anxiety. However, active sleep mechanisms are also suppressed and this effect leads to disruption of the normal sleep pattern.

Benzodiazepines are effective hypnotics: they hasten sleep onset, decrease nocturnal awakenings, increase total sleeping time and often impart a sense of deep, refreshing sleep. However, they produce changes in the relative proportion of different sleep stages. Stage 2 (light sleep) is prolonged and mainly accounts for the increased sleeping time. By contrast, the duration of SWS may be considerably reduced. REMS is also decreased; the latency to the first REMS episode is prolonged and dreaming is diminished. This abnormal sleep profile probably arises because of the unselective depression of both arousal and sleep mechanisms. The suppression of REMS may be an important factor in determining rebound effects on drug withdrawal (see below).

Mechanism of action Most of the effects of benzodiazepines result from their interaction with specific binding sites associated with postsynaptic GABA$_A$ receptors in the brain. All benzodiazepines bind to these sites, although with varying degrees of affinity, and potentiate the inhibitory actions of GABA at these sites.

GABA$_A$ receptors are multimolecular complexes that control a chloride ion channel and contain specific binding sites for GABA, benzodiazepines and several other drugs, including many non-benzodiazepine hypnotics and some anticonvulsant drugs (Haefely 1990) (Fig. 28.2). The various effects of benzodiazepines (hypnotic, anxiolytic, anticonvulsant, amnesic, myorelaxant) result from GABA potentiation in specific brain sites and at different GABA$_A$ receptor types. There are multiple subtypes of GABA$_A$ receptor which may contain different combinations of at least 18 subunits (including α_{1-6}, β_{1-3}, γ_{1-3} and others) and the subtypes are differentially distributed in the brain. Benzodiazepines bind to three or more subtypes and it appears that combination with α_2-containing subtypes mediates their anxiolytic effects, α_1-containing subtypes their sedative and amnesic effects, and α_1 as well as α_2 and α_5 their anticonvulsant effects (Rudolph et al 2001).

Zopiclone

Zopiclone, a cyclopyrrolone, is a non-benzodiazepine that nevertheless binds to benzodiazepine receptors but is said to be more selective for the α_1 subtype. It has hypnotic effects similar

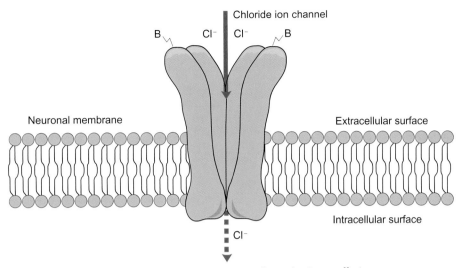

Chloride ion channel

Neuronal membrane

Extracellular surface

Intracellular surface

GABA activation of receptor opens channel gate, an effect
enhanced by benzodiazepine binding to receptor subunits

Figure 28.2 Schematic diagram of the GABA$_A$ receptor. This consists of five subunits arranged around a central chloride ion channel (one subunit has been removed in the diagram to reveal the ion channel, shown in the closed position). Some of the subunits have binding sites for benzodiazepines (B) and other hypnotics and anticonvulsants. Activation of the receptor by GABA opens the chloride channel, allowing chloride ions (Cl$^-$) to enter the cell, resulting in hyperpolarization (inhibition) of the neurone. Occupation of the benzodiazepine site, along with GABA, potentiates the inhibitory actions of GABA.

to benzodiazepines and carries the same potential for adverse effects including tolerance, dependence and abstinence effects on withdrawal. Psychiatric reactions, including hallucinations, behavioural disturbances and nightmares, have been reported to occur shortly after the first dose. This drug appears to have no particular advantages over benzodiazepines, although it may cause less alteration of sleep stages.

Zolpidem

Zolpidem is an imidazopyridine that binds preferentially to the α_1 benzodiazepine receptor subunit thought to mediate hypnotic effects. It is an effective hypnotic with only weak anticonvulsant and myorelaxant properties. Because of its short elimination half-life (2 hours) hangover effects are rare but rebound effects may occur in the later part of the night, causing early morning waking and daytime anxiety. With high doses, brief psychotic episodes, tolerance and withdrawal effects have been reported.

Zaleplon

Zaleplon is a pyrazolopyrimidine which, like zolpidem, binds selectively to the α_1 benzodiazepine receptor. It is an effective hypnotic, has a very short elimination half-life (1 hour) and appears to cause minimal residual effects on psychomotor or cognitive function after 5 hours. There is little evidence of tolerance or withdrawal effects and the drug appears suitable for use in the elderly (Doble et al 2004).

All these 'Z-drugs' are recommended for short-term use only (2–4 weeks) and are more expensive than benzodiazepines.

Other hypnotic drugs

The risk of adverse effects, including dependence and dangerous respiratory depression in overdose, generally outweighs the potential benefits of the older hypnotics, chloral derivatives, clomethiazole and barbiturates, and these drugs are best avoided. Antidepressants with sedative properties, such as amitriptyline, mirtazepine and trazodone, may be helpful if sleep disturbance is secondary to depression. Sedative antihistamines, such as promethazine, diphenhydramine and chlorphenamine, which can be purchased over the counter, have mild-to-moderate hypnotic efficacy but commonly produce hangover effects and rebound insomnia can occur after prolonged use (Drug & Therapeutics Bulletin 2004). Melatonin has been used successfully to alleviate jet lag but its place as a general hypnotic is doubtful and it is not licensed in the UK.

Adverse effects of hypnotic use

Tolerance and dependence

Tolerance to the hypnotic effects of benzodiazepines develops rapidly and may lead to dosage escalation. Nevertheless, poor sleepers may report continued efficacy and the drugs are often used long term because of difficulties in withdrawal.

Rebound insomnia

Rebound insomnia, in which sleep is poorer than before drug treatment, is common on withdrawal of benzodiazepines. Sleep latency is prolonged, intrasleep wakenings become more frequent and REMS duration and intensity are increased, with vivid dreams or nightmares which may add to frequent awakenings. These symptoms are most marked when the drugs have been taken in high doses or for long periods but can occur after only a week of low-dose administration. They are conspicuous with moderately rapidly eliminated benzodiazepines (temazepam, lorazepam) and may last for many weeks. With slowly eliminated benzodiazepines (diazepam), SWS and REMS may remain depressed for some weeks and then slowly return to the baseline, sometimes without a rebound effect. Tolerance and rebound effects are reflections of a complex homeostatic response to regular drug use, involving desensitization, uncoupling and internalization of certain GABA/benzodiazepine receptors and sensitization of receptors for excitatory neurotransmitters (Allison & Pratt 2003, Bateson 2002). These changes encourage continued hypnotic usage and contribute to the development of drug dependence.

Oversedation and hangover effects

Many benzodiazepines used as hypnotics can give rise to a subjective 'hangover' and after most of them, even those with short elimination half-lives, psychomotor performance, including driving ability and memory, may be impaired on the following day. Oversedation is most likely with slowly eliminated benzodiazepines, especially if used chronically, and is most marked in the elderly in whom drowsiness, inco-ordination and ataxia, leading to falls and fractures, and acute confusional states may result even from small doses. Chronic use can cause considerable cognitive impairment, sometimes suggesting dementia. Paradoxical excitement may occur occasionally.

Some benzodiazepines in hypnotic doses may decrease alveolar ventilation and depress the respiratory response to hypercapnia, increasing the risk of cerebral hypoxia, especially in the elderly and in patients with chronic respiratory disease.

Drug interactions

Benzodiazepines have additive effects with other central nervous system depressants. Combinations of benzodiazepines with alcohol, other hypnotics, sedative tricyclic antidepressants, antihistamines or opioids can cause marked sedation and may lead to accidents or severe respiratory depression.

Pregnancy and lactation

The regular use of benzodiazepines is contraindicated in pregnancy since the drugs are concentrated in fetal tissues where hepatic metabolism is minimal. They can cause neonatal depression, hypotonia and feeding difficulties if given in late pregnancy and infants exposed in utero to regular hypnotic maternal doses may develop withdrawal symptoms 2–3 weeks after birth (irritability, crying, muscle twitches). They also enter breast milk and long-acting benzodiazepines are contraindicated during lactation, although short- to medium-acting benzodiazepines appear to be safe.

Rational drug treatment of insomnia

A hypnotic drug may be indicated for insomnia when it is severe, disabling, unresponsive to other measures or likely to be temporary. In choosing an appropriate agent, individual variables relating to the patient and to the drug need to be considered (Table 28.2).

Patient care

Type of insomnia

The duration of insomnia is important in deciding on a hypnotic regimen. Transient insomnia may be caused by changes of routine such as overnight travel, change in time zone, alteration of shift work or temporary admission to hospital. In these circumstances a hypnotic with a rapid onset and medium duration of action and few residual effects could be used on one or two occasions.

Short-term insomnia may result from temporary environmental stress. In this case a hypnotic may occasionally be indicated but should be prescribed in low dosage for 1 or 2 weeks only, preferably intermittently on alternate nights or one night in three.

Chronic insomnia presents a much greater therapeutic problem. It is usually secondary to other conditions (organic or psychiatric) at which treatment should initially be aimed. In selected cases a hypnotic may be helpful but it is recommended that such drugs should be prescribed at the minimal effective dosage and

Table 28.2 Drug treatment in insomnia		
Type of insomnia	Choice of drugs	Administration
Transient insomnia	Benzodiazepine (temazepam, diazepam)	Once or twice only
Short-term insomnia	Benzodiazepine (medium duration of action)	1–2 weeks only, or intermittent
Chronic insomnia	1. Treat primary cause (education, sleep hygiene, pain relief, psychiatric treatment) 2. Benzodiazepine (medium duration of action) 3. Zopiclone 4. Sedative antihistamine	2–4 weeks maximum; preferably intermittent Short term (2–4 weeks) Short term (2–4 weeks)

administered intermittently (one night in three) or temporarily (not more than 2 or 3 weeks). Occasionally it is necessary to repeat short, intermittent courses at intervals of a few months.

The elderly

The elderly are especially vulnerable both to insomnia and to adverse effects from hypnotic drugs. They may have reduced metabolism of some drugs and may be at risk of cumulative effects. They are also more susceptible than younger people to central nervous system depression, including cognitive impairment and ataxia (which may lead to falls and fractures). They are sensitive to respiratory depression, prone to sleep apnoea and other sleep disorders and are more likely to have 'sociological', psychiatric and somatic illnesses which both disturb sleep and may be aggravated by hypnotics. For some of these elderly patients, hypnotics can improve the quality of life but the dosage should be adjusted (usually half the recommended adult dose) and hypnotics with long elimination half-lives or active metabolites should be avoided.

A considerable number of elderly patients give a history of regular hypnotic use going back for 20 or 30 years. In many of these patients, gradual reduction of hypnotic dosage or even withdrawal may be indicated and can be carried out successfully, resulting in improved cognition and general health with no impairment of sleep or escalation of other symptoms (Curran et al 2003, Heather et al 2004).

The young

Hypnotics are generally contraindicated for children. Where sedation is required, sedative antihistamines are usually recommended. However, a single dose of a benzodiazepine (with appropriate dosage reduction) may be more effective.

Pregnancy and lactation

Regular use of slowly eliminated hypnotics is contraindicated. If hypnotics are required, intermittent doses of relatively rapidly eliminated hypnotics may be used and have been shown to be safe during breast feeding.

Disease states

Hypnotics are contraindicated in patients with acute pulmonary insufficiency, significant respiratory depression, obstructive sleep apnoea or severe hepatic impairment. In patients with chronic pain or terminal conditions, suitable analgesics including non-steroidal anti-inflammatory agents or opiates, sometimes combined with neuroleptics, usually provide satisfactory sedation. In such patients the possibility of drug dependence becomes a less important issue and regular use of hypnotics with a medium duration of action should not be denied if they provide symptomatic relief of insomnia.

Choice of drug

There is little difference in hypnotic efficacy between most of the available agents. The main factors to consider in the rational choice of a hypnotic regimen are duration of action and the risk of adverse effects, especially oversedation and the development of tolerance and dependence. Cost may be a factor with new drugs.

Rate of elimination

Slowly eliminated drugs should be avoided because of the risk of oversedation and hangover effects. Very short-acting drugs such as zaleplon carry the risk of late-night rebound insomnia and daytime anxiety. Drugs with a medium elimination half-life (6–8 hours) appear to have the most suitable profile for hypnotic use. These may include temazepam and loprazolam, which are the drugs of first choice in most situations where hypnotics are indicated. Zopiclone is a reasonable second choice. A sedative antihistamine such as promethazine is a safe third choice and it is useful in children although it may produce daytime drowsiness.

Dosage

The minimum effective dosage should always be used as there is considerable individual variation in response and susceptibility to oversedation. It is best to start with a small dose which may be increased if necessary. Dosage should, in general, be halved in the elderly and caution exercised in the presence of respiratory or hepatic disease.

Duration and timing of administration

In order to prevent the development of tolerance and dependence, the maximum duration of treatment should be limited to 2 or 3 weeks and treatment should, where possible, be intermittent (one night in two or three). Dosage should be tapered slowly if hypnotics have been taken regularly for more than a few weeks. Doses should be taken 20 minutes before retiring in order to allow dissolution in the stomach and absorption to commence before the patient lies down in bed.

Anxiolytic drugs

As with insomnia, drugs provide only symptomatic treatment for anxiety. They may temporarily help a patient to cope with an otherwise overwhelming stress and can provide a short- or medium-term cover which allows time for more specific treatments to take effect or for natural recovery to occur but they do not cure the underlying disorder. Most anxiety states are more effectively treated in the long term by non-pharmacological interventions including counselling, psychotherapy, behavioural and cognitive methods, relaxation and anxiety management training. Essentially, all these methods involve a learning process which enables the patient to develop improved stress-coping techniques. However, these methods are time consuming, labour intensive and costly.

The ideal anxiolytic drug would selectively damp down excess activity in limbic (emotional) and somatic arousal systems, without inhibiting learning processes or producing undue sedation. The onset of action would be rapid and the drugs would be suitable for long-term use. No available drug meets all these requirements. Benzodiazepines have a rapid onset of action but impair cognitive processes and have undesirable effects if used long term. Antidepressants are effective in most types of anxiety but have a delayed onset of action; some are potentially toxic and all may be difficult to withdraw. Some of the somatic manifestations of anxiety can be alleviated by β-blockers but these drugs have little effect on subjective symptoms. Some drugs used in anxiety disorders are shown in Table 28.3.

Benzodiazepines

Benzodiazepines are still the most commonly prescribed drugs for anxiety. Over 7 million prescriptions for benzodiazepines classed as anxiolytics are issued each year in the UK and many anxious patients are also prescribed hypnotics.

Benzodiazepines have potent anxiolytic effects which are exerted at low doses that produce minimal sedation. A major advantage in acute situations is the rapid onset of action that occurs within an hour of the first effective dose. Many clinical trials have shown short-term efficacy in patients with anxiety disorders. Anxiolytic effects have also been reported in normal volunteers with high trait anxiety and in patients with anticipatory anxiety before surgery. However, in subjects with low trait anxiety and in non-stressful conditions benzodiazepines may paradoxically increase anxiety and impair psychomotor performance.

The major site of anxiolytic action is the limbic system (see above). This effect is mediated by a primary action at GABA/benzodiazepine receptors, resulting in enhancement of inhibitory GABA activity (see Fig. 28.2). There is some evidence that

Table 28.3 Profile of selected drugs used in anxiety disorders

Drug	Elimination half-life (h)[a]	Approximate anxiolytic dosage[b]
Benzodiazepines		
Alprazolam[c]	6–12	250–500 µg three times daily
Chlordiazepoxide	5–30 (36–200)	10 mg three times daily
Clonazepam[c]	18–50	250–500 µg three times daily
Diazepam	20–100 (36–200)	2–5 mg three times daily
Lorazepam	10–18	1 mg three times daily
Oxazepam	4–15	10–30 mg three times daily
Tricyclic antidepressants		
Amitriptyline	10–25 (13–93)	75–150 mg daily
Clomipramine	16–20	10–150 mg daily
Imipramine	4–18 (12–61)	75–200 mg daily
Selective serotonin reuptake inhibitors		
Fluoxetine	2–3 days (7–15 days)	20 mg daily
Fluvoxamine	15	100 mg daily
Paroxetine	20	20 mg daily
Sertraline	26 (36)	50 mg daily
Citalopram	33	20 mg daily
Escitalopram	33	10–20 mg daily
Serotonin and noradrenaline reuptake inhibitors (SNRI)		
Venlafaxine	Extended-release preparation (Efexor XL)	75 mg daily
Monoamine oxidase inhibitors[d]		
Moclobemide	1–4	300–600 mg daily
Phenelzine[c]	1	15 mg three times daily
Other anxiolytic drugs		
Buspirone	2–11	5–10 mg three times daily
Propranolol	2–4	40 mg twice daily

[a] Half-life of pharmacologically active metabolite shown in parentheses.
[b] Dosage requirements may vary and need individual titration; starting doses should be as low as possible. Dosage should be halved in the elderly.
[c] Not recommended in the UK though widely used in the US and now entering UK practices.
[d] Effects of moclobemide are reversible, but phenelzine causes irreversible enzyme inhibition and effects last 2 weeks after cessation of treatment.

patients with anxiety disorders have reduced numbers of benzodiazepine receptors in key brain areas that regulate anxiety responses (Roy-Byrne 2005). Secondary suppression of noradrenergic and/or serotonergic and other excitatory systems may also be of importance in relation to the anxiolytic effects of benzodiazepines.

Choice of benzodiazepine in anxiety Despite the drawbacks of chronic use, benzodiazepines can be valuable in the short-term management of anxiety because of their anxiolytic efficacy and rapid onset of action. The choice of an appropriate benzodiazepine, as with hypnotics, depends largely on pharmacokinetic characteristics. Potent benzodiazepines such as lorazepam and alprazolam (see Table 28.3) have been widely used for anxiety disorders but are probably inappropriate. Both are moderately rapidly eliminated and need to be taken several times daily. Declining blood concentrations may lead to interdose anxiety as the anxiolytic effect of each tablet wears off. The high potency of lorazepam (approximately 10 times that of diazepam), and the fact that it is available only in 1 and 2.5 mg tablet strengths, has often led to excessive dosage. Similarly, alprazolam (approximately 20 times more potent than diazepam) has often been used in excessive dosage, particularly in the USA. Such doses lead to adverse effects, a high probability of dependence and difficulties in withdrawal.

A slowly eliminated benzodiazepine such as diazepam is more appropriate in most cases. Diazepam has a rapid onset of action and its slow elimination ensures a steady blood concentration. It should be prescribed in the minimal effective dosage to avoid cumulative effects and it can also be used as a hypnotic, thus avoiding the need for a separate hypnotic drug. Clonazepam, although long acting, is more potent than diazepam and in practice is difficult to withdraw. It is indicated for epilepsy in the UK but is also used as an anxiolytic, especially in the USA.

However, as with hypnotics, the anxiolytic use of benzodiazepines should generally be limited to short-term (less than 4 weeks followed by tapering) or intermittent use. Parenteral administration of lorazepam or diazepam may occasionally be indicated for severely agitated psychiatric patients.

The possibility that partial benzodiazepine agonists may have anxiolytic properties with less propensity to tolerance and withdrawal effects is an area of active research (Doble et al 2004) but none has been marketed as yet.

Antidepressant drugs

Antidepressant drugs are now recognized as the drugs of first choice for the longer term treatment of anxiety disorders (Lader 2004). Trials have shown that they are as effective as benzodiazepines in generalized anxiety disorder and probably superior in panic disorder, agoraphobia and other phobias. They are of value in anxiety associated with depression and in anxiety/depression occurring in benzodiazepine withdrawal reactions. They cause little cognitive impairment and little tolerance to the anxiolytic effects. Thus, unlike benzodiazepines, they are suitable for long-term use which can be continued for several months, giving time for psychological therapies to be utilized.

The mode of action of these drugs is not fully understood but the effects are thought to be an initial increase in central serotonergic and noradrenergic activity due to inhibition of neurotransmitter reuptake at monoaminergic synapses. This may cause further anxiety but is followed after a time by downregulation of some adrenergic and serotonergic receptors in certain parts of the brain, accounting for the delayed antidepressant and anxiolytic effects.

A disadvantage of all these drugs is their slow onset of action, which may be delayed for 2–4 weeks, and they may initially exacerbate anxiety symptoms or even cause panic on the first dose. For this reason they should be started in small doses, often combined for the first 2–4 weeks with a benzodiazepine. A second disadvantage is that some antidepressants are toxic in overdose and may have many adverse effects. Third, all antidepressants can cause withdrawal reactions, especially if stopped abruptly (Table 28.4). Withdrawal should therefore be carried out gradually with tapering of dosage over several weeks.

Table 28.4 Antidepressant withdrawal symptoms

Physical symptoms	Psychological symptoms
Gastrointestinal: abdominal pain, diarrhoea, nausea, headache	Anxiety, agitation
Influenza-like: fatigue, headache, muscle pain, weakness, sweating, chills, palpitations	Crying spells Irritability
Sleep disturbance: insomnia, vivid dreams, nightmares	Overactivity, restlessness
Sensory disturbances: dizziness, light-headedness, vertigo, pins and needles, electric shock sensations	Agression Depersonalization, derealization
Motor disorders: tremor, loss of balance, muscle stiffness, abnormal movements	Memory problems Confusion
Neonatal withdrawal symptoms[a]: jitteriness, increased muscle tone, feeding difficulty, tremor, seizures and other signs	Lowered mood

[a] If taken regularly by mother during last trimester of pregnancy

Tricyclic antidepressants Tricyclic antidepressants with sedative actions such as imipramine, clomipramine and amitriptyline have been shown to be beneficial in anxiety states. The sedative action may be separate from the anxiolytic effects and is often manifested with low doses early in the treatment. This effect can be helpful if insomnia is associated with anxiety but the full anxiolytic effect may not be apparent for some weeks. These drugs block the reuptake of both noradrenaline and serotonin at central synapses. They also have anticholinergic effects and can cause dry month, blurred vision, constipation and urinary retention. Arrhythmias and heart block occasionally follow the use of tricyclic antidepressants which are contraindicated in the presence of heart disease and should be avoided in the elderly.

Selective serotonin reuptake inhibitors (SSRIs) SSRIs are preferred to tricyclic antidepressants as they are less toxic and have fewer side effects. They selectively inhibit synaptic serotonin reuptake with little effect on the reuptake of noradrenaline. The main side effects are gastrointestinal, including nausea, vomiting, dyspepsia, abdominal pain, diarrhoea, constipation, anorexia and weight loss. Sexual dysfunction is not uncommonly reported.

Serotonin and noradrenaline reuptake inhibitor (SNRI) The non-selective reuptake inhibitor venlafaxine is licensed for generalized anxiety disorder and is effective as an extended-release preparation in non-depressed patients with anxiety. Advsere effects include gastrointestinal symptoms, drowsiness and sexual dysfunction.

Monoamine oxidase inhibitor (MAOIs) The irreversible MAOI phenelzine and the reversible MAOI moclobemide are sometimes effective in phobic and panic disorders. They have a delayed onset of action, many adverse effects including drug and food interactions and withdrawal reactions. For these reasons they should be reserved for patients unresponsive to other antidepressants.

Other anxiolytic drugs

Buspirone has mixed agonist/antagonist actions at serotonergic receptors thought to be involved in anxiety. It has anxiolytic effects comparable to those of benzodiazepines but is without sedative/hypnotic, anticonvulsant or muscle relaxant effects. A major disadvantage is that the anxiolytic effects are delayed for up to 3 weeks and in some patients it produces dysphoria and increased anxiety. Furthermore, it does not alleviate anxiety associated with benzodiazepine withdrawal. Buspirone does not appear to produce dependence or a withdrawal syndrome but the drug is recommended for short-term use only.

The β-blocker propranolol can relieve somatic symptoms of anxiety such as palpitations and tremor. Used in small doses which do not induce hypotension, propranolol can be of value in acutely stressful situations or panic attacks where physical symptoms are dominant, although there is little effect on subjective symptoms. β-Blockers are commonly used by musicians to prevent tremor at concerts and by actors to combat stage fright. If used regularly, withdrawal should be gradual to prevent rebound tachycardia.

Some relatively new drugs with GABA-ergic actions appear to have anxiolytic effects, although originally developed as anticonvulsants. These include gabapentin and pregabalin which showed promise in preliminary trials in social anxiety, pain and generalized anxiety disorders (Ashton & Young 2003).

Antipsychotic drugs such as chlorpromazine and haloperidol have been used as anxiolytics but should be avoided because of the risk of inducing dyskinesias and other adverse effects (Lader 2004).

Adverse effects of anxiolytic use

Tolerance Tolerance to the anxiolytic effects of benzodiazepines seems to develop more slowly than to the hypnotic effects. In clinical use, most patients reporting initial drowsiness find that it wears off in a few days while the anxiolytic effect remains for some weeks. However, their long-term efficacy in anxiety disorders is doubtful (Lader 2004), although some argue that they maintain efficacy for many months (Doble et al 2004).

Psychomotor and cognitive impairment Although oversedation is not usually a problem in anxious patients, there is evidence that long-term use of benzodiazepines results in psychomotor impairment and has adverse effects on memory. Many patients on long-term benzodiazepines complain of poor memory and incidents of shoplifting have been attributed to memory lapses caused by benzodiazepine use. In elderly patients the amnesic effects may falsely suggest the development of dementia. There is some evidence that benzodiazepines also inhibit the learning of alternative stress-coping strategies, such as behavioural treatments for agoraphobia. Additive effects with other central nervous system depressants including alcohol occur, as with hypnotic use of benzodiazepines, and may contribute to traffic and other accidents.

Disinhibition, paradoxical effects Occasionally, benzodiazepines produce paradoxical stimulant effects. These effects are most marked in anxious subjects and include excitement, increased anxiety, irritability and outbursts of rage. Violent behaviour, including baby battering, have sometimes been attributed to disinhibition by benzodiazepines of behaviour normally suppressed by social restraints, fear or anxiety. Increased daytime anxiety can occur with rapidly eliminated benzodiazepines and is probably a withdrawal effect.

Affective reactions Chronic use of benzodiazepines can aggravate depression and provoke suicide in depressed patients and can cause depression in patients with no previous history of depressive disorder. Aggravation of depression is a particular risk in anxious patients who often have mixed anxiety/depression. Benzodiazepines are taken alone or in combination with other drugs in 40% of self-poisoning incidents. Although relatively non-toxic in overdose, they can cause fatalities as a result of drug interactions and in those with respiratory disease. According to Home Office statistics, 1810 deaths were attributed to benzodiazepine overdose in suicides, accidents and undetermined causes between 1990 and 1996. The benzodiazepine receptor antagonist flumazenil can be used to reverse benzodiazepine toxicity (usually respiratory depression) but may precipitate withdrawal symptoms in benzodiazepine-dependent patients.

Some patients on long-term benzodiazepines complain of 'emotional anaesthesia' with inability to experience either pleasure or distress. However, in some patients, benzodiazepines induce euphoria and they are increasingly used as drugs of abuse.

Dependence The greatest drawback of chronic benzodiazepine use is the development of drug dependence. It is now generally agreed that the regular use of therapeutic doses of benzodiazepines as hypnotics or anxiolytics for more than a few weeks can give rise to dependence, with withdrawal symptoms on cessation of drug use in over 40% of patients. It is estimated that there are about 1 million long-term benzodiazepine users in the UK and many of these are likely to be dependent. People with anxious or 'passive-dependent' personalities seem to be most vulnerable to dependence and withdrawal symptoms. Such individuals make up a large proportion of anxious patients in psychiatric practice, are often described as suffering from 'chronic anxiety' and are the type of patient for whom benzodiazepines are most likely to be prescribed. Such patients often continue to take benzodiazepines for many years because attempts at dosage reduction or drug withdrawal result in abstinence symptoms which they are unable to tolerate. Nevertheless, these patients continue to suffer from anxiety symptoms despite continued benzodiazepine use, possibly because they have become tolerant to the anxiolytic effects and may also suffer from other adverse effects of long-term benzodiazepine use such as depression or psychomotor impairment (Ashton 2004).

Abuse In the last 15 years there has been a growing problem with benzodiazepine abuse. Some patients escalate their prescribed dosage and may obtain prescriptions from several doctors. These tend to be anxious patients with 'passive-dependent' personalities who may have a history of alcohol misuse; they often combine large doses of benzodiazepines with excessive alcohol consumption. In addition, a high proportion (30–90%) of illicit recreational drug abusers also use benzodiazepines and some take them as euphoriants in their own right. Recreational use of most benzodiazepines has been reported in various countries; in the UK, temazepam is most commonly abused. Exceedingly large doses (over 1 g) may be taken and sometimes injected intravenously. Benzodiazepines became easily available due to widespread prescribing which favoured their entrance into the illicit drug scene. With increased prescribing, zopiclone, zolpidem and zaleplon are also being abused. Abusers become dependent and suffer the same adverse effects and withdrawal symptoms as prescribed dose users (Ashton 2002a).

Benzodiazepine withdrawal Many patients on long-term benzodiazepines seek help with drug withdrawal. Clinical experience shows that withdrawal is feasible in most patients if carried out with care. Abrupt withdrawal in dependent subjects is dangerous and can induce acute anxiety, psychosis or convulsions. However, gradual withdrawal, coupled where necessary with counselling or psychological treatments, can be successful in the majority of patients (Ashton 2004, Curran et al 2003, Heather et al 2004). The duration of withdrawal should be tailored to individual needs and may last many months. Dosage decrements may be of the order of 1–2 mg of diazepam per month. Even with slow dosage reduction, a variety of withdrawal symptoms may be experienced, including increased anxiety, insomnia, hypersensitivity to sensory stimuli, perceptual distortions, paraesthesiae, muscle twitching, depression and many others (Table 28.5). These may last for many weeks, though diminishing in intensity, but occasionally the withdrawal syndrome is protracted for a year or more. Transfer to diazepam, because of its slow elimination and availability in low dosage forms, may be indicated for patients taking other benzodiazepines (Ashton 2005). Useful guidelines for benzodiazepine withdrawal are given in the British National Formulary and detailed withdrawal schedules are also available (Ashton 2002b).

The eventual outcome does not appear to be influenced by dosage, type of benzodiazepine, duration of use, personality disorder, psychiatric history, age, severity of withdrawal symptoms or rate of withdrawal. Hence benzodiazepine withdrawal is worth attempting in patients who are motivated to stop and most patients report that they feel better after withdrawal than when they were taking the benzodiazepine. Community pharmacists may be ideally suited to advise doctors and patients on the management of benzodiazepine withdrawal.

Rational use of drugs in anxiety

It is clear that drugs do not provide a complete solution for anxiety (Table 28.6). The advantages of benzodiazepines are their immediate onset of action and high initial efficacy. Thus they are ideal for acute anxiety states such as those precipitated by stress, natural disasters and accidents, which have a high rate of spontaneous resolution.

Diazepam, prescribed in hypnotic or anxiolytic diseases (see Tables 28.2 and 28.4), depending on the circumstances, is probably the drug of choice. A single dose may be sufficient and it should not be continued for more than 1–2 weeks, followed by tapering if necessary. Lorazepam has also been widely used in such situations. Single doses of diazepam or lorazepam may also offer appropriate prophylaxis against acute stress reactions in predictably stressful situations (e.g. air travel, dental appointments in phobic patients). Benzodiazepines are not recommended, except acutely, for bereavement because their amnesic actions may hinder subsequent readjustments.

In generalized anxiety disorders, panic disorders, agoraphobia and other phobias, benzodiazepines may be prescribed initially

Table 28.5 Some common benzodiazepine withdrawal symptoms

Symptoms common to anxiety states	Symptoms relatively specific to benzodiazepine withdrawal
Anxiety, panics	Perceptual distortions, sense of movement
Agoraphobia	
Insomnia, nightmares	Depersonalization, derealization
Depression, dysphoria	Hallucinations
Excitability, restlessness	Distortion of body image
Poor memory and concentration	Tingling, numbness, altered sensation
Dizziness, light-headedness	
Weakness, 'jelly legs'	Skin prickling (formication)
Tremor	Sensory hypersensitivity
Muscle pain, stiffness	Muscle twitches, jerks
Sweating, night sweats	Tinnitus
Palpitations	Psychosis*
Blurred or double vision	Confusion, delirium*
Gastrointestinal and urinary symptoms	Convulsions*

*Usually only on rapid or abrupt withdrawal from high doses.

Table 28.6 Drug treatment in anxiety disorders*

Drug	Efficacy	Onset of therapeutic effect	Risk of withdrawal symptoms	Administration
Benzodiazepines	++	Immediate	++	Single doses, intermittent, short term 2–4 weeks
Selective serotonin reuptake inhibitors (SSRIs)	++	Delayed (2–4 weeks)	++ (most with paroxetine, least with fluoxetine)	Medium to long term (3–12 months)
Serotonin and noradrenaline reuptake inhibitors (SNRIs)	++	Delayed (2–4 weeks)	++	Medium to long term (3–12 months)
Tricyclic antidepressants	++	Delayed (2–4 weeks)	++	Medium to long term (3–12 months)
Monoamine reuptake inhibitors (MAOIs)	++	Delayed (3–6 weeks)	++	Medium to long term (3–12 months)
Buspirone	+	Delayed (2–4 weeks)	–	Short term (4 weeks)
Propranolol	+	Immediate	+	Medium term (weeks to months)

Wherever possible, psychological treatments (counselling, anxiety management training, cognitive behavioural therapy, psychotherapy) are preferred.

(about 4 weeks followed by tapering), to allow time for longer term treatments to take effect. For example, antidepressants can be prescribed concomitantly at the start of benzodiazepine treatment and arrangements made for appropriate psychological therapy. Again, diazepam is probably the benzodiazepine of first choice because of its long duration of action and relative ease of tapering. Intermittent courses of 2–4 weeks can be of value in episodic anxiety often associated with fluctuations of generalized anxiety disorder. Lorazepam, and especially alprazolam, have been promoted for use in panic disorder but are probably inappropriate. These drugs are relatively quickly eliminated and interdose anxiety frequently occurs. When prescribing benzodiazepines the aims and limitations of these drugs as treatments for anxiety and the risk of drug dependence should be explained to patients.

Longer term treatment is generally required for generalized anxiety, anxiety/depression, panic or phobic states. SSRIs or venlafaxine are the preferred drugs with tricyclic antidepressants as second choice, though not indicated for the elderly. These drugs are efficacious, can be used for several months or longer term and do not interfere with non-pharmacological therapies. However,

their therapeutic effects may be delayed for 2–4 weeks and they can initially exacerbate anxiety. For this reason they should be started in small doses which can be increased if necessary. MAOIs are effective in panic and phobic disorders but should be kept in reserve for patients unresponsive to other antidepressants. All antidepressants are associated with withdrawal effects (now euphemistically referred to as discontinuation reactions) and dosage should be tapered slowly if it is decided to terminate use.

β-Blockers are effective in controlling somatic symptoms such as palpitations and tremor and occasionally have a role as adjuvants for anxious patients in whom such symptoms are prominent. The place of newer drugs such as gabapentin needs to be established in large, long-term trials.

The most effective long-term treatment of anxiety is by psychological methods, which can include self-help groups, counselling, behavioural and cognitive techniques, anxiety management training and psychotherapy. These measures all take time to be effective; the main role of drugs is to alleviate symptoms during the learning process involved.

Some therapeutic problems in the management of insomnia and anxiety are summarized in Table 28.7.

Table 28.7 Some therapeutic problems in the management of anxiety and insomnia

Problem	Prevalence	Contributory factors	Management
Benzodiazepine overdose	Occurs in approx. 40% of all self-poisoning incidents 1810 deaths due to benzodiazepines were reported in the UK 1990–1996	Benzodiazepine often taken with other drugs with additive effects, including antidepressants, alcohol and opiates	Flumazenil (a competitive antagonist at benzodiazepine receptors) may be administered cautiously.* This reverses benzodiazepine actions and may reveal the extent to which other drugs are contributing to the patient's condition. However, in benzodiazepine-dependent patients, flumazenil may precipitate withdrawal reactions
Antidepressant overdose	Self-poisoning attempts common in anxiety disorders, especially if depression also present. Tricyclic and related antidepressants more toxic than SSRIs	Chronic benzodiazepine use may aggravate depression and increase risk of suicide. SSRIs may possibly aggravate suicidal tendencies	Symptomatic treatment, activated charcoal and general supportive measures. IV diazepam emulsion may be required for convulsions
Insomnia treated with zopiclone during or after benzodiazepine withdrawal	Many patients are prescribed zopiclone as an alternative hypnotic, since it is not a benzodiazepine, and is thought to have a different action	Patients often report that zopiclone alleviates benzodiazepine withdrawal symptoms, but tend to escalate dosage and take it during the day as well as at night	Zopiclone, zaleplon and zolpidem act on benzodiazepine receptors and cause dependence in the same way. These drugs have also been abused in escalating doses. They should not be prescribed as a substitute for benzodiazepines
Patients wishing to withdraw from lorazepam or other potent, relatively short-acting benzodiazepines	Many UK patients are still being prescribed relatively large doses of lorazepam (e.g. >7.5 mg daily)	Lorazepam is 10 times more potent than diazepam but is available in only 1mg or 2.5 mg, formulations which makes it difficult to reduce dosage gradually	If benzodiazepine withdrawal is indicated, it is usually advisable to switch to diazepam. The substitution should be carried out stepwise, replacing one dose of lorazepam at a time with the equivalent dose of diazepam. Withdrawal can then be carried out gradually at a rate of 1–2 mg diazepam every 2–4 weeks
Patients taking a combination of a benzodiazepine and an antidepressant drug	Many patients on long-term benzodiazepines are also taking a prescribed antidepressant	An antidepressant may have been prescribed for depression caused by chronic benzodiazepine use, or for patients with anxiety/depression, although this is not recommended	Gradual withdrawal from the benzodiazepine may be indicated. In this case, the patient should continue on the antidepressant drug until benzodiazepine withdrawal is complete and probably for a month or more afterwards. The advisability of continuing or slowly withdrawing the antidepressant can then be considered
Patients attending pharmacies for several months to obtain repeat prescriptions of benzodiazepines	An estimated 1 million patients in the UK are taking prescribed benzodiazepines regularly for over a year (often for many years)	A considerable proportion of these patients are likely to be at risk of adverse effects, especially if elderly	The prescriber needs to be made aware of these patients and the need to start withdrawal programmes
Benzodiazepine abuse	Well over 200000 people abuse illicitly obtained benzodiazepines in the UK	Illicit benzodiazepine abuse is common among polydrug users, alcoholics and psychiatric patients. Some of these inject benzodiazepines and are at risk of HIV and hepatitis as well as local consequences of injection	The source of most illicitly obtained benzodiazepines is stolen prescriptions, although some are now imported illegally and can be obtained on the internet. Reduction in benzodiazepine prescribing would help alleviate this problem

*Flumazenil is short acting; repeated administration may be required if a long-acting benzodiazepine has been taken in overdose.

CASE STUDIES

Case 28.1

Peter, aged 24, was hospitalized for 3 months after a serious motorcycle injury followed by painful complications. While in hospital he developed panic attacks and insomnia. He received no psychological support but was prescribed temazepam, initially in 20 mg doses but later increased to 60 mg because of continued insomnia. After discharge from hospital he continued to receive temazepam from his primary care doctor and the dosage was increased over a period of years until he was taking 80 mg temazepam each night and 40–80 mg during the day. At the age of 30, Peter was removed from the practice list of his doctor after he altered a prescription. He later attended several different primary care doctors, obtaining multiple temazepam prescriptions. When he could no longer satisfy his need from prescriptions he took to obtaining temazepam on the street, taking large and irregular doses by mouth. All this time, his anxiety levels increased. His behaviour became chaotic and he was twice imprisoned for credit card fraud but he was able to obtain temazepam and other drugs from his co-prisoners. When last heard of, Peter, aged 35, was again buying temazepam illicitly, as well as other addictive drugs, had started injecting intravenously and was involved in a court case for obtaining money under false pretences.

Question

How could this tragedy have been prevented?

Answer

Peter's downfall could have been averted at several stages.

- The hospital staff should not have allowed the temazepam dosage to escalate and should have provided psychological/psychiatric help for what was probably post-traumatic stress disorder (PTSD) or panic disorder.
- An antidepressant drug could have been prescribed, along with psychological measures, instead of prolonged treatment with excessive doses of temazepam.
- On discharge from hospital, Peter's doctor should have been warned of his temazepam intake and a slow withdrawal schedule suggested.
- The series of primary care doctors who gave Peter prescriptions should have been aware that he was likely to obtain illicit supplies and should have referred him to a withdrawal clinic or drugs unit.

Case 28.2

Ms AB, a previously well 30-year-old lady, had been treated with paroxetine for anxiety/depression which had been precipitated by a traumatic marriage break-up. After taking paroxetine for 18 months, AB's problems had mainly resolved and she was feeling well. She decided that she no longer needed the drug and stopped taking it. Within 3 days her anxiety/depression returned with insomnia and nightmares. Her mood lowered and she became irritable and found herself weeping for no reason. A week later she returned to her doctor complaining of these symptoms as well as depersonalization and strange electric shock sensations. The doctor thought the original depression had returned and reinstated paroxetine which cleared up her symptoms within a few days.

Question

What alternative explanation could there be for AB's symptoms and what other decision could the doctor have made?

Answers

- All antidepressants can cause a withdrawal ('discontinuation') reaction.
- AB's symptoms were typical of SSRI withdrawal which occur most commonly with paroxetine, perhaps partly due to its rapid rate of elimination (half-life 21 hours in chronic users).
- In this previously well lady no longer under marital stress, the doctor, after reinstating paroxetine, could have supplied a gradual tapering schedule of drug withdrawal.

Case 28.3

Mrs A, a recently widowed lady aged 65, had difficulty sleeping after her bereavement. She was prescribed nitrazepam in a bedtime dose of 5 mg, which was very effective and was continued for over 4 weeks. Mrs A lived alone but was visited occasionally by her daughter. On a visit 2 weeks after the nitrazepam was started, Mrs A seemed calm and said that she was sleeping well but the daughter noticed her mother was unsteady on her feet. A week later the daughter visited again and found her mother lying on the bedroom floor, in pain and unable to move. She said that she had lost her balance on getting out of bed. An ambulance was called and it was found in hospital that Mrs A had broken her hip.

Question

Should the doctor have prescribed nitrazepam for this lady?

Answers

- Long-acting benzodiazepines should be avoided in the elderly. The elimination half-life of nitrazepam is 15–38 hours and the recommended dose for the elderly is 2.5–5 mg. Temazepam, loprazolam or lormetazepam would have been a better choice but for short-term use only (preferably only 2 weeks).
- The elderly are particularly prone to ataxia and light-headedness with benzodiazepines and this can lead to falls and fractures.
- Benzodiazepines are not recommended, except acutely, for bereavement. Their amnesic effects may interfere with subsequent psychological adjustment.

Case 28.4

A 20-year-old man, known to have schizophrenia, was acutely admitted to a psychiatric ward in a highly agitated and disturbed state. He was panicking because of 'voices' threatening to kill him. He was aggressive and violent towards the hospital staff whom he feared were in league with the voices. He was eventually sedated by an intramuscular injection of lorazepam which was repeated 6 hours and 12 hours later and he was also given haloperidol by mouth. He remained in hospital for 4 weeks, during which time his condition was controlled with oral haloperidol and lorazepam. On discharge, he was taking haloperidol 10 mg and lorazepam 6 mg daily. His primary care doctor continued with the same drug regimen but noticed that the patient seemed drowsy and depressed over the next few months although the voices did not reappear.

Question

What would have been a better procedure for the hospital to follow?

Answer

Although lorazepam is helpful in controlling acute severe agitated states, it is not indicated for long-term use. Lorazepam dosage should have been gradually withdrawn while the patient was in hospital. It is not helpful long term in schizophrenia, and discharging the patient while he was still taking lorazepam opened the way to long-term use and the risk of adverse effects, including depression. In addition, benzodiazepines have additive effects with other sedative drugs and would have added to the drowsiness and depression which can be caused by haloperidol.

REFERENCES

Allison C, Pratt J A 2003 Neuroadaptive processes in GABAergic and glutamatergic systems in benzodiazepine dependence. Pharmacology and Therapeutics 98: 171-195

Ashton C H 2002a Benzodiazepine abuse. In: Caan W, de Belleroche J (eds) Drinks, drugs and dependence. Routledge, London, pp 197-212

Ashton C H 2002b Benzodiazepines: how they work and how to withdraw. Available online at: www.benzo.org.uk

Ashton C H 2004 Benzodiazepine dependence. In: Haddad P, Dursun S A, Deakin B (eds) Adverse syndromes and psychiatric drugs. Oxford Medical Publications, Oxford, pp 239-260

Ashton C H 2005 The diagnosis and management of benzodiazepine dependence. Current Opinions in Psychiatry 18: 249-255

Ashton C H, Young A H 2003 SSRIs, drug withdrawal and abuse: problems or treatment? In: Stanford S C (ed) Selective serotonin reuptake inhibitors. RG Landes, Austin, pp 64-80

Bateson A N 2002 Basis pharmacologic mechanisms involved in benzodiazepine tolerance and withdrawal. Current Pharmaceutical Design 8: 5-21

Curran H V, Collins R, Fletcher S et al 2003 Older adults and withdrawal from benzodiazepine hypnotics in general practice: effects on cognitive function, sleep, mood and quality of life. Psychosomatic Medicine 33: 1223-1237

Doble A, Martin I L, Nutt D 2004 Calming the brain: benzodiazepines and related drugs from laboratory to clinic. Martin Dunitz, London

Drug & Therapeutics Bulletin 2004 What's wrong with prescribing hypnotics? Drug & Therapeutics Bulletin 42: 89-93

Haefely W 1990 Benzodiazepine receptor and ligands: structural and functional differences. In: Hindmarch I, Beaumont G, Brandon S et al (eds) Benzodiazepines: current concepts. John Wiley, Chichester, pp 1-18

Heather N, Bowie A, Ashton C H et al 2004 Randomised controlled trial of two brief interventions amongst long-term benzodiazepine use: controlled trial of intervention. Addiction Research Theory 12: 141-154

Lader M 2004 Drug treatment of generalised anxiety disorder. In: Lader M (ed) Fast facts: psychiatry highlights 2003–04. Health Press Limited, Oxford, pp 43-50

Morin C M 2003 Treating insomnia with behavioural approaches: evidence for efficacy, effectiveness and practicality. In: Szuba M P, Kloss J D, Dinges D F (eds) Insomnia: principles and management. Cambridge University Press, Cambridge, pp 83-95

Roy-Byrne P P 2005 The GABA-benzodiazepine receptor complex: structure, function and role in anxiety. Journal of Clinical Psychiatry 66(suppl 2): 14-20

Rudolph U, Crestani F, Mohler H 2001 GABAA receptor subtypes: dissecting their pharmacological functions. Trends in Pharmacological Sciences 22: 188-194

Sateia M J, Nowell P D 2004 Insomnia. Lancet 364: 1959-1973

Tyrer P 1989 Choice of treatment in anxiety. In: Tyrer P (ed) The psychopharmacology of anxiety. Oxford University Press Oxford, pp 255-281

FURTHER READING

Ashton C H 1995 Protracted withdrawal from benzodiazepines: the post withdrawal syndrome. Psychiatric Annals 25: 174-179

O'Brien C P 2005 Benzodiazepine use, abuse and dependence. Journal of Clinical Psychiatry 66(suppl): 28-33

Stevens J C, Pollack M H 2005 Benzodiazepines in clinical practice: consideration of their pharmacological functions. Trends in Pharmacological Sciences 22: 188-194

29 Affective disorders

J. P. Pratt

The central feature of an affective disorder is an alteration in mood. The most common presentation is that of a low mood or depression. Less commonly, the mood may become high or elated, as in mania.

Classification

Depression

The term 'depression' can in itself be misleading. Everyone in the normal course of daily life will experience alterations in mood. Depressed mood in this context does not represent a disorder or illness; in fact, lowered mood as a response to the ups and downs of living is considered normal and termed sadness or unhappiness. Sometimes clinical depression may present in a mild form, so it is important to differentiate this from normal unhappiness.

Mania

If the mood becomes elated or irritable this may be a symptom of mania. The term 'mania' is used to describe severe cases, frequently associated with psychotic symptoms. Hypomania describes a less severe form of the disorder. In clinical practice this distinction often becomes blurred, with hypomania being seen as patients develop, or recover from, mania.

Bipolar and unipolar disorders

If a patient develops one or more severe episodes of a mood disorder which includes a manic episode, the condition may be termed a bipolar disorder. The existence of repeated manic episodes alone is sufficient to be termed a bipolar disorder. The disorder can be further categorized as bipolar I, where full-blown episodes of mania occur, and bipolar II, where depressive episodes are interspersed with less severe hypomanic episodes. The term 'manic-depressive' is now outdated. Rapid cycling describes the existence of four or more episodes within a year. Unipolar mood disorder is used to describe single episodes of depression.

Epidemiology

Differences in diagnosis, particularly of depression, make it difficult to estimate the true incidence of affective disorders. The lifetime risk of developing a bipolar I disorder is said to be about 1% (0.3–1.5%). An accurate estimate for the more broadly defined bipolar II disorder is more difficult and it may be much more common, with studies suggesting a lifetime prevalence of between 0.2% and 10.9%. The incidence of bipolar I is generally reported to be the same for both men and women, whereas some studies suggest that bipolar II may be slightly more common in women.

By comparison, the overall incidence of depression is much higher and there does appear to be a significant difference between the sexes. Studies from America and Europe, using standard assessment tools, found a lifetime prevalence of between 16% and 17%, with a 6-month prevalence of about 6%. Higher rates are consistently found in women but social, economic and ethnic factors are also likely to be influential.

Although depression may occur at any age, including early childhood, it is estimated that the average age of onset of depression is in the mid 20s. Some earlier studies found the incidence and prevalence of depression in women peaking at the age of 35–45 years. In bipolar disorder an earlier age of onset is suggested, perhaps in late adolescence, with most people experiencing their first episodes before 30 years of age.

Aetiology

Like most psychiatric disorders, the causes of affective disorders remain unknown. In depression it is likely that genetic, hormonal, biochemical, environmental and social factors all have some role in determining an individual's susceptibility to developing the disorder, with major life events sometimes, but not always, acting as a precipitant for a particular episode. Although pharmacological treatments are clearly effective, there is no simple relationship between biochemical abnormalities and affective disorders.

Genetic causes

In depression, one theory suggests that a variant of the gene responsible for encoding the serotonin transporter protein could account for early childhood experiences being translated into an increased risk of depression through stress sensitivity in adulthood. In bipolar disorder some genetic linkage has been found with chromosomal region 6q16-q21.

The incidence of affective disorder in first-degree relatives of someone with severe depression may be about 20%, which is almost three times the risk for relatives in control groups. Comparisons of the risk of affective disorder in the children of both parents with an affective disorder show a four times greater risk, and the risk is doubled in children with one parent with an affective disorder. Studies looking at twins have found fairly strong evidence for a genetic factor.

Evidence of a genetic link has also been found in studies of children from parents with affective disorder who were adopted by healthy parents. A higher incidence of affective disorder was found in the biological parents of adopted children with affective disorder than in the adoptive parents.

Environmental factors

Although environmental stresses can often be identified prior to an episode of mania or depression, a causal relationship between a major event in someone's life and the development of an affective disorder has not been firmly established. It may be that life events described as 'threatening' are more likely to be associated with depression.

The lack of prospective studies makes it difficult to interpret data linking early life events, such as loss of a parent, to the development of an affective disorder. The fact that specific environmental stresses have not been identified should not lead to the conclusion that the environment or lifestyle is irrelevant to the course or development of affective disorders. Employment, higher socio-economic status and the existence of a close and confiding relationship have been noted to offer some protection against the development of an episode.

Biochemical factors

In its simplistic form the biochemical theory of depression postulates a deficiency of neurotransmitter amines in certain areas of the brain. This theory has been developed to suggest that receptor sensitivity changes may be important. Alternative propositions suggest a central role of acetylcholine arising from dysregulation of the cholinergic and noradrenergic neurotransmitter systems.

Although many neurotransmitters may be implicated, the theory focuses on an involvement of the neurotransmitters noradrenaline (norepinephrine), serotonin (5-hydroxytryptamine) and dopamine. This theory emerged from the findings that both monoamine oxidase inhibitors (MAOIs) and tricyclic antidepressants appeared to increase neurotransmitter amines, particularly noradrenaline (norepinephrine), at important sites in the brain. When it was found that reserpine, previously used as an antihypertensive, caused both a depletion of neurotransmitter and also induced depression, this was taken as an apparent confirmation of the theory.

Although less attention has been paid to dopaminergic activity, some studies have found reduced activity in depressed patients, and an overactivity has been postulated in mania.

The concept of noradrenergic (norepinephrinergic) and serotonergic forms of depression has not gained widespread support, and there is little justification in measuring noradrenaline (norepinephrine) or serotonin metabolites in routine practice.

Endocrine factors

The endocrine system, particularly the hypothalamic-pituitary-adrenal (HPA) axis and the hypothalamic-pituitary-thyroid (HPT) axis, is felt to be implicated in the development of affective disorders. Some endocrine disorders such as hypothyroidism and Cushing's syndrome have also been associated with changes in mood. People with depression are commonly found to have increased cortisol levels, which also supports the proposition that mood disorders may be linked to dysfunction within the hypothalamic-pituitary-adrenal axis. This finding has been used as the basis for the dexamethasone suppression test in depression.

Physical illness and side effects of medication

Disorders of mood, particularly depression, have been associated with several types of medication and a number of physical illnesses (Table 29.1). Depression can affect the outcome in people with a range of physical problems. An increase in death rates has been found in those patients with co-morbid depression.

Clinical manifestations

Depression

A low mood is the central feature of depression. This is often accompanied by a loss of interest or pleasure in normally enjoyable activities. Thinking is pessimistic and in some cases suicidal. A depressed person may complain they have little or no energy. In severe cases, psychotic symptoms such as hallucination or delusion may be present.

Anxiety or agitation frequently accompany the disorder, and the so-called biological features of sleep disturbances, weight loss

Table 29.1 Drugs and physical illnesses implicated in disorders of mood

Drugs

Analgesics	Antipsychotics
Antidepressants	Benzodiazepines
Antihypertensives	Antiparkinsonism agents
Anticonvulsants	Steroids
Opiate withdrawal	Oral contraceptives
Amfetamine withdrawal	
Benzodiazepine withdrawal	

Physical illness

Viral illness	Thyroid disease
Carcinoma	Addison's disease
Neurological disorders	Systemic lupus erythematosus
Diabetes	Pernicious anaemia
Multiple sclerosis	

and loss of appetite are often present. Depressed people typically complain of somatic symptoms, particularly gastric problems, and non-specific aches are common.

Sexual drive is often reduced, and some people may lose interest in sex altogether. In some cases the biological symptoms are reversed and excessive eating and sleeping may occur. In contrast to agitation, psychomotor retardation may be a presenting feature.

Bipolar disorder

Standardized diagnostic criteria vary. For an ICD 10 diagnosis of bipolar disorder, at least two mood episodes must occur, one of which must be manic or hypomanic (Table 29.3). According to DSM IV, at least one episode of mania must have occurred for a diagnosis of bipolar I disorder to be made; depression may also occur, but it is not essential.

Mania

In mania the mood is described as elated or irritable and the accompanying overactivity is usually unproductive. Disinhibition may result in excessive spending sprees, inappropriate sexual activity and other high-risk behaviours. Driving may be particularly dangerous. Manic people may describe their thoughts as racing, with ideas rapidly changing from one topic to another. Speech may be very rapid with frequent punning and rhyming. Ideas may become grandiose with patients embarking on fantastic projects which lead nowhere and inevitably are left incomplete

Table 29.2 ICD 10 diagnostic criteria for a depressive episode (WHO 1992)

Usual symptoms

Depressed mood, loss of interest and enjoyment, and reduced energy leading to increased fatiguability and diminished activity

Common symptoms

Reduced concentration and attention

Reduced self-esteem and self-confidence

Ideas of guilt and unworthiness (even in a mild type of episode)

Bleak and pessimistic views of the future

Ideas or acts of self-harm or suicide

Disturbed sleep

Diminished appetite

In a depressive episode the mood varies little from day to day and is often unresponsive to circumstances, yet may show characteristic diurnal variation as the day goes on. The clinical picture shows marked individual variations, and atypical presentations are particularly common in adolescence. In some cases anxiety, distress and motor agitation may be more prominent at times than the depression.

For depressive episodes of all grades of severity a duration of 2 weeks is usually required for diagnosis, but shorter periods may be reasonable if symptoms are unusually severe and of rapid onset.

Mild depressive episode: For at least 2 weeks, at least two of the usual symptoms of a depressive episode plus at least two of the common symptoms listed above.

An individual with a mild depressive episode is usually distressed by the symptoms and has some difficulty in continuing with ordinary work and social activities, but will probably not cease to function completely.

Moderate depressive episode: For at least 2 weeks, at least two or three of the usual symptoms of a depressive episode plus at least three (preferably four) of the common symptoms listed above.

An individual with moderately severe depressive episode will have these symptoms to a marked degree, but this is not essential if a particularly wide variety of symptoms is present overall. They will usually have considerable difficulties in continuing with social, work or domestic activities.

Severe depressive episode: For at least 2 weeks, all three of the usual symptoms of a depressive episode plus at least four of the common symptoms listed above, some of which should be of severe intensity.

An individual with severe depressive episode may be unable or unwilling to describe many symptoms in detail, but an overall grading of severe may still be justified. They will usually show considerable distress or agitation, unless retardation is a marked feature. Loss of self-esteem or feelings of uselessness or guilt are likely to be prominent. Suicide is a distinct danger, particularly in severe cases.

Table 29.3   ICD 10 diagnostic criteria for bipolar affective disorder (WHO 1992)

Characterized by repeated (at least two) episodes in which the patient's mood and activity levels are significantly disturbed. This disturbance consisting on some occasions of an elevation in mood and increased energy and activity (mania or hypomania), and on others of a lowering of mood and decreased energy and activity (depression).

Manic episodes usually begin abruptly and last for between 2 weeks and 4–6 months (median 4 months). Depression tends to last longer (median about 6 months). Episodes of both kinds often follow stressful life events or other mental trauma, but the presence of such stress is not essential for the diagnosis.

and disjointed. Clothing is usually flamboyant, and if make-up is worn it is usually excessive and involves bright colours.

Severity

The severity of the disorder may vary from mild through moderate to severe. In most circumstances, it would be inappropriate for people with mild forms of the disorders to be seen by specialist services. In the absence of a risk of serious self-harm, people with less severe forms of the disorder should be treated by the primary healthcare team. In the UK the National Institute for Clinical Excellence (NICE) advises that a stepwise approach is taken on the management of depression.

If left untreated, it is important to remember that affective disorders carry a risk of mortality. As well as suicidal attempts by someone who is depressed, the lack of self-care and physical exhaustion resulting from mania may be life-threatening. The social and financial consequences can have a devastating effect on both the patient with mania or hypomania and their family.

Investigations

There are no universally accepted tests which will confirm the presence of an affective disorder.

Various rating scales have been developed that may help to demonstrate the severity of depressive disorder or distinguish a predominantly anxious patient from a depressed patient. Biochemical tests are generally not particularly helpful in determining the treatment plan or management of affective disorders. The dexamethasone suppression test is still used by some clinicians as an aid to diagnosis, but it must be considered as having limited value in practice.

Within the UK, mental and behavioural disorders are commonly classified using the *International Classification of Diseases*, ICD 10 (WHO 1992). The American Psychiatric Association (1994) has developed a precise system of diagnosis, based on the description of symptoms in the *Diagnostic and Statistical Manual of Mental Disorders*, now in its fourth edition (DSM IV).

A systematic approach to the diagnosis of affective disorders is important when considering the effectiveness of medication.

Although most new clinical trials for antidepressants or antipsychotics require a DSM diagnosis as an entry criterion, in the UK the ICD 10 classification is normally used, with the severity of depression determined by the presence of the number of symptoms (see Tables 29.2 and 29.3).

In the UK there are national clinical guidelines (NICE 2004) for the treatment of depression in primary and secondary care. This guidance provides a sound framework for the management of depression. It is important that people with depression are identified. A simple screening process for the presence of depression could involve asking the patient two questions about their mood and interest. For example, the patient could be asked 'During the last month, have you often been bothered by feeling down, depressed or hopeless?' and 'During the last month, have you often been bothered by having little interest or pleasure in doing things?'. If the answer to either question is 'no' it is unlikely the patient will be considered to have a depressive disorder. Patients answering 'yes' warrant further investigation.

The identification of target symptoms may be useful in evaluating the response to treatment. In routine clinical practice antidepressant medication should not generally be used to treat patients with mild depression. Non-pharmacological strategies are preferable in this group.

Rating scales

Various rating scales can be used to assist with the assessment of the severity of the disorder. Two of the more commonly used rating scales are the Beck Depression Inventory and the Hamilton Depression Rating Scale.

Beck depression inventory

This is a self-reporting scale looking at 21 depressive symptoms. The subject is asked to read a series of statements and mark on a scale of 1–4 how severe their symptoms are. The higher the score, the more severely depressed a person may be.

Hamilton depression rating scale

This rating scale is used by a healthcare professional at the end of an interview to rate the severity of the depression.

Dexamethasone suppression test

This test involves the administration of 1 mg of dexamethasone at 11 p.m., which is said to coincide with the low point of cortisol secretion. It would be expected that normally dexamethasone would suppress the secretion of cortisol for about 24 hours. Blood samples are taken the following day, at 8 a.m., 4 p.m. and 11 p.m. If it is found that serum cortisol levels are elevated between 9 and 24 hours after the administration of dexamethasone, then this is taken as a positive result, i.e. dexamethasone has failed to suppress normal cortisol secretion.

It is important to note that this test is not specific to depression, and other disorders may account for an apparent positive result. Similarly, there may be a high proportion of depressed people who show a negative result with the test.

Treatment

The aim of treatment is to prevent harm and to relieve distress or to be prophylactic. It is important to differentiate symptoms of the disorder from the premorbid personality. In general the drugs which are used to control the symptoms of mania are not specifically antimanic. These agents are also used to treat other disorders. This means the diagnosis will primarily influence the way in which these drugs are used rather than the choice of drug per se.

In the treatment of depression all the antidepressants currently available in the UK are considered to be equally effective. There is no convincing evidence from clinical trials that any one drug is faster acting or any better or any worse than any other in relieving the symptoms of depression. There are some generalizations which may help individualize the choice of antidepressant. Females may have a poorer tolerance of imipramine than males and tricyclic antidepressants are less well tolerated and more likely to be toxic in overdose than the selective serotonin reuptake inhibitors (SSRIs). Patients may prefer one drug over another based on their past experience of benefit or side effects. Overall, the major difference between antidepressant agents is in their side effect profile and toxicity in overdose. There can also be significant variations in the costs of different agents.

Treatment of depression

In moderate and severe depression, pharmacological intervention is important, but this should never be considered in isolation from the social, cultural and environmental influences on the patient. Non-pharmacological therapies are effective and in mild depression they are considered preferable to drug treatment. Non-drug treatments and antidepressant medication are not mutually exclusive and in some cases it is preferable to use both in combination.

Drug treatment

Despite the availability of many new antidepressants, the therapeutic effectiveness of these agents has changed little since the discovery of the antidepressant properties of imipramine in the late 1950s. Further research may reveal differences between antidepressants. There is limited evidence to support the notion that MAOIs are less effective than tricyclics in hospitalized inpatients, but more effective in so-called atypical depression. Overall, the SSRI antidepressants appear to be better tolerated than tricyclics. However, although less well tolerated, limited evidence suggests that venlafaxine may be more effective than SSRIs in hospital inpatients. Overall, the current evidence indicates that any claim of overall superiority of one antidepressant over another would be premature.

A strong response to placebo is found in most of the studies of antidepressants. Tolerability is therefore an important factor in the choice of drug; patients who are unable to tolerate the side effects of antidepressants are likely to discontinue these drugs. Antidepressants should be taken in adequate doses for some 4–6 weeks, and up to 12 weeks in older people, to achieve a full response. Following a single episode of depression, treatment should be continued for 6 months, at the same dose at which the patient achieved remission, before attempting withdrawal. In patients experiencing multiple episodes of depression, treatment should be continued for longer periods (2 years).

Withdrawal of antidepressants should normally be undertaken gradually. Following abrupt discontinuation patients may experience symptoms of withdrawal that include gastrointestinal symptoms, together with headache, giddiness, sweating, shaking and insomnia. In addition, extrapyramidal reactions may be associated with abrupt withdrawal from some of the SSRI antidepressants. Following successful treatment, antidepressants should be gradually reduced over a period of 4 weeks. This period should be increased if patients experience problems, or where medication has been given for extended periods.

Generally, the long half-life of fluoxetine enables the drug to be stopped without the need for tapering from the standard antidepressant dose of 20 mg. Patients taking MAOIs may experience psychomotor agitation following discontinuation.

Because patients do not experience the craving typically associated with drugs of addiction, most healthcare professionals do not class antidepressants as addictive. Patients should be warned that there is a risk of problems with abrupt discontinuation, but use of emotive words like addiction or dependence is best avoided. In moderate or severe depression the balance of risks and benefits is usually in favour of using antidepressants. Occasionally some patients report that they have become dependent on their antidepressants and feel unable to stop taking them. These concerns should not be dismissed lightly, but the focus of discussion with the patient should be on the overall risks and benefits of the treatment in the context of their individual circumstances.

As discussed earlier, there is no strong evidence for the existence of a particular biochemical subtype of depression. However, some patients do respond better to particular antidepressants. This has led to the widely held view that previous response to treatment is a strong indication to use that particular drug in the treatment of a future episode.

As well as previous response, the other important considerations to take into account when selecting an antidepressant are side effects, contraindications, toxicity in overdose, patient preference and clinician familiarity.

Generally speaking, the older drugs have a poorer side effect (Barbui et al 2001, Geddes et al 2002) and toxicity profile than the more recently introduced agents. Traditionally the antidepressant drugs are categorized by their chemical structure, e.g. tricyclic, or their predominant pharmacological action, e.g. MAOI, SSRI.

Tricyclic antidepressants A greater understanding of the pharmacology of antidepressants has given much support to the biochemical theory of depression. Although substantial data on the pharmacological effects of the tricyclic antidepressants exist, it is still not clear how the drugs relieve the symptoms of depression. This is an important point often overlooked when discussing the issue with patients. The notion that depression is a simple lack of, or imbalance of, chemicals has little basis in fact. It merely provides a useful framework from which to discuss the benefits and harms of antidepressants.

It was thought originally that the primary effect of these drugs was related to their ability to block the reuptake of noradrenaline (norepinephrine) and/or 5HT following their release and action as neurotransmitters. As this effect occurs some weeks before the antidepressant response, clearly this is not the whole story. Following chronic administration, further biochemical changes take place, particularly with pre- and postsynaptic receptor sensitivity. Reduction of presynaptic α_2-receptor sensitivity occurs, and this increases the production of noradrenaline (norepinephrine). Other effects which may be relevant include an increase in α_1 and β_1 receptor sensitivity. It is now felt that these receptor changes in the cerebral cortex and hippocampus may be more related to the antidepressant response than simple reuptake inhibition.

There are at least nine tricyclic antidepressants in current clinical use. The basic chemical structures of these compounds are similar but there are differences between them. All the tricyclic antidepressants block the reuptake of noradrenaline (norepinephrine) and 5HT to a greater or lesser degree.

Imipramine The antidepressant effect of imipramine was demonstrated around 50 years ago and it has been widely prescribed in subsequent years. Although imipramine is less sedating than other tricyclic drugs, some patients may still experience problems. As well as cardiovascular problems, significant antimuscarinic effects such as dry mouth, blurred vision and constipation occur. Females tend to tolerate imipramine less well than males.

At one time is was felt to be important that the drug should be prescribed at the full therapeutic dose. Recent analysis of clinical trials suggests this is not the case. If patients respond to lower doses, there is no rationale for increasing the dose further. Tolerance may develop to some of the unpleasant side effects, and this may be facilitated by starting with a lower dose of the drug and gradually increasing the dose over a week.

In addition to the unpleasant side effect profile, imipramine is toxic following overdose. Bearing in mind that the drug is used to treat a disorder which involves suicide, this relative lack of safety is an important disadvantage. The drug should only be used in circumstances where intentional overdose can be prevented.

Imipramine is metabolized by demethylation to an active metabolite, desipramine. Both the parent drug and its metabolite have long half-lives, of 9–20 hours and 10–35 hours respectively, that permit single daily dosing.

Amitriptyline Also developed in the late 1950s, amitriptyline has a similar poor side effect and toxicity profile to imipramine but is more sedative. Additional sedative properties are sometimes considered an advantage in selected patients.

Like imipramine, the drug and its active metabolite (nortriptyline) have long half-lives, of 9–46 hours and 18–56 hours, respectively. The dose range is similar to imipramine.

Amoxapine Although developed much later than imipramine, amoxapine does not have a significantly better side effect or toxicity profile. Like other drugs in this class, it is an effective antidepressant. In standard doses, amoxapine may be less cardiotoxic than some other tricyclics but its effects following overdose are particularly severe, with renal failure and a high rate of seizures making management difficult.

Another difference between amoxapine and the rest of the group is its dopamine-blocking effect. Theoretically it might be expected that this would result in an antidepressant drug with additional antipsychotic effects. In clinical practice this is unlikely, but the potential for antidopaminergic side effects, such as tardive dyskinesia or prolactin-related disturbance, is a significant disadvantage.

Clomipramine This was one of the first antidepressants found to be a potent 5HT reuptake inhibitor. Some clinicians believe the drug is more effective than other antidepressants, but little evidence exists to support this anecdotal view. In addition to its antidepressant effect, the drug has also been of value in obsessional states.

Data from a fatal toxicity index (Buckley & McManus 2002) show clomipramine to have a lower than expected toxicity index. It is unlikely that clomipramine is inherently less toxic than other antidepressants so this finding could be accounted for by other factors, such as the relatively high rate of prescribing in non-depressive states.

Dosulepin Although introduced over 30 years ago, this drug is widely prescribed in the UK. Guidelines for the management of depression (NICE 2004) advise that the use of dosulepin should be restricted to specialist care. Although the drug does have a slightly improved side effect profile, this is outweighed by the risks of cardiac problems and toxicity in overdose.

Doxepin Doxepin has similar effects and side effects to the traditional tricyclics. Limited evidence suggests that it may have fewer cardiac effects in patients with pre-existing cardiac disease than other traditional tricyclics. However, direct comparisons do not exist and a newer, alternative agent should be considered in preference to doxepin in patients with cardiac disease.

Lofepramine Although desipramine is a metabolite of lofepramine, the latter should not be considered purely as a prodrug. Important differences exist between lofepramine and the other traditional tricyclics. Antimuscarinic effects do occur with lofepramine, but these are less severe than with other tricyclics. In addition, despite being metabolized to desipramine, lofepramine is significantly safer than the traditional agents in overdose. This may be due to lofepramine antagonizing the cardiac effects of desipramine.

Lofepramine does not have a significant sedative effect, which may be an advantage in some patients, but in others the lack of sedation may be seen as a disadvantage. Some patients may complain of an alerting effect from lofepramine, particularly if the majority of the dose is given at bedtime. Despite a few reports of hepatic problems, given the favourable side effect profile and low toxicity in overdose, lofepramine may be considered as a reasonable option if a SSRI is ineffective or not tolerated.

Nortriptyline Nortriptyline is the major metabolite of amitriptyline, but appears to have little effect on blood pressure. Serum levels seem to show an inverted 'U' relationship with antidepressant effect. Patients respond best to intermediate serum levels of the drug (between 50 and 150 ng/mL). Levels outside this range may be associated with a poor response. Apart from these differences, nortriptyline shares many of the properties of the traditional tricyclic antidepressants.

Trimipramine This is a particularly sedative tricyclic antidepressant with few differences from the rest of the traditional tricyclics.

Monoamine oxidase inhibitors Two types of MAOI are available: the traditional MAOIs, which are both non-selective and irreversible, and moclobemide, which is a selective reversible inhibitor of monoamine-oxidase type A (RIMA).

In clinical practice the traditional MAOIs are not widely prescribed. If patients are able to tolerate adequate doses, they are effective antidepressants, particularly in patients with atypical symptoms of depression. Due to the potential for drug and food interactions, MAOIs should be reserved for use in situations where a first-line SSRI antidepressant has failed.

The potential for MAOIs to interact with other drugs and tyramine-containing foods has been well known since the 1960s. It is important that patients are made aware of the dietary restrictions and potential for serious drug interactions. These can be found in standard texts such as the British National Formulary.

Although the inhibitory effect of these drugs on monoamine oxidase is well understood, as with other antidepressants it is still not clear exactly how the MAOIs exert their antidepressant effect. MAOIs inhibit the enzymes responsible for the oxidation of noradrenaline (norepinephrine), 5HT and other biogenic amines. Two forms of monoamine oxidase have been found to exist, MAO-A and MAO-B. The traditional MAOIs are all nonselective and inhibit both forms of the enzyme.

Inhibition of MAO-A is thought to be responsible for the antidepressant effects. It is also responsible for metabolizing tyramine and producing the cheese interaction. Moclobemide is an antidepressant that acts as a reversible inhibitor of MAO-A. As tyramine is metabolized by both forms of the enzyme, if tyramine-containing foods are consumed, tyramine is metabolized by MAO-B enzymes as well as being able to reverse the inhibition of MAO-A. Unless very large quantities of tyramine are ingested, this appears to prevent the typical hypertensive reaction seen with conventional MAOIs and tyramine-containing foods.

Selegiline is a selective MAO-B inhibitor that does not seem to produce this interaction with foods, but neither does it appear to have a significant antidepressant effect.

The traditional MAOIs and moclobemide have little anticholinergic effect. Nevertheless, some patients do experience dry mouth, constipation and urinary retention. In contrast to the hypertension which follows the interaction of tyramine-rich foods with the traditional MAOIs, these drugs are liable to cause postural hypotension as a side effect. This side effect may be particularly problematic with phenelzine and may prevent adequate dosages being achieved.

Traditional MAOIs

Tranylcypromine Tranylcypromine has a structure that closely resembles amfetamine. It has a significant stimulant effect, and could be more likely to give rise to problems around dependence because of this. Unlike the other MAOIs, it does not irreversibly inhibit monoamine oxidase, which is said to recover some 5 days after withdrawal of the drug. Even so, the precautions associated with the MAOIs must still be continued for 2 weeks after discontinuing the drug.

Due to the amfetamine-like alerting effect of tranylcypromine, the last dose should not be given after about 3 p.m. The risk of severe interaction is also said to be greater with tranylcypromine than with other MAOIs.

Phenelzine Phenelzine has a hydrazine structure and because hydrazines have been associated with hepatocellular jaundice, it is recommended that phenelzine should be avoided in patients with hepatic impairment or abnormal liver function tests. In most patients, phenelzine is neither sedative nor stimulant. When considering the choice of an MAOI this distinction may be important. It is generally accepted that it is important to prescribe phenelzine at an adequate dosage (at least 1 mg/kg body weight),

although side effects such as postural hypotension often limit the dose a patient can tolerate.

Reversible inhibitors of monoamine oxidase

Moclobemide Although this is an effective antidepressant, with less propensity for interactions with tyramine-rich foods, caution should still be exercised as other drug interactions do occur. It could be considered, after a suitable wash-out period, as an option if a first-line SSRI is ineffective.

Selective serotonin reuptake inhibitors (SSRIs) These agents were developed in an attempt to reduce some of the problems associated with the tricyclic antidepressants. Unlike these drugs, the SSRIs do not share a common chemical structure, but they all selectively inhibit the reuptake of serotonin. As a group these drugs appear to be no more, but also no less, effective than the tricyclics. The major difference between these two groups of drugs is in their side effect profile. Overall, the SSRIs are better tolerated by most patients. Together with the fact that they are considerably less toxic in overdose, this means that they should be the first-line choice for the pharmacological management of moderate or severe depression. As generic versions of the drugs are available, the financial impact of using SSRIs first line has reduced in recent years. The SSRIs have a similar range of side effects, but there are variations in the intensity or duration. The degree of specificity for serotonin reuptake differs between the SSRIs, but this does not correlate with clinical efficacy. If given in adequate doses for an adequate period of time, all the drugs in this class appear equally effective.

The conclusion that the SSRIs should be considered as the first-line drug of choice (NICE 2004) is consistent with several earlier meta-analyses which showed the SSRIs were neither more nor less effective than traditional tricyclics (Anderson & Tomenson 1995, Hotopf et al 1996, Song et al 1993). They were, however, better tolerated than tricyclics as measured by fewer drop-outs from clinical trials. The NICE guideline development group considered this difference to be of sufficient importance to recommend SSRI antidepressants as the first-line drugs of choice.

Fluvoxamine This was the first SSRI available in the UK. Although patients experience few antimuscarinic side effects, other problems related to serotonergic enhancement such as nausea, headache and nervousness have been reported.

Fluoxetine The main difference between fluoxetine and the other SSRIs is the long half-lives of both the parent drug and its primary active metabolite, desmethylfluoxetine. In the initial stages of treatment some patients may experience a greater feeling of nervousness with fluoxetine than with the other SSRIs, but in most cases tolerance to this develops.

The long half-life of fluoxetine and its major metabolite is a problem if severe side effects develop. In other situations the long half-life means that the risks of discontinuation syndrome is reduced. Formulations of fluoxetine that can be taken on a weekly basis are available in some parts of the world.

Paroxetine Although all the SSRIs have been reported to cause extrapyramidal-type movements, paroxetine appears to be more commonly implicated. The problem may be particularly severe following abrupt discontinuation of high doses.

Sertraline Like the other SSRIs, sertraline is an effective antidepressant. Although doses of up to 200 mg have been used, doses of 150 mg and above should not be given for longer than 8 weeks.

Citalopram The efficacy and side effect profile of citalopram appear similar to the other agents but, like sertraline, the reduced propensity for interactions with drugs metabolized by the cyctochrome P450 2D6 isoenzyme has been suggested as a theoretical advantage.

Escitalopram Citalopram is thought to be the active enantiomer of citalopram which is a racemic mixture of R- and S-citalopram. Theoretically the use of escitalopram has been advocated on the basis that the R enantiomer has no antidepressant effect, and may even counteract some of the antidepressant effects of escitalopram. Overall, clinical studies show little difference between citalopram and escitalopram (Svensson & Mansfield 2004).

Lithium Lithium does have antidepressant properties but will be discussed in more detail in the antimanic section.

Other drugs

Trazodone In vitro, trazodone appears to operate as a mixed serotonin agonist/antagonist, but clinically it is thought to operate as a serotonin agonist. Trazodone is much safer than the tricyclics following overdose but causes pronounced sedative and hypotensive effects in some patients. Priapism has also been noted as a rare but distressing side effect. This is probably due to its potent α-receptor blocking properties.

Mianserin Mianserin was one of the first antidepressants to demonstrate an improved toxicity profile following overdose. Like many of the newer drugs, it has fewer antimuscarinic side effects than the traditional tricyclics. One drawback in using mianserin is the need for monthly blood counts during the first 3 months of treatment, due to a high reported incidence of blood dyscrasias, particularly in the elderly. Mianserin is no longer widely prescribed in the UK, and the required blood tests should not be considered a substitute for the routine clinical monitoring of the patient.

Venlafaxine Venlafaxine was reported to be the first in a new class of antidepressants, the serotonin-noradrenaline reuptake inhibitors (SNRIs). These antidepressants were developed in an attempt to improve efficacy over the standard agents. As the name suggests, they prevent the reuptake of both serotonin and noradrenaline (norepinephrine), a mechanism they have in common with the tricyclic antidepressants. It was hoped this would result in a drug with similar efficacy to the tricyclics in more severe cases but without the antimuscarinic, cardiac or toxic effects of the older drugs. A review of the safety of venlafaxine has, however, highlighted the relative increased risk of cardiac events and toxicity compared to the SSRIs. Cardiac monitoring is now required for all patients prescribed this drug. In view of the potential risks with venlafaxine, this drug is not recommended as a first- or second-line treatment for most patients with moderate or severe depression. Some patients may find that by changing to the slow-release formulation, some of the gastrointestinal problems associated with the conventional release product may be reduced.

Reboxetine Reboxetine is a specific noradrenergic (norepinephrinergic) reuptake inhibitor (NARI). Response rates appear similar to other antidepressants. This casts further doubt on the existence of particular subtypes of depression likely to respond to particular antidepressants. Patients experiencing problems with serotonergic related side effects may benefit from a switch to reboxetine.

Mirtazapine Mirtazapine is a noradrenergic and specific serotonergic antidepressant (NaSSA). It enhances both noradrenergic (norepinephrinergic) and $5HT_1$ serotonergic transmission. Specific $5HT_1$ neurotransmission is achieved as the drug also acts as a $5HT_2$ and $5HT_3$ antagonist. The receptor-specific effects of mirtazapine may explain some reduction in sexual dysfunction and nausea compared to other SSRIs. Despite this novel pharmacology, mirtazapine appears little different from other antidepressants in terms of efficacy.

Choice of antidepressant As no antidepressant has been found to be more effective than any other, the choice will be determined by other factors. In some areas, cost has become a major factor in choice. In general the SSRI drugs appear to have a better side effect profile and are less toxic following overdose. For most people with moderate-to-severe depression, the use of a SSRI as the first-line choice is appropriate. When cost is taken into account the choice is further revised to a generic SSRI such as fluoxetine or citalopram. If an SSRI is not appropriate then alternative agents include lofepramine. As long as there are no contraindications, then previous response and tolerance to a particular drug or patient preference should also be considered.

Concerns about the toxicity of dosulepin should limit this once widely prescribed antidepressant to specific patients under the supervision of specialist care. In clinical practice the identification of patients at high risk of suicide is difficult, and all patients with severe depression should be considered at risk of self-harm. The quantities of medication supplied to these patients should be carefully monitored.

Other treatments

Electroconvulsive therapy Electroconvulsive therapy (ECT) would only be considered after referral to a psychiatrist. Although it is said to have a faster onset of action, its effects are fairly short-lived and antidepressants are normally required to prevent relapse. Although the treatment itself is considered safe, there are risks from the anaesthetic agent, and some patients suffer short-term memory loss following treatment.

Non-drug treatments In addition to drug treatment, it is important to consider the patient's wider social, cultural and environmental circumstances. Although for some people the main element of treatment will be pharmacological, most patients will need help and support to cope with depression. Specific non-pharmacological interventions such as cognitive behaviour therapy (CBT) can be as effective as drug treatments. For some people a combination of antidepressants and CBT is required. Other forms of psychotherapy are also available from specialist services. For mild forms of depression non-drug strategies are generally considered as the first-line treatment.

St John's wort (*Hypericum perforatum*) Extracts of hypericum are effective in the short-term management of mild or moderately severe depression (Linde & Mulrow 2001). Hypericum may induce the metabolism of other drugs, which may lead to toxicity on discontinuation. There is currently insufficient evidence to support the use of this product in severe depression.

Treatment of mania

Valproate semisodium (divalproate) is licensed in the UK as a specific treatment for mania associated with bipolar disorder. Antipsychotics, lithium and benzodiazepines may also have a role in the management of mania. Although there is insufficient evidence to differentiate between olanzapine and divalproate, they are both considered options in the management of acute mania. Other antipsychotics which could also be considered include the atypical antipsychotics risperidone and quetiapine which have extended licensed indications to include the treatment of mania. Short-term adjunctive treatment with a benzodiazepine may be required whilst lithium may be used as an effective antimanic agent but may take longer to produce a full effect. When the potential fluctuations in physical exertion and fluid intake are also taken into account, most clinicians would not consider lithium as their first choice of antimanic treatment although it remains the drug of choice for long-term use to prevent recurrence or relapse. In time further evidence may establish the place of sodium valproate along with carbamazepine as alternatives. When used prophylactically, these agents are commonly referred to as mood stabilizers.

If an episode of mania occurs in patients taking antidepressants, these should be withdrawn. If mania occurs in patients already taking prophylactic treatment, attention should be given to maximizing the dose and, if necessary, adding a second agent.

Valproate semisodium

This is a 1:1 molar combination of sodium valproate and valproic acid. Following administration, valproate ion is released and subsequently absorbed. The therapeutic differences between sodium valproate and valproate semisodium have not been established. However, the latter is the only form of valproate licensed for the acute treatment of mania. The mechanism of action in mania is unclear but may be related to increased levels of GABA. The antimanic effects of valproate are seen within 3 days, but the full benefit of treatment may not be apparent for up to 3 weeks. Dosage should be rapidly titrated to between 1000 mg and 2000 mg per day. Routine serum levels are not necessary, but levels between 50 and 100 μg/mL are reported to be associated with optimal response.

Although the risks of liver damage are greater in young children, liver function tests should be performed prior to initiation of therapy and periodically thereafter in all patients. In addition, the patient must be instructed to report any problems, such as unexplained bruising, that may indicate abnormalities in coagulation.

Antipsychotics

All these drugs share a common effect of blocking dopamine D_2 postsynaptic receptors to some degree. The atypical antipsychotics olanzapine, risperidone and quetiapine have a marketing authorization which includes their use in the treatment of acute mania. Olanzapine's licence also extends to prophylactic use in bipolar disorder. Whether or not these licensed indications represent a real clinical distinction between the antipsychotics is unknown.

Concerns about the acute extrapyramidal effects of the traditional antipsychotics now limit the use of these drugs. Of the traditional antipsychotics, haloperidol in an appropriate dose is still commonly prescribed. It is less sedating than other antipsychotics which means it may occasionally be necessary to control severe behaviour disturbances with additional sedatives such as lorazepam, either orally or by injection. When a single agent is not considered to be effective, consideration should be given to augmenting the antipsychotic with valproate semisodium.

Dose and duration of treatment are important considerations when treating acute mania. The dose of antipsychotic should be reduced as the patient improves, and in most cases the antipsychotic can be stopped as the patient becomes euthymic. Some clinicians continue the antipsychotic for several months after the acute episode in the hope of preventing relapse. There is insufficient evidence to provide definitive guidance on the optimal duration of antipsychotic treatment of an acute episode of mania.

Lithium

Although lithium is effective in the acute management of mania, other treatments are generally preferred. This is due to the delay in response and variability of physical exertion and fluid intake which may compromise the safe use of lithium. In the acute situation lithium make take up to 10–14 days to exert an effect. Higher serum levels are also required (up to 1.2 mmol/L).

Antipsychotics or valproate semisodium, either alone or in combination, along with benzodiazepines should be considered the first-line treatment in the acute phase of mania.

Following an acute episode, lithium remains the primary consideration for prophylaxis (Baldessarini & Tondo 2000). Generally speaking, continuation therapy with a prophylactic mood stabilizer should be considered in all bipolar patients who have had two or more acute episodes within 2–4 years. It may also be reasonable to consider prophylaxis in any patient following a severe manic episode. As treatment is long term, the cooperation of the patient is essential and so a thorough explanation of the risks and benefits of the treatment is vital.

Before lithium treatment is initiated, an assessment of the patient's physical state is essential. Thyroid, renal and cardiac function should all be within normal limits. It is, however, still possible to use lithium, with caution, in patients with mild-to-moderate renal failure or cardiovascular impairment. Specialist medical advice should always be sought in such cases. Any thyroid deficiency should be corrected before lithium treatment is commenced.

Plasma levels There is a narrow therapeutic window for lithium plasma levels and variation in the reference ranges reported. Some of this variation can be accounted for by variation in dose schedules. In the main, 12-hour (post dose) levels above 1.2 mmol/L are considered to be toxic and levels below 0.4 mmol/L are not considered to be effective. If lithium plasma levels are kept in the range 0.4–0.8 mmol/L, then lithium is usually well tolerated with minimal side effects. Levels at or above 0.7 mmol/L are reported as being more effective than lower doses.

For most patients the range of 0.4–0.8 mmol/L is appropriate for prophylaxis, but if lithium is used to control the acute phase, levels may need to be around 1.0 mmol/L. To accurately interpret lithium levels, it is important that the correct schedule is followed and to establish consistent results, the 12-hour standard plasma lithium protocol has been devised. This means that lithium levels should be taken in the morning as near as possible to 12 hours after the last dose of lithium.

As the absorption and bioavailability of lithium may vary from brand to brand, it is important that patients do not inadvertently change brands or dosage forms without levels being checked.

Lithium not only has a narrow therapeutic range but is particularly toxic in overdose. It is usually well tolerated if plasma levels are kept at the lower end of the therapeutic range. Common side effects reported by patients are gastrointestinal disturbances, tremor, thirst, polyuria, weight gain and lethargy. As well as complaints of side effects, some patients prefer to remain untreated as they feel lithium 'damps down' their creativity and they miss the slight 'highs' that occur as part of their illness.

Patients taking a prophylactic mood stabilizer may occasionally stop taking their medication when they feel they no longer need it, or want to see if they can overcome the disorder without the need for drugs. Patients commonly have several trials on a mood stabilizer before they accept that the balance of risks and benefits is usually in favour of longer term treatment. There is a significant risk of relapse if lithium is discontinued abruptly.

Other anticonvulsants

Carbamazepine is generally considered as a second-line prophylactic treatment, if first-line therapy is either not tolerated or is ineffective. Emerging evidence continues to support the use of lamotrigine as an alternative in patients with bipolar depression.

Treatment combinations

In patients who cannot be controlled on a single mood stabilizer, consideration should be given to combining treatments. Although not entirely without risks, all the above drugs have been used in various combinations in resistant cases.

Patient care

In the acute phase of an affective disorder a patient will have little or no insight into his or her condition. This often makes it difficult to prescribe medication following an informed discussion on the risks and benefits of treatment. Depressed patients may say they are not worth treating; most manic patients will find it impossible to engage in meaningful dialogue, or they may insist they do not need medication and consistently refuse treatment. Thus in the initial stages of treatment some patients are treated against their will. As people respond to treatment, it is crucial that the benefits and risks of treatment are explained. This may need to be repeated and backed up by written information. Engaging the patient and including them in the choice of treatment not only supports their basic human rights but is also likely to lead to a better therapeutic outcome. The discussion should also allow the patient to record their preference for future treatment. This may include drug regimens they would prefer to receive should they relapse as well as medication they would find objectionable.

During the acute phase of their illness patients may often forget what they have been told about their medication. It is therefore important to regularly offer information or reassurance about medication, even if the patient is reported to have fully discussed the actions and effects with a healthcare professional.

Many patients are frightened by the notion of taking medication that will affect their mind. Taking an antidepressant is often felt to be a sign of failure or weakness by the patient as well as their family and friends. This often leads people to try and deal with their depression without medication. This is fine for the milder forms of the disorder and is sometimes referred to as 'watchful waiting'. In more severe cases such an approach could have life-threatening consequences for the patient.

Patients should always be offered the opportunity of discussing their medication. The use of patient information leaflets and the involvement of the family or close friends may help patients understand the risks and benefits of their treatment.

Many of the drugs used in the treatment of affective disorders have the potential to interact with other drugs that have been prescribed or purchased. Some of these are summarized in Table 29.4.

Common therapeutic problems in the management of affective disorder are outlined in Table 29.5.

Table 29.4 Examples of important drug interactions with drugs used in the management of affective disorders

Antidepressant	Interacting drug	Effect
Tricyclics	Adrenaline (epinephrine) and other directly acting sympathomimetics	Greatly enhances effect. Dangerous
	Alcohol	Enhanced sedation
	Antiarrhythmics	Risk of ventricular arrhythmias
	Anticonvulsants	Lowered seizure threshold and possible lowered tricyclic levels
	MAOIs	Severe hypertension
	Fluoxetine	Increased tricyclic serum levels
SSRIs	Anticoagulants	Enhanced effects
	MAOIs	Dangerous
	Lithium	Possible serotonin syndrome

continued

Table 29.4 (continued)

Antidepressant	Interacting drug	Effect
MAOIs	Alcohol, fermented beverages, tyramine-rich foods Antihypertensives Anticonvulsants Levodopa Sympathomimetics	Hypertensive crisis Increased effect Lowered seizure threshold Hypertensive crisis Hypertensive crisis
Antipsychotics	Anaesthetic agents Anticonvulsants Antiarrhythmics Astemizole and terfenadine	Hypotension Lowered seizure threshold Risk of ventricular arrhythmias Risk of ventricular arrhythmias
Lithium	Non-steroidal anti-inflammatory drugs (NSAIDs) SSRIs	Enhanced lithium plasma levels Possible serotonin syndrome
Diuretics	Enhanced lithium plasma levels particularly with thiazides Angiotensin-converting enzyme (ACE) inhibitors Sumatriptan	 Enhanced lithium plasma levels Possible central nervous system toxicity
St John's wort	Induces cytochrome P450 enzymes, particularly 1A2, 2C9 and 3A4 Indinavir Warfarin SSRIs Carbamazepine (and other anticonvulsants) Digoxin Oestrogens and progestogens Theophylline Ciclosporin	 Reduced plasma concentration (avoid) Reduced anticoagulant effect (avoid) Increased serotonergic effect (avoid) Reduced plasma concentrations (avoid) Reduced plasma concentration (avoid) Reduced contraceptive effect (avoid) Reduced plasma concentration (avoid) Reduced plasma concentration (avoid)

Table 29.5 Common therapeutic problems in the management of affective disorder

Problem	Possible solution
Antidepressants	
Treatment failure (30–40% of patients will not respond to first antidepressant)	Ensure adequate dose and duration of treatment Check compliance, engage the patient, develop therapeutic alliance Reassess response against target symptoms Reconfirm diagnosis and identify compounding factors, e.g. high levels of alcohol consumption
Risk of self-harm	Prescribe/dispense limited quantities. Involve family or carer in supervising medication. Avoid traditional tricyclics in unsupervised situations
Withdrawal reactions	Ensure gradual withdrawal
Relapse on discontinuation	Consider long-term treatment
Intolerance	Consider changing to a different class
Venlafaxine/dosulepin	Ensure specialist involvement in treatment plan
Antimanic agents	
Treatment failure	Ensure adequate dose, check plasma levels. Consider drug combinations
Toxicity adverse effects	Determine dose by clinical response, guided by plasma levels Ensure patient is well informed and able to recognize impending toxicity and adverse effects of treatment
Weight gain	Dietary advice; consider alternative pharmacotherapy
Lithium levels	Ensure plasma levels are 12 hours post dose, taken in the morning. Regular monitoring is important

CASE STUDIES

Case 29.1

Ms PS is a 17-year-old woman who presented to her primary care doctor with a 2-month history of difficulty in getting to sleep. She described herself as feeling generally unhappy. She had lost interest in socializing but was able to perform most of her usual daily routines. She sometimes felt as though she had little energy and was spending more time just watching the television.

Question

What diagnosis is likely to be given to Ms PS and what are the important factors to take into account when advising on treatment?

Answers

On further questioning Ms PS does not reveal any ideas of self-harm. She is in a supportive relationship and although she has some financial concerns, these are not excessive. Ms PS is likely to be diagnosed as having a depressive disorder of mild severity.

Referral to specialist services is not appropriate. The patient should be given advice on sleep hygiene, including the removal of the television from her bedroom. A watching brief should be maintained and the patient asked to attend for a follow-up appointment within 2 weeks.

Antidepressants should not be prescribed. The risk/benefit balance is generally against prescribing antidepressants in people under 18 years of age. There is also little evidence to support the use of antidepressants in patients with mild depression. A more appropriate treatment option to consider would be a structured exercise programme.

Case 29.2

Mr DD is a 50-year-old unemployed man with a long-standing history of bipolar I disorder. He was admitted, as a voluntary patient, to an acute psychiatric ward by his community psychiatric nurse (CPN). The admission followed a short period of increasingly disturbed behaviour. Mr DD's daughter had contacted the CPN when she discovered that her father had just spent over £4000 on scientific instruments from an internet auction site. Over the same period she had noticed that her father had lost interest in his self-care and become elated at the prospect of being on the verge of developing a special formula to solve the fuel crisis.

On the ward Mr DD said he felt 'fine, fine all the time'. He told staff on the ward that he didn't need to be in hospital and it was keeping him away from his top secret mission. He also told ward staff that they could not keep him on the ward and insisted he was within his rights to go home.

Mr DD's speech was sometimes very rapid, and it was sometimes difficult to understand what he was saying. His records showed that on his last admission he had been treated with haloperidol.

Question

What treatment is appropriate for Mr DD?

Answer

Before initiating treatment it is important to rule out any organic or physical causes for Mr DD's presentation. Following a thorough physical and psychiatric examination, it was established that Mr DD had been relatively well since commencing treatment with lithium almost 4 years previously.

It is important that symptoms of mania are brought under control. Haloperidol would be a suitable choice, in view of his previous response. However, a review of Mr DD's medication history revealed that he had experienced several acute dystonic reactions to haloperidol during previous admissions. His daughter also reported that her father had commented on how awful it felt being given haloperidol during his last admission. Mr DD was therefore prescribed olanzapine 15 mg daily.

When Mr DD's manic symptoms are controlled, prophylactic treatment should be discussed with him. This should include a discussion about why he had discontinued lithium several months earlier. The opportunity should be taken to provide written information with the offer of a further discussion that should include his daughter.

Mr DD had stopped lithium as he felt he no longer needed it but after discussion was prepared to restart treatment. Renal, thyroid and cardiac function should be assessed, and if within normal limits, lithium carbonate 400 mg at night may be prescribed.

One week later a 12-hour standard plasma lithium level should be performed and the dose of lithium adjusted to achieve the same lithium levels as before (0.6 mmol/L).

The side effects and signs of impending toxicity from lithium should be explained to Mr DD and if possible his daughter. He should also be reminded of the possibility of interaction with drugs he may obtain from his doctor or pharmacist in the future. The arrangements for future prescribing and monitoring of lithium should be clarified so that Mr DD's care is not compromised by moving across organizational boundaries.

Case 29.3

Mrs FA is a 40-year-old designer. She was admitted to an acute psychiatric unit from the emergency department of the local hospital. She had taken an overdose of 32 co-codamol tablets when her husband told her he was going to leave her. On the ward she told staff she hated her life, and that everything was going wrong. She was angry that she had not been successful in killing herself as there was no point in living. She could see no hope for the future and had no interest in anything, not even eating.

Question

What course of action would you advise?

Answer

Mrs FA has a severe episode of depression. Antidepressant drug treatment should be initiated immediately. In line with the NICE guidelines for the management of depression, one of the SSRIs, e.g. citalopram, should be considered as a suitable choice. Although Mrs FA may be reluctant to take medication, it should be explained that the drug does relieve the symptoms of depression. As soon as practical, the explanation should be followed up by discussing the importance of taking treatment for 4–6 weeks before the full benefit is realized and the likely time course of antidepressant treatment being in the region of 6 months. Mrs FA should also be given the opportunity to discuss any concerns she may have about becoming dependent on the antidepressant as well as a general explanation about possible side effects.

Case 29.4

Mr MA is a 49-year-old unemployed man. He was admitted to a psychiatric unit at the request of the crisis intervention team. Mr MA had been prescribed fluoxetine 20 mg 2 months ago, and after no

apparent response the prescriber in the crisis team had changed this to citalopram 4 weeks earlier. On admission he was noted to be withdrawn, lacking motivation and just gave 'yes' or 'no' in response to questioning. He reported no interests in his life, and it was noted that he had attempted to harm himself in the past.

Two weeks after admission there was no significant improvement in his symptoms.

Question

What treatment options are appropriate for Mr MA?

Answer

Before considering a change in treatment, it should be confirmed that Mr MA has regularly taken his antidepressant medication. Serum levels are not generally available, or particularly helpful. Scrutiny of the medicine charts, discussion with nursing staff, relatives, key workers and the patient will enable a reasonable judgement to be reached. A dose increase could be considered if the patient had shown a limited response. In this case, the patient had received no apparent benefit and a change in treatment was warranted.

An in-depth review of his physical condition and previous medication should be undertaken. This should include discussion with the patient about any previous antidepressant treatment he had found to be particularly effective, or troublesome.

This review revealed that Mr MA had received several different antidepressants over the past 20 years. Three years ago he was treated with venlafaxine S/R 75 mg daily. The medical records confirmed Mr MA's view that this medication had helped him in the past, but on further questioning he stated that he had not taken medication for long after discharge from hospital as he did not want to get 'hooked' on it. The importance of long-term treatment and the proposed treatment plan should be discussed with Mr MA. Particular issues to be addressed include an assessment of cardiac functioning and liaison with the primary care doctor to ensure treatment with venlafaxine would be possible under a shared care arrangement with the specialist. In view of Mr MA's concerns about dependence, particular attention should be given to discussion around this issue.

Based on Mr MA's agreement to the treatment plan, his previous response, the lack of any physical contraindication and the ability to organize regular cardiac monitoring, venlafaxine would be a reasonable treatment option.

Case 29.5

Ms YS is a 28-year-old student with a history of bipolar I disorder. She had recently moved to the area in the hope of continuing her studies. She was admitted to an acute psychiatric unit at the request of her key worker who reported that Ms YS had recently become increasingly elated and her partner was very concerned about the increased credit card bills she was incurring.

Whilst on the ward she attempted to develop sexual relationships with several young male patients.

Question

Describe the treatment options available for Ms YS.

Answer

There is insufficient information to determine whether or not Ms YS was being treated adequately with a prophylactic mood stabilizer. It is important to determine if the current episode was related to inadequate prophylactic treatment.

The current episode of hypomania must be treated. She is currently at risk through her promiscuity and the excessive use of her credit card. Both behaviours are likely to affect her ability to maintain a relationship with her partner.

As Ms YS was taking adequate contraceptive precautions and was adamant that she had no intention or desire to become pregnant, initially treatment with valproate semisodium should be considered. Olanzapine or another antipsychotic could also be considered, but Ms YS did not want to be treated with an antipsychotic. An assessment of liver function, prothrombin rate and full blood count should be performed prior to initiating therapy.

The patient should be informed of the important adverse effects of therapy. In particular, she should be advised to report any unexplained bruising and to avoid the use of salicylates. Treatment should be commenced at 250 mg three times daily and increased in accordance with response and tolerability. Benzodiazepines may also be considered as a short-term adjunct if additional sedation is required.

Following resolution of the acute episode, long-term prophylaxis must be considered. In this case Ms YS had previously been treated with lithium, but had refused to continue as this had caused significant weight gain.

In view of the patient's refusal to consider lithium, prophylactic options include carbamazepine or valproate semisodium (valproate semisodium is not licensed for prophylactic use in the UK). Little hard evidence currently exists to guide the choice. It is important to take the patient's view into account. Even though valproate does not have a UK marketing authorization for prophylaxis in bipolar disorder, on the basis of informed choice, prophylactic treatment with valproate was agreed with Ms YS.

Case 29.6

Ms AB is a 55-year-old unemployed lady with a long-standing history of depression. She has been treated with numerous antidepressants over the years and is currently under the care of the community mental health team.

The only treatment that appears to have had any effect on her depressive episodes has been dosulepin. She has taken several overdoses in the past and her psychiatrist is reluctant to prescribe this drug.

Question

What measures could be taken to enable Ms AB to be treated effectively?

Answer

Ms AB does not have treatment-resistant depression. She has been successfully treated with dosulepin in the past, but impulsively takes an overdose as a way of dealing with difficult circumstances even when she is not depressed.

Non-drug strategies by the mental health team should be directed at enabling Ms AB to find alternative ways of dealing with these difficulties. Despite the obvious risk of fatality, dosulepin could remain as the treatment of choice for Ms AB due to her previous response to this drug and the lack of response to other antidepressants. The drug will be prescribed under the direction of a consultant psychiatrist and so remains in line with the NICE guidelines for the management of depression. Practical measures of controlling the quantities of medication should be introduced such as ensuring she only receives sufficient medication for 2 or 3 days treatment.

Communication between all those involved in the care of Ms AB is crucial. When individualizing the supply of medication in this way, all those involved must be alert to the possibility that the system of supply may break down. In this case an apparently routine prescription for 1 month's supply of medication may have fatal consequences.

REFERENCES

American Psychiatric Association 1994 Diagnostic and statistical manual of mental disorders, 4th edn. American Psychiatric Association, Washington, DC

Anderson I M, Tomenson B M 1995 Treatment discontinuation with selective serotonin re-uptake inhibitors compared with tricyclic antidepressants: a meta-analysis. British Medical Journal 310: 1433-1438

Baldessarini R J, Tondo L 2000 Does lithium treatment still work? Evidence of stable responses over three decades. Archives of General Psychiatry 57: 187-908

Barbui C, Hotopf M, Freemantle N et al 2001 Selective serotonin re-uptake inhibitors versus tricyclic and heterocyclic antidepressants: comparison of drug adherence. Cochrane Review. Cochrane Library, Issue 2. Update Software, Oxford

Buckley N A, McManus P R 2002 Fatal toxicity of serotoninergic and other antidepressant drugs: analysis of United Kingdom mortality data. British Medical Journal 325: 1332-1333

Geddes J R, Freemantle N, Mason J et al 2002 Selective serotonin reuptake inhibitors (SSRIs) for depression. Cochrane Review. Cochrane Library, Issue 1. Update Software, Oxford

Hotopf M, Lewis G, Normand C 1996 Are SSRIs a cost effective alternative to tricyclics? British Journal of Psychiatry 168: 404-409

Linde K, Mulrow C D 2001 St John's wort for depression. Cochrane Review. Cochrane Library, Issue 2. Update Software, Oxford

National Institute for Clinical Excellence 2004 Management of depression in primary and secondary care. Guideline number 23. National Institute for Clinical Excellence, London. Available online at: www.nice.org.uk/pdf/cg023fullguideline.pdf

Song F, Freemantle N, Sheldon T A et al 1993 Selective serotonin re-uptake inhibitors: a meta analysis of efficacy and acceptability. British Medical Journal 306: 683-687

Svensson S, Mansfield P 2004 Escitalopram: superior to citalopram or a chiral chimera? Psychotherapy and Psychosomatics 73: 10-16

World Health Organization 1992 International classification of diseases and related health problems, 10th revision (ICD 10). World Health Organization, Geneva

FURTHER READING

Geddes J R, Burgess S, Hawton K et al 2004 Long-term lithium therapy for bipolar disorder: systematic review and meta-analysis of randomized controlled trials. American Journal of Psychiatry 161: 217-222

Gelder M, Gath D, Mayou R et al (eds) 1996 Oxford textbook of psychiatry, 4th edn. Oxford Medical Publications, Oxford

Goodwin G 2003 Evidence-based guidelines for treating bipolar disorder: recommendations from the British Association for Psychopharmacology. Journal of Psychopharmacology 17: 149-173

Kent J M 2000 SnaRIs, NaSSAs, and NaRIs: new agents for the treatment of depression. Lancet 355: 911-918

Mann J J 2005 The medical management of depression. New England Journal of Medicine 353: 1819-1834

Scottish Intercollegiate Guidelines Network 2005 Bipolar affective disorder. SIGN guideline no. 82. Available online at: www.sign.ac.uk/pdf/sign82.pdf

Walden J, Heinz G (eds) 2004 Bipolar affective disorders: etiology and treatment. Thieme Publishing Group, Stuttgart

30 Schizophrenia

D. Branford

The concept of schizophrenia can be difficult to understand. People who do not suffer from schizophrenia can have little idea of what the experience of hallucinations and delusions is like. The presentation of schizophrenia can be extremely varied, with a great range of possible symptoms. There are also many misconceptions about the condition of schizophrenia that have led to prejudice against sufferers of the illness. People with schizophrenia are commonly thought to have low intelligence and to be dangerous. In fact, only a minority show violent behaviour, with social withdrawal being a more common picture. Up to 10% of people with schizophrenia commit suicide.

Classification

Since the late 19th century there have been frequent attempts to define the illness we now call schizophrenia. Kraepelin, in the late 1890s, coined the term 'dementia praecox' (early madness) to describe an illness where there was a deterioration of the personality at a young age. Kraepelin also coined the terms 'catatonic' (where motor symptoms are prevalent and changes in activity vary), 'hebephrenic' (silly, childish behaviour, affective symptoms and thought disorder prominent), and 'paranoid' (clinical picture dominated by paranoid delusions). A few years later a Swiss psychiatrist called Bleuler introduced the term 'schizophrenia', derived from the Greek words *skhizo* (to split) and *phren* (mind), meaning the split between the emotions and the intellect.

Two systems for the classification of schizophrenia are widely used: the *Diagnostic and Statistical Manual of Mental Disorders*, 4th edition (DSM IV; American Psychiatric Association 1994) and the *International Classification of Diseases*, 10th edition (ICD 10; WHO 1992).

Symptoms and diagnosis

Acute psychotic illness

To establish a definite diagnosis of schizophrenia it is important to follow the diagnostic criteria in either DSM IV or ICD 10, but symptoms which commonly occur in the acute phase of a psychotic illness include the following:

- awkward social behaviour, appearing preoccupied, perplexed and withdrawn, or showing unexpected changes in behaviour
- initial vagueness in speech which can progress to disorders of the stream of thought or poverty of thought
- abnormality of mood such as anxiety, depression, irritability or euphoria
- auditory hallucinations, the most common of which are referred to as 'voices'; such voices can give commands to patients or may discuss the person in the third person, or comment on their actions
- delusions, of which those relating to control of thoughts are the most diagnostic; for example, patients feel that thoughts are being inserted into or withdrawn from their mind
- lack of insight into the illness.

These symptoms are commonly called positive symptoms.

Factors affecting diagnosis and prognosis

There is a reluctance to classify people as suffering schizophrenia on the basis of one acute psychotic illness, but there are a number of features which lead one to predict whether an acute illness will become chronic. These features include:

- age of onset, which, typically for schizophrenia, is late teenage to age 30 years

- reports of a childhood which indicate not mixing or a rather shy and withdrawn personality
- a poor work record
- a desire for social isolation
- being single and not seeming to have sexual relationships
- a gradual onset of the illness and deterioration from previous level of functioning
- grossly disorganized behaviour.

Treatment

There is a wide range of antipsychotic drugs available for the treatment of a psychotic illness. Although most antipsychotic drugs are equally effective in the treatment of psychotic symptoms, some individuals respond better to one drug than another.

There is controversy over how long people should remain on an antipsychotic drug following their first acute illness. Some would argue that, if the prognosis is poor, long-term therapy should be advocated. Others would want to see a second illness before advocating long-term therapy.

Chronic schizophrenia

Between 60% and 80% of patients who suffer from an acute psychotic illness will suffer further illness and become chronically affected. For these patients the diagnosis of schizophrenia can be applied.

As schizophrenia progresses, there may be periods of relapse with acute symptoms but the underlying trend is towards symptoms of lack of drive, social withdrawal and emotional apathy. Such symptoms are sometimes called negative symptoms and respond poorly to most antipsychotic drugs.

Causes of schizophrenia

Although the cause of schizophrenia remains unknown, there are many theories and models.

Vulnerability model

The vulnerability model postulates that the persistent characteristic of schizophrenia is not the schizophrenic episode itself but the vulnerability to the development of such episodes of the disorder. The episodes of the illness are time limited but the vulnerability remains, awaiting the trigger of some stress. Such vulnerability can depend on premorbid personality, social network or the environment. Manipulation and avoidance of such stress can abort a potential schizophrenic episode.

Developmental model

The developmental model postulates that there are critical periods in the development of neuronal cells which, if adversely affected, may result in schizophrenia. Two such critical periods are postulated to occur when migrant neural cells do not reach their goal in fetal development and when supernumerary neural cells slough off at adolescence. This model is supported by neuroimaging studies which show structural brain abnormalities in patients with schizophrenia.

Ecological model

The ecological model postulates that external factors involving social, cultural and physical forces in the environment, such as population density, individual space, socio-economic status and racial status, influence the development of the disorder. The evidence in support of such a model remains weak.

Genetic model

There is undoubtably a genetic component to schizophrenia, with a higher incidence in the siblings of schizophrenics. However, even in monozygotic twins there are many cases where only one sibling has developed schizophrenia.

Transmitter abnormality model

The suggestion that schizophrenia is caused primarily by an abnormality of dopamine receptors and, in particular, D_2 receptors, has largely emerged from research into the effect of antipsychotic drugs. Such a theory is increasingly being questioned.

Other factors involved in schizophrenia

Numerous other factors have been implicated in the development and cause of schizophrenia. These include migration, socio-economic factors, perinatal insult, infections, season of birth, viruses, toxins and family environment.

In reality, all of these factors may influence both the development and progression of schizophrenia. Social, familial and biological factors may lead to premorbid vulnerability and subsequently influence both the acute psychosis and the progression to chronic states. What is then likely is that the illness will feed back to influence social, familial and biological factors, thus leading to future vulnerability.

Drug treatment in schizophrenia
Mode of action of antipsychotic drugs

Although the cause of schizophrenia is the subject of controversy, an understanding of the mode of action of antipsychotic drugs has led to the dopamine theory of schizophrenia. This theory postulates that the symptoms experienced in schizophrenia are caused by an alteration to the level of dopamine activity in the brain. It is based on knowledge that dopamine receptor antagonists are often effective antipsychotics while drugs which increase dopamine activity, such as amfetamine, can either induce psychosis or exacerbate a schizophrenic illness.

At least six dopamine receptors exist in the brain, with much activity being focused on the D_2 receptor as being responsible for antipsychotic drug action. However, drugs such as pimozide, that claim to have a more specific effect on D_2 receptors, do not appear superior in antipsychotic effect when compared to other agents.

Research into the mode of action of clozapine has caused a change of attention to the mesolimbic system in the brain and to different receptors. Clozapine does not chronically alter striatal D_2 receptors but does appear to affect striatal D_1 receptors. It also appears to have more effect on the limbic system and on serotonin ($5HT_2$) receptors, which may explain its reduced risk of extrapyramidal symptoms. The term 'atypical' is used to categorize those antipsychotic drugs that, like clozapine, rarely produce extrapyramidal side effects.

Although the reason for the superiority of clozapine in schizophrenia treatment remains an enigma, a variety of theories have led to the development of a new family of antipsychotic drugs. Some mimic the impact of clozapine on a wide range of dopamine and serotonin receptors, e.g. olanzapine, others mimic the impact on particular receptors, e.g. $5HT_2/D_2$ receptor antagonists such as risperidone, others focus on limited occupancy of D_2 receptors, e.g. quetiapine, while others focus on alternative theories such as partial agonism (aripiprazole).

Rationale and mode of use of drugs

Although a variety of social and psychological therapies are helpful in the treatment of schizophrenia, drugs form the essential cornerstone. The aim of all therapies is to minimize the level of handicap and achieve the best level of mental functioning. Drugs do not cure schizophrenia and are only partially effective at eradicating some symptoms such as delusions and negative symptoms. At the same time, benefits have to be balanced against side effects and whether the need to suppress particular symptoms is important. For example, if the person has a delusion that he or she is responsible for famine in Africa, but this does not in any way influence that person's behaviour or mood, a common view would be that there would be little point in increasing antipsychotic drug therapy. However, others would argue that this 'untreated' delusion would make the person stand out or subject to social stigma and the delusion should be more aggressively treated. If, on the other hand, this delusion led to great distress, or violent or dangerous behaviour, then an increase in antipsychotic drugs would usually be indicated.

It is now accepted that antipsychotic drugs can control or modify symptoms such as hallucinations and delusions that are evident in the acute episode of illness. Except for clozapine and the other atypicals, there is little evidence for antipsychotic drugs being of value in the treatment of the negative symptoms, although the matter remains controversial. Antipsychotic drugs increase the length of time between breakdowns and shorten the length of the acute episode in most patients.

Drug selection and dose

Concerns about the side effect profile and toxicity of typical antipsychotic drugs led to calls for the 'atypicals' to be prescribed more widely. This approach was supported in national guidance (NICE 2002) which advocated that atypical antipsychotic drugs should be used for the treatment of a first illness. However, increasing concern about the side effects of the atypical antipsychotic drugs, such as weight gain, diabetes and sexual dysfunction, has led many clinicians to question the benefits of the newer and more expensive atypical antipsychotics.

Other factors that have influenced drug selection or dose are:

- withdrawal of some antipsychotic drugs from routine clinical practice and changes to the product licences of others because of concerns about cardiac toxicity
- guidelines warning about the use of high doses of antipsychotic drugs (Thompson 1994)
- introduction of intramuscular olanzapine for emergency tranquillization as an alternative to the short-term use of benzodiazepines such as lorazepam and diazepam
- introduction of rapid-release formulations, e.g. velotabs, quicktabs, etc., as alternatives to syrup formulations
- introduction of a long-acting injection formulation of risperidone
- changes to dose ranges advocated by some pharmaceutical companies, e.g. haloperidol maximum dose was reduced from 120 mg to 30 mg daily.

Another factor that has influenced prescribing practice in schizophrenia in recent years has been agreement over the role of clozapine in treatment-resistant schizophrenia.

Despite all these changes, many of the issues relevant to drug selection and dose have remained similar for the last 40 years and these include the following.

Side effects
- For older, typical antipsychotic drugs, side effects such as hypotension, extrapyramidal symptoms and anticholinergic effects are key factors in the choice of drug.
- For the newer atypical drugs, side effects such as diabetes, sexual dysfunction and weight gain affect adherence in many patients.
- Sedation remains a factor for all antipsychotic drugs.

Individual response Selection should not be based on chemical group alone since individual response to a particular drug or dose may be more important.

Polypharmacy Polypharmacy remains a matter of concern. Reasons why it occurs include:

- poor response to standard drug treatment
- unrealistic expectations about the speed of action and the extent of treatment control
- prescribers feeling inhibited about exceeding the licensed dose and resorting to prescribing two or more antipsychotic drugs to achieve control, particularly in the acute situation. Increasingly, though, prescribers are being encouraged to use clozapine at an earlier stage for patients who do not fully respond to treatment
- once control has been achieved there may be reluctance to reduce doses or the number of drugs for fear of the re-emergence of symptoms
- confusion arising between the perceived need in the ward situation for sedation and the antipsychotic effects. The sedating side effects of antipsychotic drugs may be evident within hours; they are rapid in onset but may begin to wear off after 2–3 weeks. The antipsychotic effects on thought disorder, hallucinations and delusions may take some weeks to appear, although if there has been no response within 2–3 weeks a change of antipsychotic or change of dose may be indicated.

Table 30.1 Neuroleptics/antipsychotics and their commonly associated attributes and problems

Drug group	Drug	Comments
Butyrophenones	Haloperidol	Extrapyramidal side effects of parkinsonian rigidity, dystonia, akathisia Tardive dyskinesia with long-term use Drug most associated with neuroleptic malignant syndrome Sedation common Hormonal effects common
	Benperidol	As haloperidol Claimed to reduce sexual drive
Phenothiazines Piperidines	Thioridazine	Marked anticholinergic side effects of dry mouth, blurred vision and constipation High incidence of QT abnormalities on ECG has resulted in limitations to licence Postural hypotension and falls in the elderly Low incidence of extrapyramidal side effects
	Pericyazine	Side effects similar to thioridazine
Aliphatic	Pipotiazine	As thioridazine but only available as depot formulation
	Chlorpromazine	As haloperidol but in addition postural hypotension, low body temperature, rashes and photosensitivity Increased sedative effects
	Promazine	As chlorpromazine but low potency Considered by some to have weak antipsychotic effect
	Levomepromazine (methotrimeprazine)	Very sedative and postural hypotension common Mostly used in terminal illness
Piperazine	Trifluoperazine	As chlorpromazine but greater incidence of extrapyramidal side effects and lower incidence of anticholinergic effects Some antiemetic properties
	Fluphenazine	As trifluoperazine but also available as depot formulation
	Perphenazine	As trifluoperazine
Thioxanthines	Flupentixol	Similar to fluphenazine but also available as depot formulation
	Zuclopenthixol	Similar to chlorpromazine but also available as depot formulation
Diphenylbutylpiperidines	Pimozide	As haloperidol but concerns about cardiac effects at high dose limits use
Benzamides	Sulpiride	Lower incidence of extrapyramidal effects Few anticholinergic effects Useful adjunct to clozapine in refractory illness
	Amisulpride	As sulpiride
Dibenoxazepine tricyclics	Loxapine	High incidence of extrapyramidal side effects Few anticholinergic effects
	Clozapine	Drug of choice for treatment resistant schizophrenia Low incidence of extrapyramidal side effects or tardive dyskinesia Neutropenia in 1–2% of cases Enhanced efficacy against both positive and negative symptoms Sedation, dribbling, drooling, weight gain, diabetes
Thienobenzodiazepines	Olanzapine	Sedation, weight gain and diabetes Low incidence of extrapyramidal side effects and low impact on prolactin
	Quetiapine	Low incidence of extrapyramidal side effects and low impact on prolactin
	Zotepine	Similar to olanzapine but higher rate of prolactin elevation and higher rate of drug-induced seizures
Serotonin–dopamine antagonists	Risperidone	Extrapyramidal side effects at higher doses. High rate of prolactin elevation
	Ziprasidone	As risperidone
Partial dopamine agonist	Aripiprazole	Low level of side effects but light-headedness and blurred vision common

High doses The consensus is that very high doses of antipsychotic drugs are not beneficial in improving either the speed or the overall level of response in acute psychosis.

The antipsychotic drugs in use are listed in Table 30.1, along with some of their common adverse effects.

Neuroleptic equivalence

Although antipsychotic drugs vary in potency, studies on relative dopamine receptor binding have led to the concept of chlorpromazine equivalents as a useful method of transferring dosage from one product to another. Concern has been expressed about the variation between sources for such values, in particular about the quoted chlorpromazine equivalents of the butyrophenones and the conversion of depot doses to oral (Table 30.2). Likewise, there is no agreement on the equivalent doses of the atypicals.

For research purposes the concept of proportion of the maximum dose in the British National Formulary has been developed as a standardized method for calculating average doses used in practice. However, this may not be a useful way of determining dose when transferring a patient from one antipsychotic to another.

Clozapine and refractory illness

Clozapine was developed as an antipsychotic drug during the 1960s. Unfortunately, it is associated with a 1–2% incidence of neutropenia and this initially resulted in the withdrawal of the drug from clinical practice. However, it was noted even at the early stage to be free of extrapyramidal side affects associated with other antipsychotic drugs. In the 1980s clozapine was demonstrated to have a greater efficacy than other antipsychotics and was reintroduced into clinical practice but with routine monitoring of blood mandatory.

Clozapine is now established as the drug of choice in treatment-resistant schizophrenia but it is not without problems. In addition to neutropenia, it is associated with a greater risk of seizures, particularly if doses are above 600 mg daily. Some guidelines recommend the co-prescribing of sodium valproate at such doses. Also it is associated with excessive drooling, hypotension and sedation during the early stages of treatment, requiring slow dose increases initially.

Augmentation strategies and polytherapy

Schizophrenia is a complex illness with a very varied presentation. In addition to the core symptoms, elements of other mental illnesses such as mania, depression and anxiety may predominate. Controversy remains about whether these associated symptoms should be treated separately or as a part of schizophrenia. In addition, there is debate about whether these presentations represent an alternative diagnosis, e.g. schizoaffective disorder when the mood disorder is a primary component of the presentation.

The current fashion is for these components of the illness to be treated separately, with much resulting polytherapy with SSRI antidepressants and antiepileptic drugs for mood control.

In addition to the above, complex prescriptions can arise when treatment with clozapine is perceived to be inadequate or doses are limited due to side effects. The theory behind the addition of a further drug can be either that the plasma concentration of the clozapine is enhanced or that the profile of the second drug boosts a particular receptor blocking role which may be necessary in that patient. The augmentation strategy with the best evidence to support its use is the addition of sulpiride or amisulpride to clozapine. Other strategies include the addition of risperidone, lamotrigine or ω3 fatty acids.

Prescribing guidelines

UK guidance on the use of atypical antipsychotic drugs has been published (NICE 2002) and includes the following recommendations.

- Atypical antipsychotic drugs should be considered for first-line choice for first illness patients.
- Atypical antipsychotic drugs should be considered for patients showing or reporting unacceptable adverse effects from typical antipsychotic drugs.
- Patients unresponsive to two separate treatments with antipsychotic drugs, one an atypical, should be given clozapine.
- Where more than one atypical antipsychotic drug may be suitable, the one with the lowest purchase cost should be considered.
- Depot antipsychotic medication should be considered when there are grounds to suspect the patient is unlikely to take oral drugs.
- Typical and atypical antipsychotic drugs should not be prescribed together except during changeover of medicines.

Clinical guidelines that cover psychological treatments, treatment with medicines and how best to organize mental health services to help people with schizophrenia are also available (NICE 2003).

Table 30.2 Equivalence of typical antipsychotic drugs to 100 mg chlorpromazine (from Foster 1989)

Drug	Usual dose (mg) equivalent of to 100 mg chlorpromazine	Variations in quoted dosage (mg) equivalent to 100 mg of chlorpromazine
Oral antipsychotics		
Promazine	200	100–250
Thioridazine	100	50–120
Trifluoperazine	5	3.5–7.5
Haloperidol	2	1.5–5
Sulpiride	200	–
Depot antipsychotics administered every 2 weeks (all administered as the decanoate)		
Zuclopenthixol	200	80–200
Flupentixol	40	16–40
Fluphenazine	25	10–25
Haloperidol	20	–

Long-acting formulations of antipsychotic drugs

Most long-acting (depot) formulations are synthesized by esterification of the hydroxyl group of the antipsychotic drug to a long chain fatty acid such as decanoic acid. The esters which are more lipophilic and soluble are dissolved in an oily vehicle such as sesame oil or a vegetable oil (viscoleo). Once the drug is injected into muscle, it is slowly released from the oil vehicle. Active drug becomes available following hydrolysis for distribution to the site of the action.

Although the ideal long-acting antipsychotic formulation should release the drug at a constant rate so that plasma level variations are kept to a minimum, all the available products produce significant variations (Table 30.3). This can result in increased side effects at the time of peak plasma concentrations, usually after 5–7 days, for oil-based depots and increased patient irritability towards the end of the period, as plasma concentrations decline. For many patients, though, oil-based long-acting formulations result in a very slow decline in drug availability after a period of chronic administration. When transferring a patient from depot formulations to oral administration, it may be many months before the effect of the depot finally wears off.

The long-acting risperidone injection involves a novel microsphere formulation new to clinical practice. The microsperes delay the release of risperidone for 3 weeks during which time oral supplementation is necessary. Once release has commenced, the risperidone reaches a maximum concentration 4–5 weeks after the injection with a decline over the subsequent 2–3 weeks. This more rapid decline has an advantage that by 2 months after the last injection, little of the risperidone will remain.

In addition to the principles of drug choice and dosage selection that apply to oral drugs, with depot therapy there is also a need to consider the future habitation of the patient. If the patient is to live an independent lifestyle, depot formulations are indicated, but if the person is to remain in staffed accommodation and receive other medicines via routine administration by nurses, the use of depot formulations may not be logical.

Advantages and disadvantages of long-acting formulations Non-compliance with oral medicines is a major problem in patients with any long-term illness and the administration of depot formulations guarantees drug delivery. It has been argued that, although depot injections are expensive, they have economic advantages because they reduce hospital admissions, improve drug bioavailability by avoiding the deactivating processes which occur in the gut and liver, and result in more consistent plasma levels of drug.

Depot formulations have the disadvantages of reduced flexibility of dosage, the painful nature of administration and, for the older depots, a high incidence of extrapyramidal side effects.

Anticholinergic drugs

Anticholinergic drugs are prescribed to counter the extrapyramidal side effects of typical antipsychotics, and at one time were routinely prescribed. It is generally accepted that, with the possible exception of the first few weeks of treatment with antipsychotic drugs known to have a high incidence of extrapyramidal side effects, anticholinergic drugs should only be prescribed when a need has been shown. A number of studies have looked at the discontinuation of anticholinergic agents and reported re-emergence of the symptoms. One such study reported that up to 62% of patients were affected. Between 25% and 30% of patients will have a continuing need for anticholinergic drugs.

The anticholinergic drugs are not without problems, having their own range of side effects, including dry mouth, constipation and blurred vision. Trihexyphenidyl, in particular, is renowned for its euphoric effects and withdrawal problems can include cholinergic rebound.

One of the benefits of the atypical antipsychotic drugs is the reduced need for co-prescription of anticholinergic drugs. However, extrapyramidal side effects can still occur with atypical antipsychotic drugs, particularly at high dose.

Interactions and antipsychotic drugs

There are claimed to be many interactions involving antipsychotic drugs but few appear to be clinically significant. Propranolol increases the plasma concentration of chlorpromazine, and carbamazepine accelerates the metabolism of haloperidol, risperidone and olanzapine. When tricyclic antidepressants are administered with phenothiazines, increased antimuscarinic effects such as dry mouth and blurred vision can occur and most antipsychotic drugs increase the sedative effect of alcohol. The SSRI antidepressants fluvoxamine, fluoxetine and paroxetine interact with clozapine, resulting in increases in clozapine plasma concentration.

Table 30.3 Comparison of depot antipsychotics

Drug	Ester	Vehicle	Time to peak (days) from single dose	Half-life (days)
Haloperidol	Decanoate	Sesame oil	3–9	21
Flupentixol	Decanoate	Viscoleo oil	7	17
Zuclopenthixol	Decanoate	Viscoleo oil	4–7	19
Fluphenazine	Decanoate	Sesame oil	0.3–1.5	6–9
Pipotiazine	Palmitate	Sesame oil	10–15	15
Risperidone		Microspheres	32	8–9

Adverse effects and antipsychotic drugs

There are a large number of adverse effects associated with antipsychotic drugs. Some of these effects, such as sedation, antilibido effect and weight gain, may be considered to be of value with particular patients, but the susceptibility to such adverse effects is often a major factor in determining drug choice. Prescribing guidelines (Bazire 2005, Taylor et al 2005) provide tables that show the relative likelihood of the side effects occurring with the various antipsychotic drugs. The major side effects include the following.

Sedation   Although sedation is most associated with chlorpromazine and clozapine, it is primarily related to dosage with other antipsychotics. Products claiming to be less sedating can often only substantiate such claims for low doses.

Weight gain and diabetes   Weight gain was a common feature of the first phenothiazine antipsychotics. It was originally thought that this side effect was caused by a direct effect on metabolism. This side effect has also become a feature of some of the newer atypical antipsychotic drugs, particularly olanzapine and clozapine. This re-emergence of an old side effect with the new drugs has rekindled interest in the cause, which is now thought to be more associated with loss of control of food intake, rather than a direct effect on food metabolism. In addition to weight gain, these two atypical antipsychotic drugs have also been associated with increased incidence of diabetes. Controversy remains about whether there is a link between the weight gain and onset of diabetes, and whether the development of diabetes is more associated with the illness of schizophrenia than the drugs. Whatever the link, the controversy has led to the acceptance that people with schizophrenia often suffer poor physical health in addition to poor mental health and require regular monitoring of physical health risk factors.

QT prolongation and cardiac risk   Some antipsychotic drugs are associated with changes to the QT interval measured on the ECG and, if given in high doses, may increase the risk of sudden cardiac death. Although overall the risk is low, monitoring the ECG has become a part of normal practice, especially if high doses are used.

Anticholinergic side effects   Side effects such as dry mouth, constipation and blurred vision are particularly associated with piperidine phenothiazines.

Extrapyramidal side effects   Side effects such as akathisia, dystonia and parkinsonian effects are associated with typical antipsychotic drugs and occur frequently, particularly with depot antipsychotics, piperazine phenothiazines such as trifluoperazine and fluphenazine and butyrophenones such as haloperidol. These side effects are reversible by using anticholinergic drugs or by dosage reduction. The common extrapyramidal effects include the following.

- *Akathisia* or motor restlessness. This causes patients to pace up and down, constantly shift their leg position or tap their feet.
- *Dystonia* is the result of sustained muscle contraction. It can present as grimacing and facial distortion, neck twisting and laboured breathing. Occasionally the patient may have an oculogyric crisis in which, after a few moments of fixed staring, the eyeballs move upwards and then

sideways, remaining in that position. In addition to these eye movements, the mouth is usually wide open, the tongue protruding and the head tilting backwards.
- *Parkinson-like side effects* usually present as tremor, rigidity and poverty of facial expression. Drooling and excessive salivation are also common. A shuffling gait may be seen and the patient may show signs of fatigue when performing repetitive motor activities.

Hormonal effects and sexual dysfunction   These side effects are primarily influenced by the effect on prolactin. This may result in galactorrhoea, missed menstrual periods and loss of libido. Some studies have suggested very high levels of sexual dysfunction with some antipsychotic drugs such as typical antipsychotic drugs and the atypical antipsychotics risperidone and amisulpride. However, in many of these studies the background level of such dysfunction is unclear.

Postural hypotension and photosensitivity   These are particularly associated with the aliphatic phenothiazines such as chlorpromazine.

Tardive dyskinesia   Classically the syndrome of tardive dyskinesia affects the tongue, facial and neck muscles but will often also affect the extremities. It is usual to find abnormalities of posture and movements of the fingers in addition to the oral-lingual-masticatory movements.

Epidemiological studies support the association between the prescribing of typical antipsychotic drugs and the development of tardive dyskinesia. Other factors which also appear to be associated include the duration of exposure to antipsychotic drugs, the co-prescribing of anticholinergic drugs, the co-prescribing of lithium, advanced age, prior experience of acute extrapyramidal symptoms and brain damage. Many other factors have been postulated to be associated with tardive dyskinesia such as depot formulations of antipsychotic drugs, dosage of antipsychotic drug, and antipsychotic drugs with high anticholinergic activity, but such associations remain unproven.

Although the mechanism by which tardive dyskinesia arises is unclear, the leading hypothesis is that after prolonged blockade of dopamine receptors, a paradoxical increase in the functional activity of dopamine in the basal ganglia occurs. This altered functional state is thought to come about through a phenomenon of disuse supersensitivity of dopamine receptors. The primary clinical evidence to support such a theory is that tardive dyskinesia is late in onset after prolonged exposure to antipsychotic drugs, has a tendency to worsen upon abrupt discontinuation of the antipsychotic drug and that, in terms of response to drugs, it presents as the opposite of Parkinson's disease, a disease postulated to be caused by a deficiency of dopamine in the caudate nucleus of the brain.

The attempts to treat tardive dyskinesia have been many and varied, but they include dopamine-depleting agents such as reserpine and tetrabenazine, dopamine-blocking agents such as antipsychotic drugs, interference with catecholamine synthesis such as methyldopa, cholinergic agents such as choline and lecithin, GABA mimetic agents such as sodium valproate and baclofen, and the provision of drug holidays. Such strategies are rarely successful. Most strategies currently involve a gradual withdrawal of the typical antipsychotic drug and replacement with an atypical antipsychotic drug.

Neuroleptic malignant syndrome The neuroleptic malignant syndrome (NMS) is a rare but serious complication of antipsychotic drug treatment. The primary symptoms are rigidity, fever, diaphoresis, confusion and fluctuating consciousness. Confirmation can be sought through detection of elevated creatinine kinase. The onset is particularly associated with high-potency typical drugs such as haloperidol, recent and rapid changes to dose and abrupt withdrawal of anticholinergic drugs. Treatment usually requires admission to a medical ward and withdrawal of all antipsychotic drugs.

CASE STUDIES

Case 30.1

Lee is a 20-year-old man. His childhood was disrupted by constant changes to family membership. From an early age his behaviour was difficult but despite such changes, by the age of 16 he was achieving well at school. Aged 17, he became involved with the illicit drug culture and increasingly lost interest in his studies. His parents became concerned as he appeared to undergo a change of personality, communicating with them very little. He eventually dropped out of school and took various short-term jobs. He was unable to sustain any long-term employment. He moved into a flat and seemed to live a twilight existence involving illicit drugs and all-night raves. Police were called to his flat following a violent disturbance. They found Lee living in squalor. He was surrounded by pieces of paper containing incomprehensible messages and was incoherent. He sat with a fixed stare, appearing quite inaccessible. He kept laughing and responding to imaginary people. He was very resistant to hospital admission, and had to be admitted under a section of the Mental Health Act 1983. On the ward he has remained quiet but appears to be in conversation with people who are not there.

Questions

1. Outline the drug(s) of choice for Lee and the rationale for selection.
2. What factors would influence the likely prognosis?
3. Outline the drug(s) of choice if there is the need for rapid tranquillization.

Answers

1. The first need is to ascertain whether the patient's behaviour results from abuse of illicit substances or the onset of a schizophrenic illness. If the former, he would be expected to recover within a few days with little or no drug treatment. If, however, this is the first presentation of a schizophrenic illness, the symptoms are likely to persist and it would be appropriate to prescribe an antipsychotic drug. The choice of antipsychotic drug for first-illness psychosis may partly depend on the formulation acceptable to the situation but would usually be an atypical antipsychotic drug. If oral medicines were refused the intramuscular formulation of olanzapine may be the drug of choice. If there were concerns that he may not swallow the drug, both olanzapine and risperidone are formulated as orodispersible formulations.
2. A number of factors in Lee's history indicate a poor prognosis:

   • there has been a deterioration in function
   • his age, which is typical for a first breakdown
   • his poor work record
   • grossly disorganized behaviour
   • a number of positive symptoms such as hallucinations.

3. If Lee's symptoms became such that there was a need for rapid tranquillization a decision would have to be made about whether to use antipsychotic drugs or benzodiazepines. In the past, sedative antipsychotic drugs such as chlorpromazine, haloperidol or zuclopenthixol were favoured, but increasing concern about sudden death has led to a move to use benzodiazepines such as lorazepam or diazepam. However, the introduction of intramuscular olanzapine has resulted in some swing back to using antipsychotic drugs for rapid tranquillization.

Case 30.2

Gordon has relapsed for the third time this year, the pattern for the last two relapses being the same. His positive symptoms responded rapidly on both previous occassions. On the first he suffered severe extrapyramidal side effects with 30 mg daily of haloperidol and was subsequently stabilized and discharged on sulpiride 400 mg twice daily and procyclidine 5 mg twice daily. He almost immediately stopped taking the sulpiride, claiming not to be ill. During his second relapse he was successfully treated with risperidone 4 mg daily but again stopped the medicine.

Questions

1. Was Gordon's drug treatment appropriate?
2. What strategies could be adopted to maintain Gordon in treatment?

Answers

1. Gordon's initial treatment was not according to current guidelines. The initial treatment with a large dose of haloperidol in a drug-naive patient would now be regarded as excessive. The initial choice of a low-dose typical antipsychotic followed by a second choice of an atypical after the patient suffered extrapyramidal side effects was common practice prior to the publication of national guidance (NICE 2002). Since then an atypical antipsychotic would be regarded as the drug of choice for first illness.
2. Gordon has no insight into his illness or the need for continuing treatment. This could be for a number of reasons:

   • it is part of the illness, and his failure to gain insight is symptomatic of incomplete recovery
   • he lacks a supportive environment to ensure that he takes medicines
   • he is suffering from side effects that deter him from taking the medicines.

   In most cases the use of a depot antipsychotic injection would be the easiest way to ensure compliance, although if Gordon is determined to avoid drug treatment this strategy is unlikely to be successful. In his case the history of good response to oral risperidone and severe extrapyramidal side effects with a typical antipsychotic drug would indicate that the long-acting intramuscular formulation of risperidone may be a good choice.

Case 30.3

Sharon, aged 25, has a 3-year history of schizophrenia with many admissions to hospital. Throughout the period of her illness she has received a range of different oral antipsychotic drugs including chlorpromazine, haloperidol, sulpiride, risperidone and olanzapine, as well as the depot formulations of haloperidol and zuclopenthixol. For most of this time she has had a fixed belief that she is involved with a range of mythical beasts that sexually assault her. When she is ill these beings torment her. She currently receives zuclopenthixol decanoate 500 mg by intramuscular injection every week, olanzapine

10 mg at night, carbamazepine 200 mg three times daily, haloperidol 10 mg four times daily, and procyclidine 10 mg three times daily. She has remained on the ward for the last 4 months with no sign of improvement. She has greatly increased in weight, now approaching 20 stone. The team wish to consider clozapine for Sharon.

Questions

1. Comment on the current drug therapy Sharon is receiving.
2. What action is required before Sharon can receive clozapine?

Answers

1. Although it is not uncommon for polypharmacy to occur when there has been poor response, the practice is frowned upon. Additional medicines are often added in a crisis or in the hope of achieving a greater degree of response. As in this case, the strategy is often unsuccessful. The particular issues of note with this patient's drug regimen are:

- the combination of a typical and an atypical antipsychotic drug reduces the potential benefit of using a drug with a low incidence of extrapyramidal side effects because the patient still suffers extrapyramidal side effects, requires procyclidine, and is at risk of developing tardive dyskinesia
- the very large total dose she is receiving from the combination of antipsychotic drugs

- the dose of anticholinergic drug (procyclidine) is high and likely to result in its own side effects
- the need for such frequent dosing of the intramuscular depot might not be necessary; administration at 2-week intervals would normally be appropriate
- there is little evidence to support the value of carbamazepine, either for schizophrenia or as an adjunctive treatment
- she is suffering severe weight gain
- the interaction between carbamazepine and the antipsychotic drugs may be reducing their potential efficacy.

2. The preparation for treatment with clozapine involves a number of steps. These include:

- registration with the clozapine monitoring scheme
- background blood tests to ensure that the patient is not already suffering from neutropenia or another blood disorder
- stopping the depot antipsychotic drug; this would usually occur some weeks before starting clozapine
- stopping carbamazepine as this interacts with clozapine
- slowly reducing haloperidol
- gradually stopping procyclidine.

Ideally one would want to have removed all other treatments and prescribe clozapine alone but sometimes the final step of withdrawing other medicines may occur during the initiation phase with clozapine.

REFERENCES

American Psychiatric Association 1994 Diagnostic and statistical manual of mental disorders, 4th edn. American Psychiatric Association, Washington, DC

Bazire S 2005 Psychotropic drug directory: the professionals' pocket handbook and aide memoire. Fivepin Ltd, Salisbury

Foster P 1989 Neuroleptic equivalence. Pharmaceutical Journal 243: 431-432

Jann M W, Ereshefsky L, Saklad S R 1985 Clinical pharmacokinetics of the depot antipsychotics. Clinical Pharmacokinetics 10(4): 315-333

National Institute for Clinical Excellence 2002 Guidance on the use of newer (atypical) antipsychotic drugs for the treatment of schizophrenia. Technology Appraisal Guideline 43. National Institute for Clinical Excellence, London. Available online at: www.nice.org.uk/page.aspx?o=TA043guidance

National Institute for Clinical Excellence 2003 Schizophrenia. Full national clinical guideline on core interventions in primary and secondary care. Gaskell and the British Psychological Society, London. Available online at: www.nice.org.uk/page.aspx?o=289559

Taylor D M, Kerwin R, Paton C 2005 The Maudsley 2005–2006 prescribing guidelines, 8th edn. Taylor and Francis, Abingdon

Thompson C 1994 The use of high dose antipsychotic medication. British Journal of Psychiatry 164: 448-458

World Health Organization 1992 International classification of diseases and related health problems, 10th revision (ICD 10). World Health Organization, Geneva

FURTHER READING

American Associations of Diabetes, Psychiatry, and Clinical Endocrinologists for the study of obesity 2004 Consensus development conference on antipsychotic drugs and obesity and diabetes. Journal of Clinical Psychiatry 65: 267-272

Csernansky J G, Mahmoud R, Brenner R et al 2002 A comparison of risperidone and haloperidol for the prevention of relapse in patients with schizophrenia. New England Journal of Medicine 346: 16-22

Drugs and Therapeutics Bulletin 2004 Which atypical drug for schizophrenia? Drugs and Therapeutics Bulletin 42: 57-60

Gao K, Gajwani P, Elhaj O, Calabrese J R 2005 Typical and atypical antipsychotics in bipolar depression. Journal of Clinical Psychiatry 66:1376-1385

Hunter R H, Joy C B, Kennedy E et al 2003 Risperidone versus typical antipsychotic medication for schizophrenia. Cochrane Review. Cochrane Library, Issue 2. Update Software, Oxford

Johnstone E C, Humphreys M S, Lang F H et al (eds) 1999 Schizophrenia: concepts and clinical management. Cambridge University Press, Cambridge

Kerr S 2003 Clinical aspects of schizophrenia. John Wiley, Chichester

Lieberman J A, Stroup T S, Perkins D O 2006 The American Psychiatric Publishing textbook of schizophrenia. American Psychiatric Publishing Inc., Arlington, VA

Rummel C, Hamaan J, Kissling W et al 2003 New generation antipsychotics for first episode schizophrenia. Cochrane Review. Cochrane Library, Issue 4. Update Software, Oxford

Wieck A, Haddad P M 2003 Antipsychotic-induced hyperprolactinaemia in women: pathology, severity and consequences. British Journal of Psychiatry 182: 199-204

Epilepsy 31

S. Dhillon   J. W. Sander

An epileptic seizure is a transient paroxysm of uncontrolled discharges of neurones causing an event that is discernible by the person experiencing the seizure and/or by an observer. The tendency to have recurrent attacks is known as epilepsy; by definition, a single attack does not constitute epilepsy. Epileptic seizures or attacks are a symptom of many different diseases, and the term epilepsy is loosely applied to a number of conditions that have in common a tendency to have recurrent epileptic attacks. A patient with epilepsy will show recurrent epileptic seizures that occur unexpectedly and stop spontaneously.

Epidemiology

There are problems in establishing precise epidemiological statistics for a heterogeneous condition such as epilepsy. Unlike most ailments, epilepsy is episodic; between seizures, patients may be perfectly normal and have normal investigations. Thus, the diagnosis is essentially clinical, relying heavily on eyewitness descriptions of the attacks. In addition, there are a number of other conditions in which consciousness may be transiently impaired and which may be confused with epilepsy. Another problem area is that of case identification. Sometimes the patient may be unaware of the nature of the attacks and so may not seek medical help. Patients with milder epilepsy may also not be receiving ongoing medical care and so may be missed in epidemiological surveys. Furthermore, since there is some degree of stigma attached to epilepsy, patients may sometimes be reluctant to admit their condition.

Incidence and prevalence

Epileptic seizures are common. The incidence (number of new cases per given population per year) has been estimated at between 20 and 70 cases per 100 000 persons, and the cumulative incidence (the risk of having the condition at some point in life) at 2–5%. The incidence is higher in the first two decades of life but falls over the next few decades, only to increase again in late life, due mainly to cerebrovascular diseases. Most studies of the prevalence of active epilepsy (the number of cases in the population at any given time) have estimated figures at 4–8/1000, and a rate of 5/1000 is commonly quoted. Epilepsy is most commonly developed in older age and an accurate diagnosis in the elderly is crucial. Elderly people have 2–3 times higher mortality than the general population.

Prognosis

Up to 5% of people will suffer at least one seizure in their lifetime. However, the prevalence of active epilepsy is much lower and most patients who develop seizures have a very good prognosis. About 70–80% of all people developing epilepsy will eventually become seizure free, and about half will successfully withdraw their medication. Once a substantial period of remission has been achieved, the risk of further seizures is greatly reduced. A minority of patients (20–30%) will develop chronic epilepsy and in such cases, treatment is more difficult. Patients with symptomatic epilepsy, more than one seizure type, associated learning disabilities or neurological or psychiatric disorders are more likely to have a poor outcome. Of chronic patients, fewer than 5% will be unable to live in the community or will depend on others for their day-to-day needs. Most patients are entirely normal between seizures but a small minority of patients with severe epilepsy may suffer physical and intellectual deterioration.

Mortality

There is an increased mortality in people with epilepsy, especially among younger patients and those with severe epilepsy. Most studies have given overall standardized mortality ratios between two and three times higher than that of the general population. Common causes of death in people with epilepsy include accidents, e.g. drowning, head injury, road traffic accidents, status epilepticus, tumours, cerebrovascular disease, pneumonia and suicide. Sudden unexpected death, an entity which remains unexplained, is common in chronic epilepsy, particularly among the young who have convulsive forms of epilepsy.

Aetiology

Epileptic seizures are produced by abnormal discharges of neurones that may be caused by any pathological process which affects the brain. The idiopathic epilepsies are those in which there is a clear genetic component, and they probably account for a third of all new cases of epilepsy. In a significant proportion of cases, however, no cause can be determined and these are known as the cryptogenic epilepsies. Possible explanations for cryptogenic epilepsy include as yet unexplained metabolic or biochemical abnormalities and microscopic lesions in the brain resulting from brain malformation or trauma during birth or other injury. The term 'symptomatic epilepsy' indicates that a probable cause has been identified.

The likely aetiology of epilepsy depends upon the age of the patient and the type of seizure. The commonest causes in young infants are hypoxia or birth asphyxia, intracranial trauma during birth, metabolic disturbances, congenital malformations of the brain or infection. In young children and adolescents, idiopathic seizures account for the majority of the epilepsies, although trauma and infection also play a role. In this age group, particularly in children aged between 6 months and 5 years, seizures may occur in association with febrile illness. These are usually short, generalized tonic clonic convulsions that occur during the early phase of a febrile disease. They must be distinguished from seizures that are triggered by central nervous system infections which produce fever, for example meningitis or encephalitis. Unless febrile seizures are prolonged, focal, recurrent or there is a background of neurological handicap, the prognosis is excellent and it is unlikely that the child will develop epilepsy.

The range of causes of adult-onset epilepsy is very wide. Both idiopathic epilepsy and epilepsy due to birth trauma may also begin in early adulthood. Other important causes are head injury, alcohol abuse, cortical dysplasias, brain tumours and cerebrovascular diseases. Brain tumours are responsible for the development of epilepsy in up to a third of patients between the ages of 30 and 50 years. Over the age of 50 years, cerebrovascular disease is the commonest cause of epilepsy, and may be present in up to half of patients.

Pathophysiology

Epilepsy differs from most neurological conditions as it has no pathognomonic lesion. A variety of different electrical or chemical stimuli can easily give rise to a seizure in any normal brain. The hallmark of epilepsy is a rather rhythmic and repetitive hypersynchronous discharge of neurones, either localized in an area of the cerebral cortex or generalized throughout the cortex, which can be observed on an electroencephalogram (EEG).

Neurones are interconnected in a complex network in which each individual neurone is linked through synapses with hundreds of others. A small electrical current is discharged by neurones to release neurotransmitters at synaptic levels to permit communication with each other. Neurotransmitters fall into two basic categories: inhibitory or excitatory. Therefore, a neurone discharging can either excite or inhibit neurones connected to it. An excited neurone will activate the next neurone whereas an inhibited neurone will not. In this manner, information is conveyed, transmitted and processed throughout the central nervous system.

A normal neurone discharges repetitively at a low baseline frequency, and it is the integrated electrical activity generated by the neurones of the superficial layers of the cortex that is recorded in a normal EEG. If neurones are damaged, injured or suffer a chemical or metabolic insult, a change in the discharge pattern may develop. In the case of epilepsy, regular low-frequency discharges are replaced by bursts of high-frequency discharges usually followed by periods of inactivity. A single neurone discharging in an abnormal manner usually has no clinical significance. It is only when a whole population of neurones discharge synchronously in an abnormal way that an epileptic seizure may be triggered. This abnormal discharge may remain localized or it may spread to adjacent areas, recruiting more neurones as it expands. It may also generalize throughout the brain via cortical and subcortical routes, including collosal and thalamocortical pathways. The area from which the abnormal discharge originates is known as the epileptic focus. An EEG recording carried out during one of these abnormal discharges may show a variety of atypical signs, depending on which area of the brain is involved, its progression and how the discharging areas project to the superficial cortex.

Clinical manifestations

The clinical manifestation of a seizure will depend on the location of the focus and the pathways involved in its spread. An international seizure classification scheme based on the clinical features of seizures combined with EEG data is widely used to describe seizures. It divides seizures into two main groups according to the area of the brain in which the abnormal discharge originates. If it involves initial activation of both hemispheres of the brain simultaneously, the seizures are termed 'generalized'. If a discharge starts in a localized area of the brain, the seizure is termed 'partial' or 'focal'.

Generalized seizures

Generalized seizures result in impairment of consciousness from the onset. There are various types of generalized seizures.

Tonic clonic convulsions

Often called 'grand mal' attacks, these are the commonest of all epileptic seizures. Without warning, the patient suddenly goes stiff, falls and convulses, with laboured breathing and salivation. Cyanosis, incontinence and tongue biting may occur. The convulsion ceases after a few minutes and may often be followed by a period of drowsiness, confusion, headache and sleep.

Absence attacks

Often called 'petit mal', these are a much rarer form of generalized seizure. They happen almost exclusively in childhood and early adolescence. The child goes blank and stares; fluttering of the eyelids and flopping of the head may occur. The attacks last only a few seconds and often go unrecognized even by the child experiencing them.

Myoclonic seizures

These are abrupt, very brief involuntary shock-like jerks, which may involve the whole body, or the arms or the head. They usually happen in the morning, shortly after waking. They may sometimes cause the person to fall, but recovery is immediate. It should be noted that there are forms of non-epileptic myoclonic jerks that occur in a variety of other nerve diseases and may also occur in healthy people, particularly when they are just going off to sleep.

Atonic seizures

These comprise a sudden loss of muscle tone, causing the person to collapse to the ground. Recovery afterwards is quick. They are rare, accounting for less than 1% of the epileptic seizures seen in the general population, but much commoner in patients with severe epilepsy starting in infancy.

Partial seizures

Simple partial seizures

In these seizures the discharge remains localized and consciousness is fully preserved. Simple partial attacks on their own are rare and they usually progress to the other forms of partial seizure. What actually happens during a simple partial seizure depends on the area of the discharge and may vary widely from patient to patient but will always be stereotyped in one patient. Localized jerking of a limb or the face, stiffness or twitching of one part of the body, numbness or abnormal sensations are examples of what may occur during a simple partial seizure. If the seizure progresses with impairment of consciousness, it is termed a complex partial seizure. If it develops further and a convulsive seizure occurs, it is then called a partial seizure with secondary generalization. In attacks which progress, the early part of the seizure, in which consciousness is preserved, may manifest as a sensation or abnormal feeling and is called the aura or warning.

Complex partial seizures

The patient may present with altered or 'automatic' behaviour: plucking his or her clothes, fiddling with various objects and acting in a confused manner. Lip smacking or chewing movements, grimacing, undressing, performing aimless activities, and wandering around in a drunken fashion may occur on their own or in different combinations during complex partial seizures. Most of these seizures originate in the frontal or temporal lobes of the brain and can sometimes progress to secondarily generalized seizures.

Secondarily generalized seizures

These are partial seizures, either simple or complex, in which the discharge spreads to the entire brain. The patient may have a warning, but this is not always the case. The spread of the discharge can occur so quickly that no feature of the localized onset is apparent to the patient or an observer, and only an EEG can demonstrate the partial nature of the seizure. The involvement of the entire brain leads to a convulsive attack with the same characteristics as a generalized tonic clonic convulsion.

Diagnosis

Diagnosing epilepsy can be difficult as it is first necessary to demonstrate a tendency to recurrent epileptic seizures. The one feature that distinguishes epilepsy from all other conditions is its unpredictability and transient nature. The diagnosis of epilepsy is clinical and depends on a reliable account of what happened during the attacks, if possible both from the patient and from an eyewitness, but some investigations may help and the EEG is usually one of them. However, these investigations cannot conclusively confirm or refute the diagnosis of epilepsy.

There are other conditions that may cause impairment or loss of consciousness and which can be misdiagnosed as epilepsy; these include syncope, breath-holding attacks, transient ischaemic attacks, psychogenic attacks, etc. In addition, patients may present with acute symptomatic seizures or provoked seizures as a result of other problems such as drug intake, metabolic dysfunction, infec-tion, head trauma or flashing lights (photosensitive seizures). These conditions have to be clearly ruled out before a diagnosis of epilepsy is made. Epilepsy must only be diagnosed when seizures occur spontaneously and are recurrent. The diagnosis must be accurate since the label 'suffering with epilepsy' carries a social stigma that has tremendous implications for the patient.

The EEG is often the only examination required, particularly in generalized epilepsies, and it aims to record abnormal neuronal discharges. However, EEGs have limitations that should be clearly understood. Up to 5% of people without epilepsy may have non-specific abnormalities in their EEG recording, while up to 40% of people with epilepsy may have a normal EEG recording between seizures. Therefore the diagnosis of epilepsy should be strongly supported by a bona fide history of epileptic attacks. Nevertheless, the EEG is invaluable in classifying seizures.

The chance of recording the discharges of an actual seizure during a routine EEG, which usually takes 20–30 minutes, is slight and because of this, ambulatory EEG monitoring and EEG video-telemetry are sometimes required. Ambulatory EEG allows recording in day-to-day circumstances using a small cassette recorder. EEG video-telemetry is useful in the assessment of difficult cases, particularly if surgery is considered. The patient is usually admitted to hospital and remains under continuous monitoring. This is only helpful in a very few cases, and it is best suited for patients who have frequent seizures.

Neuroimaging with magnetic resonance imaging (MRI) is the most valuable investigation when structural abnormalities such as stroke, tumour, congenital abnormalities or hydrochephalus are suspected. MRI should be carried out in anyone presenting with partial seizures or where a structural lesion on the brain may be responsible for seizures.

Treatment

NICE (2004c) issued guidance on the diagnosis and treatment of the epilepsies in adults and children in primary and secondary care. The guidance covered issues such as when a patient should be referred to a specialist centre, the special considerations concerning the care and treatment of women with epilepsy and the management of people with learning disabilities. The key points of the guidance are summarized in Table 31.1.

Treatment during seizures

Convulsive seizures may look frightening but the patient is not in pain, will usually have no recollection of the event afterwards and is usually not seriously injured. Emergency treatment is seldom necessary. Patients should, however, be made as comfortable as possible, preferably lying down (ease to the floor if sitting), cushioning the head and loosening any tight clothing or neckwear. During seizures, patients should not be moved unless

Table 31.1 Key points on the diagnosis and management of epilepsy (NICE 2004c)

- Diagnosis to be made urgently by a specialist with an interest in epilepsy

- EEG to be used to support diagnosis

- MRI[a] to be used in people who develop epilepsy as adults, in whom focal onset is suspected, or in whom seizures persist

- Seizure type(s) and epilepsy syndrome, aetiology and co-morbidity to be determined

- Initiation of appropriate treatment to be recommended by a specialist

- Treatment individualized according to seizure type, epilepsy syndrome, co-medication and co-morbidity, the individual's lifestyle and personal preferences

- The individual with epilepsy, and their family and/or carers, to participate in all decisions about care, taking into account any specific need

- Comprehensive care plans to be agreed

- Comprehensive provision of information about all aspects of condition

- Regular structured review at least once a year

- Patient to be referred back to secondary or tertiary care if:
  - Epilepsy inadequately controlled
  - Pregnancy considered or pregnant
  - Antiepileptic drug withdrawal considered

[a]Magnetic resonance imaging

they are in a dangerous place, for example in a road, by a fire or hot radiator, at the top of stairs or by the edge of water. No attempt should be made to open the patient's mouth or force anything between the teeth. This usually results in damage, and broken teeth may be inhaled, causing secondary lung damage. When the seizure stops, patients should be turned over into the recovery position and the airway checked for any blockage.

Partial attacks are usually less dramatic. During automatisms, patients may behave in a confused fashion and should generally be left undisturbed. Gentle restraint may be necessary if the automatism leads to dangerous wandering. Attempts at firm restraint, however, may increase agitation and confusion. No drinks should be given after an attack, nor should extra antiepileptic drugs (AEDs) be administered. It is commonly felt that seizures may be life threatening, but this is seldom the case. After a seizure, it is important to stay with the patient and offer reassurance until the confused period has completely subsided and the patient has recovered fully.

If a seizure persists for more than 10 minutes, if a series of seizures occur or if the seizure is particularly severe, then intravenous or rectal administration of 10–20 mg diazepam for adults, with lower doses being used in children, is advisable.

Status epilepticus

Initial management of status epilepticus is supportive and may include:

- positioning the patient to avoid injury
- supporting respiration
- maintaining blood pressure
- correcting hypoglycaemia.

Drugs used include intravenous lorazepam or diazepam. Alternative medicines include midazolam in cases where the patient has not responded to first-line drugs. Alternatively, buccal midazolam has been advocated and is increasingly being used although it is not licensed in the UK. In severe cases phenytoin, clonazepam, phenobarbital sodium or paraldehyde may be required.

Febrile convulsions

Convulsions associated with fever are termed febrile convulsions and may occur in the young. Brief febrile convulsions are managed conservatively with the primary aim of reducing the temperature of the child. Tepid sponging and use of paracetamol is usual. However, prolonged febrile convulsions lasting 10–15 minutes or longer or in a child with risk factors require active management to avoid brain damage. The drug of choice is diazepam by intravenous or rectal (rectal solution) administration. Prophylactic management of febrile convulsions may be required in some children, e.g. those with pre-existing risk factors or a history of previous prolonged seizures.

Long-term treatment

In most cases, epilepsy can only be treated by long-term, regular drug therapy. The objective of therapy is to suppress epileptic discharges and prevent the development of epileptic seizures. In the majority of cases, full seizure control can be obtained, and in other patients drugs may reduce the frequency or severity of seizures.

Initiating treatment with an antiepileptic drug is a major event in the life of a patient, and the diagnosis should be unequivocal. Treatment options must be considered with careful evaluation of all relevant factors, including the number and frequency of attacks, the presence of precipitating factors such as alcohol, drugs or flashing lights, and the presence of other medical conditions (Feely 1999). Single seizures do not require treatment unless they are associated with a progressive brain disorder or there is a clearly abnormal EEG. If there are long intervals between seizures (over 2 years) there is a case for not starting treatment. If there are more than two attacks that are clearly associated with a precipitating factor, fever or alcohol for instance, then treatment may not be necessary.

Therapy is long term, usually for at least 3 years, and, depending on circumstances, sometimes for life. A full explanation of all the implications must be given to the patient. The patient must be involved in all stages of the treatment plan. It is vital that the patient understands the implications of treatment and agrees with the treatment goals. Empowerment of patients to be actively involved in the decision-making process will encourage adherence and is essential for effective clinical management. Support for patients so that they understand the implications of the condition and why drug therapy is so important is crucial to ensure effective clinical management.

Health professionals have a key role in supporting patients with epilepsy to ensure they are able to manage their medicines appropriately. Antiepileptic treatment will fail unless the patient fully understands the importance of regular therapy and the objectives of treatment. Poor compliance is still a major factor which results in hospital admissions and poor seizure control and leads to the clinical use of multiple antiepileptic drugs.

General principles of treatment

Therapy aims to control seizures using one drug, with the lowest possible dose that causes the fewest side effects possible. The established antiepileptic drugs, carbamazepine, ethosuximide, phenytoin and sodium valproate, form the mainstay of treatment. Acetazolamide, clobazam, clonazepam, phenobarbital and primidone are also occasionally used. More recently, in the last decade new drugs such as gabapentin, lamotrigine, levetiracetam, oxcarbazepine, topiramate, tiagabine and vigabatrin have been introduced, and felbamate and zonisamide may be launched in the near future. The choice of drugs depends largely on the seizure type, and so correct diagnosis and classification are essential. Table 31.2 lists the main indications for the more commonly used antiepileptic drugs currently available, and Table 31.3 summarizes the clinical use of the newer antiepileptic drugs.

Initiation of therapy in newly diagnosed patients

The first-line antiepileptic drug most suitable for the patient's seizure type should be introduced slowly, starting with a small dose, as too rapid an introduction may induce side effects that will lose the patient's confidence. For most drugs, this gradual introduction will produce a therapeutic effect just as fast as a rapid introduction, and the patient should be reassured about this.

Table 31.2 Antiepileptic drugs for different seizure types

Seizure type	First-line treatment	Second-line treatment
Partial seizures		
Simple partial	Carbamazepine	Vigabatrin Zonisamide
Complex partial Secondarily generalized	Phenytoin Valproate Lamotrigine	Clobazam Phenobarbital Acetazolamide Gabapentin Topiramate Zonisamide
Generalized seizures		
Tonic clonic	Valproate	Vigabatrin
Tonic	Carbamazepine	Clobazam
Clonic	Phenytoin Lamotrigine	Phenobarbital
Absence	Ethosuximide Valproate	Clonazepam Lamotrigine Acetazolamide
Atypical absences	Valproate	Phenobarbital
Atonic	Clonazepam Clobazam	Lamotrigine Carbamazepine Phenytoin Acetazolamide
Myoclonic	Valproate Clonazepam	Phenobarbital Acetazolamide Topiramate

Maintenance dosage

There is no single optimum dose of any antiepileptic drug that suits all patients. The required dose varies from patient to patient, and from drug to drug. Drugs should be introduced slowly and then increased incrementally to an initial maintenance dosage. Seizure control should then be assessed, and the dose of drug changed if necessary. For most antiepileptic drugs, dosage increments are constant over a wide range. However, more care is needed with phenytoin as the plasma level–dose relationship is not linear, and small dose changes may result in considerable plasma level changes. Generic prescribing for epilepsy remains controversial. Most specialists would prefer patients to remain on the same brand of medication, and this is also preferred by the majority of patients. This is obviously important in those patients in whom the dosage has been carefully titrated to achieve optimal control.

Altering drug regimens

If the maximal tolerated dose of a drug does not control seizures, or if side effects develop, the first drug can be replaced with another first-line antiepileptic drug. To do this, the second drug should be added gradually to the first. Once a good dose of the new drug is established, the first drug should then slowly be withdrawn.

Table 31.3 Summary of newer antiepileptic agents

Antiepileptic drugs	Clinical use	Available formulation	Side effect profile
Lamotrigine	Monotherapy and adjunctive treatment of partial seizures, primary and secondary generalized tonic clonic seizure, Lennox–Gastaut syndrome	Tablets: 25 mg, 50 mg, 100 mg, 200 mg. Dispersible tablets: 5 mg, 25 mg, 100 mg	Dizziness, headache, diplopia, ataxia, nausea, somnolence, vomiting, rash. Rare: Stevens–Johnson syndrome, hematological
Vigabatrin	Adjunctive treatment of partial seizures with or without secondary generalization, monotherapy for West's syndrome	Tablets: 500 mg. Powder: 500 mg/sachet	Drowsiness, fatigue, dizziness, nystagmus, abnormal vision, agitation, amnesia, depression, psychosis, increased weight, withdrawal seizures
Gabapentin	Adjunctive treatment of partial seizures with or without secondary generalization, neuropathic pain	Capsules: 100 mg, 300 mg, 400 mg. Tablets: 600 mg, 800 mg	Somnolence, dizziness, ataxia, headache, fatigue, nystagmus, tremor, nausea, vomiting, increased weight
Felbamate	Lennox–Gastaut syndrome refractory to treatment	Tablets: 400 mg	Headache, nausea, anorexia, somnolence, insomnia, dizziness, fatigue, vomiting, rash, decreased weight. Rare: aplastic anaemia, hepatic failure, thrombocytopenia
Tiagabine	Adjunctive treatment of partial seizures with or without secondary generalization	Tablets: 5 mg, 10 mg, 15 mg	Dizziness, asthenia, nervousness, tremor, diarrhoea, depression, emotional lability, confusion, abnormal thinking, decreased weight
Topiramate	Adjunctive treatment of partial seizures with or without secondary generalization, Lennox–Gastaut syndrome, primary generalized tonic clonic seizures	Tablets: 25 mg, 50 mg, 100 mg, 200 mg. Sprinkle capsules: 15 mg, 25 mg	Dizziness, abnormal thinking, somnolence, ataxia, fatigue, confusion, impaired concentration, paresthesia, decreased weight, nephrolithiasis (1.5%)
Zonisamide	Adjunctive therapy in treatment of partial seizures with or without secondary generalization	Capsule: 25 mg, 50 mg, 100 mg	Somnolence, anorexia, dizziness, headache, nausea, agitation/irritability, confusional state, depression

Withdrawal of drugs

Antiepileptic medication should not be withdrawn abruptly, in particular for barbiturates and benzodiazepines, since rebound seizures may occur.

The withdrawal of individual antiepileptic drugs should be carried out in a slow stepwise fashion to avoid the precipitation of withdrawal seizures (e.g. over 2–3 months). This risk is particularly great with barbiturates, e.g. phenobarbital and primidone, and benzodiazepines, e.g. clobazam and clonazepam. If a drug needs to be withdrawn rapidly, for example if there are life-threatening side effects, then diazepam or another benzodiazepine can be used to cover the withdrawal phase.

Examples of withdrawal regimens are given below.

- Carbamazepine
  100 to 200 mg every 2 weeks (as part of a drug change)
  100 to 200 mg every 4 weeks (total withdrawal)
- Phenobarbital
  15 to 30 mg every 2 weeks (as part of a drug change)
  15 to 30 mg every 4 weeks (total withdrawal)
- Phenytoin
  50 mg every 2 weeks (as part of a drug change)
  50 mg every 4 weeks (total withdrawal)
- Sodium valproate
  200 to 400 mg every 2 weeks (as part of a drug change)
  200 to 400 mg every 4 weeks (total withdrawal)
- Ethosuximide
  125 to 200 mg every 2 weeks (as part of a drug change)
  125 to 200 mg every 4 weeks (total withdrawal)

Variations in the above regimens may be used in different settings. Patients must be monitored closely for any changes in seizure frequency. The pace of withdrawal may be slower if the patient is within the top end of the quoted therapeutic ranges. The pace of withdrawal may be faster if the patient is an inpatient.

When to make dose changes

Some antiepileptic drugs have long half-lives and it may therefore take some time, normally at least five half-lives, before a change in dose results in a stable blood level. For example, phenobarbital has a half-life of up to 6 days and will take more than 4 weeks to produce a stable blood level. For this reason an assessment of the effectiveness of any dose change should be undertaken several weeks after the dosage change has been made and be informed by knowledge of the half-life of the drug.

Newer antiepileptic drugs

The newer antiepileptic drugs are generally used as second-line drugs when treatment with established first-line drugs has failed. Exceptions to this are lamotrigine, topiramate and oxcarbazepine, which have indications for first-line use in the UK. However, many physicians only consider lamotrigine as a first-line option in women of child-bearing potential who have idiopathic generalized epilepsy, in view of the teratogenic profile of sodium valproate, the first-line drug for this indication. Oxcarbazepine has the same indications as carbamazepine although the latter is probably more cost-effective.

There is no evidence that the newer antiepileptic drugs are more effective than the established drugs, although it could be argued that they might be better tolerated. The chronic side effect profile of the new antiepileptic drugs has not yet been fully established and this is the main reason why use should be reserved for those cases where benefit outweighs risk. NICE (2004a) issued guidance that covered the use of the newer antiepileptic drugs in adults and their recommendations included the following.

- Newer drugs, e.g. lamotrigine, oxcarbazepine and topiramate, suitable for the type of epilepsy to be treated can be used in patients where older drugs, e.g. sodium valproate or carbamazepine, do not provide effective clinical control or cause untolerable side effects.
- Gabapentin, levetiracetam, tiagabine and vigabatrin are generally used in combination with another drug.
- Newer drugs can be used where older drugs are unsuitable for the person, e.g. liver disease, or where unwanted effects cannot be tolerated.
- The aim should be to treat people with just one antiepileptic drug where possible.

The guidance for adults was followed up by advice (NICE 2004b) for use of the newer antiepileptic drugs in children. This advice reflected that issued for adults and included the following.

- Lamotrigine, oxcarbazepine or topiramate can be given to children as sole treatment for epilepsy.
- Gabapentin, tiagabine and vigabatrin are generally used as combination therapy with another drug.
- Vigabatrin is suitable for first-line treatment of young children with a rare type of infantile spasm called West's syndrome.
- Newer drugs are indicated if older drugs are unsuitable, e.g. in liver disease, or if patients cannot tolerate unwanted effects.
- Children should be treated with just one antiepileptic drug where possible.

Follow-up and monitoring of treatment

It is essential to follow up patients in whom antiepileptic drug treatment has been started. The reason for this is essentially to monitor the efficacy and side effects of treatment, upon which drug dosage will depend, but also to encourage good compliance. This follow-up is particularly important in the early stages of treatment, when an effective maintenance dose may not have been fully established, when the importance of regular compliance may not have been recognized by the patient, and when the psychological adjustment to regular treatment may not be resolved.

Chronic epilepsy

The drug treatment of patients with established epilepsy that is uncontrolled despite initial attempts is much more difficult than that of newly diagnosed patients. Prognosis is worse, drug resistance may have developed, and there may be additional neurological, psychological or social problems.

Assessment The diagnosis of epilepsy should be reassessed before assuming seizures are intractable. A significant proportion of patients may have been incorrectly diagnosed. The aetiology of the epilepsy should also be considered, and the question of a progressive neurological condition addressed. A treatment history should be obtained and note made of previous drugs used which were helpful, unhelpful or of uncertain benefit. Plasma level measurements should be obtained where appropriate and drugs not previously tried should be identified.

Choice of drug and dosage Treatment should always be started with one antiepileptic drug appropriate for seizure type and suitable for the individual. Only when attempts at monotherapy fail should a combination of two antiepileptic drugs be tried. In the majority of patients there is no place for therapy with more than two drugs. The choice of drugs should be made according to seizure type and previous treatment history. Drugs that were helpful in the past or of uncertain benefit, or which have not been used before, should be tried if appropriate to seizure type. The use of sedative antiepileptic drugs should be minimized where possible.

Intractable epilepsy It is important to realize that there are limits to antiepileptic drug treatment and that in some patients, albeit a small group, seizure control is not possible with the drugs currently available. In such cases, the goal of drug treatment changes, and the objectives are to reduce medication to minimize toxicity while providing partial control. The sedative drugs, for example barbiturates or benzodiazepines, should be used only where absolutely necessary. In these patients surgical treatment or the use of experimental antiepileptic agents may be considered. However, only a few patients with partial epilepsy are suitable for curative surgical treatment.

Stopping treatment

Withdrawing therapy should be considered in patients who have been seizure free for a considerable period of time. In no individual case, however, can the safety of drug withdrawal be guaranteed, and the risk of relapse on withdrawal of medication in a patient who has been seizure free for more than 2 years is about 40%. The longer the patient has been free of seizures, the lower the risk of seizure recurrence when drugs are withdrawn. If a patient has a mental handicap, partial seizures or symptomatic epilepsy, neurological signs or other evidence of cerebral damage, this risk is much higher and in such cases it may be best to continue drug treatment indefinitely. Drug withdrawal should be carried out only very slowly in staged decrements, and only one drug at a time should be withdrawn.

The risks of drug withdrawal should be clearly explained to the patient, and the possible medical and social implications taken into account. There may be serious social or domestic conse-quences should seizures recur, and the attacks may be subsequently difficult to control, even if the original antiepileptic drug regimen is re-established. In the final analysis, the decision to withdraw therapy is an individual one, and a patient should be made aware of the risks and benefits of withdrawal.

Monitoring antiepileptic therapy

Therapeutic drug monitoring (TDM) involves the measurement of plasma drug levels and their pharmacokinetic interpretation. It is an integral component in the management of patients receiving phenytoin and carbamazepine but is less useful in patients receiving acetazolamide, barbiturates, benzodiazepines, ethosuximide, gabapentin, lamotrigine, levetiracetam, sodium valproate, tiagabine, topiramate and vigabatrin.

TDM is indicated:

- at the onset of therapy
- if seizure control is poor or sudden changes in seizure control occur
- if toxicity is suspected
- if poor or non-compliance is suspected
- to monitor the time-scale of drug interactions
- when changing antiepileptic drug therapy or making changes to other aspects of a patient's drug regimen that may interact with the antiepileptic drug.

The frequency of undertaking TDM varies. Stabilized patients may require their plasma levels to be checked only once or twice a year. TDM may be used more often in some patients, for one or more of the above indications. A number of the newer antiepileptic drugs do not require TDM. However, since most are used as adjuvant therapy it is useful to establish baseline levels of existing drugs before the new agent is introduced. Clinical effects should be monitored and TDM, where appropriate, carried out at 6–12 month intervals.

Drug development and action

The older, more established antiepileptic drugs were developed in animal models in which the potential antiepileptic drugs were assessed in terms of their ability to raise seizure threshold or prevent spread of seizure discharge. The animals involved in these tests would not have epilepsy but would have seizures induced by maximal electroshock and subcutaneous pentylenetetrazole. As a consequence the relevance of these models to epilepsy can be questioned.

Established therapeutic drugs such as phenytoin, phenobarbital, sodium valproate, carbamazepine, ethosuximide, clonazepam and diazepam are effective but have poor side effect profiles, are involved in many interactions and have complex pharmacokinetics. Over the past 10–15 years, there has been renewed interest in the development of new antiepileptic drugs, based on a better understanding of excitatory and inhibitory pathways in the brain. The main mechanisms of current drugs are thought to involve enhancement of the inhibitory GABA-ergic system, e.g. benzodiazepines, barbiturates, tiagabine, vigabatrin or use-dependent blockers of sodium channels, e.g. carbamazepine, oxcarbazepine, lamotrigine and phenytoin (Fig. 31.1).

The new drugs are vigabatrin, lamotrigine, gabapentin, tiagabine, topiramate, felbamate, oxcarbazepine and zonisamide. Unlike most of the older agents, vigabatrin, lamotrigine, gabapentin, tiagabine and zonisamide are devoid of significant enzyme-inhibiting or -inducing properties. Although tiagabine is extensively metabolized by cytochrome P450, it does not influence the pharmacokinetics of conventional antiepileptic drugs or interact with drugs such as theophylline, warfarin, digoxin or oral contraceptives. Topiramate and oxcarbazepine, however, induce cytochrome P450 CYP3A4 which is responsible for the metabolism of oral contraceptives (Sabers & Gram 2000).

Antiepileptic drug profiles

The maintenance doses for the more widely used antiepileptic drugs are given in Table 31.4, while their pharmacokinetic profile

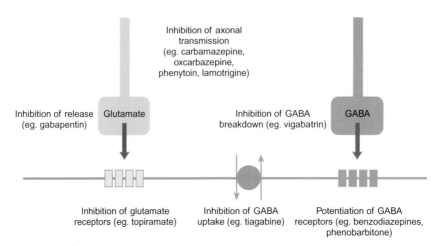

Figure 31.1 Action of antiepileptic drugs (from Duncan et al 2006).

Table 31.4 Commonly used starting and maintenance doses of antiepileptic drugs for adults

Antiepileptic drug	Starting dose (mg)	Average maintenance (total mg/day)	Doses/day
Acetazolamide	250	500–1500	2
Carbamazepine	100	600–2400	2–4 (retard 2)
Clobazam	10	10–30	1–2
Clonazepam	0.5	0.5–3	1–2
Ethosuximide	250	500–1500	1–2
Gabapentin	300	900–1200	3
Lamotrigine	50[a]	100–500[a]	2
Levetiracetam	1000	2000–3000	2
Oxcarbazepine	300	900–1800	2–3
Phenobarbital	60	60–180	1
Phenytoin	200–300	200–400	1–2
Valproate	500	2000–2500	1–2
Vigabatrin	500	2000–4000	1–2
Zonisamide	50	300–500 or 200–300[b]	2

[a] Reduce by 50% if on valproate.
[b] If patients are on enzyme inducers or have impared renal or liver function.

is presented in Table 31.5. Drug interactions are summarized in Table 31.6, and common side effects in Table 31.7.

Acetazolamide

Acetazolamide is occasionally used as an antiepileptic drug. It can be prescribed as a second-line drug for most types of seizures, but particularly for partial seizures, absence seizures and myoclonic seizures. Its intermittent use in catamenial seizures has also been suggested. Acetazolamide has only limited use as long-term therapy because of the development of tolerance in the majority of patients. Side effects include skin rashes, weight loss, paraesthesia, drowsiness and depression. Routine TDM is not available for this drug.

Carbamazepine

Carbamazepine is a drug of first choice in tonic clonic and partial seizures, and may be of benefit in all other seizure types except generalized absence seizures and myoclonic seizures. Tolerance to its beneficial effect does not usually develop. Adverse events may occur in up to a third of patients treated with carbamazepine but only about 5% of these events will require drug withdrawal, usually due to skin rash, gastrointestinal disturbances or hyponatraemia. Dose-related adverse reactions including ataxia, dizziness, blurred vision and diplopia are common. Serious adverse events including hepatic failure and bone marrow depression are extremely uncommon.

Carbamazepine exhibits autoinduction, i.e. induces its own metabolism as well as inducing the metabolism of other drugs. It should therefore be introduced at low dosage and this should be steadily increased over a period of a month. The target plasma concentration therapeutic range is 4–12 µg/mL. In addition, a number of clinically important pharmacokinetic interactions may occur, and caution should be exercised when co-medication is instituted (see Table 31.6). For patients requiring higher doses,

Table 31.5 Pharmacokinetic data of antiepileptic drugs

Drug	F (%)	T_{peak} (h)	V_d (L/kg)	Protein binding (% bound)	$T_{1/2}$ (h)	Renal excretion (%)	Active metabolite
Carbamazepine	75–85	1–5 (chronic dose)	0.8–1.6	70–78	24–45 (single), 8–24 (chronic)	<1	Yes
Diazepam	90	1–2	1–2	96	20–95	2	Yes
Clonazepam	80–90	1–2	2.1–4.3	80–90	19–40	2	–
Gabapentin	51–59	2–3	57.7	0	5–7	100	No
Lamotrigine	100	2–3	0.92–1.22	55	24–35 (induces its own metabolism)	<10	No
Ethosuximide	90–95	3–7	0.6–0.9	0	20–60	10–20	No
Phenobarbital	95–100	1–3	0.6	40–50	50–144	20–40	No

continued

Table 31.5 (continued)

Drug	Absorption			Protein binding (% bound)	Elimination		
	F (%)	T_{peak} (h)	V_d (L/kg)		$T_{1/2}$ (h)	Renal excretion (%)	Active metabolite
Phenytoin	85–95	4–7	0.5–0.7	90–95	9–40 (non-linear kinetics)	<5	No
Primidone	90–100	1–3	0.4–1.1	20–30	3–19	40	Yes
Sodium valproate	100	0.5–1.0	0.1–0.5	88–92	7–17	<5	No
Vigabatrin	60–80	2	0.6–1.0	0	5–7	100	No
Zonisamide	100	2–4	1.1–1.7	40	52–69	30	Yes

Table 31.6 Examples of drug interactions involving antiepileptic drugs

Drug affected	Effect on plasma level	Drug implicated	Possible mechanism
Carbamazepine	Increase	Sodium valproate Cimetidine Dextropropoxyphene Erythromycin Isoniazid Troleandomycin Danazol	Enzyme inhibition
	Decrease	Phenytoin Phenobarbital	Enzyme induction
Phenytoin	Increase	Sodium valproate Chloramphenicol Isoniazid Disulfiram Fluconazole Flu vaccine Amiodarone Fluoxetine	Enzyme inhibition Mechanism unclear
	Decrease	Phenobarbital Rifampicin Carbamazepine Furosemide Acetazolamide	Enzyme induction Decreased responsiveness of renal tubules Increased osteomalacia
Sodium valproate	Increase	Salicylates	Displacement from protein binding sites and possible enzyme inhibition
	Decrease	Potential enzyme inducers	Enzyme induction
Phenobarbital	Increase	Sodium valproate	Enzyme inhibition
	Decrease	Rifampicin	Enzyme induction
Lamotrigine	Increase	Sodium valproate	Enzyme inhibition
	Decrease	Phenytoin, carbamazepine	Enzyme induction
Topiramate	Decrease	Phenytoin, carbamazepine	Enzyme induction
Ethosuximide	Increase	Sodium valproate	Enzyme inhibition
	Decrease	Carbamazepine	Enzyme induction
Zonisamide	Decrease	Carbamazepine, phenytoin, phenobarbital and primidone	Enzyme induction

Table 31.7 Side effect profile of antiepileptic drugs

Drug	Dose related (predictable)	Non-dose related (idiosyncratic)
Carbamazepine	Diplopia, drowsiness, headache, nausea, orofacial dyskinesia, arrhythmias	Photosensitivity, Stevens–Johnson syndrome, agranulocytosis, aplastic anaemia, hepatotoxicity
Sodium valproate	Dyspepsia, nausea, vomiting, hair loss, anorexia, drowsiness	Acute pancreatitis, aplastic anaemia, thrombocytopenia, hepatotoxicity
Phenytoin	Ataxia, nystagmus, drowsiness, gingival hyperplasia, hirsutism, diplopia, asterixis, orofacial dyskinesia, folate deficiency	Blood dyscrasias, rash, Dupuytren's contracture, hepatotoxicity
Phenobarbital	Fatigue, listlessness, depression, poor memory, impotence, hypocalcaemia, osteomalacia, folate deficiency	Macropapular rash, exfoliation, hepatotoxicity
Ethosuximide	Nausea, vomiting, drowsinesss, headache, lethargy	Rash, erythema multiforme, Stevens–Johnson syndrome
Clonazepam	Fatigue, drowsiness, ataxia	Rash, thrombocytopenia
Lamotrigine	Headaches, drowsiness, diplopia, ataxia	Liver failure, disseminated intravascular coagulation
Gabapentin	Drowsiness, diplopia, ataxia, headache	Not reported
Topiramate	Dizziness, drowsiness, nervousness, fatigue, weight loss	Not reported
Vigabatrin	Drowsiness, dizziness, weight gain	Behavioural disturbances, severe psychosis
Zonisamide	Ataxia, dizziness, somnolence, anorexia	Hypersensitivity, weight decrease, rash, GI problems

the slow-release preparation of carbamazepine has distinct advantages, allowing twice-daily ingestion and avoiding high peak plasma concentrations. A 'chewtab' formulation is also available and pharmacokinetic studies have shown that it performs well even if inadvertently swallowed whole. Carbamazepine retard offers paediatric patients in particular a dosage form that reduces fluctuations in the peak to trough plasma levels and hence allows a twice-daily regimen, which can assist compliance.

Clobazam

Clobazam is a 1,5-benzodiazepine that is said to be less sedative than 1,4-benzodiazepine drugs such as clonazepam and diazepam. Although the development of tolerance is common, clobazam is used as an adjunctive therapy for patients with partial or generalized seizures who have proved unresponsive to other antiepileptic medication. Its intermittent use in catamenial epilepsy has also been suggested. Clobazam may produce less sedation than other benzodiazepines, but otherwise its adverse effects are similar, including dizziness, behavioural disturbances and dry mouth. Withdrawal may be difficult.

Clonazepam

Clonazepam, a 1,4-benzodiazepine, is a drug of choice for myoclonic seizures and a second-line drug for generalized tonic clonic seizures, absences, and as adjunctive therapy for partial seizures but, as with clobazam, effectiveness often wears off with time as tolerance develops. Parenteral clonazepam is useful in status epilepticus. It has an adverse effect profile similar to that of clobazam, but may be more sedating.

Diazepam

Diazepam is used mainly in the treatment of status epilepticus, intravenously or in the acute management of febrile convulsions as a rectal solution. Absorption from suppositories or following intramuscular injection is slow and erratic. The rectal solution may also be useful in status epilepticus if it is not possible to give the drug intravenously.

Ethosuximide

Ethosuximide is a drug of first choice for generalized absence seizures, and has no useful effect against any other seizure type. Tolerance does not seem to be a problem. The most commonly encountered adverse effects are gastrointestinal symptoms, which occur frequently at the beginning of therapy. Behaviour disorders, anorexia, fatigue, sleep disturbances and headaches may also occur. The therapeutic range commonly quoted is 40–100 μg/mL but some patients may require higher concentrations, sometimes as high as 150 μg/mL. The absorption of ethosuximide is complete, the bioavailability of the syrup and capsule formulations being equivalent. Increase in daily dose may lead to disproportionately higher increases in average plasma concentrations, therefore careful monitoring is indicated at high doses.

Felbamate

Felbamate may be used as a drug of last resort in patients with intractable epilepsy. It is licensed in the USA and most countries of the European Union but not in the UK. Its mechanism of action is unknown. The usual dose is between 1200 and 3600 mg/day.

Felbamate exhibits significant pharmacokinetic interactions with phenytoin, carbamazepine and valproic acid. Side effects of felbamate include diplopia, insomnia, dizziness, headache, ataxia, anorexia, nausea and vomiting. A major limiting problem is its potential to cause aplastic anaemia and liver failure, affecting up to 1 in 4000 patients exposed to the drug. It therefore seems prudent to limit its use to specialist centres and severe intractable cases.

Gabapentin

Gabapentin is a second-line treatment of partial seizures although its main use currently is for the treatment of neuropathic pain. The optimal dose remains to be established: the maximum recommended dose is currently 3600 mg/day, but the efficacy of higher doses is presently being investigated in clinical trials. In view of its pharmacokinetic profile, a three times daily dosage must be used. To date, no clinically significant interactions with other antiepileptic drugs, or other drugs, have been reported. The most frequently reported side effects are drowsiness, dizziness, diplopia, ataxia and headache. No idiosyncratic side effects have been reported so far.

Lamotrigine

Lamotrigine may be used as a first-line drug in patients with partial seizures, with or without secondary generalization, and in tonic clonic convulsions. The recommended starting dose is 50 mg when used as monotherapy, and 25 mg when used as an add-on therapy; the latter dose is given on alternate days in patients receiving concomitant sodium valproate and daily in patients receiving other antiepileptic drugs, with a maximum recommended dose of 400 mg/day in two divided doses. It should be slowly titrated as too rapid a titration may be associated with an increased incidence of skin rash. Lamotrigine does not seem to interact with other concomitantly administered antiepileptic drugs. However, hepatic enzyme inducers increase the metabolism of lamotrigine, reducing its half-life. Therefore, higher doses of lamotrigine need to be administered if it is used in conjunction with enzyme inducers such as phenytoin and carbamazepine. Inhibitors of hepatic enzymes such as sodium valproate block the metabolism of lamotrigine and reduced doses of lamotrigine need to be used if both drugs are given in combination.

Headaches, drowsiness, ataxia and diplopia, usually transient, are the most commonly reported acute adverse effects, particularly during dose escalation. A skin rash is the commonest idiosyncratic side effect of this drug and affects up to 3% of patients. There have been a few reports of fatalities due to disseminated intravascular coagulation and fulminant liver failure associated with the use of lamotrigine, but these rare events have to be seen in the context of more than 100 000 patients exposed to the drug.

Levetiracetam

Levetiracetam is indicated for the treatment of refractory partial epilepsy. Placebo-controlled trials in refractory partial epilepsy have shown a 50% seizure reduction in up to 40% of patients. In these trials 8% became seizure free compared to none on placebo. The usual dose is between 1500 and 3000 mg a day. It is usually started at 500 mg a day and the dose is titrated upwards in incremental steps of 500 mg every 1 or 2 weeks. It is well tolerated and the most frequent central nervous system adverse events are dizziness, irritability, asthenia and somnolence. No idiosyncratic adverse events have yet been reported.

Oxcarbazepine

Oxcarbazepine is an analogue of carbamazepine. It is an inactive pro-drug that is converted in the liver to the active 10-hydroxy metabolite and bypasses the 10,11-epoxide, the primary metabolite of carbamazepine. The usual dose is between 900 and 2400 mg/day. The spectrum of efficacy and side effects is broadly comparable to carbamazepine. The principal advantage of oxcarbazepine over carbamazepine is the lack of induction of hepatic enzymes, with the consequence that there is no autoinduction of the metabolism of the drug and fewer pharmacokinetic interactions. In addition, two-thirds of patients who are allergic to carbamazepine can tolerate oxcarbazepine.

Phenobarbital

Phenobarbital, a barbiturate, is a second-line drug for the treatment of tonic clonic, tonic and partial seizures. It may also be used in other seizure types. Its antiepileptic efficacy is similar to that of phenytoin or carbamazepine. Adverse effects on cognitive function, the propensity to produce tolerance and the risk of serious seizure exacerbation on withdrawal make it an unattractive option, and it should be used only as a last resort. In addition to cognitive effects, barbiturates may cause skin rashes, ataxia, folate deficiency, osteomalacia, behavioural disturbances (particularly in children) and an increased risk of connective tissue disorders such as Dupuytren's contracture and frozen shoulder. Phenobarbital is a potent enzyme inducer and is implicated in several clinically important drug interactions (see Table 31.6).

The normal adult plasma target range of 15–40 μg/mL should be interpreted with caution due to development of tolerance to some of the pharmacological effects as well as to the antiepileptic action. Decreased elimination is expected in patients with impaired renal or hepatic function. Once-a-day dosage is usually adequate in most adults because of the long half-life. However, as the steady state is not reached for 2–3 weeks, the administration of a loading dose is recommended. Routine monitoring is not necessary on initiating therapy as the dose can be adequately titrated according to the clinical response. However, monitoring is indicated if patients do not respond or exhibit toxicity.

Phenytoin

Phenytoin is a drug of first choice for tonic clonic, tonic and partial seizures, and a second-line drug for atonic seizures and atypical absences. It is not effective in typical generalized absences and myoclonic seizures. Tolerance to its antiepileptic action does not usually occur. Phenytoin has non-linear kinetics and a low therapeutic index, and in some patients frequent drug plasma level measurements may be necessary. Drug interactions (see Table 31.6) are common as phenytoin metabolism is very susceptible to inhibition by some drugs, while it may enhance the metabolism of others. Caution should be exercised when other medication is introduced or withdrawn.

Adverse events may occur in up to a half of patients treated with phenytoin, but only about 10% will necessitate drug withdrawal, most commonly due to skin rash. Dose-related adverse reactions including nystagmus, ataxia and lethargy are common. Cosmetic effects such as gum hypertrophy, hirsutism and acne are well-recognized adverse effects, and should be taken into account when prescribing for children and young women. Chronic adverse effects include folate deficiency, osteomalacia, Dupuytren's contractures and cerebellar atrophy. Serious idiosyncratic adverse events, including hepatic failure and bone marrow depression, are extremely uncommon.

Most patients require dosages from 250 to 400 mg daily. The drug shows slow and fast metabolism, hence slow metabolizers may require doses of 100–200 mg/day and fast metabolizers doses of 400–600 mg/day. The target plasma range for phenytoin is 10–20 μg/mL (although a number of patients are controlled outside the range). Once patients achieve levels within the target range, the majority require once-a-day dosage. Phenytoin is available in capsule, tablet, suspension and injection form. It is usually prescribed orally although it may be given intravenously. Oral preparations of phenytoin may present differences in bioavailability. Patients stabilized on one formulation should continue to receive the same formulation. Care is required when changing from the elixir to the capsule or tablet formulation due to the different bioavailability. Intravenous phenytoin should be administered with caution and at a rate not exceeding 50 mg/min. Intravenous phenytoin may be indicated when patients are on a nil-by-mouth regimen or require the drug for status epilepticus. Phenytoin ready-mixed parenteral formulation should not be added to intravenous fluids due to a risk of acid precipitation. The drug should never be given intramuscularly.

Pregabalin

This drug has been licensed for the adjunctive treatment of refractory partial epilepsy. It is closely related to gabapentin and a structural analogue of the neurotransmitter GABA but does not seem to affect transmitter response. It modulates calcium channels by binding to a subunit of Ca^{++} and this action is thought to be the basis of its antiepileptic mechanism.

The recommended doses for pregabalin are between 150 and 600 mg divided into two doses, although some people may respond to doses outside this range. Pregabalin would normally be started at 50 or 75 mg twice daily and increased in incremental steps of 50 mg every 2 weeks up to 600 mg according to clinical need. Pregabalin is available in 25, 50, 75, 100, 150, 200 and 300 mg tablets.

Overall, pregabalin is well tolerated and so far no idiosyncratic side effects have been described. Dizziness, drowsiness, ataxia, tremor and diplopia are the most common side effects. Weight gain, particularly with higher doses, seems to be a chronic side effect of this medication. No pharmacokinetic interactions have yet been identified.

In addition to its use in epilepsy, pregabalin has also been indicated for neuropathic pain and there are studies to suggest that it might be useful in generalized anxiety disorders.

Primidone

Primidone is principally metabolized to phenobarbital in vivo and has similar effects but a more severe side effect profile than phenobarbital. There is nothing to recommend primidone as an antiepileptic drug over phenobarbital.

Sodium valproate

Sodium valproate is a drug of first choice for the treatment of generalized absence seizures, myoclonic seizures and generalized tonic clonic seizures, especially if these occur as part of the syndrome of primary generalized epilepsy. Tolerance to its antiepileptic action does not usually occur. Drug interactions with other antiepileptic drugs may be problematic. Phenobarbital levels increase with co-medication with valproate, and a combination of these two drugs may result in severe sedation. Sodium valproate may also inhibit the metabolism of lamotrigine, phenytoin and carbamazepine. Enzyme-inducing drugs enhance the metabolism of sodium valproate, so caution should be exercised when other antiepileptic drugs are introduced or withdrawn.

Up to a third of patients may experience adverse effects, but fewer than 5% will require the drug to be stopped. Adverse effects include anorexia, nausea, diarrhoea, weight gain, alopecia, skin rash and thrombocytopenia. Confusion, stupor, tremor and hyper-ammonaemia are usually dose related. Serious adverse events, including fatal pancreatic and hepatic failure, are extremely uncommon. In children under 2 years, on other antiepileptic drugs and with pre-existing neurological deficit, the risk of this is 1/500. In adults on valproate monotherapy, the risk is 1/37 000.

The usual therapeutic range quoted is 50–100 μg/mL, although because of the lack of a good correlation between total valproate concentrations and effect, plasma level monitoring of the drug has limited use. TDM should only be performed in cases of suspected toxicity, deterioration in seizure control, to check compliance or to monitor drug interactions. Routine monitoring of this drug is not necessary.

Sodium valproate is likely to be more teratogenic than other commonly used antiepileptic drugs and should be used cautiously in women of child-bearing age.

Tiagabine

Tiagabine is a new drug with mild-to-moderate efficacy in seizure control. It is used as a second-line drug in partial seizures with or without secondary generalization. Results from controlled trials have shown that up to one-third of patients on tiagabine achieve a 50% reduction in seizure frequency, although complete remission from seizures is an infrequent occurrence. The usual dose is between 30 and 45 mg a day, and it is normally started at 10 mg/day in two divided doses, with incremental steps of 5 mg every 2 weeks. The most common adverse events are on the central nervous system and consist of sedation, tremor, headache, mental slowing, tiredness and dizziness. Confusion, irritability and depression may occur. Increases in seizure frequency and episodes of non-convulsive status have also been reported.

So far, no life-threatening idiosyncratic reactions have been reported. Use in pregnancy is not recommended although no teratogenicity has been reported in humans.

Topiramate

Topiramate is chemically unrelated to other antiepileptic drugs and is used as a second-line drug for patients with partial seizures. Usual doses are between 200 and 600 mg/day. It has to be titrated slowly, and the recommended starting dose is 25 mg once daily, titrating upwards in 25 mg/day increments every 2 weeks up to 200 mg/day in two divided doses. After that the dose should be increased by 50 mg every 2 weeks until seizure control is achieved or side effects develop. It has no clinically significant interactions with other antiepileptic drugs, although hepatic enzyme inducers accelerate its metabolism and topiramate doses need to be adjusted downwards if patients are coming off carbamazepine or phenytoin.

Side effects of topiramate include dizziness, drowsiness, nervousness, impaired concentration, paraesthesias, nephrolithiasis and fatigue. Patients starting topiramate should increase their fluid intake to reduce the risk of kidney stones. Weight loss is seen in up to 30% of patients.

Vigabatrin

Vigabatrin is an inhibitor of GABA transaminase but because of a poor safety profile, it is a last resort drug for partial seizures. Vigabatrin may also be useful in West's syndrome, particularly if associated with tuberous sclerosis. Vigabatrin does not interact with other drugs apart from decreasing phenytoin levels, probably by blocking its absorption. The most common adverse

events associated with vigabatrin are behavioural disturbances, ranging from agitation and confusion to frank psychosis and visual field defects. Other known adverse effects include drowsiness, headaches, ataxia, weight gain, depression and tremor. Careful monitoring for side effects, particularly ophthalmological, on initiation of therapy is essential. Routine TDM is not available for this drug.

Zonisamide

Zonisamide, a sulphonamide analogue which inhibits carbonic anhydrase, is a potent blocker of the spread of epileptic discharges. This effect is believed to be mediated through action at voltage-sensitive sodium channels.

It is used as a second-line drug for patients with partial seizures with or without secondary generalization. Anecdotal reports of its efficacy in other seizure types, particularly myoclonic seizures, need to be formally tested. Recommended doses are between 200 and 500 mg/day, although some patients may derive benefit from doses outside this range. The recommended starting dose for most patients is 100 mg once daily, titrating upwards every 2 weeks in 100 mg/day increments until seizure control is achieved or side effects develop. Its long elimination half-life allows once-daily dosing.

Zonisamide does not affect levels of carbamazepine, barbiturates or valproate, but may increase the plasma concentration of phenytoin by about 10–15%. Zonisamide metabolism is, however, induced by carbamazepine, barbiturates and phenytoin and higher zonisamide doses may be necessary during co-administration with these antiepileptic drugs.

Side effects of zonisamide include dizziness, drowsiness, headaches, hyporexia, nausea and vomiting, weight loss, skin rashes, irritability, impaired concentration and fatigue. These are mostly transient and seem to be related to the dose and rate of

Table 31.8 Common therapeutic problems in epilepsy

Problem	Comment
Hepatic enzyme induction	Enzyme induction occurs with carbamazepine, phenytoin, phenobarbital, primidone and topiramate. Interactions occur with a large number of drugs including oral contraceptives
Use of progesterone-only contraceptives with enzyme-inducing antiepileptic drug	Best avoided. If no acceptable alternative, patient should take at least double usual dose of progesterone-only pill
Use of combined oral contraceptive with enzyme-inducing antiepileptic drug	Preparations containing 50 µg of oestrogen should be used
Continuation of antiepileptic drug during pregnancy	Ideally review before attempting pregnancy to determine if reducing or discontinuing treatment is possible
Use of phenytoin as monotherapy	Less frequently considered first-line monotherapy due to poor side effect profile, narrow therapeutic index and saturation pharmacokinetics
Prescribing of branded antiepileptic drugs	Debate continues about whether significant differences exist between generic and branded antiepileptic drugs

titration. Nephrolithiasis has also been reported, particularly in caucasians. It is not recommended for women of child-bearing age as there are issues about its teratogenic potential.

Antiepileptic drugs in development

There are a number of potential antiepileptic compounds under-going clinical evaluation and these include rufinamide. Other drugs in development include: lacosamide, an aceto-propionamide amino acid; talamparel, an AMPA antagonist; NPS 1776, an aliphatic amide; and valrocemide, a valproryl derivative of GABA.

CASE STUDIES

Case 31.1

JB is a 31-year-old woman with a history of early morning myoclonic jerks starting at the age of 16. When she was 18 years old she had her first generalized tonic–clonic convulsive seizure. A diagnosis of juvenile myoclonic epilepsy was made and she was started on sodium valproate 1200 mg a day which controlled her seizures.

At the age of 21 the patient had a healthy baby and experienced no problems with epilepsy control. Aged 22, she had her second pregnancy and delivered a healthy baby girl. Three weeks after delivery early morning myoclonic seizures returned. The dose of sodium valproate was increased to 1500 mg to control jerks. However, 6 months later she experienced a recurrence of her convulsive attacks with no clear precipitating factor. Sodium valproate was increased to 2000 mg a day. Early morning myoclonic seizures crept back and she had further convulsive seizures. Lamotrigine was started at 200 mg daily. She has been completely seizure-free for the last 2 years and is now driving again.

JB wants to discuss her medication with you and would like to stop treatment. She has no plans to increase her family.

Question

What advice would you give JB?

Answers

JB should be advised to continue on medication. She has juvenile myoclonic epilepsy, which tends to recur when medication is withdrawn. The patient has no intention of having further children and therefore pregnancy need not be a consideration in the choice of her continued drug therapy. She is generally well and hence it would be sensible to advise her to continue with the present regimen, as sodium valproate and lamotrigine have a synergistic effect in juvenile myoclonic epilepsy. If, however, she wants to reduce medication, then a slow decrease of valproate with optimization of treatment with lamotrigine should be considered.

Case 31.2

OB is a 44-year-old man who suffers from partial epilepsy. An MRI scan shows a choroid cyst on the right temporal lobe, bilateral hippocampal sclerosis and cerebral atrophy. Seizures take the form of complex partial attacks and at night secondary generalizations

occur. He has had trials of treatment with every single drug in the book and almost every combination.

Six months ago, he was taking 225 mg of topiramate (could not tolerate more), 400 mg of phenytoin and 10 mg of clobazam each day. At this point levetiracetam was added and titrated up to 2000 mg a day. This led to a significant improvement in seizure control. Indeed, seizures have almost completely been abolished and he is only having occasional nocturnal events. He is, however, complaining of drowsiness and periods of unsteadiness.

Question

What treatment is appropriate for this patient?

Answer

Mr OB needs his drug regimen optimizing. The decision should be made to reduce either the dose of topiramate or that of phenytoin. The consensus view is that phenytoin should probably be reduced first. However, this patient had a bad experinece in the past when an attempt was made to discontinue phenytoin, at which time he had a significant increase in seizure frequency. It would therefore be more appropriate to discontinue topiramate in Mr OB.

This was done and his improvement has been mantained.

Case 31.3

Ms GD is a 28-year-old woman with a history of early morning myoclonic jerks since age 14 years. At 16 years of age she presented with her first generalized tonic clonic convulsive seizure and was referred to a hospital specialist who diagnosed juvenile myoclonic epilepsy. At that time Ms GD was started on sodium valproate 1200 mg a day and within a few weeks her seizures were totally controlled. Ms GD has since remained on the same medication and has been well controlled. However, she now wishes to start a family and is concerned about the effects of the valproate on her baby.

Question

What advice would you give Ms GD?

Answer

The available evidence indicates sodium valproate is teratogenic, with the most common malformation reported being neural tube defects. Ms GD has had no seizures for over 5 years and it must, therefore, be determined whether she still needs medication. The risk of recurrence is low since she has been fit free for well over 5 years. An important consideration is whether or not she is a driver since if she is taken off medication and has a seizure, she will be unable to hold a licence. The other issue is the effect of pregnancy on her seizure threshold as there is some evidence that up to 20% of women may experience an increase in fits during pregnancy. The options that need to be considered include change of medication. The following medicines need to be reviewed: lamotrigine, topiramate and levetiracetam.

Case 31.4

Mr TD is a 41-year-old patient who has cryptogenic partial epilepsy. He experienced his first seizure at age 14 and this was diagnosed as a secondary generalized attack, although discussing his history revealed he might have had complex partial seizures. Two years ago TD was referred for assessment but it was felt that he was not a candidate for surgery. TD was taking carbamazepine 1200 mg a day and could not tolerate higher doses. Previous trials of valproate, phenytoin, phenobarbital, vigabatrin, lamotrigine, oxcarbazepine and topiramate had demonstrated little benefit. Levetiracetam was started and increased to 2500 mg. Improvement in seizure control has been noted over the past 2 years with only two nocturnal complex partial seizures recorded. His current medication is levetiracetam 2500 mg/day and carbamazepine 1200 mg/day.

Question

What should be done next? Should Mr TD's therapy be reduced to levetiracetam monotherapy?

Answer

There is a need to discuss with TD whether he wishes to continue with his medication. Issues of relevance include a long history of epilepsy, the diagnosis and the range of drugs previously tried. It also needs to be clear whether he wishes to drive or not. If patients have been seizure free for 2 years, it is usual to review therapy.

Case 31.5

Mr PT is a 45-year-old business man who was involved in a road traffic accident and admitted to hospital with a fractured neck of femur and head trauma. He was stabilized but during his admission had two seizures and was discharged on carbamazepine 300 mg three time a day. One year on, he is reviewed by the neurology clinic and has had no further seizures. During the consultation routine blood levels are requested which include a plasma carbamazepine level. The results show that his carbamazepine level is non-detectable compared to an expected level of 6.5 mg/L. Following discussion, Mr PT explains that he stopped taking the carbamazepine 5 months ago.

Question

With regard to the carbamazepine results, what options should be discussed with Mr PT?

Answer

Mr PT requires a full neurological review. The long-term use of antiepileptics following head injury is not indicated unless the patient has a history of seizures. Mr PT has had no seizures post discharge even though his compliance has been poor. In view of the patient being well, it is likely his carbamazepine would be discontinued.

Case 31.6

DG is a 82-year-old retired bus driver who lives with his son and daughter-in-law. He has long-standing epilepsy and his current medication includes phenytoin 300 mg daily and phenobarbital 60 mg at night. DG is in general good health but suffered a recent fall and was rushed to hospital with a suspected fractured neck of femur. On admission he was stabilized and found not to have sustained a fracture. His other medication included furosemide 40 mg mane and enalapril 5 mg twice daily. Routine blood levels of the anticonvulsants revealed a toxic level of phenytoin of 50 mg/L (normal therapaeutic range 10–20 mg/L).

Question

How long will it take for the toxic levels of phenytoin to fall within the therapeutic range?

Answer

Phenytoin exhibits non-linear pharmacokinetics. Usual management will involve withholding phenytoin and monitoring plasma levels each day. One assumption that can be made is that if the hepatic enzymes are fully saturated with phenytoin then at maximum metabolic capacity, approximately 10 mg/L of the drug will be eliminated each day. Initially, however, the drug will redistribute into plasma so for the first few days phenytoin levels will fall slowly. It is usual for the levels to take 6–7 days to fall within the therapeutic range. Therapy will then need to be reviewed. On further investigation it was revealed the patient had mixed up his medications and was taking 300 mg phenytoin twice daily. The patient was counselled with regard to the correct dose and discharged.

REFERENCES

Duncan J S, Sander J W, Sisodiya S M et al 2006 Adult epilepsy. Lancet 367: 1087-1100

Feely M 1999 Drug treatment of epilepsy. British Medical Journal 318: 106-109

National Institute for Clinical Excellence 2004a New drugs for epilepsy in adults. Technology Appraisal 76. National Institute for Clinical Excellence, London. Available online at: www.nice.org.uk/download.aspx?o=ta076guidance

National Institute for Clinical Excellence 2004b Newer drugs for epilepsy in children. Technology Appraisal 79. National Institute for Clinical

Excellence, London. Available online at: www.nice.org.uk/page.aspx?o=ta079guidance

National Institute for Clinical Excellence 2004c The epilepsies: the diagnosis and management of the epilepsies in adults and children in primary and secondary care. Clinical Guideline 20. National Institute for Clinical Excellence, London. Available online at: www.nice.org.uk/page.aspx?o=CG020&c=cns

Sabers A, Gram L 2000 Newer anticonvulsants: comparative review of drug interactions and adverse effects. Drugs 60: 23-33

FURTHER READING

Brodie M J, Kwan P 2005 Epilepsy in elderly people. British Medical Journal 331: 1317-1322

Duncan J S, Shorvon S D, Fish D R (eds) 1995 Clinical epilepsy. Churchill Livingstone, Edinburgh

Perucca E 2006 Clinical pharmacokinetics of new-generation antiepileptic drugs at the extremes of age. Clinical Pharmacokinetics 45: 351-363

Sander J W A S, Shorvon S D 1996 The epidemiology of the epilepsies. Journal of Neurology, Neurosurgery and Psychiatry 61: 433-443

Tebb Z, Tobias J D 2006 New anticonvulsants – new adverse effects. Southern Medical Journal 99: 375-379

Parkinson's disease 32

D. J. Burn

KEY POINTS

- Parkinson's disease is the second most common neurodegenerative disease, affecting 1% of the population over the age of 65.
- Parkinson's disease is characterized by bradykinesia, rest tremor, rigidity and, later in the disease course, postural instability.
- Neuronal loss in the brainstem (substantia nigra) leads to a profound dopamine deficiency in the striatum. This provides the rationale for dopaminergic replacement therapies.
- Depression is common in Parkinson's disease. It is the major determinant of quality of life and is often missed. The depression of Parkinson's disease can be readily treated.
- Levodopa, coupled with a dopa-decarboxylase inhibitor, remains the most potent oral treatment for Parkinson's disease. There is debate as to whether levodopa should be deferred in biologically young patients, in an attempt to delay the onset of motor complications.
- Several other drug treatments are available for the management of Parkinson's disease. When given as adjunctive therapy to levodopa, the primary aim of these agents is to smooth out motor fluctuations.
- End-of-dose deterioration and the on–off phenomenon are motor complications synonymous with the use of levodopa, usually after a number of years. Despite advances in oral pharmacotherapy, the on–off phenomenon remains difficult to treat effectively.
- Surgical treatments of Parkinson's disease show promise, but require further evaluation.
- Advanced Parkinson's disease is difficult to manage, particularly neuropsychiatric problems. Reduction of dopaminergic therapy may be the best compromise.

Parkinson's disease is the most common cause of parkinsonism and is the second most common neurodegenerative disease, after Alzheimer's disease. Although descriptions of the condition appeared before the 19th century, it was James Parkinson's eloquent account in 1817 that fully documented the clinical features of the illness now bearing his name. The identification of dopamine deficiency in the brains of people with Parkinson's disease and the subsequent introduction of replacement therapy with levodopa represent a considerable success story in the treatment of neurodegenerative illness in general. There remain, however, a number of significant management problems in Parkinson's disease, particularly in the advanced stages of the condition.

Epidemiology

Parkinson's disease affects 1% of the population over 65 years of age, rising to 2% over the age of 80. One in 20 patients are, however, diagnosed before their 40th year. It is estimated that 110 000 people have Parkinson's disease in the UK. The condition is found worldwide, although it may be less common in China and West Africa. Most epidemiological studies have indicated a small male-to-female predominance.

Other causes of parkinsonism include the neurodegenerative conditions multiple system atrophy and progressive supranuclear palsy. Prevalences for these conditions are 4.3 and 5.0 per 100 000, respectively. Drug-induced parkinsonism is a common form of so-called 'symptomatic' parkinsonism. It affects 10–15% of individuals exposed to dopamine receptor-blocking agents (including neuroleptics and some labyrinthine sedatives).

Aetiology

Both genetic and environmental factors have been implicated as a cause of Parkinson's disease. While opinions were initially polarized, it now seems probable that in the majority of cases there is an admixture of influences, with environmental factors precipitating the onset of Parkinson's disease in a genetically susceptible individual.

Environmental factors became pre-eminent in the 1980s, when drug addicts attempting to manufacture pethidine accidently produced a toxin called MPTP (1-methyl-4-phenyl-1,2,3, 6-tetrahydropyridine). Ingestion or inhalation of MPTP rapidly produced a severe parkinsonian state, indistinguishable from advanced Parkinson's disease. Notably, not all individuals exposed to MPTP developed parkinsonism, either acutely or on subsequent follow-up, suggesting interindividual susceptibility to the toxic effects. MPTP is a relatively simple compound and is quite similar to paraquat. The demonstration that chronic systemic exposure to the pesticide rotenone can reproduce the clinical and pathological features of Parkinson's disease in rats has generated considerable interest.

In a small number of patients, genetic factors are dominant. The discovery of a mutation in the gene coding for a synaptic protein called α-synuclein provided tremendous impetus to research. Such mutations have been described in fewer than 10 families worldwide. Nevertheless, because α-synuclein is a major component of the pathological hallmark of Parkinson's disease, the Lewy body (see below), the challenge is to discover how a mutation in this protein in a tiny minority can relate to the formation of Lewy bodies in the vast majority. In recent years, eight genetic loci and a further four genes (parkin, DJ-1, PINK1 and dardarin) have been identified (Healy et al 2004). The intriguing thing is that the protein products of these genes are all involved in a cellular system called the ubiquitin-proteasomal system, which plays a crucial role in removing and recycling abnormal or damaged proteins. Current thinking is that abnormalities in the way in which the cell handles mutated or abnormal proteins may ultimately lead to its death, through increased oxidative stress and/or reduced mitochondrial energy production. The Lewy body may actually represent a defence mechanism by the cell to 'parcel up' potentially damaging proteinaceous material (Olanow et al 2004).

Pathophysiology

The characteristic pathological features of Parkinson's disease are neuronal loss in pigmented brainstem nuclei, together with the presence of eosinophilic inclusion bodies, called Lewy bodies, in surviving cells. The pars compacta of the substantia nigra in the midbrain is particularly affected. Dopaminergic neurones within this nucleus project to the striatum, which is therefore deprived of the neurotransmitter dopamine. In Parkinson's disease there is a loss of over 80% of nigral neurones before symptoms appear. There is controversy over the duration of this preclinical period, but current evidence favours a relatively short latency, of the order of 5 years.

Dopaminergic neurones are not the only cells to die within the brainstem, and a host of other nuclei and neurotransmitter systems are involved. For example, cholinergic neurones within the pedunculopontine nucleus degenerate, providing potential clinicopathological correlates with postural instability, swallowing difficulty (dysphagia) and sleep disturbance (REM sleep behavioural disturbance). The involvement of this nucleus in Parkinson's disease may explain why dopaminergic therapy is relatively ineffective in treating these particular clinical problems. Within the striatum, changes occur within γ-aminobutyric acid-positive neurones, as a consequence of nigrostriatal dopaminergic deficiency and also non-physiological dopaminergic replacement. These changes are thought to play a key role in mediating the development of involuntary movements (dyskinesias) which develop after a number of years of levodopa treatment. The loss of noradrenergic and serotonergic neurones within the locus coeruleus and the raphe nucleus, respectively, may provide a pathophysiological basis for depression, which is common in Parkinson's disease.

Clinical features

Bradykinesia is a sine qua non for parkinsonism in general. If a person does not have slowness of movement, they cannot have either parkinsonism or Parkinson's disease. Rest tremor, extra-pyramidal rigidity (so-called 'lead pipe' and/or 'cog-wheel') and postural instability comprise the remaining classic tetrad of clinical features for Parkinson's disease. Asymmetry of signs at disease onset is very common. The rest tremor is a rhythmic movement with a frequency of 4–6 Hz (cycles per second), typically noticed with the patient at rest. It is sometimes described as 'pill-rolling' in nature, from the movement of the thumb across the fingers. However, 15–20% of patients do not develop a tremor. Furthermore, up to 60% of people with Parkinson's disease may have a dominant postural tremor, worse with the arms held outstretched, which can cause diagnostic confusion with essential tremor (see

below). Postural instability is a late feature of Parkinson's disease, and comprises an impairment of righting reflexes with a tendency to fall. There may be a flexed truncal posture and loss of arm swing when walking. There is reduced blink frequency and facial expression, which, together with rather reduced volume (hypophonic) and monotonous speech, may lead to significant difficulties in communication. The patient may drool and have greasy skin (seborrhoea). Writing becomes small (micrographia) and barely legible.

Autonomic dysfunction may occur in Parkinson's disease. Urogenital difficulties, with erectile dysfunction in males and urinary urgency in both sexes, are commonly encountered. Frank incontinence is, however, rare. Constipation is invariable and is multifactorial in origin. Falling blood pressure on standing (postural hypotension) may contribute to falls later in the disease course. Depression affects approximately 40% of people with Parkinson's disease and is a major determinant of both carer stress and nursing home placement. It can be a very early feature, and may precede the onset, of Parkinson's disease. Recent studies have demonstrated that depression, above any other factor, is the most significant determinant of quality of life in the person with Parkinson's disease, yet it is generally underdiagnosed. The occurrence of dementia in Parkinson's disease is related predominantly to the age of the patient. Longitudinal community-based studies indicate that dementia may ultimately develop in nearly 80% of people with Parkinson's disease. The cognitive impairment may be accompanied by hallucinations (often visual), delusional misinterpretation (including paranoid ideation) and rapid fluctuations in attention.

Differential diagnosis

It is important to remember that, while Parkinson's disease is a common form of parkinsonism, there are numerous other degenerative and symptomatic causes. Furthermore, 'all that shakes is not Parkinson's disease'. Table 32.1 gives a differential

Table 32.1 Differential diagnosis of parkinsonism

Degenerative causes	Symptomatic causes
Parkinson's disease	Dopamine receptor blocking agents
Progressive supranuclear palsy (Steele–Richardson–Olszewski syndrome)	Cerebrovascular disease
Multiple system atrophy	Hydrocephalus (especially so-called 'normal pressure' hydrocephalus)
Alzheimer's disease Corticobasal ganglionic degeneration	Toxic (e.g. manganese, carbon monoxide, carbon disulfide, hydrocarbon, MPTP exposure) Postencephalitic parkinsonism
Wilson's disease Young-onset Huntington's disease (Westphal variant)	Dementia pugilistica ('punch drunk' syndrome)

diagnosis for causes of parkinsonism. These are separated into degenerative and symptomatic categories. The list is not exhaustive and excludes, for instance, rare parkinsonian manifestations in uncommon diseases. A detailed description of these different causes of parkinsonism is beyond the scope of this chapter, but a few points should be highlighted. Essential tremor is not included in Table 32.1, as this common condition does not cause bradykinesia. Nevertheless, it may be very difficult to differentiate from tremor-dominant Parkinson's disease. A positive family history and good response to alcohol may provide vital clues towards the diagnosis of essential tremor, although in practice these are not always reliable.

Several clinical and clinicopathological series have confirmed our fallibility in not making a correct diagnosis of Parkinson's disease. If clinical criteria, such as those produced by the UK Parkinson's Disease Brain Bank, are not applied, then the error rate (false-negative diagnosis) may be as high as 25–30%. These criteria are listed in Table 32.2. Degenerative conditions commonly masquerading as Parkinson's disease are progressive supranuclear palsy, multiple system atrophy and Alzheimer's disease.

Drug-induced parkinsonism

Perhaps the most important differential diagnosis to consider when a patient presents with parkinsonism is whether their symptoms and signs may be drug induced. This is because drug-induced parkinsonism (DIP) is potentially reversible upon cessation of the offending agent. Reports linking drug-induced parkinsonism with the neuroleptic chlorpromazine were first published in the 1950s. Since then, numerous other agents have been associated with drug-induced parkinsonism. Many of these are widely recognized,

although others are not (Table 32.3). Compound antidepressants may contain neuroleptic drugs (for example, fluphenazine is found with nortriptyline in Motival) and are not always recognized as potential culprits. Repeat prescription of vestibular sedatives and antiemetics such as prochlorperazine and cinnarizine is another commonly encountered cause of drug-induced parkinsonism. The pathogenesis of drug-induced parkinsonism is unlikely to be only due to dopamine receptor blockade. If this were the case the incidence and severity should correlate with the drug dosage and length of exposure, and this is not clearly observed.

Drug-induced parkinsonism is more common in the elderly and in women. The clinical features can be indistinguishable from Parkinson's disease, although the signs in drug-induced parkinsonism are more likely to be bilateral at the onset. Withdrawal of the offending agent will lead to improvement and resolution of symptoms and signs in approximately 80% of patients within 8 weeks of discontinuation. Drug-induced parkinsonism may, however, take up to 18 months to fully resolve in some cases. Furthermore, in other patients the parkinsonism may improve after stopping the drug, only to then deteriorate. In this situation, the drug may have unmasked previously latent Parkinson's disease. This contention is supported by a study which noted an increased risk of Parkinson's disease in subjects who had experienced a previous reversible episode of drug-induced parkinsonism.

Investigations

The diagnosis of Parkinson's disease is a clinical one and should be based, preferably, upon validated criteria. In young-onset or clinically atypical Parkinson's disease, a number of investigations may be appropriate. These include copper studies and DNA

Table 32.2 Clinical criteria for diagnosis of Parkinson's disease

Step 1 Diagnosis of parkinsonian syndrome

The patient has bradykinesia, plus one or more of the following:

(a) classic rest tremor

(b) muscular rigidity

(c) postural instability, without other explanation

Step 2 Exclusion criteria for Parkinson's disease

(a) history of repeated strokes	(i) supranuclear gaze palsy
(b) history of repeated head injury	(j) cerebellar signs
(c) history of definite encephalitis	(k) early severe autonomic involvement
(d) oculogyric crises	(l) early severe dementia
(e) dopamine receptor blocking agent exposure at onset of symptoms	(m) extensor plantar
(f) more than one affected relative	(n) cerebral tumour or hydrocephalus on CT
(g) sustained remission	(o) negative response to large doses of levodopa
(h) strictly unilateral features after 3 years	(p) MPTP exposure

---

Step 3 Supportive prospective positive criteria for Parkinson's disease (three or more required for diagnosis of definite Parkinson's disease)

(a) unilateral onset	(e) an excellent (>70%) response to levodopa
(b) rest tremor present	(f) a sustained (>5 years) response to levodopa
(c) progressive disorder	(g) severe levodopa-induced dyskinesias
(d) progressive persistent asymmetry	(h) clinical course >10 years

Table 32.3 Examples of non-neuroleptic drugs associated with drug-induced parkinsonism

Tetrabenazine
Calcium channel blockers (e.g. cinnarizine)
Amiodarone
Lithium[a]
Phenelzine[b]
Amphotericin B[c]
5-Fluorouracil[b]
Vincristine–adriamycin[b]
Pethidine[b]

[a] Lithium causes postural tremor. Reports of parkinsonism occurring with lithium have usually been in the context of prior exposure to neuroleptics.
[b] Only single case reports of drug-induced parkinsonism with these drugs.
[c] One case report of drug-induced parkinsonism in a child after bone marrow transplantation and a second in association with cytosine arabinoside therapy

testing to exclude Wilson's disease and Huntington's disease, respectively. Brain imaging by computed tomography (CT) or magnetic resonance imaging (MRI) may be appropriate to exclude hydrocephalus, cerebrovascular disease or basal ganglia abnormalities suggestive of an underlying metabolic cause. When there is difficulty in distinguishing Parkinson's disease from essential tremor, a form of functional imaging called FP-CIT SPECT (also known as DaTSCAN) may be useful, since this technique can sensitively identify loss of nigrostriatal dopaminergic terminals in the striatum (Fig. 32.1). Thus, in essential tremor the SPECT scan is normal, whereas in Parkinson's disease reduced tracer uptake is seen (Jennings et al 2004).

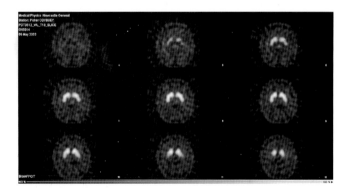

Fig 32.1 A normal FP-CIT SPECT scan image, showing symmetric tracer uptake in both striata ('mirror image commas'). In Parkinson's disease the tail of the comma is lost at an early stage, with the most severe loss being contralateral to the side most affected clinically.

The differentiation of Parkinson's disease from multiple system atrophy and progressive supranuclear palsy is a not uncommon clinical problem and may be very difficult, particularly in the early disease stages. FP-CIT SPECT cannot differentiate Parkinson's disease from these other forms of degenerative parkinsonism. Anal sphincter electromyography, tilt table testing for orthostatic hypotension and eye movement recordings may all be of some help, although they are rarely diagnostic in their own right.

Treatment

General approach

When treatment becomes necessary, it is impossible to generalize about which drug should be commenced. All currently available drugs for Parkinson's disease are symptomatic, since no agent has yet been shown, beyond reasonable doubt, to have disease-modifying or neuroprotective properties. There is no accepted algorithm for the treatment of Parkinson's disease, although a clinical management guideline has been produced (NICE 2004).

A number of factors, including age, severity and type of disease (tremor-dominant versus bradykinesia-dominant) and co-morbidity, need to be taken into account. The efficacy and tolerability of levodopa in Parkinson's disease were first described 1967, when the drug was started in low doses and gradually increased thereafter (Cotzias et al 1967). Unfortunately, despite dramatic initial benefits, the limitations of levodopa treatment were quickly realized and a phenomenon termed the 'long-term levodopa syndrome' was recognized. This syndrome comprises premature wearing off of the antiparkinsonian effects of levodopa, and response fluctuations. The wearing-off effect is the time before a patient is due their next dose of medication, during which they become increasingly bradykinetic. Response fluctuations can include dramatic swings between gross involuntary movements (dyskinesias) and a frozen, immobile state. The rapid and sudden switching between the dyskinetic state and profound akinesia is also termed the 'on–off' phenomenon. If this occurs rapidly and repeatedly, the term 'yo-yo-ing' is sometimes used. These problems emerge at a rate of approximately 10% per year, so that by 10 years into their illness all Parkinson's disease patients can expect to be experiencing such unpredictable responses. Notably, however, levodopa-induced dyskinesias and fluctuations develop earlier in younger Parkinson's disease patients than in older patients. On–off episodes may be extremely disabling and remain a major therapeutic challenge in the management of Parkinson's disease.

Current management trends have therefore shifted towards either late administration of levodopa, provided alternative treatments can give adequate symptomatic control, or the use of combination therapies, in an effort to reduce the longer term problems associated with levodopa. The evidence that such strategies benefit the patient beyond 5 years into their disease course is gradually increasing, although this remains an area of debate.

Drug treatment

Levodopa preparations

Immediate-release levodopa Irrespective of the debate regarding early or late levodopa therapy, there is no doubt that levodopa remains the most effective oral symptomatic treatment for Parkinson's disease. It is administered with the peripheral dopa-decarboxylase inhibitors carbidopa or benserazide, where carbidopa plus levodopa = co-careldopa (Sinemet) and benserazide plus levodopa = co-beneldopa (Madopar). The decarboxylase inhibitor blocks the peripheral conversion of levodopa to dopamine and thereby allows a lower dose of levodopa to be administered. Levodopa readily crosses the blood–brain barrier and is converted by endogenous aromatic amino acid decarboxylase to dopamine and then stored in surviving nigrostriatal nerve terminals.

Immediate-release levodopa is usually commenced in a dose of 50 mg per day, increasing every 3–4 days until a dose of 50 mg three times daily is reached. The patient should be instructed in the early stage of the illness to take the drug with food to minimize nausea. Paradoxically, in more advanced Parkinson's disease it may be beneficial to take levodopa 30 minutes or so before food, since dietary protein can critically interfere with the absorption of the drug.

If there is little or no response to 50 mg three times daily, the unit dose may be doubled to 100 mg. Should the patient's levodopa dose escalate to 600 mg per day with no significant response, the diagnosis of Parkinson's disease should be reviewed. Levodopa, commenced in the above way, is usually well tolerated. Nausea, vomiting and orthostatic hypotension are the most commonly encountered side effects. These adverse events may be circumvented by increasing the levodopa dose even more slowly, or co-prescribing domperidone 10 or 20 mg three times daily. Later in the illness, and in common with all antiparkinsonian drugs, levodopa may cause vivid dreams, nightmares or even a toxic confusional state.

Clinically relevant drug interactions with levodopa include hypertensive crises with monoamine oxidase type A inhibitors. Levodopa should therefore be avoided for at least 2 weeks after stopping the inhibitor. Levodopa can also enhance the hypotensive effects of antihypertensive agents and may antagonize the action of antipsychotics. The absorption of levodopa may be reduced by concomitant administration of oral iron preparations.

Controlled-release levodopa Both Sinemet and Madopar are available as controlled-release (CR) preparations. The nomenclature for Sinemet CR is confusing, as the drug is marketed as Sinemet CR (carbidopa/levodopa 50/200) and also as Half Sinemet CR (carbidopa/levodopa 25/100). Trying to prescribe Half Sinemet CR unambiguously can be difficult. If the instruction is misinterpreted and a tablet of Sinemet CR is halved, the slow-release mechanism is actually disrupted.

Levodopa in CR preparations has a bioavailability of 60–70%, which is less than the 90–100% obtained from immediate-release formulations. CR preparations have response duration of 2–4 hours, compared with 1–3 hours for immediate release.

Two large studies in early Parkinson's disease over 5 years have not shown any benefit for CR use over immediate-release levodopa in terms of dyskinesias and response fluctuation frequency. However, CR preparations may be of help in simplifying drug regimens, in relieving nocturnal akinesia, and in co-prescribing with immediate-release levodopa during the day to relieve end-of-dose deterioration.

Two commonly encountered problems with CR preparations are, first, changing the patient from all immediate release to all CR levodopa. This is poorly tolerated, as CR levodopa

has a longer latency than immediate-release levodopa to turn the patient 'on' (typically 60–90 versus 30–50 minutes), and the patient's perception is that the quality of their 'on' period is poorer. Second, CR preparations should not be prescribed more than four times a day, as the levodopa may accumulate, causing unpredictable motor fluctuations.

Duodopa A highly soluble form of levodopa has become available that is administered directly into the small bowel via the percutaneous route, using a portable electronic pump device. Through continuous delivery in this way, motor fluctuations may be significantly reduced. Although effective, this treatment modality requires careful patient selection and further evaluation.

Dopamine agonists

In theory, dopamine agonists, which stimulate dopamine receptors both post- and presynaptically, would seem to be a very attractive therapeutic option in Parkinson's disease, since they may bypass the degenerating nigrostriatal dopaminergic neurones. Unfortunately, experience to date with the oral agents available has usually shown them to be less potent than levodopa and less well tolerated. One drug in this class, apomorphine, is used in a parenteral form. It is particularly potent and is described in detail below.

Dopamine agonists differ in their affinity for a number of receptors, including the dopamine receptor family. It is not known whether these differences are clinically significant, but experience to date would suggest not. Cabergoline is a relatively new ergot dopamine agonist with a much longer plasma half-life of 63–68 hours than other agents in this class. This means that once-daily dosing is possible. Prolonged and non-pulsatile stimulation of dopamine receptors may, theoretically, be less likely to cause dyskinesias. Ropinirole and pramipexole are non-ergot derivatives. A novel transdermally administered dopamine agonist, rotigotine, will also be available in the near future (Parkinson Study Group 2003).

Four double-blind, randomized and controlled studies of up to 5 years' duration have compared the use of a dopamine agonist (cabergoline, ropinirole, pramipexole and pergolide) with levodopa in the treatment of early Parkinson's disease. Although the studies differed in a number of ways, such as levodopa supplementation not being permitted in the pergolide study, the results produced a consistent message that use of dopamine agonists in early Parkinson's disease is associated with a lower incidence of dyskinesias when compared with levodopa. Supplementary levodopa was, however, required in a significant number of patients in the cabergoline (65% of patients initially randomized to cabergoline), ropinirole (66% of patients initially randomized to ropinirole) and pramipexole (53% of patients initially randomized to pramipexole) studies, suggesting that only a subgroup of patients derive adequate benefit from agonist monotherapy alone. Further clinical follow-up will hopefully address the issue of what happens to patients receiving agonist monotherapy when they finally require levodopa. Notably, will the dyskinesia rate rapidly increase and catch up with other patients previously exposed to levodopa or will it remain at a lower frequency? Open-label 'naturalistic' extensions of several years' duration to some of the dopamine agonist studies have been undertaken, e.g. for ropinirole, and indicate that the dyskinesia rate does not seem to rapidly increase when levodopa is required. All the agonists may be used as add-on therapy to levodopa in the later stages of the disease, when motor control has become suboptimal. This may necessitate a concomitant reduction in levodopa dosage to avoid excessive dopaminergic side effects.

There have been very few comparative studies performed between the dopamine agonists, so it is not possible to be definitive as to which drug should be recommended. In practice, it is often worth changing from one agonist to another if side effects are a problem, since there is variability in a given patient's tolerance to the different drugs.

The principal side effect of the dopamine agonists are nausea and vomiting, postural hypotension, hallucinations and confusion, and exacerbation of dyskinesias. Ergot derivatives run the risk of causing pleuropulmonary fibrosis, which occurs in 2–6% of patients on long-term bromocriptine treatment. Annual monitoring with chest x-ray and erythrocyte sedimentation rate (ESR) has been suggested for patients taking ergot derivative agonists, although the utility and cost-effectiveness of this recommendation have not been established. More recently, concern has been expressed over the high frequency of cardiac valvulopathy, notably of the tricuspid valve, found in patients exposed to pergolide, another ergot derivative. It has now been withdrawn from use in many countries. Pergolide should no longer be used as a first-line agonist in Parkinson's disease and it prescribed, regular echocardiographic monitoring should be undertaken. There is also an increased risk of toxicity when erythromycin is co-prescribed with a dopamine agonist.

Ropinirole and pramipexole were previously implicated in causing 'sleep attacks', with sudden onset of drowsiness, leading to driving accidents in some cases. The term 'sleep attack' is almost certainly a misnomer, however, as patients do have warning of impending sleepiness, although they may subsequently be amnesic for up to several minutes while in this state. Excessive sleepiness attributable to antiparkinsonian drugs is actually not a new phenomenon, and is almost certainly a 'class effect' of all dopaminergic therapies. It is essential to advise patients taking all antiparkinsonian agents that they may be prone to excessive drowsiness. This may be compounded by the use of other sedative drugs and alcohol.

Catechol-O-methyl transferase inhibitors

Inhibitors of the enzyme catechol-O-methyl transferase (COMT) represent a novel addition to the range of therapies available for Parkinson's disease (Schrag 2005). Use of the first agent in this class, tolcapone, was originally suspended in the EU because of fears over hepatotoxicity, although the drug became available again in 2005, accompanied by strict prescribing and monitoring guidelines. Entacapone is also available and studies have not shown derangement of liver function with this drug.

COMT itself is a ubiquitous enzyme, found in gut, liver, kidney and brain among other sites. In theory, COMT inhibition may occur both centrally, where the degradation of dopamine to homovanillic acid is inhibited, and peripherally, where conversion of levodopa to the inert 3-O-methyldopa is inhibited, to benefit the patient with Parkinson's disease. In practice, both tolcapone and entacapone act primarily as peripheral COMT inhibitors.

Placebo-controlled studies in patients with fluctuating Parkinson's disease have confirmed the efficacy of entacapone in decreasing 'off' time, and permitting a concomitant reduction in levodopa dose. A 20% reduction in 'off' time is reported, translating into nearly 1.5 hours less immobility per day. This reduction tends to occur towards the end of the day, a time when many Parkinson's disease patients are at their worst in terms of motor function. A comparison of entacapone and tolcapone suggested that tolcapone may be the more potent COMT inhibitor, achieving up to an extra 1.5 hours of 'on' time per day.

When entacapone is prescribed, a 200 mg dose is used with each dose of levodopa administered, up to a frequency of 10 doses per day. Because of increased dyskinesias, an overall reduction of 10–30% in the daily dose of levodopa may be anticipated. Entacapone can be employed with any other antiparkinsonian drug, although caution may be needed with apomorphine. More recently, entacapone has been marketed as a compound tablet with levodopa and carbidopa (Stalevo). Although each tablet contains 200 mg of the COMT inhibitor, there are three different doses of levodopa available (50 mg, 100 mg and 150 mg), to provide flexibility. The compound tablet may help compliance by significantly reducing the total daily number of tablets a patient needs to take.

Tolcapone is prescribed as a fixed 100 mg three times a day regimen, increasing if necessary to 200 mg three times a day. It may only be used after the patient has tried and failed entacapone and where provision for 2-weekly monitoring of liver function tests for the first 12 months, reducing in frequency therafter, is available. Again, a concomitant reduction in levodopa may be necessary to offset an increase in dyskinesias.

The optimal way to use COMT inhibition is unknown. A patient experiencing end-of-dose deterioration, or generally underdosed, would seem to be the ideal candidate. However, there are few comparative studies of COMT inhibitors versus dopamine agonists available to provide guidance as to which class of drug is best to use, and when. Trials are under way to assess the potential benefits of combined treatment with levodopa and COMT inhibitors in de novo Parkinson's disease patients. These studies will address whether this combined treatment is associated with a lower incidence of motor complications.

Other than exacerbation of dyskinesias, COMT inhibitors may also cause diarrhoea, abdominal pain and dryness of the mouth. Urine discolouration is reported in approximately 8% of patients taking entacapone.

It is best to avoid non-selective monoamine oxidase inhibitors or a daily dose of selegiline in excess of 10 mg when using entacapone. In addition, the co-prescription of venlafaxine and other noradrenaline (norepinephrine) reuptake inhibitors is best avoided. Entacapone may potentiate the action of apomorphine. Patients taking iron preparations should be advised to separate this medication and entacapone by at least 2 hours.

Monoamine oxidase type B inhibitors

The propargylamines selegiline and rasagiline are inhibitors of monoamine oxidase type B. Inhibition of this enzyme slows the breakdown of dopamine in the striatum. These agents effectively have a 'levodopa-sparing' effect and may delay the onset of, or reduce existing, motor complications. Both drugs may also have an antiapoptotic effect (apoptosis is a form of programmed cell death thought to be important in several neurodegenerative conditions, including Parkinson's disease). Whether or not the drugs have a neuroprotective effect by this or some other means remains controversial and further clinical trials are planned for rasagiline to investigate this further.

A single daily dose of 5 mg or 10 mg of selegiline is prescribed. Higher doses are associated with only minimal additional inhibition of monoamine oxidase. Selegiline may also be administered as a lyophilized freeze-dried buccal preparation. The dose of rasagiline is 1–2 mg daily. Both selegiline and rasagiline may be used as de novo or adjunctive treatments in Parkinson's disease, although trial data for the latter indication are strongest for rasagiline and buccal selegiline (Rascol et al 2005).

Following publication of a study (Lees 1995) which showed excess mortality in a group of patients taking selegiline, it was suggested that the drug was best avoided in patients with falls, confusion and postural hypotension. A subsequent meta-analysis, including nine trials of selegiline, did not, however, identify any excess mortality in patients taking selegiline (Ives et al 2004). Selegiline can cause hallucinations and confusion, particularly in moderate-to-advanced disease. The withdrawal of selegiline may then be associated with significant deterioration in motor function. Unlike selegiline, rasagiline is not metabolized to amfetamine-like products, so neuropsychiatric side effects are less frequent. Selegiline should not be co-prescribed with selective serotonin reuptake inhibitors, since a serotonin syndrome, including hypertension and neuropsychiatric features, has been reported in a small minority of cases.

Amantadine

Amantadine was introduced as an antiparkinsonian treatment in the late 1960s. It has a number of possible modes of action, including facilitation of presynaptic dopamine release, blocking dopamine reuptake, an anticholinergic effect, and also as a N-methyl-D-aspartate (NMDA) receptor antagonist. Initially employed in the early stages of treatment, where its effects are mild and relatively short-lived, interest has focused more recently upon the use of amantadine as an antidyskinetic agent in advanced disease (Blanchet et al 2003).

Daily doses of 100–300 mg amantadine may be used. Some recommend even higher doses for improved antidyskinetic effect although side effects become much more frequent at higher doses. These side effects include a toxic confusional state, peripheral oedema and livedo reticularis (a persistent patchy reddish-blue mottling of the legs, and occasionally the arms). There may be significant rebound worsening of parkinsonism when amantadine is withdrawn. The mechanism for this is unknown.

Anticholinergic drugs

The availability of anticholinergic drugs such as trihexyphenidyl and orphenadrine predated the introduction of levodopa by nearly 90 years. Anticholinergic drugs have a moderate effect in reducing tremor but do not have any significant benefit upon bradykinesia.

The use of these agents has declined because of troublesome side effects, including constipation, urinary retention, cognitive impairment and toxic confusional states. In selected younger patients, an anticholinergic drug may still be helpful but close monitoring is advised. Postmortem studies have suggested that long-term anticholinergic use may have adverse disease-modifiyng effects in Parkinson's disease, by increasing cortical levels of Alzheimer-type pathology (Perry et al 2003).

Tricyclic antidepressants have anticholinergic properties, normally regarded as a disadvantage in the treatment of depression. These drugs are generally longer acting than other anticholinergic agents and may have a potential benefit in Parkinson's disease, both for their anticholinergic effects and also their effect in inhibiting monoamine reuptake at adrenergic nerve endings. A low dose of a tricyclic antidepressant, e.g. amitriptyline 10–25 mg, at night is sometimes useful in alleviating nocturnal akinesia, improving sleep and improving performance early in the morning.

Apomorphine

Apomorphine is a specialized, but almost certainly underused, drug in the treatment of Parkinson's disease. It is the most potent dopamine agonist available and is administered either by bolus subcutaneous injection or by continuous subcutaneous infusion. The drug is acidic and is generally difficult to administer in a stable form which does not lead to irritation of skin or mucosal surfaces. Alternative methods of administration, including transdermal and intranasal routes and the use of an implantable copolymer-based apomorphine matrix, are being evaluated.

The drug produces a reliable 'on' effect with short latency of action. A single bolus lasts for up to 60 minutes, depending upon the dose given. Continuous subcutaneous apomorphine may significantly improve dyskinesias in advanced Parkinson's disease, as well as lessening akinesia and rigidity. This may allow oral antiparkinsonian medications to be reduced.

Apomorphine causes profound nausea, vomiting and orthostatic hypotension. These problems are counteracted by pre-dosing for 2–3 days with domperidone 20 mg three times daily. Neuropsychiatric disturbance, probably at a lower frequency than with oral agonists, and skin reactions, including nodule formation, are other potential side effects. Apomorphine, in conjunction with levodopa, may cause a Coomb's positive haemolytic anaemia, which is reversible. It is recommended that patients be screened before beginning treatment and at 6-monthly intervals thereafter.

Surgical treatment

There has been renewed interest in the use of neurosurgical techniques for the treatment of Parkinson's disease (Walter & Vitek 2004). This has resulted not only from recognition of the shortcomings of medical treatment currently available, but also from an improved understanding of basal ganglia circuitry and better neuroimaging methods. Table 32.4 summarizes techniques currently being employed and evaluated. The functional effects of lesioning (-otomy) and the use of deep brain stimulation are similar, in that the high frequency used in stimulation is believed to act by blocking neurones. Deep brain stimulation has the advantage of being reversible but is costly, and programming the stimulator may be very time-consuming.

The subthalamic nucleus target is the current target of choice in most centres and the number of published patient-years experience with this surgical approach is rapidly increasing. An ongoing

Table 32.4 Summary of anatomical targets for surgical treatment of Parkinson's disease

Target	Bradykinesia	Tremor	Dyskinesia	Comments
Thalamus	–	+++	–	Bilateral thalamotomy is not recommended because of a high incidence of bulbar dysfunction
Globus pallidus	++	++	+++	10–15% incidence of persistent adverse events with unilateral pallidotomy; no reliable data for bilateral procedures
Subthalamic nucleus	+++	+++	++	Weight gain, contralateral dyskinesia, involuntary eyelid closure and speech disturbance reported

+ to +++ refers to the relative efficacy of the procedure for the clinical feature; – refers no benefit for the procedure for the clinical feature.
For each of the three targets listed, both ablation and stimulation procedures have been evaluated.

multicentre UK study of surgery targeted to this structure versus optimal medical therapy aims to clarify the potential benefits to be gained from deep brain stimulation of the subthalamic nucleus. Careful case selection is essential for all forms of surgical intervention for Parkinson's disease: older and less biologically fit patients, those with active cognitive and/or neuropsychiatric problems, and patients with a suboptimal levodopa response are generally regarded as poor surgical candidates.

Surgery may also play a role in neurorestorative treatments. Such approaches include stem cell and fetal cell transplantation, and also xenotransplantation (use of tissue from another species). To date, there have been conflicting results regarding the efficacy of fetal cell transplants. These differences may well reflect transplantation technique, the nature of the tissue being implanted, whether immunosuppression is prescribed, and how patients are selected and assessed. Despite the seemingly negative results from double-blind studies of embryonic cell implantation, researchers continue to explore the potential benefits from this approach.

Patient care

Table 32.5 lists some common therapeutic problems encountered in the management of people with Parkinson's disease. After diagnosis, the provision of an explanation of the condition, education and support are essential. The Parkinson's Disease Society (www.parkinsons.org.uk) produces an excellent range of literature to help the newly diagnosed patient come to terms with the condition. In accordance with advice given by the Society itself, patients who drive are advised to inform their insurance company and also the Driver and Vehicle Licensing Agency.

A doctor will record impairments in the clinic, while the patient is more concerned with their disability and handicap. Thus, a patient can be noted to have seemingly marked impairments and yet may not complain about significant disability. The converse may also be true. Not all patients, therefore, require immediate treatment. Furthermore, concomitant depression may distort the patient's perception of their disability, leading to inappropriate prescribing of antiparkinsonian therapy. In this

Table 32.5 Practice points in Parkinson's disease

Problem	Cause	Possible solution
Early-onset dyskinesias in young Parkinson's disease patients	Exposure to levodopa? Biological factors?	Delay introduction of levodopa (e.g. use a dopamine agonist)
One dose of levodopa does not last to the next ('wearing off')	Advancing disease (pre- and postsynaptic changes)	More frequent doses of levodopa; COMT inhibitor or dopamine agonist
Pain and immobility during the night	Evening dose of levodopa not lasting long enough	Use of slow-release levodopa or dopamine agonist
Freezing episodes and/or unpredictable motor fluctuations	Advancing disease (pre- and postsynaptic changes)	Apomorphine Consider Duo-dopa or surgery
Mismatch between patient's symptoms and signs	Underlying depression?	Antidepressant
Confusion and hallucinations with preserved cognition	Toxic (drug-related) psychosis	Review and reduce antiparkinsonian therapy
Confusion and hallucinations with impaired cognition	Underlying brain pathology ± drug effects	Reduce and simplify antiparkinsonian drugs as far as possible. Support team. Cholinesterase inhibitor

situation, the use of an antidepressant may be more helpful. There is no good evidence base for which antidepressant should be used, and both the tricyclic agents and selective serotonin reuptake inhibitors have their advocates.

Accurate compliance with the timing of therapy may be particularly important in patients who are beginning to develop long-term treatment complications. It can be helpful for patients to keep diary cards when they begin to experience problems with either bradykinesia or dyskinesia, so that these symptoms can be related to drug and food intake. Careful changes in timing of drug therapy or meals may initially be sufficient to reduce variation in performance. Some patients experience troublesome early morning bradykinesia. It may then be beneficial to prescribe an initial dose of a rapidly acting agent, such as dispersible oral co-beneldopa, to take on first wakening so that the patient can then get up and dress. A combination of levodopa with dopamine agonists, which are more slow acting, may be useful in the patient with motor fluctuations. A combination of levodopa and a COMT inhibitor may be more appropriate in a patient with end-of-dose deterioration.

Other factors that need to be considered in patients with Parkinson's disease are the benefits of adequate sleep and rest at night, which may be made more difficult if they have urinary frequency or problems with nocturnal bradykinesia. Judicious use of hypnotic therapy may be appropriate, while a tricyclic antidepressant may offer the dual benefit of sedation with anticholinergic effect. Low friction sheets to assist turning in bed and encouragement of mobility through physiotherapy may also be helpful. The treatment of the patient with severe disease remains one of the greatest challenges in the management of Parkinson's disease. On–off fluctuations may be refractory to oral dopaminergic therapies. Sudden freezing episodes compound failing postural stability, leading to increasing falls and injuries. In select patients, the use of apomorphine, either as a bolus injection or as a continuous subcutaneous infusion, may be helpful.

The presence of reduced dexterity in virtually all people with Parkinson's disease means that thought needs to be given to the way in which medication is dispensed and stored. If the patient is taking a complex regimen of drugs or has early cognitive problems, the use of pre-packaged therapies may improve compliance.

Patients' relatives also need emotional and social support through what can be a very demanding period. The loss of physical mobility, together with a personality change, can be very difficult for relatives to cope with. The involvement of occupational therapists and social workers in this situation is important.

Psychosis and dementia

When cognitive impairment is problematic the use of conventional antipsychotic medication is inappropriate because such drugs can precipitate a catastrophic worsening of parkinsonism. Behavioural disturbances require discussion with carers and, if possible, with the patient him- or herself. A graded withdrawal of antiparkinsonian drugs is often indicated, aiming to simplify the regimen to levodopa monotherapy. In rare cases it may be necessary to reduce the dose or even completely withdraw levodopa therapy in order to control aggressive, sexually demand-

ing or psychotic features. When reduction in dopaminergic therapy is ineffective or not tolerated because of unacceptable immobility, an atypical antipsychotic drug may be considered. In practice, the choice narrows down to quetiapine, since risperidone and olanzepine are associated with worsening parkinsonism, even in low doses. Furthermore, both risperidone and olanzepine should not be used in cognitively impaired elderly people because of an increased risk of stroke. Clozapine is difficult to use for Parkinson's disease-associated psychosis in the UK, because of the need to register the patient with a blood-monitoring programme. When quetiapine is used, it should be commenced in a low dose of 25 or 50 mg at night and increased slowly. The sedative effects may be helpful in promoting sleep.

Cholinesterase inhibitors have shown promise in treating the neuropsychiatric features of Parkinson's disease and may also have modest cognitive-enhancing benefits. Visual hallucinations, delusions, apathy and depression seem to be particularly responsive to these agents. These effects have been demonstrated for rivastigmine in dementia associated with Parkinson's disease in a large, multicentre, double-blind, placebo-controlled study (Emre et al 2004). The results of a randomized placebo-controlled study of donepezil are eagerly awaited.

Autonomic problems

Other co-existing medical complications that may need attention include disorders of gut motility, which present as constipation or difficulty with swallowing, disturbances of micturition, sometimes presenting as nocturia, and postural hypotension. Constipation can be managed in the usual way with bulking agents and, if necessary, stimulant laxatives and stool-softening agents. The management of postural hypotension includes assessment of the patient's autonomic function in order to establish whether this is primarily drug related or associated with autonomic neuropathy. If the patient is dizzy on standing, simple measures such as advice on rising slowly may be adequate. The use of elastic stockings, to reduce pooling of the blood in the lower limbs, is sometimes helpful. Pharmacological approaches include the use of fludrocortisone or occasionally midodrine (a selective α_1-adrenergic agonist). It is also important to consider other therapies the patient is receiving that might contribute to such symptoms, e.g. diuretics, and to stop these if possible.

CASE STUDIES

Case 32.1

A 70-year-old man, Mr W, was diagnosed as having mild Parkinson's disease 6 months ago. This did not require any treatment. He has no past medical history of note. He returns to clinic and it is clear that both his impairment and disability have worsened.

Questions

1. What initial treatment options should be considered for Mr W?
2. What considerations should be given to the initial drug choice?

Answers

1. There is no evidence to suggest that Mr W is depressed; a masked depression should always be considered when there is a 'mismatch' between impairment and reported disability. This was not the case here. A number of first-line antiparkinsonian drugs might therefore be considered, including immediate-release levodopa preparations, dopamine agonists and monoamine oxidase type B inhibitors.

2. Co-morbid illness or a life-shortening problem, such as cancer, usually mean that levodopa would be first choice, simply because it is most potent, with a good risk:benefit ratio. If the patient is biologically fit, then either a dopamine agonist or a monoamine oxidase type B inhibitor might be appropriate, so long as the disability is not too severe and there are no other contraindications. Dopamine agonists and selegiline, in particular, have the potential to cause or exacerbate neuropsychiatric problems and the patient and their family should be warned of such side effects. By using these 'levodopa-sparing' agents, the onset of dyskinesias may be delayed by several years.

Case 32.2

A 59-year-old gentleman, Mr X, has had Parkinson's disease for 8 years. This was initially treated with selegiline and ropinirole. Because of progressive functional disability and his wish to keep working, levodopa was introduced 5 years previously. He is now experiencing severe motor fluctuations during the day, with periods of marked dyskinesia and also increasingly unpredictable 'off' periods, during which he is stiff, immobile and anxious. Unsuccessful attempts to smooth out these fluctuations have been made by manipulating his levodopa unit dose and frequency, the use of entacapone, and changing his dopamine agonist.

Questions

1. What therapeutic options could be considered in Mr X's case?
2. What factors would influence the choice of treatment?

Answers

1. A relatively simple option that has not yet been considered is amantadine. This agent may have useful antidyskinetic effects in advanced Parkinson's disease. It is usually administered as 100 mg daily initially, increasing gradually to two or three times daily. The dose of levodopa therapy is left unchanged, to avoid worsening 'off' periods. Neuropsychiatric problems and/or a livedinous rash may complicate the use of amantadine, although younger patients are often able to tolerate the drug better. An alternative approach which may well be required is the use of continuous subcutaneous apomorphine with or without amantadine, as this may have a significant antidyskinetic effect and also effectively manage freezing episodes. Duodopa therapy, admininistered via a gastrostomy, may also be a consideration. finally, deep brain stimulation of the subthalamic nucleus may be appropriate for Mr X.

2. Patient choice, after being given the relevant options, is clearly important, as the treatments involved are potentially invasive and associated with morbidity. A previous history of neuropsychiatric problems, active psychosis or severe depression, or cognitive impairment would be relative contraindications to surgery. Severe needle phobia or the lack of an appropriately experienced and committed local nurse specialist would compromise the effective administration of apomorphine.

Case 32.3

A 63-year-old lady, Mrs Y, is referred by a colleague for consideration of deep brain stimulation surgery for her tremor-dominant Parkinson's disease which has been refractory to levodopa medication. The tremor is causing severe embarrassment and is functionally disabling. The patient also has a long history of 'dizzy turns'.

Questions

1. Which question might give additional diagnostic help in this lady's history?
2. What would be the best management?

Answers

1. Given this lady's history of 'dizzy turns', one must always be suspicious that she may have been prescribed labyrinthine sedatives. In fact, Mrs Y had been taking prochlorperazine, 15 mg three times a day, for over 8 years.

2. Discontinuation of the prochlorperazine is vital. If vertigo recurs, betahistine is safe to use in this context. A 'watch and wait' approach for 2–3 months is then reasonable, to see if Mrs Y improves. Thereafter, her levodopa medication could be gradually withdrawn over several weeks. If there is lingering doubt over the diagnosis, an FP-CIT SPECT scan can be helpful; in Parkinson's disease, the scan is abnormal whereas in drug-induced parkinsonism, because the problem is caused by postsynaptic blockade of dopamine receptors, tracer uptake will be normal. In this case, Mrs Y's tremulous parkinsonism resolved completely and she was able to come off all medication. She also avoided surgery!

Case 32.4

Mr Z has an 8-year history of Parkinson's disease. He is 77 years old. His motor symptoms are well controlled on a combination of one tablet of co-careldopa (25/100), three times a day and selegiline 10 mg daily. His wife comes to clinic with him and reports that he has recently been confused at night. Furthermore, he has been hallucinating, seeing his long-dead mother at the bottom of the bed.

Question

What should be done?

Answer

The problem here is to what extent the features of Mr Z's psychosis relates to his drugs or to the underlying disease process. Dementia associated with Parkinson's disease is more common in the older patient with long-standing disease.

A mini-mental state examination to assess cognitive function in more detail would be appropriate. Intercurrent infection and metabolic derangements, for example hypothyroidism, should also be excluded.

Selegiline is best avoided in cases like this and should be discontinued. This may lead to an improvement in Mr Z's psychotic features, without any other action being necessary. The use of an antipsychotic agent for Mr Z is absolutely contraindicated, as it will only serve to worsen his Parkinson's disease. If cognitive function is well preserved and discontinuing selegiline fails to improve the situation, then a low dose of quetiapine could be considered. If there is evidence of dementia, a cholinesterase inhibitor would be a better therapeutic choice.

REFERENCES

Blanchet P J, Verhagen-Metman L, Chase T N 2003 Renaissance of amantadine in the treatment of Parkinson's disease. Advances in Neurology 91: 251-257

Cotzias G C, Van Woert M H, Schiffer L M 1967 Aromatic amino acids and modification of parkinsonism. New England Journal of Medicine 276: 374-379

Emre M, Aarsland D, Albanese A et al 2004 Rivastigmine for dementia associated with Parkinson's disease. New England Journal of Medicine 351: 2509-2518

Healy D G, Abou-Sleiman P M, Wood NW 2004 PINK, PANK or PARK? A clinician's guide to familial parkinsonism. Lancet Neurology 3: 652-662

Ives N, Stowe R L, Marro J et al 2004 Monoamine oxidase type B inhibitors in early Parkinson's disease: meta-analysis of 17 randomised trials involving 3525 patients. British Medical Journal 329: 593-596

Jennings D L, Seibyl J P, Oakes D et al 2004 (123I)beta-CIT and single-photon emission computed tomographic imaging vs clinical evaluation in Parkinsonian syndrome: unmasking an early diagnosis. Archives of Neurology 61: 1224-1229

Lees A J, on behalf of the Parkinson's Disease Research Group of the United Kingdom 1995 Comparison of therapeutic effects and mortality data of levodopa and levodopa combined with selegiline in patients with early, mild Parkinson's disease. British Medical Journal 311:1602-1607

National Institute for Health and Clinical Excellence 2006 Parkinson's disease: diagnosis and management in primary and secondary care. Clinical Guideline 35. National Institute for Health and Clinical Excellence, London

Olanow C W, Perl D P, DeMartino G N et al 2004 Lewy-body formation is an aggresome-related disorder: a hypothesis. Lancet Neurology 3: 496-503

Parkinson Study Group 2003 A controlled trial of rotigotine monotherapy in early Parkinson's disease. Archives of Neurology 60: 1721-1728

Perry E K, Kilford L, Lees A J et al 2003 Increased Alzheimer pathology in Parkinson's disease related to antimuscarinic drugs. Annals of Neurology 54: 235-238

Rascol O, Brooks D, Melamed E et al 2005 Rasagiline as an adjunct to levodopa in patients with Parkinson's disease and motor fluctuations (LARGO, Lasting effect in Adjunct therapy with Rasagiline Given Once daily, study): a randomised, double-blind, parallel-group trial. Lancet 365: 947-954

Schrag A 2005 Entacapone in the treatment of Parkinson's disease. Lancet Neurology 4: 366-370

Walter B L, Vitek J L 2004 Surgical treatment for Parkinson's disease. Lancet Neurology 3: 719-728

FURTHER READING

Burn D J 2002 Beyond the iron mask: towards better recognition and treatment of depression associated with Parkinson's disease. Movement Disorders 17: 445-454

Lees A J 2002 Drugs for Parkinson's disease: oldies but goodies. Journal of Neurology, Neurosurgery and Psychiatry 73: 607-610

Macphee G J A 2001 Diagnosis and differential diagnosis. In: Playfer J R, Hindle J V (eds) Parkinson's disease in the older patient. Arnold, London, pp 43-76

National Institute for Health and Clinical Excellence 2006 Parkinson's disease: diagnosis and management in primary and secondary care.

Clinical Guideline 35. National Institute for Health and Clinical Excellence, London. Available online at: www.nice.org.uk/page. aspx?o=CG035

Parkinson Study Group 2004 Levodopa and the progression of Parkinson's disease. New England Journal of Medicine 351: 2498-2508

Rascol O, Goetz C, Koller W, Poewe W, Sampaio C 2002 Treatment interventions for Parkinson's disease: an evidence based assessment. Lancet 359:1589-1598

33 Pain

S. Woolfrey   D. Kapur

The International Association for the Study of Pain has defined pain as 'an unpleasant sensory and emotional experience associated with actual or potential tissue damage, or described in terms of such damage'.

Acute pain may be viewed as a symptom of a disease process and has a biological function by allowing the patient to avoid or minimize injury. Chronic pain, on the other hand, may be described more as a disease than a symptom.

Aetiology and neurophysiology

Neuroanatomy of pain transmission

The majority of tissues and organs are innervated by special sensory receptors (nociceptors) connected to primary afferent nerve fibres of different diameters. Small myelinated, Aδ fibres and unmyelinated C fibres are believed to be responsible for the transmission of painful stimuli. These afferent primary fibres terminate in the dorsal horn of the spinal grey matter.

Pain transmission onward is far more complex and understood less well. The most important parts of this process are the wide dynamic range cells that project to the thalamus and beyond in the spinothalamic tract. Modulation or inhibition also occurs at the level of the spinal cord. This process can be activated by stress or certain analgesic drugs such as morphine. When the pain modulation system is active, noxious stimuli produce less activity in the pain transmission pathway. The description of this process is the most significant contribution of the gate theory of pain. Conversely, certain factors can lead to an increased sensitivity to noxious stimuli. The most important of these is pain itself and it is clear that painful stimuli can lead to further pain from relatively trivial insults. This occurs through neurochemical and even anatomical changes within the central nervous system that have been termed central sensitization.

Neurotransmitters and pain

Various neurotransmitters found in the dorsal horn of the spinal cord may be involved in pain modulation. These include amino acids such as glutamate and γ-aminobutyric acid (GABA), monoamines such as noradrenaline and 5-hydroxytryptamine (5HT) and certain peptide molecules of which the opioid peptides are the most important. Opioid receptors are found in both the central nervous system (CNS) and the periphery; in the CNS they are found in high concentrations in the limbic system, the brainstem and the spinal cord. The natural ligands (molecules that bind to the receptor) for opioid receptors are a group of neuropeptides known as endorphins. Opioid analgesics mimic the actions of these natural ligands and exert their effect through the μ, δ and, to a lesser extent, the γ receptors. These receptors mediate the analgesic effect of morphine-like drugs.

Assessment of pain

Evaluation of pain should include a careful description of the pain and an assessment of its consequences. There should be a full history, psychosocial assessment, medication history and assessment of previous pain problems, paying attention to factors that influence the pain. Where necessary, diagnostic tests should be organized. These may include radiography, various imaging techniques, and diagnostic and prognostic nerve blocks.

Pain is a subjective phenomenon and quantitative assessment is difficult. The most commonly used instruments are visual analogue and verbal rating scales. Visual analogue scales are 10 cm long lines labelled with two extremes at each end: usually 'no pain at all' and 'worst pain imaginable'. The patient is required to mark the severity of the pain between the two extremes of the scale. Verbal rating scales use adjectival descriptors such as 'none', 'mild', 'moderate' and 'excruciating'. More elaborate questionnaires such as the McGill Pain Questionnaire help to describe other aspects of the pain, and pain diaries record the influence of activity and medication on pain.

Management

Acute pain results from noxious stimulation, such as injury. It can be managed by analgesic drugs and is often self-limiting.

Chronic pain can be defined as pain which has lasted for 6 months or more. Treatment must be comprehensive and may involve pain clinics, hospices and a multidisciplinary approach that manages medical and behavioural aspects. Initial treatment should be directed at the underlying disease process with surgery or antitumour therapy. Pain can be modulated by means other than drugs: for example, stimulation-produced analgesia such as transcutaneous electrical nerve stimulation (TENS), acupuncture and massage, or invasive procedures such as neurosurgery or neurolytic nerve blocks. Non-medical treatment such as physical therapy and various psychological techniques such as cognitive techniques, relaxation training or hypnosis may also form part of a management programme.

Analgesic ladder

The analgesic ladder (Fig. 33.1) forms the basis of many approaches to the use of analgesic drugs. There are essentially three steps: non-opioid analgesics, weak opioids and strong opioids. The analgesic efficacy of non-opioids such as non-steroidal anti-inflammatory drugs (NSAIDs), aspirin and paracetamol is limited by side effects and ceiling effects (i.e. beyond a certain dose, no further pharmacological effect is seen). Beyond the non-opioids, there are a number of drugs in the mild opioid group, such as codeine, which are of some value clinically. There may be some virtue in combining a mild opioid with a non-opioid drug although many commercial preparations contain inadequate quantities of both components and are no more effective than a non-opioid alone. Strong opioids, of which morphine is the standard, have no ceiling effect and therefore increased dosage gives increased analgesia. The relative potencies of the major opioids are summarized in Table 33.1.

Adjuvant medication

In some types of pain, such as the pain of cancer or nerve pain, the addition of non-analgesic drugs to analgesic therapy can enhance

Table 33.1 Relative potencies of opioid drugs

Drug	Potency (morphine = 1)
Codeine	0.1
Dihydrocodeine	0.1
Tramadol	0.2
Pethidine	0.1
Morphine	1
Diamorphine	2.5
Hydromorphone	7
Methadone	2–10 (with repeat dosing)
Fentanyl (transdermal)	150

pain relief. A list of adjuvant drugs is given in Table 33.2. It should be remembered that some drugs such as tricyclic antidepressants have intrinsic analgesic activity, perhaps related to their ability to affect 5HT and noradrenergic neurotransmission.

Special techniques

Patient-controlled analgesia

Patient-controlled analgesia (PCA) is a system in which the patient titrates the dose of opioid to suit individual analgesic requirements. The drug is contained in a system, usually a syringe attached to either an electronic or non-electronic pump, that delivers a preset dose when activated by the patient depressing a button. A lock-out period, during which the machine is programmed not to respond, ensures that a second dose is not delivered before the previous one has had an effect. Some devices allow an additional background infusion of drug to be delivered continuously. A maximum dose facility ensures that the machine does not deliver more than a preset dose over a given time.

Patient-controlled analgesia is a useful technique for the management of pain after surgery. The system is convenient and enjoys a high degree of patient acceptability. The traditional intermittent intramuscular injection of opioids can be effective but is less versatile than titrated intravenous administration. The subcutaneous route is subject to most of the problems associated with intramuscular administration but may be useful for pain relief in children as it avoids multiple injections if a short catheter is left in place. Opioid use via any route is associated with nausea and antiemetics should be prescribed routinely. Administration of compound preparations containing both opioids and antiemetics is not recommended as few preparations contain drugs with similar pharmacokinetic profiles and accumulation, usually of the antiemetic, may occur.

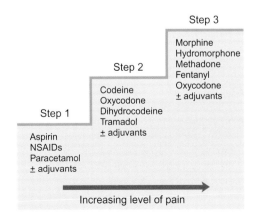

Figure 33.1 WHO three-step analgesic ladder.

Table 33.2 Adjuvant drugs used in the treatment of pain

Drug class	Type of pain	Example
Anticonvulsants	Neuropathic pain Migraine Cluster headache	Carbamazepine Sodium valproate Gabapentin Lamotrigine
Antidepressants	Neuropathic pain Musculoskeletal pain	Amitriptyline Imipramine Venlafaxine
Intravenous anaesthetic agents	Neuropathic pain Burn pain Cancer pain	Ketamine
Skeletal muscle relaxants	Muscle spasm Spasticity	Baclofen Dantrolene Botulinum toxin (type A)
Steroids	Raised intracranial pressure Nerve compression	Dexametasone Prednisolone
Antibiotics	Infection	As indicated by culture and sensitivity
Antispasmodics	Colic Smooth muscle spasm	Hyoscine butylbromide Loperamide
Hormones/ hormonal analogues	Malignant bone pain Spinal stenosis Intestinal obstruction	Calcitonin Octreotide
Bisphosphonates	Bone pain (secondary to either malignancy or osteporosis).	Pamidronate (i.v. in malignancy) Alendronate

Neural blockade

Local anaesthetic drugs injected close to a sensory nerve or plexus will block the conduction of pain impulses and provide excellent analgesia. Agents in common use are lidocaine, prilocaine and bupivacaine. Some are given with adrenaline (epinephrine) to reduce systemic toxicity and increase the duration of action.

Local anaesthetics can be applied directly to wounds or by local infiltration to produce postoperative analgesia, but will not normally block pain arising from deep internal organs. Local anaesthetic techniques are particularly useful in day-stay surgery and children. Continuous infusions via a catheter will permit prolonged analgesia. More permanent nerve blockade for the control of cancer pain is best achieved by using a neurolytic agent such as absolute alcohol or phenol.

Epidural analgesia

Epidural injections may be effective in relieving pain arising from non-malignant and malignant disease. They are very effective in postoperative and labour pain. Various combinations of local anaesthetics, opioids or steroids can be introduced into the epidural space near to the level of the pain.

Epidural local anaesthetics

Long-acting local anaesthetic drugs such as bupivacaine are most effective in relieving pain after major surgery. They work by blocking nerves in the spinal canal serving both superficial and deep tissues, and thus analgesia can be obtained in deep internal organs. Sensory nerves will be blocked and also sympathetic nerves that maintain smooth muscle tone in blood vessels. As a result, vasodilation can occur, which may result in significant hypotension. Epidural catheters allow continuous infusions and long-term therapy by this route. Adverse effects may include muscle weakness in the area supplied by the nerve and, rarely, infection and haematomas.

Epidural opioids

Effective analgesia can be obtained by adding small doses of opioids to the epidural space, because there are opioid receptors in the spinal cord. They can be given with and without long-acting local anaesthetic drugs. However, severe respiratory depression, nausea and vomiting, urinary retention and pruritus can occur after their use. Life-threatening respiratory depression can occur when additional opioids are given by other routes to patients already receiving epidural opioids, and this practice should be actively discouraged. The respiratory depression encountered soon after administration, due to intravascular absorption, is relatively common and simple to detect and treat. However, respiratory depression can occur many hours after opioid administration, particularly with the most commonly used drug, morphine, probably because of its lower lipophilicity, compared with fentanyl and diamorphine. Fentanyl has much greater stability than diamorphine and it can be used with bupivacaine in a terminally sterilized formulation with potential risk management benefits. Respiratory depression can still occur.

Stimulation-produced analgesia

TENS and acupuncture

Transcutaneous electrical nerve stimulation (TENS) machines are portable battery-powered devices that generate a small current to electrodes applied to the skin. The electrodes are placed at the painful site or close to the course of the peripheral nerve innervating the painful area, and the current is increased until paraesthesia is felt at the site of the pain.

The current stimulates the large, rapidly conducting (Aβ) fibres which close the gating mechanism in the dorsal horn cells, and this inhibits the small, slowly conducting fibres (Aδ and C). TENS may also exert an additional effect by stimulating endogenous opioids. Acupuncture also works in a similar fashion, although additional factors may be involved. Stimulation-produced analgesia can be used for trauma, postoperative pain, labour pain and various chronic pains. TENS, in particular, offers the patient a simple, non-invasive, self-controlled method of pain relief with few adverse effects.

Analgesic drugs

Non-steroidal anti-inflammatory drugs

Mode of action

Non-steroidal anti-inflammatory drugs (NSAIDs) produce their effect through cyclo-oxygenase inhibition and are used widely to relieve pain, with or without inflammation, in people with acute and chronic musculoskeletal disorders. In single doses, NSAIDs have analgesic activity comparable to that of paracetamol (Cashman 1996). In regular higher dosages they have both a long analgesic and an anti-inflammatory effect, which makes them particularly useful for the treatment of continuous or regular pain associated with inflammation. They have been shown to be suitable for the relief of pain in dysmenorrhoea, toothache and some headaches and to treat the pain caused by secondary bone tumours, many of which produce lysis of bone and release of prostaglandins.

Clinical considerations

Differences in anti-inflammatory activity between NSAIDs are small, but there is considerable variation in individual patient response as well as the incidence and type of side effects. About 60% of patients will respond to any NSAID. Of the remaining patients, those who do not respond to one NSAID may well respond to another. An analgesic effect should normally be seen within a week, whereas an anti-inflammatory effect may not be achieved, or assessable clinically, for up to 3 weeks.

The potential benefits of treatment with an NSAID must be weighed against the risks. NSAIDs are contraindicated in patients with known active peptic ulceration and should be used with caution in the elderly and in those with renal impairment or asthma.

COX-2 specific drugs

Cyclo-oxygenase exists in two forms: cyclo-oxygenase-1 (COX-1) and cyclo-oxygenase-2 (COX-2). COX-1 is a constitutive enzyme that exists under normal conditions in a variety of tissues where it catalyses the formation of essential prostaglandins. It does not have a role in nociception or inflammation. COX-2 is an inducible enzyme that appears in damaged tissues shortly after injury and leads to the formation of inflammatory prostaglandins within these tissues. COX-2 specific NSAIDs should, theoretically, inhibit the formation of inflammatory prostaglandins without affecting the activity of COX-1 in areas such as the gut. In practice use of COX-2 specific drugs is associated with reduced risks of gastrointestinal side effects when compared with non-selective drugs. However, their use has also been linked with adverse effects such as cardiotoxicity and this is now limiting their use.

Weak opioids

Drugs of this type are prescribed frequently by primary care physicians, either alone or in combination with other analgesics, for a wide variety of painful disorders. There are three major drugs in this group: codeine, dihydrocodeine and dextropropoxyphene.

They are recommended by the WHO for pain that is not responsive to non-opioid analgesics. Despite this recommendation, there are almost no modern data to show that these drugs are of any benefit in the relief of chronic pain, and it may be of more benefit to go straight to prescribing strong opioids.

Codeine

Codeine is suggested as the first-choice drug in this group. It is structurally similar to morphine and about 10% of the codeine is demethylated to form morphine, and the analgesic effect may be due to this, at least in part. It is a powerful cough suppressant as well as being very constipating. In combination with aspirin-like drugs, the analgesic effects are usually additive but the variability in response is considerable. A degree of genetic polymorphism occurs within the population such that the hepatic microsomal enzyme CYP2D6 that is responsible for the conversion of codeine to morphine does not catalyse this conversion in approximately 8% of the population. Codeine's duration of analgesic action is about 3 hours.

Dihydrocodeine

Dihydrocodeine is only available in a few countries and is chemically related to codeine. It has similar properties to codeine when used at the same dosage and is slightly more potent. It has a shorter duration of action than codeine, and this makes its value in the management of chronic pain extremely limited.

Dextropropoxyphene

Dextropropoxyphene is prescribed either alone or in combination with other analgesics such as aspirin and paracetamol. There are few data on its therapeutic value, and at least one major review has concluded that the analgesic efficacy of this drug is less than aspirin and barely more than placebo. At best, dextropropoxyphene has failed to show any superiority over paracetamol (Li Wan Po & Zhang 1997). At worst, it is a dangerous drug which has the potential for steadily developing toxicity. Patients with hepatic dysfunction and poor renal function are particularly at risk. It is associated with problems in overdosage, notably a non-naloxone reversible depression of the cardiac conducting system. Dextropropoxyphene interacts unpredictably with a number of drugs, including carbamazepine and warfarin. In 2005 the Medicines and Healthcare products Regulatory Agency (MHRA) announced concerns about the safety and effectiveness of co-proxamol (paracetamol + dextropropoxyphene) and directed that it should be withdrawn from clinical use in the UK.

Strong opioids

Morphine

Morphine is the standard strong opioid analgesic. It is available as oral, rectal and injectable formulations and has a duration of effect of about 4 hours. There is no ceiling effect when the dose is increased. A general protocol for morphine use is to obtain rapid control of acute pain with an intravenous dose of 2–5 mg titrated against relief of the patient's pain. For control of chronic pain or pain arising from malignancy, an oral regimen is appropriate using a quick-release formulation of morphine. A suitable starting dose is 5–10 mg every 4 hours, and the patient should be advised to take the same dose as often as is necessary for breakthrough pain. It may be necessary to double the dose every 24 hours until pain relief is achieved, although a slower dose escalation will often suffice. After control is achieved it is appropriate to change to an oral sustained-release preparation, which offers twice-daily dosing. Maximum daily doses of up to 1 or 2 g of morphine can be achieved if necessary, but few patients require more than about 200 mg daily. Morphine is metabolized in the liver and one metabolite, morphine 6-glucuronide, is pharmacologically active and this should be taken into consideration in patients who have renal failure.

Other strong opioids

Opioids such as pethidine and dextromoramide offer little advantage over morphine in that they are generally milder in action with a relatively short duration of action (2 hours). Dipipanone is only available in a preparation which contains an antiemetic (cyclizine), and increasing doses lead to sedation and the risk of developing a tardive dyskinesia with long-term use. Methadone has a long elimination half-life of 15–25 hours, and accumulation may occur in the early stages of use. It has a low side effect profile with long-term use and some patients who experience serious adverse effects with morphine may tolerate methadone.

Hydromorphone and oxycodone are synthetic opioids that have been used for many years in North America and more recently in Europe. They are available in both standard and sustained-release preparations. Some patients appear to tolerate hydromorphone or oxycodone better than morphine but there is no evidence to suggest which patients achieve the best effect with either of these drugs and morphine should remain the first-line treatment.

Fentanyl is now available as a sustained-release transdermal patch for long-term use. The patch is designed to release the drug continuously for 3 days. When starting the drug, existing analgesic therapy should be continued for the first 12 hours until therapeutic levels are achieved, and a short-acting opioid should be available for breakthrough pain. Patches are replaced every 72 hours.

Clinical considerations

As a general rule, strong opioids work best against visceral pain or pain arising from a somatic cause. They work moderately against sympathetically maintained pain, and poorly against neurogenic or psychogenic pain. Their use is almost universally accepted in cancer pain but many patients with chronic non-cancer pain can find considerable relief with potent opioids and barriers to their use in this setting appear to be based more on ignorance and political fashions than clinical evidence (McQuay 1997).

Agonist-antagonist and partial agonists

Most of the drugs in this category are either competitive antagonists at the μ receptor, where they can bind to the site but exert no action, or they exert only limited actions; that is to say, they are partial agonists. Those that are antagonist at the μ receptor can provoke a withdrawal syndrome in patients receiving concomitant agonist opioids such as morphine. These properties make it difficult to use these agents in the control of chronic pain, and the process of conversion from one group of drugs to another can be complex.

Pentazocine

Pentazocine is a benzomorphan derivative that is an agonist and at the same time a very weak antagonist at the μ receptor. This drug became popular in the 1960s, when it was thought that it would have little or no abuse potential. This is now known to be untrue, although its abuse potential is less than that of the conventional agonists such as morphine. It produces an analgesia that is clearly different from morphine and is probably due to agonist actions at the κ receptor. There are no detailed studies of its use in chronic pain, but its short duration of action (about 3 hours) and the high incidence of psychomimetic side effects make it a totally unsuitable drug for such use.

Buprenorphine

This drug is a semisynthetic, highly lipophilic opioid that is a partial agonist. It undergoes extensive metabolism when administered orally and to avoid this effect, it is given sublingually. It has high receptor affinity and, through this property, a duration of action of 6 hours.

A long duration of action and high bioavailability would suggest a role for buprenorphine in the management of chronic pain. However, it is difficult to find any controlled studies in the literature and the high incidence of adverse effects seems the likely reason. The incidence of nausea and vomiting appears to be substantially higher than with morphine. However, respiratory depression and constipation are less. Patients who can tolerate this drug appear to experience long-lasting effective analgesia.

Tramadol

Tramadol is a centrally acting analgesic that has opioid agonist activity and also has potent monoamine reuptake properties similar to many antidepressants. Indeed, tramadol appears to have intrinsic antidepressant activity. It is not as powerful as morphine and its value in the management of acute pain is limited by an unfavourably high risk of nausea and vomiting. Its place in the treatment of chronic pain has not been established, but it may be an acceptable alternative to the weak opioids. Its monoaminergic activity seems to be valuable in the management of neuropathic pain.

Adverse effects of opioids

The adverse effects of opioids are nearly all dose related, and tolerance develops to the majority with long-term use.

Respiratory depression Respiratory depression is potentially dangerous in patients with impaired respiratory function, but tolerance is said to develop rapidly with chronic dosing. It can be reversed by naloxone.

Sedation Sedation is usually mild and self-limiting. Smaller doses, given more frequently, may counteract the problem. Rarely, amfetamine or methylphenidate has been used to counteract this effect.

Nausea and vomiting   Antiemetics should be co-prescribed routinely with opioids for the first 10 days. Choice of antiemetic will depend upon the cause, and a single drug will be sufficient in two-thirds of patients. Where nausea is persistent, additional causes should be sought and prescribing reviewed. If another antiemetic is used it should have a different mode of action.

Constipation   Opioids reduce intestinal secretions and peristalsis, causing a dry stool and a hypotonic colon. When opioids are used on a long-term basis most patients need a stool softener and a laxative on a routine basis. A suitable routine laxative is docusate sodium. Dosage should be titrated to give a comfortable stool. High-fibre diets and bulking agents do not work very well in preventing constipation in patients on opioids. Co-danthrusate (dantron + docusate sodium) and co-danthramer (dantron + poloxamer 188) are alternative laxatives that may be effective. However, because of the potential carcinogenicity and genotoxicity of dantron, they are only indicated for use in individuals who are terminally ill.

Tolerance

Chronic drug treatment with opioids often causes tolerance to the analgesic effect although the mechanism remains unclear (Holden et al 2005). When this occurs the dosage should be increased or, alternatively, another opioid can be substituted, since cross-tolerance is not usually complete. Addiction is very rare when opioids are prescribed for pain relief.

Smooth muscle spasm

Morphine causes spasm of the sphincter of Oddi in the biliary tract and may cause biliary colic, as well as urinary sphincter spasm and retention of urine. Thus, in biliary or renal colic, it is preferable to use another opioid without these effects. Pethidine is believed to be the most effective in these circumstances but the evidence for this has been questioned (Thompson 2001).

Non-opioid analgesics

The pharmacological actions and use of the conventional non-opioids such as paracetamol, aspirin and NSAIDs are well known and will not be discussed further here.

Nefopam is a drug which is chemically related to orphenadrine and diphenhydramine. It is not an opioid, anti-inflammatory drug or an antihistamine. The mechanism of analgesic action is unclear. As a non-opioid, it is free from problems of habituation and respiratory depression. The drug has a very high number of dose-related side effects in clinical use that may be linked to its anticholinergic actions. Nefopam may be useful in asthmatic patients and in those who are intolerant of NSAIDs.

Adjuvant analgesics

To be an analgesic, a drug must relieve pain in animal models and give demonstrable and reliable pain relief in patients. Drugs such as the opioids and the NSAIDs clearly are analgesics. The evidence is less clear for the drugs in the following section, and traditional methods would not classify these drugs as analgesics, but all appear to have given some benefit in the control of chronic pain.

Anticonvulsants

The usefulness of this group of drugs is well established for the treatment of neuropathic pain (McQuay et al 1995). Conditions which may respond to anticonvulsants include trigeminal neuralgia, glossopharyngeal neuralgia, various neuropathies, lancinating pain arising from conditions such as postherpetic neuralgia and multiple sclerosis and similar pains that may follow amputation or surgery. Several classes of drugs show anticonvulsant activity. These can be broadly classed as sodium channel blockers (carbamazepine, phenytoin), glutamate inhibitors (lamotrigine, gabapentin), GABA potentiators (sodium valproate, tiagabine) or drugs showing a mixture of these effects (topiramate). Failure to respond to one particular drug does not indicate that anticonvulsants as a broad class will be ineffective. A drug with a different mechanism of action or combination therapy could be considered.

Anticonvulsants are surprisingly effective in the prophylaxis of migraine and cluster headache. Their mode of action is unclear but both of these conditions are associated with abnormal excitability of certain groups of neurones and the neuronal depression caused by anticonvulsants is probably important.

Antidepressants

Persistent chronic pain is accompanied frequently by anxiety and depression. Thus it is not surprising that the use of antidepressants and other psychoactive drugs is part of standard pain management. There is evidence that some of these drugs have analgesic properties that are independent of their psychotropic effects.

The tricyclic antidepressants (TCAs) are frequently used for the treatment of chronic pain conditions with and without the anticonvulsants, and there is a substantial body of literature about their analgesic action (McQuay et al 1996).

The biochemical activity of the tricyclic antidepressants suggests that their main effect will be on serotonergic and noradrenergic neurones. The tricyclic antidepressants inhibit the reuptake of the monoamines 5HT and/or noradrenaline at neurones in the brain and spinal cord. Through a rather complex mechanism, this causes an initial fall in the release of these transmitters followed by a sustained rise in the concentration of neurotransmitter at synapses in the pain neural pathways. This rise usually takes 2–3 weeks to develop. Since pain is a common presenting complaint of depression, it seems reasonable to assume that some relief of pain will be associated with the reversal of depression. Tricyclic antidepressants are effective analgesics in headache, facial pain, low back pain, arthritis, denervation pain and, to a lesser degree, cancer.

Clinical use of antidepressants in chronic pain

Various tricyclic antidepressants have been utilized (usually methylated tricyclics) with or without phenothiazines and anticonvulsants. Drug doses have varied considerably but most are low, of the order of 25–75 mg/day. Evidence tends to support the use of doses greater than 75 mg/day for somatic and neuropathic pain. Where depression is prominent, a full antidepressant dose schedule should be employed and in the case of amitriptyline, a target dose of 150–250 mg/day would usually be appropriate.

Tricyclic antidepressants have a wide range of adverse effects and these may cause a marked reduction in patient compliance. Newer antidepressant drugs have generally been disappointing from the analgesic perspective. However, much of the research has looked at the selective serotonin reuptake inhibitors (SSRIs). Recent work suggests that both noradrenergic and serotonergic transmission needs to be enhanced for an analgesic effect to be seen. The serotonin/noradrenaline reuptake inhibitor venlafaxine has effects on both monoamines and does appear to possess anal-gesic activity at higher dose ranges of 150 mg/day and above. A number of antidepressant compounds do not act via monoamine reuptake inhibition and do not appear to possess intrinsic analgesic activity. Examples are trazodone and mirtazepine. They are effective antidepressants and may have a place in the treatment of co-existing depression but analgesia should be tackled separately.

Ketamine

Ketamine is an intravenous anaesthetic agent with a variety of actions within the central nervous system. Many of its effects are related to its activity at central glutamate receptors although it also has actions at certain voltage-gated ion channels and opioid receptors. Low doses of ketamine (0.1–0.3 mg/kg/h via the intravenous route) can produce profound analgesia, even in situations where opioids have been ineffective, such as neuropathic pain. Despite its variable oral availability, oral administration of ketamine can be surprisingly effective (Annetta et al 2005, Mercadante 1996). Its usefulness is limited by troublesome psychotropic side effects although the simultaneous administration of benzodiazepines or antipsychotics can reduce these problems.

Neuroleptics

Phenothiazines, with the exception of methotrimeprazine, have no effect in the treatment of pain. A dose of 15 mg of methotrimeprazine has an analgesic activity equivalent to 10 mg of intramuscular morphine. Methotrimeprazine also has profound hypnotic, anxiolytic and antiemetic effects which make it a useful drug in the palliative care setting.

Anxiolytics

Benzodiazepines may be used for pain relief in conditions associated with acute muscle spasm and are sometimes prescribed to reduce the anxiety and muscle tension associated with chronic pain conditions. Many authorities believe that they reduce pain tolerance and there is good evidence that they can reduce the effectiveness of opioid analgesics although the mechanism is unclear. Clonazepam has been used in the management of neurogenic pain but some of the more modern anticonvulsants have clearer evidence of efficacy. Diazepam can be used to control painful spasticity, due to acute or spinal cord injury, but sedation may be troublesome and baclofen (see below) is probably a more suitable choice.

Antihistamines

These agents were introduced into the management of chronic pain because of their sedative muscle relaxant properties. These actions are non-specific and it is not clear whether the clinical effect is mediated centrally or peripherally. Most clinical studies have been carried out with hydroxyzine, which has shown benefit in acute pain, tension headache and cancer pain.

There is evidence that analgesic combinations of antihistamines, NSAIDs and opioids may yield greater analgesia than that provided by each drug alone.

Skeletal muscle relaxants

Drugs described in this section are used for the relief of muscle spasm or spasticity. It is axiomatic that the underlying cause of the spasticity and any aggravating factors such as pressure sores or infections should be treated. This group of drugs will usually help spasticity but this may be at the cost of decreased muscle tone elsewhere, which may lead to a decrease in the mobility of the patient and thus make matters worse.

The drug of first choice is probably baclofen, which has a peripheral site of action, working directly on the skeletal muscle. Baclofen is a derivative of the inhibitory neurotransmitter GABA and appears to be an agonist at the $GABA_B$ receptor. It is alleged that it is most effective for the treatment of spasticity caused by multiple sclerosis or other diseases of the spinal cord, especially traumatic lesions. There are reports of its use in trigeminal neuralgia and a number of painful conditions, including postherpetic neuralgia.

Dantrolene is an alternative that is effective orally and which may have fewer (but potentially more serious) adverse effects. Its effect is due to a direct effect on skeletal muscle and takes several weeks to develop.

The α_2-adrenergic agonist tizanidine has potent muscle relaxant activity and is an alternative to baclofen. It may also have some direct analgesic effects.

Botulinum toxin

The bacterium *Clostridium botulinum* produces a potent toxin that interferes directly with neuromuscular transmission. Purified preparations of the type A toxin produce long-lasting relaxation of skeletal muscle. The effect often lasts in excess of 3 months and avoids the systemic side effects of agents such as baclofen. Great care must be taken in administering this drug as spread may occur to adjacent muscle groups, producing excessive weakness. Overdosage, with systemic absorption, may lead to generalized muscle weakness and even respiratory failure.

Clonidine

The α-adrenergic agonist clonidine has been shown to produce analgesia, and there is evidence that both morphine and clonidine produce a dose-dependent inhibition of spinal nociceptive transmission that is mediated through different receptors for each drug. This may explain why clonidine has been shown to work synergistically with morphine when given intrathecally or epidurally. Clonidine also appears to work when given by other routes or even topically, but may cause severe hypotension by any route.

Cannabinoids

Cannabis has been used as an analgesic for hundreds of years. Despite the historical record, problems concerning the legal status of cannabis in most countries has hindered scientific investigation of its analgesic properties. The active ingredient in preparations made from the hemp plant, *Cannabis sativa,* is δ-9 tetrahydro-cannabinol. This compound has analgesic activity in animal models of experimental pain as well as in the clinical situation (Burns & Ineck 2006). Overall, analgesic activity appears relatively weak and it has not proved possible to separate the analgesic activity from the potent psychotropic effects characteristic of these drugs. There may be a clearer analgesic effect in neuropathic pain but the evidence for this remains anecdotal.

Treatment of selected pain syndromes

Herpetic and postherpetic neuralgia

The pain associated with herpes zoster infection is severe, continuous and often described as burning and lancinating. Antiviral therapy such as aciclovir initiated at the first sign of the rash can reduce the duration of the pain, particularly postherpetic pain, which follows the disappearance of the rash. Analgesics such as NSAIDs provide some benefit. Tricyclic antidepressants such as amitriptyline are the mainstay of treatment, commencing with a dose of 50 mg at night and increasing to 150 mg if required. They may be combined with anticonvulsants if the response is poor or incomplete. Carbamazepine is historically the most important drug of this group but modern anticonvulsant drugs (see above) have also proved useful and may be better tolerated. Recent work has suggested that direct injection of long-acting steroid preparations into the spinal fluid may help refractory cases but this remains to be confirmed.

Trigeminal neuralgia

Trigeminal neuralgia presents as abrupt, intense bursts of severe, lancinating pain, provoked by touching sensitive trigger areas on one side of the face. The disorder may spontaneously remit for periods of several weeks or months. Anticonvulsants have been used successfully. If drug therapy is ineffective, surgical techniques such as decompression of the nucleus of the fifth cranial nerve, glycerol injection or gangliolysis can be of great benefit. If surgery becomes necessary, anticonvulsants should be withdrawn gradually afterwards.

Peripheral nerve injury and neuropathy

Damage to, or entrapment of, nerves can cause pain, unpleasant sensations and paraesthesiae. Tricyclic antidepressants and anticonvulsants such as GABA have been used with some success to reduce neuropathic pain (Wiffen et al 2005). A neuroma occurs when damaged or severed nerve fibres sprout new small fibres in an attempt to regenerate. Pain develops several weeks after the nerve injury, and is often due to the neuroma growing into scar tissue, causing pain as it is stretched or mobilized. Treatment of neuroma is very difficult and few treatments are successful. Options include surgery and injections of steroid and local anaesthetic agents.

Sympathetically maintained pain

Causalgia and reflex sympathetic dystrophy are names for an important group of painful conditions that may follow trauma or damage to nerves and which are associated with overactivity of the sympathetic nervous system. Treatment is directed at blocking sympathetic overactivity, reducing pain and instituting aggressive physiotherapy to facilitate a return to normal function. Sympathetic blockade can be achieved by blocking appropriate nerves using local anaesthetics, or by injecting a dose of an α-adrenergic blocking agent such as phentolamine, which may give sufficient pain relief to permit the institution of regular physiotherapy and for recovery to take place. Other drugs that have been used successfully include oral corticosteroids, other α-adrenergic agonists and blockers, and calcium channel-blocking drugs (Kingery 1997).

Musculoskeletal (myofascial) pain

Myofascial pain is that arising from muscles and is associated with stiffness and neuralgic symptoms such as tingling and paraesthesiae. It may occur spontaneously or following trauma, such as whiplash injury. Myofascial pain syndrome is also known as myositis, fibrositis, myalgia and myofasciitis. Acute muscle injury can be treated by first aid with the application of a cooling spray or ice to reduce inflammation and spasm, followed by passive stretching of the muscle to restore its full range of motion. Injection therapy is used to disrupt sensitive muscle trigger points, and may involve injecting local anaesthetic or saline. Local injections of botulinum toxin have also been shown to be effective where muscle spasm is prolonged and severe. TENS and acupuncture have an important role to play in reducing pain and muscle spasm. Treatment of chronic myofascial syndromes should always include a programme of physical therapy.

Postamputation and phantom limb pain

The majority of amputees suffer significant stump or phantom limb pain for at least a few weeks each year. Pain will be present immediately postoperatively in the stump. This may be caused by muscle spasm, nerve injury and sensitivity of the wound and surrounding skin. As the wound heals, the pain should subside. If it does not, the reason may be vascular insufficiency or infection. Pain occurring some number of years after amputation may be caused by changes in the structure of the bones or skin in the stump, or ischaemia. For instance, reduction in the thickness of overlying tissue with age may expose nerve endings to increased stimuli.

Tricyclic antidepressants may be helpful for stump pain. Standard analgesics can be given, and surgery may be necessary to restore the vascular supply or reduce trauma to nerve endings.

Phantom pain is a referred pain which produces a burning or throbbing sensation, felt in the absent limb. Cramping sensations are caused by muscular spasm in the stump. The patient with phantom limb pain is often anxious, depressed and frightened, all of which exacerbate the pain. Analgesic drugs alone are generally not adequate for phantom pain, but tricyclic antidepressants and anticonvulsants are useful adjuvants. Other therapy which can be effective includes TENS and sympathetic blockade. These patients frequently require management at specialist pain centres.

Postoperative pain

The majority of patients suffer postoperative pain. The site and nature of surgery influence the severity of pain, although individual variations amongst patients do not allow the amount of pain to be predicted according to the type of operation.

Apart from the obvious benefit of relieving suffering, pain relief is desirable for a number of physiological reasons after surgery or any form of major tissue injury. For example, poor-quality analgesia reduces lung function, increases heart rate and blood pressure, and magnifies the stress response to surgery. The use of intermittent and patient-controlled intermittent intravenous injections of opioids has been described earlier. However, opioids themselves may delay recovery and are associated with adverse events in the postoperative period (Kehlet et al 1996). It is now common to treat postoperative pain with combinations of opioids and local anaesthetic blocks or infiltrations. In addition, NSAIDs can be used as adjuvants to opioids. Agents such as diclofenac and ketorolac are used frequently, but care must be taken because in situations where there is a possibility of renal stress, such as blood loss, the normal protective effect of prostaglandins on the kidney will be lost and renal failure may result. There is no evidence to support the use of either NSAIDs or local anaesthetic techniques pre-emptively, although there is some theoretical and clinical evidence that opioids given prior to surgery may be more effective than when given postoperatively.

Headache

Tension headaches are caused by muscle contraction over the neck and scalp. They respond well to TENS and methylated tricyclic antidepressant drugs given as a single dose at night. Propranolol and minor tranquillizers have also been used. NSAIDs may be indicated if the headache is associated with cervical spondylosis or neck injury.

Migraine

Most migraine attacks respond to simple analgesics such as aspirin or paracetamol. Soluble forms are best, as gut motility is reduced during a migraine attack and absorption of oral medication may be delayed. Migraine treatment has altered markedly in recent years with the advent of the triptan drugs such as almotriptan, eletriptan, rizatriptan, sumatriptan, naratriptan and zolmitriptan (Goadsby 2005). These are $5HT_{1B/1D}$-agonists that will often abort an attack, especially when given by the subcutaneous route. Their vasoconstrictor activity precludes their use in patients with angina or cerebrovascular disease but side effects are less serious than with the ergot derivatives they have replaced.

Prophylactic drug treatment of migraine includes α-adrenergic blockers, anticonvulsants and tricyclic antidepressants. Chronic treatment is undesirable.

Cluster headache

Cluster headache is a disabling condition characterized by severe unilateral head pain occurring in clusters of attacks varying from minutes to hours. It shares some pathological features with migraine and treatment is similar although recent high-resolution magnetic resonance imaging studies have shown specific anatomical differences in the brains of people with cluster headache. Triptans are effective in acute attacks, as is inhalation of 100% oxygen. Prophylaxis is similar to that of migraine.

Dysmenorrhoea

Dysmenorrhoea is a common cause of pelvic pain. It can be helped by the prescription of oral contraceptives, since pain is absent in anovulatory cycles. NSAIDs are effective because of their action on cyclo-oxygenase inhibition. Dysmenorrhoea due to endometriosis may require therapy with androgenic drugs such as danazol or regulators of the gonadotrophins such as norethisterone.

Burn pain

Patients with burns may require a series of painful procedures such as physiotherapy, debridement or skin grafting. Premedication with a strong opioid before the procedure coupled with intravenous opioids and the use of Entonox (premixed 50% nitrous oxide and 50% oxygen) may be necessary to control the pain. Regular, time-contingent opioids such as morphine or methadone may be useful to prevent the pain induced by movement or touch in the burn area. The anaesthetic drug ketamine (see above) has potent analgesic activity when used in subhypnotic doses. It has a short duration of action and may be used to reduce the pain of dressing changes or other forms of incident pain. Even with low doses, a significant proportion of patients will experience side effects of dysphoria or hallucinations. These can be treated with benzodiazepines or antipsychotic compounds such as haloperidol.

Pain of malignancy

The pain associated with cancer may arise from many different sources, and has the characteristics of both acute and chronic pain. It should be emphasized that the sources of the pain may change and continual assessment on a regular basis is required. Although this chapter is concerned only with the management of pain, care of the patient with a terminal illness requires management of all aspects of the patient. Cancer occurs more frequently in the elderly, who have a larger proportion of painful ailments than the general population. Pain may be arising from these sources too, and these require treatment at the same time. Pain can be treated both with drugs and other techniques such as radiotherapy and nerve blocks. Drug treatment is based on the analgesic ladder together with the use of adjuvant analgesics (Fig. 33.2). When considering non-opioid analgesics, the NSAIDs have a special role, especially in bone metastases. Some clinicians progress from non-opioid to strong opioid drugs such as morphine, omitting

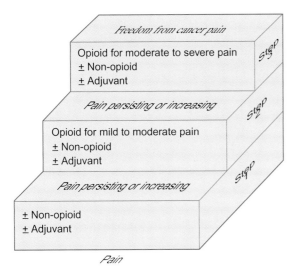

Figure 33.2 WHO analgesic ladder for cancer relief and palliative care.

the middle step of the analgesic ladder. It can be argued that the middle step of the current analgesic ladder be eliminated and that another step be added when strong opioids are not working. This would involve the use of neurolytic or neurosurgical procedures to overcome pain that is non-opioid responsive.

Strong opioids are the mainstay for the treatment of cancer pain, and virtually every form of cancer pain will respond to some degree.

Opioid use in cancer pain

Morphine is the first-line opioid in standard or sustained-release oral form but if it is not tolerated, hydromorphone or methadone, both with relatively long half-lives, may be considered. Optimal dosage is determined on an individual basis for each patient by titration against the pain. Patients on long-term sustained-release opioids should have additional oral doses of rapidly acting opioid to act as an 'escape' medicine for incident or breakthrough pain. Pain arising from malignancy may change and, as with pain arising from any source, the cause and the treatment must be subject to regular review.

Where the oral route is not available, non-oral routes of administration such as buccal, rectal, transdermal, inhaled or injection should be used. Injection means subcutaneous, intravenous or via epidural or spinal catheter. Implanted pumps and syringe drivers may be used to provide analgesia in cases where conventional opioid delivery is ineffective. The proportion of patients who need invasive forms of drug delivery is small and is confined to those who are persistently troubled with unacceptable adverse effects. Such patients can achieve pain relief with lower doses of opioid and have few problems with side effects. Long-term maintenance of indwelling lines and catheters requires training for patient, physicians and nursing teams, but excellent long-term results are possible. Morphine, oxycodone and hydromorphone are suitable for use and in the UK, diamorphine is also suitable and readily available. Diamorphine has the advantage of being very soluble, so a high dose may be given in a small volume, which reduces the frequency of changes of syringes and refills necessary to provide adequate pain relief.

Use of adjuvant drugs in cancer pain

Neuropathic pain is common in cancer. As many as 40% of patients with cancer pain may have a neuropathic component. Tricyclic antidepressants and anticonvulsants should be introduced early but where these are ineffective, ketamine has found an important role.

Methotrimeprazine, a phenothiazine with analgesic activity, is a useful alternative when opioids cannot be tolerated. It causes neither constipation nor respiratory depression and has antiemetic and anxiolytic activity. It is sedative, which may be either a virtue or a problem in palliative care.

Corticosteroids are useful in managing certain aspects of acute and chronic cancer pain. They are particularly useful for raised intracranial pressure and for relieving pressure caused by tumours on the spinal cord or peripheral nerves.

Dexametasone (16 mg/day) is the most commonly used steroid to ameliorate raised intracranial pressure in patients with brain tumours. High steroid doses given for 1 or 2 weeks do not require a reducing-dosage regimen. They also produce a feeling of well-being, increased appetite and weight gain, although the central effects are usually transient. It is axiomatic that underlying causes of pain be treated; therefore it is appropriate to use antibiotics to treat infections, radiotherapy to reduce tumour bulk or control bone pain, or surgery to achieve fracture fixation or to relieve bowel obstruction in conjunction with antispasmodics such as hyoscine butylbromide.

Pain arising from bone also responds to NSAIDs, which may be given orally or rectally. Bisphosphonates have a place in management of this problem, and new drugs in this group are being introduced into clinical practice.

Specific cancer pain syndromes

Three types of malignant pain are briefly outlined below to indicate various therapeutic approaches.

Cancer of the pancreas Pain is caused by infiltration of the tumour into the pancreas as well as by obstruction of the bowel and biliary tract and metastases in the liver. Patients will also experience anorexia, nausea, vomiting and diarrhoea, and are often depressed. Surgery, radiotherapy and chemotherapy may relieve pain for long periods, as does neurolytic blockade of the coeliac plexus. Opioid analgesics are useful and may be administered intravenously or epidurally by either bolus injection or continuous infusion.

Mesothelioma of the lung Mesothelioma causes pain when the tumour penetrates surrounding tissues such as the pleura, chest wall and nerve plexuses. The analgesic ladder should be used first, and it should be remembered that any NSAID is useful because inflammation is often a component of the chest wall involvement. Adjuvants such as tricyclic antidepressants or steroids may be helpful. As the tumour progresses, nerve blocks or neurosurgery may be necessary, and invasion of the vertebrae can lead to nerve root or spinal cord compression. In the latter case, high-dose steroids such as dexametasone may be given intravenously, but radiotherapy is also useful in reducing the size of the tumour.

Metastatic bone pain Metastatic bone pain is usually treated with courses of chemotherapy and radiotherapy, but analgesics

Table 33.3 Common therapeutic problems

Problem	Solution	Example
Neuropathic pain	Anticonvulsants	Carbamazepine Sodium valproate Gabapentin Lamotrigine
	Antidepressants	Amitriptyline Imipramine
	Intravenous anaesthetic agents	Ketamine
Malignant bone pain	Bisphosphonates	Pamidronate Calcitonin
Muscle spasm/spasticity	Skeletal muscle relaxants	Baclofen Dantrolene Botulinum toxin (type A)
Raised intracranial pressure	Corticosteroids	Dexametasone Prednisolone
Nausea with morphine	Antiemetic	Metoclopramide Domperidone
	Use an alternative route of administration	Topical or subcutaneous
Constipation	Determine if drug induced, e.g. opioids or tricyclic antidepressant. Co-prescribe a laxative	Docusate sodium
Use of antidepressants in patients with ischaemic heart disease	Use a non-cardiotoxic antidepressant	Venlafaxine
Drug interactions with carbamazepine	Use an anticonvulsant which does not affect hepatic enzymes	Gabapentin
Renal failure	Morphine accumulates; use lower dose Use a drug which is not handled renally	Fentanyl
Sedation/impaired cognition	Identify any drug-related causes and adjust dose or stop drug	

can be used. A prostaglandin-like substance has been isolated from bone metastases and therefore NSAIDs and, more recently, bisphosphonates are often used in bone pain. Steroids also interfere with prostaglandin formation and dexametasone therefore has a role, especially where there is nerve root or spinal cord compression.

CASE STUDIES

Case 33.1

A 65-year-old man presents with a 6-month history of lancinating pain in his left upper jaw that is diagnosed as trigeminal neuralgia. He is taking 600 mg of carbamazepine daily in divided doses yet still has several attacks of severe pain each day. He is becoming depressed and is unable to work.

Question

How should this patient be managed?

Answer

The blood level of carbamazepine should be measured to check adherence. If needed, an increase in the daily dose could be instituted. If side effects develop, a different anticonvulsant could be employed. If he fails to respond to adequate doses of anticonvulsant, a neurosurgical opinion would be appropriate.

Decompression of the trigeminal nucleus by posterior fossa exploration will help a substantial number of patients with trigeminal neuralgia. Other neurosurgical techniques that may benefit patients with this condition are glycerol injection and radiofrequency ablation of the trigeminal nerve.

Case 33.2

A 55-year-old lady with metastatic abdominal cancer from a probable primary in the pelvis presents with an abdominal mass. Her pain is uncontrolled despite regular prescription of oral opioids, and she has been sick for a week. Subacute bowel obstruction is present.

Question

How should this lady be managed?

Answer

Management should begin with admission and rehydration. She may be quite dehydrated and have severe electrolyte imbalance. The oral route is not available for the delivery of adequate analgesia, and consideration should be given to the use of patient-controlled analgesia. The sickness should be treated, and an underlying cause sought. This may be subacute obstruction which, in turn, may be due to constipation caused by the opioids or by the disease process. Abdominal masses that indent on palpation are faeces (not tumour). Abdominal radiographs would show fluid levels if there was obstruction rather than constipation. Other possible causes of vomiting are recent anticancer therapy, anxiety, dyspepsia from NSAIDs, raised intracranial pressure and vertigo.

Surgery may be needed to relieve the obstruction, but the need for surgery may be avoided by the use of hyoscine butylbromide, which may control colic and cause little additional sedation. Propantheline may be an alternative. If the problem is one of constipation, rectal measures may be necessary to re-establish function. These may include suppositories, enemas or digital disimpaction. Once control of her pain has been achieved and her bowel function has returned to normal, she must receive regular laxatives. The amount given should be increased as necessary every 1–2 days. A high fluid intake should be encouraged, as this will help prevent stool from becoming hard.

Attention should be paid to her emotional and spiritual needs at all times.

Case 33.3

A 28-year-old man had a crush fracture of his ankle after falling from a roof. Fixation 9 months ago is described as satisfactory, but his leg is now very painful to even small stimuli and he cannot use it or bear weight. The lower leg has muscle wasting and is much colder than the opposite limb. The skin is very sensitive to touch, shiny and has a poor circulation.

Question

What is this condition and how should this pain be treated?

Answer

This is a reflex sympathetic dystrophy. Management should be aggressive and directed towards restoration in function. Diagnostic injection of phentolamine may reduce the pain and sensitivity, which suggests that sympathetic function is increased. Longer term benefit may be achieved by the serial use of somatic or sympathetic nerve blocks using local anaesthetics. This should be associated with the use of aggressive physiotherapy. There may be a burning component to the pain, which may respond to low doses of tricyclic antidepressants such as amitriptyline (50 mg at night) or lofepramine (70 mg twice daily).

Aggressive treatment early in the course of the disease can reduce the period of time that patients have this problem, and early referral to seek specialized help is recommended. A small percentage of patients continue to have problems whatever treatment is given.

Case 33.4

An 85-year-old man is admitted to hospital after falling down a flight of stairs and landing heavily on his right side. On admission, he is in severe pain and finds breathing, and especially coughing, unbearably painful. A chest x-ray reveals that he has fractures of the 5th to 8th ribs on the right side.

Question

How should his pain be managed and what are the risks of undertreatment?

Answer

Multiple rib fractures are potentially very serious and good analgesia can prevent potentially dangerous complications. Initial analgesia should include both potent opioids and NSAIDs (unless contraindicated). Opioids should be administered parenterally in the acute situation and patient-controlled analgesia would offer the safest means of dose titration. The chest injury may well result in damage to the underlying lung and it is essential to administer unrestricted high-flow oxygen to the patient as the combination of lung injury and ventilatory suppression secondary to either pain or the effects of opioids could lead to dangerous hypoxia. TENS may also prove helpful.

Arterial oxygen saturation (and preferably arterial blood gases) should be monitored. If pain remains poorly controlled or the patient's oxygenation deteriorates, thoracic epidural analgesia using a mixture of local anaesthetic and opioid should be considered.

Failure to treat pain adequately in this situation may lead to a reduction in the patient's ability to cough and clear secretions from the chest. This can lead to respiratory failure and even death. Analgesia should be sufficient to allow regular physiotherapy in order to minimize the risk of such complications.

Case 33.5

A 45-year-old woman presents to her general practitioner with a 2-day history of back pain following a lifting injury at work. The pain is constant and aching in character with radiation into the posterior aspect of both thighs as far as the knee. Physical examination shows her to be maintaining a very rigid posture with some spasm of the large muscles of the back. Her range of movement is very poor but there are no neurological signs in the legs.

Question

Which drugs may help this lady's pain? What other advice should be given?

Answer

Acute back pain is very common and is rarely associated with serious spinal pathology. The absence of neurological signs is reassuring and indicates that early activity, possibly aided by a short course of analgesics, is the best way forward. NSAIDs, if tolerated, would be the drugs of choice. A low-dose muscle relaxant such as baclofen 20–40 mg per day in divided doses might also help although it would be unwise to continue such drugs beyond 2 weeks. If NSAIDs are contraindicated, then paracetamol can be substituted and should be given every 6 hours. The role of opioids is less clear. Short-term (7–14 days) use of a mild opioid such as codeine or tramadol is probably safe. Longer term use is less satisfactory as there is no clear evidence of their efficacy and sedative side effects may reduce the patient's capacity and motivation to remain active.

The patient should be advised to remain active and accept that some pain is likely during the recovery phase. Failure to remain active and, in particular, excessive bed rest are both associated with worse outcomes.

Case 33.6

A 50-year-old man is admitted to hospital with an acute onset of severe mid-thoracic spinal pain. He is found to be anaemic and investigations show that he has multiple myeloma with widespread bony lesions, including fresh spinal fractures.

Question

Which drugs may help this man's pain? What particular hazards may occur in this condition?

Answer

This patient is extremely ill and even with aggressive chemotherapy, he is unlikely to survive more than a few months. Most of his pain will be related to the destruction of bone and the aim should be to provide pain relief via a 'central' mechanism through the use of opioids as well as reducing the rate of bone destruction and associated inflammatory responses. A potent opioid will be required and oral morphine would usually be the drug of first choice. In this situation, a combination of a sustained-release preparation together with liberal 'as required' dosing would be appropriate. The correct dose is the dose required to produce adequate pain relief without producing excessive sedation. Inflammatory pain may be improved by the use of NSAIDs and these should be given regularly although they may be contraindicated in this condition (see below). High-dose corticosteroids may achieve a similar effect and may also reduce the hypercalcaemia that is often seen in myeloma. Bone destruction and its associated pain may be reduced by the use of bisphosphonate compounds. In this case intravenous pamidronate should be given.

Renal failure is common in myeloma. This may be due to obstruction of renal tubules by myeloma proteins or the effects of some chemotherapeutic agents. If renal impairment occurs, opioids should be used with caution so as to avoid problems with accumulation. Transdermal fentanyl may be a more appropriate drug. NSAIDs can precipitate acute renal failure in the presence of reduced renal blood flow. Finally, platelet function is often poor in patients with myeloma. This can be due to direct effects of myeloma proteins on platelets, bone marrow replacement by myeloma or the effects of chemotherapy. Use of NSAIDs may be associated with increased risk of gastrointestinal haemorrhage.

REFERENCES

Annetta M G, Iemma D, Garisto C et al 2005 Ketamine: new indications for an old drug. Current Drug Targets 6: 789-794

Burns T L, Ineck J R 2006 Cannabinoid analgesia as a potential new therapeutic option in the treatment of chronic pain. Annals of Pharmacotherapy 40: 251-260

Cashman J N 1996 The mechanisms of action of NSAIDs in analgesia. Drugs 52(suppl 5): 13-23

Goadsby P J 2005 Advances in the understanding of headache. British Medical Bulletin 73: 83-92

Holden J E, Jeong Y, Forrest J M 2005 The endogenous opioid system and clinical pain management. AACN Clinical Issues 16: 291-301

Kehlet H, Rung G W, Callesen T 1996 Postoperative opioid analgesia: time for a reconsideration? Journal of Clinical Anesthesia 8: 441-445

Kingery W S 1997 A critical review of controlled clinical trials for peripheral neuropathic pain and complex regional pain syndromes. Pain 73: 123-139

Li Wan Po A, Zhang W Y 1997 Systematic overview of co-proxamol to assess analgesic effects of addition of dextropropoxyphene to paracetamol. British Medical Journal 315: 1565-1571

McQuay H J 1997 Opioid use in chronic pain. Acta Anaesthesiologica Scandinavica 41: 175-183

McQuay H, Carroll D, Jadad A R et al 1995 Anticonvulsant drugs for management of pain: a systematic review. British Medical Journal 311: 1047-1052

McQuay H J, Tramer M , Nye B et al 1996 A systematic review of antidepressants in neuropathic pain. Pain 68: 217-227

Mercadante S 1996 Ketamine in cancer pain: an update. Palliative Medicine 10: 225-230

Thompson D R 2001 Narcotic analgesic effects on the sphincter of Oddi: a review of the data and therapeutic implications in treating pancreatitis. American Journal of Gastroenterology 96: 1266-1272

Wiffen P J, McQuay H J, Edwards J E et al 2005 Gabapentin for acute and chronic pain. Cochrane Database of Systematic Reviews 3: CD005452. Update Software, Oxford

FURTHER READING

Banks C, Mackrodt K (eds) 2004 Chronic pain management. Whurr, Chichester

Benzon H T, Raja S, Molloy R E et al (eds) 2000 Essentials of pain medicine and regional anaesthesia. Churchill Livingstone, Edinburgh

MacIntyre P (ed) 2005 Acute pain management: scientific evidence. Australian and New Zealand College of Anaethetists, Melbourne

Marcus D A (ed) 2005 Chronic pain: a primary care guide to practical management. Humana Press, USA

Moore R A, McQuay H J 2005 Prevalence of opioid adverse events in chronic non-malignant pain: systematic review of randomized trials of oral opioids. Arthritis Research and Therapy 7: R1046- R1051

Pediani R C, Counsell D J (eds) 2005 Acute pain management. Elsevier, Oxford

Wall P D, Melzack R (eds) 2000 Textbook of pain, 4th edn. Churchill Livingstone, Edinburgh

Nausea and vomiting

34

E. Mason   P. A. Routledge

KEY POINTS

- Patients must be assessed carefully, and often reassessed frequently, to identify the primary underlying cause of their nausea and/or vomiting.
- Antiemetics are symptomatic treatments only and do not treat the underlying cause.
- Drug choice is based on an understanding of the likely pathophysiology, the receptors involved, the available route of administration and drug side effects.
- In certain situations, prophylactic regimens are beneficial, e.g. motion sickness, postoperative nausea and vomiting, chemotherapy-induced nausea and vomiting.
- Simple regimens are used where possible to prevent postoperative nausea and vomiting, such as parenteral cyclizine or prochlorperazine administered at induction. These and other antiemetics can be used for rescue therapy if vomiting occurs postoperatively.
- The choice of antiemetic to use in conjunction with cytotoxic chemotherapy depends on the emetogenicity of the cytotoxic drugs used. The $5HT_3$ antagonists such as ondansetron are very effective antiemetic drugs when highly emetogenic chemotherapy is used. The addition of dexametasone may provide further benefit.
- Anticipatory emesis associated with chemotherapy can be treated with a benzodiazepine and dexametasone is useful in alleviating delayed emesis.

Nausea and vomiting are commonly (but not universally) associated symptoms. The word nausea is derived from the Greek *nautia,* meaning sea-sickness, while vomiting is derived from the Latin *vomere,* meaning to discharge. Nausea is a subjective sensation whereas vomiting is the reflex physical act of expulsion of gastric contents. Retching is defined as 'spasmodic respiratory movements against a closed glottis with contractions of the abdominal musculature without expulsion of any gastric contents, i.e. "dry heaves"' (American Gastroenterological Association 2001). It is important to differentiate vomiting from regurgitation, rumination and bulimia. Regurgitation is the return of oesophageal or gastric contents into the hypopharynx with little effort. Rumination is the passive regurgitation of recently ingested food into the mouth followed by rechewing, reswallowing or spitting out. It is not preceded by nausea and does not include the various physical phenomena associated with vomiting. Bulimia involves overeating followed by self-induced vomiting.

Epidemiology

Nausea and vomiting from all causes has significant associated social and economic costs in terms of loss of productivity and extra medical care. In the community, nausea (with or without vomiting) is most likely to be associated with infection, particularly gastrointestinal infection. Vestibular disorders may cause vomiting, as can motion sickness. Nausea and vomiting may be associated with pain, e.g. migraine and severe cardiac pain. Many medicines also cause nausea and occasionally vomiting as a common dose-related (Type A) adverse effect. This is particularly common with opioid use, for example in palliative care. Nausea and vomiting also occurs postoperatively or in association with cytotoxic chemotherapy, or radiotherapy. These and other causes of nausea and vomiting are listed in Table 34.1.

Pathophysiology

Complex interactions between central and peripheral pathways occur in the production of the clinical features of nausea and vomiting. The most important areas involved peripherally are the gastric mucosa and smooth muscle (the enteric brain) and the afferent pathways of the vagus and sympathetic nerves. Centrally the significant areas involved are the area postrema, the chemoreceptor trigger zone, the nucleus tractus solitarus (NTS) and the vomiting centre.

From a pharmacotherapeutic point of view, the most important aspect of this complex pathophysiology is the variety of receptors involved, including histaminergic (H_1), cholinergic (muscarinic M_1), dopaminergic (D2), serotonergic ($5HT_3$) and neurokinin-1 (NK_1) receptors. In the clinical situation these become targets for various drugs directed at controlling the symptoms.

There are 10^8 neurones in the intestine and a complex interaction occurs between these, the mucosa, the smooth muscle in the intestine, the parasympathetic (vagus nerve) and sympathetic nerves and the higher centres in the spinal cord and brain to result in normal gastrointestinal peristaltic activity. The enteric brain and the vagus nerve monitor stimuli from mucosal irritation and smooth muscle stretch which may result in nausea and/or vomiting.

The area postrema in the floor of the fourth ventricle contains the chemoreceptor trigger zone (CTZ) and is a special sensory organ rich in dopaminergic, serotonergic, histaminergic and muscarinic receptors. It is located outside the blood–brain barrier and it is likely that chemicals, toxins, peptides, drugs and neurotransmitters in the cerebrospinal fluid (CSF) and bloodstream

487

Table 34.1 Selected causes of nausea and vomiting (adapted from Quigley et al 2001)

Central	
i. Intracranial	Migraine
	Raised intracranial pressure (tumour, infection, haemorrhage, hydocephalus, etc.)
ii. Labyrinthine Iatrogenic	Labyrinthitis, motion sickness, Ménière's disease, otitis media
	Cancer chemotherapy
	Many other medicines (e.g. opioids)
	Radiotherapy
	Postoperative
Endocrine/ metabolic	Pregnancy, uraemia, diabetic ketoacidosis, hyperthyroidism, hyperparathyroidism, hypoparathyroidism, Addison's disease, acute intermittent porpyhria
Infectious	Gastroenteritis (viral or bacterial)
	Other infections elsewhere
Gastrointestinal disorders	Mechanical obstruction (gastric outlet or small bowel)
	Organic gastrointestinal disorders (e.g. cholecystitis, pancreatitis, hepatitis, etc.)
	Functional gastrointestinal disorders (e.g. non-ulcer dyspepsia, irritable bowel syndrome, etc.)
Psychogenic disorders	Psychogenic vomiting, anxiety, depression
Pain related	Myocardial infarction

interact with this area to cause nausea and vomiting. However, the precise mechanism is not known.

The vomiting centre is situated in the dorsolateral reticular formation close to the respiratory centre and receives impulses from higher centres, visceral efferents, the eighth (auditory) nerve (the latter two through the nucleus tractus solitarius) and from the chemoreceptor trigger zone (Fig. 34.1). It includes a number of brainstem nuclei required to integrate the responses of the gastrointestinal tract, pharyngeal muscles, respiratory muscles and somatic muscles to result in a vomiting episode. The vomiting centre may be stimulated in association with, or in isolation from, the nausea process.

The vomiting reflex can be elicited either directly via afferent neuronal connections, especially from the gastrointestinal tract and is probably dependent on the integrity of the nucleus tractus solitarius, or from humoral factors dependent on the integrity of the area postrema. The sequence of muscle excitation and inhibition necessary for the act of vomiting is probably controlled by a central pattern generator located in the nucleus tractus solitarius, and information from the chemoreceptor trigger zone and vagus nerve converges at this point.

The central causes of nausea and vomiting include increased intracranial pressure, dilation of cerebral arteries during migraine and stimulation of the labyrinthine mechanism or of the senses of sight, smell and taste.

The peripheral causes of nausea and vomiting include motion sickness, delayed gastric emptying and gastric mucosal irritation

(ulceration, NSAIDs). These mechanisms are all mediated through the vagal afferent neurones. The vomiting associated with distension or obstruction of the gastrointestinal tract is mediated through both the sympathetic and vagal afferent neurones.

Patient management

Management of the patient with nausea and vomiting is approached in three steps.

1. Recognize and correct any complications. This includes dehydration, hypokalaemia and metabolic alkalosis in the acute situation with symptoms of less than 4 weeks duration. Weight loss and malnutrition are features in chronic nausea/vomiting, i.e. when symptoms have been present for 4 weeks or longer.
2. Where possible, identify the underlying cause (see Table 34.1) and institute appropriate treatment. Here it is important to be aware that metabolic or endocrine conditions such as hypercalcaemia, hyponatraemia and hyperthyroidism can result in vomiting.
3. Implement therapeutic strategies to suppress or eliminate symptoms (these depend on the severity and clinical context). Antiemetic drugs are ideally prescribed only when the cause of the nausea and/or vomiting is known, since by suppressing symptoms, they may otherwise delay diagnosis. However, they may also be useful in situations when directly addressing the underlying cause will not bring symptom relief sufficiently rapidly.

Some scenarios illustrating common therapeutic problems in the management of nausea and vomiting are outlined in Table 34.2.

Antiemetic drugs

Several classes of antiemetic drugs are available that antagonize the neurotransmitter receptors involved in the pathophysiology of nausea and vomiting. These classes of drugs are generally distinguished from each other by the identity of their main target receptor, although some act at more than one receptor.

Antihistamines

This group of medicines includes cinnarizine, cyclizine, diphenhydramine, diphenhydrinate and promethazine. They have some efficacy in nausea and vomiting caused by a wide range of conditions, including motion sickness and postoperative nausea and vomiting (PONV). They are thought to block H_1 receptors in the chemoreceptor trigger zone and possibly elsewhere. However, several of these agents also have potent anticholinergic (M_1) receptor antagonist activity, which may contribute significantly to their efficacy as well as their adverse effect profile (see Anticholinergics below). The sedative effects of some anti-histamines may also contribute to antiemetic activity, although this property appears not to be essential and it can be a particular problem when skilled tasks, such as driving, need to be performed. Nevertheless, the newer non-sedating antihistamines, e.g. fexofenadine, are of limited value in nausea and vomiting.

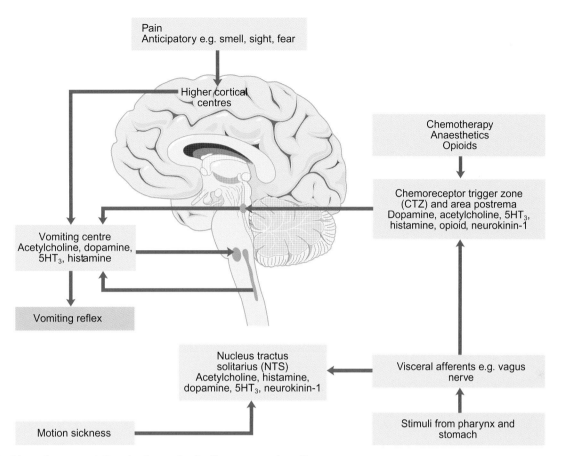

Figure 34.1 Schematic representation of pathways involved in nausea and vomiting.

Table 34.2 Common therapeutic problems in managing patients with nausea and vomiting

Problem	Possible cause/solution
Persistent nausea and vomiting despite treatment	Is the cause correctly diagnosed? Review the antiemetic agent and the dose: if both correct, change to or add a second agent
Patient with PONV is vomiting despite suitable antiemetic regimen	Check analgesia: pain may be causing nausea and vomiting, or patient-controlled analgesia may require adjustment downwards to reduce analgesic dose
Patient with bowel obstruction is passing flatus	Prokinetic drug is first-choice antiemetic. $5HT_3$ antagonists may also be effective
Patient with bowel obstruction is not passing flatus	Spasmolytic drug is first choice. Prokinetic drugs are contraindicated. Similarly, bulk-forming, osmotic and stimulant laxatives are inappropriate; phosphate enemas and faecal softeners are better
A terminally ill patient receiving diamorphine is vomiting, despite use of haloperidol	Levomepromazine given as a 24-hour subcutaneous infusion can be very effective
A patient with renal failure (uraemia) is vomiting	Consider a $5HT_3$ antagonist
A patient develops an acute dystonic reaction to metoclopramide	Give an intramuscular injection of an antihistamine. Such extrapyramidal reactions to metoclopramide are more common in young adults (especially females) and this agent is best avoided in this group

Anticholinergics

This is one of the oldest classes of antiemetics, of which many members are potent inhibitors of muscarinic receptor (M_1) activity both peripherally and centrally. Anticholinergic drugs such as atropine, hyoscine and glycopyrronium have been used preoperatively to inhibit salivation and excessive respiratory secretions during anaesthesia. Anticholinergics act by inhibition of cholinergic transmission from the vestibular nuclei to higher centres within the cerebral cortex, thereby explaining their pre-dominant use in the treatment of motion sickness. Hyoscine hydrobromide (scopolamine hydrobromide) is the most widely used agent and it can be given orally, by subcutaneous or intramuscular injection, or transdermally for motion sickness. Inhibition of peripheral muscarinic receptors can cause drowsiness, dry mouth, dilated pupils and blurred vision, decreased sweating, gastrointestinal motility and gastrointestinal secretions and difficulty with micturition. Anticholinergic agents may also precipitate closed-angle glaucoma in susceptible individuals.

Antidopaminergics

Phenothiazines and butyrophenones

Phenothiazines and butyrophenones, e.g. haloperidol, block dopamine (D2) receptors in the chemoreceptor trigger zone, but also have cholinergic (M_1) and histaminergic (H_1) receptor antagonist activity. As a consequence they share several adverse effects with antihistamines and anticholinergics, including drowsiness. In addition, the dopamine-blocking effects may be associated with acute dystonia (especially in children), and tardive dyskinesias or parkinsonism when used for prolonged periods. Prochlorperazine is less sedating and available as a buccal tablet and suppository for use when vomiting precludes oral administration. Phenothiazines are sometimes used for drug-associated emesis, including chemotherapy-induced nausea and vomiting (CINV), but like the butyrophenones, e.g. haloperidol, have in many situations been superseded by more specific agents such as metoclopramide and the selective $5HT_3$ antagonists.

Metoclopramide

At lower doses, metoclopramide acts as a selective D2 antagonist at the chemoreceptor trigger zone and its effects mirror those of the phenothiazines and butyrophenones. However, it also exerts peripheral D2 antagonism at these doses, and stimulates cholinergic receptors in gastric smooth muscle, thus stimulating gastric emptying. It may therefore be more effective than phenothiazines and butyrophenones when nausea is related to gastrointestinal or biliary disease. At higher doses, it may exert some $5HT_3$-receptor antagonism but at these doses, the incidence of acute dystonic reactions, particularly in young women, may limit its usefulness in chemotherapy-induced nausea and vomiting.

Domperidone

Although domperidone does not readily cross the blood–brain barrier (BBB), it is a selective antagonist of D2 receptors at the chemoreceptor trigger zone, which lies outside the BBB in the area postrema. It may also have peripheral effects that result in increased gastrointestinal motility and faster gastric emptying. It is used in drug-associated vomiting, including chemotherapy-induced nausea and vomiting, and is relatively non-sedating. It can be given orally or by suppository. Acute dystonic reactions occur less frequently than with metoclopramide. It prevents nausea and vomiting during treatment with apomorphine and other dopamine agonists in Parkinson's disease and is also used to treat vomiting associated with emergency hormonal contraception.

Selective $5HT_3$-receptor antagonists

Serotonin or 5-hydroxytryptamine (5HT) plays an important role in nausea and vomiting. The subtype $5HT_3$ receptors, which mediate the vomiting pathway, are located peripherally on vagal nerve endings in the gastrointestinal tract and centrally in the brain, with high concentrations found in the area postrema and nucleus tractus solitarius. Highly emetogenic agents such as cisplastin are thought to disrupt gastric mucosa and initiate the release of 5HT from enterochromaffin cells, which stimulate the $5HT_3$ receptors on afferent vagal nerve endings and thus trigger the emetic reflex. Selective $5HT_3$ receptor antagonists that act centrally and peripherally are now commonly used to treat or prevent chemotherapy-induced nausea and vomiting (with drugs of moderate to high emetogenic potential) and postoperative nausea and vomiting. They are also effective in radiotherapy-induced nausea and vomiting. Selective $5HT_3$ antagonists are generally well tolerated, with the most common adverse effects being constipation, headache, dizziness and sensation of warmth or flushing. Available agents include dolasetron, granisetron, ondansetron, palonosetron and tropisetron. They are all more expensive than antihistamines, phenothiazines, anticholinergics or dopamine antagonists.

Neurokinin-1 (NK_1) receptor antagonists

Substance P is a bioactive peptide that shares a common amino acid sequence with other bioactive peptides known as tachykinins. It appears to play an important role as a neurotransmitter in emesis as well as in pain and a number of other inflammatory processes. Substance P binds to the subtype neurokinin-1, or NK_1 receptors, which are found in the area postrema and nucleus tractus solitarius. A selective NK_1 receptor antagonist, aprepitant, is now available for use as an adjunct to dexametasone and a $5HT_3$ antagonist in preventing, but not treating, nausea and vomiting associated with moderately and highly emetogenic chemotherapy. It appears to be well tolerated but it is an inhibitor (and sometimes inducer) of cytochrome P450 (CYP3A4) and inducer of CYP2C9 and glucuronidation, so potential drug interactions with chemotherapeutic agents as well as other concomitantly administered agents may occur.

Cannabinoids

It is likely that the antiemetic activity of cannabinoids is related to stimulation of central and peripheral cannabinoid (CB1) receptors. Cannabinoids have modest antiemetic activity that is of similar magnitude to prochlorperazine in CINV, but they can cause a range of central nervous adverse effects, including drowsiness and sometimes behavioural disturbances, which may at times be severe. Thus, while the synthetic cannabinoid nabilone is indicated for nausea and vomiting caused by cytotoxic chemotherapy unresponsive to conventional antiemetics, it is recommended that it be used under close supervision, preferably in a hospital setting.

Corticosteroids

Corticosteroids are known to have antiemetic effects. Their mechanism of action is unclear but steroid receptors are thought to exist in the area postrema. As single agents, they appear to be at least as effective as prochlorperazine in preventing nausea and vomiting associated with mild to moderately emetogenic cytotoxic chemotherapy. Dexametasone, the most widely used corticosteroid in this context, improves the activity of prochlorperazine and metocloramide and may reduce some of the side effects associated with the latter. When combined with $5HT_3$ antagonists, corticosteroids are particularly effective in CINV associated with moderately emetogenic chemotherapy, or when used in delayed emesis. The same combination of dexametasone and a $5HT_3$ antagonist, and sometimes with aprepitant, may also be effective in CINV associated with highly emetogenic chemotherapy regimens.

Complementary and alternative medicines

Systematic reviews support the use of stimulating wrist acupuncture point P6 for preventing postoperative nausea and vomiting in combination with, or as an alternative to, conventional antiemetics (Lee & Done 2004). A systematic review of randomized trials has also demonstrated the efficacy of ginger (at least 1 g preoperatively) in postoperative nausea and vomiting. Ginger has also been claimed to be beneficial in motion sickness and pregnancy-associated nausea, but the evidence for each is limited to single randomized trials (Ernst & Pittler 2000).

Drug treatment in selected circumstances

Postoperative nausea and vomiting

Around 25% of patients experience postoperative nausea and vomiting within 24 hours of surgery (Gan et al 2003). The aetiology is complex and multifactorial and includes patient-, medical-, surgical- and anaesthetic-related factors. Management is multimodal and involves strategies to reduce baseline risk such as using less emetogenic induction agents, anaesthetic agents and analgesics, consideration of the use of regional rather than general anaesthesia, adequate hydration and intraoperative supplemental oxygen use and avoidance of high-dose neostigmine.

Many antiemetic agents have some efficacy in postoperative nausea and vomiting but combination therapy with drugs from different classes may be needed in patients at high risk, such as those with a previous history of postoperative nausea and vomiting or motion sickness, or after high-risk procedures, e.g. prolonged operations. Prophylactic treatments include dexametasone before induction or $5HT_3$ antagonists, antihistamines or phenothiazines at the end of surgery. Metocloramide and cannabinoids appear to be of limited value in the management of postoperative nausea and vomiting.

Premedication with opioids increases the incidence of postoperative nausea and vomiting and this may be reduced by concurrent administration of either atropine or hyoscine, which are primarily used as antisecretory drugs at premedication.

Risk scores

Prophylaxis is preferable to treatment and this can often be achieved not only by use of antiemetic drugs but also by suitable planning. For example, not all patients undergoing surgery will experience postoperative nausea and vomiting and universal prophylaxis is not cost-effective (Habib & Gan 2004). A simple risk scoring system has been devised in which the score increases relative to the presence or absence of four factors:

- female gender
- history of motion sickness or postoperative nausea and vomiting
- non-smoker
- opioid use during operation.

The incidence of postoperative nausea and vomiting with the presence of none, one, two, three or all four of these risk factors has been shown to be 10%, 20%, 40%, 60% and 80% respectively (Apfel et al 1999). Use of risk scores based on these criteria helps to appropriately tailor antiemetic use and can significantly reduce the incidence of nausea and vomiting in clinical practice (Apfel et al 2002, Pierre et al 2004).

Chemotherapy-induced nausea and vomiting

Three different types of chemotherapy-induced nausea and vomiting (CINV) have been identified: acute, delayed and anticipatory. Acute emesis begins within 1 or 2 hours of treatment and peaks in the first 4–6 hours. Delayed emesis occurs more than 24 hours after treatment, peaks at 48–72 hours and then subsides over 2–3 days. It occurs characteristically after high-dose cisplatin but may also occur after the related agent carboplatin, as well as cyclophosphamide or an anthracycline. Anticipatory emesis occurs in patients who have developed significant CINV during previous cycles of therapy. Acute CINV is often associated with an increase in plasma serotonin concentrations for the most emetogenic agents, while delayed and anticipatory vomiting seem to be mediated by serotonin-independent pathways.

Management of CINV depends on the emetogenicity of the chemotherapy regimen and the use of combinations of antiemetic drugs based on their varying target receptors. Chemotherapy agents are divided into four emetogenic levels (Table 34.3) defined by expected frequency of emesis (Kris et al 2006).

In high-level acute emesis, a single dose of a $5HT_3$ antagonist given before chemotherapy is therapeutically equivalent to a multidose regimen with these agents. Oral formulations of antiemetics are often as effective as intravenous ones. In lower level acute emesis, the cost of the $5HT_3$ antagonists is prohibitive and metocloramide or prochlorperazine are commonly used and are effective.

Dexametasone is the most extensively evaluated steroid in the management of CINV. Used alone, it is not sufficiently potent

Table 34.3 Relative emetogenicity of chemotherapy drugs (from Kris et al 2006)

Emetic risk (incidence of emesis without antiemetics)	Agent
High (>90%)	Cisplatin Mechlorethamine Streptozotocin Cyclophosphamide ≥1500 mg/m² Carmustine Dacarbazine Dactinomycin
Moderate (30–90%)	Oxaliplatin Cytarabine >1000 mg/m² Carboplatin Ifosfamide Cyclophosphamide <1500 mg/m² Doxorubicin Daunorubicin Epirubicin Idarubicin Irinotecan
Low (10–30%)	Paclitaxel Docetaxel Mitoxantrone Topotecan Etoposide Pemetrexed Methotrexate Mitomycin Gemcitabine Cytarabine ≤1000 mg/m² Flurouracil Bortezomib Cetuximab Trastuzumab
Minimal (<10%)	Bevacizumab Bleomycin Busulfan 2-Chlorodeoxyadenosine Fludarabine Rituximab Vinblastine Vincristine Vinrelbine

Table 34.4 Factors that cause nausea and vomiting in their own right and may contribute to the failure of apparently appropriate prophylactic regimens for CINV

Hypercalcaemia or other metabolic or endocrine disturbance
CNS metastases
Antibiotics such as erythromycin/clarithromycin
Gastrointestinal obstruction
Radiotherapy enteropathy

Pregnancy-associated nausea and vomiting

Pregnancy-associated nausea and/or vomiting occurs in about 70% of women during the first trimester. Risk factors for vomiting include a personal history of previous pregnancy-associated nausea/vomiting or motion sickness or migraine-associated nausea/vomiting, a family history of hyperemesis gravidarum or a large placental mass, e.g. due to multiple pregnancy. Symptoms usually begin 4 weeks after the last menses and in 80% of cases end at 12 weeks, having peaked at 9 weeks. In some women, the problem may persist until 16–20 weeks. First-trimester nausea and vomiting is not usually harmful to either the fetus or the mother and is not generally associated with a poor pregnancy outcome.

In contrast, hyperemesis gravidarum is a condition of intractable vomiting complicating between 1% and 5% of pregnancies and sometimes resulting in serious fluid and electrolyte disturbance and nutritional deficits.

In first-trimester nausea and vomiting, simple measures such as small frequent carbohydrate-rich meals and reassurance are sufficient to control symptoms. Ginger and P6 acupressure have also been advocated, although the evidence base is equivocal in early pregnancy (Jewell & Young 2003). It is important to avoid antiemetic drugs when possible, but promethazine has been recommended in severe vomiting, with prochorperazine or metoclopramide as second-line agents. In Canada and the USA a combination of pyridoxine (vitamin B_6) and an antihistamine, doxylamine, is approved for the treatment of nausea in pregnancy but this combination treatment appears to be less effective for controlling vomiting.

In hyperemesis gravidarum, drug therapy may be used, although no trials have shown clear benefit (Jewell & Young 2003). Fluid and electrolyte replacement, rest and if necessary postpyloric or parenteral feeding to provide nutritional support and vitamin (e.g. thiamine) supplementation should be considered. There are few safety or efficacy data on which to base drug selection so the agents recommended for vomiting of pregnancy mentioned above are generally used in the first instance in the UK.

Migraine

Migraine is a paroxysmal disorder with attacks of headaches, nausea, vomiting, photophobia and malaise. Treatment is directed at:

in CINV. However, it enhances the effect of other agents such as $5HT_3$ antagonists in high-risk situations and, together with metoclopramide, it also appears to be useful in treating delayed emesis.

The best management for anticipatory emesis is the avoidance of acute and delayed emesis during previous cycles. However, when anticipatory nausea and vomiting is a problem, a low dose of a benzodiazepine such as lorazepam is often effective.

When apparently appropriate antiemesis regimens fail, consideration should be given to the possibility of other underlying disease- and medication-related issues (Table 34.4).

- prophylaxis: avoid triggers, try β-blockers, pizotifen and in severe cases a $5HT_{1B/D}$-receptor agonist such as sumatriptan
- analgesia, including aspirin, paracetamol, opioids, NSAIDs
- antiemetics.

Nausea and vomiting in migraine are associated with headache intensity, and the concomitant gastric stasis aggravates the nausea and vomiting and may also delay absorption of oral analgesics. Metoclopramide and domperidone attenuate the autonomic dysfunction and promote gastric emptying. The major adverse effect of acute dystonic crisis with metoclopramide therapy should be borne in mind, especially in young women and children.

Labyrinthitis

Labyrinthine dysfunction results in vertigo, nausea and vomiting. Episodes may last a few hours or days. Causes include labyrinth viral infections, tumours and Ménière's disease. The onset of episodes is often unpredictable and disabling. Betahistine has some prophylactic effect. The anticholinergics, antihistamines, phenothiazines or benzodiazepines can be used to suppress the vestibular system. Usually hyoscine or meclozine is sufficient but if there is severe vomiting, prochlorperazine or metoclopramide may be of value.

Motion sickness

Motion sickness is a syndrome, a collection of symptoms without an identifiable cause. It is brought on by chronic repetitive movements which stimulate afferent pathways to the vestibular nuclei and lead to activation of the brainstem nuclei. Histaminergic and muscarinic pathways are involved. The symptoms include vague epigastric discomfort, headache, cold sweating and nausea which may culminate in vomiting. This is often followed by marked fatigue which can last hours or days. Onset of symptoms may be abrupt or gradual.

The anticholinergic agent hyoscine is the prophylactic drug of choice, although there is no evidence of its benefit once motion sickness is established (Spinks et al 2004). Antihistamine drugs may also be effective. The less sedating antihistamines cinnarizine or cyclizine are used. Promethazine, an antihistamine with sedative effects, is also effective but phenothiazines and $5HT_3$-receptor antagonists appear to be ineffective in this situation. Treatment should be started before travel; for long journeys, promethazine or transdermal hyoscine may be preferred for their longer duration (24 hours and 3 days, respectively). Otherwise, repeated doses will be needed.

The most important adverse effect of many drugs used is sedation, whilst for anticholinergic drugs it is blurred vision, urinary retention and constipation. In laboratory studies, the degree to which these effects impair performance, for example driving a car, is highly variable but subjects who take anti-motion sickness drugs should normally be deemed unfit for such tasks. These drugs also potentiate the effects of alcohol.

Many non-drug treatments have been advocated for alleviation, including wristbands, which act on acupuncture points, variously positioned pieces of coloured paper or card, as well as plant extracts such as ginger. The evidence base for these interventions remains very limited.

Drug-associated nausea and vomiting

As well as chemotherapeutic agents, many commonly used medications for other disorders can cause nausea and vomiting (Quigley et al 2001). Opioids are perhaps the most important group clinically, but dopamine agonists (used in Parkinson's disease), theophylline, digoxin and macrolides such as erythromycin can all cause nausea and/or vomiting, often in a dose-related manner (Type A toxicity). High-dose oestrogen, used in postcoital contraception, can produce these symptoms. Consideration should be given to altering the dose of the offending agent when possible, and administering the medication with food. With some agents, tolerance may develop. Thus tolerance to the emetic effects of opioids often develops within 5–10 days and therefore antiemetic therapy is not generally needed for long-term opioid use.

Palliative care-associated nausea and vomiting

Nausea and vomiting are common and distressing symptoms in cancer patients. In most cases the causes of nausea and vomiting are due to multiple factors such as the tumour itself, concurrent infection, drugs and metabolic disturbances such as renal failure. It is important to determine the predominant underlying cause for patients' symptoms by taking a careful history, examination and appropriate investigations so that potentially reversible causes of nausea and vomiting can be treated (Table 34.5) and the most suitable antiemetic prescribed.

Oral antiemetic therapy is effective for treatment of nausea in patients with advanced cancer but the subcutaneous route is preferred for those with severe persistent vomiting, either as a single dose injection or a continuous infusion via a syringe driver. When patients' symptoms improve, switching from subcutaneous injection to oral route might be preferable. Non-pharmacological interventions such as avoidance of certain food smells or unpleasant odours, relaxation techniques and use of acupuncture should be considered.

Table 34.5 Potentially treatable causes of nausea and vomiting in palliative care

Hypercalcaemia
Constipation
Renal failure
Raised intracranial pressure
Infection
Bowel obstruction
Peptic ulcer disease
Drugs
Anxiety

Chemotherapy-induced nausea and vomiting is described in detail elsewhere in the chapter. Strong opioids such as morphine, diamorphine, oxycodone and fentanyl cause nausea and/or vomiting in up to one-third of patients following initiation of treatment but the incidence is lower for weaker opioids such as codeine. Metoclopramide, cyclizine or haloperidol are often given for the relief of nausea and vomiting induced by opioids.

Gastroduodenal or intestinal obstructions in advanced malignancy are usually caused by occlusion to the lumen (intrinsically and/or extrinsically) or by absence of normal peristaltic propulsion. Surgery remains the definitive treatment for luminal occlusion due to cancer but this is often inappropriate for patients who are frail or with advanced malignancy. The aim of pharmacological interventions is symptom control. A prokinetic dopamine (D2) antagonist such metoclopramide or domperidone should be used for patients with nausea and vomiting associated with functional gastric or intestinal stasis. Prokinetics are also used in patients with partial gastric outlet obstruction but can worsen patients' symptoms of abdominal pain in complete gastric outlet obstruction. As prokinetics can exacerbate abdominal colicky pain associated with intestinal obstruction, their use should be avoided in that situation and antiemetics such as cyclizine or haloperidol used for symptom control.

Dexametasone has also been used for control of symptoms in malignant intestinal obstruction, not only for any antiemetic effect but also to reduce inflammatory tumour oedema around the obstructive lesion. Anticholinergics such as hyoscine butylbromide and somatostatin analogues such as octreotide have been used for symptom relief in intestinal obstruction by reducing gastrointestinal secretion and motility and thus reducing the frequency and volume of vomitus.

Biochemical disturbances such as hypercalcaemia and renal failure can be a cause of nausea and vomiting in patients with advanced malignancy. However, aggressive treatment with bisphosphonates or insertion of nephrostomy tubes respectively would not be appropriate for those who are in the terminal stages of their disease. Haloperidol and cyclizine appear to be effective for biochemical causes of nausea and vomiting. Levomepromazine has antidopaminergic, antihistaminergic, antimuscarinic and antiserotonergic activity. It is effective for most causes of nausea and vomiting and may help alleviate restlessness. It can also be given intramuscularly, intravenously or subcutaneously, including by continuous subcutaneous infusion. Unfortunately, sedation and postural hypotension can be a problem.

Summary

Nausea and vomiting are symptoms caused by a variety of underlying causes. Thorough clinical assessment and appropriate investigations should be undertaken when prescribing a therapeutic trial of an antiemetic. The choice of agent(s) should be based upon the likely cause and severity of the symptoms, the possible underlying pathophysiology, and the recommendations of evidence-based guidelines which take into account clinical effectiveness and cost-effectiveness.

CASE STUDIES

Case 34.1

A 30-year-old man presents seeking a remedy for vomiting which had an acute onset, 12 hours previously.

Question

What questions should be asked to determine the nature, cause and seriousness of these symptoms?

Answer

The cause of vomiting needs to be determined where possible to allow appropriate treatment to be initiated. The following questions should be asked.

- Are there symptoms or signs of infection, such as diarrhoea, sore throat, dysuria, photophobia, fever? (Infection, often of the gastrointestinal tract, is one of the commonest causes of vomiting.)
- Is there headache? (Raised intracranial pressure and meningitis can present with vomiting as an early symptom, usually without any nausea.)
- Is there abdominal pain? (Abdominal pain before vomiting usually means an organic gastrointestinal cause. Pain after vomiting may be due to muscle tenderness.)
- Has the patient started any new drugs (opioids, chemotherapeutic agents, digoxin, nicotine, NSAIDs, oral hypoglycaemics and some antibiotics are common causes) or drunk excess alcohol?
- Is there vertigo? (If present, this is suggestive of a labyrinthine cause.)

Case 34.2

A 19-year-old girl who is 12 weeks pregnant presents to hospital with intractable nausea and vomiting which has not responded to home therapy and which has resulted in hypotension and dehydration.

Question

List, in order of importance, the therapeutic strategies for this problem.

Answer

Treatment would normally involve:

- intravenous rehydration and electrolyte replacement
- bed rest
- antiemetics, such as promethazine; these are likely to be effective and there is little evidence to suggest that they have teratogenic effects
- postpyloric feeding
- steroids
- parenteral nutrition.

Case 34.3

A 45-year-old woman presents with ovarian carcinoma for which she is due to receive a course of cancer chemotherapy.

Question

What drugs might be appropriate, when should they be given, and what advice should be given to the patient regarding monitoring of symptoms after treatment with the chemotherapy?

Answer

This woman is likely to receive repeated cycles of emetic chemotherapy with carboplatin (moderate emetic risk) or cisplatin (high emetic risk) and therefore should be given prophylactic antiemetics before the start of chemotherapy. The choice of drug lies between metoclopramide combined with dexametasone for some moderate emetic risk situations, and one of the $5HT_3$-receptor antagonists (dolasetron, granisetron, ondansetron, palonosetron or tropisetron) for high-risk situations, with dexametasone to provide additional benefit. The monitoring of emesis and nausea both within and outside hospital for up to 5 days after treatment is a useful exercise in deciding which patients may need other therapies. It is also important to remember that patients should be given appropriate doses of antiemetics as rescue therapy to cover delayed-onset nausea.

Question

What principles for a postoperative nausea and vomiting programme should be taken into account?

Answer

The programme should contain a postoperative nausea and vomiting risk score which can be used in preoperation assessment. A simplified score has been devised, adding one point for each of the following: female gender, non-smoking status, history of postoperative nausea and vomiting, and opioid use. In low-risk individuals scoring 0 or 1 (<10% risk), prophylactic antiemetic therapy is unnecessary. Moderate-risk subjects (score 1, risk 10–30%) may require single-agent antiemetic prophylaxis, while in high-risk subjects (score 3, risk 30–60%) two agents (one of them often dexametasone) may be needed if intravenous anaesthesia is not possible. In very high-risk subjects (score 4, risk >60%) intravenous anaesthesia should be considered when possible and dexametasone and another antiemetic agent administered. Postoperative nausea and vomiting rescue therapy should be chosen depending on the postoperative clinical situation.

Case 34.4

A hospital with a large number of surgical specialties, including major inpatient thoraco-abdominal and day care procedures, wishes to update its postoperative nausea and vomiting programme.

REFERENCES

American Gastroenterological Association 2001 American Gastroenterological Association medical position statement: nausea and vomiting. Gastroenterology 20: 261-262

Apfel C C, Laara E, Koivuranta M et al 1999 A simplified risk score for predicting postoperative nausea and vomiting. Anesthesiology 91: 693-700

Apfel C C, Kranke P, Eberhart L H et al 2002 Comparison of predictive models for postoperative nausea and vomiting. British Journal of Anaesthesia 88: 234-240

Ernst E, Pittler M H 2000 Efficacy of ginger for nausea and vomiting: a systematic review of randomized clinical trials. British Journal of Anaesthesia 84: 367-371

Gan T J, Meyer T, Apfell C C et al 2003 Consensus guidelines for managing postoperative nausea and vomiting. Anesthesia and Analgesia 97: 62-71

Habib A Gan T J 2004 Evidence-based management of postoperative nausea and vomiting: a review. Canadian Journal of Anaesthesia 51: 326-341

Jewell D, Young G 2003 Interventions for nausea and vomiting in early pregnancy. Cochrane Database of Systematic Reviews, Issue 4: CD000145. John Wiley, Chichester

Kris M G, Hesketh P J, Somerfield M R et al 2006 American Society of Clinical Oncology guideline for antiemetics in oncology: update. Journal of Clinical Oncology 24: 2932-2947

Lee A, Done M L 2004 Stimulation of the wrist acupuncture point P6 for preventing postoperative nausea and vomiting. Cochrane Database of Systematic Reviews, Issue 3: CD003281. John Wiley, Chichester

Pierre S, Corno G, Benais H et al 2004 A risk score-dependent antiemetic approach effectively reduces postoperative nausea and vomiting – a continuous quality improvement initiative. Canadian Journal of Anaesthesia 51: 320-325

Quigley E M, Hasler W L, Parkman H P 2001 A technical review on nausea and vomiting. Gastroenterology 120: 263-268

Spinks A B, Wasiak J, Villanueva E V et al 2004 Scopolamine for preventing and treating motion sickness. Cochrane Database of Systematic Reviews, Issue 3: CD002851. John Wiley, Chichester

FURTHER READING

Berger A 2004 Prevention of chemotherapy-induced nausea and vomiting. PRRR Inc, New York

Gan T J 2006 Risk factors for postoperative nausea and vomiting. Anesthesia and Analgesia 102: 1884-1898

Mannix K 2006 Palliation of nausea and vomiting in malignancy. Clinical Medicine 6: 144-147

35 Respiratory infections

K. B. Saeed A. W. Berrington

KEY POINTS

- Oral cephalosporins have better clinical efficacy than penicillins in the treatment of streptococcal pharyngitis.
- There is controversy about whether otitis media should be treated with antibiotics or allowed to run its course.
- Viral respiratory tract infections are usually mild and self-limiting but influenza, including bird flu, and severe acute respiratory syndrome (SARS), can have severe consequences for individuals, for public health and for economic activity.
- Exacerbations of chronic bronchitis may be infective in origin; antibiotics are used where appropriate but other therapeutic modalities are also valuable.
- *Streptococcus pneumoniae* remains the single most common cause of community-acquired pneumonia. Reduced susceptibility to penicillin can complicate the management of serious pneumococcal infections but more significant degrees of resistance are currently not widespread among UK strains.
- Community-acquired pneumonia can be caused by a variety of pathogens and this is reflected in the antimicrobial regimens recommended for initial treatment: amoxicillin plus erythromycin is a typical regimen but newer quinolones are likely to be increasingly used for this indication.
- There are many potential causes of hospital-acquired (nosocomial) pneumonia, and each unit with patients at risk will have its own resident bacterial flora. This will strongly influence the choice of antibiotics for empiric therapy.
- *Pseudomonas aeruginosa* remains the most important respiratory pathogen in infections complicating cystic fibrosis; antibiotic treatment is targeted specifically at this organism.
- Immunocompromised patients are at risk from a variety of opportunistic respiratory infections, e.g. pneumocystis pneumonia in AIDS, invasive aspergillosis in neutropenic states, etc.

Respiratory tract infections are the most common group of infections seen in the UK. Most are viral, for which with some exceptions only symptomatic therapy is available. In contrast, bacterial infections are a major cause of treatable respiratory illness.

The respiratory tract is divided into upper and lower parts: the upper respiratory tract consists of the sinuses, middle ear, pharynx, epiglottis and larynx, while the lower respiratory tract consists of the structures below the larynx: the bronchi, bronchioles and alveoli. Although there are anatomical and functional divisions both within and between these regions, infections do not necessarily respect such boundaries. Nevertheless, it is clinically and bacteriologically convenient to retain a distinction between upper respiratory tract infections (URTIs) and lower respiratory tract infections (LRTIs).

Upper respiratory tract infections

Colds and flu

Viral upper respiratory tract infections causing coryzal symptoms, rhinitis, pharyngitis and laryngitis, and associated with varying degrees of systemic symptoms, are extremely common. These infections are usually caused by viruses from the rhinovirus, coronavirus, parainfluenza virus, respiratory syncytial virus, influenza virus and adenovirus families, although new viruses continue to be identified. For instance, in 2001 researchers in The Netherlands described a novel respiratory pathogen that has become known as human metapneumovirus (hMPV), which causes a spectrum of respiratory illness particularly in young children, the elderly and the immunocompromised (Van Den Hoogen et al 2001).

Colloquially, milder infections are usually called 'colds' while more severe infections may be known as 'flu'. This term should be distinguished from true influenza, which is reserved for infection caused by influenza virus. In general, the management of these infections is symptomatic and consists of rest, adequate hydration, simple analgesics and antipyretics. Apart from one or two exceptional situations, antiviral drugs are not indicated and in most cases are not active. Antibacterial drugs have no activity against viral infections although in the past they were widely prescribed, sometimes with spurious rationale such as prophylaxis against bacterial superinfection, sometimes simply because patients demanded them. In recent years heightened awareness of the adverse consequences of antibiotic overuse has led to national campaigns aimed at discouraging the public from seeking antibiotic treatment for viral infections.

Influenza

True influenza – that is, infection due to one of the influenza viruses (influenza A, B or rarely C) – can be a serious condition characterized by severe malaise and myalgia and potentially complicated by life-threatening secondary bacterial infections such as staphylococcal pneumonia. Coryzal symptoms are not usually a feature of influenza but the patient may have a cough. Influenza tends to occur during the winter months, providing an opportunity to offer preventive vaccination from October onwards, depending on supply. In the UK, influenza vaccine is normally targeted at three groups of individuals:

- those at risk of severe infection, e.g. people aged 65 years and over, and younger patients in special disease risk groups
- those living in long-stay care facilities in which the infection might spread particularly rapidly, and

- those in whom infection would be problematic for other reasons, such as carers and healthcare workers.

Unfortunately the virus mutates so rapidly that the circulating strains tend to change from season to season, necessitating annual revaccination against the prevailing types.

Influenza A and B infections are amenable to both prevention and treatment with neuraminidase inhibitors (NAIs) such as zanamivir and oseltamivir, although there is controversy about whether the benefits justify the costs involved. Zanamivir is administered by dry powder inhalation whereas the newer agent oseltamivir is given orally. Both are licensed for treatment and prophylaxis. National guidelines issued for the UK health service state that neuraminidase inhibitors should only be used when the number of people with flu reaches a defined threshold, i.e. influenza is known to be circulating in the community, and should only be used in patients at risk of developing complications and who can commence treatment within 48 hours of onset or exposure to influenza-like symptoms (NICE 2003a,b). Individuals at risk and eligible for treatment include those:

- with long-term chronic lung disease including asthma and chronic obstructive pulmonary disease
- with heart disease, but excluding individuals with high blood pressure who are otherwise free of cardiovascular disease
- with long-term kidney disease
- with diabetes
- experiencing immunosuppression
- aged 65 years or older.

The anti-parkinsonian drug amantadine, which has activity against influenza A virus, is also licensed for both prophylaxis and treatment but has a limited role because of toxicity and the rapid emergence of resistance.

Although they have yet to be tested in a pandemic influenza setting, the neuraminidase inhibitors almost certainly have a role and national agencies have stockpiles of the drug for use in such a situation. Pandemics (or global epidemics) of influenza A occur every 25 years or so and affect huge numbers of people. The 1918 Spanish flu pandemic is estimated to have killed 20 million people, and pandemics have taken place in 1957–58 (Asian flu), 1968–89 (Hong Kong flu) and 1977 (Russian flu). Further pandemics are thought certain to occur but their antigenic character and timing cannot be accurately predicted. Healthcare services must therefore plan carefully for such events and maintain stockpiles of antiviral drugs, and also the capacity for rapid vaccine development.

Influenza virus is not solely a human pathogen but can also infect birds and pigs. Avian influenza, caused by various serotypes of influenza A virus, is of particular economic importance in the poultry industry. Generally these viruses have not caused disease in humans but in 1997, in Hong Kong, a strain of avian influenza highly pathogenic in chickens went on to infect at least 18 people, of whom six died. Human infection was facilitated by close contact with infected birds but the virus was not able to spread from person to person, so permitting interruption of the outbreak by widespread slaughter of poultry. This is not cause for complacency, however. Transmission to humans of avian influenza continued to be reported sporadically after the 1997 outbreak, and an avian strain that emerged in South East Asia in 2003 had accounted for over 200 human cases with a case fatality of 56% by June 2006, some of which were probably acquired by person-to-person transmission. It is thought highly possible that the next human pandemic will arise in this way.

Sore throat (pharyngitis)

Causative organisms Pharyngitis is a common condition. In most cases it never comes to medical attention and is treated with simple therapy directed at symptom relief. Many cases are not due to infection at all but are caused by other factors such as smoking. Where infection is the cause, most cases are viral and form part of the colds and flu spectrum. Epstein–Barr virus (EBV), which causes glandular fever (infectious mononucleosis), is a less common but important cause of sore throat since it may be confused with streptococcal infection.

The only common bacterial cause of sore throat is *Streptococcus pyogenes*, the Lancefield group A β-haemolytic streptococcus. Infrequent causes include β-haemolytic streptococci of groups C and G, *Arcanobacterium haemolyticum*, *Neisseria gonorrhoeae*, and mycoplasmas. *Corynebacterium diphtheriae*, the cause of diphtheria, is rare in the UK but should be borne in mind when investigating travellers returning from parts of the world where diphtheria is common.

Clinical features The presenting complaint is sore throat, often associated with fever and the usual symptoms of the common cold. It is standard teaching that sore throats of different aetiology cannot be distinguished clinically. Nevertheless, more severe cases are more likely to be caused by EBV or *Strep. pyogenes* and in these patients there may be marked inflammation of the pharynx with a whitish exudate on the tonsils, plus enlarged and tender cervical lymph nodes. Previously, streptococcal infection was often accompanied by a toxin-mediated macular rash and sometimes considerable systemic illness (scarlet fever), but this presentation is now uncommon.

Group A streptococcal infection has a number of potential complications. Pharyngeal infection may occasionally give rise to disseminated infection elsewhere, but this is rare. More frequent accompaniments are otitis media, peritonsillar abscess and sinusitis. These should be distinguished from the non-suppurative compli-cations of streptococcal infection, rheumatic fever and glomeru-lonephritis, which are mediated immunologically. Discussion of these is outside the scope of this chapter but occasional cases are still seen in the UK and remain important causes of renal and cardiac disease in developing countries.

Diagnosis In most cases of pharyngitis a bacteriological diagnosis cannot be made, and these are presumed to be viral in origin. The aim of any diagnostic procedure is to distinguish the streptococcal sore throat, which is amenable to antibiotic treatment, from viral infections, which are not. If a definite bacterial diagnosis is required, a throat swab should be taken for culture and, unless the details of a particular case prompt a search for more unusual organisms, culture techniques are directed towards detecting β-haemolytic streptococci. If bacterial culture is negative and glandular fever is suspected, blood should be taken for serological confirmation, using either the non-specific 'monospot test' for atypical lymphocytes or specific tests for antibodies to EBV. Other viruses may be diagnosed by viral culture or serology but this does not usually contribute to management. Rapid bedside tests are available that detect group A streptococcal antigens in the throat, but there are concerns about their sensitivity and specificity and they have not been widely introduced in the UK.

Treatment Treatment of viral sore throat is directed at symptomatic relief, for example with rest, antipyretics and aspirin gargles. Streptococcal sore throat is usually treated with antibiotics although the extent to which they shorten the duration of symptoms and reduce the incidence of suppurative complications is modest (Del Mar et al 2004). Antibiotic treatment also reduces the incidence of non-suppurative complications, so is likely to be of greater benefit where these are common. There is also an argument that treating to eradicate streptococcal carriage might reduce the risk of relapse or later streptococcal infection at other sites.

Broadly there are three treatment strategies:

1. give antibiotics to all patients with suspected streptococcal infection and do not investigate unless symptoms persist
2. give antibiotics to all patients with suspected streptococcal infection but stop them if a throat swab is negative, or
3. wait for the results of culture before starting antibiotics.

There is no correct approach and each has its advocates, although the problem of resistance has led to increasing pressure on prescribers to restrict empirical antibiotic use, particularly for conditions that are frequently viral, of which pharyngitis is a good example.

Antibiotics effective against *Strep. pyogenes* include penicillins, cephalosporins and macrolides. Resistance to penicillins and cephalosporins has not (yet) been described in group A streptococci, although about 4% of isolates are resistant to erythromycin. Even against sensitive strains, macrolides such as erythromycin are demonstrably less effective than β-lactams.

Penicillins such as benzylpenicillin (penicillin G) or phenoxymethylpenicillin (penicillin V) have traditionally been regarded as the treatment of choice for streptococcal sore throat, but there is now convincing evidence that cephalosporins are more effective in terms of both clinical response and eradication of the organism from the oropharynx. This was summarized in a large meta-analysis of 40 studies (five unpublished) in which 10-day courses of oral cephalosporins and penicillins were compared in the management of children with streptococcal pharyngitis (Casey & Pichichero 2004). Bacteriological and clinical cure significantly favoured cephalosporins over penicillins, perhaps because penicillins are hydrolysed by β-lactamases produced by organisms such as anaerobes naturally resident in the oropharynx, whereas cephalosporins are not. The 10-day course length became accepted following earlier studies that compared the effect of different durations of penicillin treatment on bacteriological colonization. It is likely that treatment with cephalosporins and perhaps other drugs will permit shorter courses.

However, despite the therapeutic superiority, it remains controversial whether the extra expense of prescribing a cephalosporin rather than a penicillin is justified, and the two classes should be viewed jointly as first-line agents. Cefalexin is the preferred cephalosporin, penicillin V/G or amoxicillin the preferred penicillins, with the proviso that amoxicillin and other aminopenicillins should not be used unless EBV infection has been confidently excluded, since for reasons that are not understood these drugs are very likely to cause skin rashes if used in this condition.

Acute epiglottitis

Acute epiglottitis is a rapidly progressive cellulitis of the epiglottis and adjacent structures. Local swelling has the potential to cause rapid-onset airway obstruction, so the condition is a medical emergency. Previously, almost all childhood cases and a high proportion of adult cases were caused by *Haemophilus influenzae* type b (Hib), with the rest being caused by other organisms such as pneumococci, streptococci and staphylococci. With the advent of routine vaccination against *Haemophilus influenzae* type b in October 1992, this disease has become uncommon.

The typical patient is a child between 2 and 4 years old with fever and difficulty speaking and breathing. The patient may drool because of impaired swallowing. The diagnosis is made clinically and the initial management is concentrated upon establishing or maintaining an airway. This takes priority over all other diagnostic and therapeutic manoeuvres. Thereafter the diagnosis may be confirmed by visualization of the cherry-red epiglottis. Microbiological confirmation may be obtained by culturing the epiglottis and the blood.

In view of the high prevalence of amoxicillin resistance among encapsulated *H. influenzae*, the treatment of choice is a cephalosporin. It is customary to use a third-generation cephalosporin such as cefotaxime or ceftriaxone although there is no reason why the infection should not respond to a second-generation agent such as cefuroxime. If a sensitive organism is recovered, high-dose parenteral amoxicillin may be substituted.

Otitis media

Causative organisms Inflammation of the middle ear (otitis media) is a common condition seen most frequently in children under 3 years of age. Most cases are due to bacteria, although viruses such as influenza virus and rhinoviruses have been implicated in a sizeable minority. *Streptococcus pneumoniae* and *H. influenzae* are the two most commonly encountered bacterial pathogens. *Moraxella catarrhalis* and *Strep. pyogenes* account for a smaller proportion of cases, perhaps 10%, and other bacteria are seen only rarely.

Clinical features Classically, otitis media presents with ear pain, which may be severe. If the drum perforates the pain is relieved and a purulent discharge from the ear may follow. There may be a degree of hearing impairment, plus non-specific symptoms such as fever or vomiting in very young children. Complications of otitis media include mastoiditis (which is now rare), meningitis and, particularly in the case of *H. influenzae* infection, septicaemia and disseminated infection. With the advent of routine vaccination against *Haemophilus influenzae* type b, these complications have become uncommon.

Diagnosis The diagnosis of otitis media is essentially made clinically and laboratory investigations have little role to play. Unless the drum is perforated there is little sense in sending a swab of the external auditory canal, the results of which are likely to be unhelpful or misleading. For this reason a causative organism is rarely isolated and treatment has to be given empirically.

Treatment There has been much debate about whether or not antibiotics should be used for the initial treatment of acute otitis media. A meta-analysis combined seven clinical trials involving 2202 children and concluded that although antibiotics confer a modest reduction in pain at 2–7 days, they do not reduce the incidence of short-term complications such as hearing problems and they do cause side effects (Glasziou et al 2003). The benefit of antibiotic treatment may be greater in children under 2 than in older children (Damoiseaux et al 2000), but in any case about 80% of cases treated without antibiotics will resolve spontaneously within 3 days.

If treatment is to be given, it should be effective against the three main bacterial pathogens: *Strep. pneumoniae, H. influenzae* and *Strep. pyogenes*. The streptococci are both sensitive to penicillin, but penicillin is much less active against *H. influenzae* so the broader spectrum agents amoxicillin or ampicillin should be used instead. These two drugs have identical antibacterial activity but amoxicillin is recommended for oral treatment since it is better absorbed from the gastrointestinal tract. Patients with penicillin allergy may be treated with a later-generation cephalosporin (see below).

About 20% of *H. influenzae* strains are resistant to amoxicillin due to production of β-lactamase, so if there is no response to amoxicillin an alternative agent should be chosen. Both erythromycin and the earlier oral cephalosporins such as cefalexin are insufficiently active against *H. influenzae* and should not be used. Alternatives include co-amoxiclav (a combination of amoxicillin and the β-lactamase inhibitor clavulanic acid) or one of the newer oral cephalosporins such as cefixime, which possesses high activity against *H. influenzae*. Cefuroxime axetil, while active in vitro, is poorly absorbed and often causes diarrhoea.

Acute sinusitis

Causative organisms Normally the paranasal sinuses are sterile but they can become infected following damage to the mucous membrane which lines them. This usually occurs following a viral upper respiratory tract infection but is sometimes associated with the presence of dental disease. Acute sinusitis is usually caused by the same organisms which cause otitis media but occasionally other organisms such as *Staphylococcus aureus*, viridans streptococci (a term used to describe α-haemolytic streptococci other than *Strep. pneumoniae*) and anaerobes may be found. Viruses are occasionally found in conjunction with the bacteria.

Clinical features The main feature of acute sinusitis is facial pain and tenderness, often accompanied by headache and a purulent nasal discharge. Complications include frontal bone osteomyelitis, meningitis and brain abscess. The condition may become chronic with persistent low-grade pain and nasal discharge, sometimes with acute exacerbations.

Diagnosis As with otitis media, this is a clinical diagnosis and obtaining specimens for bacteriological examination is not usually practicable. In patients with chronic sinusitis, therapeutic sinus washouts may yield specimens for microbiological culture.

Treatment Since the causative organisms are the same as those found in otitis media, the same recommendations for treatment apply. Proximity to the mouth means that anaerobes are implicated quite frequently in acute sinusitis, particularly if associated with dental disease, and in such cases the addition of metronidazole may be worthwhile. Doxycycline has proved popular, particularly in chronic sinusitis, due to its broad spectrum of activity and once-daily dosage.

Lower respiratory infections

Acute bronchitis and acute exacerbations of COPD

Bronchitis means inflammation of the bronchi. It is important to distinguish between acute bronchitis, which is usually infective, and chronic bronchitis, which is a chronic inflammatory condition characterized by thickened, oedematous bronchial mucosa with mucus gland hypertrophy and usually caused by smoking. Chronic bronchitis often co-exists with emphysema, both of which lead to airflow limitation and the clinical syndrome of chronic obstructive pulmonary disease (COPD).

For the purposes of this chapter, the importance of chronic bronchitis is that it renders the patient more susceptible to acute infections and more likely to suffer respiratory compromise as a result. These acute exacerbations of COPD are a frequent cause of morbidity and admission to hospital. An exacerbation is defined as 'a sustained worsening of the patient's symptoms from his or her usual stable state that is beyond normal day-to-day variations, and is acute in onset' (NICE 2004). Common symptoms include worsening breathlessness, cough, increased sputum production and change in sputum colour. It is important to remember that not all acute exacerbations of COPD have an infective aetiology, since atmospheric pollutants are sometimes implicated.

Causative organisms In otherwise healthy patients, the causes of acute bronchitis include viruses such as rhinovirus, coronavirus, adenovirus and influenza virus, and bacteria such as *Bordetella pertussis, Mycoplasma pneumoniae* and *Chlamydophila pneumoniae* (formerly *Chlamydia pneumoniae*). The roles of bacteria such as *Strep. pneumoniae* and *H. influenzae* are uncertain because these organisms are nasopharyngeal commensals and their isolation can be misleading, but there is a presumption that they account for at least a proportion of infections.

In patients with acute exacerbations of chronic bronchitis, sputum culture frequently yields potential pathogens such as *Strep. pneumoniae, H. influenzae* and *Moraxella catarrhalis*. However, these organisms are also found in the sputum at much the same frequencies between exacerbations, so it is unclear to what extent (if at all) they play a pathogenic role. A considerable proportion of acute exacerbations is associated with viral infections such as colds or influenza, or might even be non-infective.

Clinical features The characteristic feature of acute bronchitis is a cough productive of purulent sputum, i.e. phlegm that is yellow or green, the colour reflecting the presence of pus cells, sometimes with wheezing and breathlessness. In patients with pre-existing lung disease the lack of reserve may lead to respiratory compromise, which in turn may exacerbate, or be exacerbated by, cardiac failure. Sometimes the condition progresses to frank bronchopneumonia (see below) although the dividing line between a severe exacerbation of COPD and bronchopneumonia is blurred.

Diagnosis The diagnosis of acute bronchitis or acute exacerbation of COPD is made clinically and does not depend on the results of investigations. If antibiotics are to be given, a sputum sample should be sent for bacteriology, since this will allow antibiotic sensitivity tests to be performed on potential pathogens.

Treatment   Younger patients without pre-existing respiratory disease are likely to recover rapidly and might not require specific treatment. For more severe cases, including exacerbations of COPD, the two main arms of treatment are airflow optimization and antibiotic therapy.

Airflow optimization consists of physiotherapy to aid expectoration of secretions, adjunctive oxygen if appropriate, bronchodilators and sometimes short-course corticosteroids. In severe cases a period of artificial ventilation may be required, an intervention which has become more common with the advent of non-invasive ventilation techniques.

Despite the reservation that many cases are non-infective, current guidelines recommend that antibiotics are prescribed when an exacerbation is associated with more purulent sputum. There is no unequivocal evidence that one antibiotic is better than another, so recommendations for empiric treatment are based generally upon spectrum, side effects and cost. Most authorities favour either a tetracycline such as doxycycline or an aminopenicillin such as amoxicillin, since these agents cover most strains of *Strep. pneumoniae* and *H. influenzae*. Some people argue in favour of co-amoxiclav, which covers β-lactamase producing strains of *H. influenzae* and *M. catarrhalis* that are therefore resistant to amoxicillin, but this agent is more expensive and has a greater incidence of side effects. For penicillin-allergic patients for whom tetracyclines are contraindicated, neither the macrolide erythromycin nor the earlier oral cephalosporins such as cefalexin or cefradine are sufficiently active against *H. influenzae* for empiric use. However, both clarithromycin and newer oral cephalosporins such as cefixime are active against haemophili while retaining activity against pneumococci.

The following recommendations can be made for the empiric antibiotic treatment of acute bronchitis and exacerbations of COPD. If a plausible pathogen is isolated, treatment can be modified accordingly.

First-line agents

- Doxycycline
- Amoxicillin

Second-line agents

- Co-amoxiclav
- Clarithromycin
- Cefixime

A number of other drugs are promoted for the treatment of COPD exacerbations. Of these, azithromycin is not recommended since it is less active than clarithromycin against *Strep. pneumoniae*. The activity of ciprofloxacin against *Strep. pneumoniae* is insufficient to justify its use as monotherapy against pneumococcal infections (although it has useful activity against *H. influenzae* and *M. catarrhalis*), and levofloxacin (which is the active isomer of ofloxacin) does not seem to offer any great microbiological advantage. Moxifloxacin is a newer quinolone that retains activity against Gram-negative organisms such as *Haemophilus* and *Moraxella* but has greater activity against Gram-positives such as *Strep. pneumoniae*. It has been favourably compared to standard treatment in exacerbations of COPD (Wilson et al 2004), but currently is being promoted only to secondary care where its advantages are less evident.

Bronchiolitis

Bronchiolitis is characterized by inflammatory changes in the small bronchi and bronchioles, but not by consolidation. It is particularly recognized as a disease of infants in the first year of life, in whom a small degree of airway narrowing can have a dramatic effect on airflow, but the causal organisms are equally capable of infecting adults, who may then act as reservoirs of infection. Most cases are caused by respiratory syncytial virus (RSV), which occurs in annual winter epidemics, but parainfluenzaviruses, rhinoviruses, adenoviruses and occasionally *Mycoplasma pneumoniae* have also been implicated.

Bronchiolitis is characterized by a prodrome of fever and coryzal symptoms which progresses to wheezing, respiratory distress and hypoxia of varying degrees. Aetiological confirmation may be made by immunofluorescence and/or viral culture of respiratory secretions, although increasingly the diagnosis of respiratory syncytial virus is made using rapid antigen detection tests.

The treatment of bronchiolitis is mainly supportive and consists of oxygen, adequate hydration and ventilatory assistance if required. Severe cases of respiratory syncytial virus disease may be treated with ribavirin, a synthetic nucleoside which is administered by nebulization for 12–18 hours on each of 3–7 successive days.

Babies born at less than 35 weeks of gestation or those less than 6 months of age at the onset of the respiratory syncytial virus season are at high risk of the disease. Likewise, infants under 2 years of age with a recent history of bronchopulmonary dysplasia or haemodynamically significant congenital heart disease are similarly at high risk and all are candidates for prophylactic treatment with palivizumab.

Pneumonia

Pneumonia is defined as inflammation of the lung parenchyma, i.e. of the alveoli rather than the bronchi or bronchioles, of infective origin and characterized by consolidation. Consolidation is a pathological process in which the alveoli are filled with a mixture of inflammatory exudate, bacteria and white blood cells that on chest x-ray appear as an opaque shadow in the normally clear lungs.

A wide range of organisms can cause pneumonia so it is useful to apply some kind of classification system, at least until the aetiology of a particular case has been determined. Pneumonia is often classified clinically into lobar pneumonia, bronchopneumonia or atypical pneumonia, but this does not correlate entirely with the bacteriological cause and in any case the distinctions are often blurred. It is more practical to classify pneumonia according to the nature of its acquisition, the usual terms being community-acquired pneumonia (CAP) and hospital-acquired pneumonia (HAP).

Community-acquired pneumonia

Causative organisms   The causes of community-acquired pneumonia are summarized in Table 35.1. The most common

Table 35.1 Causes of community-acquired pneumonia

Organism	Comments
Streptococcus pneumoniae	Classically causes lobar pneumonia, bronchopneumonia now common
Haemophilus influenzae	Cause of bronchopneumonia, usually non-capsulate strains
Staphylococcus aureus	Severe pneumonia with abscess formation, typically following influenza
Klebsiella pneumoniae	Friedlander's bacillus, causing an uncommon but severe necrotizing pneumonia
Legionella pneumophila	Particularly serogroup 1; causes legionnaire's disease, usually acquired from aquatic environmental sources
Mycoplasma pneumoniae	Cause of acute pneumonia in young people, respiratory symptoms often overshadowed by systemic upset
Chlamydophila pneumoniae	Mild but prolonged illness usually seen in older people, respiratory symptoms often overshadowed by systemic upset
Chlamydophila psittaci	Causes psittacosis, a respiratory and multisystem disease acquired from infected birds
Coxiella burnetii	Causes Q fever, a respiratory and multisystem disease acquired from animals such as sheep
Viruses	Several viruses can cause pneumonia in adults, including influenza, parainfluenza and varicella zoster viruses

vegetative bacterial causes are *Strep. pneumoniae*, the pneumococcus, which can cause both lobar and bronchopneumonia, and non-capsulate strains of *H. influenzae* which usually give rise to bronchopneumonia.

The so-called atypical pneumonias are a heterogeneous group of diseases which nevertheless have several clinical features in common, and which are clinically distinct from the classic picture of pneumococcal pneumonia. Aetiological agents include *Legionella pneumophila, Mycoplasma pneumoniae, Chlamydophila pneumoniae, Chlamydophila psittaci, Coxiella burnetii*, and viruses. *L. pneumophila* is the cause of legionnaire's disease, which occurs sporadically and in outbreaks often associated with contaminated air-conditioning or water systems. From 2002 to 2004 there were 300–400 new cases a year reported in England and Wales. Legionnaire's disease may be rapidly progressive with very extensive consolidation and consequent respiratory failure.

Viral infections should not be forgotten as causes of pneumonia, although in practice it is unusual to make a definitive early diagnosis so most cases are treated with antibacterials. Influenza can cause a primary viral pneumonia as well as being complicated by secondary bacterial (particularly staphylococcal) pneumonia, chickenpox can be complicated by a primary varicella pneumonia particularly in adults, and cytomegalovirus is capable of causing

a variety of infections, including pneumonia, in patients with compromised cell-mediated immunity.

Clinical features Pneumococcal lobar pneumonia presents with a cough, initially dry but later producing purulent or blood-stained, rust-coloured sputum, together with dyspnoea, fever and pleuritic chest pain. The peripheral white blood cell count is usually raised and the patient may be bacteraemic. The chest x-ray shows consolidation confined to one or more lobes (or segments of lobes) of the lungs. This classic picture is now quite rare, perhaps because the early use of antibiotics modifies the natural history of the disease. Bronchopneumonia presents more non-specifically with productive cough and breathlessness, and patchy consolidation on the chest x-ray usually in the bases of both lungs. This disease is very common and is typically seen in patients with severe COPD or in those who are frail and terminally ill (pneumonia has been described as the old man's friend because it is a relatively painless cause of death).

The atypical pneumonias are characterized clinically by fever, systemic symptoms and a dry cough, radiologically by widespread patchy consolidation in both lungs and biochemically by abnormalities in liver enzymes and perhaps evidence of inappropriate antidiuretic hormone secretion, evident as a low plasma sodium.

Despite the differences described, clinical features alone are not usually sufficient to make a confident bacteriological diagnosis, a fact that has major implications for the empirical treatment of pneumonia.

Diagnosis Sputum culture is the mainstay of diagnosis for pneumonia caused by pneumococci and *H. influenzae*. Sputum microscopy is unreliable because oropharyngeal contaminants are often indistinguishable from pathogens. The success of sputum culture is very dependent upon the quality of the specimen, which may be inadequate either because the patient is unable to expectorate or because the nature of the disease is such that sputum production is not a major feature. A more sensitive (although more invasive) technique is to perform bronchoscopy and bronchoalveolar lavage. Lavage fluid, being uncontaminated by mouth flora, is suitable for microscopy as well as culture.

In pneumococcal disease, blood cultures are frequently positive and some laboratories also perform plasma and urine testing for pneumococcal antigen. *Legionella* infection may be diagnosed by culture (if appropriate media are used) or by urinary antigen testing, but culture of *Mycoplasma* and *Chlamydophila* spp. is beyond the scope of most routine diagnostic laboratories. Viruses may be detected by immunofluorescence or by viral culture, but timely diagnosis requires a good specimen such as bronchoalveolar lavage fluid. In practice, the aetiology of atypical pneumonia is usually determined serologically (for instance, by acute and convalescent antibody testing), if at all.

Targeted treatment The treatment of choice for pneumococcal pneumonia is benzylpenicillin or amoxicillin. Erythromycin monotherapy may be used in penicillin-allergic patients but resistance rates are rising, macrolides are bacteriostatic rather than bactericidal, and the comparative efficacy of this approach is not known. There is retrospective evidence that combination therapy using both a β-lactam and a macrolide can reduce mortality in patients whose pneumonia is complicated by pneumococcal bacteraemia (Martinez et al 2003), but this awaits confirmation by prospective study.

Pneumococci with reduced susceptibility to penicillin are becoming increasingly common, particularly in continental Europe and the USA. In the UK, about 5–10% of strains express 'intermediate susceptibility' (MIC 0.1–1 mg/L), but high-level resistance (MIC >1 mg/L) remains uncommon. Intermediate susceptibility may result in treatment failure in conditions such as otitis media or meningitis, infections at sites where antibiotic penetration is reduced, but antibiotic penetration into the lungs is sufficiently good that penicillin and amoxicillin remain effective for pneumonia. Strains expressing high-level resistance are unlikely to respond to penicillins, however. Such strains are often co-resistant to macrolides and other first-line agents, and may require treatment with a later-generation cephalosporin or a glycopeptide.

The sensitivity of *H. influenzae* to antibiotics has been discussed above. Amoxicillin is the agent of choice, with co-amoxiclav, parenteral cefuroxime, cefixime or ciprofloxacin as alternatives. Erythromycin is poorly active but the newer macrolide clarithromycin and the azalide azithromycin possess more activity.

M. pneumoniae does not possess a cell wall and is therefore not susceptible to β-lactam agents. A tetracycline or a macrolide are suitable alternatives. Tetracyclines are also effective against *Chlamydophila pneumoniae*, *Chlamydophila psittaci* and *Coxiella burnetii*, but erythromycin is probably less effective. Quinolones are also highly active against these organisms.

Staphylococcal pneumonia is usually treated with flucloxacillin plus a second agent such as rifampicin, fusidic acid or gentamicin. MRSA (meticillin-resistant *Staph. aureus*) pneumonia is rarely seen outside hospital and its management demands specialist microbiological advice.

Treatment recommendations for legionnaire's disease are based on a retrospective review of the famous Philadelphia outbreak of 1976 (Fraser et al 1977), in which two deaths occurred among the 18 patients who were given erythromycin, compared to 16 deaths in 71 patients treated with penicillin or amoxicillin. This observation accords with the facts that *Legionella* is an intracellular pathogen and that macrolides penetrate more efficiently than β-lactams into cells. Azithromycin is probably the most effective of the macrolide/azalide derivatives, but clinical evidence to confirm this is lacking. Other agents with proven clinical efficacy and good intracellular activity against *Legionella* include rifampicin and quinolones. There have been no randomized controlled clinical trials, nor are there likely to be. Current practice is that legionnaire's disease is treated with high-dose erythromycin (1 g four times daily) with the addition of rifampicin in severe cases. Some experts recommend first-line use of quinolones such as ciprofloxacin, particularly in immunocompromised patients.

Empiric treatment All of the foregoing recommendations pre-suppose that the infecting organism is known before treatment is commenced. In practice, this is rarely the case and therapy will initially be empirical or best-guess in nature (Table 35.2). The most authoritative recommendations for the initial treatment of community-acquired pneumonia are those produced by the British Thoracic Society (File et al 2004). For mild disease, these recommend treatment with amoxicillin, providing activity against pneumococci and most strains of *H. influenzae*. However, for moderate or severe disease requiring admission to hospital,

Table 35.2 Treatment of community-acquired pneumonia

Scenario	Typical regimen	Comments
Mild-to-moderate pneumonia, organism unknown	Amoxicillin plus a macrolide	Amoxicillin covers *Strep. pneumoniae* and most *H. influenzae* while erythromycin provides cover against atypical pathogens. It is debatable whether clinical outcomes are improved by using antibiotics active against atypical pathogens in all-cause non-severe community-acquired pneumonia
Severe pneumonia, organism unknown	Cefuroxime (or co-amoxiclav) plus a macrolide. Quinolone with enhanced Gram-positive activity, e.g. levofloxacin or moxifloxacin	Cefuroxime provides cover against *Staph. aureus*, coliforms and β-lactamase producing haemophili while retaining the pneumococcal cover of amoxicillin. See discussion in text
Pneumococcal pneumonia	Penicillin or amoxicillin or Macrolide	High-level penicillin resistance remains uncommon in the UK. If confirmed or suspected, options include a cephalosporin such as cefotaxime or a glycopeptide such as vancomycin
H. influenzae	Non-β-lactamase producing: amoxicillin β-lactamase producing: cefuroxime or co-amoxiclav	Also sensitive to quinolones
Staphylococcal pneumonia	Non-MRSA: flucloxacillin +/– a second agent such as rifampicin or fusidic acid MRSA: vancomycin +/– a second agent	Isolation of *Staph. aureus* from sputum may reflect contamination with oropharyngeal commensals and should be interpreted cautiously. MRSA pneumonia may also be treated with linezolid
Mycoplasma pneumoniae *Chlamydophila* spp. *Legionella* spp.	A macrolide or tetracycline A tetracycline preferred A macrolide +/– rifampicin	Treat for 14 days Treat for 14 days Quinolones also active

they take the view that until the aetiology is known, treatment should cover both 'typical' causes, such as *Strep. pneumoniae* and *H. influenzae*, and atypical causes such as *M. pneumoniae*, *Chlamydophila* spp. and *Legionella*. For patients with moderate or severe community-acquired pneumonia, the guidelines therefore recommend a combination of a β-lactam drug plus a macrolide, the exact choice of agent and route being decided according to the clinical severity of the infection. In practice, this is usually interpreted as amoxicillin plus a macrolide for less severe disease, and cefuroxime plus a macrolide for more severe disease. Severity is assessed according to clinical parameters and outcome predicted by use of one of a number of assessment tools such as CURB-65, based on the onset of **C**onfusion, the serum **U**rea, the **R**espiratory rate, the **B**lood pressure and age >65 years (Lim et al 2003).

Pressure to treat pneumonia (much of which is pneumococcal and would respond to penicillin) with broad-spectrum empiric regimens has been cited as a factor in the rising incidence of *Clostridium difficile*-associated disease. Alternative treatment strategies include penicillin plus ciprofloxacin (penicillin to cover *Strep. pneumoniae*, ciprofloxacin to cover *H. influenzae* and the atypical bacteria) or even moxifloxacin alone, but these can have their own drawbacks; for instance, quinolone use is emerging as an important independent risk factor for the acquisition of MRSA, much of which is quinolone resistant.

The treatment of pneumonia illustrates many of the dilemmas and conflicting priorities of modern antimicrobial prescribing.

Hospital-acquired (nosocomial) pneumonia

Causative organisms The most frequent causes of hospital-acquired pneumonia are Gram-negative bacilli (Enterobacteriaceae, *Pseudomonas* spp. and *Acinetobacter* spp.) and *Staph. aureus* (including MRSA) (Table 35.3). However, it is important to remember that pneumococcal pneumonia may develop in hospitalized patients, and also that hospital water supplies have been implicated in outbreaks and sporadic cases of *Legionella* infection. Furthermore, it must be recognized that the common Gram-negative causes of nosocomial pneumonia will vary between hospitals and even between different units within the same hospital. This is especially true of ventilator-associated pneumonia, which for obvious reasons is usually acquired on intensive care units where broad-spectrum antibiotics are frequently used, and where there may be a particular 'resident flora' with an established antibiotic resistance pattern.

Clinical features Nosocomial pneumonia accounts for 10–15% of all hospital-acquired infections, usually presenting with sepsis and/or respiratory failure. Up to 50% of cases are acquired on intensive care units. Predisposing features include stroke, mechanical ventilation, chronic lung disease, recent surgery and previous antibiotic exposure.

Diagnosis Sputum is commonly sent for culture but is sometimes unhelpful as it may be contaminated by mouth flora. If the patient has received antibiotics, the normal mouth flora is often replaced by resistant organisms such as staphylococci or Gram-negative bacilli, making the interpretation of culture results difficult. Bronchoalveolar lavage is often more helpful. Blood cultures may be positive.

Treatment The range of organisms causing nosocomial pneumonia is very large so broad-spectrum empiric therapy is

---

Table 35.3 Causes of hospital-acquired pneumonia

Common organisms

1. Gram-negative bacteria:
   Escherichia coli
   Klebsiella spp.
   Pseudomonas aeruginosa

2. Gram-positive bacteria:
   Streptococcus pneumoniae
   Staphylococcus aureus including MRSA

Less common organisms

1. Other 'coliforms' such as *Enterobacter* spp., *Serratia marcescens*, *Citrobacter* spp., etc.
   Acinetobacter spp.
   Other *Pseudomonas* and related species, such as *Stenotrophomonas maltophilia*
   Legionella pneumophila (and other species)

2. Anaerobic bacteria

3. Fungi:
   Candida albicans (and other species)
   Aspergillus fumigatus (particularly following prolonged episodes of neutropenia)

4. Viruses:
   Cytomegalovirus
   Herpes simplex virus

---

indicated. The choice of antibiotics will be influenced by preceding antibiotic therapy, the duration of hospital admission, and above all by the individual unit's experience with hospital bacteria. The combinations shown in Table 35.4 have all been used at some time and all have advantages and disadvantages. Several of the combinations include an aminoglycoside and this may not be desirable in all patients. Single-agent therapy is attractive for ease of administration and three agents, ceftazidime, piperacillin-tazobactam and meropenem, have suitably broad spectra that include activity against *Pseudomonas aeruginosa*. Unfortunately, treatment failures have been recorded when ceftazidime is used alone due to the emergence of resistance while the patient is on treatment. In all cases erythromycin would be added if legionnaire's disease was suspected and, except for the regimens containing clindamycin or meropenem, metronidazole would be required for suspected anaerobic infection. β-Lactam agents are inactive against MRSA, which would require specialist management advice.

Prevention General strategies for minimizing the incidence of hospital-acquired pneumonia include early postoperative mobilization, analgesia and physiotherapy, and promotion of rational antibiotic prescribing.

A strategy proposed for the prevention of ventilator-associated pneumonia is selective decontamination of the digestive tract (SDD), which is based on the premise that the infecting organisms initially colonize the patient's oropharynx or intestinal tract (Kallett & Quinn 2005). By administering non-absorbable antibiotics such as an aminoglycoside or colistin to the gut, and applying a paste containing these agents to the oropharynx, it is thought that the potential causative organisms will be eradicated

Table 35.4   Treatment regimens for hospital-acquired pneumonia

Regimen	Comments
Ureidopenicillin plus aminoglycoside (e.g. piperacillin plus gentamicin)	Good activity against Gram-negative bacilli such as *P. aeruginosa* and also against pneumococci. Combination of piperacillin with the β-lactamase inhibitor tazobactam, currently the only ureidopenicillin product marketed in the UK, extends the spectrum to include *Staph. aureus* (not MRSA), anaerobes and some strains of *E. coli*, *Klebsiella*, etc. that are resistant to piperacillin alone
Cephalosporin plus an aminoglycoside (e.g. cefuroxime plus gentamicin)	Good activity against Gram-negative bacilli such as *E. coli*, *Klebsiella*, and Gram-positive organisms, but poor against *P. aeruginosa* and anaerobes
Clindamycin plus aminoglycoside	Good activity against Gram-positive organisms and anaerobes but much less so against Gram-negatives. Favoured in the USA where metronidazole is unpopular for the treatment of anaerobic infections
Ciprofloxacin plus glycopeptide (vancomycin or teicoplanin)	Ciprofloxacin provides good activity against most Gram-negative bacilli including *P. aeruginosa*. Glycopeptide provides activity against *Staph. aureus* (including MRSA) and pneumococci, although its penetration into the respiratory tract is relatively poor
Ceftazidime (monotherapy)	Convenient and avoids risk of aminoglycoside toxicity. Very active against Gram-negative bacilli including *Pseudomonas* but less so against Gram-positive organisms and anaerobes
Meropenem (monotherapy)	Broad-spectrum agent but expensive; not active against MRSA. Newer carbapenem agent ertapenem does not cover *Pseudomonas* spp. or *Acinetobacter* spp. so is unsuitable
Linezolid combinations	It is increasingly necessary to cover MRSA in empiric or targeted treatment of hospital-acquired pneumonia. Traditional options include glycopeptides and, where the prevailing strains are sensitive, aminoglycosides, but there are concerns about penetration into the lung. Linezolid, an oxazolidenone, provides reliable activity

and the incidence of pneumonia thereby reduced. In some centres an antifungal agent such as amphotericin B has been added; others have added a systemic broad-spectrum agent such as cefotaxime.

The role of selective decontamination of the digestive tract remains controversial. It has never been particularly popular in the UK, and concerns have been expressed about cost and the promotion of antibiotic resistance. A number of clinical trials have been performed and several meta-analyses published. Generally, these have shown that there is a reduction in pneumonia but no consistent benefit on mortality. While it seems likely that selective decontamination of the digestive tract is of some benefit to some patients, these variables require more rigorous definition before it can be routinely adopted.

Another suggestion is that the prophylactic administration of aerosolized antibiotics to ventilated patients (and perhaps other patients at risk) might reduce the incidence of infection. Agents suitable for aerosolized delivery and with the appropriate antimicrobial spectrum include aminoglycosides, particularly tobramycin, and the polymyxin drug colistin. Trials are in progress to assess the benefits and risks of this approach, and until the results are available it cannot be universally recommended.

Aspiration pneumonia

One further condition which may be seen either in hospital or in the community is aspiration pneumonia, caused by inhalation of stomach contents contaminated by bacteria from the mouth. Risk factors include alcohol, hypnotic drugs and general anaesthesia, all of these being factors that may make a patient vomit while unconscious. Gastric acid is very destructive to lung tissue, causing

severe tissue necrosis and infection often with abscess formation. Anaerobic bacteria are particularly implicated but these are often accompanied by aerobic organisms such as viridans streptococci. Treatment with metronidazole plus amoxicillin is usually adequate, or metronidazole plus cefuroxime if there are reasons to suspect a Gram-negative infection, for instance if the patient has been in hospital or previously exposed to antibiotics.

Severe acute respiratory syndrome

In February 2003 an antibiotic-resistant community-acquired pneumonitis of apparently viral origin was reported in Vietnam, Hong Kong and Singapore. In retrospect, the first cases had appeared in November 2002 in China. The illness, named severe acute respiratory syndrome (SARS), appeared to be transmitted by aerosol inhalation and perhaps by contaminated objects, infected faeces and skin contact. It spread rapidly to a number of other countries in North America, South America, Europe and Asia. The causative agent was subsequently identified (Drosten et al 2003) as a coronavirus and is now called SARS-associated coronavirus (SARS CoV). According to the WHO (2003), a total of 8096 cases was identified, of whom 774 died.

Clinical features   Following an incubation period of about 2–7 days, the illness started with a prodrome of fever with or without rigors, headache, an overall feeling of discomfort, and occasionally diarrhoea. A few days later the lower respiratory phase began, with a dry cough and/or dyspnoea, sometimes progressing to hypoxia. About 20% of patients with clinically recognized infection progressed to develop adult respiratory distress syndrome requiring intubation and ventilatory support. Elderly patients had the highest mortality.

Management Various methods of diagnosis were successfully explored during the outbreak, including detection of SARS-associated coronavirus RNA, virus culture, and serological detection of specific antibody. Treatment was largely supportive. Antiviral agents such as ribavirin were used in some cases but without much success. Prevention of secondary cases was achieved by strict isolation of cases and contacts. The outbreak had been terminated by July 2003, but since then there has been a small cluster of community-acquired cases in China, and several laboratory-associated cases. Many experts predict that SARS will re-emerge.

Cystic fibrosis

Cystic fibrosis (CF) is an inherited, autosomal recessive disease which at the cellular level is due to a defect in the transport of ions in and out of cells. This leads to changes in the consistency and chemical composition of exocrine secretions, which in the lungs is manifest by the production of very sticky, tenacious mucus which is difficult to clear by mucociliary action. The production of such mucus leads to airway obstruction with resulting infection. Repeated episodes of infection lead eventually to bronchiectasis and permanent lung damage, which in turn predisposes the patient to further infection.

Infecting organisms In infants and young children *Staph. aureus* is the most common pathogen. *H. influenzae* is sometimes encountered, but from the age of about 5 years onwards *Pseudomonas aeruginosa* is seen with increasing frequency until, by the age of 18, most patients are chronically infected with this organism, which once present is never completely eradicated. An important feature of those *Pseudomonas aeruginosa* strains which infect CF patients is their production of large amounts of alginate, a polymer of mannuronic and glucuronic acid. This seems to be a virulence factor for the organism in that it inhibits opsonization and phagocytosis and enables the bacteria to adhere to the bronchial epithelium, thus inhibiting clearance. It does not confer additional antibiotic resistance. Strains which produce large amounts of alginate have a wet, slimy appearance on laboratory culture media and are termed 'mucoid' strains.

Occasionally other Gram-negative bacteria are seen, such as *Escherichia coli*, which interestingly may also produce alginate in these patients, a characteristic which is otherwise very rare, or *Stenotrophomonas maltophilia*. Many centres worldwide have also experienced problems with members of the *Burkholderia cepacia* complex, which previously were known as plant pathogens. The most frequent culprits are *B. cenocepacia* (formerly *B. cepacia* genomovar III) and *B. multivorans* (formerly *B. cepacia* genomovar II). These organisms are often exceptionally resistant to antibiotics, and their acquisition may be associated with rapidly progressive respiratory failure, so patients colonized with *B. cepacia* complex should be isolated from other CF patients.

Clinical features Cystic fibrosis is characterized by persistent cough and copious sputum production. Many patients are chronically breathless. At times acute exacerbations occur in which there is fever, increased cough with purulent sputum, and increased dyspnoea. Systemic sepsis, however, is very rare. Eventually, chronic pulmonary infection leads to respiratory insufficiency, cardiac failure and death.

Treatment Although this section will concentrate on antibiotic therapy, it should not be forgotten that other means of treatment such as physiotherapy play a vital part, while lung transplantation can be life-saving. Even regarding antibiotics, there are fundamental questions that remain to be addressed; for instance, it is not known whether it is best to give antibiotics according to a planned, regular schedule or in response to exacerbations, and practice varies.

Table 35.5 Antipseudomonal antibiotics

Antibiotic	Comment
Ticarcillin	One of the first β-lactam agents effective against *Pseudomonas* but now considered insufficiently active. In combination with the β-lactamase inhibitor clavulanic acid it may be active against some otherwise resistant strains
Ureidopenicillins	Piperacillin, formulated in combination with the β-lactamase inhibitor tazobactam, is the only one of these agents now available in the UK. It should be given in combination with an aminoglycoside, with which it is synergistic
Cephalosporins	Ceftazidime is the most active antipseudomonal cephalosporin and is very active against other Gram-negative bacilli. It has rather lower activity against Gram-positive bacteria. *Pseudomonas* may develop resistance during treatment
Aminoglycosides	Gentamicin and tobramycin have very similar activity against *Pseudomonas*; tobramycin is perhaps slightly more active. Netilmicin is less active, while amikacin may be active against some gentamicin-resistant strains
Quinolones	Ciprofloxacin can be given orally and parenterally but as with ceftazidime, resistance can develop while the patient is on treatment. Other quinolones such as ofloxacin, its L-isomer levofloxacin, and moxifloxacin have better Gram-positive spectrum but concomitantly less activity against *Pseudomonas*
Polymyxins	These peptide antibiotics are considered too toxic for systemic use in all but the most desperate cases, but colistin (polymyxin E) can be given by inhalation
Carbapenems	Broad-spectrum agents with good Gram-negative activity. Imipenem was the first of these drugs but CNS toxicity and its requirement for combination with the renal dipeptidase inhibitor cilastatin have largely led to its replacement by meropenem. A third drug, ertapenem, has poor activity against *P. aeruginosa*

The treatment of infection in a child with cystic fibrosis will probably be directed against staphylococci, for which the usual anti-staphylococcal antibiotics such as flucloxacillin or erythromycin can be used. Once the patient is colonized by *Pseudomonas aeruginosa*, treatment depends on early and vigorous therapy with antipseudomonal antibiotics (see Table 35.5). A β-lactam/aminoglycoside combination such as ceftazidime plus gentamicin is usually used. Agents such as meropenem or a quinolone are usually reserved for treatment failures or when resistant organisms are encountered. The prolonged use of ceftazidime or ciprofloxacin alone should be avoided if possible since strains of *Pseudomonas aeruginosa* and some other Gram-negative bacilli may become resistant to these agents while the patient is receiving treatment. Other treatment modalities are emerging: in a multicentre, randomized controlled trial, long-term low-dose azithromycin was associated with improvements in lung function in patients chronically infected with *P. aeruginosa* (Saiman et al 2003).

Interestingly, patients with cystic fibrosis have a more rapid clearance of some antibiotics than other patients. This is particularly noticeable with the aminoglycosides, and larger doses are often required to achieve satisfactory plasma levels.

Children with cystic fibrosis are admitted to hospital very frequently, sometimes for long periods of time, and it is not surprising that some of these children develop an intense dislike of hospitals. This has encouraged the use of long-term indwelling central venous cannulae to allow administration of intravenous antibiotics at home by the parents. Ciprofloxacin can be given orally and offers the possibility of treatment for less severe exacerbations at home, perhaps after a brief time in hospital for parenteral therapy.

B. cepacia is often very difficult to treat, and strains may be resistant to all available antibiotics. Under these circumstances combination therapy is often used; there is some evidence with this organism that in vitro resistance does not always correlate with treatment failure in the patient.

The use of inhaled (usually nebulized) antibiotics as an adjunct to parenteral therapy has attracted some attention, both for treatment of acute exacerbations and for longer term use in an attempt to reduce the pseudomonas load. Agents which have been administered in this way include colistin, gentamicin and other aminoglycosides, carbenicillin and ceftazidime. The best evidence that long-term administration can be beneficial comes from a large multicentre trial of nebulized tobramycin (Moss 2001) in which 520 patients were randomized to receive once-daily nebulized tobramycin or placebo in on–off cycles for 24 weeks, followed by open label tobramycin to complete 2 years of study. Nebulized tobramycin was safe and well tolerated, and was

Table 35.6   Basic causes, defects and infections in immunocompromised individuals

Principal defect	Causative illnesses, diseases or agents	Pathogens causing chest problem (defect related)			
		Bacteria	Viruses	Fungi	Others
Phagocytes	Acute leukaemia, bone marrow failure and chronic granulomatous disease	Staphylococci, aerobic Gram-negative bacilli, *Nocardia asteroides*		*Candida* and *Aspergillus* species	
Antibody (B-cell) immunity	X-linked agammaglobulin-aemia, multiple myeloma, Waldenstrom's macroglobulinaemia and chronic lymphocytic leukaemia	Encapsulated bacteria such as *Strep. pneumoniae*, *H. influenzae*, *Staph. aureus*		*Pneumocystis jiroveci*	
Complement system		Encapsulated bacteria, and *N. meningitidis*			
Cell-mediated (T-cell) immunity	Di George syndrome, lymphoma, hairy cell leukaemia, medications (ciclosporin, steroids), AIDS, CMV and EBV infection	Intracellular micro-organisms, e.g. mycobacteria, *Nocardia asteroides*	Varicella zoster virus, herpes simplex virus, cytomegalovirus, EBV	*Cryptococcus neoformans*, *Histoplasma capsulatum*, *Pneumocystis jiroveci*	*Toxoplasma gondii*
Defects caused by splenectomy or hyposplenism		Encapsulated bacteria such as *Strep. pneumoniae*, *H. influenzae*, *N. meningitidis* and *Capnocytophaga canimorsus*			

Most agents currently used in mainstay immunosuppression regimens to prevent graft rejection, in organ transplantation, interfere with discrete sites in the T- and B-cell activation cascades.

Table 35.7 Common therapeutic problems

Problem	Comments
No pathogens isolated on sputum culture	Possibilities include an inadequate specimen such as saliva, non-infected or sterilized sputum, or a pathogen that cannot be cultured on routine media such as *Chlamydophila pneumoniae* or *Mycobacterium tuberculosis*. Pneumococci are susceptible to autolysis and may fail to grow even from a well-taken specimen, particularly if transport to the laboratory is delayed
Staphylococcus aureus isolated (including MRSA)	*Staph. aureus* pneumonia is a severe disease with characteristic clinical features, often associated with bacteraemia. However, the organism is frequently isolated from the sputum of patients with bronchitis or bronchopneumonia. In these instances it usually reflects contamination of the specimen with oropharyngeal commensals although some patients undoubtedly have a clinical infection requiring antistaphylococcal antibiotics
Candida spp. isolated	Unless there are reasons to suspect *Candida* pneumonia (as a consequence of neutropenia, for example), the isolation of yeasts is likely to reflect oropharyngeal contamination of the specimen. Yeasts can be carried commensally in the mouth, particularly in the presence of dentures, but a search for clinically apparent mucocutaneous candidiasis should be made
Aspergillus spp. isolated	Invasive aspergillosis, allergic bronchopulmonary aspergillosis and aspergilloma should be considered. Alternatively the finding might reflect inconsequential oropharyngeal carriage
Penicillin-resistant pneumococci isolated	Respiratory infections caused by strains with low-level resistance (MIC 0.1–1 mg/L) may be treated with penicillins. Strains with high-level resistance should be treated according to their sensitivity profile, for example using a later-generation cephalosporin
Coliforms isolated	Significance depends on the clinical context: unlikely to be responsible for community-acquired infection unless there is bronchiectasis, but may be relevant to hospital-acquired infections particularly if present in pure culture
Failure of a chest infection to respond to antibiotics	Consider poor compliance, inadequate dosage, viral or otherwise insensitive aetiology. Remember that β-lactam drugs are ineffective against *Chlamydophila*, *Mycoplasma* and *Legionella* infections
Sore throat, no pathogens isolated	Consider viral aetiology, particularly glandular fever in teenagers and young adults
Persistent illness following treatment for pneumococcal pneumonia	Consider the possibility of an empyema (pus in the pleural space), a condition which usually requires surgical drainage

associated with a reduction in hospitalization and improvements in lung function. This was at the expense of a degree of tobramycin resistance, although this did not seem to be clinically significant.

Respiratory infection in the immunocompromised

Increased use of immunosuppressive agents and, to a lesser extent (in the UK at least), the spread of AIDS have caused populations of immunocompromised hosts to expand. Respiratory tract infections in general, and pneumonia in particular, are frequent complications. Morbidity and mortality are high, so rapid recognition, accurate diagnosis and correct treatment are of prime importance. Diagnosis may be complicated by the sheer number of potential pathogens, the problem of distinguishing infection from non-infective conditions such as malignant infiltration or radiation pneumonitis, and non-specific or delayed presentation. The nature, duration and severity of the underlying immune defect, together with specific epidemiologic or environmental factors, influence the risk of infection by different organisms. These are summarized briefly in Table 35.6.

CASE STUDIES

Case 35.1

A 19-year-old male presented to his primary care medical doctor complaining of headache, sore throat, tiredness and difficulty in swallowing. On examination he had fever, tonsillitis and enlarged lymph nodes in his neck. The doctor took blood samples for full blood count and heterophile antibodies (monospot), and a throat swab. A course of oral cefalexin was prescribed.

Questions

1. What is the differential diagnosis?
2. Why was this antibiotic chosen?

   Two days later the culture results are negative and the monospot test is positive.

3. What is the final diagnosis?

Answers

1. The main differential diagnosis is between streptococcal infection, usually group A streptococci, although groups C and G streptococci

can cause a similar illness, and infectious mononucleosis typically due to EBV infection. HIV seroconversion may produce similar features.

2. Cefalexin was a good choice in this situation because it is effective against streptococcal infection (probably more so than penicillin), and did not risk causing the rash that almost inevitably occurs when amoxicillin is given to patients with glandular fever.

3. The monospot test is a test for atypical lymphocytes and is highly suggestive that the patient has infectious mononucleosis, probably caused by EBV, less likely cytomegalovirus. The precise aetiology could be confirmed by specific EBV and cytomegalovirus serology, but in this case this is not necessary. Once the diagnosis had been made, the antibiotics were discontinued and the patient advised on conservative management.

Case 35.2

During the winter, an elderly lady was found collapsed and unresponsive, and an ambulance was summoned. When paramedics arrived, she was in a state of cardiopulmonary arrest and they were unable to resuscitate her. The lady had a history of COPD and a few days previously had visited her doctor for antibiotics, having complained of a cough, malaise and increased breathlessness. Postmortem evaluation showed interstitial pneumonia, and a lung swab was positive for influenza A virus by rapid immunofluorescence and later by viral culture. The previous autumn she had refused the offer of influenza vaccine.

Questions

1. What were this patient's risk factors for serious complications of influenza?
2. What measures might have prevented this outcome?

Answers

1. Risk factors in this patient include her age and her underlying COPD. Other risk factors include chronic renal impairment, heart disease and liver disease.

2. If she had accepted her influenza vaccine this might have protected her against infection in the first place. Provided she presented early enough to her doctor (within 48 h of symptom onset), there may have been an opportunity to prescribe one of the neuraminidase inhibitors, zanamivir or oseltamivir. Whether the doctor would be able to routinely prescribe a neuraminidase inhibitor is normally determined by the public health authority/Chief Medical Officer. Prescribing is permitted during the influenza season when circulating influenza has been confirmed and the number of reported cases have exceeded a predefined threshold.

Case 35.3

A 35-year-old male was referred to hospital with pneumonia. He had recently returned from Spain. On examination he was febrile and tachypnoeic, but haemodynamically stable. Sputum, blood cultures, plasma for atypical pathogens and urine for *Legionella* antigen were sent, and pending these results he was started on oral amoxicillin 500 mg 8 hourly plus erythromycin 500 mg twice daily.

Questions

1. What are the differential diagnosis and the likely infecting organisms? The following day he was no better. His blood cultures were positive for

an organism that the microbiologists strongly suspected would prove to be *Streptococcus pneumoniae*.

2. How does this affect the management?

The organism was confirmed to be *Streptococcus pneumoniae*. Its sensitivity profile revealed that it expressed intermediate susceptibility to penicillin (MIC = 0.5 mg/L).

3. How does this new information affect the management?

Answers

1. He has a community-acquired pneumonia of moderate severity. The most likely causes include *Streptococcus pneumoniae*, *Mycoplasma pneumoniae*, *Chlamydophila pneumoniae*, *Legionella pneumophila* and viruses.

2. Isolation of pneumococcus from blood cultures effectively confirms that this organism is responsible for the pneumonia. At this point some practitioners would stop the erythromycin on the grounds that he no longer needs treatment for atypical bacteria. However, there is some evidence in favour of dual therapy in pneumococcal bacteraemia. In any case, the fact that he is bacteraemic and still unwell should prompt a review of the antibiotic dose and route of administration. He should be changed to high-dose intravenous penicillin or amoxicillin.

3. Pneumonia and bacteraemia caused by strains of pneumococcus with intermediate susceptibility to penicillin (MIC 0.12–1 mg/L) can be successfully treated with high-dose penicillin, so provided he begins to improve this need not lead to a further change of therapy. If, on the other hand, he was suffering from meningitis, this would be an indication to change to another drug, e.g. cefotaxime and/or vancomycin, according to sensitivities, in order to achieve satisfactory activity at the site of infection.

Case 35.4

A 6-month-old baby girl presented in January with a respiratory infection. She was off her feed, tachypnoeic and had a cough. On day 3 of this illness she was admitted to hospital where she was found to be cyanosed. Crackles were audible throughout her chest. Chest x-ray revealed bilateral hyperaeration with patchy atelectasis. She was treated with artificial ventilation for a few days, but a week later was back to normal.

Questions

1. What is the most likely cause of this infant's illness?
2. How would you establish the diagnosis?
3. What is the most appropriate specific therapy?

Answers

1. Although almost any respiratory infection could present like this in an infant, the most likely diagnosis at this time of year would be respiratory syncytial virus (RSV) causing acute bronchiolitis.

2. Respiratory syncytial virus can be rapidly detected in the laboratory from respiratory specimens by direct immunofluorescence, or more commonly using immunochromatographic kits. The virus can also be cultured.

3. Management is aimed at maintaining oxygen saturations, initially using airway suction and supplemental oxygen. Bronchodilators are of limited benefit. Artificial ventilation may be necessary in severe cases. The antiviral drug ribavirin, given by aerosolization or nebulization, is sometimes used in severe cases.

Case 35.5

A 48-year-old man was admitted to an intensive care unit with severe pneumonia. He gave a short history of abdominal pain and episodes of loose stool, but had become confused over the previous 24 hours. He was febrile, tachycardic and a little jaundiced. The chest x-ray showed extensive bilateral pulmonary infiltrates. He had recently returned from a Mediterranean cruise. Initial laboratory findings were white blood cell count elevated, plasma sodium reduced, liver enzymes deranged.

Questions

1. What is the likely diagnosis?
2. How could this be confirmed?
3. What antibiotic treatment would you give in this situation?
4. What is the natural habitat of this organism and how do people contract it?

Answers

1. This presentation is strongly suggestive of *Legionella pneumophila* pneumonia. The abdominal symptoms, liver involvement and mental confusion are characteristic (and can overshadow any respiratory symptoms), and a low plasma sodium is commonly seen as a consequence of inappropriate secretion of antidiuretic hormone.
2. The urinary antigen test is very rapid and accessible, with about 90% sensitivity and 100% specificity. Sputum culture, on buffered charcoal yeast extract medium, is definitive but can take up to 14 days. Other tests include direct fluorescence assay of the sputum or bronchoalveolar lavage, and serology.
3. Legionellosis should be treated with a macrolide, e.g. clarithromycin, with or without rifampicin. It also responds to fluoroquinolones.
4. *Legionella* is ubiquitous in the natural environment, where it parasitizes aquatic amoebae. Human infection usually follows exposure to aerosolized, contaminated water, and has been acquired via bathroom plumbing, whirlpool spas and cooling towers throughout the world. The well-recognized association with foreign travel probably reflects exposure to poorly designed or maintained air-conditioning systems.

REFERENCES

Casey J R, Pichichero M E 2004 Meta-analysis of cephalosporin versus penicillin treatment of Group A streptococcal tonsillopharyngitis in children. Pediatrics 113: 866-882

Damoiseaux R A M, Van Balen F A M, Hoes A W et al 2000 Primary care based randomised, double blind trial of amoxicillin versus placebo for acute otitis media in children aged under 2 years. British Medical Journal 320: 350-354

Del Mar C B, Glasziou P P, Spinks A B 2004 Antibiotics for sore throat. Cochrane Library, Issue 2. Update Software, Oxford

Drosten C, Gunther S, Preiser W et al 2003 Identification of a novel coronavirus in patients with severe acute respiratory syndrome. New England Journal of Medicine 348: 1967-1976

File T M, Garau J, Blasi F et al 2004 Guidelines for empiric antimicrobial prescribing in community-acquired pneumonia. Chest 125: 1888-1901. Available online at: www.brit-thoracic.org.uk/guidelines

Fraser D W, Tsai T R, Orenstein W et al 1977 Legionnaire's disease: description of an epidemic of pneumonia. New England Journal of Medicine 297: 1189-1197

Glasziou P P, Del Mar C B, Sanders S L et al 2003 Antibiotics for acute otitis media in children. Cochrane Library, Issue 2. Update Software, Oxford

Kallet R H, Quinn T E 2005 The gastrointestinal tract and ventilator-associated pneumonia. Respiratory Care 50: 910-923

Lim W S, Van Der Eerden M M, Laing R et al 2003 Defining community acquired pneumonia severity on presentation to hospital: an international derivation and validation study. Thorax 58: 377-382

Martinez J A, Horcajada J P, Almeda M et al 2003 Addition of a macrolide to a beta-lactam based empirical antibiotic regimen is associated with lower in-hospital mortality for patients with bacteraemic pneumococcal pneumonia. Clinical Infectious Diseases 36: 389-395

Moss R B 2001 Administration of aerosolized antibiotics in cystic fibrosis patients. Chest 120: 107-113

National Institute for Health and Clinical Excellence 2003a Guidance on the use of zanamivir, oseltamivir and amantadine for the treatment of influenza. Technology Appraisal 58. National Institute for Health and Clinical Excellence, London. Available online at: www.nice.org.uk

National Institute for Health and Clinical Excellence 2003b Guidance on the use of oseltamivir and amantadine for the prophylaxis of influenza. Technology Appraisal 67. National Institute for Health and Clinical Excellence, London. Available online at: www.nice.org.uk

National Institute for Health and Clinical Excellence 2004 Management of chronic obstructive pulmonary disease in adults in primary and secondary care. Clinical Guidance 12. National Institute for Health and Clinical Excellence, London. Available online at: www.nice.org.uk

Saiman L, Marshall B C, Mayer-Hamblett N et al 2003 Azithromycin in patients with cystic fibrosis chronically infected with pseudomonas aeruginosa. Journal of the American Medical Association 290: 1749-1756

Van Den Hoogen B G, De Jong J C, Groen J et al 2001 A newly discovered human pneumovirus isolated from young children with respiratory tract disease. Nature Medicine 7: 719-724

Wilson R, Allegra L, Huchon G et al 2004 Short-term and long-term outcomes of moxifloxacin compared to standard antibiotic treatment in acute exacerbations of chronic bronchitis. Chest 125: 953-964

World Health Organization 2003 Summary of probable SARS cases with onset of illness from 1 November 2002 to 31 July 2003. Based on data as of the 31 December 2003. Available online at: www.who.int/csr/sars/country/table2004_04_21/en

FURTHER READING

Bartlett J G (ed) 2001 Management of respiratory tract infections. Lippincott, Williams and Wilkins, Philadelphia

Brook I (ed) 2006 Atlas of upper respiratory and head and neck infections. Current Medicine Group, London

Hoare Z, Lim W S 2006 Pneumonia: update on diagnosis and management. British Medical Journal 332: 1077-1079

Nightingale C H, Ambrose P G, File T M (eds) 2003 Community-acquired respiratory infections: antimicrobial management. Taylor and Francis, Abingdon

Pedro-Botet L, Yu V L 2006 Legionella: macrolides or quinolones? Clinical Microbiology and Infection 3(suppl): 25-30

Santiago E, Mandell L, Woodhead M et al 2006 Respiratory infections. Hodder Education, London

Useful website: Health Protection Agency. Available at: www.hpa.org.uk/topics/index.htm

36 Urinary tract infections

N. J. B. Carbarns

The term urinary tract infection (UTI) usually refers to the presence of organisms in the urinary tract together with symptoms, and sometimes signs, of inflammation. However, it is more precise to use one of the following terms.

- *Significant bacteriuria:* defined as the presence of at least 100 000 bacteria per mL of urine. A quantitative definition such as this is needed because small numbers of bacteria are normally found in the anterior urethra and may be washed out into urine samples. Counts of fewer than 1000 bacteria per mL are normally considered to be urethral contaminants unless there are exceptional clinical circumstances, such as a sick immunosuppressed patient.
- *Asymptomatic bacteriuria:* significant bacteriuria in the absence of symptoms in the patient.
- *Cystitis:* a syndrome of frequency, dysuria and urgency, which usually suggests infection restricted to the lower urinary tract, i.e. the bladder and urethra.

- *Urethral syndrome:* a syndrome of frequency and dysuria in the absence of significant bacteriuria with a conventional pathogen.
- *Acute pyelonephritis:* an acute infection of one or both kidneys. Usually the lower urinary tract is also involved.
- *Chronic pyelonephritis:* a potentially confusing term used in different ways. It can refer either to continuous excretion of bacteria from the kidney; or to frequent recurring infection of the renal tissue; or to a particular type of pathology of the kidney seen microscopically or by radiographic imaging, which may or may not be due to infection. Although chronic infections of renal tissue are relatively rare, they do occur in the presence of kidney stones and in tuberculosis.
- *Relapse and reinfection:* recurrence of urinary infection may be due to either relapse or reinfection. Relapse is recurrence caused by the same organism that caused the original infection. Reinfection is recurrence caused by a different organism, and is therefore a new infection.

Epidemiology

Babies and infants

Urinary tract infection is a problem in all age groups, although its prevalence varies markedly. In infants up to the age of 6 months symptomatic UTI has a prevalence of about two cases per 1000, and is much more common in boys than in girls. In boys the rate of asymptomatic UTI is much more common than this, at around 2% in the first few months of life.

Children

In preschool children UTI becomes more common and the sex ratio reverses, such that the prevalence of bacteriuria is 4.5% in girls and 0.5% in boys. In older children, the prevalence of bacteriuria falls to 1.2% among girls and 0.03% among boys. Overall, about 3–5% of girls and 1–2% of boys will experience a symptomatic UTI during childhood. However, in girls about two-thirds of UTIs are asymptomatic. The occurrence of bacteriuria during childhood appears to lead to a higher incidence of bacteriuria in adulthood.

Adults

When women reach adulthood, the prevalence of bacteriuria rises to between 3% and 5%. Each year about a quarter of these bacteriuric women clear their infections spontaneously and are replaced by an equal number of newly infected women, who are often those with a history of previous infections. On average, about one in eight adult women has a symptomatic UTI each year and over half of adult women report that they have had a symptomatic UTI at some time, 20% recurrently, with the peak age incidence in the early 20s. UTI is uncommon in young healthy men, with 0.5% of adult men having bacteriuria. The rate of symptomatic UTI in men rises progressively with age, from 1% annually at age 18 to 4% at age 60.

Elderly

In the elderly of both sexes the prevalence of bacteriuria rises dramatically, reaching 20% among women and 10% among men. In hospitals, a major predisposing cause of UTI is urinary catheterization. With time, even with closed drainage systems and scrupulous hygiene, almost all catheters become infected.

Aetiology and risk factors

In acute uncomplicated UTI acquired in the community, *Escherichia coli* is by far the most common causative bacterium, being responsible for about 80% of infections. The remaining 20% are caused by other Gram-negative enteric bacteria such as *Klebsiella* and *Proteus* species, and by Gram-positive cocci, particularly enterococci and *Staphylococcus saprophyticus*. The latter organism is almost entirely restricted to infections in young, sexually active women.

UTI associated with underlying structural abnormalities, such as congenital anomalies, neurogenic bladder and obstructive uropathy, is often caused by more resistant organisms such as *Pseudomonas aeruginosa*, *Enterobacter* and *Serratia* species. Organisms such as these are also more commonly implicated in hospital-acquired urinary infections, including those in patients with urinary catheters.

Rare causes of urinary infection, nearly always in association with structural abnormalities or catheterization, include anaerobic bacteria and fungi. Urinary tract tuberculosis is an infrequent but important diagnosis that may be missed through lack of clinical suspicion. A number of viruses are excreted in urine and may be detected by culture or nucleic acid amplification methods, but symptomatic infection is confined to immunocompromised patients, particularly children following bone marrow transplantation, in whom adenoviruses and polyomaviruses such as BK virus are associated with haemorrhagic cystitis.

Pathogenesis

There are three possible routes by which organisms might reach the urinary tract: the ascending, blood-borne and lymphatic routes. There is little evidence for the last route in humans. Blood-borne spread to the kidney can occur in bacteraemic illnesses, most notably *Staphylococcus aureus* septicaemia, but by far the most frequent route is the ascending route.

In women, UTI is preceded by colonization of the vagina, perineum and periurethral area by the pathogen, which then ascends into the bladder via the urethra. Uropathogens colonize the urethral opening of men and women. That the urethra in women is shorter than in men, and the urethral meatus is closer to the anus, are probably important factors in explaining the preponderance of UTI in females. Furthermore, sexual intercourse appears to be important in forcing bacteria into the female bladder, and this risk is increased by the use of diaphragms and spermicides, which have both been shown to increase *E. coli* growth in the vagina. Whether circumcision reduces the risk of infection in adult men is not known, but it markedly reduces the risk of UTI in male infants.

The organism

E. coli causes most UTIs and although there are many serotypes of this organism, only a few of these are responsible for a disproportionate number of infections. While there are as yet no molecular markers that uniquely identify uropathogenic *E. coli*, some strains possess certain virulence factors that enhance their ability to cause infection, particularly infections of the upper urinary tract. Recognized factors include bacterial surface structures called P-fimbriae, which mediate adherence to glycolipid receptors on renal epithelial cells, possession of the iron-scavenging aerobactin system, and increased amounts of capsular K antigen, which mediates resistance to phagocytosis.

The host

Although many bacteria can readily grow in urine, and Pasteur used urine as a bacterial culture medium in his early experiments, the high urea concentration and extremes of osmolality and pH inhibit growth. Other defence mechanisms include the flushing mechanism of bladder emptying, since small numbers of bacteria finding their way into the bladder are likely to be eliminated when the bladder is emptied. Moreover, the bladder mucosa, by virtue of a surface glycosaminoglycan, is intrinsically resistant to bacterial adherence. Presumably, in sufficient numbers, bacteria with strong adhesive properties can overcome this defence. Finally, when the bladder is infected, white blood cells are mobilized to the bladder surface to ingest and destroy invading bacteria. The role of humoral immunity in defence against infection of the urinary tract remains unclear.

Abnormalities of the urinary tract

Any structural abnormality leading to the obstruction of urinary flow increases the likelihood of infection. Such abnormalities include congenital anomalies of the ureter or urethra, renal stones and, in men, enlargement of the prostate. Renal stones can become infected with bacteria, particularly *Proteus* and *Klebsiella* species, and thereby become a source of 'relapsing' infection. Vesicoureteric reflux (VUR) is a condition caused by failure of physiological valves at the junction of the ureters and the bladder which allows urine to reflux towards the kidneys when the bladder contracts. It is probable that VUR plays an important role in childhood urinary tract infections that lead to chronic renal damage (scarring) and persistence of infection. If there is a diminished ability to empty the bladder such as that due to spinal cord injury, there is an increased risk of bacteriuria.

Clinical manifestations

Most UTIs are asymptomatic. Symptoms, when they do occur, are principally the result of irritation of the bladder and urethral mucosa. However, the clinical features of UTI are extremely variable and to some extent depend on the age of the patient.

Babies and infants

Infections in newborn babies and infants are often overlooked or misdiagnosed because the signs may not be referable to the urinary tract. Common but non-specific presenting symptoms include failure to thrive, vomiting, fever, diarrhoea and apathy. Furthermore, confirmation may be difficult because of problems in obtaining adequate specimens. UTI in infancy and childhood is a major risk factor for the development of renal scarring, which in turn is associated with future complications such as chronic pyelonephritis in adulthood, hypertension and renal failure. It is therefore vital to make the diagnosis early, and any child with a suspected UTI should receive urgent expert assessment.

Children

Above the age of 2, children with UTI are more likely to present with some of the classic symptoms such as frequency, dysuria and haematuria. However, some children present with acute abdominal pain and vomiting, and this may be so marked as to raise suspicions of appendicitis or other intra-abdominal pathology. Again, however, it is extremely important that the diagnosis of UTI is made promptly to pre-empt the potential long-term consequences.

Adults

In adults the typical symptoms of lower UTI include frequency, dysuria, urgency and haematuria. Acute pyelonephritis (upper UTI) usually causes fever, rigors and loin pain in addition to lower tract symptoms. Systemic symptoms may vary from insignificant to extreme malaise. Importantly, untreated cystitis in adults rarely progresses to pyelonephritis, and bacteriuria does not seem to carry the adverse long-term consequences that it does in children.

In about 40% of women with dysuria, urgency and frequency the urine sample contains fewer than 100 000 bacteria per mL. These patients are said to have the urethral syndrome. Some have a true bacterial infection but with relatively low counts (100–1000 bacteria per mL). Some have urethral infection with *Chlamydia trachomatis*, *Neisseria gonorrhoeae*, mycoplasmas or other 'fastidious' organisms, any of which might give rise to symptoms indistinguishable from those of cystitis. In others no known cause can be found by conventional laboratory techniques. It is important to consider the possibility of urinary tract tuberculosis, as special methods are necessary for its detection. Sometimes the symptoms are of non-infectious origin, such as menopausal

oestrogen deficiency or allergy. However, most cases of urethral syndrome will respond to standard antibiotic regimens as used for treating confirmed UTI.

Elderly

Although UTI is frequent in the elderly, the great majority of cases are asymptomatic, and even when present, symptoms are not diagnostic because frequency, dysuria, hesitancy and incontinence are fairly common in elderly people without infection. Furthermore, there may be non-specific systemic manifestations such as confusion and falls, or alternatively the infection may be the cause of deterioration in pre-existing conditions such as diabetes mellitus or congestive cardiac failure, whose clinical features might predominate. UTI is one of the most frequent causes of admission to hospital among the elderly.

Investigations

The key to successful laboratory diagnosis of UTI lies in obtaining an uncontaminated urine sample for microscopy and culture. Contaminating bacteria can arise from skin, vaginal flora in women and penile flora in men. Patients therefore need to be instructed in how to produce a midstream urine sample (MSU). For women, this requires careful cleansing of the perineum and external genitalia with soap and water. Uncircumcised men should retract the foreskin. This is followed by a controlled micturition in which about 20 mL of urine from only the middle portion of the stream is collected, the initial and final components being voided into the toilet or bedpan. Understandably, this is not always possible and many so-called MSUs are in fact clean-catch specimens in which the whole urine volume is collected into a sterile receptacle and an aliquot transferred into a specimen pot for submission to the laboratory. These are more likely to contain urethral contaminants. In very young children, special collection pads for use inside nappies or stick-on bags are useful ways of obtaining a urine sample. Occasionally, in-and-out catheterization or even suprapubic aspiration directly from the bladder is necessary.

For primary care doctors located at some distance from the laboratory, transport of specimens is a problem. Specimens must reach the laboratory within 1–2 hours or should be refrigerated, otherwise any bacteria in the specimen will multiply and might give rise to a false-positive result. Methods of overcoming bacterial multiplication in urine include the addition of boric acid to the container and the use of dip-slides, in which an agar-coated paddle is dipped into the urine and submitted directly to the laboratory for incubation. Both of these alternatives have difficulties. For the boric acid technique, it is important that the correct amount of urine is added to the container to achieve the appropriate concentration of boric acid (1.8% w/v), as the chemical has significant antibacterial activity when more concentrated. When the dip-slide is used, no specimen is available on which to do cell counts.

Concerns about the relative expense and slow turn-around time of urine microscopy and culture have stimulated interest in alternative diagnostic strategies. Some advocate a policy of empirical antimicrobial treatment in the first instance, and reserve investigation only for those cases that do not respond. Others are in favour of using cheaper, more convenient screening tests, for example urine dipsticks. Urine microscopy and culture remain the standard by which other investigations are measured.

Dipsticks

Dipsticks for rapid near-patient testing for urinary blood, protein, nitrites and leucocyte esterase are usually used, although there are concerns that these are reliable only when applied to fresh urine samples tested at the point of care. Assessment of colour changes on dipsticks can be subjective and automated reading systems have been developed to assist interpretation. Generally the negative predictive value is better than the positive predictive value, so their preferred use is as screening tests to identify those specimens which are least likely to be infected and which therefore do not require culture. A perfectly valid alternative is just to hold the specimen up to the light: specimens that are visibly clear are very likely to be sterile (Bulloch et al 2000).

The leucocyte esterase test detects enzyme released from leucocytes in urine and is approximately 90% sensitive at detecting white blood cell counts of >10 per mm³. It will be positive even if the cells have been destroyed due to delays in transport to a laboratory. However, vitamin C and antibiotics in the urine such as cephalosporins, gentamicin and nitrofurantoin may interfere with the reaction. The nitrite test (also called the Griess test) detects urinary nitrite made by bacteria that can convert dietary nitrate used as a food preservative to nitrite. Although the coliform bacteria that commonly cause UTI can be detected in this way, some organisms cannot, e.g. enterococci, group B streptococci, *Pseudomonas*, because they do not contain the converting enzyme. In addition, the test depends on sufficient nitrate in the diet and on allowing enough time, at least 4 hours, for the chemical conversion to occur in the urine. The inability of the test to detect group B streptococci makes it a relatively inappropriate test for screening for asymptomatic bacteriuria in pregnancy.

Although a negative dipstick test for leucocytes and nitrites can quite accurately predict absence of infection, it does not necessarily predict response to antibiotic treatment and further research is needed on this (Richards et al 2005). An algorithm for the use of dipstick testing in uncomplicated UTI in adult women is set out in Figure 36.1.

There are other rapid methods for detecting bacteriuria, such as tests for interleukin-8, and no shortage of data concerning their sensitivity and specificity, but the optimal strategy will always be a compromise between accuracy, speed, convenience and cost, and is likely to be very different for different settings and populations.

Microscopy

Microscopy is the first step in the laboratory diagnosis of UTI, and can be readily performed in practice. A drop of uncentrifuged urine is placed on a slide, covered with a coverslip and examined under a ×40 objective. Excess white cells are usually seen in the urine of patients with symptomatic UTI, and more than five per high-power field is abnormal. It should be noted that there are other methods in common use, and laboratories may report white cell counts per microlitre (cubic millimetre) of urine or even per millilitre.

It is important not to be too rigid in the interpretation of the white cell count: UTI may occur in the absence of pyuria, particularly at the extremes of age, in pregnancy and in pyelonephritis. Red blood cells may be seen, as may white cell casts, which are suggestive of pyelonephritis. As a rule of thumb, the presence of at least one bacterium per field correlates with 100 000 bacteria per mL. Automated machinery for microscopy of urine is increasingly used and offers increased precision and handling capacities of over 100 specimens per hour. Although there is a substantial capital cost to such equipment, it is offset by savings in labour and bacterial culture materials.

Culture

Bladder urine is normally sterile but when passed via the urethra it is inevitable that some contamination with the urethral bacterial flora will occur. This is why it is important that laboratories quantify the number of bacteria in urine specimens. In work carried out over 40 years ago it was demonstrated that patients with UTI usually have at least 100 000 bacteria per mL, while in patients without infection the count is usually below 1000 bacteria per mL. Between these figures lies a grey area, and it should be appreciated that the MSU is not an infallible guide to the presence or absence of urinary infection. True infections may be associated with low counts, particularly when the urine is very dilute because of excessive fluid intake or where the pathogen is slow-growing. Most genuine infections are caused by one single bacterial species; mixed cultures usually suggest contamination. If a patient is taking an antibiotic when a urine specimen is obtained for culture, growth of bacteria may be inhibited. The laboratory may perform a test to detect antimicrobial substances in the urine and this may be useful information to clarify circumstances in which the culture is negative but a significant pyuria is present.

Treatment

Although many, and perhaps most, cases would clear spontaneously given time, symptomatic UTI usually merits antibiotic treatment to eradicate both symptoms and pathogen. Asymptomatic bacteriuria may or may not need treatment depending upon the circumstances of the individual case. Bacteriuria in children and in pregnant women requires treatment because of the potential complications. On the other hand, in non-pregnant, asymptomatic bacteriuric adults without any obstructive lesion, screening and treatment are probably unwarranted in most circumstances (Nicolle et al 2005). A number of the common management problems are summarized in Table 36.1.

Non-specific treatment

Advising patients with UTI to drink a lot of fluids is common practice on the theoretical basis that more infected urine is

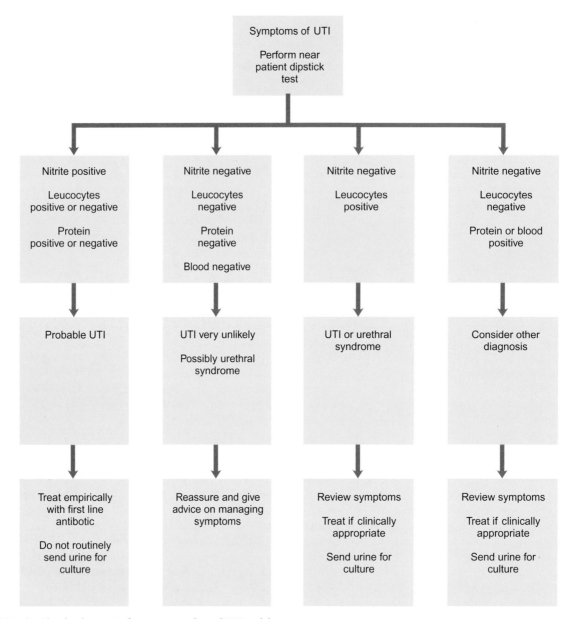

Figure 36.1 Algorithm for diagnosis of acute uncomplicated UTI in adult women.

removed by frequent bladder emptying. This is plausible, although not evidence based. Some clinicians recommend urinary analgesics such as potassium or sodium citrate, which alkalinize the urine, but these should be used as an adjunct to antibiotics. They should not be used in conjunction with nitrofurantoin, which is active only at acidic pH.

Antimicrobial chemotherapy

The principles of antimicrobial treatment of UTI are the same as those of treating any other infection: from a group of suitable drugs chosen on the basis of efficacy, safety and cost, select the agent with the narrowest possible spectrum and administer it for the shortest possible time. In general, there is no evidence that bactericidal antibiotics are superior to bacteriostatic agents in treating UTI, except perhaps in relapsing infections. Blood levels of antibiotics appear to be unimportant in the treatment

of lower UTI; what matters is the concentration in the urine. However, blood levels probably are important in treating pyelonephritis, which may progress to bacteraemia. Drugs suitable for the oral treatment of cystitis include trimethoprim, the β-lactams, particularly amoxicillin and co-amoxiclav, oral cephalosporins, fluoroquinolones such as ciprofloxacin, norfloxacin and ofloxacin, and nitrofurantoin. Where intravenous administration is required, suitable agents include β-lactams such as amoxicillin and cefuroxime, quinolones such as ciprofloxacin, and aminoglycosides such as gentamicin.

In renal failure it may be difficult to achieve adequate therapeutic concentrations of some drugs in the urine, particularly nitrofurantoin and quinolones. Furthermore, accumulation and toxicity may complicate the use of aminoglycosides. Penicillins and cephalosporins attain satisfactory concentrations and are relatively non-toxic, and are therefore the agents of choice for treating UTI in the presence of renal failure.

Table 36.1 Common management problems

Problem	Comments
Asymptomatic infection	Asymptomatic bacteriuria should be treated where there is a risk of serious consequences (e.g. in childhood), where there is renal scarring, and in pregnancy. Otherwise treatment is not usually required
Catheter in situ, patient unwell	Systemic symptoms may result from catheter-associated UTI, and should respond to antibiotics although the catheter is likely to remain colonized. Local symptoms such as urgency are more likely to reflect urethral irritation than infection
Catheter in situ, urine cloudy or smelly	Unless the patient is systemically unwell, antibiotics are unlikely to achieve much and may give rise to resistance. Interventions of uncertain benefit include bladder wash-outs or a change of catheter
Penicillin allergy	Clarify 'allergy': vomiting or diarrhoea are not allergic phenomena and do not contraindicate penicillins. Penicillin-induced rash is a contraindication to amoxicillin but cephalosporins are likely to be tolerated. Penicillin-induced anaphylaxis suggests that all β-lactams should be avoided
Symptoms of UTI but no bacteriuria	Exclude urethritis, candidosis, etc. Otherwise likely to be urethral syndrome, which usually responds to conventional antibiotics
Bacteriuria but no pyuria	May suggest contamination. However, pyuria is not invariable in UTI and may be absent particularly in pyelonephritis, pregnancy, neonates, the elderly, and *Proteus* infections
Pyuria but no bacteriuria	Usually the patient has started antibiotics before taking the specimen. Rarely, a feature of unusual infections (e.g. anaerobes, tuberculosis, etc.)
Urine grows *Candida*	Usually reflects perineal candidosis and contamination. True candiduria is rare, and may reflect renal candidosis or systemic infection with candidaemia
Urine grows two or more organisms	Mixed UTI is unusual – mixed cultures are likely to reflect perineal contamination. A repeat should be sent unless this is impractical (e.g. frail elderly patients), in which case best-guess treatment should be instituted if clinically indicated
Symptoms recur shortly after treatment	May represent relapse or reinfection. A repeat urine culture should be performed

UTI, urinary tract infection.

Antibiotic resistance

Coliform bacteria of many species that produce extended-spectrum β-lactamase (ESBL) enzymes have emerged worldwide in recent years, particularly as a cause of UTI in community-based patients. These strains are clinically important as they produce enzymes that destroy almost all commonly used β-lactams except the carbapenem class, rendering penicillins and cephalosporins largely useless in clinical practice. In addition, many ESBL producers are multiresistant to non-β-lactam antibiotics too, such as quinolones, aminoglycosides and trimethoprim, narrowing treatment options. Some strains cause outbreaks both in hospitals and in the community. Empirical treatment strategies may need to be reviewed in settings where ESBL-producing strains are prevalent and it may be considered appropriate to use a carbapenem in seriously ill patients until an infection has been proved not to involve an ESBL producer.

Uncomplicated lower UTI

Adults

Therapeutic decisions should be based on accurate, up-to-date antimicrobial susceptibility patterns. Interim data have been published from a European multicentre survey that examined the prevalence and antimicrobial susceptibility of community-acquired pathogens causing uncomplicated UTI in women (Kahlmeter 2000). Among the first 1163 *E. coli* isolates, the resistance rates were 29.9% for amoxicillin, 15.6% for trimethoprim, 2.9% for ciprofloxacin, 2.3% for cefadroxil, 2.1% for co-amoxiclav, and 1.4% for nitrofurantoin. These figures are lower than most routine laboratory data would suggest, but it should be remembered that the experience of diagnostic laboratories is likely to be biased by the overrepresentation of specimens from patients in whom empirical treatment has already failed. It is important to be aware of local variations in sensitivity pattern and to balance the risk of therapeutic failure against the cost of therapy. The preference for best-guess therapy would seem to be a choice between trimethoprim, an oral cephalosporin such as cefalexin, co-amoxiclav or nitrofurantoin, with the proviso that therapy can be refined once sensitivities are available. The quinolones are best reserved for treatment failures and more difficult infections, since overuse of these important agents is likely to lead to an increase in resistance, as has already been seen in countries such as Spain and Portugal. These recommendations are summarized in Table 36.2.

Other drugs that have been used for the treatment of UTI include co-trimoxazole, pivmecillinam and earlier quinolones such as nalidixic acid. Co-trimoxazole is now recognized as a

Table 36.2 Oral antibiotics used for lower urinary tract infections

Antibiotic	Dose (adult)	Side effects	Contraindications	Comments
Amoxicillin	250–500 mg three times a day	Nausea, diarrhoea, allergy	Penicillin hypersensitivity	High levels of resistance in *E. coli*
Co-amoxiclav	375–625 mg three times a day	See amoxicillin	See amoxicillin	Amoxicillin and clavulanic acid
Cefalexin	250–500 mg four times a day	Nausea, diarrhoea, allergy	Cephalosporin hypersensitivity, porphyria	
Trimethoprim	200 mg twice a day	Nausea, pruritus, allergy	Pregnancy, neonates, folate deficiency, porphyria	
Nitrofurantoin	50 mg four times a day	Nausea, allergy, rarely pneumonitis, pulmonary fibrosis, neuropathy	Renal failure, neonates, porphyria, G6PD deficiency	Modified-release form may be given twice daily
Ciprofloxacin	100–500 mg twice a day	Rash, pruritus, tendinitis	Pregnancy, children	Reserve for difficult cases

G6PD, glucose 6-phosphate dehydrogenase.

cause of bone marrow suppression and other haematological side effects, and in the UK its use is greatly restricted. Furthermore, despite superior activity in vitro, there is no convincing evidence that it is clinically superior to trimethoprim alone in the treatment of UTI. Pivmecillinam is metabolized to mecillinam, a β-lactam agent with a particularly high affinity for Gram-negative penicillin binding protein 2 and a low affinity for commonly encountered β-lactamases, and which therefore has theoretical advantages in the treatment of UTI. Pivmecillinam has been extensively used for cystitis in Scandinavian countries, where it does not seem to have led to the development of resistance, and for this reason there have been calls for wider recognition of its usefulness. Finally, older quinolones such as nalidixic acid and cinoxacin were once widely used, but generally these agents have given ground to the more active fluorinated quinolones.

Duration of treatment

The question of duration of treatment has received much attention. Traditionally, a course of 7–10 days has been advocated, and this is still the recommendation for treating men, in whom the possibility of occult prostatitis should be borne in mind. For women, though, there has been particular emphasis on the suitability of short-course regimens such as 3-day or even single-dose therapy. The consensus of an international expert working group was that 3-day regimens are as effective as longer regimens in the cases of trimethoprim and quinolones. β-Lactams have been inadequately investigated on this point but short courses are generally less effective than trimethoprim and quinolones, and nitrofurantoin requires further study before conclusions can be drawn (Warren et al 1999). Single-dose therapy, with its advantages of cost, compliance and the minimization of side effects, has been used successfully in many studies but in general is less effective than when the same agent is used for longer. This view may be challenged in future by the advent of newer fluoroquinolones.

In the urethral syndrome, it is worth trying a 3-day course of one of the agents mentioned above. If this fails, a 7-day course of tetracycline could be tried to deal with possible chlamydia or mycoplasma infection.

Children

In children, the risk of renal scarring is such that UTI should be diagnosed and treated promptly, even if asymptomatic. The drugs of choice include β-lactams, trimethoprim and nitrofurantoin. Quinolones are relatively contraindicated in children because of the theoretical risk of causing cartilage and joint problems. Children should be treated for 7–10 days.

Renal scarring occurs in 5–15% of children with UTI, who should be identified so that appropriate treatment can be instituted. Unfortunately, the subgroup at high risk cannot be predicted and for this reason many clinicians choose to investigate all children with UTI, for example using ultrasound and radioisotope scanning.

Acute pyelonephritis

Patients with pyelonephritis may be severely ill and if so, will require admission to hospital and initial treatment with a parenteral antibiotic. Suitable agents with good activity against *E. coli* and other Gram-negative bacilli include cephalosporins such as cefuroxime and ceftazidime, some penicillins such as co-amoxiclav, quinolones, and aminoglycosides such as gentamicin (Table 36.3). A first-choice agent would be parenteral cefuroxime, gentamicin or ciprofloxacin. When the patient is improving, the route of administration may be switched to oral therapy, typically using a quinolone. Conventionally, treatment is continued for 10–14 days.

Patients who are less severely ill at the outset may be treated with an oral antibiotic, and possibly with a shorter course of treatment. The safety of this approach has been demonstrated

Table 36.3 Parenteral antibiotics used for pyelonephritis

Antibiotic	Dose (adult)	Side effects	Contraindications	Comments
Cefuroxime	750 mg three times a day	Nausea, diarrhoea, allergy	Cephalosporin hypersensitivity, porphyria	
Ceftazidime	1 g three times a day	*See* cefuroxime	*See* cefuroxime	
Co-amoxiclav	1.2 g three times a day	Nausea, diarrhoea, allergy	Penicillin hypersensitivity	
Gentamicin	80–120 mg three times a day gravis or 5 mg/kg once daily	Nephrotoxicity, ototoxicity	Pregnancy, myasthenia	Monitor levels
Ciprofloxacin	200–400 mg twice a day	Rash, pruritus, tendinitis	Pregnancy, children	
Meropenem	500 mg three times a day	Nausea, rash, convulsions		Reserve for difficult cases

in a study of adult women with acute uncomplicated pyelonephritis (Talan et al 2000). Among 113 patients treated with oral ciprofloxacin 500 mg twice daily for 7 days (+/- an initial intravenous dose), the cure rate was 96%.

In hospital-acquired pyelonephritis, there is a risk that the infecting organism may be resistant to the usual first-line drugs. In such cases it may be advisable to start a broad-spectrum agent such as ceftazidime, ciprofloxacin or meropenem.

Relapsing UTI

The main causes of persistent relapsing UTI are renal infection, structural abnormalities of the urinary tract and, in men, chronic prostatitis. Patients who fail on a 7–10-day course should be given a 2-week course and if that fails, a 6-week course can be considered. Structural abnormalities may need surgical correction before cure can be maintained. It is essential that prolonged courses (i.e. more than 4 weeks) are managed under bacteriological control, with monthly cultures. In men with prostate gland infection, it is appropriate to select antibiotics with good tissue penetration such as trimethoprim and the fluoroquinolones.

Catheter-associated infections

In most large hospitals 10–15% of patients have an indwelling urinary catheter. Even with the very best catheter care, most will have infected urine after 10–14 days of catheterization, although most of these infections will be asymptomatic. Antibiotic treatment will often appear to eradicate the infecting organism but as long as the catheter remains in place, the organism, or another more resistant one, will quickly return. The principles of antibiotic therapy for catheter-associated UTI are therefore as follows:

- do not treat asymptomatic infection
- if possible, remove the catheter before treating symptomatic infection.

Although it often prompts investigation, cloudy or strong-smelling urine is not per se an indication for antimicrobial therapy. In these situations, saline or antiseptic bladder wash-outs are often performed, but there is little evidence that they make a difference.

Similarly, encrusted catheters are often changed on aesthetic grounds, but it is not known whether this reduces the likelihood of future symptoms.

Following catheter removal, bacteriuria may resolve spontaneously but more often it persists and may become symptomatic. In a study of women with catheter-associated infection, asymptomatic bacteriuria resolved spontaneously within 2 weeks in only 15 of 42 patients (Godfrey et al 1991). However, those with persistent and symptomatic bacteriuria responded well to single-dose treatment.

Antimicrobial catheters

Several different types of novel catheters with anti-infective properties have been developed with the aim of reducing the ability of bacteria to adhere to the material, which should lead to a decreased incidence of bacteriuria and symptomatic infection. Several studies of the effect of incorporating antibiotics such as rifampicin and minocycline (Darouchie et al 1999) or silver-based alloys (Newton et al 2002) into the catheter have shown benefit. Although clearly more costly than standard catheters, economic evaluation shows silver alloy catheters to be cost-efficient when used in patients needing catheterization for several days (Plowman et al 2001). The effect of these catheters on clinical outcomes such as bacteraemia remains to be determined.

Bacteriuria of pregnancy

The prevalence of asymptomatic bacteriuria of pregnancy is about 5%, and about a third of these women proceed to develop acute pyelonephritis, with its attendant consequences for the health of both mother and pregnancy. Furthermore, there is evidence that asymptomatic bacteriuria is associated with low birth weight, prematurity, hypertension and pre-eclampsia. For these reasons it is recommended that screening is carried out, preferably by culture of a properly taken MSU, which should be repeated if positive for confirmation (National Collaborating Centre for Women's and Children's Health 2003).

Rigorous meta-analysis of published trials (Smaill 2000) has shown that antibiotic treatment of bacteriuria in pregnancy is effective at clearing bacteriuria, reducing the incidence of pyelonephritis and reducing the risk of preterm delivery. The drugs of choice are amoxicillin, cefalexin or nitrofurantoin, depending on the sensitivity profile of the infecting organism. Co-amoxiclav is cautioned in pregnancy because of lack of clinical experience in pregnant women, as is ciprofloxacin. Trimethoprim is contraindicated (particularly in the first trimester) because of its theoretical risk of causing neural tube defects through folate antagonism. There are insufficient data concerning short-course therapy in pregnancy, and 7 days of treatment remains the standard. Patients should be followed up for the duration of the pregnancy to confirm cure and to ensure that any reinfection is promptly addressed.

Prevention and prophylaxis

There are a number of folklore and naturopathic recommendations for the prevention of UTI. Most of these have not been put to statistical study, but at least are unlikely to cause harm.

Cranberry juice

Cranberry juice (*Vaccinium macrocarpon*) has long been thought to be beneficial in preventing UTI, and this has been studied in a number of clinical trials. Cranberry is thought to inhibit adhesion of bacteria to urinary tract cells on the surface of the bladder. In sexually active women, a daily intake of 750 mL cranberry juice was associated with a 40% reduction in the risk of symptomatic UTI in a double-blinded 12-month trial (Stothers 2002). Many studies have been criticized for methodological flaws and currently there is only limited evidence that cranberry juice is effective at preventing recurrent UTI (Jepson et al 2004). There have been no randomized controlled trials of its use in the treatment of established infection, or comparing it with established therapies such as antibiotics for preventing infection.

A hypothetical benefit in using cranberry instead of antibiotics for this purpose is a reduced risk of the development of antibiotic-resistant bacteria. A significant hazard is an interaction of cranberry with warfarin, with a risk of bleeding episodes, and available products are not available in standardized formulations. Furthermore, cranberry juice is unpalatable unless sweetened with sugar and therefore carries a risk of tooth decay, although ironically it is reported to prevent dental caries by blocking adherence of plaque bacteria to teeth.

Antibiotic prophylaxis

In some patients, mainly women, reinfections are so frequent that long-term antimicrobial prophylaxis with specific antibiotics is indicated. If the reinfections are clearly related to sexual intercourse, then a single dose of an antibiotic after intercourse is appropriate. In other cases, long-term, low-dose prophylaxis may be beneficial. One dose of trimethoprim (100 mg) or nitrofurantoin (50 mg) at night will suffice. These drugs are unlikely to lead to the emergence of resistant bacteria, although breakthrough infection with strains intrinsically resistant to the chosen prophylactic antibiotic is possible.

Children

In children, recurrence of UTI is common and the complications potentially hazardous, so many clinicians recommend antimicrobial prophylaxis following documented infection. The evidence in favour of this practice is not strong (Le Saux et al 2000), and although it has been shown to reduce the incidence of UTI, it has not been shown to reduce the incidence of renal complications. Furthermore, important variables remain to be clarified, such as when to begin prophylaxis, which agent to use, and when to stop.

CASE STUDIES

Case 36.1

Two days after transurethral resection of the prostate, a 75-year-old man becomes unwell with rigors, fever and loin pain. Microscopy of his urine shows over 200 white cells/mm³. Blood cultures are taken and rapidly become positive, with Gram-negative bacilli seen in the Gram film.

Question

What antibiotic therapy is indicated?

Answer

The patient should be started on intravenous antibiotic therapy for presumed pyelonephritis and consequent bacteraemia. The antibiotic should cover Gram-negative organisms found in the hospital environment such as *Klebsiella*, *Enterobacter* and *Pseudomonas*. Appropriate agents would be ceftazidime, ciprofloxacin or meropenem. An alternative would be an aminoglycoside such as gentamicin, provided the patient has satisfactory renal function.

Case 36.2

A pregnant woman aged 26 years is found to have bacteriuria at her first antenatal visit. There are no white or red cells seen in her urine. Urine culture demonstrates *E. coli* at a count of more than 100 000 bacteria per mL, sensitive to trimethoprim, nitrofurantoin and cefalexin but resistant to amoxicillin. Other than a degree of urinary frequency, which she ascribes to the pregnancy itself, the patient does not complain of any urinary symptoms.

Question

Does this patient need antibiotic treatment, and if so, which drugs could be safely used?

Answer

The patient may be correct that her urinary frequency is a consequence of pregnancy. However, because of the consequences of untreated infection during pregnancy, even asymptomatic bacteriuria should be treated. A repeat urine specimen should be obtained to confirm the finding, and treatment started with either cefalexin or nitrofurantoin for 7 days. Trimethoprim should be avoided during early pregnancy because of its theoretical risk of teratogenicity. Following treatment, she should be reviewed throughout the pregnancy to ensure eradication of the bacteriuria, and to permit early treatment of any relapse or reinfection.

Case 36.3

A boy aged 2 is admitted to hospital with vomiting and abdominal pain. His mother reports that he was treated for urinary tract infection 6 months previously, but was not investigated further at the time. A clean catch urine sample shows over 50 white cells/mm³ and bacteria are seen on microscopy.

Question

What action should be taken?

Answer

It seems that this child is suffering from a recurrent urinary tract infection. An intravenous antibiotic such as cefuroxime should be started, since the child will not tolerate oral antibiotics at present. If the organism proves to be sensitive to amoxicillin, the treatment could be changed accordingly. Further investigations, for example ultrasonography and radioisotope scan, should be carried out to determine any underlying cause of the infection and to look for already established renal scarring. The child may require long-term prophylaxis to prevent recurrence.

Case 36.4

An elderly lady on an orthopaedic ward is catheterized because of incontinence. She is afebrile but has been confused since her hip replacement 5 days earlier, and remains on cefuroxime, which was started as prophylaxis at the time of the operation. The urine in her catheter bag is cloudy, has a high white cell count, and grows *Enterococcus faecalis* sensitive to amoxicillin but resistant to cephalosporins.

Question

How should this patient be managed?

Answer

The patient's confusion may have a number of causes, including her recent surgery, sleep disturbance, drug toxicity, deep venous thrombosis

or infection. If, following clinical examination and investigation which should include blood cultures, her catheter-associated infection is thought to be contributing to her systemic problems, it should be treated with amoxicillin. If possible the catheter should be removed, even if this is inconvenient for the nursing staff. Unless it has another indication, the cefuroxime is achieving nothing and may be stopped.

Case 36.5

A woman aged 45 suffers from recurrent episodes of cystitis. Examination is unremarkable. On the occasions when a specimen has been sent, the urine has contained few white cells and no significant growth of organisms.

Question

How should the patient be managed?

Answer

This patient is suffering from the urethral syndrome, in which symptoms of infection are not associated with objective evidence of urinary tract infection. It may be felt necessary to investigate her to exclude causes of urethritis such as *Chlamydia trachomatis*, *Neisseria gonorrhoeae* and *Mycoplasma hominis*. Otherwise, her symptoms are likely to respond to conventional courses of antibiotics.

Case 36.6

During an admission for the investigation of long-standing confusion, an elderly man is found to have a heavy mixed growth of organisms in his urine.

Question

Should he be treated with an antibiotic, and if so, which one?

Answer

The question cannot be fully addressed using the available information, but mixed cultures are usually the result of contamination. Unless his clinical condition demands urgent antimicrobial therapy, his urine culture should be carefully repeated in the first instance with attempts to avoid contamination.

REFERENCES

Bulloch B, Bauscher J C, Pomerantz W J et al 2000 Can urine clarity exclude the diagnosis of urinary tract infection? Pediatrics 106: E60

Darouiche R O, Smith J A Jr, Hanna H et al 1999 Efficacy of antimicrobial-impregnated bladder catheters in reducing catheter-associated bacteriuria: a prospective, randomized, multicenter clinical trial. Urology 54: 976-981

Godfrey K M, Lindsay E N, Ronald A R et al 1991 How long should catheter-acquired urinary tract infection in women be treated? Annals of Internal Medicine 114: 713-719

Jepson R G, Mihaljevic L, Craig J 2004 Cranberries for preventing urinary tract infections. Cochrane Database of Systematic Reviews, Issue 2. Update Software, Oxford

Kahlmeter G 2000 The ECOSENS project: a prospective, multinational, multicentre epidemiological survey of the prevalence and antimicrobial

susceptibility of urinary tract pathogens. Interim report. Journal of Antimicrobial Chemotherapy (Suppl. S1): 15-22

Le Saux N, Pham B, Moher D 2000 Evaluating the benefits of antimicrobial prophylaxis to prevent urinary tract infections in children: a systematic review. Canadian Medical Association Journal 163: 523-529

National Collaborating Centre for Women's and Children's Health 2003 Antenatal care: routine care for the healthy pregnant woman. Royal College of Obstetricians and Gynaecologists Press, London, pp 79-81

Newton T, Still J M, Law E 2002 A comparison of the effect of early insertion of standard latex and silver-impregnated latex Foley catheters on urinary tract infections in burn patients. Infection Control and Hospital Epidemiology 23: 217-218

Nicolle L E, Bradley S, Colgan R et al 2005 Infectious Diseases Society of America guidelines for the diagnosis and treatment of asymptomatic bacteriuria in adults. Clinical Infectious Diseases 40: 643-654

Plowman R, Graves N, Esquivel J et al 2001 An economic model to assess the cost and benefits of the routine use of silver alloy coated urinary catheters to reduce the risk of urinary tract infections in catheterized patients. Journal of Hospital Infection 48: 33-42

Richards D, Toop L, Chambers S et al 2005 Response to antibiotics of women with symptoms of urinary tract infection but negative dipstick urine test results: double blind randomised controlled trial. British Medical Journal 331:143-146

Smaill F 2000 Antibiotics for asymptomatic bacteriuria in pregnancy (Cochrane Review). Cochrane Library, Issue 4. Update Software, Oxford

Stothers L 2002 A randomized trial to evaluate effectiveness and cost effectiveness of naturopathic cranberry products as prophylaxis against urinary tract infection in women. Canadian Journal of Urology 9: 1558-1562

Talan D A, Stamm W E, Hooton T M 2000 Comparison of ciprofloxacin (7 days) and trimethoprim-sulfamethoxazole (14 days) for acute uncomplicated pyelonephritis in women: a randomized trial. Journal of the American Medical Association 283: 1583-1590

Warren J W, Abrutyn E, Hebel J R et al 1999 Guidelines for antimicrobial treatment of uncomplicated acute bacterial cystitis and acute pyelonephritis in women. Clinical Infectious Diseases 29: 745-758

FURTHER READING

Anonymous 2005 Cranberry and urinary tract infection. Drug and Therapeutics Bulletin 43:17-19

Bonnet R 2004 Growing group of extended-spectrum β-lactamases: the CTX-M enzymes. Antimicrobial Agents and Chemotherapy 48: 1-14

Fihn S D 2003 Clinical practice: acute uncomplicated urinary tract infection in women. New England Journal of Medicine 349: 259-266

Finer G, Landau D 2004 Pathogenesis of urinary tract infections with normal female anatomy. Lancet Infectious Diseases 4: 631-635

Sobel J D, Kaye D 2004 Urinary tract infections. In: Mandell G L, Bennett J E, Dolin R D (eds) Principles and practice of infectious diseases. Elsevier, London, pp 875-905

Stamm W E 2003 Urinary tract infections. Infectious Disease Clinics of North America 17: 227-471

Stamm W E 2005 Urinary tract infections and pyelonephritis. In: Kasper D L, Braunwald E, Fauci A S et al (eds) Harrison's principles of internal medicine. McGraw-Hill, New York, pp 1715-1721

Gastrointestinal infections 37

J. W. Gray

KEY POINTS

- There are many different microbial causes of gastrointestinal infections.
- Gastroenteritis is the most common syndrome of gastrointestinal infection, but some gastrointestinal pathogens can cause systemic infections.
- Fluid and electrolyte replacement is the mainstay of management of gastroenteritis.
- Most cases of gastroenteritis that occur in developed countries are mild and self-limiting, and do not require antibiotic therapy.
- Antibiotic therapy should be considered for patients with underlying conditions that predispose to serious or complicated gastroenteritis, or where termination of faecal excretion of pathogens is desirable to prevent further spread of the infection.
- Antibiotic therapy is essential for life-threatening systemic infections, such as enteric fever.
- Where possible, antibiotic therapy should be delayed until a microbiological diagnosis has been established.
- The fluoroquinolones, e.g. ciprofloxacin, are currently the most useful antibiotics for treating bacterial gastrointestinal infections, but resistance rates are increasing in many pathogens.
- Antibiotic resistance in gastrointestinal pathogens is an escalating problem.

Gastrointestinal infections represent a major public health and clinical problem worldwide. Many species of bacteria, viruses and protozoa cause gastrointestinal infection, resulting in two main clinical syndromes. Gastroenteritis is a non-invasive infection of the small or large bowel that manifests clinically as diarrhoea and vomiting. Other infections are invasive, causing systemic illness, often with few gastrointestinal symptoms. *Helicobacter pylori*, and its association with gastritis, peptic ulceration and gastric carcinoma, is discussed in Chapter 12 (Peptic ulcer disease).

Epidemiology and aetiology

In Western countries the average person probably experiences one or two episodes of gastrointestinal infection each year. Infections are rarely severe and the vast majority never reach medical attention. In the UK, *Campylobacter*, followed by non-typhoidal serovars of *Salmonella enterica*, are much the most common reported causes of bacterial gastroenteritis. Gastroenteritis due to viruses such as rotaviruses, adenoviruses and noroviruses is also common. Cryptosporidiosis is the most commonly reported parasitic infection. In developing countries the incidence of gastrointestinal infection is at least twice as high and the range of

common pathogens is much wider. Infections are more often severe and represent a major cause of mortality, especially in children.

Gastrointestinal infections can be transmitted by consumption of contaminated food or water or by direct faecal–oral spread. Air-borne spread of viruses that cause gastroenteritis also occurs. The most important causes of gastrointestinal infection, and their usual modes of spread, are shown in Table 37.1. In developed countries, the majority of gastrointestinal infections are food-borne. Farm animals are often colonized by gastrointestinal pathogens, especially *Salmonella* and *Campylobacter*. Therefore, raw foods such as poultry, meat, eggs and unpasteurized dairy products are commonly contaminated and must be thoroughly cooked in order to kill such organisms. Raw foods also represent a potential source of cross-contamination of other foods, through hands, surfaces or utensils that have been inadequately cleaned. Food handlers who are excreting pathogens in their faeces can also contaminate food. This is most likely when diarrhoea is present but continued excretion of pathogens during convalescence also represents a risk. Food handlers are the usual source of *Staphylococcus aureus* food poisoning, where toxin-producing strains of *Staph. aureus* carried in the nose or on skin are transferred to foods. Bacterial food poisoning is often associated with inadequate cooking and/or prolonged storage of food at ambient temperature before consumption.

Water-borne gastrointestinal infection is primarily a problem in countries without a sanitary water supply or sewerage system, although outbreaks of water-borne cryptosporidiosis occur from time to time in the UK.

Spread of pathogens such as *Shigella* or enteropathogenic *Escherichia coli* by the faecal–oral route is favoured by overcrowding and poor standards of personal hygiene. Such infections in developed countries are most common in children and can cause troublesome outbreaks in paediatric wards, nurseries and residential children's homes.

Treatment with broad-spectrum antibiotics alters the bowel flora, creating conditions that favour superinfection with micro-organisms (principally *Clostridium difficile*) that can cause diarrhoea. *C. difficile* infection may be associated with any antibiotic but clindamycin, ampicillin and the cephalosporins are most commonly implicated. *C. difficile*-associated diarrhoea is more common in patients with serious underlying disease and in the elderly. Although some sporadic cases are probably due to overgrowth of endogenous organisms, person-to-person transmission also occurs in hospitals and nursing homes, sometimes resulting in large outbreaks. The dramatic rise in the incidence of health-care-associated *C. difficile* infection over the past decade, and

Table 37.1 Important causes of gastrointestinal infection, their modes of spread and pathogenic mechanisms

Causative agent	Chief mode(s) of spread	Pathogenic mechanisms
Bacteria		
Campylobacter	Food, especially poultry, milk	Mucosal invasion Enterotoxin
Salmonella enterica, non-typhoidal serovars	Food, especially poultry, eggs, meat	Mucosal invasion Enterotoxin
Salmonella enterica serovars Typhi and Paratyphi	Food, water	Systemic invasion
Shigella	Faecal–oral	Mucosal invasion Enterotoxin
Escherichia coli		
Enteropathogenic	Faecal–oral	Mucosal adhesion
Enterotoxigenic	Faecal–oral, water	Enterotoxin
Enteroinvasive	Faecal–oral, food	Mucosal invasion
Verotoxin-producing	Food, especially beef	Verotoxin
Staphylococcus aureus	Food, especially meat, dairy produce	Emetic toxin
Clostridium perfringens	Food, especially meat	Enterotoxin
Bacillus cereus		
Short incubation period	Food, especially rice	Emetic toxin
Long incubation period	Food, especially meat and vegetable dishes	Enterotoxin
Vibrio cholerae O1, O139	Water	Enterotoxin
Vibrio parahaemolyticus	Seafoods	Mucosal invasion Enterotoxin
Clostridium difficile	Uncertain – nosocomial transmission common	Cytotoxin Enterotoxin
Clostridium botulinum	Inadequately heat-treated canned/preserved foods	Neurotoxin
Protozoa		
Giardia lamblia	Water	Mucosal invasion
Cryptosporidium	Water, animal contact	Mucosal invasion
Entamoeba histolytica	Food, water	Mucosal invasion
Viruses	Food, faecal–oral, respiratory secretions	Small intestinal mucosal damage

the apparent emergence of strains with greater virulence, are of considerable concern.

Pathophysiology

Development of symptoms after ingestion of gastrointestinal pathogens depends on two factors. First, sufficient organisms must be ingested and then survive host defence mechanisms, and second, the pathogens must possess one or more virulence mechanisms in order to cause disease.

Host factors

Healthy individuals possess a number of defence mechanisms that protect against infection by enteropathogens. Therefore,

large numbers of many pathogens must be ingested for infection to ensue; for example, the infective dose for *Salmonella* is typically around 10^5 organisms. Other species, however, are better able to survive host defence mechanisms; for example, infection with *Shigella* or verotoxin-producing *E. coli* (VTEC) can result from ingestion of fewer than 100 organisms. VTEC (principally *E. coli* O157) are especially important because of the risk of a life-threatening complication, haemolytic uraemic syndrome (HUS).

Gastric acidity

Most micro-organisms are rapidly killed at normal gastric pH. Patients whose gastric pH is less acid, as for example following treatment with antacids or ulcer-healing drugs, are more susceptible to gastrointestinal infections.

Intestinal motility

It is widely held that intestinal motility helps to rid the host of enteric pathogens, and that antimotility agents are therefore potentially hazardous in patients with infective gastroenteritis. However, there is little evidence for this belief and self-medication with antidiarrhoeals in otherwise healthy individuals is considered safe.

Resident microflora

The resident microflora of the lower gastrointestinal tract, largely composed of anaerobic bacteria, help to resist colonization by enteropathogens.

Immune system

Phagocytic, humoral and cell-mediated elements are important in resistance to different pathogens. Individuals with inherited or acquired immunodeficiencies are therefore susceptible to specific gastrointestinal infections, depending on which components of their immune system are affected.

Organism factors

The symptoms of gastrointestinal infection can be mediated by several different mechanisms (see Table 37.1).

Toxins

Toxins produced by gastrointestinal pathogens can be classified as enterotoxins, neurotoxins and cytotoxins. Enterotoxins act on intestinal mucosal cells to cause net loss of fluid and electrolytes. The classic enterotoxin-mediated disease is cholera, the result of infection with toxigenic serotypes of *Vibrio cholerae*. Many other bacteria produce enterotoxins, including enterotoxigenic *E. coli* and *Clostridium perfringens*.

The emetic toxins of *Staph. aureus* and *Bacillus cereus* are neurotoxins that induce vomiting by an action on the central nervous system. The symptoms of botulism are mediated by a neurotoxin that blocks release of acetylcholine at nerve endings. Cytotoxins cause mucosal destruction and inflammation (see below). Verotoxins are potent cytotoxins that cause direct damage to small vessel endothelial cells, which is exacerbated by stimulation of production of inflammatory mediators by non-endothelial cells. This causes multiorgan microvascular injury, expressed most commonly as haemorrhagic colitis and haemolytic uraemic syndrome.

Mucosal damage

Cytotoxins are important in mediating mucosal invasion but other mechanisms are also involved. Enteropathogenic *E. coli* causes diarrhoea by adhering to the intestinal mucosa and damaging microvilli. Organisms such as *Shigella* and enteroinvasive *E. coli* express surface proteins that facilitate mucosal invasion. Diarrhoea due to mucosal damage may be due to reduction in the absorptive surface area or the presence of increased numbers of immature enterocytes which are secretory rather than absorptive.

Systemic invasion

The lipopolysaccharide outer membrane and possession of an antiphagocytic outer capsule are important virulence factors in invasive *Salmonella* infections.

Clinical manifestations

Many cases of gastrointestinal infection are asymptomatic or cause subclinical illness.

Gastroenteritis is the most common syndrome of gastrointestinal infection, presenting with symptoms such as vomiting, diarrhoea and abdominal pain. The term 'dysentery' is sometimes applied to infections with *Shigella* (bacillary dysentery) and *Entamoeba histolytica* (amoebic dysentery), where severe colonic mucosal inflammation causes frequent diarrhoea with blood and pus. Table 37.2 shows the most important causes of

Table 37.2   Characteristic clinical features of various causes of gastroenteritis

Causative agent	Incubation period	Symptoms (syndrome)
Campylobacter	2–5 days	Bloody diarrhoea Abdominal pain Systemic upset
Salmonella	6–72 h	Diarrhoea and vomiting Fever; may be associated bacteraemia
Shigella	1–4 days	Diarrhoea, fever (bacillary dysentery)

Escherichia coli
  Enteropathogenic
  Enterotoxigenic
  Enteroinvasive
  Verotoxin-producing
	
	12–72 h
	1–3 days
	1–3 days
	1–3 days
		
		Infantile diarrhoea
		Traveller's diarrhoea
		Similar to *Shigella*
		Bloody diarrhoea (haemorrhagic colitis)
		Haemolytic uraemic syndrome

continued

Table 37.2 (continued)

Causative agent	Incubation period	Symptoms (syndrome)
Staphylococcus aureus	4–8 h	Severe nausea and vomiting
Clostridium perfringens	6–24 h	Diarrhoea
Bacillus cereus Short incubation period Long incubation period	 1–6 h 6–18 h	 Vomiting Diarrhoea
Vibrio cholerae O1, O139	1–5 days	Profuse diarrhoea (cholera)
Vibrio parahaemolyticus	12–48 h	Diarrhoea, abdominal pain
Clostridium difficile	Usually occurs during/just after antibiotic therapy	Diarrhoea, pseudomembranous enterocolitis
Giardia lamblia	1–2 weeks	Watery diarrhoea
Cryptosporidium	2 days–2 weeks	Watery diarrhoea
Entamoeba histolytica	2–4 weeks	Diarrhoea with blood and mucus (amoebic dysentery), liver abscess
Viruses	1–2 days	Vomiting, diarrhoea Systemic upset

gastroenteritis together with a brief description of the typical illness that each causes. However, the symptoms experienced by individuals infected with the same organism can differ considerably.

Gastrointestinal manifestations of infection with verotoxin producing *E. coli* range from non-bloody diarrhoea to haemorrhagic colitis. In addition, verotoxin-producing *E. coli* are the most important cause of haemolytic uraemic syndrome (HUS), a serious complication which is most common in young children and the elderly. Haemolytic uraemic syndrome is defined by the triad of microangiopathic haemolytic anaemia, thrombocytopenia and acute renal dysfunction. The mortality is about 5% and up to half of survivors suffer long-term renal damage.

The clinical spectrum of infection with *C. difficile* ranges from asymptomatic carriage to life-threatening pseudomembranous colitis (so called because yellow-white plaques or membranes consisting of fibrin, mucus, leucocytes and necrotic epithelial cells are found adherent to the inflamed colonic mucosa).

Enteric fever, resulting from infection with *Salmonella enterica* serovars Typhi and Paratyphi, presents with symptoms such as headache, malaise and abdominal distension after an incubation period of 3–21 days. During the first week of the illness the temperature gradually increases but the pulse characteristically remains slow. Without treatment, during the second and third weeks the symptoms become more pronounced. Diarrhoea develops in about half of cases. Examination usually reveals splenomegaly, and a few erythematous macules (rose spots) may be found, usually on the trunk. Serious gastrointestinal complications such as haemorrhage and perforation are most common during the third week. Symptoms begin to subside slowly during the fourth week. In general, paratyphoid fever is less severe than typhoid fever.

Botulism typically presents with autonomic nervous system effects, including diplopia and dysphagia, followed by symmetrical descending motor paralysis. There is no sensory involvement.

Gastrointestinal infections are often followed by a period of convalescent carriage of the pathogen. This usually lasts for no more than 4–6 weeks but can be for considerably longer, especially for *Salmonella.*

Investigations

Many cases of gastroenteritis outside hospital are mild and short-lived, and microbiological investigation may not be necessary. However, investigations are always recommended where antibiotic therapy is being considered (Fig. 37.1), where there are public health concerns (for example, if the sufferer works in the food industry) and for gastrointestinal infections in hospitalized patients. The mainstay of investigation of diarrhoeal illness is examination of faeces. Bacterial infections are usually diagnosed by stool culture. Various selective culture media designed to suppress growth of normal faecal organisms and/or enhance the growth of a particular pathogen are used. When sending specimens to the laboratory it is important that details of the age of the patient, the clinical presentation and recent foreign travel are provided, so that appropriate media for the likely pathogens can be selected.

Various other procedures are sometimes useful in investigating patients with suspected bacterial gastroenteritis. Blood cultures should be taken from patients with severe systemic upset. In *Staph. aureus* and *B. cereus* food poisoning the pathogen can sometimes be isolated from vomitus. In cases of food poisoning, suspect foods may also be cultured. In general, serological

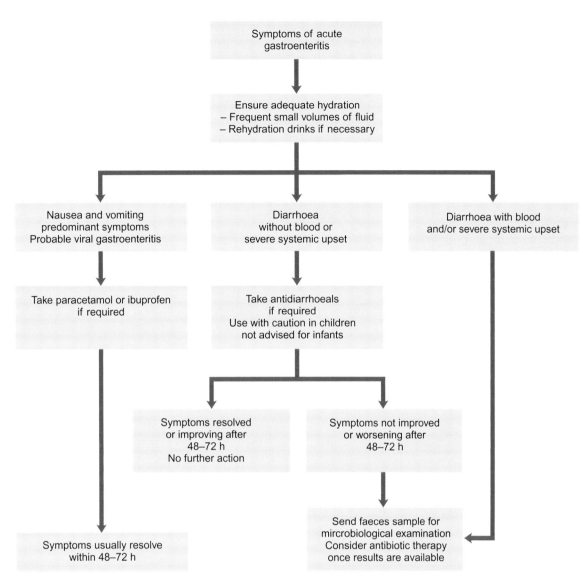

Figure 37.1 Pathway for the investigation and management of patients outside hospital with symptoms of acute gastroenteritis.

investigations are of little value in the diagnosis of bacterial gastroenteritis. However, demonstration of serum antibodies to *E. coli* O157 can be helpful in retrospectively determining the cause of the haemolytic uraemic syndrome. Parasitic infestations are usually detected by microscopic examination of faeces. Electron microscopy has been largely superseded by immunological and molecular-based detection techniques for detection of enteric viruses.

Tests are available for detection of *C. difficile* toxin in faeces, while sigmoidoscopy may be helpful in diagnosing pseudomembranous colitis. Suspected enteric fever is usually investigated by culture of blood and faeces; urine and bone marrow cultures may also be positive. Serological tests for typhoid and paratyphoid fever are available but the results must be interpreted with caution. Botulism is diagnosed by demonstration of toxin in serum.

Treatment

Many gastrointestinal infections are mild and self-limiting and never reach medical attention. Where treatment is required, there are three main therapeutic considerations. Fluid and electrolyte replacement is the cornerstone of treatment of diarrhoeal disease. Most patients can be managed with oral rehydration regimens but severely dehydrated patients require rapid volume expansion with intravenous fluids. Symptomatic treatment with antiemetics and antidiarrhoeal agents is occasionally prescribed but the efficacy and safety of these agents in infective gastroenteritis are uncertain. Antimicrobial agents may be useful both in effecting symptomatic improvement and in eliminating faecal carriage of pathogens and therefore reducing the risk of transmitting infection to others.

Antiemetics and antidiarrhoeal drugs are discussed in Chapters 34 (Nausea and vomiting) and 14 (Constipation and diarrhoea), respectively. This chapter focuses on the place of antibiotic therapy in gastrointestinal infections.

Antibiotic therapy

The requirement for antibiotic treatment in gastrointestinal infection depends on the causative agent, the type and severity of symptoms, and the presence of underlying disease. Antibiotics are ineffective in some forms of gastroenteritis, including bacterial intoxications and viral infections. For many other infections, such as salmonellosis and campylobacteriosis, effective agents are available but antimicrobial therapy is often not clinically necessary. Serious infections such as enteric fever always require antibiotic therapy.

Conditions for which antibiotic therapy is not available or not usually required

The symptoms of *Staph. aureus* and short incubation period *B. cereus* food poisoning and botulism are usually caused by ingestion of preformed toxin and therefore antibiotic therapy would not influence the illness. Pathogens such as *C. perfringens*, *V. parahaemolyticus* and enteropathogenic *E. coli* usually cause a brief self-limiting illness that does not require specific treatment.

None of the presently available antiviral agents are useful in viral gastroenteritis. While most viral infections are self-limiting, chronic rotavirus diarrhoea can occur in immunocompromised patients. Immunoglobulin-containing preparations, administered orally or directly into the duodenum via a nasogastric tube, have been reported to be effective in such circumstances. As well as human serum immunoglobulin, antibodies from other species (e.g. immunized bovine colostrum) have been used. Immunotherapy of rotavirus infection remains experimental and dosages and frequency of administration of immunoglobulin preparations cannot be recommended (Mohan & Haque 2003). A new rotavirus vaccine is undergoing clinical trials; a previous rotavirus vaccine was withdrawn from the USA due to an association with intussusception (Ward 2005).

Conditions for which antimicrobial therapy should be considered

The place for antibiotics in the management of uncomplicated gastroenteritis due to organisms such as *Salmonella*, *Campylobacter* and *Shigella* is not clear-cut. Certain antibiotics are reasonably effective in reducing the duration and severity of clinical illness and in eradicating the organisms from faeces. However, many microbiologists are cautious about the widespread use of antibiotics in diarrhoeal illness because of the risk of promoting antibiotic resistance (Sack et al 1997). Another difficulty with respect to antibiotic prescribing is that it is not usually possible to determine the aetiological agent of diarrhoea on clinical grounds, and stool culture takes at least 48 hours. Patients with severe illness, especially systemic symptoms, may require antibiotic therapy before the aetiological agent has been established. In such circumstances a fluoroquinolone antibiotic such as ciprofloxacin would usually be the most appropriate empiric agent, at least in adults. Otherwise, it is reasonable to limit antibiotic use to microbiologically proven cases where there is serious underlying disease and/or continuing severe symptoms. Antibiotics may also be used to try to eliminate faecal carriage, for example in controlling outbreaks in institutions, or in food handlers who may be prevented from returning to work until they are no longer excreting gastrointestinal pathogens.

Campylobacteriosis Erythromycin is effective in terminating faecal excretion of *Campylobacter*. Some studies have shown that treatment commenced within the first 72–96 hours of illness can also shorten the duration of clinical illness, especially in patients with severe dysenteric symptoms. The recommended dosage for adults is 250–500 mg four times a day orally for 5–7 days, and for children 30–50 mg/kg/day in four divided doses. The newer macrolide antibiotics such as azithromycin and clarithromycin are also effective but are only recommended where the patient is unable to tolerate erythromycin. Ciprofloxacin, at a dose of 500 mg twice daily orally for adults, may also be effective in *Campylobacter* enteritis. However, whereas resistance rates to erythromycin have generally remained below 5%, resistance to ciprofloxacin has emerged rapidly, exceeding 10% in the UK and 50% in some countries (Dingle et al 2005).

Salmonellosis Most cases of *Salmonella* gastroenteritis are self-limiting and antibiotic therapy is unnecessary. However, antimicrobial therapy of salmonellosis is routinely recommended for young infants and immunocompromised patients, who are susceptible to complicated infections. Most antibiotics, even those with good in vitro activity, do not alter the course of uncomplicated *Salmonella* gastroenteritis. However, the fluoroquinolones, such as ciprofloxacin, can often shorten both the symptomatic period and the duration of faecal carriage. Ciprofloxacin resistance is now seen in up to 10% of non-typhoidal serovars of *S. enterica* in some coutries but is rarely seen in the UK (Murray et al 2005). The recommended dose of ciprofloxacin for adults is 500 mg twice daily orally for 1 week. Fluoroquinolones are not licensed for this indication in children, although there is increasing evidence that they can safely be given to children. The recommended dose of ciprofloxacin in childhood is 7.5 mg/kg twice daily orally. Trimethoprim at a dose of 25–100 mg twice daily orally may be used in children if it is preferred not to use a fluoroquinolone.

Ciprofloxacin given orally at a dose of 500–750 mg twice daily in adults (7.5–12.5 mg/kg twice daily in children) or 200 mg intravenously twice daily in adults (5–7.5 mg/kg twice daily in children) is recommended for invasive salmonellosis. Alternative agents include ampicillin or amoxicillin, trimethoprim or chloramphenicol (see under enteric fever). However, resistance to these agents is more common than resistance to ciprofloxacin.

Enteric fever Fluoroquinolones are now widely regarded as the drugs of choice for typhoid and paratyphoid fevers. The clinical response is at least as rapid as with the older treatments, there is a lower relapse rate, and convalescent faecal carriage is shortened. Moreover, multidrug-resistant *S. enterica* serovar Typhi (MDRST) that are resistant to co-trimoxazole, chloramphenicol and ampicillin now account for a large proportion of isolates in some parts of the Indian subcontinent, from where most infections seen in the UK originate. Doses of ciprofloxacin are as outlined for non-typhoidal salmonellosis. The usual dose of chloramphenicol is 50 mg/kg/day in four divided doses, and for ampicillin 100 mg/kg/day in four divided doses. Two weeks of antibiotic therapy is usually recommended, although shorter courses of ciprofloxacin (7–10 days) may be as effective.

During the late 1990s isolates of *S. enterica* serovar Typhi with reduced susceptibility (but usually not complete resistance) to ciprofloxacin began to emerge. Clinical outcomes of such cases treated with conventional ciprofloxacin dosage regimens have been reported to be less good, prompting the suggestion that higher doses and/or longer courses of fluoroquinolone treatment should be used (Kadhiravan et al 2005). Alternative agents that have been reported to be successful in treating infections with MDRST that also have reduced susceptibility to ciprofloxacin include imipenem, meropenem, intravenous ceftriaxone (75 mg/day; maximum dose 2.5 g/day) and oral azithromycin at a dose of 20 mg/kg/day (maximum 1000 mg) for at least 5 days. Time taken for clearance of bacteraemia may be longer with azithromycin but the relapse rate appears to be lower than with β-lactam antibiotics such as ceftriaxone.

Chronic carriers of Salmonella Patients may become chronic carriers after *Salmonella* infection, especially in the presence of underlying biliary tract disease. Oral ciprofloxacin 500–750 mg twice daily continued for 2–6 weeks is usually effective in eradicating carriage, and has largely superseded the use of oral amoxicillin at a dose of 3 g twice daily.

Shigellosis *Shigella sonnei*, which accounts for most cases of shigellosis in the UK, usually causes a mild self-limiting illness. Although often not required on clinical grounds, antibiotic therapy of shigellosis is usually recommended in order to eliminate faecal carriage, and therefore prevent person-to-person transmission. In contrast to salmonellosis, a number of antibiotics are effective in shortening the duration of illness and terminating faecal carriage. These include oral trimethoprim at a dose of 200 mg twice daily in adults (25 mg twice daily for infants aged 2–5 months; 50 mg twice daily for children aged 6 months to 5 years, and 100 mg twice daily for children aged 6–12 years) or amoxicillin 250–500 mg three times daily in adults (62.5–125 mg three times daily in children). However, resistance to these agents is increasing throughout the world. The fluoroquinolones are also highly active in shigellosis and may now be the treatment of choice, at least in adults. The dose of ciprofloxacin is 500 mg twice daily orally in adults (7.5 mg/kg twice daily in children). Antibiotic therapy is usually given for a maximum of 5 days. Azithromycin is increasingly recommended as an alternative agent for shigellosis, especially in children (Jain et al 2005).

Cholera Fluid and electrolyte replacement is the key aspect of the management of cholera. However, antibiotics do shorten the duration of diarrhoea, and therefore reduce the overall fluid loss, and also rapidly terminate faecal excretion of the organism. Effective agents include tetracyclines, erythromycin, trimethoprim, ampicillin or amoxicillin, chloramphenicol, ciprofloxacin and furazolidine. However, antibiotic resistance is being increasingly seen and, in particular, *V. cholerae* O139 is intrinsically resistant to furazolidine and trimethoprim. Choice of antibiotics is therefore governed by knowledge of local resistance patterns. Tetracycline 250 mg four times daily, or doxycycline 100 mg once daily by mouth, is probably the most widely used therapy in adults. Ampicillin, amoxicillin or erythromycin are the generally preferred agents for children. Although clinical cure can be achieved after a single dose of antibiotics, treatment is

usually given for 3–5 days to ensure eradication of *V. cholerae* from faeces.

E. coli infections While most infections with enteropathogenic *E. coli* can be managed conservatively, small trials suggest that trimethoprim may be effective, especially in controlling nursery or hospital outbreaks. On the basis that enteroinvasive *E. coli* are closely related to *Shigella*, and cause a similar clinical syndrome, similar therapy may be appropriate. Antibiotic therapy for enterotoxigenic *E. coli* infection is often unnecessary but troublesome symptoms will often respond to a single dose of ciprofloxacin or azithromycin, the need for further doses depending on clinical response. Alternatively, a 3–5 day course of trimethoprim may be given, although resistance is becoming increasingly common in some areas. Rifaximin is a new non-absorbable antibiotic that is available in a number of countries. It appears to be as effective as ciprofloxacin in treating *E. coli*-predominant traveller's diarrhoea but is ineffective in patients with inflammatory or invasive enteropathogens (Robins & Wellington 2005). The dose is 200 mg three times per day for 3 days.

At least one study has found that the risk of haemolytic uraemic syndrome in children with diarrhoea due to verotoxin-producing *E. coli* was much higher in those who received antibiotics (Wong et al 2000). On that basis it is advised in the UK that antibiotics are contraindicated in children with verotoxin-producing *E. coli* infection.

C. difficile infection In antibiotic-associated diarrhoea, current antibiotic therapy should, if possible, be stopped. Although mild cases may resolve without specific therapy, treatment of all hospitalized patients with diarrhoea due to *C. difficile* is recommended, both to shorten the duration of illness and to reduce environmental contamination and therefore the risk of nosocomial transmission. However, treatment of asymptomatic individuals is not usually necessary. Oral metronidazole 400 mg three times daily for 10 days is the treatment of choice. Oral vancomycin is no more effective, is around 200-fold more expensive, and its use may be an important factor in the emergence and spread of vancomycin-resistant enterococci (Brar & Surawicz 2000). Oral vancomycin 125–500 mg four times daily (there is little evidence that higher doses are more effective) should therefore be reserved for those who cannot tolerate or have not responded to metronidazole. Vancomycin is sometimes also preferred for severe potentially life-threatening cases, although clear evidence of greater efficacy is lacking. In patients unable to take oral medication, either drug can be administered via a nasogastric tube. Metronidazole suppositories may be used, and vancomycin has been instilled into the rectum and caecum via a tube. Intravenous therapy should be a last resort.

Recurrence of symptoms occurs in about 20% of patients treated for *C. difficile* infection. Although some recurrences are due to germination of spores that have persisted in the colon since the original infection, it is now recognized that many of these cases are due to reinfection, rather than relapse caused by the original strain (Loo et al 2004). Most recurrences respond to a further 10–14 day course of metronidazole or vancomycin but a few patients experience repeated recurrences. There is no reliable means of managing these patients. Recognizing that recurrences may be due to repeated reinfections, enhanced infection control precautions may be the most important measure. Prolonged, tapered or pulsed antibiotic therapy is effective in some cases. Experimental therapeutic options that have shown potential include use of probiotics, such as the yeast *Saccharomyces boulardi*, and immunotherapy with antibodies to *C. difficile* toxin.

Cryptosporidiosis Cryptosporidiosis in immunocompetent individuals is generally self-limiting. However, in immunosuppressed patients, severe diarrhoea can persist indefinitely and can even contribute to death. HIV-infected patients on highly active antiretroviral therapy (HAART) now have a much lower incidence of cryptosporidiosis due to immune reconstitution, and possibly a direct anti-cryptosporidium effect of protease inhibitors. There is no reliable antimicrobial therapy. There have been a number of reports of successful treatment of individual patients using azithromycin at a dose of 500 mg once daily (10 mg/kg once daily in children). Treatment should be continued until *Cryptosporidium* oocysts are no longer detectable in faeces (typically 2 weeks), to minimize the risk of relapse post treatment. Occasionally therapy has to be continued indefinitely to prevent relapse. Most other agents, e.g. nitazoxanide, spiramycin, paromomycin and letrazuril, that have been investigated for treatment of cryptosporidiosis are unlicensed in the UK (Smith & Corcoran 2004).

Giardiasis Metronidazole is the treatment of choice for giardiasis (Vesy & Peterson 1999) Various oral regimens are effective, for example 400 mg three times daily (children 7.5 mg/kg) for 5 days, or 2 g/day (children 500 mg to 1 g) for 3 days. Alternative treatments are tinidazole 2 g as a single dose, or mepacrine hydrochloride 100 mg (children 2 mg/kg) three times daily for 5–7 days. Nitazoxanide is a new thiazolide antiparasitic drug that has been licensed for treatment of giardiasis in some countries, but is not currently available in the UK. A single course of treatment for giardiasis has a failure rate of up to 10%. A further course of the same or another agent is often successful. Sometimes repeated relapses are due to reinfection from an asymptomatic family member. In such cases all affected family members should be treated simultaneously.

Amoebiasis The aim of treatment in amoebiasis is to kill all vegetative amoebae and also to eradicate cysts from the bowel lumen. Metronidazole is highly active against vegetative amoebae and is the treatment of choice for acute amoebic dysentery and amoebic liver abscess. The dose for adults is 800 mg (children 100–400 mg) three times daily for 5–10 days. To eradicate cysts, metronidazole therapy is followed by a 5-day course of diloxanide furoate 500 mg three times daily (20 mg/kg daily in three divided doses for children).

Asymptomatic excretors of cysts living in areas with a high prevalence of *E. histolytica* infection do not merit treatment because most individuals would quickly become reinfected. However, asymptomatic excretors of cysts in Europe or North America are usually treated with diloxanide furoate for 5–10 days, sometimes combined with metronidazole.

Patient care

Prevention of person-to-person transmission of gastrointestinal infections

People excreting gastrointestinal pathogens are potentially infectious to others. Liquid stools are particularly likely to contaminate the hands and the environment. All cases of gastrointestinal infection should be excluded from work or school at least until the patients are symptom free; hospitalized patients should be isolated in a single room. Patients should be advised on general hygiene, and in particular on thorough handwashing and drying after visiting the toilet and before handling food.

In most countries many gastrointestinal infections are statutorily notifiable. Following notification, the authorities will judge whether the implications for public health merit investigation of the source of infection, contact screening or follow-up clearance stool samples from the original case.

Common therapeutic problems in the management of gastrointestinal infection are summarized in Table 37.3.

Table 37.3 Common therapeutic problems in the management of gastrointestinal infections

Infection	Antibiotic	Common problems	Resolution
Campylobacteriosis	Erythromycin	Not always effective, especially if commenced >72 h after onset of symptoms	Reserve therapy for cases where symptoms are severe or worsening at time of diagnosis
	Ciprofloxacin[a]	Up to 50% of strains are resistant	Use only as a second-line agent for isolates that have been shown to be sensitive
Salmonellosis	Ciprofloxacin[a]	Not always effective

Resistance is increasing | Reserve therapy for cases where symptoms are severe or worsening at time of diagnosis |
Enteric fever	Ciprofloxacin[a]	Resistance is increasing	Alternative therapies must be guided by antibiotic sensitivities of the isolate
	Ampicillin or amoxicillin	Resistance to these agents now common	Ciprofloxacin[a] now generally regarded as treatment of choice
	Chloramphenicol	Higher incidence of chronic carriage and relapse than with ciprofloxacin	

Table 37.3 (continued)

Infection	Antibiotic	Common problems	Resolution
Shigellosis	Trimethoprim	Resistance is increasing	Therapy should be guided by antibiotic sensitivities of the isolate. Most trimethoprim-resistant strains are ciprofloxacin sensitive
Clostridium difficile	Metronidazole	Relapse rate up to 20%	Repeat course of treatment Enhanced infection control precautions to prevent reinfection
	Vancomycin	Comparable efficacy to, but much more expensive than, metronidazole	Generally reserved as a second-line agent, e.g. where no response to metronidazole, or occasionally for patients with severe infection
		Risk of promoting emergence and spread of vancomycin-resistant enterococci	
Cryptosporidiosis	Azithromycin	Not always effective. Recommended only for patients who are immunocompromised or have unusually severe or protracted symptoms	Long-term therapy may be required to control symptoms Possible alternative agents are not licensed in UK

 a Ciprofloxacin is not licensed for general paediatric use; it is widely used to treat gastrointestinal infections in children.

CASE STUDIES

Case 37.1

A 7-year-old girl is admitted to hospital with a history of fever, weight loss and malaise 1 week after returning from visiting relatives in Pakistan. Whilst there she was diagnosed as having typhoid fever, and although details are sketchy it seems that she received treatment with chloramphenicol for a few days. Twenty-four hours after admission *Salmonella enterica* serovar Typhi is isolated from a blood culture.

Questions

1. Give three reasons why she might not have responded fully to the treatment given in Pakistan.
2. Which antibiotic would now be most appropriate as empirical therapy?

Answers

1. (i) Chloramphenicol resistance is common in *Salmonella enterica* serovar Typhi in the Indian subcontinent.
(ii) Even if the strain of *Salmonella enterica* serovar Typhi had been chloramphenicol sensitive, the dose and/or duration of therapy may have been inadequate.
(iii) The young girl may have experienced a relapse despite adequate therapy in Pakistan.
2. Fluoroquinolones (usually ciprofloxacin) are generally regarded as the treatment of choice for enteric fever. Fewer than 10% of *Salmonella enterica* serovar Typhi are resistant to ciprofloxacin.

Case 37.2

A chef returns from holiday in Tunisia with diarrhoea. He follows the policy of the restaurant by staying off work and submitting a stool sample for microbiological examination. After 48 hours the laboratory telephones to report that it has detected both *Campylobacter* and non-typhoidal *Salmonella*. The patient still has diarrhoea and will not be allowed to return to work until he is asymptomatic and has been shown to be free of enteric pathogens.

Question

What are the treatment options for this patient?

Answer

Fluoroquinolones, such as ciprofloxacin, are the only antibiotic group that in salmonellosis can hasten resolution of diarrhoea and clearance of the pathogen from stool. Fluoroquinolones are also effective in camplylobacteriosis but resistance rates in *Campylobacter* exceed 50% in some countries. However, compared with *Salmonella*, prolonged excretion of *Campylobacter* is uncommon. Therefore, in this case it would be reasonable to commence treatment with a fluoroquinolone, regardless of the results of antibiotic susceptibility testing on the *Campylobacter*.

Case 37.3

A businessman is planning a short trip to India. During previous visits to the area he has experienced troublesome diarrhoea despite being careful about what he ate and drank. Although the diarrhoea has not made him seriously unwell, it has caused him considerable inconvenience.

Question

Are there any antimicrobials that he could take to prevent this problem?

529

Answer

Although traveller's diarrhoea is not usually serious it can cause considerable inconvenience whether the sufferer is travelling for leisure or business reasons. The are two approaches to antibiotic use. Either the drug can be taken prophylactically to try to prevent development of diarrhoea, or treatment can be commenced with the onset of diarrhea. The latter approach is generally preferred because it limits unnecessary exposure to antibiotics and the reponse to treatment is usually rapid. However, there are instances such as this case where the inconvenience of even short-lived diarrhoea may be great enough to justify use of prophylaxis.

The choice of antibiotics for traveller's diarrhoea has been made more complicated by the increasing prevalence of antibiotic resistance in many developing countries. A fluoroquinolone, such as ciprofloxacin, still represents a reasonable first choice, with azithromycin as a possible alternative in areas where fluoroquinolone resistance is known to be common. For travellers from countries where it can be prescribed, rifaximin may be the agent of choice.

Case 37.4

An 80-year-old woman on a geriatric ward develops profuse diarrhoea 5 days after commencing therapy with cefuroxime for a respiratory tract infection. *Clostridium difficile* **toxin is detected in a stool sample. An increasing number of other patients on the ward have been developing** *C. difficile*-**associated diarrhoea during the past 6 months, which appears to have coincided with an increase in antibiotic prescribing.**

Questions

1. How should this patient be managed?
2. What measures might be taken to try to reduce the number of cases of *C. difficile*-associated diarrhoea on the ward?

Answers

1. If possible, treatment with cefuroxime should be discontinued. If further antibiotic therapy for her respiratory tract infection is required, an antibiotic that is less likely to disturb the bowel flora should be prescribed. Metronidazole is the preferred treatment for infection with *C. difficile*. The patient should be isolated to reduce the risk of spread of the infection.
2. There are two elements to control of *C. difficile* in hospitals. First, strict infection control precautions and improved standards of environmental cleanliness can reduce the risk of patients being exposed to the bacterium. Second, the antibiotic policy on the ward should be reviewed with a view to both minimizing the use of antibiotics in general and, where antibiotic therapy is essential, selecting agents that have least effect on the bowel flora.

REFERENCES

Brar H S, Surawicz C M 2000 Pseudomembranous colitis: an update. Canadian Journal of Gastroenterology 14: 51-56

Dingle K E, Clarke L, Bowler I C 2005 Ciprofloxacin resistance among human *Campylobacter* isolates 1991–2004: an update. Journal of Antimicrobial Chemotherapy 55: 395-396

Jain S K, Gupta A, Glanz B et al 2005 Antimicrobial-resistant *Shigella sonnei*: limited antimicrobial treatment options for children and challenges of interpreting in vitro azithromycin susceptibility. Pediatric Infectious Disease Journal 24: 494-497

Kadhiravan T, Wig N, Kapil A et al 2005 Clinical outcomes in typhoid fever: adverse impact of infection with nalidixic acid-resistant *Salmonella typhi*. Biomed Central Infectious Diseases 5: 37

Loo V G, Libman M D, Miller M A et al 2004 *Clostridium difficile*: a formidable foe. Canadian Medical Association Journal 171: 47-48

Mohan P, Haque K 2003 Oral immunoglobulin for the prevention of rotavirus infection in low birth weight babies (review). Cochrane Database of Systematic Reviews: CD003740. John Wiley, Chichester

Murray A, Coia J E, Mather H et al 2005 Ciprofloxacin resistance in non-typhoidal *Salmonella* serotypes in Scotland, 1993–2003. Journal of Antimicrobial Chemotherapy 56: 110-104

Robins G W, Wellington K 2005 Rifaximin: a review of its use in the management of traveller's diarrhea. Drugs 65: 1697-1713

Sack R B, Rahman M, Yunus M et al 1997 Antimicrobial resistance in organisms causing diarrheal disease. Clinical Infectious Diseases 24 (suppl 1): S102-S105

Smith H V, Corcoran G D 2004 New drugs and treatment for cryptosporidiosis. Current Opinion in Infectious Disease 17: 557-564

Vesy C J, Peterson W L 1999 Review article: the management of giardiasis. Alimentary Pharmacology and Therapeutics 13: 843-850

Ward R L 2005 Rotavirus vaccines: is the second time the charm? Current Opinion in Investigational Drugs 6: 798-803

Wong C S, Jelacic S, Habeeb R L et al 2000 The risk of hemolytic-uremic syndrome after antibiotic treatment of *Escherichia coli* O157:H7 infections. New England Journal of Medicine 342: 1930-1936

FURTHER READING

Aslam S, Hamill R J, Musher D M 2005 Treatment of *Clostridium difficile*-associated disease: old therapies and new strategies. Lancet Infectious Diseases 5: 549-557

Bhan M K, Bahl R, Bhatnagar S 2005 Typhoid and paratyphoid fever. Lancet 366: 749-762

DuPont H L 2005 What's new in enteric infectious diseases at home and abroad. Current Opinion in Infectious Disease 18: 407-412

Starr J 2005 *Clostridium difficile* associated diarrhoea: diagnosis and treatment. British Medical Journal 331: 498-501

Townes J M 2004 Acute infectious gastroenteritis in adults. Seven steps to management and prevention. Postgraduate Medicine 115: 11-19

Wilson J 2000 Clinical microbiology. An introduction for health care professionals. Baillière Tindall, London

Infective meningitis 38

J. W. Gray

KEY POINTS

- The causative agents of meningitis are related to the age of the patient and the presence of underlying disease.
- The most common cause of early-onset neonatal meningitis is the group B streptococcus. Other important causes of neonatal meningitis include *Escherichia coli* and *Listeria monocytogenes*.
- Outside the neonatal period, *Neisseria meningitidis* and *Streptococcus pneumoniae* are the major causes of infective meningitis, accounting for around 75% of confirmed cases.
- Antibiotic treatment of meningitis requires attainment of adequate concentrations of bactericidal antibiotics in the cerebrospinal fluid (CSF).
- Suitable therapies for neonatal meningitis are ampicillin or amoxicillin, combined with either an aminoglycoside or a cephalosporin such as cefotaxime or ceftazidime.
- Increasing resistance to penicillins and concerns about the toxicity of chloramphenicol have led to the widespread use of cefotaxime or ceftriaxone as empiric therapy for meningitis outside the neonatal period.
- Because of the potentially rapid progression of the disease, patients with suspected meningococcal infection should receive emergency therapy with penicillin before admission to hospital.
- Close contacts of patients with meningococcal, and in some circumstances *Haemophilus influenzae* type b, disease should receive chemoprophylaxis.
- Introduction of vaccines against *H. inflenzae* type b and *N. meningitidis* group C has markedly reduced the incidence of meningitis due to these bacteria.

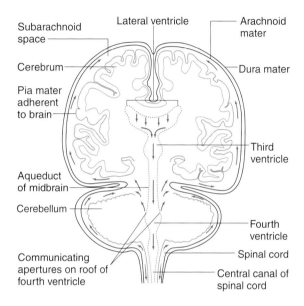

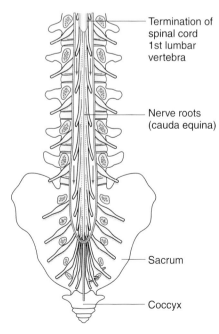

Figure 38.1 The meninges covering the brain and spinal cord and the flow of cerebrospinal fluid (arrowed) (modified from Ross & Wilson (1981), by permission of Churchill Livingstone).

The brain and spinal cord are surrounded by three membranes, which from the outside inwards are the dura mater, the arachnoid mater and the pia mater. Between the arachnoid mater and the pia mater, in the subarachnoid space, is found the cerebrospinal fluid (CSF) (Fig. 38.1). This fluid, of which there is approximately 150 mL in a normal individual, is secreted by the choroid plexuses and vascular structures which are in the third, fourth and lateral ventricles. CSF passes from the ventricles via communicating apertures to the subarachnoid space, after which it flows over the surface of the brain and the spinal cord (see Fig. 38.1). The amount of CSF is controlled by resorption into the bloodstream by vascular structures in the subarachnoid space, called the arachnoid villi. Infective meningitis is an inflammation of the arachnoid and pia mater associated with the presence of bacteria, viruses, fungi or protozoa in the CSF. Meningitis is one of the most emotive of infectious diseases. Even today, infective meningitis is associated with significant mortality and serious morbidity.

Aetiology and epidemiology

In the UK, 3500–4000 cases of meningitis are notified annually. Overall, two organisms, *Neisseria meningitidis* and *Streptococcus pneumoniae,* account for about 75% of cases. However, the pattern of micro-organisms causing meningitis is related to the age of the patient and the presence of underlying disease. Although bacterial meningitis occurs in all age groups, it is predominantly a disease of young children, with 40–50% of all cases occurring in the first 4 years of life. The incidences of meningitis due to *N. meningitidis* and *Strep. pneumoniae* by age group are shown in Figure 38.2.

In the neonatal period, group B streptococci are the most common cause of bacterial meningitis. Other causes of neonatal meningitis include *Escherichia coli* and other Enterobacteriaceae, *Listeria monocytogenes* and enterococci. In most cases infection is acquired from the maternal genital tract around the time of delivery, but transmission between patients can also occur in hospitals.

N. meningitidis is the most common cause of bacterial meningitis from infancy through to middle age, with peaks of incidence in the under-5 year age group and in adolescents. There are several serogroups of *N. meningitidis,* including A, B, C, W135 and Y. In the late 20th century, serogroups B and C accounted for 60–65% and 35–40% of infections in the UK, respectively. However, with the introduction of vaccination against *N. meningitidis* serogroup C (MenC) into the routine immunization programme in 1999, serogroup B now accounts for around 85% of all meningococcal disease. There is currently no vaccine available for *N. meningitidis* serogroup B. Serogroups A and W135 predominate in Africa and the Middle East. A tetravalent vaccine against serogroups A, C, W135 and Y is available to protect travellers to countries of risk. *Strep. pneumoniae* is the most common cause of meningitis in adults aged over 45 years, but almost half of all cases of pneumococcal meningitis occur in children aged under 5 years. It has a poorer outcome than meningococcal meningitis. A vaccine against the seven most common serotypes of *Strep. pneumoniae* has been licensed for routine use in children aged less than 5 years in the United States, but pneumococcal vaccination in the UK is currently recommended only for children and adults at increased risk of invasive pneumococcal disease. *Haemophilus influenzae* type b (Hib) was once the major cause of bacterial meningitis in children aged 3 months to 5 years, but introduction of routine immunization in 1992 has almost eliminated Hib disease in the UK and other developed countries.

Although patients with meningococcal or Hib meningitis are potentially infectious, most cases of meningitis due to these bacteria are acquired from individuals who are asymptomatic nasopharyngeal carriers. People living in the same household as a case of meningococcal disease have a 500 to 1200-fold increased risk of developing infection if they do not receive chemoprophylaxis (see later). Susceptible young children who are household contacts of a case of Hib disease have a similarly increased risk of becoming infected. Epidemics of meningococcal disease sometimes occur. In developed countries these take the form of clusters of cases among people living in close proximity (for example, in schools or army camps) or in a particular geographical area. In Africa, large epidemics with many thousands of cases occur, usually during the dry season.

Meningitis can also occur as a complication of neurosurgery, especially in patients who have ventriculoatrial or ventriculoperitoneal shunts. Coagulase-negative staphylococci are the major causes of shunt-associated meningitis but other bacteria are important, including Enterobacteriaceae and *Staphylococcus aureus.* Meningitis due to *Staph. aureus* may also be secondary to trauma, or local or haematogenous spread from another infective focus. Meningitis may also be a feature of multisystem bacterial diseases such as syphilis, leptospirosis and Lyme disease. *L. monocytogenes* is an occasional cause of meningitis in immunocompromised patients.

The decline in the incidence of tuberculous meningitis in developed countries has mirrored the fall in the incidence of tuberculosis in these countries. Tuberculous meningitis may occur as part of the primary infection or as a result of recrudescence of a previous infection.

Enteroviruses such as echoviruses and coxsackieviruses account for about 70% of cases of viral meningitis in the UK. Other agents include mumps virus, herpes viruses and human immuno-deficiency viruses.

In Europe, fungal meningitis is rare in individuals without underlying disease. *Candida* species are an occasional cause of shunt meningitis. *Cryptococcus neoformans* has emerged as an important cause of meningitis in patients with late-stage HIV infection and other severe defects of T-cell function. With greater use of fluconazole for oral candidiasis, and especially the advent of highly active antiretroviral therapy, cryptococcosis has become much less common in developed countries. However, in sub-Saharan African countries with the highest HIV prevalence, cryptococcus is the leading cause of infective meningitis. In certain other areas of the world, infections with fungi such as *Coccidioides immitis* and *Histoplasma capsulatum* are endemic.

Pathophysiology

Most cases of bacterial meningitis are preceded by nasopharyngeal colonization by the causative organism. In most colonized individuals, infection will progress no further but in susceptible individuals, local invasion occurs, leading to bacteraemia and meningeal invasion. Other routes by which micro-organisms can reach the meninges include:

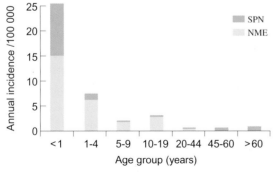

Figure 38.2 Approximate annual incidence of meningitis due to *Neisseria meningitidis* (NME) and *Streptococcus pneumoniae* (SPN) in the UK by age group.

- direct spread from the nasopharynx
- blood-borne spread from other foci of colonization or infection
- abnormal communications with the skin or mucous membranes, for example skull fractures, anatomical defects or a meningocoele
- spread from an infected adjacent focus, for example brain abscess, tuberculoma, infected paranasal air sinus or infection of the middle ear.

Once in the subarachnoid space, the infection spreads widely. The cerebral tissue is not usually directly involved although cerebral abscess may complicate some types of meningitis.

The micro-organisms that most frequently cause meningitis are capable of doing so because they have a variety of virulence factors, including mechanisms for:

- attachment to host mucosal surfaces
- evasion of phagocytosis and other host defences
- meningeal invasion
- disruption of the blood–brain barrier
- induction of pathophysiological changes in the CSF space
- secondary brain damage.

Both *H. influenzae* and *N. meningitidis* have pili that mediate attachment to specific host cell surface receptors. Most bacteria and fungi causing meningitis are encapsulated, which helps them resist neutrophil phagocytosis and complement-mediated bactericidal activity. Other surface structures may protect bacteria from antibody and complement-mediated bacteriolysis.

Virulence factors that facilitate access of micro-organisms into the CSF, and disruption of the blood–brain barrier, are less well understood but components of the cell envelope, including fimbriae and outer membrane proteins, are probably important. Inflammatory mediators such as interleukin-1, tumour necrosis factor, prostaglandins and platelet-activating factor released by the host in response to microbial components also contribute to mucosal invasion and disruption of the blood–brain barrier. Cell wall components, such as teichoic acid in Gram-positive bacteria and lipo-oligosaccharides and lipopolysaccharides from Gram-negative bacteria, are potent inducers of the inflammatory response. Pneumolysin is a cytolysin produced by *Strep. pneumoniae* that causes inflammation and apoptosis.

Cranial nerves may be damaged by the presence of inflammatory exudate. The local inflammatory response can cause obstruction of blood vessels and cerebral oedema, leading to impaired CSF flow, increased intracranial pressure, reduced cerebral blood flow and a risk of cerebral infarction. Brain damage may also be due to reactive oxygen species, nitric oxide and excitatory amino acids.

Clinical manifestations

Acute bacterial meningitis usually presents with sudden-onset headache, neck stiffness, photophobia, fever and vomiting. On examination, Kernig's sign may be positive. This is resistance to extension of the leg when the hip is flexed, due to meningeal irritation in the lumbar area. Where meningitis is complicated by septicaemia, there may be septic shock. The presence of a haemorrhagic skin rash is highly suggestive, but not pathognomic,

of meningococcal infection. Untreated, patients with bacterial meningitis deteriorate rapidly, with development of seizures, focal cerebral signs and cranial nerve palsies. Finally, obtundation and loss of consciousness herald death.

In infants with meningitis the early physical signs are usually non-specific and include fever, diarrhoea, lethargy, feeding difficulties and respiratory distress. Focal signs such as seizures or a bulging fontanelle usually only occur at a late stage.

Viral meningitis usually presents with acute onset of low-grade fever, headache, photophobia and neck stiffness. Unless they develop encephalitis, patients usually remain alert and oriented.

Although tuberculous and fungal meningitis sometimes present acutely, these infections typically have a more indolent course. The early stages of the diseases are dominated by general symptoms such as malaise, apathy and anorexia. As they progress, symptoms and signs more typical of meningitis usually appear.

Diagnosis

The definitive diagnosis of meningitis is established by detection of the causative organism and/or demonstration of biochemical changes and a cellular response in CSF. CSF is obtained by lumbar puncture, where a needle is inserted between the posterior space of the third and fourth lumbar vertebrae into the subarachnoid space. Before performing lumbar puncture, the possibility of precipitating or aggravating existing brain herniation in patients with intracranial hypertension must be considered; patients are increasingly being investigated beforehand by computed tomography or other imaging techniques.

In health, the CSF is a clear colourless fluid which, in the lumbar region of the spinal cord, is at a pressure of 50–150 mmH$_2$O. There may be up to 5 cells/μL, the protein concentration is up to 0.4 g/L, and the glucose concentration is at least 60% of the blood glucose (usually 2.2–4.4 mmol/L). Table 38.1 shows how the cell count and biochemical measurements can be helpful in determining the type of aetiological agent in meningitis.

In bacterial meningitis, organisms may be visible in Gram-stained smears of the CSF. The common causes of bacterial meningitis are easily distinguished from each other by their Gram stain appearance. Special stains, such as the Ziehl–Neelsen method, are necessary to visualize mycobacteria. However, only small numbers of mycobacteria are present in the CSF in tuberculous meningitis and direct microscopy is often unrevealing. Although cryptococci can be visualized by Gram staining, they are often more easily seen with India ink staining, which highlights their prominent capsules.

Regardless of the microscopic findings, CSF should be cultured to try to confirm the identity of the causative organism and to facilitate further investigations such as antibiotic sensitivity testing and typing. Special cultural techniques are required for mycobacteria, fungi and viruses. Cultures of other sites are sometimes helpful. In suspected bacterial meningitis, blood for culture should always be obtained. Bacteraemia occurs in only 10% of patients with meningococcal meningitis but is more commonly associated with some other forms of meningitis. CSF and blood cultures may be negative in patients with meningococcal disease, especially if antibiotics have been administered prior to the cultures being taken. Cultures from sites where antibiotic

Table 38.1 Cellular and biochemical responses in different forms of infective meningitis

Type of meningitis	Cell count	Protein (g/L)	Glucose
Bacterial	Predominantly polymorphs, 500–2000 µL (lymphocytes may predominate in early or partially treated cases)	1–3	<50% blood glucose
Tuberculous	Predominantly lymphocytes, 100–600 µL	1–6	<50% blood glucose
Viral	Predominantly lymphocytes, 50–500 µL	0.5–1	Usually normal
Cryptococcal	Predominantly lymphocytes, 50–1000 µL	1–3	<50% blood glucose

penetration is less good, for example haemorrhagic skin lesions and the nasopharynx, may be helpful in such cases.

Non-culture based methods may also be helpful in determining the aetiology of meningitis. Techniques include antigen detection and detection of microbial genomic material using molecular methods such as polymerase chain reaction (PCR). Polymerase chain reaction is now established as a standard investigation in suspected meningococcal meningitis and may be the only positive test in up to 50% of cases. Polymerase chain reaction is increasingly being used to diagnose pneumococcal meningitis, and nucleic acid amplification techniques are also widely available for detection of *M. tuberculosis* and several viruses, including herpes simplex virus and enteroviruses. Serum antibodies to *N. meningitidis* and various viruses may be detected but these investigations usually depend on demonstration of seroconversion between two samples collected a week or more apart, and therefore have no role in the early diagnosis of infections. Patients with tuberculous meningitis may have a positive Mantoux test.

Drug treatment

Acute bacterial meningitis is a medical emergency that requires urgent administration of antibiotics. Other considerations in some forms of meningitis include the use of adjunctive therapy such as steroids, and the administration of antibiotics to prevent secondary cases. The antimicrobial therapy of meningitis requires the attainment of adequate levels of bactericidal agents within the CSF. The principal route of entry of antibiotics into CSF is by the choroid plexus; an alternative route is via the capillaries of the central nervous system into the extracellular fluid and thence into the ventricles and subarachnoid space (see Fig. 38.1). The passage of antibiotics into CSF is dependent on the degree of meningeal inflammation and integrity of the blood–brain barrier created by capillary endothelial cells, as well as the following properties of the antibiotic:

- lipid solubility (the choroidal epithelium is highly impermeable to lipid-insoluble molecules)
- ionic dissociation at blood pH
- protein binding
- molecular size
- the concentration of the drug in the serum.

Antimicrobials fall into three categories according to their ability to penetrate the CSF:

- those that penetrate even when the meninges are not inflamed, for example chloramphenicol, metronidazole, isoniazid and pyrazinamide
- those that generally penetrate only when the meninges are inflamed, and used in high doses, for example most β-lactam antibiotics, the quinolones and rifampicin
- those that penetrate poorly under all circumstances, including the aminoglycosides, vancomycin and erythromycin.

Clinical urgency determines that empirical antimicrobial therapy will usually have to be prescribed before the identity of the causative organism or its antibiotic sensitivities are known. Consideration of the epidemiological features of the case, together with microscopic examination of the CSF, is often helpful in identifying the likely pathogen. However, there is a trend towards the use of broad-spectrum antimicrobial therapy to cover all likely pathogens, at least until definite microbiological information is available. For the purpose of selecting empirical antimicrobial therapy, patients with acute bacterial meningitis can be categorized into four broad groups: neonates and infants aged below 3 months; immunocompetent older infants, children and adults; immuno-compromised patients; and those with CSF shunts.

Meningitis in neonates and infants aged below 3 months

The most important pathogens in neonates include group B streptococci, *E. coli* and other Enterobacteriaceae, and *L. monocytogenes*. In many centres a third-generation cephalosporin such as cefotaxime or ceftazidime, along with amoxicillin or ampicillin, is the empiric therapy of choice for neonatal meningitis (Harvey et al 1999). Cephalosporins penetrate into CSF better than aminoglycosides, and their use in Gram-negative bacillary meningitis has contributed to a reduction in mortality to less than 10%. Other centres continue to use an aminoglycoside, such as gentamicin, together with benzylpenicillin, ampicillin or amoxicillin as empiric therapy. This approach remains appropriate, especially in countries such as the UK where group B streptococci are by far the predominant cause of early-onset neonatal meningitis. Whichever empiric regimen is used, therapy can be altered as appropriate once the pathogen has been identified. Suitable dosages are shown in Table 38.2.

In infants outside the immediate neonatal period, the classic neonatal pathogens account for a decreasing number of cases of meningitis and the common bacteria of meningitis in childhood

Table 38.2 Suitable antibiotic regimens for treatment of acute bacterial meningitis in different age groups

Age group	First-choice antibiotic therapy	Alternative therapies
Neonates, aged ≤7 days	Ampicillin, 50 mg/kg twice daily or amoxicillin 25 mg/kg twice daily and cefotaxime 50 mg/kg twice daily or ceftazidime 50 mg/kg twice daily	Benzylpenicillin 50 mg twice daily and ampicillin 50 mg/kg twice daily or amoxicillin 25 mg/kg twice daily and gentamicin 2.5 mg/kg twice daily
Neonates, aged 8–28 days	Ampicillin 50 mg/kg four times daily or amoxicillin 25 mg/kg three times daily and cefotaxime 50 mg/kg three times daily or ceftazidime 50 mg/kg three times daily	Benzylpenicillin 50 mg three or four times daily or ampicillin 50 mg/kg three or four times daily or amoxicillin 25 mg/kg three times daily and gentamicin 2.5 mg/kg three times daily
Infants, aged 1–3 months	Ampicillin 50 mg/kg four times daily or amoxicillin 25 mg/kg three times daily and cefotaxime 50 mg/kg three times daily or ceftriaxone 75–100 mg/kg once daily	
Infants and children aged >3 months[a]	Cefotaxime 50 mg/kg three times daily or ceftriaxone 75–100 mg/kg once daily	Ampicillin 50 mg/kg four times daily or amoxicillin 25 mg/kg three times daily or benzylpenicillin[b] 30 mg/kg 4-hourly and chloramphenicol[c] 12.5–25 mg/kg four times daily
Adults	Cefotaxime[d] 2 g three times daily or ceftriaxone[d] 2–4 g once daily	Benzylpenicillin 2.4 g 4-hourly or ampicillin 2–3 g four times daily or amoxicillin 2 g three or four times daily and chloramphenicol[c] 12.5–25 mg/kg four times daily

[a] Calculated doses for children should not exceed maximum recommended doses for adults.
[b] Benzylpenicillin is inactive against *H. influenzae* and should therefore not be used in children aged <5 years.
[c] Monitoring of serum chloramphenicol levels is recommended, especially in children aged ≤4 years.
[d] Add ampicillin or amoxicillin to cover *L. monocytogenes* in elderly patients or where Gram-positive bacilli seen in CSF.

(see below) become increasingly important. Amoxicillin or ampicillin plus cefotaxime or ceftriaxone is the recommended treatment. Therapy with amoxicillin or ampicillin and gentamicin is unsuitable for this age group because it provides inadequate cover against *H. influenzae*.

Meningitis in older infants, children and adults

Antimicrobial therapy has to cover *Strep. pneumoniae*, *N. meningitidis* and, in children aged below 5 years, *H. influenzae* (Yogev & Guzman-Cottrill 2005). Achievable antibiotic CSF concentrations are compared with the susceptibilities of the common agents of meningitis in Table 38.3. The third generation cephalosporins cefotaxime and ceftriaxone are now widely used in place of the traditional agents of choice, chloramphenicol, ampicillin, amoxicillin and penicillin (see Table 38.2). This change has stemmed from concern over the rare but potentially serious adverse effects of chloramphenicol and the emergence of resistance to penicillin, ampicillin and chloramphenicol among *Strep. pneumoniae* and *H. influenzae* in particular. Chloramphenicol resistance and reduced susceptibility to penicillin have also been reported in *N. meningitidis*. Cefotaxime and ceftriaxone have a broad spectrum of activity that encompasses not only the three classic causes of bacterial meningitis but also many other bacteria that are infrequent causes of meningitis. However, cephalosporins are inactive against *L. monocytogenes*, and amoxicillin or ampicillin should be added where it is possible that the patient may have listeriosis, for example in elderly patients, or where Gram-positive bacilli are seen on Gram stain. Although earlier generation cephalosporins such as cefuroxime achieve reasonable CSF penetration and are active against the agents of meningitis in vitro, they do not effectively sterilize the CSF and should not be used to treat meningitis.

In meningitis due to *N. meningitidis* and *H. influenzae*, prompt administration of chemoprophylaxis to eliminate nasopharyngeal carriage can reduce the risk of secondary cases in close contacts of the case.

Neisseria meningitidis

In view of the potentially rapid clinical progression of meningococcal disease, treatment should begin with the emergency administration of benzylpenicillin. General practitioners should give penicillin while arranging transfer of the patient to hospital. The dose is normally 1200 mg for adults and children aged 10 years and above, 600 mg for children aged 1–9 years, and 300 mg for children aged below 1 year. Ideally this should be given intravenously. The intramuscular route is less likely to be effective in shocked patients but can be used if venous access cannot be obtained. The only contraindication is allergy to penicillin, where cefotaxime (1 g for adults, 50 mg/kg for children aged <12 years) or chloramphenicol (1.2 g for adults, 25 mg/kg for children aged <12 years) may be given, if available.

Strains of *N. meningitidis* with reduced sensitivity to penicillin are well known and presently account for 5–10% of isolates in Europe and the USA. In general these cases respond to treatment with adequate doses of benzylpenicillin, and failure of penicillin treatment has rarely been reported. Nevertheless, cefotaxime and ceftriaxone are now widely used in preference to benzylpenicillin or chloramphenicol.

Streptococcus pneumoniae

Benzylpenicillin was once widely regarded as the treatment of choice for pneumococcal meningitis. However, pneumococci

Table 38.3 Achievable CSF concentrations of antibiotics in meningitis and MIC values for common CNS pathogens

Antibiotic	CSF: serum ratio	Peak CSF level (mg/L)	MIC$_{90}$ (mg/L) values for:		
			N. meningitidis	*H. influenzae*	*Strep. pneumoniae*
Ampicillin	1:10	10	0.02	0.25	0.05
Benzylpenicillin	1:20	1.5	0.02	1.0	0.02
Cefotaxime	1:20	10	0.01	0.06	0.25
Ceftriaxone	1:15	15	0.01	0.06	0.12
Chloramphenicol	1:2	15	1.0	1.0	2.5
Ciprofloxacin	1:5	0.6	0.004	0.015	1.0
Gentamicin	1:40	<0.5	2.0	0.5	16
Imipenem	1:15	2.0	0.1	1.0	0.05
Linezolid	1:1.25	5.0	>8.0	>8.0	2.0
Meropenem	1:15	4.0	0.03	0.1	0.1
Rifampicin	1:20	1.0	0.5	1.0	2.0
Vancomycin	1:40	1.0	>4.0	>4.0	0.2

MIC$_{90}$, minimum concentration of antibiotic that is inhibitory for 90% of isolates; CSF, cerebrospinal fluid.

that are resistant to penicillin have emerged across the world, presenting a major therapeutic challenge in view of the severity of pneumococcal meningitis.

Although currently only about 5% of pneumococci in the UK are penicillin resistant, the frequency of resistance is increasing and resistance rates of more than 50% have been reported in other countries, including Spain, Hungary and South Africa. Penicillin resistance in pneumococci is defined in terms of the minimum inhibitory concentration (MIC) of penicillin. Most strains have a MIC value of 0.1–1.0 mg/L and are defined as having moderate resistance; strains with an MIC value of 2 mg/L or more are considered highly resistant. This distinction is relevant for less serious infections with moderately resistant strains, which may still respond to adequate doses of some β-lactam antibiotics, such as cefotaxime, ceftriaxone or a carbapenem. However, the clinical outcome of meningitis with penicillin-resistant pneumococci treated with a β-lactam antibiotic as monotherapy is less good. For this reason, many guidelines, including those produced by the Infectious Diseases Society of America, now recommend therapy with a combination of a third-generation cephalosporin and vancomycin (McIntosh 2005). This approach has not been adopted universally in the UK but would certainly appear justified at least for patients who might have acquired their infection in a location where the incidence of penicillin resistance is high. Because of concern over limited CSF penetration of vancomycin, it has been suggested that trough serum levels of 15–20 mg/L should be aimed for, rather than the target of 5–10 mg/L often used for other infections. Another problem is the emergence of pneumococci that are tolerant to vancomycin (that is, they are able to survive, but not proliferate, in the presence of vancomycin).

Although such strains are uncommon, the outcome of meningitis treated with vancomycin is poor.

Other antibiotics may be useful in treating pneumococcal meningitis. Use of rifampicin in combination with a cephalosporin and/or vancomycin is sometimes recommended but there are few data confirming this can improve the response rate in either penicillin-sensitive or -resistant pneumococcal meningitis. The dose of rifampicin is 600 mg twice daily in adults or 10 mg/kg (maximum 600 mg) twice daily in children. Chloramphenicol is a suitable alternative to penicillin for treatment of meningitis due to penicillin-sensitive strains, for example in patients who are penicillin allergic. However, chloramphenicol is not recommended for treating penicillin-resistant pneumococcal meningitis. Although isolates may appear sensitive to chloramphenicol on routine laboratory testing, bactericidal activity is often absent and the clinical response is usually poor. Although rare, meningitis caused by *Strep. pneumoniae* that are both penicillin resistant and vancomycin tolerant presents a major therapeutic difficulty (Cottagnoud & Tauber 2004). Moxifloxacin is a new-generation quinolone antibiotic with enhanced activity against Gram-positive bacteria, including *Strep. pneumoniae,* which has shown promise in experimental pneumococcal meningitis. Linezolid has excellent CSF penetration but does not have bactericidal activity, and clinical experience in treating meningitis has been variable (Rupprecht & Pfister 2005). Daptomycin has potent bactericidal activity and in experimental meningitis with penicillin-resistant pneumococci has been found to give a better clinical outcome than ceftriaxone with vancomycin.

Because of the unpredictable nature of the response to therapy of penicillin-resistant and/or vancomycin-tolerant pneumococcal meningitis, patients require close observation during treatment, for example monitoring of C-reactive protein (CRP) and repeated examination of CSF during therapy.

Haemophilus influenzae

A third-generation cephalosporin such as cefotaxime or ceftriaxone is generally the treatment of choice for *H. influenzae* menin-gitis. These agents have superseded the traditional therapy where chloramphenicol and ampicillin or amoxicillin were used in combination until the sensitivities of the organism were known and therapy could be rationalized to a single agent.

Other bacteria

Meningitis in immunocompetent individuals is rarely due to other bacteria. The definitive treatment for these individuals should be determined on an individual basis in the light of careful clinical and microbiological assessment.

Chemoprophylaxis

In meningococcal meningitis, spread between family members and other close contacts is well recognized; these individuals should receive chemoprophylaxis as soon as possible, preferably within 24 hours. Sometimes chemoprophylaxis may be indicated for other contacts but the decision to offer prophylaxis beyond household contacts should only be made after obtaining expert advice (Table 38.4). Of the antibiotics conventionally used to treat meningococcal infections, only ceftriaxone reliably eliminates nasopharyngeal carriage; where another antibiotic has been used for treatment, the index case also requires chemoprophylaxis. A number of antibiotics are suitable as prophylaxis (Table 38.5).

Ciprofloxacin is now widely recommended for adults because of the convenience of single-dose administration and, unlike rifampicin, it does not interact with oral contraceptives and is readily available in community pharmacies. Although anaphylactoid reactions have been reported to occur in individuals receiving ciprofloxacin as chemoprophylaxis, none of these reactions has been fatal. If the strain is confirmed as group C (or A, W135 or Y), vaccination is normally offered to contacts who were given prophylaxis. There is no need to vaccinate the patient. There is currently no vaccine that protects against group B disease, which accounts for about 70% of cases of meningococcal disease in Europe.

Chemoprophylaxis against Hib infection is usually only indicated where there is an unimmunized child in the vulnerable age group in the household (see Table 38.4). Only rifampicin has been proved to be effective in eliminating nasopharyngeal carriage (see Table 38.5). Unimmunized household contacts aged below 4 years should also receive Hib vaccine. The index case should also receive rifampicin in order to eliminate nasopharyngeal carriage, and should be immunized, irrespective of age.

Meningitis in the immunocompromised host

In the immunocompromised neutropenic patient the meninges can become infected. Possible causes of meningitis include Enterobacteriaceae and *Pseudomonas aeruginosa,* as well as the classic bacterial causes of meningitis. The choice of therapy is governed by the need to attain broad-spectrum coverage, using agents with good CSF penetration. Meropenem may now be the drug of choice for meningitis in this setting, although many other regimens are also appropriate.

Patients with cellular immune dysfunction are vulnerable to meningitis due to *L. monocytogenes* and *C. neoformans.* Ampicillin or amoxicillin, along with cefotaxime or ceftriaxone, is recommended as empirical antibacterial therapy for meningitis in these patients. Definitive treatment of listeria meningitis is normally with high-dose ampicillin (3 g four times daily) or amoxicillin (2 g four times daily), with the addition of gentamicin

---

Table 38.4   Indications for chemoprophylaxis in contacts of cases of infection with *N. meningitidis* or *H. influenzae* type b

Neisseria meningitidis
Household and other close contacts: prophylaxis usually initiated as soon as possible by clinicians caring for the case
• Persons who have slept in the same house as the patient at any time during the 7 days before the onset of symptoms
• Boy/girl friends of the case
• Unless treated with ceftriaxone (which reliably eliminates nasopharyngeal carriage), the index case should also receive antibiotic prophylaxis as soon as he or she is able to take oral medication
Healthcare workers: prophylaxis should only by initiated after consultation with hospital infection control team or public health doctor

• Individuals who have administered mouth-to-mouth resuscitation or had some other form of prolonged close face-to-face contact with the patient
Other contacts: prophylaxis should be initiated by a public health doctor

• Schools, nurseries, universities and other closed communities where two or more linked cases have occurred

Invasive *Haemophilus influenzae* type b infection
Household and other close contacts: prophylaxis usually initiated as soon as possible by clinicians caring for the case

• Indicated only where there is another child aged less than 4 years who has not been immunized in the same household as the index case. In such circumstances prophylaxis should be given to all household contacts aged 1 month or older, unless there are contraindications. The index case should also receive antibiotic prophylaxis as soon as he or she is able to take oral medication

Other contacts: prophylaxis very rarely necessary and should only be initiated by a public health physician

Table 38.5 Recommended prophylactic regimens for contacts of cases of infection with *N. meningitidis* or *H. influenzae* type b

Meningococcal infection

Rifampicin (oral)

Children aged <1 year	5 mg/kg twice daily on 2 consecutive days
Children aged 1–12 years	10 mg/kg (max 600 mg) twice daily on 2 consecutive days
Adults[b]	600 mg twice daily on 2 consecutive days

Ciprofloxacin[a] (oral)

Children aged 5–12 years	250 mg as a single dose
Adults[b]	500 mg as a single dose

Ceftriaxone[a] (intramuscular)

Children aged <12 years	125 mg as a single dose
Adults[b]	250 mg as a single dose

Invasive *Haemophilus influenzae* type b infection

Rifampicin (oral)

Children aged 1–3 months	10 mg/kg once daily for 4 days
Children aged >3 months	20 mg/kg once daily (max 600 mg) for 4 days
Adults[b]	600 mg once daily for 4 days

[a] Not licensed for this indication.
[b] For pregnant women, obtain expert advice.

in order to obtain a synergistic effect. The most appropriate treatment for patients who are penicillin allergic, or in the rare circumstance of infection with a strain that is ampicillin resistant, is uncertain and specialist microbiological advice should be sought. Specific therapies for cryptococcal meningitis are described in detail below.

Splenectomized patients are susceptible to invasive infections with encapsulated bacteria, including *Strep. pneumoniae* and Hib. Standard therapy with either cefotaxime or ceftriaxone is appropriate.

Shunt meningitis

Patients who have a shunt are at increased risk of meningitis. Shunt infections are classified according to the site of initial infection. Internal infections, where the lumen of the shunt is colonized, constitute the majority of cases. External shunt infections involve the tissues surrounding the shunt. Most internal shunt infections are caused by coagulase-negative staphylococci. *Staph. aureus* and Enterobacteriaceae account for most external infections. It is generally held that management of shunt infections should include shunt removal, as well as antibiotic therapy (Infection in Neurosurgery Working Party 2000). However, recent work suggests that infections with coagulase-negative staphylococci can at least sometimes be successfully managed without shunt removal. Appropriate antimicrobial regimens are shown in Table 38.6.

Tuberculous meningitis

The outcome in tuberculous meningitis relates directly to the severity of the patient's clinical condition on commencement of therapy. A satisfactory response demands a high degree of clinical suspicion such that appropriate chemotherapy is initiated early, even if tubercle bacilli are not demonstrated on initial microscopy. Most currently used antituberculous agents achieve effective concentrations in the CSF in tuberculous meningitis. Detailed discussion of antituberculous therapy is given in Chapter 40 (tuberculosis). Adjunctive steroid therapy is of value in patients with more severe disease, particularly those who

Table 38.6 Antimicrobial regimens for treatment of shunt meningitis

Type of infection	First-choice antibiotic regimen	Other antibiotic regimens	Duration of therapy before reshunting
Internal shunt infection caused by Gram-positive bacteria	Intraventricular vancomycin + intravenous or oral rifampicin	Substitute flucloxacillin or intravenous vancomycin for rifampicin in cases of rifampicin resistance, except in the case of enterococci, where an aminoglycoside (e.g. gentamicin) should be used	7–10 days intravenous
External shunt infection caused by *Staph. aureus*	As above, with the addition of intravenous flucloxacillin	Substitute intravenous vancomycin for flucloxacillin in the case of methicillin resistance (MRSA)	12–14 days
Enterobacteriaceae	Intravenous cefotaxime ± an aminoglycoside + intraventricular aminoglycoside	Substitute ceftazidime or meropenem for cefotaxime in the case of cefotaxime resistance	14 days
Polymicrobial ventriculoperitoneal shunt infections	Intravenous amoxicillin, metronidazole, cefotaxime ± an aminoglycoside + intraventricular aminoglycoside	Seek specialist advice	14 days
Candida	Intravenous amphotericin B + flucytosine	Intravenous fluconazole	10–14 days (antifungal fungal therapy should continue for 1 week after reshunting)

suddenly develop cerebral oedema soon after starting treatment or who appear to be developing a spinal block. However, routine use of steroids is not recommended. They may suppress informative changes in the CSF and interfere with antibiotic penetration by restoring the blood–brain barrier. Early neurosurgical management of hydrocephalus by means of a ventriculoperitoneal or ventriculoatrial shunt is also important in improving the prospects for neurological recovery.

Steroids as adjunctive therapy in the management of bacterial meningitis

In pharmacological doses, adrenal corticosteroids regulate many components of the inflammatory response and also lower CSF hydrostatic pressure. However, by reducing inflammation and restoring the blood–brain barrier, they may reduce CSF penetration of antibiotics. The benefits of steroids in the initial management of meningitis due to *M. tuberculosis* and Hib are well recognized. In Hib meningitis dexametasone commenced early at a dose of 0.6–1.5 mg/kg/day in four divided doses for 4 days significantly reduces sensorineural hearing loss and possibly other long-term sequelae. Recent evidence suggests that dexametasone is also of benefit in pneumococcal meningitis, provided that it is commenced early (before or with the first dose of antibiotics). There is no evidence of benefit from steroids in meningococcal meningitis (McIntyre 2005).

Cryptococcal meningitis

The standard treatment of cryptococcal meningitis is amphotericin B, given intravenously at a dose of 0.7–1.0 mg/kg/day, together with flucytosine 100 mg/kg/day, for 6–10 weeks. Lipid formulations of amphotericin B, such as liposomal amphotericin B, at doses of 4–6 mg/kg/day have comparable efficacy to conventional amphotericin B at a dose of 0.7 mg/kg. As an alternative to prolonged therapy with two potentially toxic drugs, 2 weeks' therapy with amphotericin B and flucytosine may be given, followed by consolidation therapy with fluconazole 400 mg/day for at least 10 weeks. Patients with HIV infection treated for cryptococcal meningitis should then receive fluconazole indefinitely, or at least until immune reconstitution occurs. The dose of fluconazole may be reduced to 200 mg/day, depending on the patient's clinical condition (Bicanic & Harrison 2004).

Side effects are common with both amphotericin B and flucytosine. Side effects of amphotericin B include fever, nausea, vomiting, local thrombophlebitis, anaemia, hypokalaemia and impairment of renal function. These are much less common with lipid formulations of amphotericin B. Side effects of flucytosine include deranged liver function and bone marrow depression. Regular haematological and biochemical monitoring is recommended during treatment, along with measurement of serum concentrations of flucytosine (which should not exceed 80 mg/L).

The azole drugs itraconazole and fluconazole are generally well tolerated in high doses, and exhibit excellent dose-dependent in vitro activity against *C. neoformans*. Fluconazole offers excellent CSF penetration and has been found to be superior to itraconazole as initial and maintenance therapy for cryptococcal meningitis. However, use of fluconazole alone is not recommended as induction therapy, because with conventional doses the clinical and microbiological responses are slower than with amphotericin B. Fluconazole 400–800 mg/day together with flucytosine 150 mg/kg/day for 6 weeks is an alternative to amphotericin B-based regimens but the toxicity of this regimen is surprisingly high. Itraconazole 200–400 mg/day is a suitable alternative to fluconazole as maintenance therapy in patients unable to tolerate fluconazole.

The clinical response to treatment of cryptococcal meningitis is slow and it often takes 2 or 3 weeks to sterilize the CSF. Monitoring of intracranial pressure is essential, with large-volume CSF drainage indicated if the opening pressure reaches 250 mmHg. Serial CSF cultures are occasionally helpful in following the response to treatment but monitoring of cryptococcal antigen titres in serum or CSF is of little value.

Intrathecal and intraventricular administration of antibiotics

Intrathecal administration, i.e. administration into the lumbar subarachnoid space, of antibiotics was once widely used to supplement levels attained by concomitant systemic therapy. However, there is little evidence for the efficacy of this route of delivery and it is now rarely used. In particular, it produces only low concentrations of antibiotic in the ventricles and therefore does little to prevent ventriculitis, one of the most serious complications of meningitis. Direct intraventricular administration of antibiotics in meningitis is important in certain types of meningitis, especially where it is necessary to use an agent, e.g. vancomycin or an aminoglycoside, that penetrates CSF poorly (Shah et al 2004). The most common situation is in shunt-associated meningitis, where multiple antibiotic-resistant coagulase-negative staphylococci are the major pathogens.

There are considerable differences in recommended doses of antibiotics for intrathecal or intraventricular administration. A dose of 20 mg vancomycin per day is recommended for treatment of shunt-associated meningitis in patients of all ages with an extraventricular drain (CSF volumes in babies with hydrocephalus are at least as high as in adults). Lower success rates have been found with doses of less than 20 mg (Infection in Neurosurgery Working Party 2000). Recommended doses of antibiotics are otherwise largely based on anecdotal experience (Table 38.7).

Viral meningitis

It is fortunate that most cases of viral meningitis are self-limiting since none of the currently available antiviral agents

Table 38.7 Daily doses (mg) of gentamicin and vancomycin for intraventricular administration

Antibiotic	Adult	Child ≥2 years	Child <2 years
Gentamicin	5	2.5	1.0
Vancomycin	20	10[a]	10[a]

[a]20 mg/day is recommended for children of all ages with shunt-associated meningitis and an extraventricular drain.

Table 38.8 Common therapeutic problems in infective meningitis

Infection	Antibiotic	Common problems	Resolution
Bacterial meningitis	Chloramphenicol	Risk of serious toxicity, especially in neonates	Avoid use if possible Close monitoring of serum levels where use essential
Neonatal meningitis	Aminoglycosides (e.g. gentamicin)	Poor CSF penetration provides unreliable activity against Gram-negative bacteria Unpredictable neonatal pharmacokinetics (especially preterm neonates)	Substitute with, or add, an antibiotic with better CSF penetration (e.g. a cephalosporin) Close monitoring of serum levels
Strep. pneumoniae meningitis	Penicillin Cefotaxime or ceftriaxone Vancomycin (intravenous)	Resistance is increasing Treatment failure in meningitis due to penicillin-resistant strains Unreliable CSF penetration	Use cefotaxime or ceftriaxone ± vancomycin as empiric therapy Add rifampicin or vancomycin Consider one of the newer antibiotics with good activity against multiresistant Gram-positive bacteria
Listeria monocytogenes meningitis	Any	Relapse rate up to 10% after short courses of therapy	Give prolonged therapy (usually 3–4 weeks)
Cryptococcal meningitis	Amphotericin B Flucytosine Fluconazole	High incidence of side effects, e.g. fever, nausea, vomiting, anaemia, hypokalaemia, impaired renal function Risk of side effects, e.g. deranged liver function, bone marrow depression Low cure rate when used as monotherapy (except as consolidation therapy)	Change to lipid-based preparation of amphotericin B, or replace with fluconazole Close monitoring of serum levels Combine with flucytosine

has useful activity against the viruses that commonly cause this condition. CNS infections with herpes simplex viruses tend to present as encephalitis rather than meningitis. Herpes simplex meningoencephalitis is treated with high-dose aciclovir, 10 mg/kg three times daily.

Patient care

Prevention of person-to-person transmission of meningitis

Patients with meningitis may be infectious to others. Neonates with meningitis usually have generalized infections, and the causative organisms can often be isolated from body fluids and faeces. Babies with meningitis should therefore be isolated to prevent infection spreading to other patients. Patients with meningococcal or Hib meningitis should be isolated until after at least 48 hours of antibiotic therapy. Contacts of these patients may be asymptomatic carriers and potentially infectious to others and/or at risk of developing invasive infection themselves. Chemoprophylaxis and vaccination can reduce these risks (see above). Patients with most other types of meningitis do not represent a significant infectious hazard, and enhanced infection control precautions are not usually necessary.

Common problems in the treatment of meningitis are set out in Table 38.8.

CASE STUDIES

Case 38.1

A 3-week-old boy presents with a 24-hour history of poor feeding, fever and increasing drowsiness. Lumbar puncture reveals 1200 WBC/μL (80% of which are polymorphs), and low glucose and elevated protein levels. No organisms are seen on a Gram-stained smear of the CSF. The diagnosis is acute purulent meningitis.

Question

How should this patient be managed?

Answer

At 3 weeks of age the possible causes include neonatal pathogens (group B streptococci, *Escherichia coli* and *Listeria monocytogenes*) as well as the usual causes of meningitis in older infants (especially *Neisseria meningitidis* and *Streptococcus pneumoniae*). Cefotaxime or ceftriaxone will provide adequate cover for most of these pathogens, but addition of ampicillin or amoxicillin is required to cover *L. monocytogenes*. Ampicillin or amoxicillin should be given along with cefotaxime or ceftriaxone. Although the differential diagnosis includes pneumococcal meningitis, which might be pencillin resistant, it is not usual to include vancomycin in the empiric therapy for meningitis where the aetiological agent is unknown.

Case 38.2

A 70-year-old man is being treated for meningitis due to *Streptococcus pneumoniae* that is moderately resistant to penicillin (MIC value 0.75 mg/L). Despite 7 days' treatment with intravenous vancomycin and cefotaxime, there has been little improvement in his clinical condition. A CT scan has shown meningeal inflammation consistent with meningitis, but no evidence of intracranial complications that might explain his poor clinical response. The most recent trough (predose) serum vancomycin concentration was 5.3 mg/L.

Questions

1. Why might there have been no response to treatment with cefotaxime and vancomycin?
2. What options are there to modify his antimicrobial therapy?

Answers

1. CSF penetration of vancomycin is poor and the serum vancomycin concentration in this case was at the lower end of the normal therapeutic range of 5–15 mg/L. Alternatively, the infection may be due to a vancomycin-tolerant strain of *Strep. pneumoniae*. Tolerant strains appear fully sensitive to vancomycin by routine laboratory antimicrobial susceptibility sensitivity testing.
2. If the strain of *Strep. pneumoniae* is not vancomycin tolerant then the infection may respond to increasing the dose of vancomycin together with addition of rifampicin. Alternatively, or if the infecting strain is vancomycin tolerant, one of the newer antibiotics active against resistant Gram-positive bacteria such as linezolid could be used instead of vancomycin.

Case 38.3

A 2-year-old girl from a large family living in poor social circumstances presents with meningitis. An urgent Gram stain of the CSF shows Gram-negative bacilli with the morphological appearance of *Haemophilus influenzae*. On further questioning of the family, it appears that the patient and other children in the family did not receive all their routine immunizations.

Questions

1. What treatment would you give this child immediately?
2. What other immediate action would you take?
3. What further treatment will the patient require?

Answers

1. One of the third-generation cephalosporins, cefotaxime or ceftriaxone, is the first-choice treatment for *H. influenzae* (Hib) meningitis. In addition, the benefits of early steroid adjunctive therapy in Hib meningitis are well established and a 4-day course of dexametasone should be commenced along with, or as soon as possible after, the first dose of antibiotics.
2. If there is another child aged less than 4 years in the household who has not been immunized, prophylaxis with rifampicin should be given to all household contacts aged 1 month or older, unless there are contraindications. Unimmunized household contacts aged below 4 years should also receive Hib vaccine.
3. The patient should receive prophylaxis with rifampicin as soon as she is able to take oral medication, and should also be immunized against Hib.

Case 38.4

A 46-year-old renal transplant recipient has received 18 days treatment with amphotericin B and flucytosine for cryptococcal meningitis. His clinical condition has improved significantly, but his renal function is deteriorating seriously.

Question

What could be done to address this patient's deteriorating renal function?

Answer

There are two options. A lipid preparation of amphotericin B could be used to complete the planned course of treatment. Alternatively, amphotericin B could be replaced by fluconazole. However, dose adjustment of immunosuppressive drugs may be required because of interactions with fluconazole. If fluconazole is preferred, given that the patient has already received more than 2 weeks therapy and has recovered well, it would be appropriate to use it as monotherapy.

REFERENCES

Bicanic T, Harrison T S 2004 Cryptococcal meningitis. British Medical Bulletin 72: 99-118

Cottagnoud P H, Tauber M G 2004 New therapies for pneumococcal meningitis. Expert Opinion on Investigational Drugs 13: 393-401

Harvey D, Holt D E, Bedford H 1999 Bacterial meningitis in the newborn: a prospective study of mortality and morbidity. Seminars in Perinatology 23: 215-218

Infection in Neurosurgery Working Party of the British Society for Antimicrobial Chemotherapy 2000 The management of neurosurgical patients with postoperative bacterial or aseptic meningitis or external ventricular drain-associated ventriculitis. British Journal of Neurosurgery 14: 7-12

McIntosh E D 2005 Treatment and prevention strategies to combat pediatric pneumococcal meningitis. Expert Review of Antiinfective Therapy 3: 739-750

McIntyre P 2005 Should dexamethasone be part of routine therapy of bacterial meningitis in industrialized countries? Advances in Experimental Medicine and Biology 568: 189-197

Ross J S, Wilson K J W 1981 Foundations of anatomy and physiology, 5th edn. Churchill Livingstone, Edinburgh, pp172-173

Rupprecht T A, Pfister H W 2005 Clinical experience with linezolid for the treatment of central nervous system infections. European Journal of Neurology 12: 536-542

Shah S, Ohlsson A, Shah V 2004 Intraventricular antibiotics for bacterial meningitis in neonates. Cochrane Database of Systematic Reviews: CD004496. Update Software, Oxford

Yogev R, Guzman-Cottrill J 2005 Bacterial meningitis in children: critical review of current concepts. Drugs 65: 1097-1112

FURTHER READING

Chang L, Phipps W, Kennedy G, Rutherford G 2005 Antifungal interventions for the primary prevention of cryptococcal disease in adults with HIV. Cochrane Database of Systematic Reviews: CD004773. John Wiley, Chichester

Chavez-Bueno S, McCracken G H Jr 2005 Bacterial meningitis in children. Pediatric Clinics of North America 52: 795-810

Correia J B, Hart C A 2004 Meningococcal disease. Clinical Evidence 12: 1164-1181

Law M R, Palomaki G, Alfirevic Z et al 2005 The prevention of neonatal group B streptococcal disease: a report by a working group of the Medical Screening Society. Journal of Medical Screening 12: 60-68

Lutsar I, Friedland I R 2000 Pharmacokinetics and pharmacodynamics of cephalosporins in cerebrospinal fluid. Clinical Pharmacokinetics 39: 335-343

Roos K L 2004 Neurologic infectious diseases. McGraw-Hill, New York

Wilson J 2000 Clinical microbiology. An introduction for health care professionals. Baillière Tindall, London

Surgical antibiotic prophylaxis

J. C. Graham

Infection at the site of incision is a common but avoidable complication of a surgical procedure. The term surgical site infection (SSI) encompasses not only infection at the site of incision but also infections of implants, prosthetic devices and adjacent tissues involved in the operation. Precise definitions are used to allow comparison of infection rates. The importance of surgical site incision as a healthcare-associated infection is demonstrated by the recent introduction in England of mandatory surveillance for surgical site incision in orthopaedic surgery.

Surgical infections result in significant morbidity; a recent estimate of additional attributable hospital costs of surgical site incision ranged from £959 to £6103 per patient (Coello et al 2005). There are a number of costs associated with these infections (Fig. 39.1). Antibiotic prophylaxis is one component of a preventive strategy that is based on good surgical technique, strict asepsis in the operating theatre and control of infection within the hospital or primary care medical practice. The decision to use antibiotics to prevent infection in an individual patient depends upon the patient's risk of surgical infection, the severity of the consequences of SSI, the effectiveness of prophylaxis in that operation and adverse consequences of prophylaxis for that patient. Administration of these agents should be monitored to ensure a quality standard is met (Dellinger et al 1994).

Hence, the goals of antibiotic prophylaxis are to:

- reduce the incidence of SSI
- use antibiotics in a manner that is supported by evidence of effectiveness
- minimize the effect on the patient's normal flora

- minimize adverse effects
- cause minimal alteration of the host defences.

Despite numerous guidelines on antimicrobial prophylaxis, the recommendations made are not always followed and it has been suggested that three performance measures can be monitored to improve the quality of prophylaxis (Bratzler & Houck 2004):

1. the proportion of patients who have parenteral antibiotics administered within 1 h before surgical incision
2. the proportion of patients who have prophylactic antimicrobials consistent with currently published guidelines
3. the proportion of patients who have antibiotics discontinued within 24 h after the end of surgery.

Risk factors for infection

Following the initial development of antibiotics in the 1940s, it was believed that these agents would be effective in reducing SSI; however, early studies suggested otherwise (Fry 1988). This was due to inconsistent timing of antibiotic administration and methodological problems as relatively clean procedures were compared with procedures where bacterial contamination was likely. This led to the stratification system outlined in Table 39.1 (Managram et al 1999). Other factors affect the incidence of SSI, including the following.

Insertion of prosthetic implants

All implants have a detrimental effect on host defences and therefore a lower bacterial inoculum is required to initiate infection. Hence there is a greater risk of infection of the wound and surgical site.

Duration of surgery

The longer the operation, the greater the risk of wound infection; this risk is additional to that of the classification of the operation.

Co-morbidities

The American Society of Anesthesiology (ASA) preoperative risk score is based on the co-morbidities at time of operation. A score greater than 2 (Table 39.2) is associated with an increased risk of wound infection (additional to classification of operation and duration). A risk index can be ascertained for an individual patient based on the presence of a co-morbidity (ASA score

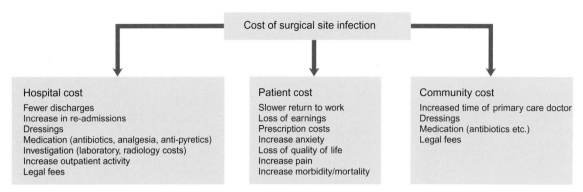

Figure 39.1 Example of factors that may contribute to the cost of surgical site incision infection.

Table 39.1 Classification of surgical procedures by risk of infection (Managram et al 1999)

Type of procedure	Definition	Wound infection rate (%)	Need for prophylaxis
Clean	Atraumatic; no inflammation encountered, no break in technique; gastrointestinal, genitourinary and respiratory tracts not entered	1.5–4.2	Not usually required
Clean-contaminated	Gastrointestinal or respiratory tract entered but without spillage; oropharynx, appendectomy, sterile genitourinary or biliary tract entered; minor break in technique	<10	Usually required
Contaminated	Acute inflammation; infected bile or urine; gross spillage from gastrointestinal tract; major lapse in technique; fresh traumatic wound	10–20	Always required
Dirty and infected	Established infection; transection of clean tissues to enable collection of pus; traumatic wound with retained devitalized tissue; faecal contamination; delayed treatment	20–40	Therapy required

Table 39.2 American Society of Anesthesiology (ASA) classification of physical status

ASA score	Physical status
1	A normal healthy patient
2	A patient with mild systemic disease
3	A patient with a severe systemic disease that limits activity but is not incapacitating
4	A patient with an incapacitating systemic disease that is a constant threat to life
5	A moribund patient that is not expected to survive 24 hours with or without operation

Table 39.3 Risk index based on presence of co-morbidity and duration of operation

Risk index 0 = when neither risk factor is present
Risk index 1 = when either one of the risk factors is present
Risk index 2 = when both risk factors are present

Patient risk factors

- Advanced age
- Malnutrition
- Obesity
- Concurrent infection
- Diabetes mellitus
- Liver impairment.
- Renal impairment
- Immune deficiency states
- Prolonged preoperative stay
- Blood transfusion

Operative risk factors

- Tissue ischaemia
- Lack of haemostasis
- Tissue damage, e.g. crushing by surgical instruments

>2) and duration of operation (>75th percentile). As the index increases, the risk of infection rises as it does from clean to contaminated surgery (Table 39.3).

There are a number of other risk factors that may contribute to the risk of SSI for an individual patient but have not been classified as well as above.

- Presence of necrotic tissue
- Presence of foreign bodies including surgical materials

Benefits and risk of antibiotic prophylaxis

The prophylactic use of antibiotics has important implications. It requires a risk–benefit analysis which is distinct from that used when antibiotics are given to treat active infections. On the risk side, patients without an immediate need for therapy are potentially exposed to dose-related toxicity, drug interactions and idiosyncratic toxic reactions, including potentially fatal allergic responses. More generally, the routine and widespread use of antibiotics in hospitals is a powerful ecological pressure in favour of bacterial antibiotic-resistance genes, threatening the therapy of real infections. The financial costs of antibiotics are a complex additional consideration; the prophylaxis chosen must be cost-effective and significant savings can be made by not prolonging antibiotic prophylaxis.

An additional potential problem is *Clostridium difficile* infection. *C. difficile*-associated diarrhoea is related to antibiotic usage, typically third-generation cephalosporins, although recent data suggest fluoroquinolones may also be important (Pepin et al 2005). *C. difficile* infection increases morbidity and mortality and prolongs hospital stay, leading to an overall increase in healthcare costs.

Individual patients whose infections have been prevented will benefit although who these patients are can never be known with certainty. At a more subtle level, other patients may also benefit from prevented infections in fellow patients, since an opportunity for transmission of infection from patient to patient will have been avoided.

It is important to be aware of the definitions used in wound infection studies and caution should be the watchword when comparing infection rates between studies, hospitals or surgeons. The Centers for Disease Control in the USA have published guidelines that define wound infections from both clinical and microbiological criteria, which may allow comparison of wound infection rates (Table 39.4). Similarly, one must recognize that surgical site infection may present following discharge; in fact, using the National Nosocomial Infection Surveillance (NNIS) data, 16% are detected through postdischarge surveillance with a further 38% identified on readmission (Gaynes et al 2001).

Table 39.4   Centers for Disease Control (CDC) definitions of surgical site (wound) infections (Horan et al 1992)

Incisional surgical site infection

Superficial incisional surgical site infection

BOTH:

- Infection involves only the skin or subcutaneous tissue of incision
- Occurs within 30 days of operation

AND AT LEAST ONE OF THE FOLLOWING:

- Purulent drainage from the incision
- Organisms isolated from an aseptically taken culture of fluid or tissue from the superficial incision
- At least one of the following signs:
  - Pain or tenderness
  - Localized swelling, redness or heat
- Diagnosis of superficial surgical site infection by a clinician

Exclusion from the definitions include:

- Suture abscess (minimal inflammation and discharge confined to the points of suture penetration)
- Infected burn wound
- Surgical site infection that extends into the fascial and muscle layers (these are deep surgical site infections)

Deep incisional surgical site infection

BOTH:

- Infection involves deep soft tissues (fascial and muscle layers)
- Occurs within 30 days of an operation if no non-human derived implantable foreign body is left in place OR within 1 year if an implant is left in place and infection is related to operative procedure

AND AT LEAST ONE OF THE FOLLOWING:

- Purulent drainage from deep incision but not from organ/space component of the surgical site
- A deep microbiological culture-positive incision that spontaneously dehisces or is deliberately opened surgically in the presence of one or more of the following features:
  - Pyrexia >38°C
  - Local pain
- Objective evidence of abscess formation or other forms of infection in the deep part of the incision
- Diagnosis of deep incisional surgical site infection by a clinician

continued

Table 39.4 (continued)

Organ/space surgical site infection

BOTH:

- Infection involves any part of the anatomy (organs or spaces) opened or manipulated during the operation other than the incision
- Occurs within 30 days of operation if no non-human derived implantable foreign body is left in place OR within 1 year if an implant is left in place and infection is related to operative procedure

AND AT LEAST ONE OF THE FOLLOWING:

- Purulent drainage from drain placed in the organ/space
- Organism isolated from an aseptically obtained culture of fluid or tissue from the organ/space
- Objective evidence of abscess formations or other forms of infection in the organ/space
- Diagnosis of organ/space surgical site infection by a clinician

Pathogenesis

It is not surprising that the most frequent infectious complication of surgery is local wound infection. The epithelial surfaces of the body act as efficient boundaries between the sterile contents of the body and the bacteria-rich external world. Epithelial surfaces include not only the skin but also the conjunctiva, tympanic membranes and the mucosal surfaces of the respiratory, gastrointestinal and genitourinary tracts. Topologically, the external world includes the luminal contents of these tracts. Any surgical operation will breach at least one of these surfaces and allow entry of bacteria. Whether an infection follows depends on the ability of the other defences to kill the invading bacteria. Important host mechanisms include antibodies, complement and phagocytic cells.

Organisms and sources

The identities and quantities of bacteria entering a wound are important factors in determining outcome, and to a large extent these depend on the nature of the operation (Table 39.5). In some circumstances bacteria will have already entered sterile tissues before the patient reaches hospital – when an appendix perforates into the peritoneal cavity or bacteria are introduced into soft tissues in a road traffic accident, for example. In the former, many different species of normal bowel flora including enterococci, coliforms and anaerobes will be involved, potentially in massive numbers. In the latter, organisms not normally associated with the human body will have entered the wound from the external environment.

Many surgical operations involve incision of the skin. This will permit the inoculation of Gram-positive skin flora, including *Staphylococcus aureus*, coagulase-negative staphylococci and *Corynebacterium* spp. Some skin sites, the groin for example, carry both typical skin flora and gut bacteria and this extended spectrum of organisms needs to be considered when constructing prophylaxis protocols. Skin diseases such as eczema and psoriasis, although not of infectious origin, support abnormally large populations of skin bacteria including *Staph. aureus.* Patients with these diseases, regardless of whether or not the surgical incision involves diseased skin, are at increased risk of wound infection simply because of heavy skin colonization. In all patients a vital step in prevention of wound infection is preoperative skin disinfection. This both dilutes the number of bacteria and kills many of those remaining.

The upper gastrointestinal tract supports the growth of few bacteria. The acid environment of the stomach and alkaline and bile salt content of the small bowel create an unfavourable environment for the survival of most bacteria. However, gastric disease such as cancer and drugs inhibiting acid production can allow gastric overgrowth with coliforms. In contrast, the large bowel is heavily colonized with a wide range of bacteria. While they are contained within the lumen of the colon, they have a broadly beneficial role. However, if they are released into the peritoneal cavity by disease or surgery they can cause fulminating

Table 39.5 Most likely pathogens in postoperative wound infections

Category of surgery	Most likely pathogen(s)
Clean	
Cardiac/vascular	Coagulase-negative staphylococci, Staph. aureus, Gram-negative bacilli
Breast	Staph. aureus
Orthopaedic	Coagulase-negative staphylococci, Staph. aureus, coliforms
Dialysis access	Coagulase-negative staphylococci, Staph. aureus
Neurological	Coagulase-negative staphylococci, Staph. aureus, coliforms
Clean-contaminated	
Burn	Staph. aureus, Pseudomonas aeruginosa
Head and neck	Staph. aureus, streptococci spp., anaerobes (from oral cavity)
Gastrointestinal tract	Coliforms, anaerobes (Bacteroides fragilis)
Urogenital tract	Coliforms, enterococci spp.
Dirty	
Ruptured viscera	Coliforms, anaerobes (Bacteroides fragilis)
Traumatic wound	Staph. aureus, Streptococcus pyogenes, Clostridium spp.

sepsis. Elective bowel surgery is usually preceded by attempts to physically reduce bowel contents with enemas and purgatives so that there is less potential for spillage during surgery. Even so, colonic and rectal surgery frequently result in significant wound contamination, making prophylaxis a prime concern.

The vagina and, in both sexes, the urethra are normally colonized with organisms drawn from large bowel flora. For the vagina this is especially so in both the prepubertal and postmenopausal age groups. In the intervening years the vaginal pH is kept acid by the action of lactobacilli and this keeps the growth of coliforms in check. Although bladder urine is normally sterile, most urological operations are associated with disease that predisposes to infected bladder urine. Incisions of the urinary epithelium in such circumstances can permit rapid and large amounts of bacterial bloodstream invasion, with a high risk of septicaemia.

The upper respiratory tract supports large and complex communities of bacteria, which may infect both local pharyngeal and respiratory tract wounds. Aerosol transmission may result in contamination of more distant wounds. The nares can be heavily colonized by *Staph. aureus*. Measures to reduce this in renal dialysis patients have been followed by a decline in skin wound infection rates.

An important advance in surgery was the recognition that the skin and respiratory tract flora of the surgical team can cause postoperative infection. This understanding is the basis for hand disinfection, gloves, gowns and masks for operators.

Contamination by organisms from the environment can occasionally occur within the operating theatre, for example if there is a breakdown in the decontamination of surgical equipment or if the theatre ventilation system is not functioning properly. Characteristically, such sources are only uncovered after several patients have been infected with the same organism. Finally, disinfectants have been contaminated during preparation and have acted as sources of infection.

Although many species of bacteria may enter wounds, only a small range is commonly associated with infections. This may be partly due to poor recognition of some organisms, but it is undoubtedly true that bacteria such as *Staph. aureus* are better adapted to reproduction in human wounds and will outgrow many other species.

Consequences of infection

So far this chapter has not drawn a distinction between the consequences of wound infections at different sites. It is important to do so. Skin and superficial soft tissue infections are generally readily amenable to antibiotic therapy. However, they can impair the aesthetic quality of the surgical scar, which may be of major importance to the patient. Deeper soft tissue infections can progress to cellulitis and abscess formation, both of which can prolong hospital stay, and in some cases can be fatal. Infection of bone and joint prostheses can cause long-term disability and may necessitate further operations. Cardiac valve infection can result in sudden and catastrophic dysfunction or chronic ill health, again forcing additional operations. Eye infections can produce irreversible blindness. Central nervous system infections results in meningitis, brain or spinal abscess formation.

In skin and soft tissue infections the responsible organisms are usually major pathogens such as *Staph. aureus*, β-haemolytic

streptococci and anaerobes. Their antibiotic susceptibilities are usually easily predictable and to an extent they are more readily controlled than other less commonly involved organisms, such as coagulase-negative staphylococci, enterococci, *Corynebacterium* spp., *Pseudomonas* spp. and *Acinetobacter* spp., which are often antibiotic resistant.

It can be appreciated that organisms that are of little importance to a general surgeon may be of grave concern to a neurosurgeon. Hence, when considering the value of surgical antibiotic prophylaxis, there is a need to consider the surgical downside, i.e. what is the worst outcome of infection?

Choice of antibiotic regimen for prophylaxis

Antibiotic regimens consist of not only the antibiotic (or antibiotics) but also the dose, route and timing of administration. The choice of a particular regimen is the product of scientific principles, practical considerations, empiricism and cost. One obvious principle is that the antibiotic should be active against the organisms most likely to cause infection. Early approaches were to give antibiotics at a dose that would exceed the minimum inhibitory concentration (MIC), an in vitro measurement of the lowest concentration of a particular antibiotic required to inhibit growth of a particular organism. This parallels the approach to therapy of active infections. Apart from the presumption that such doses were required for effective prophylaxis, there was a fear that lower doses would lead to the development of antibiotic resistance. The assumption that all organisms should be covered is now less favoured. Several studies have shown that infections by mixed flora can be lessened or prevented by targeting just one component of the bacterial population.

Although regimens may be recommended by national bodies local treatment policies may have to be altered on the basis of local incidence of resistant bacteria. Similarly, many regimens do not offer alternatives for patients with a history of anaphylaxis or urticaria immediately following penicillin therapy for whom β-lactams are contraindicated.

The timing of administration is one of the most important aspects of prophylaxis regimens. Animal studies and latterly clinical observational studies have shown that prophylaxis is most effective when given immediately before an operation (within 30 minutes of induction of anaesthesia), so that antibiotic activity is present for the duration of the operation and for about 4 hours afterwards (Classen et al 1992). Antibiotics given too early are associated with prophylaxis failure, presumably because of elimination of the drug before the end of wound contamination. Conversely, one study showed an increasing rate of wound infection for each hour that antibiotic administration was delayed after the start of the operation, suggesting that bacterial replication, once commenced, could no longer be eliminated by antibiotic regimens designed for prophylaxis. The microbiological basis for these observations is likely to be that bacterial reproduction at a logarithmic rate follows a lag phase of relatively little increase in bacterial population. The lag phase for wound infection bacteria lasts typically 3–4 hours. If bacteria inoculated into a wound can be killed or inhibited by antibiotics given early, the immune system has a relatively easier job moping up remaining organisms. If antibiotics are given only when the growth curve has entered the logarithmic phase, the chances of successful prophylaxis are reduced.

As a net result of this research, the duration of many prophylaxis regimens has been curtailed. Formerly protocols extended for several postoperative days. Now single-dose schedules are increasingly common. Greater emphasis is being placed on ensuring immediate preoperative administration. Since surgery may be delayed at short notice, sometimes between the time the patient leaves the ward and arrives at the theatre, it is sensible to take the responsibility for giving antibiotics away from ward staff and transfer it to the operating team, when prophylaxis can be given at induction of anaesthesia.

The adoption of short-course protocols obviates the need for dosage adjustment in patients with reduced ability to excrete the drug, usually due to renal failure, for it is unlikely that small numbers of doses will have significant dose-related adverse effects, and idiosyncratic reactions are dose independent. Although the half-life of many drugs used is relatively short (1–2 hours in normal volunteers), surgical patients often have slower clearance of antibiotics from the blood. However, additional doses may be needed when there is significant blood loss (>1500 mL) as plasma is effectively diluted by intraoperative transfusions and fluid replacement. Long operations may also need extra antibiotic doses during the operation but additional doses postoperatively do not provide an additional prophylactic benefit. Therefore any decision to continue must be explicit and supported by an evidence base.

Antibiotic administration by hospital theatre staff has practical implications for the route of administration. Ward-based prophylaxis could be given orally, if appropriate preparations exist, but this route is impractical in sedated or unconscious patients. The oral route tends to suffer from variable absorption, especially in the presence of anaesthetic premedication, and this also makes it unsatisfactory. The intravenous route is the most reliable way of ensuring effective plasma levels and is the only route supported by a substantial body of evidence.

Several protocols using local application of antibiotics have been tested. Although some of these approaches have been effective, they have generally been seen as unnecessarily complicated when compared with intravenous antibiotics. However, there remains a role for local antibiotic applications in specialties such as ophthalmic surgery where the addition of antibiotics to irrigation fluid is common practice. Preoperative antibiotic drops are used by some eye surgeons but the value of these is debatable.

Antibiotics have also been incorporated into foreign bodies implanted at surgery, including the cement used to secure joint prostheses. However, there has been concern that antibiotics leaching from the cement leave a surface that allows easier subsequent bacterial colonization. Some neurosurgeons advocate rinsing ventriculoperitoneal shunts in antibiotic solutions before insertion.

Once scientific principles and practical considerations have indicated a limited range of potentially useful regimens, the next step should be to compare them empirically against current best practice in the form of a randomized clinical trial. There are many pitfalls at this stage and criteria for judging antibiotic trials include the following:

- trials should be prospective, blinded and randomized with control groups
- selection and exclusion criteria for patients should be specified
- regimens should be clearly specified
- operative practices and procedures should be standardized as much as possible; this is especially important when more than one centre is involved
- the period of postoperative follow-up should be defined, and should be long enough to realistically detect most infections
- reasons for patient failure to complete the study protocol should be given; high exclusion and failure rates render a trial clinically unrealistic
- appropriate statistical analyses should be performed
- sufficient numbers of patients must be enrolled to avoid the appearance of a difference when none exists (type 1 error) or of no apparent difference when one does exist (type 2 error).

The greatest problem is recruiting a large enough number of similar patients to show a statistically meaningful difference. This is especially the case for surgical specialties with low wound infection rates, but is especially important when such infections have dire outcomes, for example meningitis in neurosurgery. Multicentre trials may be necessary to enrol large enough patient groups. Ideally, any conclusions should be applicable to similar patients undergoing treatment elsewhere, but this cannot be assumed.

An increasingly important complication in the application of clinical trial data is the risk of infection by multiple-resistant bacteria, e.g. meticillin-resistant *Staph. aureus* (MRSA). This is more likely when a patient has had a prolonged preoperative inpatient stay. Antibiotic prophylaxis protocols that were once effective may be invalidated by such developments.

A final hurdle is calculating the cost of prophylaxis and setting this against potential savings from prevented infection. Perhaps fortunately, postoperative infections are so expensive that nearly all clinically effective regimens are also financially effective.

Prophylaxis protocols in practice

This section describes a number of approaches to antibiotic prophylaxis in selected surgical specialties. A recurrent feature will be that there is often little objective evidence to show that prophylaxis is effective in many situations, and consequently there is often wide variation in the approach to prophylaxis. Two extremes can be discerned. One approach is to cover all possible bacteria by using broad-spectrum antibiotics, the other is a minimalist approach, which concentrates on a few key pathogens, for example *Staph. aureus*. It is often not certain which approach is best.

Gastrointestinal surgery

The medical management of peptic ulcer disease has led to a reduction in gastric and duodenal surgery for complications of ulcers. However, many operations are still performed for malignancies involving the oesophagus and stomach, and these are associated with an infection rate of nearly 20%. Contributing factors to this high rate include overgrowth of the stomach and oesophagus by Gram-negative bacteria and poor patient physical condition leading to immunosuppression. Anaerobic bacteria from the mouth may also contribute to infection. Consequently, first- and second-generation cephalosporins with or without metronidazole have been chosen to reduce infection rates. A single preoperative dose of ciprofloxacin has been compared with a single dose of cefuroxime and was shown to be as effective, even when the ciprofloxacin was given orally (Kogler et al 1989). Whether an oral route is useful or appropriate has been discussed already.

Small bowel surgery is uncommon but when it is necessary, the luminal flora often resemble large bowel conditions both in number and species, and so broad-spectrum cover with a second-generation cephalosporin and metronidazole is appropriate.

Biliary tract surgery (open) has infection rates of around 10%. Frequent causes of postoperative infections include enterococci and Enterobacteriaceae. Aminoglycosides have been frequently used as prophylaxis and their success, despite poor bile levels, indicates the importance of high tissue and blood antibiotic levels. Quinolones do reach high bile levels and have also been shown to give good protection against infections. Oral preparations make them useful for endoscopic manipulations of the biliary tract, but opiate premedication reduces bioavailability and so other premedications would need to be used. Antibiotic prophylaxis is not recommended for laparoscopic cholecystectomy.

Surgery for appendicitis has an overall wound infection rate of around 16% in the absence of prophylactic antibiotics. Antibiotics reduce infection rates when the appendix is gangrenous or perforated, but there is little difference between prophylaxis and no prophylaxis groups when the appendix is normal or mildly inflamed. Unfortunately, it is difficult to predict the severity of inflammation preoperatively and prophylaxis is recommended in all cases, especially in adults, who have higher postoperative infection rates than children Although prophylaxis against both aerobes and anaerobes is usual, using a first- or second-generation cephalosporin and metronidazole, there is evidence that a single preoperative dose of metronidazole alone is as effective as cefuroxime/metronidazole together, even in perforated appendicitis.

Colorectal surgery requires antibiotic prophylaxis beyond all doubt. However, there are many regimens in use. Several preoperative days of antibiotics given orally, for example parenteral aminoglycosides combined with oral erythromycin, tetracyclines and metronidazole, have been employed to reduce absolute bacterial numbers in the large bowel. These protocols expose the patient to antibiotics for a relatively long time and increase the risk of unwanted effects. Newer antibiotics allow single-agent parenteral prophylaxis, for example perioperative cefoxitin or co-amoxiclav, both of which have activity against meticillin-sensitive *Staph. aureus,* Enterobacteriaceae and bowel anaerobes. Combinations of metronidazole with amoxicillin, second generation cephalosporins such as cefuroxime, or aminoglycosides have all been used with some success. Cefuroxime and metronidazole has become a frequent combination, at least in the UK. More emphasis is now concentrated on appropriate timing of prophylaxis. Administration as the peritoneum is opened, so that

maximum tissue concentrations coincide with the period of maximum contamination, has been advocated, with top-up doses as dictated by the length of the operation. It should also be noted that laparoscopic or non-laparoscopic hernia repair without mesh insertion does not require antibiotic prophylaxis.

Minimally invasive surgery

Endoscopic techniques have dramatically changed approaches to general surgery. Many procedures, including cholecystectomies, appendicectomies and hernia repairs, can now be performed using laparoscopes. The minimal trauma associated with endoscopic surgery has led to faster postoperative recovery. Reduced tissue damage and smaller incisions also appear to reduce wound infection rates, although such figures may be biased by exclusion from laparoscopic surgery of patients with conditions that make such surgery difficult, for example peritoneal adhesions. Surgeons performing laparoscopic surgery must therefore reassess the need for prophylaxis. It is possible that antibiotic usage is no longer justified in at least some types of operations. Good-quality trials are urgently required in this area, so that the full benefits of this technique can be delivered.

Cardiac surgery

The most important thoracic infectious complications of cardiac surgery are endocarditis, mediastinitis and sternal wound infection. Sternal wound infection is a consequence of around 5% of cardiac operations and is frequently due to staphylococcal infection, both coagulase-negative staphylococci and *Staph. aureus.* Enterobacteriaceae have also been implicated in sternal infections. The severe consequences of sternal infections are sufficient incentive to use antibiotics prophylactically, and several trials of antibiotic regimens have shown them to be effective. Antibiotics are recommended for permanent pacemaker insertion, open heart surgery including coronary artery bypass grafting and prosthetic valve insertion. Cephalosporins including cefazolin and cefuroxime have been used to cover meticillin-sensitive staphylococci and Enterobacteriaceae. However, the increasing proportion of infections due to resistant coagulase-negative staphylococci and *Staph. aureus* in some hospitals has reduced the effectiveness of this class of antibiotics.

Consequently there has been a divergence of opinions in the approach to prophylaxis in this type of surgery, with some groups advocating broad antibiotic cover against Gram-positive organisms with glycopeptides such as teicoplanin, while others suggest using flucloxacillin either alone or with antibiotics such as aminoglycosides, which are active against Gram-negative organisms. Leg veins may be used to replace blocked coronary arteries and incisions made to harvest veins can also become infected, although these are generally prevented by the antibiotics chosen to prevent sternal infections

Urological surgery

The most important determinant of infectious complications of urological surgery is the presence or absence of bacteria in the urine. A level higher than 10^5 organisms/mL in a midstream specimen of urine is indicative of infection although lower amounts may be significant. Any bacteria in urine collected aseptically from the bladder, ureters or pelvis of the kidneys is abnormal and should be taken into account when considering prophylaxis. Common causes of infected urine are Enterobacteriaceae, especially *Escherichia coli*, and also enterococci and *Pseudomonas aeruginosa*. The last is frequent in patients who are catheterized and who have received antibiotics. Patients with abnormal structure or function of the urinary tract leading to residual urine post voiding are also at increased risk of Gram-negative urinary tract infections.

The great danger of operating on a urinary tract containing infected urine is bacteraemia leading to septic shock. This is especially dangerous when Gram-negative organisms are involved. Ideally, urine samples should be cultured a few days before a planned procedure so that appropriate antibiotics can be chosen. Such antibiotics should reach good blood and tissue levels, and it is an advantage if they are excreted renally. If preoperative culture is not possible, broad-spectrum antibiotics likely to be effective against all Gram-negative bacteria should be used, for example aminoglycosides or quinolones, possibly in conjunction with antibiotics such as amoxicillin, which is active against enterococci. In the absence of urine culture results, antibiotics are recommended for transrectal prostate biopsy, shock-wave lithotripsy and transurethral resection of the prostate but not transurethral resection of bladder tumours.

Obstetrics and gynaecology

Most births in developed countries are unaccompanied by significant infections, which is remarkable given the high levels of faecal organisms around the perineum. This was not always the case. Puerperal sepsis was a leading cause of death in women until the need for good hygiene practices was appreciated. However, there is no indication for routine antibiotic prophylaxis for either normal vaginal deliveries or forceps deliveries. If an episiotomy or tear extends to include the rectum then infection rates are increased and antibiotics need to be considered although there are no randomized controlled trials to support their routine use in this situation (Buppasiri et al 2005).

Infection rates following caesarean sections vary considerably depending on the population studied. Mothers with iron deficiency anaemia, from poor social backgrounds and those with obstetric complications are more likely to develop infections. Women having a caesarean section should be offered prophylactic antibiotics; a single dose of a first-generation cephalosporin or ampicillin, to reduce the risk of postoperative infection such as endometritis, urinary tract or wound infection, which occurs in about 8% of women, is recommended by the National Collaborating Centre for Women's and Children's Health (2004). It should also be noted that ampicillin is not reliably active against *Staph. aureus* and that in most trials antibiotic prophylaxis has been administered intravenously after clamping of the cord and not at induction of anaesthesia.

Gynaecological procedures are also subject to infection by the range of organisms detailed above. Infections can occur at the suture line of the vaginal cuff and extend into the tissues of the pelvis. An abdominal hysterectomy can additionally be complicated by skin incision infections. It is likely that wound infection rates are decreased by prophylaxis, and the antibiotics usually employed are indicated for both vaginal and abdominal hysterectomy and induced abortion.

Vascular surgery

Wound infection rates vary with body site. Surgery performed on vessels of the neck or upper limbs carries a low risk of infection and prophylaxis is usually not necessary. Operations involving groin incisions have the highest rate of infection and prophylaxis is indicated here as well as with abdominal and lower limb procedures. Organisms often involved are *Staph. aureus* and Enterobacteriaceae. However, the worst complication of postoperative infection in vascular surgery is infection of the implanted graft. Once grafts are infected they are almost impossible to sterilize with antibiotic therapy and often require removal. This may jeopardize the survival of the limb or the patient. Frequent causes of graft infections are coagulase-negative staphylococci and *Corynebacterium* spp. The antibiotic susceptibilities of these organisms are unpredictable. Other organisms such as the Enterobacteriaceae and enterococci are also likely to cause infections of grafts implanted through abdominal and groin incisions. The range of potential pathogens precludes the use of narrow-spectrum antibiotics and many regimens have been proposed. Aminoglycosides with antistaphylococcal penicillins, several cephalosporins, and penicillins combined with β-lactamase inhibitors have all been used. The optimum duration of prophylaxis is unclear. Courses lasting for up to 14 days have been given, but 24 hours of antibiotics is probably adequate. Amputations also require prophylaxis to be given.

Neurosurgery

Any postoperative infection of the central nervous system can have devastating consequences. Avoidance of infection in neurosurgery should therefore always be a high priority. Using microbiological principles, an appropriate antibiotic would be one which is active against the most common causes of neurosurgical infection, namely *Staph. aureus*, which accounts for half of all postoperative infections, coagulase-negative staphylococci (15%), streptococci (9%) and Gram-negative rods (16%). Unfortunately this is a wide range and if they are all to be countered, either a single broad-spectrum antibiotic or a combination of at least two antibiotics would be required. Some surgeons use vancomycin and an aminoglycoside such as gentamicin. However, there are concerns that broad-spectrum cover may promote antibiotic multiresistant bacteria. Additionally, both of these antibiotics penetrate the blood–brain barrier only poorly. At the other extreme, narrow-spectrum cover with benzylpenicillin, which penetrates the uninflamed blood–brain barrier poorly, or rifampicin has been used with apparent success. Intermediate alternatives, predominantly cephalosporins, have been suggested. The need for repeated intraoperative doses during operations of more than 3 hours duration has also been advocated (British Society for Antimicrobial Chemotherapy 1994).

Similar obstacles and considerations apply to the use of antibiotics in cerebrospinal fluid shunt implantation surgery. Recent reports indicate an infection rate of around 10%, although children less than 6 months old at the time of the operation have a higher rate than older children (15.7% versus 5.6% in one report). Approximately 70% of shunt infections present within 2 months of surgery, indicating that the causative organisms are introduced into the cerebrospinal fluid at the time of operation. Half of the infections are due to coagulase-negative staphylococci, the remainder are predominantly caused by enterococci, *Staph. aureus* and Enterobacteriaceae. Less common causes are *Pseudomonas* spp. and *Candida* spp. Again, there is no consensus as to appropriate regimens. It has been suggested that gentamicin and vancomycin should be instilled into the ventricles during the operation (British Society for Antimicrobial Chemotherapy 1995). This approach would presumably not reduce contamination of that part of the wound outside the brain, and perhaps should be supplemented by a single, immediately preoperative dose of gentamicin and/or vancomycin, although intravenous cephalosporins could also be used as an alternative.

Several studies have emphasized the importance of surgical technique in reducing shunt infection rates. A French study presented a protocol that considered preoperative preparation, intraoperative precautions and postoperative care (Choux et al 1992). When this protocol was implemented, the infection rate dropped from 7.75 to 0.17%. Although this study was unable to define the relative values of the various elements of their protocol, it is clear that antibiotic prophylaxis is only part of the approach to reducing the incidence of shunt infections.

Orthopaedic surgery

Fractures

Open fractures, those where a break in the bone is accompanied by a skin wound, are associated with an infection rate that is proportional to the extent of soft tissue damage. Fractures with little soft tissue injury and a small wound less than 1 cm long have infection rates of less than 10%. When skin is missing or badly torn, or when there is extensive vascular damage and muscle injury that makes it difficult to cover the fracture, infection rates can be as high as 55%. Fixation of the fractures has been associated with increased infection rates when compared to those fractures not requiring fixation, although this may reflect the severity of the injury and may not be an independent risk factor.

Despite high infection rates in severe injuries, the lack of well-conducted prospective trials of prophylaxis means that their efficacy remains uncertain. However, there is increasing evidence that antibiotics active against *Staph. aureus* reduce the rate of wound infection. The additional presence of coliforms and anaerobes in extensively damaged wounds would suggest that patients with such injuries should receive broader spectrum antibiotics, but there is little trial evidence to support this.

When soft tissue coverage of the fracture is difficult there is a likelihood that the wound will become infected with hospital environment flora, which may be antibiotic resistant. Broadspectrum antibiotics may hasten this. When prophylaxis is given there is a tendency for it to be continued for up to 10 days. Where duration of prophylaxis has been studied, 24 hours' duration has been as effective as 5 days.

Fractures that remain closed at the time of injury may be opened in the operating theatre to allow fixation, placement of prosthetic devices or osteosynthesis. Because the wound is made in a controlled, aseptic fashion the infection rate is low, usually below 10%. However, good evidence has accumulated that supports the role of prophylaxis in such surgery. A single preoperative dose of ceftriaxone has been shown to significantly reduce the rate of both wound infections and other types of nosocomial infections, including respiratory and urinary tract infections.

Joint replacement surgery

Elective hip and knee prosthesis surgery is now a major part of orthopaedic surgery. One of the most serious and common complications is infection of the bone and soft tissue surrounding the implant. This can result from intraoperative contamination, which accounts for early infections, and haematogenous seeding, which can occur years later. Early infections can be significantly reduced by the ultrafiltration of operating theatre air, laminar air-flow ventilation, whole-body exhaust suits and strict theatre discipline to reduce movement in the theatre to the absolute minimum. Antibiotics also appear to reduce infection rates. It is not clear whether theatre effects and antibiotics are independent, and so cumulative when combined, or whether the use of one makes the other redundant.

The cause of early infection is usually *Staph. aureus* and any prophylaxis should be active against this organism. Short courses of antibiotics lasting for 12–24 hours seem to be as effective as courses lasting 7 or 14 days. An optimal approach would be to combine ultra-clean air theatres and short courses of antibiotics, for example flucloxacillin. An alternative, or additional, approach to chemoprophylaxis is to incorporate antibiotics, for example gentamicin or cefuroxime, in the bone cement. The limited available data do not suggest a clear role for routine prophylaxis in elective joint replacement surgery.

Late infections are predominantly caused by coagulase-negative staphylococci, which are usually assumed to infect the joint following haematogenous spread. Other bacterial species can also cause late infections, so it is important that patients with prosthetic joints receive prompt appropriate treatment for infections at any site. Currently there is little else that can be done to avoid late infections. In particular, risk–benefit analyses show that patients with joint prostheses undergoing dental treatment should not be given prophylactic antibiotics.

Oral and maxillofacial surgery

The oral cavity is heavily colonized with aerobic α-haemolytic streptococci, anaerobic streptococci and anaerobic Gram-negative rods. Nevertheless, minor oral surgery, including most dentoalveolar surgery, has an infection rate of less than 1% and wound infection prophylaxis in healthy individuals is not indicated. However, endocarditis prophylaxis may be indicated. More invasive and extensive surgery has a higher infection rate, about 10–15%, and penicillin has been advocated as a suitable agent for prophylaxis when the transoral approach is used. When the incision involves the skin, either alone or in combination with an oral mucosa incision, staphylococcal infections are more likely and flucloxacillin could be added. In prolonged surgery additional antibiotic doses should be administered but there is no evidence to support prolonged postoperative courses of prophylaxis. In general, prophylaxis is recommended for contaminated/clean-contaminated head and neck surgery but not clean procedures, nose or sinus surgery or tonsillectomy.

Hand surgery

An investigation of infection rates following a wide range of hand surgical procedures revealed overall rates of 10.7% in elective operations and 9.7% in emergency operations. Further analysis showed that elective surgery patients who had received prophylactic antibiotics did not have a significantly lower wound infection rate compared with the no prophylaxis elective surgery patients. However, patients undergoing emergency surgery were at greater risk of wound infection if they were not given antibiotics prophylactically compared with emergency patients receiving antibiotics. Emergency procedures were 13.4 times more likely to become infected if the original trauma had left significant contamination, crush injuries or devascularization of tissues. *Staph. aureus* was the organism most frequently isolated from infected wounds.

Wound infections following hand surgery can have grave effects on subsequent recovery of dexterity, and it is legitimate to use prophylaxis in these situations even to achieve a small benefit. Appropriate circumstances have included elective or emergency surgery involving percutaneous K-wires, joint prostheses and operations of 2 hours or more duration, and all emergency hand surgery on dirty wounds, open fractures or where a delay of 6 hours or more has occurred between trauma and surgery. It is possible that patients with systemic disease, such as diabetes, or local disease, including rheumatoid arthritis or eczema, would benefit from prophylactic antibiotics for all types of hand surgery.

Appropriate antibiotics are flucloxacillin, or clindamycin if penicillin allergic, given before tourniquet inflation (tourniquets are used to reduce bleeding that would otherwise obscure the surgical site). One dose should be adequate for elective surgery.

It may be justifiable to give treatment for 48 hours or longer if the wound is grossly contaminated, and in these circumstances there is the possibility of infection due to anaerobic organisms, especially if a bite or similar wound. In this event infection could be prevented by adding metronidazole or by using co-amoxiclav as a single agent.

Improving antibiotic prophylaxis

Errors in prescribing and administering antimicrobial prophylaxis for surgery are one of the most frequent medication errors in hospitals (Burke 2001). Optimal use including case selection, agent used, dose, route of administration, timing and duration should be audited. Results of these audits need to be fed back to the whole surgical unit as appropriate use of antimicobial prophylaxis may involve several disciplines (pharmacists, nurses, anaesthetists, operating department assistants) and not just the prescriber. As well as assessing the process of administration of antibiotic(s), other objective measures such as surgical site infection rate or other adverse outcomes such as *C. difficile* infection should be measured. Computer-based expert systems may improve prescribing. In one study its use was associated with an improvement in the timeliness of prophylaxis and a shortening in prophylaxis duration. Measures to improve compliance include educational interventions and use of pre-printed stickers (Ritchie et al 2004).

Alternative approaches

Despite optimal antibiotic prophylaxis, surgical wound infections still occur and alternative strategies have been developed. Warming patients using either a forced-air warming blanket or a non-contact radiant heat dressing has been shown to reduce infection rates in clean surgery (Melling et al 2001).

Table 39.6 Common therapeutic problems in surgical antibiotic prophylaxis

Problem	Background	Management
Antibiotic given too soon	An adequate concentration of antibiotic is required at the site of the operation to be effective	Most surgical prophylaxis is given at induction of anaesthesia
Antibiotics continued for prolonged periods after the operation	This increases hospital costs, promotes the emergence of resistant bacteria and may cause complications such as *Clostridium difficile* infection	Antibiotic prophylaxis should be prescribed for a fixed duration. Administration of antibiotics should be audited
Operations involving insertion of prosthetic material	All implants have a detrimental effect on host defences and a lower bacterial inoculum is required to initiate infection	Rigorous adherence to antibiotic prophylaxis
Repeated surgical explorations	Patients exposed to antibiotics may have a bacterial flora that is resistant to the standard antibiotic prophylaxis regimens	Generally a more broad-spectrum agent is used but the choice depends on the nature of the operation and knowledge of current local resistance patterns
Patient gives clear history of allergy to β-lactam antibiotics	Unable to use commonly prescribed regimens due to risk of anaphylaxis to penicillins and cephalopsorins	Choice of agent will depend on type of surgery, clindamycin, aminoglycosides, glycopetides or fluoroquinolnes may be used.

CASE STUDIES

Case 39.1

A patient who is due to undergo coronary artery bypass grafting is found to be colonized with meticillin-sensitive *Staphylococcus aureus* (MSSA). Routine nose and throat swabs are taken at the preadmission clinic to determine the appropriate prophylactic regimen. Standard antibiotic prophylaxis on the unit is normally intravenous cefuroxime.

Question

Should any modifications be made to the prophylaxis protocol employed?

Answer

No, both flucloxacillin and cefuroxime are active against MSSA. Patients undergoing coronary artery bypass grafting are at risk of surgical site infection due to *Staph. aureus* carried on the patient's skin. Many units screen patients for the carriage of MRSA for infection control purposes; the presence of resistant bacteria needs to be considered when deciding on the most appropriate antibiotic prophylaxis. If this patient were colonized with MRSA then vancomycin or teicoplanin would be appropriate agents to use. All patients should receive prophylaxis for this surgery.

Case 39.2

A negative urine culture result is recorded for a patient with a prosthetic heart valve admitted for a transurethral resection of the prostate. The hospital protocol states that antibiotic prophylaxis is not recommended in this situation as the urine is sterile and, therefore, there is little risk of infection.

Question

Should this patient receive antibiotic prophylaxis?

Answer

Although the urine is sterile and there is little risk of infection arising from the genitourinary tract, if an infection were to arise it could have serious consequences for the patient. For example, it is possible for organisms from the urinary tract to spread through the bloodstream to the prosthetic valve and precipitate endocarditis. Therefore, although the patient does not meet the definition of someone requiring prophylaxis, he has an additional risk factor and therefore prophylaxis is indicated. Intravenous amoxicillin and gentamicin should be given at induction; vancomycin or teicoplanin and gentamicin may be given if the patient is penicillin allergic. Infection of the prosthetic valve with *Enterococcus* spp. is of particular concern. Coliforms are rarely implicated in endocarditis. Finally, some endocarditis prophylaxis regimens include clindamycin but this antibiotic is poorly active against enterococci and should not be used in this situation.

Case 39.3

A patient known to be colonized with glycopeptide-resistant enterococci (GRE) is to undergo a liver transplant. Standard antibiotic prophylaxis on the unit is amoxicillin, cefuroxime and metronidazole.

Question

Should any modification be made to the standard antibiotic prophylaxis?

Answer

This is a difficult question to answer. The glycopeptide-resistant enterococcus may well be resistant to amoxicillin (enterococci are intrinsically resistant to cephalosporins) and therefore the regimen chosen would not cover the colonizing gut flora of the patient. A significant postoperative infection due to glycopeptide-resistant enterococci would be difficult to treat and if an intra-abdominal abscess developed, surgical drainage would be required too. Although there is a concern that these isolates may become more resistant if antibiotic chemoprophylaxis is used inappropriately, on the balance of risks an appropriate antibiotic such as synercid or linezolid should be used, in conjunction with appropriate Gram-negative cover, for this liver transplant.

Case 39.4

You discover that a hospital surgeon routinely gives all his patients gentamicin for 24 hours before theatre to ensure that adequate tissue levels are achieved.

Question

Is this appropriate prophylaxis?

Answer

No, the pharmacokinetics of gentamicin mean that the peak plasma concentration is reached 30–120 minutes after an intramuscular injection or 20–30 minutes after an intravenous infusion. Therefore a regimen such as this may not guarantee that peak levels are achieved at the time of surgery. Prolonged administration of antibiotic prior to surgery is not recommended as it may select out resistant bacteria that may make treatment of any postoperative infection more difficult. The risk of nephro- and ototoxicty associated with aminoglycoside therapy is related to treatment duration and this protocol results in unnecessary prolonging of the preoperative duration of antibiotics. Finally, if for whatever reason the surgery is postponed or cancelled then the patient has been unnecessarily exposed to an antibiotic.

Case 39.5

Mr B is a neurosurgical patient who has been given cefuroxime for 6 days postoperatively because he has an external ventricular drain in place.

Question

Is such treatment part of standard antibiotic prophylaxis? Are there any adverse consequences of this regimen?

Answer

Most surgical antibiotic prophylaxis is given perioperatively. However, because of Mr B's external ventricular drain the antibiotic has to be continued. Although cefuroxime is used in this context to prevent infection, it has been suggested that there is no reduction in infection rates (Alleyne et al 2000). Prolonged administration of antibiotics results in an alteration of host microbial flora; bacteria that are resistant to cefuroxime are selected out (such as MRSA or *P. aeruginosa*). Therefore, if the patient's external ventricular drain becomes infected or he develops a hospital-acquired pneumonia it is likely to be due to a more resistant organism. Widespread use of antibiotics in this manner is costly and contributes to the emergence of resistant organisms within hospitals. The patient may also develop complications of antibiotic use such as *C. difficile* infection.

Case 39.6

A patient with an infected prosthetic knee joint is having the joint replaced.

Question

Is it appropriate to use standard antibiotic prophylaxis for this procedure?

Answer

No, the standard (short course) of antibiotics is not appropriate as the surgeon is operating on an infected joint; therefore a therapeutic course of antibiotics is required. Often in this situation, a two-stage procedure is performed where the infected joint is removed, a 6-week course of antibiotics is given (based on relevant microbiology results), and then a new prosthetic joint inserted at the end of 6 weeks as long as there is a good clinical response.

REFERENCES

Alleyne C H, Hassan M, Zabramski J M 2000 The efficacy and cost of prophylactic and periprocedural antibiotics in patients with external ventricular drains. Neurosurgery 5: 1124-1129

Bratzler D W, Houck P M for the Surgical Infection Prevention Guidelines Writers Workgroup 2004 Antimicrobial prophylaxis for surgery: an advisory statement from the National Surgical Infection Prevention Project. Clinical Infectious Diseases 38: 1706-1715

British Society for Antimicrobial Chemotherapy 1994 Report of Infections in Neurosurgery Working Party: antimicrobial prophylaxis in neurosurgery and after head injury. Lancet 344: 1547-1551

British Society for Antimicrobial Chemotherapy 1995 Report of a working party on the use of antibiotics in neurosurgery: treatment of infections associated with shunting for hydrocephalus. British Journal of Hospital Medicine 53: 368-373

Buppasiri P, Lumbiganon P, Thinkhamrop J et al 2005 Antibiotic prophylaxis for fourth-degree perineal tear during vaginal birth. Cochrane Database of Systematic Reviews. Available online at: www.mrw. interscience.wiley.com/cochrane/clsysrev/articles/CD005125/frame.html

Burke J P 2001 Maximizing appropriate antibiotic prophylaxis for surgical patients: an update from LDS hospital, Salt Lake City. Clinical Infectious Diseases 33 (suppl 2): S78-S83

Choux M, Genitori L, Lang D et al 1992 Shunt implantation: reducing the incidence of shunt infection. Journal of Neurosurgery 77: 875-880

Classen D C, Evans R S, Pestotnik S L et al 1992 The timing of prophylactic administration of antibiotics and the risk of surgical-wound infection. New England Journal of Medicine 326: 281-286

Coello R, Charlett A, Wilson J et al 2005 Adverse impact of surgical site infections in English hospitals. Journal of Hospital Infection 60: 93-103

Dellinger E P, Gross P A, Barrett T L et al 1994 Quality standard for antimicrobial prophylaxis in surgical procedures. Clinical Infectious Diseases 18: 422-427

Fry D E 1988 Antibiotics in surgery: an overview. American Journal of Surgery 155(5A): 11-15

Gaynes R P, Culver D H, Horan T C et al and the National Nosocomial Infections Surveillance System 2001 Surgical site infection (SSI) rates in the United States, 1992–1998: The National Nosocomial Infections Surveillance System basic SSI risk index. Clinical Infectious Diseases 33 (suppl 2): S69-S77

Horan T C, Gaynes R P, Martone W J et al 1992 CDC definitions for nosocomial surgical site infections, 1992: a modification of CDC definitions of surgical wound infections. Infection Control and Hospital Epidemiology 13: 606-608

Kogler J, Hancke E, Marklein G et al 1989 Ciprofloxacin for single shot prophylaxis during cholecystectomy. Infection 17: 174-175

Managram A J, Horan T C, Pearson M L et al 1999 Guideline for prevention of surgical site infection, 1999. Hospital Infection Control Practices Advisory Committee. Infection Control and Hospital Epidemiology 20: 247-278

Melling A C, Ali B, Scott E M et al 2001 Effect of preoperative warming on the incidence of wound infection after clean surgery: a randomized controlled trial. Lancet 358: 876-880

National Collaborating Centre for Women's and Children's Health 2004 Caesarean section. NICE Clinical Guideline 13.Available online at: www. rcog.org.uk/resources/public/ pdf/cs_summary_of_guideline.pdf

Pepin J, Saheb N, Coulombe M A et al 2005 Emergence of fluoroquinolones as the predominant risk factor for Clostridium-difficile-associated diarrhoea: a cohort study during an epidemic in Quebec. Clinical Infectious Diseases 41: 1254-1260

Ritchie S, Scanlon N, Lewis M et al 2004 Use of a preprinted sticker to improve the prescribing of prophylactic antibiotics for hip fracture surgery. Quality and Safety in Health Care 13: 384-387

FURTHER READING

Gould F K, Elliott T S, Foweraker J et al 2006 Guidelines for the prevention of endocarditis: report of the Working Party of the British Society for Antimicrobial Chemotherapy. Journal of Antimicrobial Chemotherapy 57: 1035-1042

Groselj Grenc M, Derganc M, Trsinar B et al 2006 Antibiotic prophylaxis for surgical procedures on children. Journal of Chemotherapy 18: 38-42

Martone W J, Nicholls R L 2001 Recognition, prevention, surveillance and management of surgical site infections. Clinical Infectious Diseases 33 (suppl 2): S67-106

Schaeffer E M 2006 Prophylactic use of antimicrobials in commonly performed outpatient urologic procedures. Nature Clinical Practice Urology 3: 24-31

Scottish Intercollegiate Guidelines Network 2000 (reviewed 2006) Antibiotic prophylaxis in surgery. Scottish Intercollegiate Guidelines Network, Edinburgh. Available online at: www.sign.ac.uk

Swedish-Norwegian Consensus Group 1998 Antibiotic prophylaxis in surgery: summary of a Swedish-Norwegian consensus conference. Scandinavian Journal of Infectious Diseases 30(6): 547-557

Trampuz A, Zimmerli W 2006 Antimicrobial agents in orthopaedic surgery: prophylaxis and treatment. Drugs 66: 1089-1105

Tuberculosis 40

L. K. Nehaul

Tuberculosis (TB) is an important public health problem worldwide. An increase in reported cases of tuberculosis in countries across all continents led the World Health Organization (WHO) to declare tuberculosis a global emergency in 1993.

Of additional concern has been the increase in multidrug-resistant tuberculosis, with outbreaks in different parts of the world. This has been attributed to both human immunodeficiency virus (HIV) infection and inappropriate or inadequate treatment.

The increase in tuberculosis in the UK, since the late 1980s, has affected principally the larger conurbations in England. A TB Action Plan for England was published in 2004 and sets out key actions for bringing tuberculosis under control.

Adequate and effective treatment is essential, both clinically for patients and to control the spread of tuberculosis. The success of this depends on a close working collaboration between clinical, microbiological, infection control and public health teams in managing patients and their contacts, and a shared understanding with primary care teams as to the role of all health professionals involved in tuberculosis.

Guidance for the diagnosis and clinical management of tuberculosis and measures for its prevention and control have been published (NICE 2006), replacing that of the British Thoracic Society (2000).

Epidemiology

Tuberculosis causes about 2 million deaths worldwide each year, and one-third of the world's population is infected with the tubercle bacillus. It is becoming the leading cause of death among HIV-positive people.

Globally over 4 million cases of tuberculosis disease are notified annually although the estimated number of new cases is put at 9 million. The majority of cases occur in poor countries in the southern hemisphere but TB is re-emerging in Eastern Europe, which experiences over a quarter of a million cases each year.

The numbers of cases reported, and estimated to have occurred, in 2004, globally and by WHO region, are presented in Table 40.1.

In the UK, there have been changes in the epidemiology of tuberculosis since the late 1980s. Following a decrease in notifications over decades, cases of tuberculosis started to increase again from the late 1980s. A total of 6837 cases were reported to the Enhanced Tuberculosis Surveillance system in England, Wales and Northern Ireland in 2003 (Tuberculosis Section, Health Protection Agency Centre for Infection 2005). The overall rate across all population groups was 12.5 per 100 000 population. Of all cases, 45% occurred in the London region, where the rate was 41.3 per 100 000 population. Rates of tuberculosis outside London varied between 3.3 per 100 000 (Northern Ireland) and 15.2 per 100 000 (West Midlands). Of these cases, 70% were born abroad. The tuberculosis rate was higher in those born abroad than among those born in the UK (90.1 compared with 3.8 per 100 000). This reflected higher rates of tuberculosis in people from high-incidence countries, mainly South-East Asia. The risk of tuberculosis is highest in the 5 years after arrival in the UK. Tuberculosis can also occur as a travel-related disease in UK residents from high-incidence countries, who return to visit their country of birth and are exposed to tuberculosis there. The numbers of cases, by region, in England, Wales and Northern Ireland, in 2003, are shown in Table 40.2.

Table 40.1 Case notifications and rates, and estimated cases of tuberculosis and incidence rates by WHO region 2004 (Source: WHO)

WHO region	Case notifications 2004	Case notification rates per 100 000 population 2004	Estimated number of new cases 2004	Estimated incidence rate per 100 000 population 2004
Africa	1 105 952	153	2 572 988	356
Americas	221 358	25	363 246	41
Eastern Mediterranean	235 797	45	644 531	122
Europe	290 772	33	444 777	50
South-East Asia	1 609 891	99	2 967 328	182
Western Pacific	1 061 520	61	1 925 332	111
Global	4 525 290	71	8 918 203	140

Table 40.2 Tuberculosis case reports and rates by UK region/country, England, Wales and Northern Ireland, 2003

UK region/country	Number of cases	Rate per 100 000 population
London	3049	41.3
West Midlands	810	15.2
North West	592	8.7
Yorkshire and the Humber	547	10.9
East Midlands	475	11.2
South East	455	5.6
East of England	328	6.0
South West	205	4.1
North East	147	5.8
Wales	172	5.9
Northern Ireland	57	3.3

Source: Tuberculosis Section, Health Protection Agency Centre for Infections, Enhanced Tuberculosis Surveillance MycobNet (Mycobacterial Surveillance Network)

Aetiology

Tuberculosis infection is caused by tubercle bacilli, which belong to the genus *Mycobacterium*. These form a large group but only three relatives are obligate parasites that can cause tuberculosis disease. They are part of the *Mycobacterium tuberculosis* complex and include *M. tuberculosis, M. bovis* and *M. africanum*. However, generally only the first two are found in isolates from people with tuberculosis diagnosed in the UK, with *M. tuberculosis* accounting for over 98% of isolates.

The vast majority of the other members of the genus *Mycobacterium* are saprophytes and have been found in soil, milk and water. They are often referred to as atypical or mycobacteria other than tuberculosis (MOTT). Only about 15 are recognized as pathogenic to humans and some cause pulmonary disease resembling tuberculosis. Public health action is not required for infections caused by atypical mycobacteria, as there is no evidence of person-to-person transmission.

Infection with tubercle bacilli occurs in the vast majority of cases by the respiratory route. The lung lesions caused by infection commonly heal, leaving no residual changes except occasional pulmonary or tracheobronchial lymph node calcification (Heymann 2004). About 5% of those initially infected will develop active primary disease (Begg et al 2005). This can include pulmonary disease, through local progression in the lungs, or by lymphatic or haematogenous spread of bacilli, to pulmonary, meningeal or other extrapulmonary involvement, or lead to disseminated disease (miliary TB). In the other 95%, the primary lesion heals without intervention but in at least one half of patients, the bacilli survive in a latent form, which may then reactivate later in life. Infants, adolescents and immunosuppressed people are more susceptible to the more serious forms of tuberculosis such as miliary or meningeal tuberculosis.

Pulmonary (respiratory) tuberculosis is more common than extrapulmonary (non-respiratory) tuberculosis, accounting for about 70% of cases in the UK. Sites of extrapulmonary tuberculosis can include the pleura, lymph nodes, pericardium, kidneys, meninges, bones and joints, larynx, skin, intestines, peritoneum and eyes. In practice, in the UK the lymph nodes are the most common site for extrapulmonary disease.

Progressive pulmonary tuberculosis arises from exogenous reinfection or endogenous reactivation of a latent focus remaining from the initial infection. If untreated, about 65% of patients will die within 5 years, the majority of these within 2 years. Completion of chemotherapy using drugs to which the tubercle bacilli are sensitive almost always results in a cure, even with HIV infection (Heymann 2004).

Symptoms include fatigue, fever, night sweats and weight loss, which may occur early, while localizing symptoms of cough, chest pain, haemoptysis and hoarseness become prominent in the later stages.

Abnormal chest radiographs with pulmonary infiltration, cavitation and fibrosis can occur before clinical manifestations.

Transmission

Transmission occurs through exposure to tubercle bacilli in airborne droplet nuclei produced by people with pulmonary or respiratory tract tuberculosis during expiratory efforts such as coughing or sneezing. Laryngeal tuberculosis is highly contagious, but rarely seen in the UK.

Most infections are acquired from adults with post-primary pulmonary tuberculosis. Between 90% and 95% of cases of tuberculosis in children are non-infectious (Davies 2003). Tuberculosis cannot be acquired from individuals with latent TB infection.

Incubation period

The incubation period from infection to demonstrable primary lesion or significant tuberculin reaction ranges from 2 to 10 weeks. Latent infection may persist for a lifetime. HIV infection appears to shorten the interval for the development of clinically apparent tuberculosis.

Infectious forms of tuberculosis

Patients should be considered infectious if they have sputum smear-positive pulmonary disease (that is, where they produce sputum containing sufficient tubercle bacilli to be seen on direct sputum examination) or laryngeal tuberculosis. Patients with smear-negative pulmonary disease (three sputum samples) are less infectious than those who are smear positive. The relative transmission rate from smear-negative compared with smear-positive patients has been estimated to be 0.22 (British Thoracic Society 2000).

Risk groups

Certain groups are at increased risk of latent TB infection, and possibly tuberculosis disease if exposed. These include:

- close contacts of patients with tuberculosis, especially those with sputum smear-positive pulmonary disease
- casual contacts (e.g. work colleagues) if they are immunosuppressed
- people from countries with a high incidence of tuberculosis (40/100 000 population or greater).

People with certain medical conditions are at increased risk of developing active tuberculosis if they have latent TB infection. These medical risk factors are set out in Table 40.3.

Impact of HIV infection

People with HIV infection have an increased risk of developing tuberculosis if exposed to infection. The estimated annual risk

Table 40.3 Groups at increased risk of developing active tuberculosis if infected

HIV positive
Injecting drug users
Have had solid organ transplantation, jejunoileal bypass or gastrectomy
Have a haematological malignancy, e.g. leukaemia and lymphomas
Have chronic renal failure or are receiving haemodialysis
Are receiving anti-TNF-α treatment
Have silicosis

Source: NICE: Tuberculosis, Quick Reference Guide

of tuberculosis in those with HIV infection and tuberculosis co-infection is 2–13% as opposed to a 10% lifetime chance in someone infected with tuberculosis, but not HIV.

Most cases of tuberculosis in patients with HIV infection are likely to result from the reactivation of previously acquired infection, but reinfection may be important in populations with a high prevalence of tuberculosis.

Diagnosis

An essential step in the early diagnosis of tuberculosis is awareness of the possibility of tuberculosis in people presenting with lower respiratory tract symptoms, e.g chronic cough or 'chest infections' not responding to antibiotics. This is particularly important for individuals at higher risk, e.g. those from high incidence countries, or contacts of respiratory tuberculosis. Early diagnosis, especially of pulmonary tuberculosis, followed by prompt commencement of treatment can reduce the period of infectivity to other people, especially susceptible contacts, who might be at risk of the more serious forms of tuberculosis disease. Awareness of the possibility of tuberculosis at the earliest possible stage after admission to hospital of people from higher risk groups with lower respiratory tract symptoms is also important. Placement of patients with respiratory tuberculosis, especially those with potential drug-resistant disease, in appropriate facilities and strict attention to infection control procedures will prevent transmission of infection to other vulnerable groups, in particular immunosuppressed individuals.

The preliminary diagnosis of tuberculosis disease is based on the symptoms and signs in the patient, in conjunction with microscopy of sputum (for acid-fast bacilli) followed by culture, chest radiography and tuberculin skin testing.

Notification of tuberculosis

Tuberculosis disease is a statutorily notifiable communicable disease in the UK. Cases should be notified on clinical suspicion to the 'Proper Officer' for communicable disease control of the local authority where the patient resides. This is usually the local Consultant in Communicable Disease Control. Notification enables public health action to be initiated; that is, the investigation of individuals who might be at risk of infection, mainly household contacts. It may also enable the source of the infection to be found and treated. Latent TB infection is not notifiable.

Investigations

Investigations are essential for confirming a clinical diagnosis of tuberculosis. Microbiological tests are crucial, especially for pulmonary disease, as they facilitate both the clinical and public health management of tuberculosis and ensure the appropriate implementation of infection control procedures for cases managed in healthcare settings.

Microbiological investigations

Microbiological investigations are necessary to assess the infectious state of the patient, and distinguish between infection with mycobacteria causing tuberculosis and other mycobacteria. They also determine the drug susceptibility patterns of the infecting organisms, to ensure that the drugs prescribed will be effective in treating the individual patient. They comprise microscopy, culture, drug susceptibility testing, and strain typing.

Direct microscopy of sputum using the Ziehl–Neelsen or other fluorescent stain is the simplest and quickest method of detecting the infectious patient, by looking for acid-fast bacilli. A minimum of three sputum samples, one of which should be early morning, should be collected from patients with suspected respiratory tuberculosis.

Direct microscopy is not as useful in non-pulmonary disease as the diagnosis depends more on culture.

If conventional culture methods are used, such as the Lowenstein–Jensen medium, growth may take up to 6 weeks. However, modern liquid cultures can produce results in 1–2 weeks. Bacteria of the *M. tuberculosis* complex and atypical mycobacteria can be distinguished by gene probe. This facilitates the clinical and public health management of tuberculosis, especially for potentially infectious tuberculosis cases in schools and other institutions. Commercial polymerase chain reaction (PCR) based tests can also detect *M. tuberculosis* complex in clinical specimens. A rapid test is available for assessing rifampicin resistance in individuals thought to have drug-resistant tuberculosis. A 'positive' result indicates the need to assess susceptibility to other first-line anti-tuberculosis drugs.

DNA fingerprinting is useful in determining whether cases might be linked, i.e. to distinguish between sporadic cases and clusters/outbreaks. It also helps to detect cross-contamination in laboratories. A new method, mycobacterial interspersed repetitive unit/variable number of tandem repeats (MIRU/VNTR) typing, has recently been introduced for routine use in the UK. It is available in regional centres for mycobacteriology, where specialist microbiological tuberculosis tests are routinely undertaken.

Two new blood-based immunological tests, T-spot TB and Quantiferon, have been introduced in a limited number of UK centres. These tests can distinguish between tuberculosis infection and previous BCG vaccination. The NICE tuberculosis

guideline recommends criteria for their use. Their usefulness in the diagnosis and control of tuberculosis is yet to be fully assessed.

Tuberculin testing

Tuberculin testing is used to detect latent tuberculosis infection. The Heaf (multiple puncture) test is no longer available in the UK. However, the Mantoux test is used but should only be undertaken by someone trained and experienced in its use. The standard Mantoux test in the UK consists of an intradermal injection of 2TU of Statens Serum Institute (SSI) tuberculin RT23 in 0.1 mL solution for injection. In this test 0.1 mL of the appropriate solution is injected intradermally so that a bleb of at least 6 mm is produced. The results should be read 48–72 hours later. A positive result consists of induration with a transverse diameter of at least 6 mm.

The interpretation of the test will depend on the clinical circumstances, including a past history of tuberculosis or exposure to tuberculosis. In the absence of specific risk factors for tuberculosis, a reaction of between 6 and 15 mm is more likely to be due to BCG vaccination or infection with environmental mycobacteria, but does not rule out the possibility of latent TB infection. An induration of more than 15 mm is unlikely to be due to BCG vaccination or exposure to environmental bacteria. Details can be found on the UK immunization website (www.immunisation.nhs.uk).

Chest radiography

The earliest change is the appearance of an ill-defined opacity or opacities, usually seen in one of the upper lung lobes. In the more advanced stages of the disease, the opacities are larger and more widespread and may be bilateral. Occasionally there is extensive patchy shadowing involving the whole lobe. An area or areas of translucency within the opacities indicates cavitation. The presence of cavitation in an untreated case usually indicates that disease is active.

Radiological changes of a pleural effusion or pneumothorax may also be seen.

Diagnosis of tuberculosis in people with HIV

Tuberculosis can occur early in the course of HIV infection and may therefore be diagnosed before the patient is known to be HIV positive. The possibility of HIV infection in people with tuberculosis should therefore be considered and testing for the virus should be undertaken after appropriate counselling in those with risk factors for HIV. In the USA, tuberculin testing is recommended for patients with newly diagnosed HIV. Chemoprophylaxis is recommended for those who have a positive tuberculin reaction.

Early in the course of HIV disease, before serious immunodeficiency occurs, tuberculosis usually presents with upper zone changes on chest radiography, with or without cavitation, and the tuberculin test is usually positive. Acid-fast bacilli may also be seen on microscopy.

As the immunodeficiency state worsens, the presentation of tuberculosis can become increasingly non-specific and atypical.

Acid-fast bacilli are rarely seen on sputum microscopy and mycobacterial culture is often negative. Chest radiographs may be unusual, with lower zone changes and diffuse or miliary shadowing; cavitation is seen less often.

One of the key features of tuberculosis in patients with HIV infection is the tendency to extrapulmonary disease, usually with pulmonary involvement.

Patients may appear relatively well for the degree of abnormality shown on radiography, but if the shadowing is not felt to be associated with non-mycobacterial infections or Kaposi's sarcoma, then anti-tuberculous treatment may have to be started empirically pending results of the cultures, and the clinical process monitored.

Treatment

Anti-tuberculosis drugs have two main purposes:

* to cure people with tuberculosis, provided the bacilli are drug sensitive
* to control tuberculosis, by either preventing the development of infectious forms or reducing the period of infectivity of people with infectious disease.

Tuberculosis had started to decline in the UK before the advent of chemotherapy, probably due to improved nutrition and social conditions. With the advent of effective anti-tuberculosis chemotherapy, it became apparent that patients no longer needed sanatorium treatment. Results with regimens containing isoniazid together with p-aminosalicylate (PAS) or ethambutol, and sometimes streptomycin, gave excellent results. Treatment was required for 18–24 months if relapse was to be prevented. The availability of pyrazinamide and, more importantly, rifampicin made shorter courses of treatment a possibility.

Most regimens in the developed world now contain isoniazid and rifampicin, which are the two most important drugs. These are prescribed together with pyrazinamide or possibly with another agent, such as ethambutol.

In order to eradicate the bacteria in an individual, combination anti-tuberculosis chemotherapy is always used. The choice of drug regimen is based on a number of factors, including a need to reduce the risk of resistance emerging and improve patient adherence.

In most developed countries there are guidelines for the treatment of tuberculosis and contacts of cases. The WHO has expanded its Directly Observed Treatment Short course (DOTS) programme to promote a systematic approach to tuberculosis treatment and control (WHO 2005).

Bacterial characteristics

There are four environments in which tubercle bacilli live. The activities of anti-tuberculosis agents in these environments will influence the choice of regimen. Open pulmonary cavities have a plentiful supply of oxygen and will have large numbers of rapidly growing organisms. However, bacilli in closed lesions will be oxygen starved and therefore slow growing or dormant. Intracellular tubercle bacilli will be slow growing due to the low intracellular pH and lack of oxygen. Some bacilli may also grow intermittently as their environment changes.

The anti-tuberculosis agents differ in their ability to kill these different populations of bacilli. Isoniazid, which is considered bactericidal, is effective against intracellular organisms. Rifampicin, also bactericidal, is most effective against intermittently dividing bacilli. Dormant bacilli are usually found in closed lesions hidden from the effects of both the immune system and the action of drugs. These bacilli are usually eradicated from the body by encapsulation (closing off of pathological lesions within the body and fibrosis over time).

Treatment of tuberculosis

Treatment guidelines in the UK were published by the Joint Tuberculosis Committee of the British Thoracic Society in 1998. The guidelines are summarized in Table 40.4 and the evidence-based gradings are detailed in Table 40.5. Updated

Table 40.4 Dosages of first-line anti-tubercular agents[a]

Drug	Forms available	Dosage				Reduce dose in	
		Adults daily	Adults intermittent (doses per week)	Children daily	Children intermittent (doses per week)	Renal failure	Liver failure
Rifampicin	Capsules 150 mg, 300 mg[b] Liquid 100 mg in 5 mL Injection for infusion 300 mg	450 mg/kg (<50 kg) 600 mg (>50 kg)	600–900 mg (3)	10 mg/kg	15 mg/kg (3)	No	Only in severe liver failure
Isoniazid	Tablets 100 mg[b] Injection 100 mg Mixture[c]	300 mg	15 mg/kg	5–10 mg/kg	10–15 mg/kg (3)	Only in severe liver failure	Impatients with acute or chronic liver disease

continued

Table 40.4 (continued)

Drug	Forms available	Dosage				Reduce dose in	
		Adults daily	Adults intermittent (doses per week)	Children daily	Children intermittent (doses per week)	Renal failure	Liver failure
Ethambutol[xx]	Tablets 100 mg 400 mg[b] Mixture[c]	15 mg/kg[d]		As adult dose	30 mg/kg (3)	Yes	No
Pyrazinamide	Tablets 500 mg	1.5 g (<50 kg) 2.0 g (≥50 kg)	2.0 g[d] (<50 kg) (3) 2.5 g[a] (≥50 kg)	35 mg/kg		Yes	No
Streptomycin	Injection 1 g	750 mg (<50 kg) 1 g (<50 kg)	750 mg–1 g[e]	15 mg/kg		Yes	No

a   Some of the doses quoted are not licensed but have been recommended by the British Thoracic Society.
b   Also available as combined oral preparations (see British National Formulary).
c   Mixture may be prepared extemporaneously.
d   Doses refer to patients under 50 kg. Reduce by 500 mg for patients weighing less than 50 kg.
e   Drug levels should be monitored to prevent toxicity.
xx Acute calculation is required to reduce the risk of toxicity.

Table 40.5 Grading of recommendations (British Thoracic Society 1998)

Grade	Recommendations
A	Requires at least one randomized controlled trial as part of the body of literature of overall good quality and consistency addressing the specific recommendation
B	Requires availability of well conducted clinical studies but no randomized clinical trials on the topic of recommendation
C	Requires evidence from expert committee reports or opinions and/or clinical experience of respected authorities, but indicates absence of directly applicable studies of good quality

recommendations for the treatment of tuberculosis in the UK (NICE 2006) are summarized below. These cover the regimens to be used in tuberculosis of different sites, but do not include details of dosage or other pharmaceutical details.

For fully drug-sensitive cases, tuberculosis is treated in two phases: an initial phase (using at least three drugs) and a continuation phase (using two drugs). Combination drugs (rifampicin, isoniazid, pyrazinamide and ethambutol, and rifampicin and isoniazid) are available for use in the 2-month initial and 4-month continuation phases, respectively. The doses in the combination tablets are set for a daily drug-taking regimen. Combination tablets have the advantage of preventing accidental or inadvertent single drug therapy, which can lead to acquired drug resistance within weeks in active tuberculosis. In view of the similarity in names between several anti-tuberculous drugs in the UK, great care should be taken when prescribing and dispensing. Doses should always be checked for both daily dosing and intermittent (thrice-weekly) directly observed treatment.

Patients with suspected drug reactions should always be referred back to the specialist physician supervising their treatment. Treatment should not be changed by a primary care doctor (general practitioner) without first consulting with the physician.

Drug-resistant tuberculosis should be treated by a specialist physician with experience in such cases, and where there are appropriate facilities for infection control.

Respiratory tuberculosis

Respiratory tuberculosis is defined as active tuberculosis affecting any of the following:

- lungs
- pleural cavity
- mediastinal lymph nodes
- larynx

In the UK, a 6-month regimen is recommended, consisting of rifampicin, isoniazid, pyrazinamide and ethambutol for the initial 2 months (initial phase), followed by a further 4 months of rifampicin and isoniazid (continuation phase), for respiratory disease.

Individuals who are known or suspected to be HIV positive, or who have had previous treatment, or are recent arrivals, such as immigrants or refugees from high-incidence countries, whatever their ethnic group, have a higher risk of resistance to isoniazid and other drugs. Patients should be commenced on the four-drug combination unless there are strong contraindications to the use of any one of these drugs.

The doses of all drugs which should be given in a single daily dose are shown in Table 40.4.

Intermittent (directly observed therapy) regimens

Directly observed therapy (DOT) is not needed for most cases of active tuberculosis. It is recommended that a risk assessment for treatment adherence is undertaken in all patients, and supervised intermittent DOT regimens should be considered where non-adherence to treatment might be a problem, for example in street- or shelter-dwelling homeless people with active tuberculosis and patients with a history of non-adherence. This latter group includes individuals with chronic alcohol or other social problems. If intermittent regimens are to be effective, they need to be organized in a systematic way, with input from the TB team, primary healthcare professionals, including pharmacists, as well as the patient and their family. This ensures that everyone involved is clear about the process and their responsibilities.

Trials of intermittent regimens have shown that a course of treatment is as effective when given intermittently as given daily. Regimens may be fully or partially intermittent. In the latter, four drugs (isoniazid, rifampicin, pyrazinamide and either ethambutol or streptomycin) are given daily for 2 months followed by rifampicin and isoniazid two or three times weekly for the subsequent 4 months. For most drugs the doses are increased when given intermittently and these are shown in Table 40.4. NICE (2006) recommends the thrice-weekly regimen.

Meningeal tuberculosis (tuberculous meningitis)

Patients with active meningeal TB should be treated with rifampicin and isoniazid for 12 months together with pyrazinamide, and a fourth drug, for example, ethambutol, for the first 2 months. Ethambutol (and streptomycin, where used) only reaches cerebrospinal fluid through inflamed meninges. However, care must be exercised when ethambutol is used in unconscious patients as visual acuity cannot be assessed. Meningeal tuberculosis is a serious disease and treatment must be started promptly. The stage at which the disease is diagnosed, and treatment started, most affects prognosis. Therefore it is often justified to start a therapeutic trial of anti-tuberculosis drugs in the absence of a definite diagnosis. Glucocorticoids are also recommended (see below).

Tuberculosis of peripheral lymph nodes

Trials have shown that 6 months of treatment are just as effective as 9 months, and the 6-month regimen is therefore recommended.

Bone and joint tuberculosis

Bone and joint tuberculosis is treated effectively with standard agents such as isoniazid and rifampicin for 6 months, together with pyrazinamide and a fourth drug, usually ethambutol in the initial phase (for 2 months). The spine is the most common site for bone tuberculosis. Occasionally surgery may be needed to either relieve spinal cord compression or correct spinal deformities.

Disseminated tuberculosis

Generalized (disseminated or miliary) tuberculosis must be treated promptly as there is appreciable mortality from delayed diagnosis and treatment. Standard regimens are used containing both isoniazid and rifampicin, with pyrazinamide and ethambutol in the first 2 months. If there is evidence of CNS involvement, treatment should be the same as for meningeal tuberculosis.

Pericardial tuberculosis

Although tuberculosis of the pericardium accounts for less than 4% of non-respiratory disease in the UK, it is potentially important because of the possibility of cardiac tamponade and constrictive pericarditis. These have significant morbidity and mortality. The standard 6-month treatment regimen is recommended for patients with active pericardial disease. Glucocorticoids should also be prescribed (see below).

Genitourinary tuberculosis and active tuberculosis of sites other than those above

The standard 6-month regimen is recommended.

Treatment of tuberculosis in special circumstances

Tuberculosis in children

The doses of drugs used in children are shown in Table 40.4. Doses are generally estimated to facilitate prescription of easily administered volumes of syrup or tablets of appropriate strength. Ethambutol should not routinely be used in young children, who would be unable to report visual disturbances should they occur. However, it might need to be used if there is toxicity or resistance to other agents.

Pregnancy

Pregnant women should be given standard therapy, although streptomycin should not be used as it may be ototoxic to the fetus. Although the other first-line drugs are not known to be teratogenic, they are either contraindicated or must only be used with caution. It is considered safe for mothers to breast feed while taking anti-tuberculosis agents.

Patients should be warned of the reduced effectiveness of oral or injectable contraceptives in regimens containing rifampicin.

Renal disease

Patients with renal disease may be given isoniazid, rifampicin and pyrazinamide in standard doses as these drugs are predominantly eliminated by non-renal routes. Ethambutol undergoes extensive renal elimination and therefore dose reduction is needed. Monitoring serum concentrations has been suggested but this is not readily available in many centres. Streptomycin must be used with considerable caution to prevent toxicity and is best avoided in renal failure. Rifampicin may be given in standard doses to patients on dialysis. However, doses of the other agents need to be modified and a number of different regimens have been suggested.

Liver disease

Monitoring of liver enzymes is recommended in patients with liver failure or in alcoholics because rifampicin, isoniazid and pyrazinamide are all potentially hepatotoxic. However, increases in transaminases at the start of anti-tuberculous treatment occur frequently. These are usually transient and not a reason for stopping treatment unless frank jaundice or hepatitis develops, in which case all drugs should be stopped. It is usually possible to restart treatment when transaminases have returned to pre-treatment levels.

Immunocompromised patients

Patients who are immunocompromised, including those with HIV infection, should be treated with normal first-line agents unless multidrug-resistant tuberculosis is suspected. Theoretically these patients have a greater risk of relapse and may need to be treated for longer than the normal 6 months. Current evidence indicates that on the completion of treatment, lifelong chemoprophylaxis with isoniazid should be instituted.

Glucocorticoids

Glucocorticoids (corticosteroids) have long been used in the treatment of tuberculosis, chiefly for their anti-inflammatory properties. They are recommended for use in meningeal and pericardial tuberculosis, to be commenced at the same time as anti-tuberculous drugs. Consideration should be given to their gradual withdrawal within 2–3 weeks of initiation. The decision on when to do this should be taken by the physician responsible for the care of the patient. The recommended doses are as follows.

Meningeal tuberculosis

- Adults: equivalent to prednisolone 20–40 mg if on rifampicin, otherwise 10–20 mg
- Children: equivalent to prednisolone 1–2 mg/kg, maximum 40 mg

Pericardial tuberculosis

- Adults: a glucocorticoid equivalent to prednisolone at 60 mg per day
- Children: a glucocorticoid equivalent to prednisolone 1 mg/kg/day (maximum 40 mg/day)

Drug-resistant tuberculosis

Drug-resistant tuberculosis is a considerable problem worldwide but is not often seen in the UK. It is an important issue in the management of tuberculosis, as it may compromise the effectiveness of treatment and prolong the period during which patients are infectious to others. Resistance to tuberculosis drugs is defined as a level of resistance to four times or greater the concentration of drug required to inhibit a fully susceptible organism. Isoniazid is the most usual agent to which resistance is seen. MDR tuberculosis is high-level resistance to both rifampicin and isoniazid with or without resistance to other drugs. It is important because there is loss of both the main bactericidal drug (isoniazid) and the main

sterilizing drug (rifampicin). Patients who are sputum smear positive are infectious for much longer than those with (drug) susceptible bacteria, and have a higher death rate from, and a lower cure rate for, their tuberculosis. Their treatment has to be individualized, requires a complex regimen involving the use of multiple reserve drugs of toxicity, and can cost at least £50 000 to £70 000 each to treat (Table 40.6).

It is recommended that treatment is only carried out:

- by physicians with substantial experience in drug-resistant tuberculosis
- in hospitals with appropriate isolation facilities (negative pressure rooms)
- in close conjunction with the Health Protection Agency (HPA) regional centres for mycobacteriology/the Wales Centre for Mycobacteriology.

The fluoroquinolones, especially ciprofloxacin and ofloxacin, have been used in patients with drug resistance, as has rifabutin.

Monitoring treatment

In pulmonary tuberculosis, sputum examination and culture are the most sensitive markers of treatment success. Patients taking regimens containing rifampicin and isoniazid should be non-infective within 2 weeks. If a patient does not become culture negative, it may be due to either drug resistance or non-adherence, the latter being more likely. Chest radiographs provide only limited information as to the progress of treatment. Good adherence is essential if treatment is to be successful and checking this can be difficult, especially when a patient is unco-operative.

Monitoring treatment outcomes

In 1999 the Enhanced Tuberculosis Surveillance system was established to collect epidemiological information on tuberculosis in England, Wales and Northern Ireland. It now includes a section to document treatment outcomes for each notified patient.

Drugs used and toxicities

In the UK, the first-line drugs for the treatment of tuberculosis are rifampicin, isoniazid, pyrazinamide, ethambutol and streptomycin. Other agents such as amikacin, capreomycin, cycloserine, newer macrolides (e.g. azithromycin) and quinolones (e.g. moxifloxacin) are reserved for use when first-line agents fail, usually due to resistance.

The major adverse reactions of the first-line drugs are shown in Table 40.7.

With the exception of streptomycin, first-line agents are usually administered orally. There is a liquid preparation of rifampicin available for patients who cannot take tablets or capsules. There are no commercial sources of liquid isoniazid, ethambutol or pyrazinamide in the UK although there is a BPC formulation for isoniazid elixir available on special order. Extemporaneous formulations for all three drugs have been used. The manufacturers or local medicine information centres are probably the best sources of information for these individual formulations. In patients who are severely ill and cannot take oral medication, rifampicin may be given intravenously, and isoniazid by both the

Table 40.6 Reserve drugs: dosages and side effects (British Thoracic Society 1998)

Drug (once daily)	Children	Adults	Main side effects
Streptomycin	15 mg/kg	15 mg/kg (max dose 1 g daily)	Tinnitus, ataxia, vertigo, renal impairment
Amikacin	15 mg/kg	15 mg/kg	As for streptomycin
Capreomycin		15 mg/kg	As for streptomycin
Kanamycin		15 mg/kg	As for streptomycin
Ethionamide or prothianamide	15–20 mg/kg	<50 kg, 375 mg twice a day ≥50 kg, 500 mg twice a day	Gastrointestinal, hepatitis; avoid in pregnancy
Cycloserine		250–500 mg twice a day	Depression, fits
Ofloxacin		400 mg twice a day	Abdominal distress, headache, tremulousness
Ciprofloxacin		750 mg twice a day	As ofloxacin plus drug interactions
Azithromycin		500 mg	Gastrointestinal upset
Clarithromycin		500 mg twice a day	As for azithromycin
Rifabutin		300–450 mg	As for rifampicin; uveitis can occur with drug interactions e.g. macrolides. Often cross-resistance with rifampicin
Thiacetazone	4 mg/kg	150 mg	Gastrointestinal, vertigo, conjunctivitis, rash. Avoid if HIV positive (Stevens–Johnson syndrome)
Clofazimine		300 mg	Headache, diarrhoea, red skin discolouration
PAS[a] sodium	300 mg/kg	10 g every morning or 5 g twice a day	Gastrointestinal, hepatitis, rash, fever

[a] PAS, p-aminosalicylate.

Table 40.7 Major adverse reactions of first-line anti-tuberculous drugs

Drug	Common reaction	Uncommon reaction
Isoniazid		Hepatitis, cutaneous hypersensitivity, peripheral neuropathy
Rifampicin		Hepatitis, cutaneous reactions, gastrointestinal reactions, thrombocytopaenic purpura, febrile reactions, 'flu syndrome'
Pyrazinamide	Anorexia, nausea, flushing	Hepatitis, vomiting, arthralgia, hyperuricaemia, cutaneous hypersensitivity
Ethambutol		Retrobulbar neuritis, arthralgia

intravenous and intramuscular routes. Although not commercially available, ethambutol injection has been used and may be available on request from the manufacturer.

Rifampicin, isoniazid and pyrazinamide are all potentially hepatotoxic. Transient increases in transaminases and bilirubin commonly occur at the start of treatment. However, there is no need to routinely monitor liver function in patients who have normal liver function at the start of treatment. If frank jaundice or hepatitis occurs, all drugs should be stopped and liver function allowed to return to normal, at which time treatment should be recommenced one drug at a time. Clinical hepatitis is rare although patients may complain of vague symptoms such as abdominal pain and malaise which may indicate impending hepatitis. Rifampicin will colour the urine red within approximately 4 hours of a dose.

Isoniazid may also cause a dose-dependent peripheral neuropathy, probably due to depletion of vitamin B_6. This reaction is rare at recommended doses but certain patient groups, e.g. the poorly nourished, alcoholics, diabetics, uraemic patients and pregnant women, are at greater risk and should receive pyridoxine supplementation at a dose of 10–20 mg per day.

Hypersensitivity reactions or rashes may occur with any of the drugs. However, the most important, although rare, is caused by rifampicin and can be quite severe. It is more prevalent during intermittent treatment and presents as a flu-like syndrome, sometimes with abdominal pain and respiratory symptoms. This usually resolves on reverting to a daily dosage. However, if more serious effects, such as renal impairment or haematological abnormalities, occur the drug should be stopped and never restarted.

Rashes can occur with isoniazid, pyrazinamide and streptomycin.

Ocular toxicity is by far the most important side effect of ethambutol. It occurs in fewer than 2% of patients at the usual dosage of 15 mg/kg but is more common in the elderly and people with renal impairment. Patients may complain of changes in colour vision or visual field which may appear suddenly. The effect is usually reversible on discontinuation of treatment but permanent damage may occur if the drug is continued. It is important that visual acuity is checked before treatment. Regular visual checks should be performed. However, as the majority of patients only receive the drug for 8 weeks, many clinicians do not consider this is necessary in adults, preferring to counsel patients to report any changes in visual acuity. However, this side effect precludes its use in those who are unable to report such changes, e.g. young children and the severely ill.

Tuberculosis control

The WHO recommends the DOTS treatment strategy. However, the administration of treatment is only one aspect of the WHO's strategy to control tuberculosis, especially in resource-poor countries. There are five components to DOTS.

1. Sustained political commitment to increase human and financial resources and make tuberculosis control a nationwide activity and an integral part of the national health system.
2. Access to quality-assured tuberculosis sputum microscopy for case detection among persons presenting with symptoms of tuberculosis. Screening of individuals with prolonged cough by sputum microscopy and special attention to case detection among HIV-infected people and other high-risk groups, e.g. people in institutions.
3. Standardized short-course chemotherapy to all cases of tuberculosis under proper case management conditions.
4. Uninterrupted supply of quality-assured drugs with reliable drug procurement and distribution systems.
5. Recording and reporting systems to allow outcome measurement of each patient and assessment of overall programme performance.

Chemoprophylaxis

Chemoprophylaxis is recommended routinely for everyone who may have recently acquired infection. These include:

- tuberculosis contacts who have demonstrated tuberculin conversion on testing as part of contact tracing
- individuals identified through screening as being tuberculin positive
- healthcare workers.

Prophylaxis is usually with isoniazid alone for 6 months or rifampicin and isoniazid for 3 months. NICE specifies the situations in which isoniazid versus rifampicin and isoniazid should be used.

The groups requiring prophylaxis and the drug regimen to be used are detailed in the new NICE TB guideline.

BCG vaccine

BCG vaccine contains a live, attenuated strain derived from *M. bovis*. It does not protect against infection but it prevents the more serious forms of disease such as miliary tuberculosis and meningeal tuberculosis. In 2005 the Joint Committee on Vaccination and Immunization recommended changes to the UK BCG vaccination policy. These were accepted by all four UK country health departments and the main changes are detailed below.

- The Schools BCG Programme ceased from the beginning of September 2005.
- A focus on the protection of individuals at higher risk of tuberculosis.
- The maximum age at which BCG can be given without prior tuberculin testing was raised to under 6 years of age, subject to certain conditions.

Full details of the changes can be found in the TB chapter of the 'Green Book' (*Immunization against Infectious Disease*) available on the Department of Health website (www.dh.gov.uk).

Patient care

It is possible to cure virtually all patients with tuberculosis infection or disease provided that an adequate regimen, to which the bacilli are susceptible, is prescribed and the patient complies with treatment. By far the largest cause of treatment failure is non-adherence by the patient. Non-adherence has serious consequences: treatment may fail and disease may relapse, in some cases with resistant organisms. If a non-adherent patient remains infectious they will also be a public health hazard.

Factors affecting adherence

A number of studies have shown that adherence falls as the number of tablets to be taken per day increases, and falls still further if doses have to be taken frequently through the day. Ideally, the least number of tablets should be given.

Patients may fail to adhere because they feel better and do not appreciate the need to continue with their medication. Lack of clarity of instructions, written, verbal or other, may compromise adherence, particularly if the patient is confused by conflicting advice from different healthcare professionals. Finally, adverse effects, or symptoms perceived to be adverse effects, may reduce adherence.

Improving patient adherence

Anti-tuberculosis therapy should be prescribed once a day using as few tablets as possible. Single daily dosing enables patients to fit their medication into their daily routine. Rifampicin and isoniazid are both well absorbed when taken on an empty stomach. However, absorption is reduced and delayed when taken with or after food. It is therefore recommended that both are taken 1 hour before food to achieve rapid high blood levels. It is usually recommended that patients take their medication before breakfast. Cueing tablet taking to a regular activity may improve adherence in some patients.

The number of tablets to be taken each day may be reduced by using combination preparations. There are a number of combination preparations available. Some, for example Rifater, contain ratios of drugs that differ slightly from the dosages recommended by the British Thoracic Society. This difference in dosage is probably not clinically significant and is far preferable to potential undertreatment due to non-adherence. Combination preparations may not be suitable for use in children as the required dose regimens differ from those of adults.

Patient education

Written instructions and/or patient information leaflets may be offered to support verbal counselling if there is any doubt as to the patient's understanding. It should be emphasized that the disease will be cured but this will take some months and the tablets will need to be taken as prescribed even if the patient feels better. Some patients will adhere initially while they are unwell but will fail to adhere later as they begin to feel better.

The occurrence of some adverse effects may require discontinuation of a drug, but others are harmless. The patient should be told which side effects to expect and which require referral to a member of the healthcare team. Again, written instructions may be helpful.

A number of patients from abroad with tuberculosis have a poor command of English. It may still be possible to give written instructions on dosage as some pharmaceutical companies are able to provide pictorial material and dosage sheets in a number of languages.

Counselling points

Patients taking rifampicin should be told that the drug will cause a harmless discoloration of their urine and other body fluids, for example sweat and tears. The staining of tears is important if the patient uses soft contact lenses as these may be permanently stained. Gas-permeable and hard lenses are unaffected. Women using the oral contraceptive pill should be advised to use other non-hormonal methods of contraception for the duration of rifampicin treatment and for 8 weeks afterwards.

Although ocular side effects are rare when ethambutol is taken in normal dosages, patients should be warned of this potentially serious side effect. They should be advised to stop the drug and report to their doctor if they notice any changes in vision, such as a reduction in visual acuity or changes in colour vision. This is especially important because visual changes are usually reversible on discontinuation of the drug but may be permanent if the drug is not stopped.

CASE STUDIES

Case 40.1

A man in his mid-30s is admitted to hospital with a cough productive of sputum and a fever. A chest x-ray indicates bilateral pneumonia with apical involvement. A sputum smear reveals the presence of acid, alcohol-fast bacilli. The patient is transferred to a side room and commenced on anti-tuberculosis therapy.

Soon after admission, a history of drug misuse comes to light. The man 'absconds' from hospital on two occasions. He sometimes leaves his room and enters the general medical ward, coming into contact with other patients.

Questions

1. What form of tuberculosis does this patient have?
2. Should he be kept in hospital for treatment, and should he be compelled to stay in hospital?
3. Does he need any other healthcare?

Answers

1. This man has sputum smear-positive pulmonary tuberculosis, the infectious form of the disease.
2. As he wanders onto the general ward, and in view of his habit of absconding from hospital, he poses a risk to others, particularly susceptible individuals. Therefore, he should preferably be kept in hospital for at least 2–3 weeks to help ensure adherence with treatment so that he becomes non-infectious.

   If encouragement to comply with treatment and to avoid the main ward or leaving hospital fails, legal measures could be considered. These are set out in the Public Health (Control of Diseases) Act 1984 for England and Wales. Transfer to a specialist infectious diseases hospital or unit may be necessary.
3. Referral to a psychiatrist specializing in substance misuse could help. Where a patient presenting with tuberculosis has other health problems, it is important that all their health needs are addressed, as this may help encourage adherence with treatment.

Case 40.2

A woman in her 40s is admitted to hospital with shortness of breath. She has lived in sub-Saharan Africa. She subsequently develops a non-productive cough. Bronchial washings are smear negative for acid-fast bacilli but *M. tuberculosis* is isolated from the sample. Early sputum samples are smear negative but later samples are smear positive.

Questions

1. What form of tuberculosis does this patient have?
2. Should she be in isolation?
3. What treatment should she receive for her tuberculosis?
4. Is she at low or high risk for drug-resistant tuberculosis?
5. What further microbiological investigations would be essential?

Answers

1. She has pulmonary tuberculosis, indicated by her symptoms and chest x-ray.
2. She should be in isolation in a side room.
3. She should be commenced on standard quadruple therapy, comprising rifampicin and isoniazid, supplemented with pyrazinamide and ethambutol for the first 2 months.
4. A history of residence in sub-Saharan Africa suggests she could be at risk of drug-resistant tuberculosis, in particular multiple drug-resistant tuberculosis. The change in sputum smear status, despite being on standard quadruple therapy, would certainly suggest drug resistance.
5. A PCR test should be done on the isolate to determine whether her infecting strains of tubercle bacilli are resistant to rifampicin. Tests should also be done to assess susceptibility to other drugs. If she is confirmed as having multiple drug-resistant tuberculosis, she should

be transferred to a negative pressure room under the care of a specialist tuberculosis physician.

Case 40.3

A woman in her mid-20s is diagnosed as having sputum smear-negative pulmonary tuberculosis. Although she initially takes her anti-tuberculous drugs, she does not attend follow-up clinics and her condition deteriorates. Her primary care physician collects a sputum sample from her and persuades her to attend the chest clinic. The sputum smear is now positive and it is found she has been continuing in her job.

Questions

1. What type of treatment regimen should be offered to this patient?
2. Who should be involved in planning this treatment regimen, and what arrangements should be put in place to ensure this works?
3. Should the patient's work contacts be screened?

Answers

1. Patients like this should receive supervised treatment three times a week in a convenient setting, such as at home.
2. There needs to be close collaboration between the physician responsible for treatment, the patient's primary care physician, the public health team and the healthcare professionals (often district nurses or health visitors in the UK) who will supervise treatment. The patient needs to be involved in discussions about these arrangements, as treatment will not be successful without her co-operation.

   The physician will need to adjust the treatment dosage in line with the thrice-weekly regimen, inform the primary care physician and ensure the correct prescriptions are issued. Those supervising treatment need a clear explanation of what is expected of them, including details of the drugs and dose, and duration of treatment. They also need to know what to do if the patient does not adhere.
3. The question of whether work contacts should be screened must be dealt with on an individual case basis. This usually involves the public

health team informing the patient of the need to inquire into work contacts, and getting the patient's agreement to approach a supervisor or manager in the workplace. A telephone conversation will provide initial information on the working environment and should be followed up by a visit if initial inquiries indicate a possible need to screen workplace contacts.

Case 40.4

A 65-year-old man with a chest infection resulting in cough with sputum production does not improve after two courses of antibiotics prescribed empirically.

Questions

1. What investigations should be done?
2. In this patient, all three sputum specimens came back as smear (AFB) positive. Does this mean the patient has tuberculosis?
3. Should the patient be notified to the local public health team (communicable disease control)?

Answers

1. Three early morning sputum specimens should be collected and sent to the microbiology laboratory for microscopic examination for AFB, culture for *M. tuberculosis* and *M. bovis*. In this case, as the patient has failed to respond to antibiotic treatment, a diagnosis of tuberculosis should be considered.
2. Not necessarily. He may have an atypical mycobacterial infection. He should be sent to the chest clinic for further clinical assessment of symptoms and a chest x-ray. Some atypical mycobacterial infections cause pulmonary disease resembling tuberculosis. The chest physician will make a judgement on the most likely clinical diagnosis.
3. Only if the clinician thinks the most likely diagnosis is tuberculosis. If unsure, but the patient is commenced on anti-tuberculous therapy, then he should be notified as having tuberculosis. If the culture subsequently indicates infection with atypical mycobacteria, the case can be de-notified.

ACKNOWLEDGEMENT

Permission to use material prepared for the first edition by P. J. Barker is gratefully acknowledged, as is the help from consultant physician colleagues in Gwent for the case studies.

REFERENCES

Begg N, Blair I, Reintjes R et al 2005 Communicable disease control handbook. Blackwell, Oxford

British Thoracic Society 1998 Joint Tuberculosis Committee. Chemotherapy and management of tuberculosis in the United Kingdom: recommendations 1998. Thorax 53: 536-548

British Thoracic Society 2000 Control and prevention of tuberculosis in the United Kingdom: Code of Practice 2000. Thorax 55: 887-901

Davies P D O 2003 Clinical tuberculosis, Arnold, London

Heymann D L (ed) 2004 Control of communicable diseases manual. American Public Health Association, Washington DC

National Institute for Clinical Excellence/National Collaborating Centre for Chronic Conditions. Tuberculosis 2006 Clinical diagnosis and management of tuberculosis and measures for its prevention and control. Royal College of Physicians, London. Available online at: www.nice.org.uk/page.aspx?o= 297929

Tuberculosis Section, Health Protection Agency Centre for Infection 2005 Annual report on tuberculosis cases reported in England, Wales and Northern Ireland in 2003. Health Protection Agency, London. Available online at: www.hpa.org.uk/infections/topics_az/tb/pdf/2003_Annual_Report.pdf

World Health Organization 2005 DOTS. World Health Organization, Geneva. Available online at: www.who.int/tb/dots/whatisdots/en/print.html

Useful websites

WHO fact sheet on tuberculosis, 2005: www.who.int/mediacentre/factsheets/fs104/en/print.html

Global data on tuberculosis: www.who.int/tb/publications/global_report/2006/pdf/annex_2_en.pdf.

FURTHER READING

Department of Health 2004 Stopping tuberculosis in England: an action plan from the Chief Medical Officer. Department of Health, London

Interdepartmental Working Group on Tuberculosis 1998 The prevention and control of tuberculosis in the United Kingdom. Department of Health, Scottish Office, Welsh Office, London. Available online at: www.doh.gov.uk/Ebguide.htm

Veen J, Raviglione M, Rieder H L et al 1998 Standardised tuberculosis treatment outcome monitoring in Europe. Recommendations of a Working Group of the World Health Organization (WHO) and the European Region of the International Union Against Tuberculosis and Lung Disease (IUATLD) for uniform reporting of cohort analysis of treatment outcome in tuberculosis patients. European Respiratory Journal 12: 505-510

41 HIV infection

H. Leake Date   M. Fisher

KEY POINTS

- Untreated infection with the human immunodeficiency virus (HIV) leads to a progressive deterioration in the cellular immune response. After initial seroconversion, the infected individual may appear asymptomatic for a number of years, before developing symptomatic disease and/or acquired immune deficiency syndrome (AIDS).
- Complications arising from HIV infection can manifest in a variety of ways, usually as opportunistic infections or malignancies that are uncommon in the immunocompetent population.
- The aim of the treatment of HIV infection is to reconstitute, or prevent further deterioration of, the immune system, with the intention of improving the quality and quantity of life. Management of HIV-related complications primarily involves the treatment and prophylaxis of opportunistic diseases.
- Currently available antiretroviral agents are classified by their mechanism of actions as: nucleoside or nucleotide analogue reverse transcriptase inhibitors (NRTIs), non-nucleoside reverse transcriptase inhibitors (NNRTIs), protease inhibitors (PIs) and entry inhibitors.
- Antiretroviral agents are given in combination, usually of at least three agents, to improve efficacy and reduce the development of viral resistance.
- Treatment regimens are frequently complex and many of the drugs have significant toxicities and interactions with other drugs and with food. A high level of adherence to therapy is vital to ensure efficacy and prevent the emergence of resistant virus.

The acquired immune deficiency syndrome (AIDS) is the state of profound immunosuppression produced by chronic infection with the human immunodeficiency virus (HIV).

Epidemiology

In June 1981, five cases of *Pneumocystis jiroveci* (formerly known as *carinii*) pneumonia (PCP) were described in homosexual men in the USA. Reports of other unusual conditions, such as Kaposi's sarcoma (KS), followed shortly. In each of these patients there was found to be a marked impairment of cellular immune response, and so the term acquired immune deficiency syndrome or AIDS was coined. In 1984 a new human retrovirus, subsequently named human immunodeficiency virus (HIV), was isolated and identified as the cause of AIDS.

Although initially described in homosexual men, it soon became apparent that other population groups were affected, including intravenous drug users and haemophiliacs. During the first decade the epidemic grew and the importance of transmission via heterosexual intercourse and from mother to child (vertical transmission) was increasingly recognized. In the UK since 1999, the number of new HIV diagnoses has been higher in heterosexuals than in men who have sex with men (MSM). The majority of heterosexuals with HIV have acquired their infection in countries of high prevalence, whilst the majority of ongoing transmission within the UK is still amongst men who have sex with men. The impact of treatment advances on the mortality from AIDS-related illnesses has been significant, although current data indicate that rates may now have plateaued, possibly due to the failure to diagnose HIV infection amongst the asymptomatic population. As the use of antiretroviral therapy has become more widespread, reports of primary HIV resistance (people initially infected with virus already resistant to one or more drugs) have been increasingly common. Rates of primary resistance vary widely and differ from country to country, but rates of up to 20% have been reported in the UK.

In the developing world, particularly sub-Saharan Africa, South-East Asia, South America and Eastern Europe, numbers continue to increase and prevalence rates of up to 40–50% have been reported in certain communities in Botswana and South Africa. Major efforts are being made to provide antiretroviral therapies in these settings, although choice of agents and facilities for monitoring may be limited and locally produced generic formulations are often used.

The virus has been isolated from a number of body fluids, including blood, semen, vaginal secretions, saliva, breast milk, tears, urine, peritoneal fluid and cerebrospinal fluid (CSF). However, not all of these appear to be important in the spread of infec-tion and the predominant routes of transmission remain: sexual intercourse (anal or vaginal); sharing of unsterilized needles or syringes; blood or blood products in areas where supplies are not screened or treated; and vertical transmission in utero, during labour or through breast feeding.

Pathogenesis

HIV, in common with other retroviruses, possesses the enzyme reverse transcriptase and consists of a lipid bilayer membrane surrounding the capsid (Fig. 41.1). Its surface glycoprotein molecule (gp120) has a strong affinity for the CD4 receptor protein found predominantly on the T-helper/inducer lymphocytes. Monocytes and macrophages may also possess CD4 receptors in low densities and can therefore also be infected. The process of HIV entry is more complex than originally thought and, in addition to CD4 attachment, subsequent binding to co-

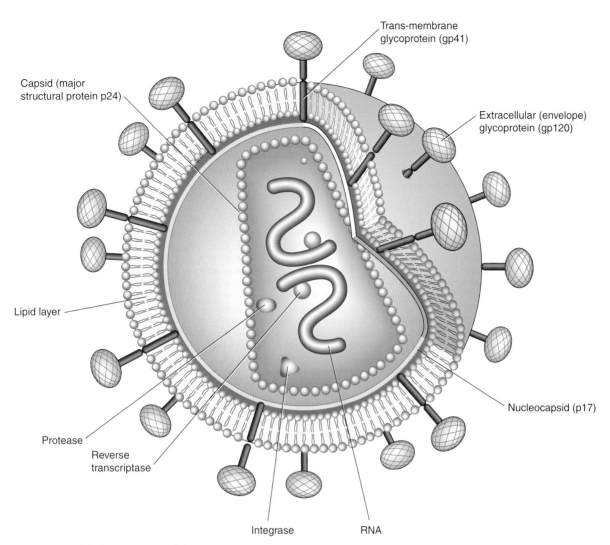

Figure 41.1 Structure of the human immunodeficiency virus (HIV).

receptors such as CCR-5 or CXCR-4 and membrane fusion also occur (Fig. 41.2).

After penetrating the host cell, the virus sheds its outer coat and releases its genetic material. Using the reverse transcriptase enzyme, the viral RNA is converted to DNA using nucleosides. The viral DNA is then integrated into the host genome in the cell nucleus, where it undergoes transcription and translation, enabling the production of new viral proteins. New virus particles are then assembled and bud out of the host cell, finally maturing into infectious virions under the influence of the protease enzyme.

Immediately after infection there is a very high rate of viral turnover, after which equilibrium is reached. At this stage the infection may appear to be clinically latent but in fact, as many as 10 000 million new virions are produced each day.

Over time, as chronic infection ensues, cells possessing CD4 receptors, particularly the T-helper lymphocytes, are depleted from the body. The T-helper cell is often considered to be the conductor of the 'immune orchestra' and thus, as this cell is depleted, the individual becomes susceptible to myriad infections and tumours. The rate at which this immunosuppression progresses is variable and the precise interaction of factors affecting it is still not fully understood. It is well recognized that some

individuals rapidly develop severe immunosuppression whilst others may have been infected with HIV for many years whilst maintaining a relatively intact immune system. It is likely that a combination of viral, host and environmental factors contributes to this variation.

Outside the body, HIV is inactivated by physical and chemical agents, including household bleach in a 1:10 dilution, hydrogen peroxide, glutaraldehyde, ethyl and isopropyl alcohols and heat of 56°C for 10 minutes.

Clinical manisfestations

The sequelae of untreated HIV infection can be broadly considered in four categories:

- opportunistic infections, i.e. infections that would not normally cause disease in an immunocompetent host, e.g. *Pneumocystis jiroveci pneumonia* and cytomegalovirus (CMV)
- infections that can occur in immunocompetent patients but tend to occur more frequently, more severely and often atypically in the context of underlying HIV infection, e.g. *Salmonella*, herpes simplex and *Mycobacterium tuberculosis*

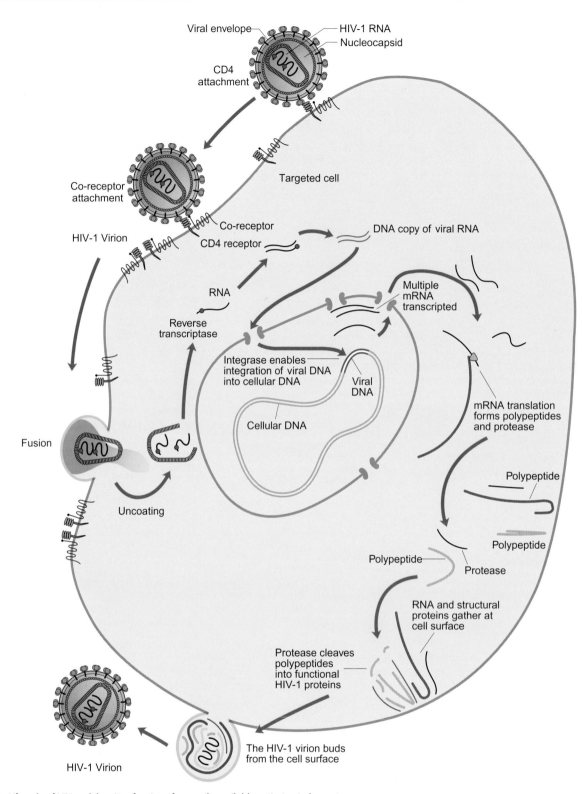

Figure 41.2 Lifecycle of HIV and the site of action of currently available antiretroviral agents.

- malignancies, particularly those that occur rarely in the immunocompetent population, e.g. Kaposi's sarcoma and non-Hodgkin's lymphoma
- direct manifestations of HIV infection per se, e.g. HIV encephalopathy, HIV myelopathy and HIV enteropathy.

In addition, approximately 70% of individuals develop a flu-like illness at seroconversion. This primary HIV infection is characterized by fever, arthralgia, pharyngitis, rash and lymphadenopathy. Rarely, the degree of associated CD4 count depletion may be sufficient to result in development of an opportunistic illness such as oropharyngeal/oesophageal candidiasis or *Pneumocystis jiroveci* pneumonia.

Opportunistic infections generally fall into two categories:

- DNA viruses, e.g. cytomegalovirus and JC virus
- intracellular pathogens, e.g. *Pneumocystis jiroveci*, *Toxoplasma gondii* and *Mycobacterium avium*.

Although the clinical course of HIV disease varies with each individual, there is a fairly consistent and predictable pattern that enables appropriate interventions and preventive measures to be adopted. Patients can be classified into one of three groups according to their clinical status: asymptomatic, symptomatic or AIDS. Symptomatic disease is characterized by non-specific symptomatology such as fevers, night sweats, lethargy and weight loss, or by complications including oral candidiasis, oral hairy leucoplakia, and recurrent herpes simplex or herpes zoster infections. AIDS is defined by the diagnosis of one or more specific conditions including *Pneumocystis jiroveci* pneumonia, *M. tuberculosis* infection and cytomegalovirus disease.

The most common manifestations currently seen in the UK are outlined below.

Investigations and monitoring

Current and previous infections

The initial diagnosis of HIV infection is made by the detection of antibodies against HIV. However, it may take up to 3 months after infection with the virus for antibodies to be detected. After confirmation of HIV infection, the patient is usually tested for prior exposure to a number of potential pathogens, including syphilis, hepatitis A, B and C, cytomegalovirus, varicella zoster (VZV) and *T. gondii*. This can enable subsequent treatment (in the case of undiagnosed syphilis), vaccination (if no prior exposure to hepatitis B) and prevention (if no prior exposure to *Toxoplasma* and cytomegalovirus), prophylaxis (if previous exposure to *Toxoplasma*), and aid subsequent diagnosis (according to cytomegalovirus or status).

CD4 count

The level of immunosuppression is most easily estimated by monitoring a patient's CD4 count. This measures the number of CD4-positive T-lymphocytes in a sample of peripheral blood. The normal range can vary between 500 and 1500 cells/mm^3. As HIV disease progresses, the number of cells falls. Particular complications of HIV infection usually begin to occur at similar CD4 counts (Fig. 41.3), which can assist in differential diagnoses

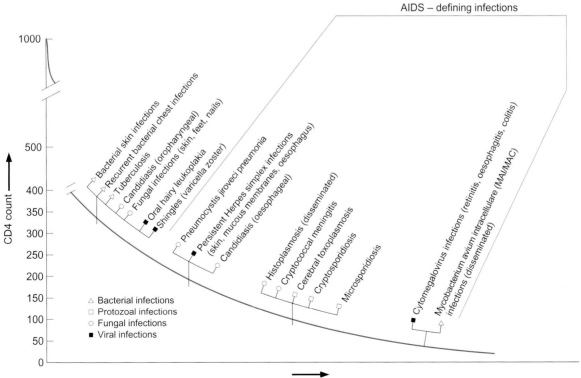

Figure 41.3 Opportunistic complications of HIV infection and the CD4 count ranges at which they commonly occur.

and enable the use of prophylactic therapies. For example, patients with a CD4 count of less than 200 cells/mm³ should always be offered prophylaxis against *Pneumocystis jiroveci* pneumonia. Similarly, both patient and clinician are likely to use the CD4 count as one indicator of when to consider starting antiretroviral therapy and how effective such therapy is.

Viral load

The measurement of plasma HIV RNA (viral load) estimates the amount of circulating virus in the blood plasma. This has been proven to correlate with prognosis, with a high viral load predicting faster disease progression (Mellors et al 1997). Conversely, a reduction in viral load after commencement of antiviral therapy is associated with clinical benefit. This measure, in combination with the CD4 count, allows patients and clinicians to make informed decisions regarding when to start and when to change antiviral therapies, enabling the more effective use of such agents.

Resistance testing

Due to significant rates of primary resistance, it is recommended that all patients have a genotype performed after diagnosis; this will ensure that appropriate initial therapy is selected. Further resistance tests should be performed at any subsequent virological failure to direct therapy choice.

Drug treatment

The drug treatment of HIV disease can be classified as antiretroviral therapy, the management of opportunistic infections or malignancies, and symptom control. For the first decade of the epidemic, most of the available drugs and therapeutic strategies were aimed at treating or preventing opportunistic complications and alleviating HIV-related symptoms. Whilst these are still important, there has been a shift in emphasis towards treatment aimed at reducing the HIV viral load and restoring immune function. The three main factors contributing to this change have been increased understanding of the pathogenesis of HIV infection, the increasing number of agents and classes of agents to combat HIV, and the many clinical trials that have demonstrated the superiority of highly active antiretroviral therapy (HAART), i.e. the benefit of triple therapy over dual or monotherapy.

Due to the speed at which new antiretroviral agents are being developed, comprehensive data on drug interactions, side effects, etc. are often lacking. Thus the ability to apply general pharmacological and pharmacokinetic principles, together with common sense, is required.

The treatment of many of the opportunistic complications of HIV comprises an induction phase of high-dose therapy, followed by indefinite maintenance and/or secondary prophylaxis using lower doses. This is due to the high rate of relapse or progression after a first episode of diseases such as *Pneumocystis jiroveci* pneumonia, cerebral toxoplasmosis (toxoplasmic encephalitis), systemic cryptococcosis and cytomegalovirus retinitis. Where a cost-effective agent with an acceptable risk/benefit ratio exists, primary prophylaxis may be offered to individuals who are deemed to be at high risk of developing a particular opportunistic infection, e.g. *Pneumocystis jiroveci* pneumonia prophylaxis. Discontinuation of prophylaxis, both primary and secondary, is now usually possible in individuals who demonstrate immunological restoration on HAART.

Paradoxically, this immunological restoration may result in apparent clinical deterioration with opportunistic infections during the first few weeks after initiation of HAART. This is known as immune reconstitution inflammatory syndrome (IRIS).

The goals of therapy in HIV-positive individuals are to:

- improve the quality and duration of life
- prevent deterioration of immune function and/or restore immune status
- treat and/or prevent opportunistic infections
- relieve symptoms.

Antiretroviral therapy

Antiretroviral therapy is currently one of the fastest evolving areas of medicine. The specific details of treatment will therefore continue to change as new drugs emerge, although it is likely that the following general principles will remain.

- A combination of three antiretroviral agents, selected on the basis of treatment history and resistance tests, should be prescribed to increase efficacy and reduce the development of drug-resistant virus.
- Wherever possible, a regimen should contain a drug that penetrates the central nervous system and confers protection against HIV-related encephalopathy/dementia.
- Treatment strategies should be adopted that sequence drug combinations, being mindful of potential cross-resistance and future therapy options.
- Given the crucial importance of a high level of adherence to these therapies, the regimen adopted for a particular individual should, wherever possible, be tailored to suit their daily lifestyle.

Many organizations, such as the British HIV Association (BHIVA) and the International AIDS Society, produce regularly updated guidelines on the use of antiretroviral therapy (e.g. Gazzard et al 2005). These guidelines include the most up-to-date considerations of:

- when to start therapy
- what to start with
- how to monitor, including use of therapeutic drug monitoring (TDM) and resistance testing
- when to switch therapy
- what to switch to
- treating individuals who have been highly exposed to multiple agents
- managing individuals with significant comorbidities (e.g. tuberculosis or hepatitis B/C).

In the absence of a definitive evidence base, and given the rapidly developing nature of this field of medicine, such guidelines should be integrated wherever possible into routine patient care.

Most studies evaluating triple combinations of antiretrovirals have been designed with so-called 'surrogate marker' endpoints, measuring the effect on laboratory parameters such as CD4 count and HIV viral load. These trials are generally smaller and shorter in duration than clinical endpoint studies that are powered to measure the impact on survival and disease progression. The first large clinical endpoint trial that demonstrated the superiority of a triple combination over dual therapy was undertaken by Hammer et al (1997). Following the results of this trial, the standard approach, where treatment is indicated, has been to use a combination of at least three agents. The reduction in morbidity and mortality associated with HAART has been confirmed in routine clinical practice, as well as in other trials (Palella et al 1998, Smit et al 2006). Subsequent clinical trials have largely been for licensing purposes and/or have served to refine therapeutic choices rather than to change the paradigm of treatment.

Postexposure prophylaxis

Postexposure prophylaxis (PEP) involves the use of antiretroviral drugs to prevent infection with HIV after possible exposure, which may be recommended after occupational injuries (DH 2004) or sexual exposure (Fisher et al 2006). Whilst PEP is a largely unproven and unlicensed indication for the drugs used, it is supported by animal model data and case control studies. Where recommended in guidelines, PEP is usually commenced as a 3–5 day starter regimen of two nucleoside/nucleotide analogues (NRTIs) and a protease inhibitor (PI), followed by an ongoing course for a total of 4 weeks post exposure. It is believed this will reduce the likelihood of infection by at least 80%, although toxicity issues are not insignificant and so the decision to prescribe or take PEP must reflect a careful risk/benefit evaluation.

Choosing and monitoring therapy

The majority of individuals are currently commenced on a combination of two NRTIs and a non-nucleoside reverse transcriptase inhibitor (NNRTI) or two NRTIs and a boosted protease inhibitor. The term 'boosted protease inhibitor' refers to a combination of one protease inhibitor combined with a low dose (usually 100–200 mg once or twice daily) of ritonavir, another protease inhibitor. The ritonavir is used as a pharmacokinetic enhancer of the other protease inhibitor, generally by increasing the maximum plasma concentration, C_{max}, and extending the half-life, $t_{1/2}$, and does not directly add to the antiretroviral activity of the regimen. Triple nucleoside (NRTI) therapy is no longer recommended, as it is associated with unacceptable rates of virological failure. Alternative strategies, such as NRTI-sparing regimens and boosted protease inhibitor monotherapy, are currently only routinely recommended in a research setting.

The aim of initial therapy is to achieve viral load suppression in the plasma to levels below the detection limits of available assays (40 copies/mL). Such virological suppression is almost invariably accompanied by an elevation in CD4 count and clinical evidence of immune reconstitution. Whilst sustained suppression over many years is possible, viral rebound may occur and is usually accompanied by the development of resistance to one or more agents in the combination. Upon confirmed virological failure, a resistance test is usually performed which will help to identify which agents the virus may have adapted to and the extent to which any such resistance mutations may confer cross-resistance to other available drugs. A second-line regimen is then constructed, wherever possible utilizing a new class of drug to which the individual has not previously been exposed. Upon virological failure of subsequent regimens, the therapeutic options available become increasingly limited and the aims of such 'salvage regimens' may not always be to achieve complete virological suppression but rather to gain immunological and clinical benefit within acceptable tolerability and toxicity limits.

Many of the antiretrovirals, particularly the protease inhibitors and NNRTIs, exhibit a wide range of interactions, especially with other drugs that are metabolized by the cytochrome P450 enzyme system. There is a need to ensure that significant interactions, including with herbal medicines, are avoided and the timing and frequency of doses are compatible with the patient's lifestyle. General prescribing guidelines for antiretrovirals are presented in Table 41.1 whilst details of common side effects and interactions of the currently available agents are summarized in Tables 41.2, 41.3 and 41.4.

Table 41.1 General prescribing and monitoring information for antiretroviral agents

- The Summary of Product Characteristics, BNF and national guidelines should be consulted when managing the treatment of an HIV positive patient.

- Interaction and side effect data on drugs that are on trial, compassionate release or newly licensed are often limited and are frequently updated.

- Adverse events should be reported to the MHRA. With greater exposure and long-term use it is likely that more adverse events will be recognized. Some of these may be class effects associated with particular groups of antiretrovirals and should therefore be monitored even in new agents within a class. Examples include dyslipidaemia and diabetes mellitus with protease inhibitors; mitochondrial myopathy and lipoatrophy with NRTIs; rash with NNRTIs.

- Many of the newer antiretroviral agents have not been studied extensively in individuals with renal or hepatic insufficiency. Data are also limited in patients with other significant co-morbidities such as diabetes and cardiac disease. Caution should therefore be exercised when prescribing for such patients and all their medical conditions should be closely monitored.

- There are limited data on the safety of many antiretroviral drugs when taken during pregnancy, or their long term effects on babies/children. Efavirenz has been shown to be teratogenic in animal studies, but comparable data are not available for the other antiretrovirals. Caution should therefore be exercised with all agents. Treatment of women who are planning conception or who are pregnant must be discussed with the relevant experts. All pregnant women who are treated with antiretrovirals should be reported prospectively to the Antiretroviral Pregnancy Register.

Table 41.2 General prescribing points for nucleoside/nucleotide analogue reverse transcriptase inhibitors (NRTIs)

Drug	Dose and formulation	Administration	Side effects	Drug interactions and pharmacokinetic information
Abacavir Ziagen⌒	300 mg bd 600 mg od 300 mg tablets 20 mg/mL oral solution	Can be taken with or without food	– usually well tolerated – most common side effects are rash, headache, nausea and vomiting, diarrhoea, reduced appetite – hypersensitivity (5% incidence). Patient must NEVER be rechallenged if abacavir has to be withdrawn due to suspected hypersensitivity. – lactic acidosis	Metabolism of methadone may be altered Mycophenolate mofetil may increase abacavir levels
Combivir⌒ (Zidovudine + Lamivudine)	One tablet bd	Tablet contains 300 mg zidovudine + 150 mg lamivudine	See entries for individual drugs	See entries for individual drugs
Didanosine (ddl) Videx⌒	If >60 kg: 400 mg od (with tenofovir: 250 mg od) If <60 kg: 250 mg od (with tenofovir: 200 mg od) 400 mg, 250 mg, 200 mg & 125 mg e/c capsules Suspension	Must be taken on an empty stomach: Capsules: no food for ≥2 h either side of dose Suspension: to be taken >30 mins before and >2 h after food N.B. No food restrictions when taken with tenofovir	– nausea, bloating, diarrhoea – dry mouth – pancreatitis (incidence <1%): caution in patients with high alcohol intake or history of pancreatitis – peripheral neuropathy (incidence <10%) – hyperuricaemia – lactic acidosis	Reduce dose in renal impairment Co-administration with tenofovir causes an increase in didanosine levels Ganciclovir and valganciclovir increase didanosine levels leading to ≠ risk of pancreatitis. Take at least 2 h apart from valganciclovir Ribavirin may increase didanosine levels leading to ≠ risk of toxicity Take dapsone and other drugs adsorbed by antacids at least 2 h before or after didanosine suspension. No interaction with didanosine e/c caps Take indinavir >1 h after didanosine suspension (can take with didanosine e/c caps) Caution with drugs associated with pancreatitis such as iv pentamidine
Emtricitabine (FTC) Emtriva⌒	200 mg od 200 mg capsules	Can be taken with or without food	– headache most common – also nausea, diarrhoea, dizziness; harmless skin discoloration, especially in darker skins – lactic acidosis	No clinically significant interactions noted Reduce dose in renal impairment Do not use with lamivudine Also active against hepatitis B
Kivexa⌒ (Abacavir + Lamivudine)	One tablet od	Tablet contains 600 mg abacavir + 300 mg lamivudine	See entries under individual drugs Patients who have had a hypersensitivity reaction to abacavir must NEVER be rechallenged with abacavir or Kivexa®	See entries under individual drugs
Lamivudine (3TC) Epivir⌒	150 mg bd 300 mg od 150 mg & 300 mg tablets Oral solution (10 mg/mL)	Can be taken with or without food	Generally well tolerated – GI disturbances, headache, anaemia and neutropenia have been reported but not common – lactic acidosis	Reduce dose in renal impairment Increased risk of neutropenia with high-dose co-trimoxazole and ganciclovir/valganciclovir Increases trimethoprim levels Do not use with emtricitabine Also active against hepatitis B

Table 41.2 (continued)

Drug	Dose and formulation	Administration	Side effects	Drug interactions and pharmacokinetic information
Stavudine (D4T) Zerit⌒	If >60 kg: 40 mg bd If <60 kg: 30 mg bd 30 mg & 40 mg capsules Oral solution (1 mg/mL)	Can be taken with or without food	– peripheral neuropathy; following discontinuation symptoms may worsen before improvement noted – pancreatitis – lactic acidosis – lipoatrophy – hyperlipidaemia	Caution with drugs associated with peripheral neuropathy such as isoniazid Avoid use with didanosine where possible Do not use with zidovudine
Tenofovir (TDF) Viread™	300 mg od Tenofovir disoproxil 245 mg tablet is equivalent to tenofovir disoproxil fumarate 300 mg	Can be taken with or without food	– diarrhoea, nausea and vomiting, flatulence and headache most common (incidence >10%) – renal impairment and hypophosphataemia reported; Fanconi's syndrome rare; monitor serum creatinine and phosphate	Reduce dose in renal impairment Mostly eliminated unchanged in the urine Minor inducer of CYP450 1A Possible interactions with nephrotoxic drugs or drugs that are excreted renally, e.g. ganciclovir, cidofovir, probenecid Co-administration with didanosine causes an increase in didanosine levels (↑ ddI dose) Co-administration with Kaletra® causes ↑ in Kaletra® levels and ≠ in tenofovir
Trizivir⌒	One tablet bd	Tablet contains abacavir 300 mg, lamivudine 150 mg and zidovudine 300 mg	See entries under individual drugs Patients who have had a hypersensitivity reaction to abacavir must NEVER be rechallenged with abacavir or Trizivir	See entries under individual drugs
Truvada⌒	One tablet od	Tablet contains emtricitabine 200 mg, tenofovir disoproxil 245 mg	See entries under individual drugs	See entries under individual drugs
Zidovudine (AZT) Retrovir⌒	Usual dose 250 mg bd (300 mg bd in Combivir & Trizivir) 100 mg, 250 mg capsules 50 mg/5 mL syrup	Can be taken with/after food to reduce GI side effects	– nausea, vomiting, headache, fatigue and muscle pain more common in first few weeks and usually wear off – haematological toxicities, e.g. neutropenia, anaemia, may develop after approximately 6 weeks – myopathy may be associated with long-term therapy (>12 months) – lipoatrophy lactic acidosis	Take >1 hour apart from clarithromycin (can ↑ zidovudine absorption) Monitor phenytoin levels Myelotoxic drugs, e.g. ganciclovir/valganciclovir and high-dose co-trimoxazole, may worsen neutropenia Fluconazole and probenecid may ≠ zidovudine levels Do not use with stavudine

od, once daily; bd, twice daily; e/c, enteric coated; GI, gastrointestinal; caps, capsules

Table 41.3 General prescribing points for non-nucleoside reverse transcriptase inhibitors (NNRTIs)

Drug	Dose and formulation	Administration	Side effects	Drug interactions and pharmacokinetic information
Efavirenz (EFV) Sustiva⌒	600 mg od usually at night – oral solution has lower bioavailability than tabs or caps: equivalent dose 720 mg od (24 mL) – increase to 800 mg od with rifampicin 600 mg tablets 200 mg capsules 30 mg/mL oral solution	Can be taken with or without food. Taking with fatty food may increase bioavailability and toxicity. Taken at night to minimize sedative effect, but can be taken during the day if preferred	– CNS disturbances ranging from sedation, feeling[6] stoned[3], dizzy and impaired concentration to vivid dreams, mood swings and hallucinations. Warn patients about not driving if affected – caution in patients with previous or current psychiatric illness – rash in about 18% of adults, mostly in first 2 weeks, usually mild; severe rash rare – raised LFTs more common if hepatitis B or C co-infected – hyperlipidaemia: monitor cholesterol – avoid in early pregnancy; animal studies show teratogenic effects; effective contraception must be used	Caution on stopping efavirenz - containing regimen due to long half-life Recommend switching efavirenz to an agent with a shorter $t_{1/2}$ for 4 weeks before stopping entire regimen Mixed inhibitor and inducer of CYP3A4 (usual net effect is induction) Inhibits 2B6 and 3A4 (plus 2C9 & 2C19) in vitro. Caution with other drugs metabolized by or inducers of these enzymes; use alternatives wherever possible. TDM required on potentially affected drugs where indicated, e.g. phenytoin, Do not co-administer with St John's wort, carbamazepine or voriconazole Increases levels of midazolam. Avoid or start with low doses and titrate and monitor carefully; do not use in outpatients, caution in day case attenders. (Manufacturer says contra-indicated) Methadone dose may require increase monitor closely May increase levels of amfebutamone/bupropion May affect warfarin levels; monitor INR
Nevirapine (NVP) Viramune⌒	200 mg od for first 14 days then 200 mg bd 400 mg od (only after ≥6 wks to reduce risk of liver toxicity) - unlicensed dose 200 mg bd initially if switching from efavirenz (unlicensed dose) 200 mg tablets 50 mg/5 mL oral suspension	Can be taken with or without food. If dosing interrupted for >7 days NVP must be restarted at lead-in dose (200 mg od for 2 weeks)	– rash in about 20%; most common in first 6 weeks, can often treat through; do NOT ≠ dose if patient has rash – raised LFTs/hepatitis; check every 2 weeks for first 2 months – caution on restarting nevirapine if previously discontinued due to rash or hepatitis/raised LFTs – also nausea, headache, sedation, fatigue – caution: greater risk of rash-associated hepatic events if starting in women with CD4 >250 cells/mm³ or men with CD4 >400 cells/mm³; avoid in these patients	Caution on stopping a nevirapine-containing regimen due to long half-life Recommend switching nevirapine to an agent with a shorter $t_{1/2}$ for 4 weeks before stopping entire regimen CYP450 inducer. Caution with drugs metabolized by or inducers of CYP3A4 & 2B6 Do not co-administer with St John's wort as it reduces nevirapine levels Methadone dose may require alteration: monitor closely May reduce levels of erectile dysfunction agents sildenafil, tadalafil, vardenafil May reduce levels of amfebutamone/bupropion May affect warfarin levels; monitor INR May reduce efficacy of hormonal contraception Perform TDM with Kaletra® (May require increase in PI dose, especially PI resistance). may decrease levels of other perform TDM and adjust dose accordingly Rifampicin decreases nevirapine levels TDM on potentially affected drugs

od, once daily; bd, twice daily; TDM, therapeutic drug monitoring; LFTs, liver function tests; INR, international normalized ratio; $t_{1/2}$, plasma half-life

Table 41.4 General prescribing points for protease inhibitors and fusion inhibitors

Drug	Dose and formulation	Administration	Side effects	Drug interactions and pharmacokinetic information
Protease inhibitors				
Atazanavir Reyataz[3]	300 mg with 100 mg ritonavir od 400 mg with 100 mg ritonavir od with enzyme inducers 400 mg od if without ritonavir (not recommended) 200 mg capsules 150 mg capsules	Take with or after food to enhance bioavailability	Most common: nausea, diarrhoea, headache, rash, jaundice Also – hyperbilirubinaemia – raised LFTs more common in hepatitis B or C co-infection – does not appear to ↑ lipids – ECG changes – other protease inhibitor class side effects, e.g. lipodystrophy syndrome	Mainly metabolized by CYP450 3A4 (rifampicin contraindicated, avoid St John's wort) in vitro – moderate inhibitor of CYP 3A4. Also competitively inhibits CYP1A2 & CYP2C9. Caution with other drugs metabolized by this route as may get ≠ in levels Do NOT co-administer with simvastatin, triazolam and ergotamines. Increases levels of midazolam; avoid or start with low dose and titrate and monitor carefully; do not use in outpatients, caution in day case attenders. Manufacturer advises avoid May increase levels of corticosteroids, including inhaled/intranasal steroids (avoid fluticasone) May require dose alteration of: warfarin (monitor INR), methadone, amfebutamone/bupropion H₂-antagonists and proton pump inhibitors significantly decrease atazanavir. Avoid antacids within 2 hours of atazanavir dose No data yet on co-administration with nevirapine; avoid if possible May reduce efficacy of hormonal contraception Caution with erectile dysfunction agents sildenafil, tadalafil and vardenafil: reduce initial dose (e.g. max. dose sildenafil 25 mg in 48 h) If boosted, see ritonavir for full list of potential interactions
Darunavir (TMC-114) Prezista®	600 mg bd with ritonavir 100 mg bd 300 mg tablets	Take with food to improve bioavailability	Most common: nausea, vomiting diarrhoea, constipation, abdominal pain, headache, hyperlipidaemia Also – raised LFTs – other protease inhibitor class side effects, e.g. lipodystrophy syndrome	Metabolized by CYP450 3A4 (rifampicin contraindicated, avoid St John's wort, carbamazepine) Inhibitor of CYP450 3A4; caution with other drugs metabolized by this route as may get ≠ in levels. Do NOT co-administer with simvastatin, triazolam, ergotamines Increases levels of midazolam; avoid or start with low dose and titrate and monitor carefully; do not use in outpatients, caution in day case attenders. Manufacturer advises avoid May increase levels of corticosteroids, including inhaled/intranasal steroids; avoid fluticasone

continued

Table 41.4 (continued)

Drug	Dose and formulation	Administration	Side effects	Drug interactions and pharmacokinetic information
Darunavir (TMC-114) Prezista® (continued)				Increases rifabutin levels; reduce rifabutin dosing to 3 times a week May require dose alteration of: warfarin (monitor INR); methadone; amfebutamone/bupropion No dose adjustment of darunavir required with efavirenz or nevirapine Until further information available, avoid co-administration with Kaletra®, saquinavir; caution with pravastatin, SSRIs May reduce efficacy of hormonal contraception Caution with erectile dysfunction agents sildenafil, tadalafil and vardenafil; reduce initial dose (e.g. max. dose sildenafil 25 mg in 48 h) See ritonavir for full list of potential interactions
Fosamprenavir Telzir⌒	700 mg bd with 100 mg bd ritonavir Unlicensed doses for PI-experienced – 1400 mg od with 200 mg od ritonavir – 1400 mg bd unboosted 700 mg tablets 50 mg/mL oral suspension	Can be taken with or without food	Most common: nausea & vomiting, diarrhoea, rash, fatigue Also – raised LFTs – hyperlipidaemia – other protease inhibitor class side effects, e.g. lipodystrophy syndrome	Metabolized by CYP450 3A4 (rifampicin contraindicated, avoid St John's wort) Inhibitor of CYP450 3A4; caution with other drugs metabolized by this route as may get ≠ in levels. Do NOT co-administer with simvastatin, triazolam, ergotamines, amiodarone Increases levels of midazolam; avoid or start with low dose and titrate and monitor carefully; do not use in outpatients, caution in day case attenders. Manufacturer advises avoid May increase levels of corticosteroids, including inhaled/intranasal steroids; avoid fluticasone May require dose alteration of: warfarin (monitor INR); methadone; amfebutamone/bupropion Co-administration of efavirenz and nevirapine may reduce levels; TDM recommended Complex interaction with Kaletra®, recommend starting dosefosamprenavir 700 mg with ritonavir100 mg bd plus standard Kaletra® dose; TDM at 2 weeks May reduce efficacy of hormonal contraception. Caution with erectile dysfunction agents sildenafil and tadalafil; reduce initial dose (e.g. max. dose sildenafil 25 mg in 48 h); avoid vardenafil If boosted, see ritonavir for full list of potential interactions
Indinavir Crixivan⌒	800 mg 8 hourly With ritonavir: 800 mg with 100 or 200 mg ritonavir bd; or 400 mg with 400 mg	Best on an empty stomach >1 hour before food or >2 hours after meals May take with light, low fat (<5 g fat) snacks (diet booklet available)	– nephrolithiasis – hyperbilirubinaemia – increase in LFTs – rash, dry skin, pruritus, hair loss	Metabolized by CYP450 3A4 (rifampicin contraindicated, avoid St John's wort, carbamazepine) Inhibits CYP450 3A4 and may increase levels of

Drug	Dose	Food/storage	Side effects	Interactions/cautions
ritonavir bd ↑ dose in hepatic insufficiency 200 mg & 400 mg capsules	No food restrictions if with ritonavir Store with desiccant Drink >1.5 L water per day even if taking with ritonavir	– ingrown toenails – taste perversion – haemolytic anaemia – other protease inhibitor class side effects, e.g. lipodystrophy syndrome	other drugs metabolized by this system Do NOT co-administer with: simvastatin, triazolam, ergotamines Increases levels of midazolam; avoid or start with low dose and titrate and monitor carefully; do not use in outpatients, caution in day case attenders. Manufacturer advises avoid May increase levels of corticosteroids, including inhaled/intranasal steroids; avoid fluticasone May require dose alteration of: warfarin (monitor INR); methadone; amfebutamone/bupropion Ketoconazole and itraconazole ≠ indinavir levels Interaction with rifabutin; halve rifabutin dose, ≠ indinavir to 1000 mg 8 hourly Co-administration of efavirenz and nevirapine may reduce levels Administer indinavir and didanosine tablets at least 1 hour apart (OK to take with e/c caps) Caution with erectile dysfunction agents sildenafil and tadalafil; reduce initial dose (max. dose sildenafil 25 mg in 48 h); avoid vardenafil If boosted, see ritonavir for full list of potential interactions	
Kaletra⌐ Lopinavir/ ritonavir	2 tablets bd 3 tablets bd + TDM if with NNRTI and PI resistance 4 tablets (if no PI resistance and not with NNRTI) unlicensed dose 3 capsules bd 4 capsules bd with efavirenz and nevirapine Tablets: 200 mg lopinavir with 50 mg ritonavir Capsules: 133.3 mg lopinavir co-formulated with 33.3 mg ritonavir 400/100 mg lopinavir/ritonavir in 5 mL oral solution	Tablets: no food restrictions Capsules and liquid: take with or after food Capsules do not contain ethanol, unlike ritonavir caps Oral solution has high alcohol content; do not administer with disulfiram or metronidazole Store capsules and liquid in refrigerator (stable at <25°C for 6 weeks) Tablets: store at room temperature	Most common: diarrhoea, nausea, vomiting, bloating, headache, dyslipidaemias – raised LFTs – other protease inhibitor class side effects, e.g. lipodystrophy syndrome Contains low-dose ritonavir so potentially the same range of side effects, though less severe	Metabolized by CYP450 3A4 (rifampicin contraindicated, avoid St John's wort, carbamazepine) Lopinavir is a moderate inhibitor of CYP 3A4, ritonavir is a potent inhibitor of CYP3A4 and also affects other isoenzymes. Caution with other drugs metabolized by this route as may get ≠ in levels. Do NOT co-administer with simvastatin, triazolam, ergotamines Increases levels of midazolam; avoid or start with low dose and titrate and monitor carefully; do not use in outpatients, caution in day case attenders. Manufacturer advises avoid May increase levels of corticosteroids, including inhaled/intranasal steroids; avoid fluticasone Increases rifabutin levels; reduce rifabutin dosing to 3 times a week May require dose alteration of: warfarin (monitor INR); methadone; amfebutamone/bupropion Nevirapine and efavirenz reduce lopinavir levels (increase dose of Kaletra®)

continued

Table 41.4 (continued)

Drug	Dose and formulation	Administration	Side effects	Drug interactions and pharmacokinetic information
Kaletra ® Lopinavir/ ritonavir (continued)				May reduce efficacy of hormonal contraception Caution with erectile dysfunction agents sildenafil, tadalafil and vardenafil; reduce initial dose (e.g. max. dose sildenafil 25 mg in 48 h) See ritonavir for full list of potential interactions
Nelfinavir (NFV) Viracept	1250 mg bd 750 mg tds 250 mg tablets	Take with or after food to increase bioavailability (up to 2 hours after full meal or with/just after small meal/snack)	Most common: diarrhoea and flatulence, nausea Also: – hyperglycaemia/ diabetes – other protease inhibitor class side effects, e.g. lipodystrophy syndrome	Metabolized by CYP450 3A4 (also 2C9, 2C19 & 2D6) (rifampicin contraindicated, avoid St John's wort, carbamazepine) Weak CYP450 inhibitor; caution with other drugs metabolized by this route as may get ≠ in levels. Do NOT use with triazolam, ergotamines, amiodarone and quinidine Increases levels of midazolam; avoid or start with low dose and titrate and monitor carefully; do not use in outpatients, caution in day case attenders. Manufacturer advises avoid May increase levels of corticosteroids, including inhaled/intranasal steroids; avoid fluticasone May require dose alteration of: warfarin (monitor INR); methadone; amfebutamone/bupropion Halve rifabutin dose Caution with erectile dysfunction agents sildenafil and tadalafil; reduce initial dose (max. dose sildenafil 25 mg in 48 h); avoid vardenafil May reduce efficacy of hormonal contraception
Ritonavir (RTV) Norvir	600 mg bd Escalate dose over 2 weeks to ↑ side effects, e.g. 300 mg bd 4 days, 400 mg bd 4 days, 500 mg bd 4 days, then 600 mg bd thereafter Normally used to boost other protease inhibitors at doses of 100–200 mg od-bd 100 mg capsules, 400 mg/5 mL oral solution	Do not administer liquid formulation with disulfiram or metronidazole due to high alcohol content; caps OK with metronidazole Take with or after food if possible to reduce GI intolerance. May mix oral solution with chocolate milk within 1 h of dosing Store capsules in refrigerator (stable at <25°C for up to 28 days) Solution stored at room temperature	– asthenia, – nausea, vomiting – diarrhoea, – anorexia – abdominal pain – taste perversion, – circumoral and peripheral paraesthesiae – other protease inhibitor class side effects, e.g. lipodystrophy syndrome	Metabolized by CYP450 3A4 & 2D6 (rifampicin contraindicated, avoid St John's wort) Ritonavir can cause increases or decreases in the level of other drugs; induces CYP450 1A2. Caution with theophylline due to potential for decreased levels Its inhibitory effect is commonly used to pharmacokinetically enhance ('boost') other inhibitors. Care should be taken when stopping ritonavir to ensure that this does not result in subtherapeutic levels of other drugs Potent inhibitor of CYP 450 3A4, 2D6, 2C9 and 2C19. Caution with other drugs metabolized by this route. Due to potential for ≠ levels, do NOT co-administer with simvastatin, rifabutin, pethidine, amiodarone, dextropropoxyphene, piroxicam, triazolam, ergotamines and amphetamines (including ecstasy).

continued

Drug	Dose	Administration	Side effects	Interactions
				Caution with diazepam, azole antifungals, and clarithromycin Increases levels of midazolam; avoid or start with low dose and titrate and monitor carefully; do not use in outpatients or day case attenders. Manufacturer advises avoid May increase levels of corticosteroids, including inhaled/intranasal steroids; avoid fluticasone May require dose alteration of: warfarin (monitor INR); methadone; amfebutamone/bupropion Caution with erectile dysfunction agents sildenafil, tadalafil and vardenafil; reduce initial dose (e.g. max. dose sildenafil 25 mg in 48 h) May reduce efficacy of hormonal contraception
Saquinavir (SQV) Invirase⌒	1000 mg with 100 mg ritonavir bd – 400 mg with 400 mg ritonavir bd – 1500–2000 mg od with 100 mg ritonavir od 200 mg capsules, 500 mg tablets	Take with or after food (up to 2 h after a full meal)	– diarrhoea – nausea – abdominal discomfort/wind – raised LFTs – other protease inhibitor class side effects, e.g. lipodystrophy syndrome	Metabolized by CYP450 3A4 (rifampicin contraindicated, avoid St John's wort, carbamazepine, phenytoin, rifabutin) Inhibits CYP450 3A4 so can ≠ levels of drugs metabolized by this system. Do NOT use with simvastatin, ergotamines. May raise levels of dapsone, clindamycin, calcium channel blockers, quinidine Increases levels of midazolam; avoid or start with low dose and titrate and monitor carefully; do not use in outpatients, caution in day case attenders May increase levels of corticosteroids, including inhaled/intranasal steroids (avoid fluticasone) May require dose alteration of: warfarin (monitor INR); methadone; bupropion (Zyban) Co-administration of clarithromycin, ketoconazole, ranitidine or cimetidine may increase levels of saquinavir May reduce efficacy of hormonal contraception Caution with erectile dysfunction agents sildenafil, tadalafil and vardenafil; reduce initial dose (e.g. max. dose sildenafil 25 mg in 48 h) If boosted, see ritonavir for full list of potential interactions
Tipranavir Aptivus⌒	500 mg bd: co-administer with 200 mg bd ritonavir 250 mg capsules	Take with or after food to improve GI tolerance Store in refrigerator; once opened, container may be stored below	– diarrhoea – nausea, vomiting – fatigue – headache	Metabolized by CYP450 3A4 (rifampicin contraindicated, avoid St John's wort) Do not use without ritonavir. Do not use in combination with any other protease inhibitor

Table 41.4 (continued)

Drug	Dose and formulation	Administration	Side effects	Drug interactions and pharmacokinetic information
Tripanavir Aplivus (continued)		30°C for 60 days	– elevated LFTs – other protease inhibitor class side effects, e.g. lipodystrophy syndrome	Tipranavir co-administered with low-dose ritonavir inhibits CYP450 3A (2D6 to a lesser extent). Caution with other drugs metabolized by this route as may get ≠ in levels Do NOT co-administer with simvastatin, triazolam and ergotamines Increases levels of midazolam; avoid or start with low dose and titrate and monitor carefully; do not use in outpatients, caution in day case attenders. Manufacturer advises avoid May increase levels of corticosteroids, including inhaled/intranasal steroids; avoid fluticasone May require dose alteration of: warfarin (monitor INR); methadone; amfebutamone/bupropion May reduce efficacy of hormonal contraception Caution with erectile dysfunction agents sildenafil, tadalafil and vardenafil; reduce initial dose (e.g. max. dose sildenafil 25 mg in 48 h) See ritonavir for full list of potential interactions
Fusion inhibitors				
Enfuvirtide (T-20) Fuzeon⌐	90 mg bd Ideally every 12 h but dosing interval of 8–16 h allowed, i.e. 4 h flexibility for each dose 90 mg/mL powder and solvent for solution for s/c injection Each vial contains 108 mg enfuvirtide 1 mL of reconstituted solution contains 90 mg enfuvirtide	Single-use vials: reconstitute with 1.1 mL water for injection (may take up to 45 minutes to dissolve powder, do not shake vial) Once reconstituted, can be stored in fridge for 24 h (i.e. can make up more than 1 dose at once)	– injection site reactions very common and include pain/discomfort, erythema, nodules and cysts but do not usually require discontinuation – other common side effects: insomnia, headache, lymphadenopathy, eosinophilia – increased rate of bacterial infections (especially pneumonia) reported – hypersensitivity reactions requiring discontinuation reported, but rare	No clinically significant pharmacokinetic interactions expected

od, once daily; bd, twice daily; tds, three times daily; s/c, subcutaneous; INR, international normalized ratio; TDM, therapeutic drug monitoring; e/c, enteric coated; ECG, electrocardiogram

The BHIVA does not advocate the routine use of therapeutic drug monitoring but recommends that blood levels of protease inhibitors and NNRTIs should be measured in selected patients, e.g. during pregnancy, where there is liver impairment, and where there are concerns regarding potentially interacting drugs (Gazzard et al 2005).

HIV mutates readily and resistance to antiretrovirals develops rapidly in the face of suboptimal treatment, e.g. monotherapy or subtherapeutic blood levels. A high level of adherence to the prescribed regimen is therefore of major importance.

Treatment interruptions

For many reasons, including toxicity, cost and adherence, patients and clinicians have been interested in considering' drug holidays' or treatment interruptions. However, it is recognized that there are dangers with this approach because of CD4 decline and disease progression, and viral load rebound which is associated with increased transmission risk and a seroconversion-like syndrome. Furthermore, since different anti-HIV medications have different half-lives there may be a risk of functional monotherapy, particularly with NNRTIs, and the development of resistance if combinations are stopped abruptly in an unplanned fashion.

Nucleoside and nucleotide analogue reverse transcriptase inhibitors

NRTIs are phosphorylated intracellularly and then inhibit the viral reverse transcriptase enzyme by acting as a false substrate. Nucleotide analogues only require two intracellular phosphorylations, whereas activation of nucleoside analogues is a three-stage process. The NRTIs licensed in the UK include:

- abacavir (Ziagen)
- didanosine (ddI, Videx)
- emtricitabine (FTC, Emtriva)
- lamivudine (3TC, Epivir)
- stavudine (d4T, Zerit)
- tenofovir (Viread)
- zidovudine (AZT, Retrovir).

In addition, there are a number of combination formulations of NRTI's that may be used to reduce the number of tablets/capsules to be taken each day:

- abacavir plus lamivudine (Kivexa)
- emtricitabine plus tenofovir (Truvada)
- zidovudine plus lamivudine (Combivir)
- zidovudine plus lamivudine plus abacavir (Trizivir).

Most antiretroviral regimens will include two NRTIs, together with a protease inhibitor and/or a NNRTI. The most commonly prescribed NRTIs as first-line therapy are the combination formulations, with Kivexa and Truvada having the benefits of once-daily administration and an improved toxicity profile compared to other therapies. A number of combinations should be avoided. These include zidovudine and stavudine (intracellular competition resulting in antagonism); stavudine and didanosine (unacceptable toxicity); tenofovir and didanosine (unacceptable rates of virological failure and potential for CD4 decline).

Non-nucleoside reverse transcriptase inhibitors

NNRTIs inhibit the reverse transcriptase enzyme by binding to its active site. They do not require prior phosphorylation and can act on cell-free virions as well as infected cells. The NNRTIs available include:

- efavirenz (Sustiva)
- nevirapine (Viramune).

Resistance to NNRTIs occurs rapidly in incompletely suppressive regimens and it is therefore essential that they are prescribed with at least two NRTIs or a combination of NRTIs and protease inhibitors. Cross-resistance between these agents is high and therefore a number of second-generation NNRTIs are currently under development which may possess a different resistance profile. Efavirenz and nevirapine both have much longer plasma half-lives than protease inhibitors and NRTIs, so when stopping an NNRTI-containing combination, consideration should be given to either continuing the other agents for a period after cessation of the NNRTI or switching to a boosted protease inhibitor prior to regimen discontinuation. Second-generation NNRTIs e.g. etravirine that are active against virus resistant to the currently available agents are in clinical development.

Protease inhibitors

Protease inhibitors bind to the active site of the HIV-1 protease enzyme, preventing the maturation of the newly produced virions so that they remain non-infectious. The following protease inhibitors are currently available:

- atazanavir (Reyataz)
- darunavir (Prezista)
- fosamprenavir (Telzir)
- indinavir (Crixivan)
- lopinavir and ritonavir (Kaletra)
- nelfinavir (Viracept)
- ritonavir (Norvir)
- saquinavir (Invirase)
- tipranavir (Aptivus).

The use of ritonavir boosted protease inhibitors has superseded use of single protease inhibitors, due to better pharmacokinetic profiles, superior efficacy data and reduced likelihood of resistance development. Protease inhibitors may be used in multiple combinations but drug interactions can be complex and unpredictable. Newer second-generation protease inhibitors such as tipranavir and darunavir are effective against viruses resistant to many of the earlier protease inhibitors.

Entry inhibitors

There are currently two types of entry inhibitors – fusion inhibitors and CCR-5 inhibitors – with one agent available in each class. Enfuvirtide (T-20, Fuzeon), a fusion inhibitor, is administered subcutaneously and is largely used in heavily treatment-experienced patients, with the best results seen when it is used with at least two other active agents. Whilst the main side effect is injection site reactions, these do not usually lead to treatment discontinuation. Maraviroc is the first CCR-5 inhibitor to become available (currently unlicensed) but the place of this group of agents remains unclear.

New classes of antiretroviral agents and approaches to therapy

Various new classes of drugs are currently in both clinical and preclinical stages of development and are likely to increase the anti-HIV armamentarium over the next few years. These include:

- attachment blockers
- integrase inhibitors (e.g. raltegravir)
- maturation inhibitors.

In addition, newer strategies for treating HIV are likely to be more widely studied, including:

- immunomodulatory therapies (including interleukin-2 [IL-2], granulocyte macrophage colony stimulating factor [GM-CSF] and pegylated interferon α)
- adjunctive therapeutic vaccines.

Toxicity of antiretroviral therapies

As more antiretroviral agents have become available and the number of patient-years of exposure to them has increased, our understanding of their various toxicities has grown significantly.

Whilst there are many individual drug toxicities (see Tables 41.2, 41.3 and 41.4), there are also a number of class-specific or therapy-related toxicities (Carr & Cooper 2000).

Mitochondrial toxicity Mitochondrial toxicity is increasingly recognized in patients with prolonged exposure to nucleoside analogue antiretrovirals, particularly stavudine, didanosine and, to a lesser extent, zidovudine, and is thought to explain such side effects as peripheral neuropathy, myopathy, pancreatitis and lactic acidosis. If these problems should arise, management is to switch the likely causative agent, if possible (McComsey & Lonergan 2004).

Rash and hepatitis These are both recognized side effects of the NNRTI class, although the incidence and severity appear greatest with nevirapine, particularly in patients with a higher CD4 count (>250 cells/mm^3 for women and >400 cells/mm^3 for men). Management is either close observation (in mild-to-moderate cases) or withdrawal of the causative agent (in severe cases). An abacavir hypersensitivity reaction is well characterized and historically occurs in approximately 6–8% of individuals who receive abacavir. It typically presents in the first 6 weeks of therapy as a progressive illness with fevers, rash and flu-like symptoms. Fatalities have been reported where the drug has subsequently been reintroduced in patients with a prior history of hypersensitivity reaction. Management has traditionally been to withdraw the agent and never reintroduce. However, the use of newer pharmacogenomic techniques, e.g. HLA B*5701 testing, and subsequent prescription of abacavir only to those who are B*5701 negative have dramatically reduced the incidence of hypersensitivity reaction.

Lipodystrophy Lipodystrophy has been well reported in individuals on HAART. This is characterized by one or both of: lipoatrophy (fat loss, particularly from the face, upper limbs and buttocks) and lipohypertrophy (abnormal fat deposition, particularly affecting the abdomen and neck). Whilst these body shape changes are associated with drug therapy, predominantly stavudine and zidovudine for lipoatrophy and protease inhibitors for lipohypertrophy, it is likely that host and disease factors also play a role in aetiology (Carr 2003, Lichtenstein 2005). Management at present is to avoid or switch away from the causative agent(s) and or to use cosmetic approaches (fillers or liposuction).

Metabolic disturbances Hypercholesterolaemia and hypertriglyceridaemia in particular are frequently seen in patients receiving HAART. Again, the aetiology of these toxicities is likely to represent a combination of drug and host factors but they are particularly associated with protease inhibitors, with the possible exception of atazanavir, and stavudine. Whilst it is likely that this hyperlipidaemia contributes to an increased cardiovascular disease risk, this needs to be considered in the context of traditional risk factors, e.g. smoking, which may be present in this patient group. Management is to reduce all modifiable risk factors and either switch away from the likely causative agent to one more metabolically friendly or consider adjunctive lipid-lowering therapy, taking into consideration potential drug–drug interactions (Schambelan et al 2002).

Renal impairment and, rarely, Fanconi's syndrome have been reported with tenofovir. Creatinine clearance should be calculated prior to starting therapy with this agent and renal function must be monitored regularly and the dose adjusted appropriately.

Opportunistic infections and malignancies

Selected drugs used to treat opportunistic infections are summarized in Table 41.5.

Fungal infections

***Pneumocystis jiroveci* pneumonia** This remains one of the most common causes of morbidity and mortality in HIV-positive individuals. Classically, patients present with an insidious onset of a non-productive cough, shortness of breath on exertion and an inability to take a deep breath. Fever, anorexia and weight loss are common accompanying symptoms. Patients are usually markedly immunosuppressed, with CD4 counts less than 200 cells/mm^3. Diagnosis is supported by the presence of exercise-induced oxygen desaturation and the typical chest radiographic appearance of bilateral interstitial shadowing, though in mild cases the chest x-ray may be normal. The diagnosis is confirmed by demonstration of the organism by immunofluorescence or silver staining of samples obtained by sputum induction (by nebulization of hypertonic sodium chloride) or bronchoalveolar lavage.

Treatment is instigated in patients with a proven diagnosis, or empirically where there is a suspicion prior to confirmation. Oxygen is essential for patients with compromised respiratory function. First-line therapy is high-dose co-trimoxazole (120 mg/kg/day in divided doses), orally in mild cases and intravenously in moderate-to-severe disease. Nausea and vomiting commonly occur and may be best managed pre-emptively by administration of a prophylactic antiemetic.

Table 41.5   Selected drugs to treat opportunistic infections in HIV disease

Drug	Indication	Dosage: route, frequency, duration	Common or significant side effects include:	Significant interactions	Monitoring	Comments
Aciclovir	Herpes simplex	5–10 mg/kg i.v. three times daily for 5–10 days 200–400 mg po five times daily for 5–10 days	Nausea, vomiting, abdominal pain, diarrhoea Skin rash, abnormal LFTs, extravasation (i.v.), renal impairment (i.v.)	Ciclosporin, mycophenolate mofetil, tacrolimus, probenecid	Renal function (when administered i.v.)	Higher dose and longer duration for herpes encephalitis or varicella zoster Patients on HAART with CD4 >300 may be treated as for non-immunocompromised Intravenous infusion diluted to 0.5% w/v and infused over at least 1 h to reduce likelihood of renal toxicity
	Herpes zoster	10 mg/kg i.v. three times daily for 5–10 days 800 mg po five times daily for 7 days				
	Prophylaxis/suppression of herpes infections	200–400 mg po twice daily				
Amphotericin A. sodium deoxycholate complex B. liposomal C. sodium cholesteryl sulfate complex D. lipid complex	Cryptococcal meningitis and other severe fungal infections	A. 0.25–1 mg/kg (increased over 3–5 days as tolerated) i.v. once daily B. 1–3 mg/kg (increased over 2–3 days) i.v. once daily C. 1–4 mg/kg (increased over 2–3 days) i.v. once daily D. 5 mg/kg i.v. once daily 2–6 weeks	Fever, chills, nausea and vomiting, headache, anorexia, weight loss, malaise, myalgia, thrombophlebitis, epigastric pain, diarrhoea, renal impairment, hypokalaemia, hypomagnesaemia, anaemia	Nephrotoxic drugs, antineoplastics, corticosteroids	Renal function, FBC, U+Es	Test dose required before first infusion with any parenteral amphotericin All i.v. preparations administered in 5% glucose Pre- and posthydration with 0.9% sodium chloride may decrease nephrotoxicity Liposomal, colloidal cholesteryl sulfate and lipid complex formulations generally better tolerated
Atovaquone suspension	Treatment of mild-to-moderate PCP Prophylaxis of PCP[a] Treatment of toxoplasmosis[a]	750 mg po twice daily with food for 3 weeks 750 mg bd 1.5 g po twice daily for at least 6 weeks[b]	Nausea, rash, diarrhoea, vomiting, headache, insomnia, fever, increased LFTs, decreased sodium, anaemia, neutropenia	Indinavir, metoclopramide, rifampicin, rifabutin, tetracycline[b]	LFTs, U+Es, FBC	Absorption improved by taking with food (especially high-fat food); absorption reduced by diarrhoea
Azithromycin	Atypical *Mycobacterium* infections[a], toxoplasmosis[a] and PCP (adjunctive therapy or part of combination regimen)	500 mg po daily for MAI treatment or PCP prophylaxis; 1250 mg po once weekly for MAI prophylaxis[b], 1200–1250 mg daily for toxoplasmosis treatment[b]	Nausea, vomiting, abdominal discomfort, anorexia, dyspepsia, flatulence, diarrhoea, constipation, raised LFTs. Rare: ototoxocity	Antacids, theophylline, coumarins[a] ciclosporin artemether/lumefantrine, ergot derivatives, digoxin, bromocriptine, cabergoline, reboxetine, oestrogens	LFTs, hearing (if on long-term or high-dose therapy)	Less significant drug interactions than with the other macrolides
Cidofovir	Cytomegalovirus retinitis	5 mg/kg weekly for two doses then every 2 weeks thereafter	Renal impairment, neutropenia, ocular hypotony, iritis/uveitis, nausea, vomiting	Other nephrotoxic drugs, agents that are contraindicated with probenecid, tenofovir	Renal function (including urine protein), neutrophils	Co-administer with probenecid and intravenous fluids Caution with handling Avoid if on tenofovir

continued

Table 41.5 (continued)

Drug	Indication	Dosage: route, frequency, duration	Common or significant side effects include:	Significant interactions	Monitoring	Comments
Clindamycin	Treatment of PCP Toxoplasmosis treatment Toxoplasmosis maintenance	600 mg i.v./po four times daily for 3 weeks 600 mg i.v./po four times daily for at least 6 weeks 1.2 g po daily in 3–4 divided doses	Diarrhoea, abdominal discomfort, oesophagitis, nausea, vomiting, rash, abnormal LFTs, thrombophlebitis (i.v.).Rarely: pseudomembranous colitis, blood dyscrasias	Non-depolarizing muscle relaxants, suxamethonium, oestrogens, pyridostigmine, neostigmine, erythromycin	LFTs, renal function, FBC, diarrhoea	Taken with primaquine for PCP Taken with pyrimethamine for toxoplasmosis Higher doses may be used if previous failure of co-trimoxazole (for PCP) or sulfadiazine (for toxoplasmosis)[b]
Co-trimoxazole (trimethoprim + sulfamethoxazole)	Treatment of PCP Prophylaxis of PCP	120 mg/kg i.v/po in 2–4 divided doses for 3 weeks 480 or 960 mg daily or 960 mg three times per week (960 mg daily if on rifampicin)	Nausea, diarrhoea, headache, rash, hyperkalaemia, vomiting. Rare: drug fever, blood dyscrasias, serious skin reactions, e.g. Stevens–Johnson syndrome	Amiodarone, oestrogens, pyrimethamine, rifampicin, ciclosporin, lamivudine, phenytoin, azathioprine, mercaptopurine, methotrexate, sulfonylureas	FBC, renal function, LFTs, rash	For infusion dilute each 480 mg with 125 mL of glucose 5% or sodium chloride 0.9% and infuse over 1.5–3 h If fluid restricted, 480 mg in 75 mL of glucose 5% Caution in G6PD deficiency
Dapsone	Prophylaxis of PCP Treatment of PCP[a]	100 mg po daily (with trimethoprim) 15 mg/kg/day in divided doses for PCP treatment)	Anorexia, nausea, vomiting, rash Rare: blood dyscrasias including methaemoglobinaemia; dapsone syndrome	Rifamycins, probenecid, oestrogens, antacids	FBC, LFTs	Caution in G6PD deficiency
Famciclovir	Treatment of herpes zoster Treatment of genital herpes	Doses for immunocompromised patients: zoster use 500 mg three times daily for 10 days; genital herpes all episodes use 500 mg twice daily for 7 days, for suppression 500 mg twice daily	Rare: headache and nausea	Probenecid	Renal function	Patients on HAART with CD4 >300 may be treated as for non-immunocompromised
Fluconazole	Oesophageal candidiasis Oropharyngeal candidiasis Cryptococcal meningitis treatment Cryptococcal meningitis prophylaxis	100 mg po daily for 2 weeks 50 mg po daily for 7–14 days 400 mg i.v./po daily for ≥8 weeks 200 mg po daily	Headache, rash, abdominal pain, diarrhoea, flatulence, nausea, abnormal LFTs, hepatotoxicity	Coumarins, midazolam, sulfonylureas, rifabutin, rifampicin, phenytoin, tacrolimus, ciclosporin, theophylline, zidovudine	Renal function, LFTs	Higher doses have been used for treatment and prophylaxis of candida and cryptococcus infections (depending on clinical response and antifungal sensitivities) i.v. route only necessary if patient nil by mouth
Flucytosine	Cryptococcal meningitis treatment	100 mg/kg daily po/i.v. in four divided doses for 2 weeks (with i.v. amphotericin)	Nausea, vomiting, diarrhoea, rash. Rare: blood dyscrasias, hepatotoxicity	Cytarabine	Renal function, FBC, LFTs	Oral formulation is no longer licensed in the UK but can be imported on named-patient basis
Foscarnet	Cytomegalovirus retinitis treatment	180 mg/kg/day i.v. in 2–3 divided doses (adjust	Renal impairment, alterations in serum calcium, potassium,	Nephrotoxic drugs, drugs that inhibit renal	Renal function, LFTs, plasma magnesium,	Good hydration, prompt correction of electrolyte abnormalities & dose

Drug	Indication	Dose	Side effects	Interactions	Monitoring	Comments
	Cytomegalovirus retinitis maintenance	according to renal function) over 2 hours for 3 weeks 60–120 mg/kg i.v. once daily over 2 hours for 7 days each week	magnesium and other minerals, headache, rash, convulsions, thrombophlebitis, genital ulceration, anaemia, nausea, vomiting, diarrhoea	tubular secretion (e.g. probenecid), i.v. pentamidine	potassium, calcium and phosphate, FBC, U&Es	adjustment for renal function vital. Wash genital area after micturition to reduce risk of ulceration. Give centrally to prevent phlebitis. If infusion-related side effects, reduce rate. Adjust maintenance dose for disease state, drug tolerability and renal function
	Mucocutaneous herpes simplex infection	40 mg/kg i.v. three times daily for 2–3 weeks				
Ganciclovir	Cytomegalovirus induction treatment	5 mg/kg i.v. twice daily for 3 weeks	Blood dyscrasias, anorexia, renal impairment, abnormal LFTs, central nervous system effects, fatigue, nausea, vomiting, flatulence, abdominal pain, dysphagia, dyspepsia, constipation, ear pain, injection site reactions	Zidovudine, didanosine, imipenem-cilastatin, probenecid, mycophenolate mofetil, nephrotoxic drugs, bone marrow suppressive agents	FBC, Renal function, LFTs	Give over 1 h, preferably via central venous access Caution with handling
	Cytomegalovirus retinitis maintenance	5 mg/kg i.v. once every day or 6 mg/kg once daily for 5 days each week				
Peg-interferon α	Hepatitis C (ideally in combination with ribavirin)	See product literature for dose as it varies by brand Weekly s/c injection Usual duration 48 weeks	Anorexia, nausea, influenza-like symptoms, lethargy, depression, ocular side effects, rash, myelosuppression, hypertriglyceridaemia	Theophylline	Lipids, renal function, LFTs, TFTs, U+Es, FBC, blood glucose	Longer duration of treatment in HIV co-infected patients
Pentamidine isetionate	PCP treatment	4 mg/kg i.v. once daily for 3 weeks (+600 mg nebulized for first 3 days)	Intravenous: renal impairment, postural hypotension, leucopenia, hypo/hyperglycaemia, pancreatitis, electrolyte disturbances, nausea, vomiting. Nebulized: cough, bronchospasm	Nephrotoxic drugs, foscarnet, drugs that prolong QT interval, e.g. quinolones, erythromycin	I.V., Renal function, blood glucose, blood pressure, U+Es	Infuse over 1 h with patient supine Caution with handling Pretreat with bronchodilator if nebulized and use special nebulizer
	Mild PCP treatment	600 mg nebulized daily for 3 weeks				
	PCP prophylaxis	300 mg nebulized every 4 weeks				
Primaquine	PCP treatment	15–30 mg po daily for 3 weeks	Nausea, vomiting, anorexia, abdominal pain Rare: methaemoglobinaemia, haemolytic anaemia	Bone marrow suppressive drugs, artemether/ lumefantrine	FBC	Avoid in G6PD deficiency No longer licensed in UK but obtained on named patient barb.
Pyrimethamine	Toxoplasmosis treatment	100 mg on day 1 then 50 mg po once daily for at least 6 weeks	Anaemia, leucopenia, thrombocytopenia, rash	Bone marrow suppressive drugs, antimalarials, methotrexate, antacids, lorazepam, kaolin, highly protein-bound drugs (e.g. coumarins)	FBC	Combined with sulfadiazine or clindamycin. Higher dose can be used if previous treatment failure. Recommend folinic acid 15 mg od to reduce bone marrow suppression.
	Toxoplasmosis maintenance	25 mg po once daily				

continued

Table 41.5 (continued)

Drug	Indication	Dosage: route, frequency, duration	Common or significant side effects include:	Significant interactions	Monitoring	Comments
Ribavirin	Hepatitis C treatment	Dose depends on product, patient weight and hepatitis C genotype	Anaemia, neutropenia, thrombocytopenia. For other side effects reported in combination with peg-interferon α, see above	Stavudine, zidovudine, didanosine, abacavir	FBC, LFTs, renal function	Given with peg-interferon α Colony-stimulating factor support may counteract haematological side effects without requiring dose reduction Teratogenic
Rifabutin	MAI prophylaxis	300 mg od	Abnormal LFTs, nausea, vomiting, bone marrow suppression, arthralgia, myalgia, jaundice Rare: uveitis, risk increased with concomitant administration of drugs that increase rifabutin levels	Coumarins, aripiprazole, atovaquone, dapsone, efavirenz, erythromycin, clarithromycin, protease inhibitors, sirolimus, oral hypoglycaemics, azole and triazole antifungals, disopyramide, quinidine, carbamazepine, oestrogens, progestogens	LFTs, renal function	Combine with at least one other drug for MAI treatment TDM of both agents may be useful when given with Kaletra
	MAI treatment	300–450 mg po once daily with other drugs 150 mg 3 times a week with Kaletra[b]				
Sulfadiazine	Toxoplasmosis treatment[a] Toxoplasmosis maintenance[a]	1–1.5 g i.v./po four times daily for at least 6 weeks 2 g po daily in divided doses	Nausea, vomiting, rash, bone marrow suppression, crystalluria (also see under co-trimoxazole)	Bone marrow suppressive drugs, ciclosporin, oestrogens, coumarins, methenamine	Renal function, LFTs, FBC	Use with pyrimethamine Prevent crystalluria by ensuring good fluid input/output. Alkalinizing urine with sodium bicarbonate may help if crystals formed
Valaciclovir	Herpes zoster treatment Herpes simplex treatment	1 g po three times daily for 7 days 500 mg po twice daily for 5–10 days (initial) or 5 days (recurrent episodes)	Mild headache and nausea (more serious events reported in transplant patients on 8 g/day long term)	Ciclosporin, mycophenolate mofetil, tacrolimus, probenecid	Renal function	Interactions more likely to be significant if renal impairment
Valganciclovir	CMV retinitis	Induction treatment: 900 mg twice a day with food for 3 weeks Maintenance: 900 mg once daily	See ganciclovir; similar potential for side effects except those associated with intravenous administration, e.g. injection site reactions	As for ganciclovir	FBC, renal function, LFTs	

[a] Unlicensed treatment indication in UK; [b] unlicensed dose in UK. FBC, full blood count; U+Es, urea and electrolyte levels; LFTs, liver function tests; MAI, *Mycobacterium avium intracellulare*; G6PD, glucose-6-phosphate dehydrogenase; PCP, *Pneumocystis jiroveci* pneumonia; TFTs, thyroid function tests; CMV, cytomegalovirus; po, oral; i.v., intravenous.

In cases of co-trimoxazole intolerance, several alternative therapies are available. For mild *Pneumocystis jiroveci* pneumonia, a combination of oral trimethoprim (10–15 mg/kg/day in two divided doses) with dapsone (100 mg daily) may be effective. For moderate-to-severe disease a combination of clindamycin (600 mg four times a day, intravenous or oral, depending on severity) and primaquine (30 mg once a day, oral) is often used. Intravenous pentamidine (4 mg/kg/day) is another alternative, though its use may be associated with more significant adverse reactions. Pentamidine should also be given in nebulized form (600 mg) via a suitable nebulizer, e.g. Respirgard II, for the first 3 days, to ensure prompt attainment of adequate lung tissue levels. Oral atovaquone suspension (750 mg twice daily) can be used for mild-to-moderate *Pneumocystis jiroveci* pneumonia but must be taken with food, particularly fatty food, to be effective.

For cases of moderate-to-severe *Pneumocystis jiroveci* pneumonia, adjunctive corticosteroid therapy is recommended, e.g. prednisolone 75 mg daily for 5 days, 50 mg for 5 days then 25 mg for 5 days. Ventilatory support should be considered for patients in whom the underlying prognosis is good, e.g. those presenting for the first time with *Pneumocystis jiroveci* pneumonia, those without severe co-existing medical complications, and those with remaining effective antiretroviral options.

It has been clearly demonstrated that prophylactic therapy reduces both the incidence and severity of *Pneumocystis jiroveci* pneumonia in patients with either prior disease or those at risk of a first episode, and that this intervention significantly improves survival. Primary prophylaxis is recom-mended for those individuals with a previous AIDS-defining illness, markedly symptomatic disease or a CD4 count of less than 200–300 cells/mm^3.

Co-trimoxazole is the gold standard and also confers protection against toxoplasmosis and some other bacterial infections. The optimum dose remains to be determined but commonly used regimens with proven efficacy are 960 mg daily or three times a week or 480 mg daily. The incidence of adverse reactions to co-trimoxazole in HIV-positive individuals is higher than in the general population, although many patients who are intolerant of high-dose treatment do not experience problems at prophylactic doses. In cases of intolerance, several alternative approaches may be adopted. Desensitization may be attempted or other agents may be used. Dapsone 100 mg daily, with or without pyrimethamine, according to *Toxoplasma* status, is effective, as is nebulized pentamidine at a dose of 300 mg every month or 150 mg every 2 weeks via an appropriate nebulizer, with prior nebulized or inhaled β$_2$-agonist to prevent bronchospasm.

Oropharyngeal candidiasis Candidiasis is a frequent mani-festation of HIV infection and may occur early in the disease. Clinically, it is usually characterized by white plaques on the oral mucosa, but may present as erythematous patches or as angular cheilitis. If swallowing is difficult (dysphagia) or painful (odynophagia), oesophageal involvement may be suspected.

First-line therapy for mild oral candidiasis is topical and includes nystatin suspension or pastilles, amphotericin lozenges or suspension, with miconazole gel recommended for patients with dentures. Good oral hygiene, including smoking cessation, should be stressed and adjunctive therapies may be helpful, e.g. chlorhexidine or hydrogen peroxide mouthwashes. For severe cases, or for those who have failed topical therapy, systemic agents, such as fluconazole (50 mg daily) or itraconazole (200 mg once daily), are recommended.

In cases of oesophageal candida, which is an AIDS-defining illness, systemic therapy is necessary using higher doses of the above agents for a longer duration, e.g. fluconazole 100 mg once daily for 2 weeks. Continuous azole therapy or frequent courses of these drugs predispose to the development of azole resistance. In such instances an alternative azole or caspofungin may be used, or occasionally higher than usual doses of the original agent, e.g. fluconazole 400 mg daily. In intractable cases intravenous amphotericin may be required. With the use of HAART such complications are rarely seen.

Cryptococcus neoformans This causes a disseminated infection, usually with meningeal involvement, in individuals with HIV infection. Patients present with fever and headaches, often without the characteristic symptoms of meningism such as photophobia and neck stiffness. Diagnosis is normally made on the basis of cerebrospinal fluid analysis, though serum cryptococcal antigen and blood cultures may also be indicative.

For patients who are moderately or severely unwell, intravenous amphotericin B or a lipid complex/liposomal formulation, with flucytosine (100 mg/kg/day in divided doses, oral or intravenous) is the first-line therapy. Conventional amphotericin is generally administered in 500 mL or 1L of buffered glucose 5% over 4–8 hours. The dose is increased from 0.25 mg/kg to 0.7–1 mg/kg as soon as tolerated. Renal function and serum electrolytes, particularly potassium and magnesium, should be monitored closely and any abnormalities addressed promptly. 'Sodium loading' (pre- and post-amphotericin infusions of sodium chloride 0.9%) may help to reduce nephrotoxicity. Administration of corticosteroids and/or antihistamines may reduce the severity of infusion-related reactions. The usual duration of amphotericin and flucytosine treatment is 2 weeks, after which high-dose fluconazole (400 mg daily orally) should be continued for a further 10 weeks. Subsequent maintenance therapy with fluconazole 200 mg daily has been shown to be efficacious in reducing the incidence of relapse and should be continued for life or until immune function is restored.

In milder cases, fluconazole may be given for the entire duration of treatment. There are a number of liposomal or lipid-complexed formulations of amphotericin available, which are more expensive but less nephrotoxic, and which may be considered in cases of amphotericin intolerance or pre-existing renal impairment. Itraconazole has been used for both treatment and maintenance, but may be less effective than fluconazole.

Protozoal infections

Toxoplasmosis *Toxoplasma gondii* is a frequent cause of central nervous system disease in patients with AIDS. Individuals may present with headaches, fever, confusion, seizures or focal neurological symptoms and signs. Diagnosis is usually based on the appearance of ring enhancing lesion(s) on computed tomography (CT scan). Definitive diagnosis is based on brain biopsy, which is rarely performed, but is generally made presumptively after response to therapy.

First-line treatment is with sulfadiazine and pyrimethamine, with folinic acid to prevent myelosuppression. Alternatives include clindamycin and pyrimethamine with folinic acid, atovaquone, clarithromycin or doxycycline, although there is limited evidence for the latter two agents. Adjunctive therapy with corticosteroids or anticonvulsants may be used in cases of severe oedema or seizures, respectively.

Cryptosporidiosis *Cryptosporidium parvum* is a ubiquitous organism and a common cause of diarrhoea in immunocompetent individuals. In patients who are immunocompromised, persistent infection may occur characterized by abdominal pain, weight loss and severe diarrhoea. Diagnosis is generally based on stool analysis.

Although many agents have been investigated for the treatment of cryptosporidiosis, the majority of results have been disappointing. The optimal treatment for cryptosporidiosis (and indeed the majority of chronic opportunistic infections) is to increase immunological function with HAART. The mainstay of management in patients who are not able or willing to take HAART remains symptomatic control with nutritional supplementation, adequate hydration and antidiarrhoeal agents. The use of octreotide or total parenteral nutrition (TPN) in this patient group remains controversial.

Bacterial infections

Bacterial infections are common in the context of HIV infection. Recurrent bacterial pneumonia, particularly *Streptococcus pneumoniae*, and diarrhoeal illnesses associated with *Salmonella*, *Shigella* or *Campylobacter* are particularly common. In general, these are treated the same as in immunocompetent individuals, although recurrent infections and/or septicaemia occur more frequently.

Mycobacteria In HIV-positive individuals *M. tuberculosis* (TB) is characterized by: increased likelihood of reactivation of latent disease; more rapid progression to clinical disease following acquisition; more frequent extrapulmonary manifestations of tuberculosis, and more rapid progression of HIV disease (if the individual is not receiving HAART). Overall, there is no increase in infectivity of tuberculosis compared with HIV-negative patients.

Definitive diagnosis is reliant on culture of the organism from biological specimens, but may be complicated by atypical clinical features and reduced response to tuberculin testing; it is often necessary to initiate treatment empirically.

Treatment for pulmonary and extrapulmonary tuberculosis should follow conventional guidelines for immunocompetent individuals. Meningitis is an unusual but significant complication of tuberculosis. The use of primary and secondary prophylaxis remains controversial but may be appropriate in high-incidence groups. The increased incidence of multidrug-resistant tuberculosis (MDRTB) is a cause for concern, raises many infection control issues and highlights the need for antibiotic therapy driven by bacteriological sensitivities.

Managing tuberculosis and HIV co-infection is further complicated by drug–drug interactions between anti-tuberculous and antiretroviral agents, overlapping toxicities, and the risk of

development of immune reconstitution disease (see below). This is a complex area and is the subject of guidance (Pozniak et al 2005). One of the most frequent concerns is the question of when to initiate therapy for HIV in an individual receiving tuberculosis treatment. This decision is based upon the risk of developing other opportunistic infections in the medium term. HAART is usually started after 2 weeks of tuberculosis treatment in those with severe immunosuppression (CD4 <100 cells/mm³), after 2 months if the CD4 is between 100 and 200 cells/mm³, and on completion of tuberculosis treatment or at 6 months if the CD4 is greater than 200 cells/mm³.

Mycobacterium avium intracellulare (MAI or MAC) infection was historically a frequent manifestation of late-stage HIV disease, but is rarely seen now that HAART is widely used. Patients with disseminated infection classically present with fevers, weight loss, diarrhoea and hepatosplenomegaly. Diagnosis is sometimes made presumptively but is usually based on culture of the organism(s). In vitro sensitivities may not be good predictors of response to therapy. Therapy may need to be tailored to account for drug interactions with concomitant antiretrovirals, but usually includes rifabutin, azithromycin and ethambutol. Alternative agents include the quinolones and amikacin. Corticosteroids may be useful for symptomatic control. Although rifabutin, clarithromycin and azithromycin have all been demonstrated to be effective agents for primary prophylaxis against MAI, their cost–benefit remains controversial and use is not widespread in the UK.

Viral infections

Cytomegalovirus CMV is a herpes virus that is acquired by approximately 50% of the general population and over 90% of homosexual men. Like other herpes viruses, once infection has occurred the virus remains dormant thereafter but in individuals with advanced immunosuppression, reactivation may occur and cause disease. In the context of HIV infection, the most common sites of disease are the retina and gastrointestinal tract, though neurological involvement and pneumonitis are well reported.

Diagnosis of cytomegalovirus retinitis is based on clinical appearance; it may be detected in asymptomatic individuals but usually presents with symptoms of blurred vision, visual field defects or 'floaters'. Untreated cytomegalovirus retinitis progresses rapidly to blindness and treatment substantially reduces the morbidity associated with this condition. Although previously lifelong treatment had been recommended, where immunological restoration occurs discontinuation may be possible. Conventional therapeutic approaches are based upon an initial induction period of high-dose therapy for 2–3 weeks, until the retinitis is quiescent, followed by lower dose maintenance treatment, with reinduction if disease progression occurs.

The most commonly used agent for induction therapy in the UK is ganciclovir, which can be given intravenously or orally, as the pro-drug valganciclovir. It is usually administered (5 mg/kg) via a central line over 1 hour and should be handled as a cytotoxic agent. Valganciclovir is well absorbed and a dose of 900 mg twice daily has been shown to be as effective as intravenous ganciclovir for induction therapy. Significant side effects encountered with these agents include neutropenia, which may require colony stimulating factor support, and thrombocytopenia. Maintenance treatment may also be given either intravenously (6 mg/kg on 5 days a week) or orally (valganciclovir 900 mg once daily). Intravenous maintenance therapy requires the insertion of a permanent indwelling catheter and is therefore usually used only when oral administration is not possible. Intravitreal administration of ganciclovir is possible, but rarely used, as this does not confer any systemic protection.

An alternative agent to ganciclovir is foscarnet. It has a less favourable toxicity profile and is thus usually reserved for cases of therapeutic failure with ganciclovir. Its main adverse effects are electrolyte abnormalities, nephrotoxicity that requires dose adjustment or cessation of therapy, and ulceration, particularly of the genitals, which may be prevented by assiduous attention to personal hygiene after micturition. No effective oral formulation is currently available.

Cidofovir requires less frequent administration: two doses at weekly intervals for induction and fortnightly for maintenance, though intravenous administration is again required and nephrotoxicity and other metabolic disturbances are well recognized. A strict regimen of intravenous hydration and oral probenecid (2 g given 3 hours prior to infusion and 1 g 2 hours and 8 hours post cidofovir) must be followed. The risk of nephrotoxicity is increased if cidofovir is co-administered with agents such as tenofovir that are excreted via the same renal tubular anion transporter.

Cytomegalovirus disease of the gastrointestinal tract usually affects the oesophagus or colon, causing dysphagia and abdominal pain with diarrhoea, respectively. Diagnosis is based upon histological analysis of biopsy specimens. Treatment is as for cytomegalovirus retinitis induction therapy; maintenance therapy is not usually given unless relapses occur. Neurological disease may present in a variety of ways, is difficult to diagnose and frequently carries a poor prognosis, even with treatment. The optimal agent, dosage and duration of therapy remain undetermined.

Wasting syndrome

Many patients with advanced HIV disease historically reported significant weight loss, and no underlying pathogen could be identified. True wasting syndrome is characterized by loss of greater than 10% of body weight with diarrhoea and/or fever for which no other cause is found. Putative pathogenic mechanisms include hypermetabolism, hormonal imbalance and HIV infection of enterocytes, though in many cases reduced oral intake is sufficient to explain the degree of weight loss. A variety of therapeutic interventions including appetite stimulants, e.g. megestrol, medroxyprogesterone acetate, nabilone, anabolic agents and recombinant human growth hormone have been used alongside intensive nutritional support, but now the mainstay of management is effective antiretroviral therapy.

Impact of HAART on opportunistic infections

The widespread use of HAART has had a dramatic effect on the incidence, prognosis and clinical aspects of opportunistic infections.

Decreased incidence of opportunistic infections HAART has resulted in a major reduction in the vast majority of opportunistic infections and a consequent reduction in mortality rates and requirement for hospital admissions.

Withdrawal of prophylaxis The rise in CD4 count associated with HAART has lead to an improvement in functional immunity. Clinical trials have suggested that the withdrawal of both primary and secondary prophylaxis against *Pneumocystis jiroveci* pneumonia is safe, and similar results are thought to be likely for cryptococcosis, toxoplasmosis, *Mycobacterium avium intracellulare* and cytomegalovirus. Most would consider withdrawing prophylaxis in individuals on successful HAART if the CD4 count is consistently greater than 200 cells/mm^3 (*Pneumocystis jiroveci* pneumonia, toxoplasmosis, cryptococcosis) or 100 cells/mm^3 (*Mycobacterium avium intracellulare* and cytomegalovirus).

Successful treatment of opportunistic infections Some previously difficult to treat infections, notably cryptosporidiosis and microsporidiosis, appear to resolve with significant CD4 count improvements associated with HAART. However, in up to 30% of individuals initiation of HAART can be associated with a clinical deterioration known as immune reconstitution inflammatory syndrome or IRIS. This typically occurs in the first 2–6 weeks after starting HAART and presents as fevers and localized symptoms pertaining to a recently treated or previously undiagnosed opportunistic pathogen. It is most frequently seen with mycobacteria (lymphadenitis with both *Mycobacterium tuberculosis* and *Mycobacterium avium intracellulare*) and cytomegalovirus (vitritis, iritis and retinal oedema), but has been reported for most infections. Diagnosis is difficult as the signs and symptoms mimic those of resistant disease, non-adherence and comorbidity. No management strategy is proven but corticosteroids, NSAIDs and immunomodulatory therapies (IL-2 and GM-CSF) have all been used.

Cancers

Although there are a number of malignancies associated with HIV infection, the most common are Kaposi's sarcoma and lymphoma.

Kaposi's sarcoma This is the most common malignancy in people with HIV infection and may be triggered by infection with human herpes virus 8 (HHV-8). The majority of lesions affect the skin and appear as raised purple papules. These may be single or multiple and in severe cases may result in oedema, ulceration and infection. Visceral involvement is not uncommon but rarely causes clinically significant disease.

In some cases, no therapeutic intervention is necessary and cosmetic camouflage may be sufficient. Indeed, treatment of HIV with antiretroviral therapy usually results in improvement, and in most cases complete resolution, of Kaposi's sarcoma. When individual lesions are troublesome, local radiotherapy or intralesional chemotherapy, e.g. vincristine, can be beneficial. Newer approaches using topical agents, e.g. retinoic acid derivatives, remain largely investigational. In cases of widespread cutaneous disease or significant visceral involvement, systemic chemotherapy is used, though this is typically withheld until the potential benefits of HAART have been established. The liposomal formulations of doxorubicin and daunorubicin have superseded the combination of vincristine and bleomycin, being more effective and less toxic. Etoposide and paclitaxel have also been used in recalcitrant or recurrent cases.

Lymphomas   The most common lymphomas in patients with HIV infection are high-grade B-cell (non-Hodgkin's) types. Primary central nervous system lymphomas, which are extremely rare in the general population, are more common in individuals with HIV infection but tend to occur only in those with severe immunosuppression. Diagnosis of lymphoma is usually based upon histological confirmation from biopsy specimens. This may not be possible for primary central nervous system disease. The advent of HAART has dramatically reduced the incidence of all lymphomas. However, whilst it has similarly improved the outcome for most cases, this is unfortunately not true for primary central nervous system lymphomas. Lymphoma of the central nervous system is associated with an extremely poor outcome, and in many cases even palliative radiotherapy or corticosteroids confer little benefit.

The optimal therapy for HIV-associated lymphomas has yet to be determined. For non-central nervous system disease, a regimen involving cyclophosphamide, doxorubicin, vincristine (Oncovin) and prednisolone (CHOP) was previously used, but more recent approaches have included cyclophosphamide, doxorubicin and etoposide (CDE). The outcome for patients with relatively preserved immune function or those receiving HAART is comparable to that in the general population. However, many individuals are unable to tolerate treatment without dose modification. Drug interactions between antiretrovirals and chemotherapeutic agents need to be considered to minimize the risk of treatment-limiting toxicities, whilst the proactive use of colony-stimulating factors may enable optimal dosing.

Cervical intraepithelial neoplasia and anal intraepithelial neoplasia   CIN and AIN are both associated with human papillomavirus infection, are more common in individuals with HIV infection and may progress to cervical cancer and anal cancer respectively. It is currently believed that HAART reduces the progression of CIN but this does not appear to be true of AIN and there are concerns that the incidence of this malignancy may increase with improvements in HIV survival.

The optimal management is a combination of early diagnosis, surgery, chemotherapy and/or radiotherapy. It is possible that screening by smear tests and early treatment with imiquimod may reduce the need for such aggressive treatment approaches.

Neurological manifestations

Neurological symptoms may be due to opportunistic infections, tumours or the primary neurological effects of HIV.

HIV encephalopathy or AIDS dementia complex (ADC) is believed to result from direct infection of the central nervous system with HIV itself. Individuals who may otherwise be physically well can be debilitated by profound cognitive dysfunction and amnesia. Although psychometric test results are usually suggestive of the underlying aetiology, it is wise to rule out any other cause with brain scanning and CSF analysis.

The incidence of AIDS dementia complex has reduced dramatically with the use of HAART, and similarly, the use of HAART has been anecdotally associated with an improvement in outcome in many cases. Whilst it is known that the central nervous system penetration of some antiretroviral agents is better than others,

the beneficial effects on AIDS dementia complex do not appear to be limited to those agents which penetrate well. Nonetheless, many clinicians would choose to include at least one agent with good penetration of the central nervous system in most HAART regimens, particularly in individuals with cognitive impairment.

Progressive multifocal leucoencephalopathy (PML) is caused by JC virus and may, at presentation, appear similar to a cerebrovascular accident but will have characteristic white matter lesions on an MRI scan, with or without the presence of JC virus in the cerebrospinal fluid. In many cases the introduction of HAART prevents progression of disease, but it is unlikely to reverse the functional deficit at presentation. The role of adjunctive cidofovir in treatment remains controversial.

Hepatitis B co-infection

There are a number of ways in which HIV can impact on hepatitis B (HBV) infection.

- Hepatitis B vaccination is less successful.
- Hepatitis B is less likely to be cleared and hence more likely to become chronic.
- Hepatitis B infection is likely to be associated with higher hepatitis B DNA levels.
- Progression to cirrhosis is more rapid.
- Hepatocellular carcinoma is more common.

Although many individuals with HIV will have hepatitis B serological markers suggestive of previous infection, only 6–10% in most series have active hepatitis B infection.

Management requires an understanding of both viruses and is complicated by immunosuppression and the availability of drugs with dual HIV and hepatitis B activity (Brook et al 2004). Where treatment of hepatitis B (but not HIV) is indicated, interferon α or adefovir should be used. If treatment of both viruses is indicated, then the HAART regimen should include two agents with anti-hepatitis B activity, usually tenofovir with either emtricitabine or lamivudine. If HIV develops resistance to these agents, they can still be continued for their anti-hepatitis B activity.

Hepatitis C co-infection

HIV also impacts on hepatitis C infection in a number of ways.

- Hepatitis C is less likely to be cleared spontaneously.
- Higher levels of hepatitis C RNA are seen.
- Hepatitis C progresses to cirrhosis more rapidly.
- Hepatocellular carcinoma occurs more frequently.
- Response to hepatitis C therapy is poor.

In the UK, approximately 5–10% of individuals are co-infected with hepatitis C. In Eastern Europe, where the predominant route of HIV transmission is needle sharing, co-infection rates of over 50% are reported.

The management of hepatitis C/HIV co-infection is complicated (Nelson et al 2004). If treatment for hepatitis C is needed for someone on HAART, the antiretrovirals used must be compatible with hepatitis C therapy (pegylated α interferon and ribavirin). Didanosine, abacavir, stavudine and zidovudine should be avoided. It is commonplace to treat individuals with co-infection for a longer duration, for example, 48 weeks rather than 24 weeks for individuals with genotype 2 and 3 hepatitis C. Side effects of hepatitis C therapy tend to be more frequent and severe in the co-infected population. The proactive use of the colony-stimulating factors erythropoietin and G-CSF may enable optimal dosing of hepatitis C therapy and thereby improve outcome.

Women with HIV

The issues for women with HIV are complex and the following general points should be borne in mind:

• viral load and CD4 results may need to be interpreted differently
• there is a need for regular cervical screening to check for gynaecological manifestations of HIV
• drug toxicity may manifest in different ways or occur with different frequencies, e.g. nevirapine hypersensitivity reaction occurs at a lower CD4 count in women whilst lipodystrophy syndrome may also present differently, with breast hypertrophy commonly seen.

Pregnancy and contraception impact on the medicines prescribed for women of child-bearing potential. The factors that need to be taken into account include the following.

• There may be interactions with oral and injectable/depot contraceptive agents. (Note: barrier methods should also be recommended in addition to hormonal contraception, to prevent transmission of HIV and other sexually transmitted infections.)
• Potential teratogenicity of the drugs prescribed.
• Possible increased toxicity of the drugs prescribed to both mother and child.
• The use of antiretroviral agents to reduce vertical (mother-to-child) transmission of HIV.

The use of combination antiretroviral therapy, with or without caesarean section, with zidovudine as postexposure prophylaxis to the neonate, together with a non-breast feeding strategy has reduced vertical transmission rates from 35% to less than 1% where HIV status is known and where antiretroviral therapies are widely available.

Nonetheless, questions remain regarding the optimal therapies to use, the risk of transmission of resistant virus to the neonate, and the risk of toxicity from antiretroviral agents administered during pregnancy, particularly in the first trimester. Ideally, all HIV-positive women should be counselled regarding these issues before they become pregnant so they can make informed decisions regarding both therapy and timing of pregnancy.

Guidelines are available that set out the management of HIV infection in pregnant women and the prevention of mother-to-child transmission (Blott et al 2005). In general, intervention reflects a risk/benefit evaluation between the efficacy of reducing transmission and the potential harmful effects to the mother and fetus. Where HAART is clinically indicated for the mother herself, this should utilize a regimen of optimal efficacy with a favourable safety profile. Where therapy is initiated to reduce transmission, this may be a HAART regimen if the viral load is moderate to high but could be zidovudine monotherapy if the viral load is low. In the latter situation, therapy is initiated after the first and usually at the beginning of the third trimester. Adjunctive caesarean

section is recommended where monotherapy is used or there is a detectable viral load prior to delivery, but may not be essential if the mother is on fully suppressive HAART. Breast feeding should be avoided and antiretroviral therapy is usually administered to the newborn for 4 weeks after birth. In the developing world, different strategies may be adopted. For example, single-dose nevirapine monotherapy is effective in reducing transmission but may be associated with the development of resistance, and exclusive breast feeding, with or without antiretrovirals for the baby, may be recommended where water safety is poor.

Ethnicity

It is now recognized that ethnicity as well as gender can affect drug handling and response to treatment. This is due, in part, to epidemiological differences in gene expression. For example, reduced activity of cytochrome P450 2B6, one of the key enzymes involved in the metabolism of NNRTIs, appears to be more common amongst Africans than Caucasians. These drugs, therefore, have a significantly longer plasma half-life in those affected, which may impact on efficacy, toxicity and treatment interruptions. The prevalence of the HLA*B5701 gene, associated with abacavir hypersensitivity, also varies in different ethnic groups, though the clinical implications of this have yet to be fully researched.

As pharmacogenomics becomes more widely incorporated into clinical trials and routine patient care it is hoped that a greater understanding will be gained of differences in response to treatment, enabling treatment strategies to be individualized and optimized.

Patient care

AIDS is a multisystem disorder that presents numerous challenges to the infected individual, their partner and family and their healthcare workers. In addition, patients have other specific needs or characteristics to take into consideration, e.g. homosexual men, haemophiliacs, injecting drug users, asylum seekers, people who do not have English as a first language, women and children. The management of HIV-infected children differs significantly from adults and is not addressed in this chapter.

Regardless of the manner in which they acquired HIV, all infected people should be treated as individuals, recognizing the various lifestyle factors that may affect their choice of treatment and ability to adhere to it, such as lack of childcare facilities which may prevent some women from accessing services or entering clinical trials. They should be given appropriate information to empower them to participate in their own healthcare decision-making processes and adhere to the chosen treatment regimen. They should also be monitored regularly for signs of treatment failure, low adherence and drug toxicity and be given appropriate advice regarding prevention of transmission and reinfection (e.g. safer sex, safer drug use).

Patients with advanced AIDS may be managed at home, in a hospice or in hospital, depending on the services available. The same principles of palliative/terminal care apply in this patient population as in any other. However, the notable difference in HIV infection is that patients may continue with a number of active or prophylactic therapies until they are very close to death. Common examples are with HAART itself, valganciclovir to prevent blindness due to cytomegalovirus retinitis and co-trimoxazole to prevent *Pneumocystis jiroveci* pneumonia. The decision to stop treatment, particularly with antiretrovirals, should be made in consultation with the patient.

The pharmaceutical care needs of HIV-positive individuals overlap significantly with other groups such as the elderly, oncology and transplant patients, and can be summarized by the acronym PANDA:

- Polypharmacy
- Adverse drug reactions
- New drugs
- Drug interactions
- Adherence.

Antiretrovirals, particularly protease inhibitors and NNRTIs, interact with a large number of other agents including prescribed, herbal and recreational drugs, with the attendant risks of treatment failure or increased toxicity. People with HIV have also been reported to suffer a higher incidence of adverse reactions than the general population. In addition, the widespread use of new or experimental agents, or the prescribing of unusual doses or using drugs for unlicensed indications, raises the likelihood of a previously unreported adverse event occurring.

A high level of adherence to treatment is crucial to the sustained, successful outcome of antiretroviral regimens and has been the subject of much research. For example, in one study of people taking their first regimen containing nelfinavir, it was found that at least 95% adherence was required to achieve a sustained response in the majority (78%) of patients. The chances of treatment success declined as the level of adherence dropped, such that 80% of patients whose adherence was below 80% experienced virological failure. Virological success was also found to correlate with a better clinical outcome in terms of fewer hospitalizations, opportunistic infections and deaths (Paterson et al 2000). Such clinical trial data have also been supported by clinical experience in the UK and elsewhere, although it has yet to be established if the level of adherence required is the same for all regimens and every patient.

In other medical conditions, low adherence has been shown to increase with the number of prescribed medications and to be more common in patients suffering from confusion or dementia. Compliance devices such as pill boxes, timers and medication record cards may be helpful in enabling patients or their carers to manage their medicines safely and appropriately. However, some of the drugs have particular storage requirements and may require refrigeration or storage with a desiccant. Significant progress has been made over recent years in reducing some of the physical burden of therapy, for example with the development of combination tablets and the use of strategies such as ritonavir boosting to reduce dietary restrictions and dosing frequency. However, practical issues are not the only barriers to adherence and consideration should be given to addressing the individual's health beliefs and motivation, particularly around HIV and antiretroviral therapy, before treatment is commenced, as these are likely to have a significant impact on outcome (Horne et al 2004).

Although there is little evidence to demonstrate what the optimal interventions to improve adherence are, multidisciplinary and multiagency approaches (many involving pharmacists) appear to be most useful (Poppa et al 2003).

CASE STUDIES

Case 41.1

Ms A is a 35-year-old heterosexual woman, who was recently diagnosed HIV positive following a hospital admission with *Pneumocystis jiroveci* pneumonia. She has a history of previous injecting drug use and is currently maintained on a methadone programme via the local substance misuse service. Her most recent CD4 count was 50 cells/mm³, with a plasma HIV RNA (viral load) of 500 000 copies/mL. Her current therapy is: co-trimoxazole 480 mg once a day, Cilest 1 daily, multivitamin BPC 1 daily and methadone mixture 1 mg/mL 50 mg daily. On questioning, the patient also reports occasionally buying St John's wort from a health food store, although she is not currently taking it. The patient presents to the pharmacy with her first prescription for antiretrovirals: Truvada 1 daily and efavirenz 600 mg one at night, with metoclopramide 10 mg twice daily for the first 2–4 weeks.

....

Question

1. What are the actual and potential pharmaceutical care issues that should be addressed at this stage? Outline the main counselling points for Ms A's new drugs.

....

Answer

1. Ms A has been newly diagnosed with HIV so may be feeling rather overwhelmed with the implications of her diagnosis and the amount of information she has been given, particularly around antiretroviral therapy. The main issues presenting here are to counsel her on her new medication and to resolve a number of potential drug interactions. Medication counselling should include:

- what the medication is and how to take it
- potential side effects and how to prevent them, what to do, who to contact about them, particularly with the central nervous system side effects such as dizziness and vivid dreams with efavirenz. She also needs to be advised not to drive if affected
- relevant drug interactions, including effects of recreational drugs and alcohol, need to be discussed along with counselling to avoid St John's wort as it may decrease efficacy of efavirenz and the oral contraceptive pill. The need for additional barrier contraception should be discussed along with the need to liaise closely with the HIV team and substance misuse service regarding her methadone dose, in case it requires adjustment
- what to do if she misses or is late with a dose, or if she vomits soon after taking a dose
- the importance of a high level of adherence for successful treatment, outlining services that are available to support her, such as provision of compliance aids.

Two weeks later the patient rings the clinic saying she feels her methadone is wearing off after about 18 hours and she feels shivery, achy, etc., but the substance misuse service have refused to increase her methadone dose. She is also feeling dizzy, having difficulty concentrating while she is awake and is having nightmares and disturbed sleep. She is not sure she can continue with therapy if this carries on.

Questions

2. What are the problems here and what are the possible management options? Outline your preferred course of action.
3. If Ms A subsequently confides in you that she was hoping to become pregnant at some stage, what issues would you want to consider and what advice would you give her?

Answers

2. The likely causes of Ms A's distress may include:

- symptoms of methadone withdrawal before the next dose is due because of accelerated hepatic metabolism caused by efavirenz
- CNS side effects of efavirenz.

Possible courses of action include the following.

- Liaise with the substance misuse team to explain the methadone interaction. If patients are not on a programme of supervised administration, they may be able to manage the interaction by keeping the same total dose of methadone but splitting the administration times, e.g. taking 30 mg twice daily instead of 60 mg once daily. If they are on a supervised consumption programme they will only be able to receive their dose once a day and will not be allowed to keep part of the dose until later. A dose increase is the most appropriate course of action in this case. Explain to the patient that her methadone requirements will not continue to increase and that she will soon be restabilized on a suitable dose.
- The central nervous system side effects of efavirenz tend to be most pronounced in the first month of therapy and generally improve markedly after that. Therefore, if Ms A is able to persevere for another couple of weeks, she should notice an improvement in her symptoms, so simple reassurance may be sufficient. It may be that by resolving the problem of methadone withdrawal, Ms A will be able to persevere with the other symptoms she is experiencing. However, other palliative options might include the short-term use of a short-acting hypnotic (which may, paradoxically, help counteract the sleep disturbances, though these might also improve with the methadone dose increase). Taking the efavirenz earlier in the evening may help to reduce the 'hangover' effect the next day (particularly if the effects do not begin until several hours after taking the dose).

3. There are many complex issues to consider if Ms A is contemplating pregnancy and it would be very important for her to discuss them with her HIV physician and/or a specialist in the care of pregnant women with HIV. Issues to consider include:

- the efficacy of the oral contraceptive pill may be reduced by her efavirenz (efavirenz increases ethinyloestradiol levels but there are limited data on the interaction with progestogens), so until she is planning to conceive, she should use a barrier method as well. This will also protect her and her partner from acquiring new strains of HIV infection from each other (including drug-resistant HIV) as well as other sexually transmitted infections
- the status of her partner (if he is HIV negative, she may be advised to conceive by artificial insemination, to prevent him becoming infected)
- her drug therapy: whilst antiretrovirals in the later stages of pregnancy and labour can reduce the transmission of HIV from mother to baby, the potential long-term effects on the fetus/baby of many of the drugs are unknown. Efavirenz has been shown to be teratogenic in cynomolgus monkeys, so women are advised not to conceive whilst taking this drug. However, similar teratogenicity studies have not been done on all the other antiretrovirals and up-to-date 'real-life' data should be obtained (e.g. from the Antiretroviral Pregnancy Register). In view of the complexity of the issues and the seriousness of the ramifications, Ms A would be strongly advised to discuss this with her HIV physician.

Case 41.2

In 1996, a 44-year-old man, who had been diagnosed HIV positive 6 years earlier, presented with pneumonia which was later confirmed to be *Pneumocystis jiroveci* pneumonia. He made a good response to treatment with high-dose co-trimoxazole and was subsequently commenced on dual combination therapy with zidovudine and lamivudine. He remained on this regimen until 1998 when, after experiencing a fall in his CD4 count with a corresponding rise in viral load, he was switched to triple therapy with stavudine, didanosine and efavirenz, on which he remained until 2005. At this time his latest surrogate markers showed a CD4 count of 648 cells/mm^3 and a viral load below the limits of detection (<50 copies/mL). He presented to the HIV department with a 6-week history of feeling generally unwell, with nausea and vomiting for the past 5 days. His examination and initial investigations were unremarkable, except for some mild epigastric tenderness and a slightly elevated urea. His serum amylase was normal. A provisional diagnosis of gastroenteritis was given and he was asked to return 3–5 days later if there was no improvement. He reattended 36 hours later following further clinical deterioration with ongoing vomiting and anorexia. On this occasion, his amylase remained normal and his urea slightly elevated. Arterial blood gases were performed which revealed a metabolic acidosis (pH 7.2 and serum bicarbonate 12 mmol/L).

Questions

1. What was the most likely diagnosis?
2. What tests would confirm the diagnosis?
3. List three stages in the immediate management of this patient.
4. Are there any additional therapeutic interventions that should be considered?
5. What recommendation should be made regarding future antiretroviral therapy?

Answers

1. Lactic acidosis secondary to nucleoside analogue therapy. This is believed to be a relatively rare though increasingly recognized complication of long-term nucleoside analogue therapy resulting from mitochondrial toxicity.
2. The serum lactate would be elevated. Ideally a lactate/pyruvate ratio should be done but this is difficult to perform in most laboratories.
3. i. There is a need to admit to hospital as this is a potentially fatal condition that can be complicated by multiorgan failure, including hepatic steatosis.
   ii. Stop nucleoside analogue therapy. In cases of simple hyperlactataemia it may be advisable to monitor carefully and continue therapy, but where acidosis is present, discontinuation is recommended.
   iii. Supportive therapy with rehydration and possibly intravenous bicarbonate. Haemodialysis and haemofiltration have been used though the place of this in routine practice is unclear.
4. The following agents have been used as adjuvant therapies in this setting, although evidence for a definite therapeutic benefit is limited.

- Riboflavin 50 mg once daily
- Nicotinamide: use vitamin B compound strong tablets and/or Pabrinex injection
- Pabrinex (intravenous high-potency vitamins B and C)

- Sodium dichloroacetate: this is only available as a laboratory-grade chemical, that is not intended for human pharmaceutical use although favourable results have been reported
- Acetylcarnitine 1 g twice or three times a day

Although lactic acidosis may be associated with all NRTIs, the combination of stavudine and didanosine is most strongly linked. A new regimen should be selected on the basis of previous treatment and any resistance test results that are available. A nucleoside-sparing regimen may be used. Alternatively NRTIs which are less likely to cause mitochondrial toxicity, e.g. abacavir, tenofovir, may be preferred.

Case 41.3

Mr C is a 53-year-old homosexual man who was diagnosed HIV positive 20 years previously but has never had any AIDS-defining illnesses. He received 16 months of zidovudine monotherapy during 1993–4 as part of a study but subsequently remained off therapy until 1996 when, following a fall in his CD4 count to 240 cells/mm³, he was commenced on stavudine, lamivudine and indinavir. His response was excellent, with a rise in his CD4 count to 520 cells/mm³ and a viral load below detection (<50 copies/mL) but in 1999 the indinavir was changed to Kaletra, following an admission to hospital with indinavir-induced nephrolithiasis. In 2003, when his viral load was still undetectable, the stavudine was switched to tenofovir because of marked facial and peripheral lipoatrophy. The facial wasting was successfully treated with a course of polylactic acid (New Fill®) injections and there has been a small, gradual natural recovery of subcutaneous limb fat. He has been on pravastatin 40 mg once daily and fenofibrate 160 mg once daily since 2000.

His most recent surrogate markers remain excellent with a CD4 count of 1100 cells/mm³ and a viral load of <50 copies/mL. However, his lipid control is not ideal with a fasting total cholesterol 5.9 mmol/L and triglycerides 3.3 mmol/L. His calculated creatinine clearance (Cockcroft & Gault) is 45 mL/min (was >50 when last checked 3 months ago).

Questions

1. What are the options for managing his hyperlipidaemia?
2. What other relevant information would you want to know and what general health promotion advice would you offer?
3. What is the likely explanation for his worsening renal function and what action would you advise?

Answers

1. Although pravastatin was probably chosen as the lipid-lowering agent because of a lack of interactions with protease inhibitors, it is not the most potent agent for reducing cholesterol and Mr C is being prescribed the maximum dose. Simvastatin is contraindicated with boosted protease inhibitors as ritonavir inhibits its metabolism, resulting in significant muscle toxicity. Atorvastatin and rosuvastatin may be used cautiously, starting at their lowest recommended dose. Dosing of fenofibrate should be adjusted according to renal function. Ezetimite may be considered.

   Some boosted protease inhibitors, e.g. atazanavir/ritonavir, appear to have less of an impact on plasma lipids than Kaletra, so this would be another option to consider. The potential risks and benefits of any change in therapy must be carefully weighed up and discussed with the patient before a decision is made.
2. The usual recommendations regarding reduction in other cardiovascular disease risk factors are equally relevant in people with HIV, i.e. smoking cessation, dietary advice, and exercise. Mr C should be questioned about these factors and advised accordingly. His weight

and blood pressure should be monitored. Other non-modifiable risks, e.g. family history, should also be taken into account when calculating his likely risk of cardiovascular disease.
3. The deterioration in renal function could be due to tenofovir. More detailed renal investigations, such as fractional excretion of phosphate, creatinine clearance calculated from 24-hour urine collection, paired plasma and urine osmolality, should be carried out to ascertain the cause. The patient should be questioned about, and advised against, the use of other potentially nephrotoxic drugs such as NSAIDs. The tenofovir dose should be adjusted in renal impairment in accordance with the Summary of Product Characteristics. If no other cause for the deterioration in renal function is found and if it persists/worsens a change in antiretrovirals would be advised, where suitable alternative options to tenofovir exist.

Case 41.4

Mrs D is a 25-year-old nurse, originally from Zimbabwe, who has just been diagnosed HIV positive during routine antenatal screening. Her husband and their 3-year-old child have yet to be tested. She is 13 weeks pregnant and has a CD4 count of 450 cells/mm³ and a viral load of 15 000 copies/mL. She has no HIV-related symptoms and is very shocked by the diagnosis.

Questions

1. From the perspective of the HIV infection, what recommendations should be made for the management of Mrs D's pregnancy and delivery, and for the care of her newborn baby?
2. Outline the pharmaceutical care issues for Mrs D during her pregnancy, delivery and immediate postnatal period.
3. If Mrs D's husband tests negative for HIV, what advice should be given to them regarding future family planning and HIV prevention?

Answers

1. The latest recommendations from the BHIVA Pregnancy Guidelines should be followed.

   - Mrs D does not require HAART for herself, so a 3-month course of antiretrovirals throughout the final trimester of her pregnancy would be recommended. With a viral load of 15 000 copies/mL, zidovudine monotherapy would not be advised. A boosted protease inhibitor-based combination would be recommended. A CD4 count >250 cells/mm³ precludes use of nevirapine and stopping an NNRTI-based combination is complex, due to the long half-life. None is licensed for this indication but there is increasing anecdotal experience with, for example, Kaletra. The nucleoside backbone with which there is most experience in pregnancy is zidovudine/lamivudine (Combivir). The combination of didanosine and stavudine should not be used because of the increased risk of lactic acidosis in pregnant women. Tenofovir should also be avoided because of theoretical concerns about adverse effects on fetal bone development.
   - If Mrs D has an undetectable HIV viral load (<50 copies/mL) at her last antenatal appointment and the delivery of her previous child was uncomplicated, it may be appropriate for her to opt for a normal vaginal delivery. However, if the viral load is detectable and/or her previous delivery was long/complicated, an elective caesarean section, performed at about 36 weeks, may be advised. She should receive intravenous zidovudine prior to and during labour.
   - Her newborn baby should be given a 1-month course of zidovudine liquid (4 mg/kg twice daily), starting within 12 hours of birth, and she should be advised not to breast feed.

2. Pharmaceutical care issues will include the following.

- Counselling about the rationale for and aims of treatment during her pregnancy, as well as practical issues relating to the combination, e.g. how to take, side effects, drug interactions, what to do if problems such as missed, late or vomited dose occur, and more general points, e.g. how resistance develops and the importance of a high level of adherence.

- Consider the need for therapeutic drug monitoring of the protease inhibitor component of the regimen and dose adjustment if appropriate.

- Ensure the maternity unit has clear guidelines on the management of Mrs D's antiretrovirals, including preparation and infusion of intravenous zidovudine, and that drug supplies for mother and baby are available, including the possibility of unplanned/premature labour.

- Ensure Mrs D understands the rationale for giving her baby a 1-month course of zidovudine and that she has sufficient information and practical support to enable her to do this.

3. If Mr D is HIV negative, the couple should use a barrier method of contraception to prevent him from becoming infected. They should also be advised about the availability of postexposure prophylaxis following sexual exposure (PEPSE) in the event of a condom breakage. If they wish to have more children they should be advised to discuss the matter with a specialist assisted conception unit. Artificial insemination would usually be advised, to prevent the risk of Mr D becoming infected with HIV. If the couple wished to try to conceive at a stage when Mrs D was taking HAART, the risks and benefits of conceiving whilst taking antiretrovirals must also be discussed with her. The choice of HAART would also be informed by her wishes regarding future pregnancies and the need to avoid efavirenz if she intended to have another child.

REFERENCES

Blott M, Clayden P, de Ruiter A et al 2005 Guidelines for the management of HIV infection in pregnant women and the prevention of mother-to-child transmission of HIV. British HIV Association. Available online at: www.bhiva.org

Brook G, Gilson R, Wilkins E et al 2004 BHIVA guidelines. HIV and chronic hepatitis: co-infection with HIV and hepatitis B virus infection. British HIV Association. Available online at: www.bhiva.org

Carr A 2003 HIV lipodystrophy: risk factors, pathogenesis, diagnosis and management. AIDS 17 (suppl 1): S141-S148

Carr A, Cooper D A 2000 Adverse effects of antiretroviral therapy. Lancet 356: 1423-1430

Department of Health 2004 HIV post-exposure prophylaxis: guidance from the UK Chief Medical Officers' Expert Advisory Group on AIDS. Department of Health, London. Available online at: www.advisorybodies. doh.gov.uk/eaga/publications.htm

Fisher M, Benn P, Evans B et al 2006 UK guideline for the use of post-exposure prophylaxis for HIV following sexual exposure. International Journal of STD and AIDS 17: 81-92

Gazzard B on behalf of the BHIVA Writing Committee 2005 British HIV Association (BHIVA) guidelines for the treatment of HIV-infected adults with antiretroviral therapy. HIV Medicine 6 (suppl 2):1-61. Available online at: www.bhiva.org

Hammer S M, Squires K E, Hughes M D et al 1997 A controlled trial of two nucleoside analogues plus indinavir in persons with human immunodeficiency virus infection and CD4 cell counts of 200 per cubic millimeter or less. New England Journal of Medicine 337: 725-733

Horne R, Buick D, Fisher M et al 2004 Doubts about necessity and concerns about adverse effects: identifying the types of beliefs that are associated with non-adherence to HAART. International Journal of STD and AIDS 15: 38-44

Lichtenstein K A 2005 Redefining lipodystrophy syndrome: risks and impact on clinical decision making. Journal of Acquired Immune Deficiency Syndrome 39: 395-400

McComsey G, Lonergan J T 2004 Mitochondrial dysfunction: patient monitoring and toxicity management. Journal of Acquired Immune Deficiency Syndrome 37: S30-S35

Mellors J W, Munoz A, Giorgi J V et al 1997 Plasma viral load and CD4 lymphocytes as prognostic markers of HIV-1 infection. Annals of Internal Medicine 126: 946-954

Nelson M, Matthews G, Brook G et al 2004 British HIV Association (BHIVA) guidelines for treatment and management of HIV and hepatitis C coinfection. British HIV Association. Available online at: www.bhiva.org

Palella F J Jr, Delaney K M, Moorman A C et al 1998 Declining morbidity and mortality among patients with advanced human immunodeficiency virus infection. New England Journal of Medicine 338: 853-860

Paterson D L, Swindells S, Mohr J et al 2000 Adherence to protease inhibitor therapy and outcomes in patients with HIV infection. Annals of Internal Medicine 133: 21-30

Poppa A, Davidson O, Deutsch J et al 2003 British HIV Association (BHIVA)/British Association for Sexual Health & HIV (BASHH) guidelines on provision of adherence support to individuals receiving antiretroviral therapy. British HIV Association. Available online at: www.bhiva.org

Pozniak A L, Miller R F, Lipman M C I 2005 BHIVA treatment guidelines for TB/HIV infection. British HIV Association. Available online at: www.bhiva.org

Schambelan M, Benson C A, Carr A et al 2002 Management of metabolic complications associated with antiretroviral therapy for HIV-1 infection: recommendations of an International AIDS Society-USA Panel. Journal of Acquired Immune Deficiency Syndrome 31: 257-275

Smit C, Geskus R, Walker S et al 2006 Effective therapy has altered the spectrum of cause-specific mortality following HIV seroconversion. AIDS 20: 741-749

FURTHER READING

Bhagani S, Sweny P, Brook G et al 2005 Guidelines for kidney transplantation in patients with HIV disease. British HIV Association. Available online at: www.bhiva.org

Department of Health 2005 HIV infected health care workers: guidance on management and patient notification. Department of Health, London. Available online at: www.advisorybodies.doh.gov.uk/ eaga/publications. htm

Geretti A M, Brook G, Cameron C et al 2006 Immunisation guidelines for HIV-infected adults. British HIV Association. Available online at: www. bhiva.org

Gupta S K, Eustace J A, Winston J A et al 2005 Guidelines for the management of chronic kidney disease in HIV-infected patients: recommendations of the HIV Medicine Association of the Infectious Diseases Society of America. Clinical Infectious Diseases 40: 1559-1585

O'Grady J, Taylor C, Brook G et al 2005 Guidelines for liver transplantation in patients with HIV infection. British HIV Association. Available online at: www.bhiva.org

USEFUL WEBSITES

British Association for Sexual Health and HIV: www.bashh.org

British HIV Association: www.bhiva.org

United States national HIV guidelines (antiretroviral treatment, management of opportunistic infections, co-infections and post-exposure prophylaxis): www.aidsinfo.nih.gov/guidelines/

UK-based community provider of wide range of HIV-related information (including drug/treatment updates, conference reports and daily news items): www.aidsmap.com

US-based medical website with HIV specialty home page: www.medscape.com

University of California San Francisco: www.hivinsite.ucsf.edu

University of Liverpool HIV Pharmacology Group: www.hiv-druginteractions.org

www.hivpharmacology.com

Johns Hopkins University: www.hopkins-aids.edu

Toronto General Hospital HIV clinic: www.tthhivclinic.com

Fungal infections 42

Stephen J. Pedler

KEY POINTS

- The triazole antifungals fluconazole and itraconazole provide effective, orally available treatment for oral and vaginal candidiasis, which were previously treatable only by topical therapy.
- Itraconazole and terbinafine are efficacious, non-toxic alternatives to griseofulvin when systemic treatment of dermatophytosis is required.
- Most therapy for deep-seated fungal infection in the immunocompromised host is empirical in nature due to the difficulties in reaching rapid, accurate diagnosis of systemic fungal infection.
- Lipid-complexed formulations of amphotericin offer a less toxic alternative to conventional amphotericin in the treatment of systemic fungal infection; of these, liposomal amphotericin appears to give the best combination of efficacy and lack of toxicity.
- Published studies have not convincingly shown greater clinical efficacy for lipid preparations of amphotericin B compared to the conventional form.
- Fluconazole may be used to treat systemic candidiasis in non-neutropenic patients, but concerns exist about the increasing prevalence of fluconazole-resistant *Candida* species.
- While itraconazole may be useful as a second-line agent in the treatment of aspergillosis, it should not be regarded as a first-line treatment for this condition. It is, however, an excellent choice for the prophylaxis of fungal infection in neutropenic patients.
- Voriconazole appears to be an effective alternative to amphotericin in the treatment of invasive aspergillosis.
- Caspofungin is an alternative agent to amphotericin for invasive aspergillosis and may have a role to play in the empirical treatment of febrile neutropenic patients.

Fungi are extremely common organisms which are widely distributed in nature. Fortunately, only a tiny minority cause human disease although many others are plant or animal pathogens. Human infections fall into two groups: superficial infections of skin or mucosal surfaces and deep (or systemic) infections.

Fungi of medical importance can be divided into four groups (Table 42.1). Yeasts are unicellular organisms with round or oval cells, while the moulds or filamentous fungi (such as those which grow on decaying organic material) produce hyphae. The hyphae grow and intertwine together, producing the familiar fluffy material which is often seen on rotten food; this mass of hyphae is known as a mycelium. The yeast-like fungi are similar to yeasts but occasionally produce hyphae-like structures (pseudohyphae) as well. This group includes the most common human fungal pathogen, *Candida albicans*. Finally, there is a group of 'dimorphic' fungi which can exist either as yeasts at 37°C in the body or as

moulds. This chapter will focus on those organisms which are the common causes of fungal infections in the United Kingdom, and for this reason the dimorphic fungi will be mentioned only briefly.

There are a number of differences between fungi and bacteria. Fungal cells have true nuclei, which bacteria do not; they differ from bacteria in their cell wall and cell membrane constituents; and many produce hyphae which are long, branching tubular structures. In addition, yeasts reproduce by budding, a process in which the daughter cell grows as a small bud on the side of the parent, whereas bacteria reproduce by binary fission, giving rise to two daughter cells of equal size. These differences are important because they mean that fungi are resistant to the action of most antibacterial agents. Fungal cells are closer to mammalian cells than are bacteria, which also reduces the ease of development of drugs with selective toxicity towards fungal rather than mammalian cells.

Superficial infections

Superficial *Candida* infections

Epidemiology

Candida albicans is a very common yeast-like fungus which is found as part of the normal flora of the gastrointestinal tract of almost all healthy people. When infection occurs it is usually endogenous (i.e. the source of the organism is the patient's own flora) although cross-infection leading to outbreaks of candidiasis have been described in hospitals. In addition, there are a number of other species in the genus *Candida*, such as *C. glabrata, C. krusei, C. tropicalis,* etc., which, although less common, are important as some of them have inherent resistance to antifungal agents such as fluconazole.

Superficial candidiasis usually presents as an infection of mucous membranes, especially in the mouth or vagina, and is commonly referred to as oral or vaginal thrush, respectively. Skin infection and occasionally nail infection may also occur. Predisposing factors for oral candidiasis include the presence of dentures and the use of inhaled steroids for the treatment of asthma. Patients with the acquired immunodeficiency syndrome (AIDS) also have a high incidence of oral candidiasis which may extend to the oesophagus, a potentially severe condition. Antibiotics which remove the normal vaginal flora and allow colonization by *Candida*, diabetes mellitus, pregnancy and oral contraceptives are predisposing factors for vaginal thrush. Candidiasis of the skin usually occurs in moist areas, for example in nappy rash, in the

Table 42.1 Classification of the fungi of medical importance

Group	Examples	Diseases caused
True yeasts	Crypotococcus neoformans	Meningitis
		Pulmonary and cutaneous infection
	Saccharomyces cerevisiae	Rarely systemic infection in immunocompromised patients
Yeast-like fungi	Candida albicans and other Candida species	Superficial: mucositis of the mouth and vagina (thrush); cutaneous and nail infection
		Deep: bloodstream infection and a wide variety of other deep-seated infections
Dimorphic fungi	Histoplasma capsulatum Coccidioides immitis Blastomyces dermatidis Paracoccidioides brasiliensis	Specific conditions such as histoplasmosis, coccidioidomycosis, etc. which are more common in immunocompromised patients, especially those with AIDS, but may also cause disease in otherwise healthy individuals
Moulds	Aspergillus fumigatus and other Aspergillus species	Systemic infection in immunocompromised patients, especially invasive pulmonary disease and central nervous system infection
	Mucor, Absidia, Rhizopus	Mucormycosis, mainly in neutropenic patients and those with diabetic ketoacidosis
	A wide variety of other filamentous fungi	See the further reading list for more information

perianal region and in intertriginous areas such as skinfolds and under the breasts.

Clinical presentation

The usual presentation of oral thrush is a sore mouth, particularly on eating. Examination shows white patches of the fungus on the oral mucosa and tongue which can be scraped away, leaving a raw, tender, often bleeding surface behind.

Vaginal candidiasis usually presents as a vaginal discharge which classically is thick and creamy in nature, often accompanied by itching, which may be severe. Infection of the sexual partner may occur which may be asymptomatic or lead to a balanitis (inflammation of the glans penis).

Infection of the skin causes an inflamed, itching area of skin with pustules, maceration and fissuring of the skin. Nail involvement may present as infection of the subcutaneous tissue around and under the nail (Candida paronychia), which is often seen in people whose hands are frequently immersed in water, or as infection of the nail itself (onychomycosis).

More severe mucosal infection may occur in immunocompromised patients, particularly in patients with AIDS in whom oesophageal candidiasis is common. This condition presents with difficulty and pain on swallowing, and endoscopy is usually required to confirm the diagnosis.

Diagnosis

The diagnosis of oral or vaginal candidiasis is usually made clinically but can be confirmed easily by taking a swab of the affected area. Microscopy of the specimen shows large numbers of yeast cells and pseudohyphae, and culture will readily yield the organism. Skin and nail infections may be confused with other infections and conditions such as eczema, and culture should always be performed. For superficial infections in immuno-competent hosts, further species differentiation and

antifungal sensitivity testing are not usually required but in immunodeficient patients or those who have been previously exposed to antifungals, this may be required in case the infecting strain possesses intrinsic or acquired resistance, particularly to fluconazole.

Treatment

Oral and vaginal candidiasis may be treated by either topical or systemic antifungal agents. The drugs currently available for topical use fall into two groups: the polyenes, of which only amphotericin and nystatin are used clinically, and the imidazoles such as econazole, clotrimazole, miconazole and fenticonazole. These agents are essentially identical in their antifungal activity and the only reasons to choose between them are price and differing preparations. The two systemic agents are both triazoles (fluconazole and itraconazole) and can be given by mouth. Skin infections may also be treated topically but nail infections are unlikely to respond to a topical antifungal agent and require systemic treatment. Oesophagitis will invariably require systemic treatment.

Topical treatment The polyenes are broad-spectrum antifungal agents that are virtually insoluble in water and which are not absorbed from the gastrointestinal tract or from skin or mucous membranes. Both nystatin and amphotericin (but particularly nystatin) are available in a wide range of formulations including pessaries, creams, gels, tablets, pastilles, etc. The choice of formulation clearly depends on the site of infection and patient preference. Nystatin is also available in combination with steroids, which may be useful in relieving associated inflammation and itching in skin infections, and antibiotics such as tetracycline and bacitracin.

Very little in the way of unwanted effects occurs with these agents, but in mixed formulations the effects of the other components must also be taken into account. They are safe for use in pregnancy.

The imidazoles also have a broad antifungal spectrum. They too are available in a wide variety of formulations and may be combined with steroids. Absorption when taken by mouth or from mucosal surfaces is minimal, but detectable plasma levels are present after oral administration, particularly with miconazole. Unwanted effects are few; the imidazoles are fetotoxic in high doses in laboratory animals but this has never been shown to occur in pregnant women.

Overall, for the treatment of oral thrush, the polyenes and the imadazoles seem equally efficacious. In vaginal candidiasis, although there are no direct comparisons in clinical trials, the imidazoles seem to be more effective; cure rates of 90% versus 80% for the polyenes have been quoted.

Systemic treatment Two triazole agents are available for the systemic treatment of oral and vaginal candidiasis. These compounds, fluconazole and itraconazole, are discussed below.

Fluconazole is highly effective in vaginal candidiasis, giving similar cure rates to topical therapy. However, many patients find oral fluconazole preferable to topical therapy for reasons of convenience, as it is given as a single dose of 150 mg. Itraconazole is also effective in vaginal candidiasis, given as two oral doses of 200 mg 12 hours apart. Both drugs are effective in oral candidiasis, although systemic therapy would usually be considered only after failure of topical therapy or in difficult clinical conditions such as patients with human immunodeficiency virus (HIV) infection. Typical doses would be fluconazole 50–100 mg daily for 7–14 days or itraconazole 100–200 mg daily for 15 days.

Candida balanitis can also be treated with topical polyenes or imidazoles, or with systemic fluconazole in the same dose as for vaginal infection. It is sometimes stated that when treating a woman with vaginal candidiasis, the male partner should be treated simultaneously in order to prevent reinfection. Although there is no evidence to support this approach, it may be considered in women who suffer from repeated vaginal candidiasis.

Dermatophytosis

Epidemiology and causative organisms

Dermatophytosis, or tinea, is a condition caused by three genera of dermatophyte fungi: *Trichophyton, Epidermophyton* and *Microsporum*. Unlike *Candida*, these are moulds which have a predilection for keratinized tissue such as skin, nail and hair. These fungi are very widely distributed throughout the world and may be acquired from the soil, from animals or from humans infected with the fungus.

Clinical features

The classic clinical presentation of dermatophyte infection of the skin is ringworm, a circular, inflamed lesion with a raised edge and associated skin scaling. However, presentation is influenced by the site of infection and by the actual species of fungus causing the infection. In general, less severe lesions are produced by human fungal strains, while those acquired from animals can produce quite intense inflammatory reactions.

Dermatophytosis of the nail results in thickened, discoloured nails while in the scalp infection presents with itching, skin scaling and inflammation, and patchy hair loss (alopecia).

Diagnosis

The diagnosis of dermatophyte infection is confirmed by collecting appropriate specimens such as material from infected nails and skin. The fungi can be seen microscopically and specimens may also be cultured, but antifungal susceptibility testing is not required.

Treatment

As with superficial *Candida* infections, dermatophytosis can be treated either topically or systemically.

Topical therapy This is most appropriate for small or medium areas of skin infection. Larger areas or nail or hair infection should be treated with a systemic agent. The most commonly used topical agents are the imidazoles, of which a wide variety is available, including clotrimazole, ecoazole, miconazole, sulconazole and tioconazole. There is little to choose between these agents, all of which are usually applied two or three times daily, continuing for up to 2 weeks after the lesions have healed. Side effects are uncommon and usually consist of mild skin irritation. Other topical agents include amorolfine, terbinafine and tolnaftate.

Griseofulvin The first orally administered treatment for dermatophytosis was griseofulvin, which has now been available for over 40 years. Griseofulvin is active only against dermatophyte fungi and is inactive against all other fungi and bacteria. In order to exert its antifungal effect, it must be incorporated into keratinous tissue, where levels are much greater than plasma levels, and therefore it has no effect if used topically.

The usual adult dose is 500–1000 mg daily, given in one dose or divided doses if required. The higher dose is recommended for severe infection and should be reduced once clinical response occurs. Griseofulvin is well absorbed and absorption is enhanced if taken with a high-fat meal. In children it may be given with milk. A 1000 mg dose produces a peak plasma level of about 1–2 mg/L after 4 hours, with a half-life of at least 9 hours. An ultra-fine preparation of griseofulvin exists which is almost totally absorbed and permits the use of lower doses (typically 330–660 mg daily). This preparation is not available in the UK. Elimination is mainly through the liver and inactive metabolites are excreted in the urine. Less than 1% of a dose is excreted in urine in the active form but some active drug is excreted in the faeces.

The duration of treatment with griseofulvin is dependent entirely on clinical response. Skin or hair infection usually requires 4–12 weeks' therapy but nail infections respond much more slowly; 6 months treatment is often required for fingernails, a year or more for toenail infections. Unfortunately, the rate of treatment failure or relapse in nail infection is high, and may reach up to 60%.

Because of this high failure rate, other agents have been sought. Itraconazole at a dose of 200 mg daily for 1 week and terbinafine (250 mg daily for 2 weeks) have been shown to be effective, well-tolerated treatments for dermatophyte skin infections (Hay 2005). Terbinafine and itraconazole (see below) are now preferred to griseofulvin for the treatment of nail infections, since shorter treatment courses with greater efficacy are possible. 'Pulse' therapy with itraconazole for nail infections has also been used in which 7-day courses of 200 mg twice daily are prescribed at 21-day intervals. Two courses are recommended for fingernail infections, or three courses for toenail infections, which are more difficult to treat. Unfortunately, itraconazole and terbinafine are not licensed in the UK for hair infection (tinea capitis), for which griseofulvin remains the treatment of choice.

Terbinafine   Terbinafine is the first member of a new class of antifungal agents, the allylamines, to become available for systemic use. These agents act by inhibition of the fungal enzyme squalene epoxidase, an enzyme involved in the synthesis of ergosterol, an essential component of the fungal cytoplasmic membrane. Although terbinafine has a very broad antifungal spectrum in the laboratory, its in vivo efficacy does not correspond to its in vitro activity and it is used only for the treatment of dermatophyte infection.

Table 42.2   Examples of major drug interactions with antifungal agents

Drug	Interaction with	Result
Cyclo-oxygenase 2 inhibitors	Fluconazole	Increased plasma concentration of the analgesic
Terfenadine, mizolastine	Itraconazole	Increased plasma concentration of terfenadine and mizolastine, leading to cardiac arrhythmias
Any nephrotoxic agent	Amphotericin B	Enhanced nephrotoxicity
Cimetidine	Terbinafine	Increased plasma concentration of terbinafine
Ciclosporin	Griseofulvin	Reduced concentration of ciclosporin
	Triazoles	Increased ciclosporin concentration due to reduced ciclosporin metabolism
Didanosine	Itraconazole	Reduced absorption of itraconazole (avoid simultaneous administration)
Digoxin	Amphotericin	Increased digoxin toxicity due to hypokalaemia
	Itraconazole	Increased plasma digoxin concentration
Ergot alkaloids	Triazoles	Increased risk of ergotism
Midazolam	Fluconazole, itraconazole	Increased plasma midazolam concentration leading to prolonged sedation
Omeprazole	Voriconazole	Increased plasma concentration of omeprazole
Oral contraceptives	Griseofulvin, triazoles	Reduced contraceptive efficacy caused by induction of liver enzymes which metabolize the oral contraceptive
Phenytoin	Fluconazole	Increased plasma concentration of phenytoin
	Voriconazole	Increased plasma concentration of phenytoin, reduced concentration of voriconazole
Quinidine	Itraconazole, voriconazole	Increased plasma concentration of quinidine leading to an increased risk of arrhythmias
Rifabutin	Triazoles	Increased plasma concentration of rifabutin leading to an increased risk of uveitis Rifabutin may reduce the plasma concentration of voriconazole
Rifampicin	Triazoles, terbinafine	Reduced plasma triazole and terbinafine concentrations (rifampicin induces more rapid metabolism)
Simvastatin and other statins	Triazoles (especially itraconazole)	Increased risk of myopathy
Sulfonylureas	Triazoles	Enhanced effects of sulfonylureas
Tacrolimus	Triazoles	Inhibition of metabolism of tacrolimus leading to increased plasma concentration
Warfarin	Griseofulvin	Reduced anticoagulant effect; induces liver enzymes which metabolize warfarin
	Triazoles	Enhanced anticoagulant effect; may displace warfarin from plasma albumin binding sites and inhibit metabolism of warfarin
Zidovudine	Fluconazole	Inhibition of metabolism of zidovudine leading to increased plasma concentration

About 70% of an oral dose is absorbed and the drug appears in high concentrations in the skin. The half-life is about 16–17 hours and therefore the drug can be given once per day. Terbinafine is metabolized in the liver and the metabolites are excreted in the urine, so that hepatic or renal dysfunction will prolong the elimination half-life. The usual dose is 250 mg once daily; the duration of treatment will vary depending on the site of infection, but as with itraconazole, in the treatment of nail infections shorter courses of treatment can be given compared to griseofulvin. It is not licensed for the treatment of dermatophytosis of the scalp and hair (tinea capitis) although clinical trial evidence would indicate that it is at least as effective as griseofulvin.

The main drug interactions with these agents are shown in Table 42.2. Side effects are shown in Table 42.3. Griseofulvin is teratogenic in animals and is contraindicated in pregnancy (and pregnancy should be avoided for 1 month after treatment) and in severe liver disease. It is also recommended that males who have taken griseofulvin should not father children within 6 months of treatment because the drug has been shown to induce sperm abnormalities in animal studies.

Pityriasis versicolor

Causative organism

This is a common skin infection caused by a yeast-like fungus, *Malassezia furfur*. The organism is a member of the normal skin flora and lives only on the skin because it has a growth requirement for medium-chain fatty acids present in sebum.

Clinical features

The condition usually appears as patches scattered over the trunk, neck and shoulders. These patches produce scales and may be pigmented in light-skinned individuals, appearing light brown in colour. In dark-skinned patients, the lesions may lose pigment and appear lighter than normal skin.

In some patients, this yeast is also associated with dandruff and seborrhoeic dermatitis, although the exact role of the yeast in causing this condition remains uncertain. In AIDS patients, seborrhoeic dermatitis may be quite extensive and sudden in onset.

Diagnosis

The diagnosis is made by microscopy of scrapings from the lesion. The specimen is examined for the presence of yeast cells and short hyphae. Culture is not usually required for diagnosis and, since it requires special culture media, is not routinely attempted.

Treatment

Pityriasis versicolor is treated with a topical agent such as 2% selenium sulfide, topical terbinafine or a topical imidazole such as clotrimazole, econazole or miconazole. Relapses are common and treatment may need to be repeated. In severe cases, oral itraconazole (200 mg once daily for 7 days) may be given.

Table 42.3 Side effects of antifungal agents

Drug	Side effects
Griseofulvin	Mild: headache, gastrointestinal side effects. Hypersensitivity reactions such as skin rashes, including photosensitivity
	Moderate: exacerbation of acute intermittent porphyria; rarely, precipitation of systemic lupus erythematosus. Contraindicated in both these conditions, also in pregnancy, and in the presence of severe liver disease
Terbinafine	Usually mild: nausea, abdominal pain; allergic skin reactions; loss and disturbance of sense of taste. Not recommended in patients with liver disease
Amphotericin	Immediate reactions (during infusion) include headache, pyrexia, rigors, nausea, vomiting, hypotension; occasionally these can be severe Thrombophlebitis after the infusion is very common Nephrotoxicity and hypokalaemia Anaemia due to reduced erythropoiesis Peripheral neuropathy (rare) Cardiac failure (this is exacerbated by hypokalaemia due to nephrotoxicity) Immunomodulation (the drug can both enhance and inhibit some immunological functions)
Flucytosine	Mild: gastrointestinal side effects (nausea, vomiting). Occasional skin rashes Moderate: myelosuppression (dose related), hepatotoxicity
Fluconazole	Mild: nausea, vomiting and occasional skin rashes; occasionally elevated liver enzymes (reversible) Moderate or severe: rarely, hepatotoxicity and severe cutaneous reactions, especially in AIDS patients
Itraconazole	Mild: nausea and abdominal pain; occasional skin rashes Moderate or severe: rarely, hepatotoxicity
Voriconazole	Similar to fluconazole and itraconazole Mild, reversible visual disturbances are common with voriconazole (about 30% of patients)
Caspofungin	Mild: gastrointestinal side effects; occasional skin rashes

Fungal ear infection

Fungi sometimes infect the external auditory canal, causing otitis externa, the most common causative organisms being various species of *Aspergillus* (such as *A. niger* and *A. fumigatus*) and *Candida albicans* and other *Candida* species. A variety of other fungi found in the environment can also cause this condition. The use of topical antibacterial agents in the ear may predispose to local fungal infection.

Clinical features

Fungal infection of the ear usually presents as pain and itching in the auditory canal, sometimes with a reduction in hearing due to blockage of the canal. There may be an associated discharge from the ear. Clinical examination shows a swollen red canal, and the fungal mycelium is sometimes visible as an amorphous white or grey mass.

Diagnosis

The diagnosis of a fungal infection of the external canal can be made by microscopy and culture of material obtained from the ear.

Treatment

Aural toilet with removal of obstructing debris is very important in the management of this condition. A topical antifungal agent such as nystatin or amphotericin, or an imidazole can also be applied.

Deep-seated fungal infections

Most deep-seated or systemic fungal infections seen in the UK are the result of some breakdown in the normal body defences, which may be due to disease or medical treatment. There are, however, a group of fungi, often referred to rather misleadingly as the 'pathogenic' fungi, which are able to cause systemic infection in a previously healthy person. These infections, which are usually due to 'dimorphic' fungi, include diseases such as histoplasmosis, blastomycosis and coccidioidomycosis. They are rare in the UK but rather more common in the USA and some other parts of the world.

Fungal infections in the compromised host

Epidemiology and predisposing factors

There are a large number of conditions which may predispose the individual to systemic or deep-seated fungal infection. These are summarized in Table 42.4. A breach in the body's mechanical barriers may predispose to fungal infection. For example, fungal infection of the urinary tract occurs most commonly in catheterized patients who have received broad-spectrum

Table 42.4 Conditions predisposing to systemic or deep-seated fungal infection

Infection	Predisposing conditions
Systemic candidiasis	Neutropenia from any cause (disease or treatment) Use of broad-spectrum antibiotics which eliminate the normal body flora Indwelling intravenous cannulae, especially when used for total parenteral nutrition Haematological malignancy Organ transplantation AIDS (particularly associated with severe mucocutaneous infection) Intravenous drug abuse Cardiac surgery and heart valve replacement, leading to *Candida* endocarditis Gastrointestinal tract surgery
Aspergillosis	Neutropenia from any cause, especially if severe and prolonged Acute leukaemia Organ transplantation Chronic granulomatous disease of childhood (defect in neutrophil function) Pre-existing lung disease (usually leads to aspergillomas; fungus balls form in the lung rather than invasive or disseminated infection)
Cryptococcosis	AIDS Systemic therapy with corticosteroids Renal transplantation Hodgkin's disease and other lymphomas Sarcoidosis Collagen vascular diseases
Mucormycosis	Diabetic hyperglycaemic ketoacidosis (leading to rhinocerebral infection) Severe, prolonged neutropenia Burns (leading to cutaneous infection)

antibiotics, while total parenteral nutrition (TPN) is strongly associated with fungaemia, sometimes with unusual fungi such as *Malassezia furfur*. This is due to the use of TPN infusions containing lipids, which are a growth requirement of this organism. Most cases of systemic fungal infection, however, are associated with a defect in the patient's immune system and the nature of the organisms encountered is often related to the nature of the immunosuppression. Neutropenia, for example, is usually associated with *Candida* species, *Aspergillus* and mucormycosis, while defects of cell-mediated immunity, e.g. HIV infection, are strongly associated with infection due to *Cryptococcus neoformans*.

Causative fungi

Many different fungi have been described as causing systemic fungal infection but the most common organisms encountered and the conditions they cause are listed in Table 42.5. Of these, *Candida* and *Aspergillus* are by far the most common in the UK.

Clinical presentation

Deep-seated fungal infection can present in a large number of different ways, which are listed in Table 42.6. The most common presentation is as a fungaemia, with fever, low blood pressure and sometimes the other features of septic shock. Relatively low-grade fungaemia (for example, those associated with TPN) often present only with fever.

Diagnostic measures

Unfortunately, the diagnosis of deep-seated fungal infection is difficult and is often only made post mortem. Systemic candidiasis may be diagnosed by isolation of the organism from blood culture and culture of other appropriate specimens. *Cryptococcus neoformans* grows readily on laboratory media and can be isolated from blood and cerebrospinal fluid; a simple test for the detection of cryptococcal antigen in CSF and plasma is also available. Aspergillosis is rarely, if ever, diagnosed from blood culture but the organism can occasionally be isolated from sputum; however, bronchoalveolar lavage and open lung biopsy are the best techniques for the diagnosis of pulmonary aspergillosis.

Table 42.5 Common causes in the UK of systemic and deep-seated fungal infection

Condition/organism	Common clinical presentations
Candidiasis (*Candida albicans, C. glabrata, C. krusei, C. tropicalis,* other *Candida* species)	Fungaemia Colonization of intravenous cannulae Pneumonia Meningitis Bone and joint infections Endocarditis Endophthalmitis Peritonitis in chronic ambulatory peritoneal dialysis
Aspergillosis (*Aspergillus fumigatus, A. flavus,* other *Aspergillus* species)	Invasive pulmonary aspergillosis Disseminated aspergillosis Aspergilloma Endocarditis
Cryptococcosis (*Cryptococcus neoformans*)	Meningitis Pneumonia Cutaneous infection
Mucormycosis (various species of the genera *Rhizopus, Absidia* and *Mucor*)	Rhinocerebral infection Pulmonary mucormycosis
Malassezia furfur	Cutaneous infection (especially in burns patients) Fungaemia associated with total parenteral nutrition

Table 42.6 Clinical presentation of systemic fungal infection

Condition	Clinical presentation
Fungaemia (the presence of fungi in the bloodstream), usually due to *Candida* species	Fever, low blood pressure and sometimes other features of septic shock, especially in neutropenic patients. Relatively low-grade fungaemias such as those associated with colonized intravenous cannulae often present only with fever Disseminated infection to multiple organ systems is quite common with *Candida* species, leading to central nervous system disease, endocarditis, endophthalmitis, skin infections, renal disease and bone and joint infection
Pneumonia, most frequently due to *Aspergillus* species	Fever, chest pain and cough which may be non-productive. May progress rapidly, especially with *Aspergillus* infection, to severe respiratory distress, necrosis of the lung and pulmonary haemorrhage
Meningitis and other central nervous system infection	*Candida* infection may present as a typical meningitis, although it is often more insidious. Aspergillosis is associated with headache, confusion and focal neurological signs due to the presence of brain infarcts. Cryptococcosis most frequently presents as a chronic, insidious meningitis with headache and alteration in mental state
Mucormycosis	The most common presentation of mucormycosis is as rhinocerebral infection. Initially an infection of the sinuses, it then spreads locally to the palate, orbit and eventually into the brain, leading to encephalitis

Other diagnostic methods

Despite a great deal of work in recent years on the diagnosis of both candidiasis and aspergillosis by detection of circulating antigens or metabolites, or the use of molecular biology techniques such as the polymerase chain reaction (PCR), these techniques are not yet available for use in routine microbiology laboratories, and even when available from reference laboratories, the results are often disappointing. Mucormycosis is most readily diagnosed by histological examination of tissue biopsies since the organism is rarely cultured from clinical specimens.

Drug treatment

The difficulties in making the diagnosis of deep fungal infection are accompanied by a relative lack of effective antifungal agents for systemic use, at least when compared to the plethora of antibacterial agents. Two new agents, voriconazole and caspofungin, have become established for the treatment of deep fungal infection and these are discussed below. Details of drug interactions with these agents can be found in Table 42.2 and their side effects in Table 42.3.

Amphotericin B

General properties

Amphotericin is a member of the polyene group of antibiotics, which are obtained from various species of *Streptomyces*. There are a number of different polyenes but for various reasons, such as lack of stability or solubility, or excessive toxicity, only amphotericin is used systemically. Nystatin is available for topical use.

The chemical structure of amphotericin is that of a large carbon ring containing 37 carbon atoms and closed by a lactone bond. The molecule contains seven carbon-to-carbon double bonds (hence the name 'polyene' for this group of compounds) which are all situated on one side of the molecule while the other side contains seven hydroxyl groups. The molecule is therefore amphipathic (or amphoteric) in nature and this may be of some importance in the mode of action of all the polyenes. These agents all have very limited solubility in water and organic non-polar solvents such as acetone, but will readily dissolve in organic polar solvents such as dimethylsulfoxide. In water, amphotericin forms a colloidal suspension of micelles, which is rendered more stable if a surfactant such as sodium desoxycholate is added.

Mode of action The mode of action of the polyenes is to increase the permeability of the cytoplasmic membrane, leading to leakage of the cell contents and eventually death. This action is dependent on binding of the antibiotic to sterols present in the cell membrane, and organisms such as bacteria which do not contain sterols are inherently resistant to the polyenes. The different polyenes have differing affinities for sterols, and amphotericin has a higher affinity for ergosterol present in fungal cytoplasmic membranes than cholesterol, which is found in mammalian cell membranes. This fact presumably explains the selective toxicity of amphotericin for fungal cells.

Spectrum of activity Amphotericin is active against the vast majority of the fungi which cause systemic mycoses in the UK. It is synergistic in vitro with other agents such as flucytosine and rifampicin and in some cases, e.g. amphotericin plus flucytosine in candidiasis or cryptococcosis, this synergistic interaction appears to be of clinical significance. The results of combination with other antifungal agents are less certain, and both synergy and antagonism have been described. Acquired resistance to amphotericin during or following treatment is rarely a clinical problem, although it has been described, and only a few fungi are inherently resistant to this agent.

Conventional amphotericin B

Pharmacokinetics The pharmacokinetics of amphotericin are unusual. A 50 mg dose produces a peak plasma level of 0.5–3.5 mg/L, but clinical response cannot be related to the plasma level. Amphotericin penetrates poorly into cerebrospinal fluid (CSF) and is heavily (99%) protein bound. Initial elimination of the drug occurs with a half-life of 24–48 hours, but this is followed by very slow elimination (half-life about 2 weeks) and the drug may take several weeks to disappear completely. This may result from strong binding to cell membranes with a gradual elution over a period of weeks. Repeated doses of the drug do not cause accumulation in plasma. A small fraction, perhaps 3%, of a dose is excreted in the urine, so that renal dysfunction does not affect plasma levels, and the rest appears to be inactivated in the body. The measurement of plasma levels of amphotericin is not clinically helpful.

Administration Amphotericin is administered by slow intravenous infusion. If the drug is added to electrolyte solutions or solutions with a low pH it will precipitate out, so it must always be given in 5% dextrose. Since some commercial dextrose solutions have a surprisingly low pH, presumably due to slight caramelization of the dextrose during manufacture, it may be advisable to add a small amount of a buffer to dextrose solutions before adding amphotericin. Several different dosage schedules have been suggested; the two schedules given in Table 42.7 have been used successfully. The doses shown are for adults and would need to be modified for children. Although the need for a test dose has been disputed, the manufacturers currently recommend that before commencing treatment, a 1 mg test dose be given in 50 mL of 5% dextrose over a 1–2 hour period and the patient monitored for serous side effects such as fever, rigors and hypotension, during that time.

If the patient tolerates the test dose, there are two options. The first is designed to minimize serious side effects by a gradual build-up to the usual maximum daily dose of 1 mg/kg body weight. This is satisfactory if the infection is not immediately life-threatening but would be inappropriate for fulminating infections. In such cases the dose is increased rapidly with careful monitoring of the patient by medical staff.

It is also possible to give amphotericin intrathecally in very small doses (0.1–0.5 mg) although this is rarely done since the advent of the triazoles for the treatment of fungal infections of the CNS. In catheterized patients with fungal urinary tract infection, treatment is usually not indicated unless the patient is symptomatic but, if required, amphotericin can be given as a bladder wash-out in a concentration of 50 mg/L.

Table 42.7 Suggested dosage schedules for conventional (not lipid-complexed formulations) amphotericin B

Dose	Volume of infusion	Day	Duration of infusion
Regimen 1: For use in a patient with a non-life-threatening, deep-seated infection			
1 mg (test dose)	50 mL	1	2 hours
If no intolerable side effects or anaphylactic reaction, follow 2 hours later with:			
10 mg	500 mL	1	6 hours
Then on each successive day, increase dose by 10 mg to standard 50 mg daily dose:			
20 mg	500 mL	2	6 hours
30 mg	1000 mL	3	6 hours
40 mg	1000 mL	4	6 hours
50 mg	1000 mL	5 et seq.	6 hours
Regimen 2: For use in a compromised patient with a life-threatening infection			
1 mg (test dose)	50 mL	1	2 hours
If no intolerable side effects or anaphylactic reaction, follow 2 hours later with:			
25 mg	1000 mL	1	6 hours
Leave a 6-hour interval then administer the remainder of the 50 mg daily dose:			
25 mg	1000 mL	1	6 hours
50 mg	1000 mL	2 et seq.	6 hours

Notes

1. 50 mg represents a dose of about 0.7 mg/kg for a 70 kg adult. It may not be possible to achieve this dose, depending on the side effects. In this case the highest dose which does not produce unacceptable side-effects should be given.
2. Alternate-day treatment with a higher unit dose (up to a maximum unit dose of 1.5 mg/kg) may be given. This has the advantage of allowing the patient to attend for outpatient therapy. If the patient is still in hospital it will reduce the amount of time needed for amphotericin administration, which otherwise makes heavy use of intravenous access time that may be needed for other purposes.

Adverse effects Amphotericin is associated with a long list of toxic effects (see Table 42.3). It is possible to try to minimize the immediate side effects during the infusion by administering 25–50 mg of hydrocortisone, and antiemetics and an antihistamine may also be given. Nephrotoxicity is the most serious side effect of amphotericin and is almost invariable in patients given a full course of treatment. Renal function should be monitored regularly at least every other day and if the plasma creatinine exceeds 250 μmol/L the drug should be discontinued until the creatinine level falls below this limit. Hypokalaemia is also a problem and may be severe, necessitating replacement therapy. Fortunately, renal function returns to normal in most patients unless very large total doses have been given. There is little experience of the use of amphotericin in pregnancy, but what there is indicates that the risk of fetal toxicity is small.

Duration of treatment The duration of therapy is guided by clinical response. There is some evidence that the total dose administered is of some importance in determining response,

and for an established deep-seated infection a total dose of 1.5–2 g would be appropriate. This represents at least 6 weeks of therapy at 50 mg/day. The patient may be well enough to attend for treatment on an outpatient basis, in which case the drug can be given in a higher unit dose on alternate days. However, a maximum alternate daily dose of 1.5 mg/kg should not be exceeded. For fungaemia due to infected intravenous cannulae, the main therapeutic action is removal of the cannula, since the use of antifungal agents cannot be relied upon to eliminate the fungus from the cannula. However, they should still be given to prevent disseminated infection elsewhere in the body. There is no consensus about the length of therapy in such patients but 1 week's treatment at full dose has been suggested.

Amphotericin B lipid formulations

As a result of the toxicity of amphotericin B, considerable work has been carried out in the development of delivery systems in which amphotericin is encapsulated in liposomes or as a complex with lipid molecules. The advantages of these methods of delivery are that a higher unit dose may be given and there is a reduction in toxic effects. Three such preparations are currently available: liposomal amphotericin B (AmBisome), amphotericin B lipid complex (Abelcet) and amphotericin B colloidal dispersion (Amphocil).

Liposomal amphotericin B In liposomal amphotericin B (AmBisome), the drug is contained in small vesicles each consisting of a phospholipid bilayer enclosing an aqueous environment. This permits the delivery of higher doses (3 mg/kg is recommended, but doses up to 10 mg/kg have been used in some centres) compared to conventional amphotericin, with very little of the immediate toxicity which is such a problem with the conventional formulation. Higher peak plasma concentrations are obtained with the liposomal formulation compared to equivalent doses of the conventional drug, although it is not certain if this is clinically relevant. Liposomal amphotericin is concentrated mainly in the liver and spleen, where it is taken up by cells of the reticuloendothelial system. Concentrations in the lung and kidneys are much lower, which may or may not be clinically important.

There is reduced nephrotoxicity with this formulation, and some of the renal dysfunction which has been described in clinical trials of liposomal amphotericin may have been due to concomitant drugs. Three randomized, comparative clinical trials of liposomal amphotericin versus conventional amphotericin B have shown reduced toxicity due to the liposomal preparation, and there is additional evidence for this from open studies. It is this comparative lack of toxicity which accounts for much of the popularity of this agent, despite its expense. These studies also indicate that this agent performs as well as the conventional preparation in febrile neutropenic patients.

Amphotericin B lipid complex and amphotericin B colloidal dispersion Amphotericin B lipid complex (Abelcet) is not a liposomal formulation, but consists of large sheets of amphotericin combined with phospholipids. This formulation gives lower peak plasma levels compared to the conventional drug because it is rapidly taken up by tissue macrophages, while concentrations in the lungs and the liver are much higher. Patients seem to experience more immediate side effects than with liposomal amphotericin. There is less clinical trial evidence for the use of this agent compared to the liposomal preparation. Amphotericin B colloidal dispersion (Amphocil) is a formulation consisting of tiny discs of amphotericin and cholesterylsulfate. Like the lipid complex, it too produces low peak plasma levels but high liver concentrations compared to the conventional drug. There is less clinical experience with this preparation than with the liposomal preparation and it appears to have a higher incidence of certain adverse reactions than conventional amphotericin.

Choosing a lipid preparation It is unclear which of these agents should be chosen for routine use and whether the newer preparations should be used in preference to conventional amphotericin. Unfortunately, there are limited comparative trial data between the different lipid formulations. At present the greatest clinical experience is with liposomal amphotericin B and by reason of this and the reduced incidence of side effects, it is the preferred agent of the three in many centres in the UK. In an ideal world all patients requiring amphotericin would receive the conventional preparation initially, being changed to a lipid formulation only if they fail to respond to or cannot tolerate the side effects of the conventional form. However, the incidence of side effects and difficulty in administration of conventional amphotericin have in practice led to its replacement in most centres with a lipid formulation.

Flucytosine

Mode of action and spectrum of activity

Flucytosine (5-fluorocytosine) is a synthetic fluorinated nucleotide analogue. The mode of action is twofold. Following uptake by the cell, which is dependent on the presence of cytosine permease, flucytosine is deaminated to 5-fluorouracil by cytosine deaminase. This in turn is incorporated into fungal RNA in place of uracil, leading to impairment of protein synthesis. Further metabolism of 5-fluorouracil leads to a metabolite which inhibits the enzyme thymidylate synthetase, leading to inhibition of DNA synthesis. Mammalian cells have absent or weak cytosine deaminase activity which accounts for the selective toxicity of flucytosine

For all practical purposes, flucytosine is only active against yeasts and yeast-like fungi. Inherent resistance occurs in perhaps 10% of clinical isolates of *Candida* species and acquired resistance develops rapidly if the drug is used alone. There are several resistance mechanisms, some of which result from a single-step mutation giving a high frequency of acquired resistance in organisms exposed to the drug. For this reason flucytosine should always be given in combination with another agent such as amphotericin, with which it is synergistic.

Pharmacokinetics

Flucytosine is highly soluble in water and over 90% of an oral dose is absorbed from the gastrointestinal tract. Virtually all of the absorbed dose is excreted unchanged in the urine by glomerular filtration. The elimination half-life is about 4 hours, but this is greatly prolonged in renal failure and dosage modification is required in patients with renal dysfunction. The degree of protein binding is very low and flucytosine penetrates well into all tissues, including the aqueous humour of the eye, where about 10% of the plasma level is achieved, and the CSF, where about 80% of the plasma level is achieved.

Administration

Flucytosine is given orally or by a short intravenous infusion and the dose by either route in patients with normal renal function is 100–200 mg/kg/day in four divided doses. This must be reduced in renal failure, but the degree of reduction depends on the degree of renal impairment and it is obligatory to monitor the plasma levels of flucytosine. Unfortunately, flucytosine assay is now rarely carried out in routine laboratories in the UK and is usually performed in a reference laboratory, which is a practical obstacle to its use. Flucytosine is usually given in conjunction with amphotericin which will probably cause some degree of renal dysfunction, so requiring modification of the flucytosine dose. To avoid dose-related marrow toxicity, the peak plasma level, obtained at 1 hour after an intravenous dose or 2 hours after an oral dose, should be maintained in the range 70–80 mg/L and should not be allowed to exceed 100 mg/L.

Side effects

The side effects of flucytosine are given in Table 42.3. The most important toxic effect is a dose-related myelosuppression with neutropenia and thrombocytopenia. This is usually reversible and can be avoided by monitoring plasma levels of flucytosine and adjusting the dose accordingly. Hepatotoxicity is also probably a result of high plasma levels, and liver function tests should be performed regularly. The drug is teratogenic in some animals and is not recommended in pregnant women for relatively trivial infections such as a fungal urinary tract infection. In cases of a life-threatening fungal infection, which is very rare in pregnancy, the potential benefits of flucytosine must be weighed against the possible risks.

Imidazoles

The imidazoles clotrimazole, econazole, fenticonazole, sulconazole and tioconazole are now principally used for the local treatment of vaginal candidiasis and for dermatophyte infections. One imidazole, ketoconazole, is still available for systemic use but even this agent has been superseded by the triazoles.

Triazoles

Three triazoles are licensed in the UK: fluconazole, itraconazole and voriconazole. They differ substantially from one another in their physical properties and antifungal activity (Table 42.8) and their main side effects are listed in Table 42.3.

The basic chemical structure of the triazoles is the azole ring, a five-membered ring containing three nitrogen atoms. Their principal mode of action is inhibition of the synthesis of ergosterol, which is an important component of the cytoplasmic membrane in fungal but not in mammalian cells. One of the nitrogen atoms of the azole ring binds to the iron atom of cytochrome P450 and inhibits its activation. Ergosterol synthesis is dependent on cytochrome P450 activation and as a result, its production is impaired.

Table 42.8 Properties of the triazoles

Property	Fluconazole	Itraconazole	Voriconazole
Water solubility	High	Very low	Low; intravenous preparation complexed with cyclodextrin to increase solubility
Oral absorption	Very good	Capsule preparation incompletely absorbed, but is improved by presence of food; new liquid formulation is better absorbed and not affected by food	Very good
Bioavailability	90%	55% (capsules), 75% (liquid); may be reduced in patients with renal dysfunction, those with reduced gastric acid production, and in AIDS patients	96%
Typical peak plasma concentration	1.0 mg/L	0.2 mg/L (capsules), 0.5 mg/L (liquid); steady-state levels are only achieved after about 2 weeks of treatment	2.0 mg/L
Protein binding	10%	99%	58%
CSF penetration	60% of plasma levels achieved	Very low	Up to 50% of blood levels
Excretion in urine	90% excreted as unchanged drug	<1% as unchanged drug	<2% as unchanged drug
Liver metabolism	Negligible	Extensive; metabolites appear in bile and urine	Extensive; majority excreted as metabolites in urine

This mode of action does, however, result in a considerable number of drug interactions with these agents.

Fluconazole

Clinical use Fluconazole is available both orally and parenterally and is used only in the treatment and prophylaxis of infections due to yeasts and yeast-like fungi. It is not used for the treatment of infections due to moulds. It is highly effective in the treatment of *Cryptococcus* infection, but the first-line treatment of cryptococcosis of the central nervous system is the combination of amphotericin B plus flucytosine for CNS infection due to this organism (Perfect 2005). This may be followed by fluconazole, which in HIV-infected patients will be required for life as suppressive treatment to prevent relapse. In immunocompetent hosts, fluconazole may be used as the primary treatment for disease not involving the CNS, such as pulmonary infection.

The role of fluconazole in systemic candidiasis is not quite so clear-cut. In patients with candidaemia due to colonized intravenous cannulae, the most important treatment is removal of the infected cannula, but it is common practice to give a short course of antifungal therapy to prevent disseminated infection elsewhere. Fluconazole is suitable for this purpose (Kramer et al 1997). In non-neutropenic patients, studies have shown fluconazole and caspofungin to be as efficacious as, and less toxic than, conventional amphotericin B (Edwards 2005, Mora-Duarte et al 2002). In such patients, where the infecting organism and its susceptibility to fluconazole are known, it would be reasonable to commence treatment with fluconazole;

caspofungin is a potential alternative. In neutropenic patients, and in patients infected with fluconazole-resistant organisms, amphotericin continues to be the treatment of choice (Edwards 2005). Fluconazole has also been successfully used as prophylaxis against *Candida* infections in neutropenic patients and patients with AIDS, but this in turn has been associated with an increasing incidence of systemic infections with fluconazole-resistant strains.

Resistance Some units which use fluconazole extensively have noted the increasing isolation of yeasts resistant to the drug, and the prevalence of resistance is related to the extent of the use of fluconazole. Resistance in *Candida* species is mainly seen in patients who are given long-term prophylactic fluconazole, which selects out those *Candida* species (such as *C. krusei* and *C. glabrata*) that are inherently less susceptible to fluconazole. Resistance in *C. albicans*, the most common species infecting humans, is seen mainly in AIDS patients, partly due to the extensive use of fluconazole in treating severe oral and pharyngeal candidiasis in such patients and partly due to the very large numbers of yeasts in the oropharynx of AIDS patients with candidiasis, which increases the chance of resistance due to spontaneous mutation.

Itraconazole

Itraconazole is available both orally and intravenously. The drug was originally available in capsules but a newer liquid formulation gives better absorption than the original capsule preparation, leading to significantly greater bioavailability and higher plasma levels. This is a broad-spectrum antifungal which is effective against yeasts, dermatophytes, the 'pathogenic' fungi and some filamentous fungi, such as *Aspergillus*.

Clinical use In deep-seated infection, itraconazole is used to treat infections due to the 'pathogenic' fungi, but there is less published evidence of its use in the treatment of systemic candidiasis and it cannot be recommended for this purpose (Maertens & Boogaerts 2005). However, it may be useful in patients who are infected with strains resistant to fluconazole, some of which may remain sensitive to itraconazole, and in patients who are for some reason unable to tolerate fluconazole. It has also been used to treat cryptococcosis, despite its poor CSF penetration, and in that condition it is an alternative to fluconazole for patients who cannot take the latter drug. However, one study comparing fluconazole and itraconazole as maintenance treatment for cryptococcosis (Saag et al 1999) was discontinued due to the high rate of relapse in the itraconazole arm.

There is now considerable evidence to support the use of itraconazole as a prophylactic agent in immunocompromised patients. It has been shown to be effective in reducing the incidence of systemic fungal infection compared to placebo, and to be more effective than fluconazole, although this is due to a greater reduction in infections due to filamentous fungi, including *Aspergillus* (Glasmacher & Prentice 2005).

A particular area of interest has been the treatment of aspergillosis, since itraconazole would be a less toxic and orally available alternative to amphotericin. Unfortunately, the difficulty of performing clinical trials in aspergillosis, which is not a common condition and which invariably occurs in seriously ill patients, means that there is relatively little published work. One open prospective multicentre study (Denning et al 1998) evaluated cases of invasive aspergillosis in cancer patients, and concluded that there was no difference between initial treatment with amphotericin B (conventional or lipid formulations) and itraconazole. However, a small study in heart transplant recipients indicated that treatment with amphotericin was superior (Nanas et al 1998). At the present time the published evidence suggests that itraconazole should probably not be used as the first-line treatment for this condition (Maertens & Boogaerts 2005).

Voriconazole

This is the latest triazole to be licensed for use in the UK and it is available both orally and intravenously. It has advantages over itraconazole in that its absorption from the gastrointestinal tract is significantly better and is not affected by reductions in gastric acidity due to disease or concomitant medication. Its spectrum of activity is similar to that of itraconazole but it is more active against *Fusarium* species, a mould which causes superficial infection of the nails and cornea, and occasionally systemic infection in immunocompromised patients.

Clinical use The main clinical indication for the use of voriconazole is aspergillosis. Studies have shown improved efficacy compared to conventional amphotericin B in systemic *Aspergillus* infection (Herbrecht et al 2005). Unfortunately, comparative studies with liposomal or other lipid-based preparations of amphotericin are not available. One particular indication is cerebral aspergillosis. Although rare, this carries a very high mortality rate (90% or higher) and one study has shown

this to be reduced by voriconazole, presumably due to its better penetration into the central nervous system (Potter 2005).

In addition to aspergillosis, voriconazole is also licensed in the UK for the treatment of *Fusarium* infection and for the management of patients infected with strains of *Candida* which are resistant to fluconazole. It has been shown to be as efficacious as amphotericin B followed by fluconazole in the treatment of candidaemia in patients who were not neutropenic but it is not licensed for this indication. At present, there is insufficient evidence to recommend voriconazole as the first-line agent for the empirical treatment of suspected fungal infection.

Caspofungin

Caspofungin is the first of the echinocandins to become available for routine use, although others, such as micafungin and anidulafungin, are under development. These agents interfere with the production of the fungal cell wall by inhibiting the synthesis of an important component, 1,3-β-D-glucan. This is a target which does not exist in mammalian cells, providing selective toxicity against fungi. Caspofungin has a significant advantage over the triazoles in that it does not inhibit the cytochrome P450 system and therefore is not associated with such a wide range of drug interactions.

Susceptible fungi

The drug has a rather unusual spectrum of activity. It is active against most species of *Candida*, although some are less susceptible than others, but *Cryptococcus* is resistant. The commonly encountered species of *Aspergillus* are susceptible, but the drug is inactive against the dermatophytes and activity against other fungi is variable.

Clinical use

Caspofungin is only available via the intravenous route and does not penetrate into the cerebrospinal fluid. Due to its spectrum of activity, caspofungin is indicated only for candidiasis and aspergillosis. A comparative study showed caspofungin to be as efficacious as conventional amphotericin B in invasive candidiasis (Mora-Duarte et al 2002). It has been shown to be effective in patients with aspergillosis who failed to respond to, or who could not tolerate, other antifungal agents (Maertens et al 2004). Finally, caspofungin was also shown to be as effective as liposomal amphotericin B in the empirical treatment of fungal infection in neutropenic patients, and had a lower incidence of unwanted effects (Walsh et al 2004). In the UK, the drug is therefore also licensed for this condition.

Choice of treatment

The overall picture of the treatment of deep-seated fungal infection is constantly changing. At the present time, amphotericin B, perhaps in its liposomal form, remains the gold standard for the treatment of deep-seated infections due to filamentous fungi such as *Aspergillus*, and for systemic candidiasis in neutropenic patients. However, this may soon change, with voriconazole and caspofungin replacing amphotericin in these respective roles. Amphotericin, usually in one of the lipid preparations, is the most frequent choice for the empirical treatment of fungal infection in febrile neutropenic patients but again, caspofungin may become the first-line agent for this purpose.

In immunocompetent patients, fluconazole is the primary treatment for cryptococcosis outside the CNS, and also possibly also for invasive candidiasis. Voriconazole and caspofungin would be potential alternative agents in known or suspected infection with strains of *Candida* resistant to fluconazole. Itraconazole is a useful agent in infections due to the pathogenic fungi and possibly as a second-line agent in aspergillosis, although this role is rapidly being superseded by voriconazole and caspofungin.

Table 42.9 **Practice points**	
Drug toxicity in systemic antifungal agents	
Infusion-related side effects	• Particularly with conventional amphotericin B • Lipid-based preparations also show these, but to a lesser extent
Nephrotoxicity	• Particularly with conventional amphotericin B • Results in renal dysfunction • Cessation of treatment may be required • Drug level monitoring is not helpful in prevention • Potassium loss and hypokalaemia is a serious complication • Renal toxicity may be potentiated by concomitant nephrotoxic agents
Hepatotoxicity	• Associated with the azole antifungals • Was particularly severe with ketoconazole • The newer triazoles may also cause serious liver damage
Bone marrow suppression	• Associated with flucytosine • Dose-related problem, so drug level monitoring may help to prevent it • Tends to preclude the use of flucytosine in patients whose marrow is already damaged (e.g. in haematological malignancy or following bone marrow transplant)
Drug interactions	• Associated particularly with the azoles • Due to their mode of action in inhibiting the cytochrome P450 system • A wide range of drugs may be affected, some with serious interactions
Difficulties in drug administration	
Drug precipitation	• Amphotericin B will precipitate out if given in electrolyte-containing infusions • This may also happen in 5% dextrose due to acidity resulting from the manufacturing process
Need for a test dose	• Required for all amphotericin B preparations
Long infusion times and/or large infusion volumes	• A particular problem with conventional amphotericin • Long infusion times mean reduced access to intravenous cannulae for other purposes • Large infusion volumes may be undesirable in patients with renal or cardiac dysfunction
Variable absorption when taken by mouth	• A known problem with itraconazole • Absorption is reduced in the presence of raised gastric pH (e.g. following the use of antacids or drugs such as omeprazole) • Absorption is increased in the presence of food or if taken with a cola drink • Subtherapeutic levels may occur due to poor absorption • Therapeutic drug monitoring is recommended to avoid low levels
Resistance to antifungal agents	

Amphotericin B	• Usually seen as a very broad-spectrum antifungal but inherent resistance is seen in several clinically significant species:
	    Aspergillus terreus
	    Candida lusitaniae
	    Scedosporium apiospermum
	• Acquired resistance developing during treatment is very uncommon
	• Lipid preparations have identical in vitro antifungal activity to the conventional form

Flucytosine	• Acquired resistance during treatment is very common in *Candida* species • Monotherapy promotes the rapid development of resistance • Combination therapy with amphotericin will reduce the possibility of acquired resistance developing during treatment

Fluconazole	• Some species of *Candida* are inherently resistant or less susceptible to fluconazole:
	    C. krusei
	    C. glabrata
	• Long-term use of fluconazole may result in increased infections with these more resistant strains
	• Long-term use may also result in reduced susceptibility in strains of *C. albicans*

Itraconazole has an additional role in the prophylaxis of systemic fungal infection, where it is probably the agent of choice at present.

A recent development has been the use of combinations of antifungal agents to try to improve on the results from single agents. At the present time, there is little firm evidence to support the use of such combinations. Amphotericin B plus flucytosine in the treatment of cryptococcosis is the only combination where evidence exists of increased efficacy over either agent alone. However, faced with a seriously ill patient not responding to single agents, it is not surprising that many clinicians attempt the use of a combination of antifungals, even though the evidence is that the results are no better than with monotherapy (Cuenca-Estrella 2004).

CASE STUDIES

Case 42.1

A 14-year-old girl is diagnosed with acute myeloblastic leukaemia (AML). She receives induction chemotherapy which renders her very neutropenic (peripheral white blood cell count less than 1×10^9/L). Three days later she develops a high fever and feels very unwell, although there are no clinical signs of septic shock. She receives treatment with broad-spectrum antibacterials but after 72 hours is clinically no better, and blood cultures have not yielded an infecting organism. At this point the haematologist wishes to add an antifungal agent as empirical treatment.

Question

What would be the most appropriate agent in this case?

Answer

The problem of 'febrile neutropenia' is an extremely common one in patients such as this and the causes are imperfectly understood. It is presumed that the majority are due to infection, but a microbial cause is often never identified. A failure to respond to antibacterial agents in a very vulnerable neutropenic patient will almost invariably require empirical antifungal therapy – that is, treatment given even though the infecting organism is not known. Waiting until the diagnosis becomes certain is not an option since by that time the patient may have died. In this case the identity of a possible infecting fungus is unknown but many studies have shown that by far the most frequent organisms in this condition are either *Candida albicans* or related species, or a species of *Aspergillus*. Many other fungi have been isolated from such patients but these two organisms must be covered by any empirical therapy.

The possible alternatives in this case are few. The current 'gold standard' is still amphotericin B since this is a broad-spectrum agent which is active against most, but not all, fungi of medical importance, including the two organisms which must be included. This immediately poses the question of whether conventional amphotericin or a lipid preparation should be used. In terms of efficacy, published evidence has not convincingly shown a greater clinical response rate for any of the lipid preparations. However, there are disadvantages to using the conventional form as first-line treatment. The patient may be unable to tolerate the side effects or the development of renal dysfunction may preclude its use beyond a certain length of treatment. In addition, these patients may be receiving other nephrotoxic drugs, which may interact with amphotericin to worsen the renal function still further. From a patient management perspective, conventional amphotericin is not an easy drug

to administer. One particular disadvantage is the length of time required for infusion (up to 6 hours) which may delay the administration of other medication or blood products. Finally, patients may require multiple courses of amphotericin over the duration of their treatment, which may have a permanent effect on renal function.

In this case, it was decided to avoid these complications and use liposomal amphotericin B, accepting the significantly greater cost as justified by the avoidance of complications, which might themselves require considerable expenditure to treat further along the course of treatment for the leukaemia.

Case 42.2

A 54-year-old man is involved in an industrial accident which causes a severe burn injury. He has a prolonged hospital stay complicated by multiple episodes of sepsis with multiresistant healthcare-associated bacteria, for which he receives several courses of broad-spectrum antibiotics. Six weeks after admission he undergoes another septic episode, with accompanying septic shock, and this time a blood culture is taken which after 24 hours' incubation shows the presence of yeast cells on microscopy. The unit policy in suspected or proven systemic yeast infection is to use fluconazole as first-line treatment, on the basis that the most likely infecting organism is *Candida albicans*, which is usually susceptible to fluconazole.

Fluconazole is commenced but after 24 hours the patient's condition worsens and he is gravely ill. The results of fungal identification and susceptibility testing are not yet available. Amphotericin B is prescribed but the patient cannot tolerate the side effects following infusion and it is discontinued. The clinician is now asking for advice on alternative treatment.

Question

What advice would you give the clinician?

Answer

This case illustrates the difficulty in treating an apparently straightforward condition – fungal sepsis in a non-neutropenic (but still vulnerable) patient. Fluconazole is an attractive choice for presumed yeast infections due to its ease of use and low toxicity, but not all *Candida* species are susceptible to it. For this reason, in a patient who is particularly unwell, which would include a patient in septic shock, it may not be the most appropriate choice. In this case it was suspected that the organism was resistant to fluconazole and the choices then are clear: either amphotericin B or caspofungin. Both have shown efficacy in treating infection due to fluconazole-resistant yeasts (which in this case was eventually identified as *Candida krusei*, a species known to be resistant to fluconazole). Since the patient could not tolerate amphotericin, which in any case might be contraindicated in a patient with shock and developing renal failure, caspofungin was the better choice.

Case 42.3

A 27-year-old woman visits her doctor complaining that her toenails have become distorted and discoloured. Since it looks unattractive, she would like it corrected before her summer beach holiday. The primary care doctor makes the clinical diagnosis of 'tinea unguium' (dermatophytosis of the nail) which is confirmed by laboratory culture of nail scrapings. The doctor knows that this condition is unlikely to respond to topical treatment and therefore consults the British National Formulary for a systemic agent. There he finds that griseofulvin, terbinafine and itraconazole are all available for this condition. However, the situation is complicated by the fact that his patient tells him that she is trying to get pregnant and does not want to take anything which might harm a baby. At this point the doctor seeks specialist advice.

Question

What is the most appropriate (and safe) treatment in this patient?

Answer

This is a difficult issue. Griseofulvin is contraindicated, due to its known teratogenicity in animals. In addition, this drug decreases the effectiveness of oral contraceptives, so it would not be appropriate to give it along with an oral contraceptive agent to prevent pregnancy during its use. It is also recommended that oral contraception be continued for at least a month after discontinuing griseofulvin, so in this patient it is not an appropriate choice.

The position of itraconazole is a little different. Like griseofulvin, it has the US Food & Drugs Administration (FDA) category C (studies show fetal harm in animals but evidence in human beings is lacking) but there is at least one report of almost 200 women given itraconazole in the first trimester of pregnancy without evidence of fetal harm. In the current state of knowledge, however, it would be difficult to recommend itraconazole to this patient.

Terbinafine carries FDA category B (no evidence in animal studies of fetal harm but studies proving safety in pregnant women are not available). Therefore it could be given to the patient if the benefit outweighs the risk, but since this is not a serious condition this approach would be difficult to justify.

After some discussion the patient decided that she wanted the condition treated more than she wanted to become pregnant, so she opted to take a course of terbinafine but return to using her oral contraceptives until the course was complete.

REFERENCES

Cuenca-Estrella M 2004 Combinations of antifungal agents in therapy – what value are they? Journal of Antimicrobial Chemotherapy 54: 854-869

Denning D W, Marinus A, Cohen J et al 1998 An EORTC multicentre prospective survey of invasive aspergillosis in haematological patients: diagnosis and therapeutic outcome. EORTC Invasive Fungal Infections Cooperative Group. Journal of Infection 37: 173-180

Edwards J E 2005 Candida species. In: Mandell G L, Bennett J E, Dolin R (eds) Principles and practice of infectious diseases, 6th edn. Elsevier/Churchill Livingstone, Philadelphia, pp 2938-2957

Glasmacher A, Prentice A G 2005 Evidence-based review of antifungal prophylaxis in neutropenic patients with haematological malignancies. Journal of Antimicrobial Chemotherapy 56 (suppl S1): i23-i32

Hay R J 2005 Dermatophytosis and other superficial mycoses. In: Mandell G L, Bennett J E, Dolin R (eds) Principles and practice of infectious diseases, 6th edn. Elsevier/Churchill Livingstone, Philadelphia, pp 3051-3062

Herbrecht R, Nivoix Y, Fohrer C et al 2005 Management of systemic fungal infections: alternatives to itraconazole. Journal of Antimicrobial Chemotherapy 56 (suppl S1): i39-i48

Kramer K M, Skaar D J, Ackerman B H 1997 The fluconazole era: management of hematogenously disseminated candidiasis in the nonneutropenic patient. Pharmacotherapy 17: 538-548

Maertens J, Boogaerts M 2005 The place for itraconazole in treatment. Journal of Antimicrobial Chemotherapy 56 (suppl S1): i33-i38

Maertens J, Raad I, Petrikkos G et al 2004 Efficacy and safety of caspofungin for treatment of invasive aspergillosis in patients refractory to or intolerant of conventional antifungal therapy. Clinical Infectious Diseases 39: 1563-1571

Mora-Duarte J, Betts R, Rotstein C et al 2002 Comparison of caspofungin and amphotericin B for invasive candidiasis. New England Journal of Medicine 347: 2020-2029

Nanas J N, Saroglou G, Anastasiou-Nana M I et al 1998 Itraconazole for the treatment of pulmonary aspergillosis in heart transplant recipients. Clinical Transplantation 12: 30-34

Perfect J R 2005 Cryptococcus neoformans. In: Mandell G L, Bennett J E, Dolin R (eds) Principles and practice of infectious diseases, 6th edn. Elsevier/Churchill Livingstone, Philadelphia, pp 2997-3012

Potter M 2005 Strategies for managing systemic fungal infection and the place of itraconazole. Journal of Antimicrobial Chemotherapy 56 (suppl S1): i49-i54

Saag M S, Cloud G A, Graybill J R et al 1999 A comparison of itraconazole versus fluconazole as maintenance therapy for AIDS-associated cryptococcal meningitis. National Institute of Allergy and Infectious Diseases Mycoses Study Group. Clinical Infectious Diseases 28: 291-296

Walsh T J, Teppler H, Donowitz G R et al 2004 Caspofungin versus liposomal amphotericin B for empirical antifungal therapy in patients with persistent fever and neutropenia. New England Journal of Medicine 351: 1391-1402

FURTHER READING

Barrett J P, Vardulaki K A, Conlon C et al 2003 A systematic review of the antifungal effectiveness and tolerability of amphotericin B formulations. Clinical Therapeutics 25: 1295-1320

Letscher-Bru V, Herbrecht R 2003 Caspofungin: the first representative of a new antifungal class. Journal of Antimicrobial Chemotherapy 51: 513-521

Richardson M D 2005 Changing patterns and trends in systemic fungal infection. Journal of Antimicrobial Chemotherapy 56 (suppl S1): i5-i11

Richardson M D, Jones B L 2003 Therapeutic guidelines in systemic fungal infections, 3rd edn. Current Medical Literature, London

Richardson M D, Warnock D W 2003 Fungal infection: diagnosis and management, 3rd edn. Blackwell Publishing, Oxford

43 Thyroid and parathyroid disorders

M. D. Page

KEY POINTS

- When diagnosing thyroid conditions, the possibility of drug-induced disease should always be considered.
- The treatment of hypothyroidism requires lifelong thyroxine therapy and monitoring. Written advice should be given to the patient.
- Thyroxine replacement therapy should be introduced cautiously in the elderly, particularly those with cardiac disease.
- Thyrotoxicosis can be treated with thionamide therapy, radioiodine or surgery; the choice will largely be determined by patient age, the cause of the thyrotoxicosis, the severity of the condition, co-morbidity and patient preference.
- Patients treated with thionamide therapy require careful counselling about the symptoms and management of agranulocytosis, and written guidance.
- Hypoparathyroidism can occur after thyroid surgery. It is managed with vitamin D analogues and requires lifelong monitoring.
- Surgery for hyperparathyroidism is only required in a minority of patients.

The Thyroid

The thyroid gland consists of two lobes and is situated in the lower neck. The gland synthesizes, stores and releases two major metabolically active hormones: tetra-iodothyronine (thyroxine, T_4) and tri-iodothyronine (T_3). Regulation of hormone synthesis is by the secretion of the glycoprotein thyroid-stimulating hormone (TSH) from the anterior pituitary. In turn, TSH is regulated by hypothalamic secretion of the tripeptide thyrotrophin-releasing hormone (TRH) (Fig. 43.1). Low circulating levels of thyroid hormones initiate the release of TSH, and probably also TRH. Rising levels of TSH promote increased iodide trapping by the gland and a subsequent increase in thyroid hormone synthesis. The increase in circulating hormone levels feeds back on the pituitary and hypothalamus, shutting off TRH, TSH and further hormone synthesis.

Both T_4 and T_3 are produced within the follicular cells in the thyroid. The stages in synthesis are shown in Figure 43.2.

- Thyroglobulin and thyroid peroxidase are synthesized by follicular cells.
- Hydrogen peroxide (H_2O_2) is synthesized at the luminal membrane.
- Dietary inorganic iodide is trapped from the circulation and transported to the follicular lumen where it is oxidized by H_2O_2.
- Iodine is then transferred onto the tyrosine residues in thyroglobulin by iodinase enzymes, forming mono-iodotyrosine (MIT) and di-iodotyrosine (DIT).

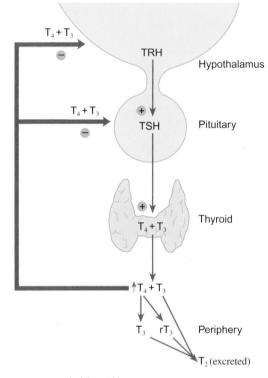

Figure 43.1   Control of thyroid hormone secretion.

- Subsequently the formation of T_4 occurs as a result of the coupling of two DIT residues and of T_3 by coupling a DIT and a MIT residue. The hormones are then stored within the gland until their release into the circulation.
- Finally thyroglobulin is resorbed into the follicular cell, hydrolysed and the amino acids and remaining iodide reused.

The ratio of $T_4:T_3$ secreted by the thyroid gland is approximately 10:1. Consequently the gland secretes approximately 80–100 μg of T_4 and 10 μg of T_3 per day. However, only 10% of circulating T_3 is derived from direct thyroidal secretion, the remaining 90% being produced by peripheral conversion from T_4. T_4 can therefore be considered a pro-hormone that is converted in peripheral tissues (liver, kidney and brain) either to the active hormone T_3 or to the biologically inactive reverse T_3 (rT_3). In the circulation, the hormones exist in both the active free and inactive protein bound forms. T_4 is 99.98% bound, with only 0.02% circulating free. T_3 is slightly less protein bound (99.8%), resulting in a considerably higher circulating free fraction (0.2%). Details of protein binding are shown in Table 43.1.

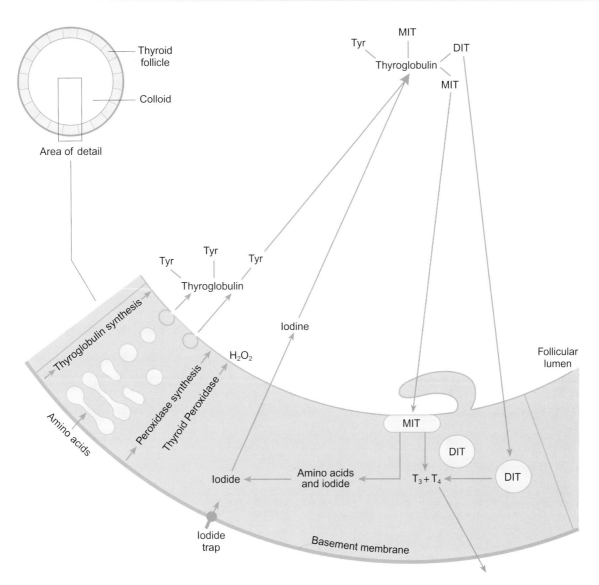

Figure 43.2 Synthesis of thyroid hormones.

Table 43.1 Plasma protein binding of thyroid hormones

Carrier protein	Plasma concentration	Percent T_4 & T_3 bound
Thyroid-binding globulin (TBG)	15 mg/L	75
Transthyretin (formerly thyroid-binding prealbumin)	250 mg/L	10
Albumin	40 g/L	15

The hormones are metabolized in the periphery (kidney, liver and heart) by deiodination. T_4 and T_3 are also eliminated by biliary secretion of their glucuronide and sulfate conjugates (15–20%). The half-life of T_4 in plasma is about 6–7 days and that of T_3 24–36 hours in euthyroid adults. The apparent volume of distribution for T_4 is about 10 litres and for T_3 about 40 litres.

Hypothyroidism

Hypothyroidism is the clinical state that results from decreased production of thyroid hormones or, very rarely, from tissue resistance.

Epidemiology

Accurate assessment of the prevalence and incidence of hypothyroidism is difficult due to the variation in definitions and population samples. The prevalence of previously undiagnosed, spontaneous, overt hypothyroidism has been estimated to be between 2 and 4 per 1000 of the total population worldwide. However, if all cases of previously diagnosed hypothyroidism and the effects of previous thyroid surgery and radioiodine treatment are included, this prevalence rises to approximately 10 per 1000. Primary hypothyroidism in the UK is common, with reports of new cases of hypothyroidism being 3 per 1000 women. Total prevalence is of the order of 14 per 1000 women and <1 per 1000 men (Tunbridge et al 1977). Thus, hypothyroidism occurs 10–20 times more frequently in women than in men. Despite these data, population screening for autoimmune hypothyroidism is thought probably not cost-effective unless incorporated into a screening programme for other conditions. Although the disease may occur at any age, most patients present between 30 and 60 years of age.

Aetiology

Primary hypothyroidism accounts for more than 95% of adult cases and is due to a failure of the thyroid gland itself as a result of autoimmune destruction, or the effects of treatment of thyrotoxicosis. Hypothyroidism may also be drug induced by agents such as amiodarone and lithium which cause hypothyroidism in around 10% of patients treated. Secondary disease is due to hypopituitarism, and tertiary disease due to failure of the hypothalamus. Peripheral hypothyroidism is due to tissue insensitivity to the action of thyroid hormones. A more extensive classification is shown in Table 43.2.

Iodides may produce hypothyroidism in patients who are particularly sensitive to their ability to block the active transport pump of the thyroid gland. Iodine absorption from topical iodine-containing antiseptics has been shown to cause hypothyroidism in neonates. This is potentially very dangerous at a critical time of neurological development in the newborn infant. Transient hypothyroidism may be seen in 25% of iodine-exposed infants.

Clinical manifestations

The clinical features of hypothyroidism can affect multiple body systems, are mainly non-specific and gradual in onset (Table 43.3). Symptoms, especially in the early stages, are frequently vague. It is common for symptoms to be incorrectly attributed by patients and their relatives to increasing age. The reverse is also common in that patients who have read about or have friends/family with hypothyroidism will assume that hypothyroidism is responsible for their symptoms of fatigue and weight gain. Thus hypothyroidism is often confused with obesity and depression. Mercifully, simple thyroid function tests give accurate diagnoses in all cases (see below).

The most common symptoms reported by patients are weakness, lethargy, cold intolerance, slowness, constipation, memory loss and weight gain. The skin becomes dry and flaky, head hair thins and is dry and the patient may have noticed a change in voice, with deepening or gruffness.

The most useful clinical signs are myotonic (slow relaxing) tendon reflexes, bradycardia, hair loss and cool, dry hands. Effusions may occur into pericardial, pleural, peritoneal or joint spaces. Mild anaemia of a macrocytic type is quite common and responds to thyroxine replacement. Pernicious anaemia is a frequent concomitant finding in hypothyroidism. Other, organ-specific autoimmune diseases such as Addison's disease may be associated.

Myxoedema coma   Myxoedema coma is a rare but potentially fatal complication of severe, untreated hypothyroidism. Coma can be precipitated by hypothermia, stress, infection, trauma and certain drugs, notably β-blockers and respiratory depressants, including anaesthetic agents, narcotics, phenothiazines and hypnotics. The condition is a medical emergency and should be treated rapidly and aggressively.

Table 43.2   Classification of hypothyroidism

Primary hypothyroidism

Congenital hypothyroidism
  Agenesis
  Inherited enzyme defects

Immune
  Hashimoto's thyroiditis
  Spontaneous hypothyroidism in Graves' disease
  Postpartum hypothyroidism

Iatrogenic
  Postoperative hypothyroidism
  Hypothyroidism after radioactive iodine
  External neck irradiation
  Drugs, e.g. antithyroid thionamides, amiodarone, lithium, elemental iodide

Iodine deficiency

Subacute (viral)

Secondary/tertiary hypothyroidism

Hypopituitarism (any cause)

Hypothalamic disease

Peripheral hypothyroidism

Insensitivity to thyroid hormones

Table 43.3   Signs and symptoms of hypothyroidism

Skin and appendages	Dry, cool, flaking, thickened skin Reduced sweating Yellowish complexion Puffy facies and eyes Sparse, coarse, dry hair Brittle nails
Neuromuscular system	Slow speech Poor memory and reduced cognitive function Somnolence Carpal tunnel syndrome Psychiatric disturbance Hearing loss Depression Muscle pain and weakness Delayed deep tendon reflexes
Metabolic abnormalities	Raised total and LDL cholesterol Macrocytic anaemia
Gastrointestinal	Weight gain with decreased appetite Abdominal distension and ascites Constipation
Cardiovascular	Reduced cardiac output Bradycardia Cardiac enlargement

The term 'myxoedema' used to be synonymous with hypothyroidism. It is now reserved for advanced disease in which there is swelling of the skin and subcutaneous tissues.

Investigations

The laboratory investigation of hypothyroidism is extremely simple. Usually clinical assessment, combined with a single estimation of thyroid hormones and TSH, is sufficient to make the diagnosis. In primary disease, the levels of free T_4 and T_3 are low and the TSH level rises markedly. Some laboratories offer only TSH as a first-line test of thyroid function. This can result in delayed diagnosis of secondary or tertiary hypothyroidism, which should be suspected on the basis of a low free T_4 along with low TSH levels.

Elevation of the TSH level occurs early in the course of thyroid failure and may be present before overt clinical manifestations appear. It is important to appreciate that hypothyroidism is not one disease but a spectrum. Early hypothyroidism may be asymptomatic or the symptoms less obvious and non-specific but a normal TSH with normal free T_4 effectively excludes the diagnosis.

A chest radiograph may detect the presence of effusions, and an electrocardiogram (ECG) is useful, especially in patients with angina or coronary heart disease, in whom replacement therapy needs to be introduced gradually.

Testing thyroid function As already indicated, a clinical assessment and measurement of free T_4 and TSH is usually all that is necessary to arrive at an accurate diagnosis of thyroid status. All modern TSH assays now employ double antibody immunometric techniques, which are robust and highly reliable. Moreover, these assays are now so sensitive that they are able to identify thyrotoxic patients with TSH levels below the normal euthyroid range. Commercial free T_4 and free T_3 assays, however, are all indirect methods and are subject to interference from drugs and other disease states. As such, both T_3 and to a lesser extent T_4 can be decreased as a non-specific consequence of systemic illness (sick euthyroid syndrome) and depression along with a host of drugs (Surks & Sievert 1995), which can interfere with thyroid hormone metabolism and free hormone assays (Table 43.4). These patients require specialist assessment and collaboration with the local laboratory to rule out confounding disease and pituitary failure.

Treatment

The aims of treatment with thyroxine are to ensure that patients receive a dose that will restore well-being and which usually returns the TSH level to the lower end of the normal range (Vanderpump et al 1996). It is important to avoid both under- and overtreatment. All patients with symptomatic hypothyroidism require replacement therapy. T_4 is usually the treatment of choice except in myxoedema coma, where T_3 may be used in the first instance. Before commencing T_4 replacement, the diagnosis of glucocorticoid deficiency must be excluded in order to prevent precipitation of a hypoadrenal crisis. If in doubt, hydrocortisone replacement should be given concomitantly until cortisol deficiency is excluded.

Table 43.4 Drug effects on thyroid function

	Clinical/biochemical effects
Decrease TSH secretion Dopamine Glucocorticoids Octreotide	Hypothyroidism (rarely clinically important)
Alter thyroid hormone secretion Iodide (amiodarone, contrast agents) Lithium	Both hyper- and hypothyroidism Hypothyroidism
Decrease T_4 absorption Colestyramine/colestipol Aluminium hydroxide Ferrous sulfate Sucralfate	Increased thyroxine dose requirement

Alter T_4 and T_3 metabolism
Increased hepatic metabolism
    Phenobarbital
    Phenytoin
    Rifampicin
    Carbamazepine
	Low T_4 and T_3 levels.
	Normal or increased TSH

Reduce conversion of T_4 to T_3 β-Blockers Propylthiouracil Amiodarone Glucocorticoids	Lower T_3 levels Normal or increased TSH
Reduce T_4 and T_3 binding Furosemide Salicylates and NSAIDs Heparin	Increased measured free T_4 in some assays
Increase thyroglobulin levels Oestrogen and tamoxifen Opiates and methadone	Increased total T_4
Others Cytokines, e.g. interferon and interleukin-2	Thyroiditis. Can produce hypothyroidism and thyrotoxicosis

Hypothyroidism is very rarely life-threatening and adverse effects such as osteoporosis and atrial fibrillation may result from prolonged overtreatment. The initial dose of T_4 will depend on the patient's age, severity and duration of disease, and the co-existence of cardiac disease.

In young, healthy patients with disease of short duration, T_4 may be commenced in a dose of 50–100 μg daily. As the drug has a long half-life it should only be given once daily. The most convenient time is usually in the morning. After 6 weeks on the same dose, thyroid function tests should be checked. The TSH concentration is the best indicator of the thyroid state and this should be used for further dosage adjustment. Clearly, a raised TSH concentration indicates either inadequate treatment or poor compliance. The majority of patients will be controlled with doses of 100–200 μg daily, with few patients requiring more than 200 μg. In adults, the median dose required to suppress TSH to normal is 125 μg daily. In the majority of patients, once the appropriate dose has been established it remains constant. During pregnancy, an increase in the dose of thyroxine, often by 50 μg daily, is needed to maintain normal TSH levels.

In elderly patients, particularly those with cardiac disease, treatment should be introduced more cautiously. Some 5% of patients with long-standing hypothyroidism either complain of angina at presentation or develop it during treatment with thyroxine. Exacerbation of myocardial ischaemia, infarction and sudden death are all well-recognized complications of T_4 replacement therapy. Patients with coronary heart disease may be unable to tolerate full replacement doses because of palpitations, angina or heart failure. Treatment should be started with 25 μg daily and increased slowly by 25 μg every 4–6 weeks. Some authorities recommend starting with 5 μg of T_3. The proposed advantage is that if adverse effects occur, these will be alleviated more rapidly due to the shorter half-life of T_3. During this time the patient's clinical progress should be carefully monitored. In some patients T_4 may be better tolerated if a β-blocker such as propranolol is given concomitantly.

There has been considerable recent interest in the risks of overtreatment with T_4. Although T_4 exerts an effect on many organs and tissues, it is probably the effects on bone and the heart that give the greatest cause for concern. There is evidence that bone density may be reduced in patients taking T_4 replacement therapy (Faber & Galloe 1994, Uzzan et al 1996), and that atrial fibrillation is more common if TSH is suppressed (Sawin et al 1994). In order to minimize the risk of development of these complications, the dose should be carefully tailored to the needs of each individual patient. Some patients will have undetectable serum TSH levels while taking thyroxine and may complain of recurrent fatigue if the dose is reduced to permit the TSH to rise. In these patients, it may be permissible to leave the dose unchanged if levels of free T_4 and T_3 are normal, after a discussion of the relative risks and benefits with the patient.

Myxoedema coma The treatment of myxoedema coma has been poorly studied and the optimal regimen remains to be defined. Thyroid hormone replacement is usually commenced by giving 5–10 μg of T_3 parenterally twice daily. Possible adrenal underactivity should be treated with parenteral hydrocortisone 100 mg three times daily. Heart failure and arrhythmias should be treated if they arise. Sources of infection should be actively sought, particularly chest or urinary infections, and treated aggressively. The body temperature should be monitored rectally and allowed to rise slowly by keeping the patient in a warm room and wrapped in a 'space blanket' that retains heat. Urea, electrolyte and haematological assessments must be made and corrected as necessary. Even with this kind of management approach, the mortality rate exceeds 50%.

Patient care

The treatment of hypothyroidism requires lifelong treatment with T_4. Patients on long-term drug therapy are well recognized to have a low adherence with their medication regimen and these patients are no exception. Treatment with T_4 is often terminated because patients feel well and think that treatment is no longer

required. Patients should be educated to understand the effects of drug holidays on their health and thyroid function tests and should know that a normal TSH indicates adequate dosage. Written advice should be provided before discharge to primary care and monitoring of dosage should continue annually.

Prevention At present nothing can be done to prevent autoimmune thyroid failure from developing. However, much can be done to ensure early detection and treatment. Careful follow-up of patients who have undergone iodine[131] treatment or subtotal thyroidectomy or completed a course of treatment for thyrotoxicosis is essential, along with monitoring of those prescribed amiodarone and lithium. The earliest biochemical change is an increase in TSH with normal concentrations of T_3 and T_4. These should be used to diagnose hypothyroidism before the patient becomes symptomatic. Table 43.5 shows the prevalence of hypothyroidism after treatment for thyrotoxicosis.

Hyperthyroidism

Hyperthyroidism is defined as the production by the thyroid gland of excessive amounts of thyroid hormones. Thyrotoxicosis refers to the clinical syndrome associated with prolonged exposure to elevated levels of thyroid hormone. This distinction is important when evaluating thyroid function tests (Table 43.6)

Epidemiology

Hyperthyroidism is a common condition. It has been estimated that there are 4.7 per 1000 women with active disease. When previously treated cases were included, the population prevalence rose to 20 per 1000 in women. As with hypothyroidism, it is much less common in men, with a lifetime prevalence of around 2 per 1000 (Tunbridge et al 1977).

Aetiology

Hyperthyroidism is a disorder of various aetiologies. In clinical terms, thyrotoxicosis is the result of persistently elevated levels of thyroid hormones.

Graves' disease Graves' disease is the most common cause of thyrotoxicosis. It is an autoimmune condition resulting from production of an abnormal immunoglobulin. This

---

Table 43.5 Prevalence of hypothyroidism after treatment for thyrotoxicosis

Thyroidectomy
- 6–75% hypothyroidism over their lifetime, dependent on the amount of remnant tissue
- Risk highest during first year after surgery

Antithyroid drugs (>6 month course)
- 43% relapse in the first year
- 13–21% relapse in the next 4 years

^{131}I therapy
- 24–90% develop hypothyroidism over their lifetime, depending on dose given

Table 43.6 Aetiology of hyperthyroidism

Condition	Frequency	Clinical features	I^{131} uptake
Thyrotoxicosis (increased hormone synthesis)			
Graves' disease	70%	Antibody mediated (TRABs) 90% are young women Diffuse goitre Ophthalmopathy (30%) Pretibial myxoedema Acropachy Transmissible to neonate	Increased
Multinodular goitre	20%	Benign autonomous nodules Often secrete T_3 Older women Always relapse after withdrawal of thionamides	Increased
Toxic single adenoma	5%		Increased
Iodine induced	<1%	Increased urine iodine	Variable
HCH induced	Rare	Molar pregnancy or choriocarcinoma	Increased
TSH dependent	Rare	Pituitary tumour	Increased
Thyroid destruction (leakage of stored thyroid hormones)			
Acute	2%	Probably viral Neck pain often severe	Absent
Silent	2%	Viral Autoimmune	Absent
Amiodarone induced	<1%	Increased urine iodine	Absent

TRAB, thyroid receptor antibody

immunoglobulin is able to occupy the TSH receptor on the thyroid follicular cell where it mimics the effect of TSH, causing cell division and stimulating thyroid hormone secretion. They are therefore known as thyroid receptor antibodies (TRABs). Rarely the TRAB is inhibitory to the receptor, resulting in hypothyroidism.

Ninety percent of patients with Graves' disease are young women. There is often a family history of the condition. In addition to the effects of thyrotoxicosis, patients (30%) may develop additional features including a congestive ophthalmopathy which is thought to result from antibody-mediated inflammation of orbital contents. Pretibial myxoedema, gynaecomastia and thyroid acropachy are rare manifestations.

The maternal IgG immunoglobulin can pass through the placenta to the fetus resulting in transient neonatal thyrotoxicosis.

Nodular disease Toxic multinodular goitre is also a common form of thyrotoxicosis often affecting older women. An euthyroid nodular goitre may have been pesent for many years. Individual nodules become autonomous, producing T_4 and/or T_3. The thyrotoxicosis is generally less severe and more gradual in onset. Often only T_3 levels are elevated, though the TSH will be suppressed in all cases. Thyrotoxicosis may also be caused by single autonomous thyroid adenomas. These are benign, well-differentiated tumours that secrete excessive amounts of thyroid hormones.

Thyroiditis If the thyroid is inflamed by viral or rapid autoimmune attack, the resulting follicular cell death will lead to the release of preformed thyroid hormones. This can result in a brief period of thyrotoxicosis before thyroid hormone

levels fall to subnormal. Often the period of thyrotoxicosis is not clinically apparent and in any event is brief, but it is common for patients to be prescribed thionamides, which compound the ensuing hypothyroidism. It is therefore necessary to be aware of these conditions. Any suspicion of neck pain should prompt the clinician to request an iodine uptake scan. Iodine uptake is absent in hyperthyroidism associated with thyroiditis.

Clinical manifestations

Thyrotoxicosis is characterized by increased metabolism of all body systems due to excessive quantities of thyroid hormones. There is a wide spectrum of clinical thyroid hormone excess. The clinical signs and symptoms reflect increased adrenergic activity, especially in the cardiovascular and neurological systems (Table 43.7). Not all manifestations will be seen in every patient. Additional clinical features will depend on the underlying cause of the thyrotoxicosis (see Table 43.6).

The diagnosis of thyrotoxicosis in the elderly may not be so easily made. Signs and symptoms of cardiovascular disturbance tend to predominate. Atrial fibrillation is frequent, and the patient may be in congestive cardiac failure. Unexplained heart failure after middle age should always arouse suspicion of thyrotoxicosis.

The extrathyroidal manifestations of Graves' disease deserve separate mention. Most frequent is ophthalmopathy due to inflammation and expansion of the contents of the orbit. The eye is pushed forward (proptosed) such that white sclera appears

Table 43.7 Signs and symptoms of thyrotoxicosis

Skin and appendages	Warm, moist skin Thinning or loss of hair Increased sweating Heat intolerance
Nervous system	Insomnia Irritability, nervousness Lid retraction – staring eyes Symptoms of an anxiety state Psychosis
Musculoskeletal	Tremor Proximal muscle weakness Rapid deep tendon reflexes Osteoporosis
Gastrointestinal	Weight loss despite increased appetite Thirst Diarrhoea
Cardiovascular	Palpitations, tachycardia Shortness of breath on exertion Atrial fibrillation Congestive cardiac failure Worsening angina

between the iris and the lower lid. Congestive changes develop including periorbital oedema, conjunctival swelling and redness. The extraocular muscles are swollen and become tethered, leading to failure of movement of the globe of the eye and thus diplopia. Severe disease causes pressure in the orbit, which can compress the optic nerve, leading to blindness. The cutaneous features of Graves' disease include thickening of the pretibial skin (myxoedema), onycholysis (separation of the nail from the nail bed) and acropachy (similar to finger clubbing).

Investigations

In any patient with suspected thyrotoxicosis it is good practice to document the diagnosis with at least two sets of thyroid function tests. If the diagnosis is in doubt, treatment should be withheld. Unless severe, thyrotoxicosis can usually be safely observed while investigations are carried out. Plasma free T_4 (and/or T_3) levels are clearly elevated in more than 90% of patients with thyrotoxicosis. The TSH level is suppressed to subnormal levels in all causes of thyrotoxicosis, except the exceptionally rare cases of TSH-secreting pituitary adenomas.

In the overwhelming majority of patients the combination of the clinical findings and simple investigations is sufficient to make a firm diagnosis. Radioactive iodine uptake scans will differentiate those patients with thyroiditis. Measurement of TRABs will identify Graves' disease patients. If the diagnosis is still equivocal the clinical findings should be reassessed, and particular attention paid to the patient's drug history. There are a number of drugs that may modify the clinical features or interfere with the tests (Table 43.4).

Treatment

A number of factors need to be considered when choosing the most appropriate form of therapy for an individual patient (Table 43.8). There are usually a number of therapeutic options available and the patient should be involved in deciding on treatment. The decision may also be influenced by physician preference, which in turn can depend on the facilities available. Three forms of therapy available are antithyroid drugs, surgery and radioactive iodine. There is no general agreement as to the specific indications for each form of therapy and none of them is ideal, all being associated with both short- and long-term sequelae. Neither surgery nor radioactive iodine should be given until the patient has been rendered euthyroid due to the risk of inducing a thyroid crisis.

In children, surgery may be difficult and the complication rate is higher. Radioiodine is generally avoided due to concerns about the potential development of thyroid malignancy. In pregnancy radioiodine is not used due to the likelihood of producing a hypothyroid neonate. Surgery should be deferred until the second trimester if possible but most patients can be controlled with drugs. However, doses should be kept as low as possible, especially in the last 2 months of pregnancy, as excessive treatment may produce goitre in the fetus. Aplasia cutis is said to occur after carbimazole therapy so propylthiouracil is usually used in pregnancy. Pregnant patients with thyrotoxicosis should be under the care of a specialist endocrine unit.

Table 43.8 Treatments available for thyrotoxicosis

	Adverse effects (%)	Contraindications	Cautions
Thionamides Carbimazole Propylthiouracil	Rash/arthropathy (5%) Agranulocytosis (0.3%) Hepatitis (rare)	Previous allergy Cross-reactivity in 10%	Pregnancy: PTU preferred. Do not use block/replace regimens
Radioiodine	Hypothyroidism requiring lifelong T_4	Pregnancy	Ensure euthyroid first Ophthalmopathy may deteriorate
Surgery	Hospital stay Neck scar Surgical/anaesthetic risk 10% require T_4		Ensure euthyroid first Ophthalmopathy may deteriorate

Acute management of thyrotoxocosis Patients need to have their symptoms addressed and their thyrotoxicosis controlled. β-blockers in standard antihypertensive doses are effective within hours and should be given to all non-asthmatics with severe thyrotoxicosis. Carbimazole (40 mg o.d.) or propylthiouracil (300 mg b.d.) will render most patients euthyroid within 6 weeks. Adjunctive treatment of cardiac disease and anxiety/sleeplessness may also be required.

Graves' disease A proportion (40–50%) of patients with Graves' disease will achieve a long-lasting remission after a period of euthyroidism on thionamides. The optimal duration of antithyroid treatment is unknown and remains a controversial issue (Maugendre et al 1999), but in most units the length of the treatment course has fallen from 2 years in the 1970s to between 6 and 12 months. Remission of Graves' disease is much less likely in those with very large goitres, those who require high-dose thionamide treatment to maintain euthyroidism, those with high TRAB titres and patients who have relapsed once after a course of drug treatment. Such patients should therefore be rendered euthyroid and then have a discussion about either surgical or radioiodine thyroid ablation.

Nodular thyroid disease As the nodules function autonomously and thyrotoxicosis will always recur when drugs are stopped, there is no value in attempting to achieve a remission of nodular thyroid disease using prolonged courses of thionamides. Patients should be rendered euthyroid with drugs and then have a discussion about ablative therapy.

Antithyroid drugs The thionamides, propylthiouracil (PTU), thiamazole (methimazole) and its precursor carbimazole, are equally effective pharmacological therapies for thyrotoxicosis. In the UK, carbimazole is usually used. These drugs prevent thyroid hormone synthesis by inhibiting the oxidative binding of iodide and its coupling to tyrosine residues. PTU, but not carbimazole, inhibits the peripheral deiodination of T_4 to T_3. In addition, the thionamides are also thought to have an immunosuppressive action.

Adverse effects The most common adverse effect of antithyroid treatment is rash and arthropathy (5%) and less commonly agranulocytosis, hepatitis, aplastic anaemia and lupus-like syndromes (Table 43.9). Overall, serious effects such as these occur in approximately 0.3% of patients treated. These side effects usually occur during the first 6 weeks of treatment but this is not invariable. Cross-sensitivity between carbimazole and propylthiouracil is around 10% and the patient can often be safely changed to the alternative agent if an adverse event occurs.

Regular monitoring of white cell counts has been advocated, but is not warranted. Agranulocytosis is a rare event and even if it does occur, it happens rapidly and even routine monitoring of white cell counts may miss it. At the time of prescription, all patients should be warned about the possible implication of sore throat, mouth ulcers and pyrexia, and instructed to seek an urgent (within hours) full blood count. This verbal information should be backed up by written advice, along with advice on where to go for the blood test. An abnormal white cell count should prompt urgent admission under a specialist team.

Treatment regimens Carbimazole is usually given initially at a dose up to 40–60 mg daily, depending on the severity of the condition. It can be given as a single daily dose in multiples of 20 mg tablets to aid adherence. Although the plasma half-life is

Table 43.9 Adverse effects of thionamides

	Adverse effect	Comments
Skin	Pruritic, maculopapular rash	Most common in first 6 weeks May disappear spontaneously with continued treatment Can be treated with an antihistamine Change to alternative agent Occurs in 5% of patients
	Urticarial rash with systemic symptoms, i.e. fever, arthralgia	Discontinue drug Alternative treatment required
Haematological	Agranulocytosis	Most common in first 6 weeks Incidence increases with age Discontinue drug Reversible Consider alternative treatment Occurs in 0.3% of patients
	Leucopenia	Transient Continue treatment Does not predispose to agranulocytosis
Other	Hepatitis Vasculitis Hypoprothrombinaemia Aplastic anaemia Thrombocytopenia	Rare Discontinue drug

short (4–6 hours) the biological effect lasts longer (up to 40 hours). T_4 concentrations are checked at 6-week intervals until the patient is clinically euthyroid and the T_4 and T_3 levels are normalized. TSH remains suppressed for up to 4 weeks after resolution of significant thyrotoxicosis so TSH levels are unhelpful in the early stages of treatment.

At this point a decision is made about the ongoing treatment. It is simplest to continue a high dose of carbimazole to suppress endogenous thyroid hormone production and to give a standard replacement dose of thyroxine to maintain euthyroidism. This is the 'block and replacement' regimen. This combination results in a more steady thyroid state and reduces the need for blood monitoring and hospital attendances. Since adverse drug effects are allergic and not dose related, it is no more risky than tailored dose regimens.

Pregnancy is a specific situation in which tailored-dose propylthiouracil should be used. Both the immunoglobulins, which cause Graves' disease, and thionamide drugs cross the placenta and will affect the fetal thyroid but maternal thyroxine is not able to reach the fetus. Thus the lowest possible dose of propylthiouracil, which is preferred to carbimazole in pregnancy, should be used and the fetus closely monitored for heart rate and growth. Breast feeding is considered to be safe when mothers are taking thionamides.

Patient counselling Patients should be advised of the importance of regular clinic attendance. This is necessary to monitor both therapeutic outcome and the development of adverse effects. As indicated above, the development of skin rashes, mouth ulcers or a sore throat should be immediately investigated and a full blood count performed. It may be dangerous to treat these symptoms with over-the-counter medication before carrying out further investigations.

It is important for the patient to understand the difference between specific antithyroid therapy and symptomatic treatment. The patient should also be advised about the timing of doses to aid adherence. Following completion of a course of treatment, the patient should understand that relapse may occur, and medical help should be sought if the initial symptoms recur (Table 43.10).

Thyroid ablative therapy Thyroid ablation is required for all patients with toxic multinodular goitres, those who have relapsed or are likely to relapse after drug therapy for Graves' disease and those who are allergic to thionamides. Thyroid ablation can be achieved by radioiodine or surgery.

Radioactive iodine Radioiodine therapy is extremely easy to administer and very effective for a majority of patients. It is contraindicated in pregnancy and breast feeding and is usually avoided in children. It is known to make ophthalmopathy worse in some patients with Graves' disease, but giving prednisolone 0.5 mg/kg for 3 weeks and commencing thyroxine replacement early can mitigate this. Despite public concern in relation to radioactivity, accumulated experience over 60 years has not demonstrated any discernible risk of genetic, leukaemic or lymphoma risk (Vanderpump et al 1996). The very slight apparent increase in risk of thyroid cancer in patients treated with ^{131}I is solely due to underlying disease rather than to the radioiodine.

The most common complication is the development of hypothyroidism. Using doses sufficient to cause thyrotoxicosis to remit will result in virtually 100% of patients given radioiodine for Graves' disease becoming hypothyroid compared to around 50% of those treated for multinodular disease. Patients should expect to have to commence thyroxine treatment after radioiodine therapy.

If antithyroid drugs have been used they should be withdrawn at least 4 days before radioiodine is given and should not be restarted for at least 3 days afterwards, otherwise the isotope will not be trapped by the thyroid. Drug therapy can then be withdrawn periodically to assess the effects of the radioiodine.

The patient receiving radioiodine treatment is effectively radioactive for 6 weeks without ill effect. It seems inherently unlikely therefore that the public faces any risk at all to health. Nevertheless, there are regulations governing exposure to radiation, which must be followed. After a standard 555 MBq dose, for 14 days a patient must avoid close contact (2 metres) with other persons for periods of more than 1 hour, undertake to be careful in disposing of urine, and must not work. For 24 days they must avoid close contact with children and pregnant women. In practice, it is these regulations and the concerns they engender in the patient that result in a proportion of patients preferring a surgical approach.

Surgery Surgery is required for those patients with very large goitres, patients who cannot be persuaded of the safety of radioiodine and those who have reacted adversely to both thionamides in pregnancy. The hyperthyroid patient to be treated surgically should first be rendered biochemically euthyroid whenever possible but occasionally surgery needs to be performed as a semi-urgent procedure. This may require a combination of antithyroid drugs and β-blockers, and iodide given as Lugol's solution. Iodide usually exerts a transient inhibitory effect on the ability of the gland to trap iodide and it may also reduce the vascularity of the gland. Lithium has also been used in patients hypersensitive to iodides. In doses of 800–1200 mg/day, lithium has actions similar to iodides. Lithium levels should be monitored to minimize toxicity. The dose of β-blockers should be titrated to reduce the pulse rate to below 80 beats per minute. This is usually continued for 1 week postoperatively. It is imperative that treatment is given right up to the time of operation and the operation deferred if the pulse rate is not adequately controlled. Inadequate pretreatment can result in the occurrence of thyroid crisis.

Complications of surgery are the generic ones of anaesthetic risk, bleeding, thromboembolic disease and infection. Specific risks of thyroid surgery include damage to recurrent laryngeal nerves, which may be particularly important to actors, singers and teachers, and hypoparathyroidism as a result of interference of the blood supply to the parathyroids or their inadvertent removal during surgery. Tetany will begin within 48 hours of the operation and treatment should be initiated with intravenous calcium gluconate. All patients who have undergone partial thyroidectomy should have plasma calcium estimates done 3 months after operation since the development of hypoparathyroidism can be delayed. Later complications of thyroidectomy include hypothyroidism and recurrent thyrotoxicosis.

Treatment of complications

Ophthalmopathy In most patients with Graves' disease, no specific treatment is required for the eyes. The most common complaint is of 'grittiness', which can be treated with hypromellose eye drops. If lid retraction is severe the inadequate lid closure can result in early morning soreness. This can be alleviated by the short-term use of 5% guanethidine eye drops instilled each night and morning. The eyes should be monitored for any signs of infection, and treated appropriately.

Fortunately, severe eye involvement occurs in less than 2% of patients with Graves' disease. Progressive ophthalmopathy

Table 43.10 Counselling points for patients on antithyroid drugs
Carbimazole can be given as a single daily dose
Identify anticipated duration of treatment
Explain block and replacement regimen
Explain use of adjuvant therapy, e.g. β-blockers
Encourage reporting of skin rashes, sore throat or mouth ulcers. Provide written guidance
Ensure patient understands need for regular review
Outline management of relapse

producing severe complications from proptosis, diplopia or visual failure should be treated with high-dose steroid therapy (prednisolone 60 mg daily) until symptoms resolve. Failure to respond is an indication for orbital irradiation or surgical decompression, but such patients should be under the care of a highly specialized ophthalmic surgeon.

Localized myxoedema Myxoedema is usually localized to small areas and is asymptomatic. More extensive disease causes difficulty in walking and considerable discomfort. Probably the most effective therapy is the nightly topical application of steroid creams, such as betametasone, under occlusive polythene dressings.

Thyroid crises This condition can develop in any patient with significant untreated thyrotoxicosis but is most common in those with severe Graves' disease. It is precipitated in such patients by infection, injury, trauma, anaesthetics, surgery and radioiodine. There is rapidly progressive tachycardia, muscle weakness including cardiomyopathy, hyperthermia, sweating and vomiting compounding hypotension with ensuing circulatory collapse. In addition, patients are extremely anxious and often psychotic. It should be managed as a medical emergency in a high care area. In addition to supportive measures, specific antithyroid therapy is required along with drugs, which inhibit deiodination of T_4 to T_3. Propylthiouracil which inhibits deiodinase is given orally or via a nasogastric tube in high dose along with Lugol's iodine. Glucocorticoids should be given intravenously as they also inhibit deiodinase. Effective β-blockade is required by intravenous infusion, with propranolol the preferred agent as it also inhibits deiodinase.

Calcium and parathyroid hormone

Most individuals possess four parathyroid glands situated along the posterior surface of the thyroid. Calcium is 50% bound to albumin. It is the unbound ionized plasma calcium levels which regulate the secretion of parathyroid hormone (PTH), increased levels suppressing secretion and low levels stimulating it. PTH is an 84 amino acid straight chain polypeptide that acts on hormone-specific receptors on target tissue cells. PTH acts on the renal tubular transport of calcium and phosphate and also stimulates the renal synthesis of 1,25-dihydroxycholecalciferol. PTH increases distal tubular reabsorption of calcium and decreases proximal and distal tubular reabsorption of phosphate. The effects of PTH on bone are complex. The two major cell types in bone are osteoblasts and osteoclasts. Osteoblasts are responsible for the synthesis of extracellular bone matrix and priming of its subsequent mineralization. Osteoclasts decalcify and digest the protein matrix of bone, liberating calcium. PTH stimulates osteoclast-mediated bone resorption in addition to anabolic effects on bone, with an increase in osteoblast number and function. PTH and vitamin D act to maintain plasma calcium levels within the normal range.

Hypoparathyroidism

Hypoparathyroidism is the clinical state which may arise either from failure of the parathyroid glands to secrete parathyroid hormone (PTH) or from failure of its action at the tissue level.

Aetiology

Hypoparathyroidism most commonly occurs as a result of surgery for thyroid disease or neck exploration and resection of adenoma causing hyperparathyroidism. In experienced hands, the incidence of permanent hypoparathyroidism is less than 1% for all thyroid and parathyroid surgery. Other causes include autoimmune parathyroid destruction either as an isolated idiopathic disorder or as part of a multiple endocrine deficiency. The latter is an autosomal recessive disorder characterized by hyposecretion of many endocrine glands. Transient hypoparathyroidism with symptomatic hypocalcaemia can occur in neonates. The condition pseudohypoparathyroidism occurs in patients with defects of the PTH receptor such that although PTH levels are normal, calcium is low.

Clinical manifestations

Most of the clinical features of hypoparathyroidism are due to hypocalcaemia. The decrease in plasma calcium levels leads to increased neuromuscular excitability. The major signs and symptoms are shown in Table 43.11.

Investigations

Hypocalcaemia associated with undetectable or low plasma PTH levels is consistent with hypoparathyroidism. Total plasma calcium levels should always be corrected for any abnormality in the plasma albumin concentration (see Chapter 6).

Hyperphosphataemia is often present. It should be noted that there are many other causes of hypocalcaemia (Table 43.12). Pseudohypoparathyroidism is easily distinguished, as it is associated with excessive PTH secretion and reduced target organ responsiveness. Drugs that may produce hypocalcaemia include calcitonin, plicamycin, phosphate, bisphosphonates, phenytoin, phenobarbital, colestyramine. cisplatin, 5-fluorouracil (5FU), and high-dose i.v. citrate or lactate.

Table 43.11 Signs and symptoms of hypocalcaemia

Numbness and tingling in the extremities

Numbness and tingling around the mouth

Muscle spasm (tetany)

Epilepsy

Irritability

Cataracts (prolonged hypocalcaemia)

Positive Chvostek's sign (facial spasm on tapping the 7th cranial nerve)

Positive Trousseau's sign (spasm of hand when BP cuff inflated above systolic pressure)

Table 43.12   Causes of hypocalcaemia

Hypoparathyroidism

Pseudohypoparathyroidism

Vitamin D deficiency/malabsorption/insensitivity

Acute and chronic renal failure

Chronic alcoholism

Hypomagnesaemia

Drug induced

Acute pancreatitis

Treatment

Severe, acute hypocalcaemia with tetany should be treated with intravenous calcium gluconate. Initially, 10 mL of 10% calcium gluconate is given by slow intravenous injection, preferably with ECG monitoring. If the patient can swallow, oral therapy should then be commenced. If further parenteral therapy is required, 20 mL of 10% injection should be added to each 500 mL of intravenous fluid and given over 6 hours. The plasma magnesium level should always be measured in patients with hypocalcaemia and, if low, magnesium therapy instituted.

For chronic treatment, PTH therapy is not currently a practical option as the hormone has to be administered parenterally, and the current high cost is prohibitive. Maintenance treatment for hypoparathyroidism is easily achieved with a vitamin D preparation to increase intestinal calcium absorption, often in conjunction with calcium supplementation. Details of the preparations available are given in Table 43.13. Ergocalciferol (vitamin D_3) can be difficult to use. It has a long pharmacological and biological half-life, takes 4–8 weeks to restore normocalcaemia, and its effect persists for 6–18 weeks following withdrawal. In contrast, calcitriol and its synthetic analogue alfacalcidol are much easier to use. Alfacalcidol restores normocalcaemia within 1 week and its effect only persists for 1 week following withdrawal, permitting greater flexibility in dosage manipulation. The usual daily dose is 0.5–2 µg. Patients need close monitoring initially until stable normocalcaemia is achieved and thereafter at a minimum of 6-monthly intervals indefinitely.

Hyperparathyroidism

Hyperparathyroidism is the clinical state that results from increased production of PTH by the parathyroid gland. Primary hyperparathyroidism causes hypercalcaemia; secondary hyperparathyroidism reflects a physiological response to hypocalcaemia or hyperphosphataemia.

Epidemiology

Recent studies in the USA and Europe indicate an incidence rate for primary hyperparathyroidism of 25 cases per 100 000 of the population per year. The incidence is two to three times higher in women than in men, and the disease most commonly presents between the third and fifth decades.

Aetiology

Primary hyperparathyroidism is due to the development of either parathyroid adenomas or four-gland hyperplasia. It may occur as part of the dominantly inherited multiple endocrine neoplasia (MEN) syndromes.

There are several conditions associated with secondary hyperparathyroidism, including chronic renal failure and vitamin D deficiency. Chronic renal failure is the most common cause and in the early stages of the disease, a rise in the plasma phosphate concentration causes stimulation of PTH release. In more advanced renal impairment, reduced 1α-hydroxylation of vitamin D results in reduced intestinal calcium absorption, hypocalcaemia and further stimulation of the parathyroid glands.

Table 43.13   Vitamin D preparations

Drug	Preparations	Activity
Ergocalciferol (calciferol, vitamin D_2)	Calciferol injection 7.5 mg (300 000 units/mL) Calciferol tablets 250 µg (10 000 units) and 1.25 mg (50 000 units) Calcium and ergocalciferol tablets (2.4 mmol of calcium + 400 units of ergocalciferol)	Requires renal and hepatic activation
Colecalciferol (vitamin D_3)	A range of preparations containing calcium (500–600 mg) and colecalciferol (200–440 units)	Requires renal and hepatic activation
Alfacalcidol (1α-hydroxycolecalciferol)	Alfacalcidol capsules 250 ng, 500 ng and 1 µg Alfacalcidol injection 2 µg /mL	Requires hepatic activation
Calcitriol (1,25-dihydroxycolecalciferol)	Calcitriol capsules 250 ng and 500 ng Calcitriol injection 1 µg /mL	Active
Dihydrotachysterol	Dihydrotachysterol oral solution 250 mg/mL	Requires hepatic activation

Tertiary hyperparathyroidism occurs in a minority of patients with end-stage renal disease, when hyperplastic parathyroid glands become autonomous and secrete PTH in levels which raise calcium levels above normal.

Pathophysiology

Primary hyperparathyroidism can result from a parathyroid adenoma, hyperplasia or carcinoma. Solitary adenoma is the most common, occurring in over 90% of cases. Four-gland hyperplasia accounts for most other cases. Carcinoma is rare, occurring in approximately 1–2%.

Clinical manifestations

The clinical features of primary hyperparathyroidism are shown in Table 43.14. These are related to the effects of hypercalcaemia itself, plus the effects of mobilization of calcium from the skeleton and excretion in the urine. With increasingly early recognition of the biochemical abnormalities of primary hyperparathyroidism, largely due to automated measurement of plasma calcium, most cases are identified at the stage of mild or asymptomatic disease. The classic presenting features of bone disease and renal stones are now relatively uncommon. Recent studies indicate that over 50% of cases are asymptomatic at the time of diagnosis. Although radiological evidence of bone disease is now rare in these patients, measurement of bone mineral content usually indicates that bone loss is accelerated. Thus, the risk of osteoporotic fractures later in life may be increased.

Investigations

Hypercalcaemia is the primary biochemical abnormality in primary hyperparathyroidism. Phosphate levels are often decreased. PTH levels are either inappropriately normal in the face of hypercalcaemia or elevated. In a patient with borderline elevation

Table 43.14 Signs and symptoms in hyperparathyroidism

Anorexia, weight loss
Polydipsia, polyuria
Mental changes – poor concentration and memory
Fatigue
Nausea, dyspepsia and vomiting
Constipation
Hypertension
Renal stones
Conjunctival and corneal deposits
Bone pain and deformity
Pathological fractures

of calcium and a normal or only marginally elevated PTH, the condition familial hypocalciuric hypercalcaemia (FHH) must be excluded. Urine calcium excretion is increased in primary hyperparathyroidism and low in FHH.

It should be noted that there are many other causes of hypercalcaemia, including malignancy and myeloma, drugs such as thiazides and excess vitamin D, thyrotoxicosis, immobilization and sarcoidosis. The most common cause of symptomatic hypercalcaemia is that associated with malignancy and this diagnosis must always be excluded.

Localization of parathyroid tumours is only required in those listed for neck exploration. Most parathyroid surgeons request a neck ultrasound prior to performing a neck exploration. Isotope scanning, CT, MRI and selective venous sampling are reserved for those patients (approximately 1%) in whom the adenoma cannot be located at the first operation.

Treatment

Surgical removal of the adenoma or removal of all hyperplastic tissue is the only curative treatment for primary hyperparathyroidism. However, the natural history of hyperparathyroidism is poorly documented. Some studies have indicated that over 50% of untreated patients with primary hyperparathyroidism show no deterioration over 5 years, although the longer term effects on renal function and bone mass remain unknown. In practice, many patients are observed and their specific problems separately addressed. Thus patients receive bisphosphonates for osteoporosis, antihypertensives, proton pump inhibitors and laxatives.

The main indications for surgical treatment are persistent hypercalcaemia (>2.85 mmol/L), symptomatic hypercalcaemia, renal impairment, recurrent renal stones and progression of osteoporosis. Postoperatively temporary hypocalcaemia ('hungry bones') is common. In patients with bone disease, treatment with alfacalcidol and calcium supplements should be started on the day before the operation. Approximately 10% develop permanent hypoparathyroidism.

Severe hypercalcaemia is a common medical emergency. It must be corrected whilst investigation continues to identify the cause. Table 43.15 shows the common treatments available. In

Table 43.15 Treatment of hypercalcaemia

Mechanism	Treatment
Increase urinary calcium excretion	Normal saline plus loop diuretic
Reduce bone resorption	Bisphosphonates Calcitonin Gallium, plicamycin
Reduce GI absorption	Glucocorticoids in calcitriol-dependent (vitamin D excess, sarcoid and lymphoma) patients
Chelation	Intravenous EDTA or phosphate
Dialysis	

practice rehydration and parenteral bisphosphonates, e.g. pamidronate 60 mg in 250 mL normal saline over 30 minutes, will normalize calcium over 72 hours in most patients.

CASE STUDIES

Case 43.1

Miss SM is a 25-year-old patient with known Graves' disease. She was initially treated with carbimazole but developed a severe urticarial rash, which necessitated withdrawal of the drug. A similar rash occurred within 2 weeks of starting propylthiouracil. She is overtly thyrotoxic with a blood pressure of 160/60 mmHg, a pulse of 110 beats per minute and a very large thyroid gland with a vascular bruit. Laboratory results show an elevated free T$_4$ and an undetectable TSH. It is decided that thyroid surgery is indicated.

Questions

1. What are the indications for surgery in patients with thyrotoxicosis?
2. What adjunctive therapy would you recommend to help alleviate some of Miss SM's symptoms prior to surgery?
3. What preoperative thyroid preparation is needed for Miss SM prior to surgery?
4. What postoperative complications are associated with thyroidectomy?

Answers

1. Surgery is considered the treatment of choice when malignancy is suspected, when the patient has features of local compression, e.g. difficulty swallowing, respiratory stridor, for cosmetic removal of a large goitre, when patients cannot receive radioiodine treatment (pregnancy, childhood) and when thionamides have caused side effects.
2. β-Blockers are effective in relieving many of the symptoms of thyrotoxicosis, particularly tremor, palpitations and anxiety, probably because many of these symptoms mimic sympathetic overactivity. Long-acting agents such as atenolol or long-acting formulations of shorter acting agents such as propranolol are particularly useful, as a once-daily regimen may improve compliance. In addition, propranolol inhibits peripheral conversion of T$_4$ to T$_3$.
3. Subtotal thyroidectomy is effective and safe provided that the patient is adequately prepared for surgery. Ideally all patients should be euthyroid at the time of surgery to avoid a rapid postoperative rise in T$_4$ levels and precipitation of thyroid crisis, which carries high morbidity and mortality. Generally thionamides and propranolol are used. Miss SM cannot be given thionamides due to allergy but with the exception of these agents, her preoperative preparation is essentially the same as management of thyroid crisis. She should be admitted for supervised treatment prior to urgent thyroidectomy. She should receive oral iodide (Lugol's solution) and high-dose β-blockade. Iodides reduce thyroid hormone output in the short term and decrease the vascularity of the gland, which facilitates the surgical procedure. β-Blockers alleviate symptoms and protect against the sympathetic nervous system crisis, which is a major feature of thyroid crisis. Treatment should be continued for 10–14 days before surgery is performed.
4. In addition to the risks of anaesthesia and the surgery itself, postoperative complications include hypoparathyroidism, adhesions, laryngeal nerve damage, infection and poor wound healing. The risks of hypothyroidism are higher during the first year after surgery, although there is an insidious rise in incidence over the following 10 years. The incidence of hypothyroidism ranges from 6% to 75% and is inversely related to the amount of remnant tissue left behind.

Case 43.2

Mrs EA is a 66-year-old woman. She has recently been complaining of tiredness, lethargy and weight gain. Her primary care doctor performed routine thyroid function tests and found she has primary hypothyroidism. She has had congestive cardiac failure for 5 years.
Her doctor now wishes to commence her on T$_4$ replacement therapy. Her current drug therapy includes:

- **ramipril 5 mg daily**
- **furosemide 80 mg in the morning.**

Questions

1. What are the therapeutic objectives in this patient?
2. How should T$_4$ therapy be instituted?
3. How should the replacement therapy be monitored?

Answers

1. The therapeutic objectives should be to relieve the symptoms (tiredness, lethargy and weight gain) of hypothyroidism, suppressing the elevated TSH towards the lower limit of the normal range, without producing an exacerbation of her congestive cardiac failure.
2. Thyroxine replacement therapy should be introduced cautiously in this patient. The low circulating levels of thyroid hormones and the resulting slow metabolic rate may be protecting her heart by reducing the demand upon it. Mrs EA should be commenced on T$_4$ 25 μg daily. If this is well tolerated and there is no deterioration of angina or heart failure, the dose can be gradually increased every 4–6 weeks. Older patients usually require lower maintenance doses than their younger counterparts, possibly due to a decrease in clearance of T$_4$ in the elderly. In older patients the daily maintenance dosage of T$_4$ is usually 100 μg or less.

   It has been suggested that T$_3$ should be used as replacement therapy in patients with cardiac disease as T$_3$ has a shorter half-life than T$_4$. Thus if adverse effects do develop, they will last for a shorter period of time. Against this, T$_3$ is more biologically active than T$_4$ and therefore potentially more cardiotoxic. Most physicians would simply introduce T$_4$ slowly.
3. Replacement therapy should be monitored both clinically and biochemically by means of the TSH assay. Symptomatic improvement of hypothyroidism should occur within 2–3 weeks of starting therapy, but maximal benefit may take considerably longer. The clinical assessment should include both symptoms of hypothyroidism and congestive cardiac failure, of which the most critical is the latter.

   The patient should be questioned about the development of any symptoms suggestive of cardiac failure, for example ankle swelling or shortness of breath. If there is a clear exacerbation of the heart failure, the T$_4$ should be discontinued or the dose reduced. A temporary increase in the dose of diuretic and/or angiotensin converting enzyme inhibitor may be required. If all these precautions are adhered to and the dose is increased slowly, it is usually possible to render the patient euthyroid.

Case 43.3

Mr BC is 66 years old. He has recently been commenced on thyroxine at a dose of 50 μg daily. He is now collecting his first repeat prescription for T$_4$. In addition, he has a long-standing prescription for carbamazepine 200 mg three times daily, and ferrous sulphate 200 mg in the morning.

Question

What issues would you need to cover when counselling Mr BC about his medicines?

Answer

First, there are two potential drug interactions within Mr BC's medication regimen. Ferrous sulfate has been shown to cause a reduction in the effect of thyroxine in patients with hypothyroidism. The mechanism is not fully understood but may be the result of the production of a poorly absorbable iron–thyroxine complex within the gastrointestinal tract. Mr BC should be advised to separate his doses of thyroxine and ferrous sulfate by 2 hours.

In addition, there have been isolated reports that the anticonvulsants carbamazepine and phenytoin increase the metabolism of thyroid hormones and decrease their serum concentrations. However, as it is normal clinical practice to monitor T_4 replacement by measurement of T_3 and T_4 concentrations, this is unlikely to be of any clinical significance. The importance of attending for regular monitoring should be stressed. It should be explained to the patient that it may be several weeks or even months before the symptoms are fully controlled. He is not yet receiving a full maintenance dose; the dose should not be increased any more frequently than every 4 weeks owing to the long half-life of T_4. Consequently, it may be several months before a full maintenance dose is achieved. Mr BC will also need to understand the need for lifelong therapy. It is particularly important to reinforce this when the patient has become asymptomatic from his thyroid disease.

Case 43.4

Mrs EH, aged 55 years, has been attending the anticoagulant clinic for several years. She is on long-term anticoagulant therapy following a prosthetic heart valve replacement 3 years ago. Recently, her anticoagulant control has been difficult and she has required decreasing doses of warfarin to maintain a therapeutic international normalized level (INR). Other recent symptoms include diarrhoea and weight loss, which have been investigated by her primary care doctor, as a result of which she has been found to have thyrotoxicosis. Her current drug therapy is warfarin 2 mg daily.

Questions

1. How may thyroid disease influence warfarin dosage?
2. What will happen to Mrs EH's warfarin requirements when her thyrotoxicosis is treated?

Answers

1. Thyroid dysfunction can alter the metabolism of both oral anticoagulants and vitamin K-dependent clotting factors. The net circulating levels of vitamin K-dependent clotting factors are not usually altered in hyperthyroid patients because both the biosynthesis and catabolism of these factors are decreased. However, an enhanced anticoagulant response is seen when the warfarin-induced decrease in clotting factor synthesis is combined with thyrotoxicosis-induced increase in clotting factor catabolism.

   It can be predicted that patients with thyrotoxicosis will require less warfarin to produce a therapeutic INR than euthyroid patients.
2. When Mrs EH's thyrotoxicosis is treated, her warfarin requirements will increase. The time to stabilization will depend on which form of treatment is used. Warfarin requirements would be expected to change quickly after surgery. If drug therapy is used it usually takes

several months to achieve euthyroidism but if radioactive iodine therapy is used this time period could be much longer.

Regardless of which form of treatment is used, frequent tests of anticoagulant control will need to be performed and the dose of warfarin adjusted accordingly.

Case 43.5

Mr CJ, 64 years old, visits his primary care doctor complaining of increasing lethargy and tiredness. On further questioning he has also put on 5 kg in weight over the last few months, without any change in appetite or exercise patterns. Six months ago he had a myocardial infarction and subsequently developed a ventricular tachyarrhythmia. This is now controlled on amiodarone 200 mg daily. The doctor does some thyroid function tests, which subsequently show a low free T_4 and a high TSH, indicating a diagnosis of hypothyroidism.

Questions

1. How common is amiodarone-induced hypothyroidism and what is the mechanism for its development?
2. The preferred management of drug-induced thyroid disease is to stop the responsible agent. If it were possible to stop the amiodarone, what would be the anticipated pattern of recovery?
3. In Mr CJ it is not possible to stop the amiodarone. How should the hypothyroidism be managed?

Answers

1. The reported incidence of amiodarone-induced hypothyroidism varies widely, but may be as high as 13% in countries such as the UK with a high dietary iodine intake. The risk of developing hypothyroidism is independent of the daily or cumulative dose of amiodarone but is increased in elderly and female patients. This is to be expected as autoimmune thyroid disease is the main risk factor for the development of hypothyroidism and is particularly common in these patient groups.

   Amiodarone contains pharmacological amounts of iodine and the most likely explanation for the development of hypothyroidism is an inability of the thyroid gland to escape from the acute inhibitory effects of this iodine load on thyroid hormone release and synthesis. This may reflect an unmasking of underlying thyroid disease, as hypothyroidism is a well-recognized outcome in patients with subclinical disease who are given excess iodine. In these patients, the hypothyroidism occurs relatively soon (3–12 months) after starting treatment with amiodarone.
2. The ideal approach to the treatment of this patient's hypothyroidism is to stop the amiodarone. If that is possible, many patients without pre-existing thyroid disease will become euthyroid within 2–4 months of stopping the drug although it may take longer in some patients. However, permanent hypothyroidism requiring thyroxine replacement is common in patients with thyroid antibodies.
3. In practice, amiodarone is often used in high-risk patients or when other agents have failed to control the symptoms. In Mr CJ amiodarone is being used to treat a life-threatening arrhythmia and stopping the drug is unlikely to be a therapeutic option. The safest, quickest and most reliable treatment is to continue the amiodarone and add in T_4. This should be done in the same way as for any other patient, increasing the dose at 6-week intervals until the TSH concentration is in the normal range and the patient's symptoms have resolved.

Case 43.6

Mrs HP, a 46-year-old teacher, is assessed for osteoporosis risk. She has no symptoms but is found to have a serum calcium of

2.92 mmol/L (normal range 2.19–2.37) with an elevated PTH. She is taking a combined HRT preparation having experienced a menopause at age 41. Her mother suffers from osteoporosis. A bone scan reveals subnormal bone mineral density suggestive of osteopenia. She is not keen on the idea of neck surgery.

Questions

1. What investigations are required to identify the cause of hypercalcaemia?
2. What advice should Mrs HP be given and what monitoring is indicated?
3. What are the indications for neck exploration in primary hyperparathyroidism?

Answers

1. The most likely diagnosis in a woman this age is primary hyperparathyroidism. An elevated PTH level along with demonstration of hypercalciuria and exclusion of thyrotoxicosis will confirm the diagnosis. A renal scan should be arranged to rule out nephrocalcinosis. An older patient would require exclusion of malignancy and myeloma by checking immunoglobulins, Bence Jones protein, full blood count and biochemical profile and a CXR.
2. Mrs HP should be warned that the calcium is at a level that would warrant a surgical approach, and the condition is likely to predispose to a deterioration of osteoporosis despite the HRT preparation. In addition, Mrs HP's calcium is likely to rise further. She should be counselled that surgery is appropriate. If this is still refused the calcium and blood pressure should be measured 6 monthly and the bone scan (DEXA) repeated every 2–3 years. A bisphosphonate should be considered for the osteoporosis either alongside or instead of the HRT.
3. As well as renal stone disease and progressive osteoporosis, hypercalcaemic symptoms and a calcium >3 mmol/L would be considered definite indications for neck exploration. Relative indications include any patient with a calcium >2.8 mmol/L with these or other features of hyperparathyroidism.

Case 43.7

Mrs EY is 62 years old when she is admitted to hospital after a grand mal convulsion. She is found to have a serum calcium of 1.15 mmol/L (normal range 2.19–2.37) and an undetectable PTH. She has taken thyroxine 100 μg daily since she had a thyroidectomy 30 years previously. Her TFTs are normal.

Questions

1. What is the likely cause of her hypocalcaemia? Does she require any additional tests?
2. How should she be treated?
3. What monitoring does she require?

Answers

1. Mrs EY has hypoparathyroidism probably related to her previous neck surgery. Though hypoparathyroidism commonly occurs in the weeks after such surgery, the presentation can be very delayed and presumably occurs as a result of postsurgical scarring affecting the blood supply to the parathyroid glands. No further tests are required to establish the diagnosis, but her magnesium levels should be checked. Hypomagnesaemia is a frequent association with such severe hypocalcaemia, makes the hypocalcaemia more difficult to correct and may therefore require specific treatment in its own right.
2. In addition to magnesium, the emergency treatment of hypocalcaemia involves regular intravenous infusions of 10% calcium gluconate. Mrs EY will then need oral vitamin D analogues plus calcium supplements to maintain her calcium in the normal range. 1α-Cholecalciferol is an effective and convenient preparation and the dose required ranges from 0.5 to 2 μg daily.
3. Once her calcium has been normalized she will need biochemical monitoring at a minimum of 6-month intervals. She should never be discharged. In some patients the calcium can drift above the normal range. If this is not identified, renal stone disease and renal failure can develop.

REFERENCES

Faber J, Galloe M 1994 Changes in bone mass during prolonged treatment of subclinical hyperthyroidism due to L-thyroxine treatment: a meta analysis. European Journal of Endocrinology 130: 350-356

Maugendre D, Gatel A, Campion L et al 1999 Antithyroid drugs and Graves' disease: prospective randomised assessment of long-term treatment. Clinical Endocrinology 50: 127-132

Sawin C T, Geller A, Wolf P A et al 1994 Low serum thyrotropin concentrations as a risk factor for atrial fibrillation in older persons. New England Journal of Medicine 331: 1249-1252

Surks M I, Sievert R 1995 Drugs and thyroid function. New England Journal of Medicine 333: 1688-1694

Tunbridge W M, Evered D C, Hall R et al 1977 The spectrum of thyroid disease in a community: The Wickham survey. Clinical Endocrinology 7: 481-493

Uzzan B, Campos J, Cicherat M et al 1996 Effects on bone mass of long-term treatment with thyroid hormones: a meta-analysis. Journal of Clinical Endocrinology and Metabolism 81: 4278-4289

Vanderpump M P J, Alquist J A O, Franklyn J A et al 1996 Consensus statement for good practice and audit measures in the management of hypo and hyperthyroidism. British Medical Journal 313: 539-544

FURTHER READING

Abraham P, Avenell A, Watson W A et al 2005 Antithyroid drug regimen for treating Graves' hyperthyroidism. Cochrane Metabolic and Endocrine Disorders Group. Cochrane Database of Systematic Reviews 4.

Beckerman P, Silver J 1999 Vitamin D and the parathyroid. American Journal of the Medical Sciences 317: 363-369

Brown A J 1998 Vitamin D analogues. American Journal of Kidney Diseases 32(2 suppl 2): S25-39

Hanna F W F, Lazarus J H, Scanlon M F 1999 Controversial aspects of thyroid disease. British Medical Journal 319: 894-899

Helfand M, Redfern C 1998 Clinical guideline – part 2. Screening for thyroid disease: an update. Annals of Internal Medicine 129: 144-158

Lourwood D L 1998 The pharmacology and therapeutic utility of bisphosphonates. Pharmacotherapy 18: 779-789

MacFarlane I 2000 Thyroid disease. Pharmaceutical Journal 265: 240-244

Marx S J 2000 Hyperparathyroid and hypoparathyroid disorders. New England Journal of Medicine 343: 1863-1875

Newman C M, Price A, Davies D W et al 1998 Amiodarone and thyroid: a practical guide to the management of thyroid dysfunction induced by amiodarone therapy. Heart 79: 121-127

Woeber K 2000 Update on the management of hyperthyroidism and hypothyroidism. Archives of Internal Medicine 160: 1067-1071

Diabetes mellitus 44

Elizabeth A. Hackett   Stephen M. Thomas

KEY POINTS

- Diabetes is a chronic, incurable condition with an estimated 1.8 million individuals diagnosed in the UK, equivalent to 3% of the population. An estimated 1.5 million have type 2 disease, 0.3 million type 1 disease and another 1 million are probably undiagnosed.
- The cost of treating diabetes and its related complications is approximately 5% of the total NHS budget. It is estimated that this spend will rise to 10% of the NHS budget by 2011.
- Effective control of diabetes (glycaemic levels, blood pressure, dyslipidaemia) can reduce the risk of developing long-term complications, and save both lives and money.
- Abdominal fat is metabolically different from subcutaneous fat and is implicated in the development of insulin resistance and type 2 diabetes.
- Extreme hyperglycaemia and hypoglycaemia may lead to diabetic emergencies, both of which carry mortality risks.
- There is a wide variety of insulins and delivery devices available, allowing regimens to be tailored to individual need.
- Dietary modifications and oral medicines may maintain adequate glycaemic control in type 2 diabetes but in time many patients will eventually require insulin.
- People with diabetes require education and support to enable them to effectively manage their disease, diet and lifestyle.

Table 44.1   Aetiological classification of diabetes mellitus

Type 1 (β-cell destruction, usually leading to absolute insulin deficiency)

    Autoimmune

    Idiopathic

Type 2   (may range from predominantly insulin with relative insulin deficiency to a predominantly secretory defect with or without insulin resistance)

Other specific types

    Genetic defects of β-cell function
    Genetic defects in insulin action
    Diseases of the exocrine pancreas
    Endocrinopathies
    Drug or chemical induced, e.g. nicotinic acid, glucocorticoids, high-dose thiazides, pentamidine, interferon-α
    Infections
    Uncommon forms of immune-mediated diabetes
    Other genetic syndromes sometimes associated with diabetes
    Gestational diabetes

Diabetes mellitus is the most common endocrine disorder. It is a chronic condition, characterized by hyperglycaemia due to impaired insulin secretion with or without insulin resistance. Diabetes mellitus may be classified according to aetiology, the most common types being type 1 and type 2 diabetes (Table 44.1). More than 1.8 million people in the UK have diabetes and by the end of the decade this may rise to 3 million.

Type 1 diabetes (formerly referred to as insulin-dependent diabetes mellitus or IDDM) is a disease that causes destruction of the insulin-producing pancreatic β-cells, the development of which is either autoimmune T-cell mediated destruction (type 1A) or idiopathic (type 1B). In over 90% of cases, β-cell destruction is associated with autoimmune disease. Type 1 diabetes usually develops in the young (below the age of 30), although it can develop in older adults and is usually associated with a faster onset of symptoms leading to dependency on extrinsic insulin for survival.

Type 2 diabetes (formerly referred to as non-insulin dependent diabetes mellitus or NIDDM) is more common above the age of 40, with a peak age of onset in developed countries of between 60 and 70 years, although it is being increasingly seen in younger people and even children. It is caused by a relative insulin deficiency and/or insulin resistance. Symptoms are generally slower in onset and less marked than those of type 1. Type 2 diabetes may be an incidental finding, particularly when patients present with complications associated with the disease (e.g. heart disease). Type 2 disease often progresses to the extent whereby extrinsic insulin is required to maintain blood glucose levels. The differences between type 1 and type 2 diabetes are highlighted in Table 44.2.

Two other varieties of non-typical diabetes that may be seen are latent autoimmune diabetes in adults (LADA) and maturity-onset diabetes of the young (MODY). Latent autoimmune diabetes in adults occurs in younger, leaner individuals who appear to have type 2 diabetes as they do not become ketotic and may manage without insulin for a time. Antiglutamic acid decarboxylase (GAD) antibodies may be present and the individual usually progresses to insulin more rapidly than those with other varieties of type 2 diabetes. Maturity-onset diabetes of the young was noted over 20 years ago and described a subset of type 2 diabetes of young onset, often with a positive family history. Genetic studies have now identified this to be a monogenic form of diabetes. MODY related to the glucokinase gene typically causes a resetting of the glucose level with a 'mild' non-progressive hyperglycaemia in which diet treatment is usually sufficient. Another type of MODY is related to mutations in the

Table 44.2 Differences between type 1 and type 2 diabetes

Type 1 diabetes	Type 2 diabetes
β-cell destruction	No β-cell destruction
Islet cell antibodies present	No islet cell antibodies present
Strong genetic link	Very strong genetic link
Age of onset usually below 30	Age of onset usually above 40
Faster onset of symptoms	Slower onset of symptoms
Insulin must be administered	Diet control and oral hypoglycaemic agents often sufficient control
Patients usually not overweight	Patients usually overweight
Extreme hyperglycaemia causes diabetic ketoacidosis	Extreme hyperglycaemia causes hyperosmolar non-ketotic hyperglycaemia

hepatocyte nuclear factor-1 α gene and usually develops during adolescence or the early 20s. Pharmacological treatment is required but sulfonylureas are extremely effective and insulin can usually be avoided.

Epidemiology

The incidence of type 1 diabetes is increasing worldwide, for unknown reasons. However, it is speculated that environmental changes may cause modification to the diabetes-associated alleles. Also, since the introduction of insulin in the 1930s, an increasing number of people with type 1 diabetes have had children. There are major ethnic and geographical differences in the prevalence and incidence of type 1 diabetes. Figures are highest in caucasians (especially Scandinavians) while the disorder is rare in Japan and the Pacific area. In northern Europe the prevalence is approximately 0.3% in those under 30 years of age. Type 1 diabetes may present at any age but there is a sharp increase around the time of puberty and a decline thereafter. Approximately 50–60% of patients with type 1 will present before 20 years of age.

Type 2 diabetes is much more common than type 1, accounting for 80–85% of people with diabetes. It usually occurs in those over the age of 40 years. Estimates in the UK suggest that type 2 diabetes currently affects approximately 1.5 million people, and up to another million are thought to be undiagnosed. The incidence of type 2 rises with age and with increasing obesity. As with type 1, there are major ethnic and geographical variations. In general, in non-obese populations the prevalence is 1–3%. In the more obese societies, there is a sharp increase in prevalence with estimates of 6–8% in the USA, increasing to values as high as 50% in the Pima Indians of Arizona. Diabetes is five times more common among Asian immigrants in the UK than in the indigenous population. World studies of immigrants have suggested that the chances of developing type 2 are

between two and 20 times higher in well-fed populations than in lean populations of the same race.

Aetiology

Genetic and environmental factors are both relevant in the development of type 1 diabetes but the exact relationship between the two is still unknown. There is a strong immunological component to type 1 and a clear association with many organ-specific autoimmune diseases. Circulating islet cell antibodies (ICAs) are present in more than 70% of those with type 1 at the time of diagnosis. Family studies have shown that the appearance of islet cell antibodies often precedes the onset of clinical diabetes by as much as 3 years. Type 1 has been widely believed to be a disease of clinically rapid onset, but the development is related to a slow process of progressive immunological damage. However, it is not currently possible to use screening methods to identify patients who will develop diabetes in the future. The final event that precipitates clinical diabetes may be caused by sudden stress such as an infection when the mass of β-cells in the pancreas falls below 5–10%.

Studies have been carried out in which patients with newly diagnosed type 1 have been treated with immunosuppressive therapies such as ciclosporin, azathioprine, prednisolone and antithymocyte globulin. When started soon after diagnosis, these therapies showed transient improvements in clinical measures and increased the rate of remissions in which insulin was not required. However, their use is limited in an otherwise healthy and young population due to potential toxicity and the risks associated with immune suppression.

Studies have investigated the use of anti-CD3 monoclonal antibodies. When newly diagnosed type 1 patients are treated with short courses of anti-CD3 monoclonal antibodies, smaller insulin doses are required. This relates to better preservation of β-cell function.

Type 2 diabetes also has a strong genetic predisposition. Identical twins have a concordance rate approaching 100%, suggesting the relative importance of inheritance over environment. If a parent has type 2, the risk of a child eventually developing type 2 is 5–10% compared with 1–2% for type 1. Type 2 diabetes occurs because of the progressive development of insulin resistance and β-cell dysfunction. About 80% of people with type 2 diabetes are obese. This highlights the clear association between type 2 and obesity, with obesity causing insulin resistance. In particular, central obesity, where subcutaneous fat is deposited intra-abdominally, is associated with most risk. Body mass index (BMI) has been used as an indicator for predicting type 2 risk; however, it does not take fat distribution into account so waist circumference measurements are now being increasingly used.

Pathophysiology

The islets of Langerhans are the endocrine component of the pancreas, constituting 1% of the total pancreatic mass. Insulin is synthesized in the pancreatic β-cells, initially as a polypeptide precursor, preproinsulin. The latter is rapidly converted in the pancreas to proinsulin. This forms equal amounts of insulin and C-peptide through removal of four amino acid residues. Insulin consists of 51 amino acids in two chains (the A chain contains 21 amino acids and B chain contains 30), connected by two disulfide bridges. In the islets, insulin and C-peptide (and some proinsulin) are packaged into granules. Insulin associates spontaneously into a hexamer containing two zinc ions and one calcium ion.

Glucose is the major stimulant to insulin release. The response is triggered both by the intake of nutrients and the release of gastrointestinal peptide hormones. Following an intravenous injection of glucose, there is a biphasic insulin response. There is an initial rapid response in the first 2 minutes, followed after 5–10 minutes by a second response which is smaller but sustained over 1 hour. The initial response represents the release of stored insulin and the second phase reflects discharge of newly synthesized insulin. Glucose is unique; other agents, including sulfonylureas, do not result in insulin biosynthesis, only release. Once released from the pancreas, insulin enters the portal circulation. The liver rapidly degrades it and only 50% reaches the peripheral circulation. In the basal state, insulin secretion is at a rate of approximately 1 unit per hour. The intake of food results in a prompt five- to tenfold increase. Total daily secretion is approximately 40 units.

Insulin circulates free as a monomer, has a half-life of 4–5 minutes and is primarily metabolized by the liver and kidneys. In the kidneys, insulin is filtered by the glomeruli and reabsorbed by the tubules and degraded. In both renal and hepatic disease, there is a decrease in the rate of insulin clearance, which may necessitate dosage reduction for those using insulin. Peripheral tissues such as muscle and fat also degrade insulin but this is of minor quantitative significance.

The interaction of insulin with the receptor on the cell surface sets off a chain of messengers within the cell. This opens up transport processes for glucose, amino acids and electrolytes.

In type 1 diabetes there is an acute deficiency of insulin that leads to unrestrained hepatic glycogenolysis and gluconeogenesis with a consequent increase in hepatic glucose output. Also, glucose uptake is decreased in insulin-sensitive tissues, hence hyperglycaemia ensues. Either as a result of the metabolic disturbance itself or secondary to infection or other acute illness, there is increased secretion of the counterregulatory hormones glucagon, cortisol, catecholamine and growth hormone. All of these will further increase hepatic glucose production.

In type 2 diabetes the process is usually less acute, since insulin production decreases over a sustained period of time. Hyperinsulinaemia is able to maintain glucose levels for a period of time but eventually β-cell function deteriorates and hyperglycaemia ensues. If this cycle is not interrupted, type 2 diabetes develops. Impaired glucose tolerance (IGT) and hyperinsulinaemia may be detected before overt diabetes develops and if so a strict diet and exercise regimen, leading to weight loss, may delay or even prevent the onset of diabetes. At the time of diagnosis those with type 2 diabetes may have already lost about 50% of their β-cell function. Irrespective of treatment, β-cell function continues to decline with time, often leading to the need for regular insulin therapy.

Type 2 diabetes is also associated with the metabolic syndrome (or syndrome X), although the real existence of this 'syndrome' continues to be debated in the literature (Khan et al 2005). The metabolic syndrome is a group of risk factors commonly found in those with type 2 diabetes, including insulin resistance, glucose intolerance (type 2 diabetes or impaired glucose tolerance), hyperinsulinaemia, hypertension, dyslipidaemia, central obesity, atherosclerosis and increased levels of procoagulant factors, e.g. plasminogen activator inhibitor-1 and fibrinogen.

Pathophysiology of insulin resistance

Abdominal fat, found in abundance in the majority of those with type 2 diabetes, is metabolically different from subcutaneous fat and can cause 'lipotoxicity'. Abdominal fat is resistant to the antilipolytic effects of insulin, resulting in the release of excessive amounts of free fatty acids, which in turn lead to insulin resistance in the liver and muscle. The effect is an increase in gluconeogenesis in the liver and an inhibition of insulin-mediated glucose uptake in the muscle. These both result in increased levels of circulating glucose. Furthermore, excess fat itself may contribute to insulin resistance because when adipocytes become too large they are unable to store additional fat, resulting in fat storage in the muscles, liver and pancreas, causing insulin resistance in these organs.

Adipose tissue causes the oversecretion of some cytokines (adipokines or adipocytokines) associated with inflammation, endothelial dysfunction and thrombosis. Examples of such adipokines include plasminogen activator inhibitor-1 (which is prothrombotic), tumour necrosis factor-α and interleukin-6 (which are proinflammatory) and resistin (which causes insulin resistance). The atherosclerosis associated with insulin resistance is due to hypercoagulability, impaired fibrinolysis and the toxic combination of endothelial damage (caused by chronic, subclinical inflammation), oxidative stress and hyperglycaemia. Adipose tissue is also thought to cause undersecretion of a beneficial adipokine called adiponectin. Adiponectin suppresses the attachment of monocytes to endothelial cells, thereby protecting against vascular damage. People with type 2 diabetes have lower levels of adiponectin than those without diabetes and weight reduction increases adiponectin levels.

Clinical manifestations

The symptoms of both type 1 and type 2 diabetes are similar but they usually vary in intensity. Those associated with type 1 diabetes are more severe and faster in onset. Common symptoms include polyuria (increased urine production), nocturia (the need to urinate during the night) and polydipsia (increased thirst). These are all a consequence of osmotic diuresis secondary to hyperglycaemia. These symptoms are frequently accompanied by fatigue (due to inability to utilize glucose) and marked weight loss (due to breakdown of body protein and fat as an alternative energy source to glucose). Blurred vision (caused by a change in lens refraction) may occur and patients should be advised that as glucose levels are normalized, vision should improve. Patients may also experience a higher infection rate, especially Candida, and urinary tract infections due to increased circulating glucose levels.

Type 1 diabetes

The main problem with developing type 1 diabetes is that if the symptoms of hyperglycaemia are not recognized, life-threatening diabetic ketoacidosis (DKA) may develop. About one-third of those who develop type 1 diabetes present with diabetic ketoacidosis.

Type 2 diabetes

Many patients with type 2 diabetes have an insidious onset of hyperglycaemia, with few or no classic symptoms. This is particularly true in obese individuals, whose diabetes may only be detected after glycosuria or hyperglycaemia is found during routine investigation. Some patients are unaware of the disease even with marked classic symptoms as they begin so gradually and over such a long period of time. Recurring infections, e.g. urinary tract, chest, soft tissue, are common because sustained hyperglycaemia can result in severe impairment of phagocyte function and raised glucose levels provide a growth medium for bacteria. Generalized pruritus and symptoms of vaginitis, which may be due to candidal infection, are frequently the initial complaints of women with type 2. Patients often present when the complications of sustained hyperglycaemia have already developed, (e.g. cardiovascular disease or renal disease). Retinopathy may be detected on routine ophthalmological examination. Alternatively, a combination of neuropathy, peripheral vascular disease and infection may manifest as foot ulceration or gangrene. In some cases patients present with hyperosmolar non-ketotic hyperglycaemia (HONK) where glucose levels in excess of 35 mmol/L are measured and excessive dehydration has occurred. Occasionally patients with type 2 diabetes present with diabetic ketoacidosis, especially in severe infection or in those of African/Caribbean descent.

Diagnosis

In June 2000, the UK formally adopted the World Health Organization criteria for diagnosing diabetes mellitus (WHO 1999).

1. Diabetes symptoms (i.e. polyuria, polydipsia and unexplained weight loss) plus:
   • a random venous plasma glucose concentration ≥11.1 mmol/L
   • or a fasting plasma glucose concentration 7.0 mmol/L (whole blood = 6.1 mmol/L)
   • or plasma glucose concentration ≥11.1 mmol/L 2 hours after 75 g anhydrous glucose in an oral glucose tolerance test.

2. With no symptoms, diagnosis should not be based on a single glucose determination but requires confirmatory plasma venous determination. At least one additional glucose test result, on another day with the value in the diabetic range, is essential, either fasting, from a random sample or from the 2-hour postglucose load. If the fasting or random values are not diagnostic, the 2-hour value should be used.

Current recommendations are that the diagnosis is confirmed by a glucose measurement performed in an accredited laboratory on a venous plasma sample. A diagnosis should never be made on the basis of glycosuria or a stick reading of a finger prick blood glucose alone, although such tests are being examined for screening purposes. Glycated haemoglobin (HbA_{1c}) is also not currently recommended for diagnostic purposes.

Diabetic emergencies

Hypoglycaemia and extreme hyperglycaemia, causing diabetic ketoacidosis or hyperosmolar non-ketotic hyperglycaemia, constitute the three acute emergencies associated with diabetes.

Hypoglycaemia

Hypoglycaemia occurs both with insulin treatment and in those taking oral agents, especially the longer-acting sulfonylureas, e.g. chlorpropamide and glibenclamide. Hypoglycaemia in diabetes is defined as a blood sugar level of 3.5 mmol/L or less. Symptoms can occur at different blood glucose levels in different individuals. Symptoms may be categorized into autonomic symptoms, caused by the release of adrenaline (epinephrine), or neuroglycopenic effects, which occur as the brain becomes affected (Table 44.3). At blood glucose levels of 3.5 mmol/L some people start to experience symptoms. Other people may not experience symptoms of hypoglycaemia until their blood glucose levels drop lower. Autonomic symptoms are a normal physiological response to hypoglycaemia and alert the person to consume carbohydrates. However, if the person does not act on these symptoms or if they are unaware of them, blood glucose levels may drop further, causing neuroglycopenic symptoms. Neuroglycopenic symptoms occur when the brain is starved of glucose. Often the patient becomes confused and may not be able to correct the hypoglycaemia without assistance. A normal

Table 44.3 Symptoms of hypoglycaemia

Autonomic
Sweating
Trembling
Tachycardia
Palpitations
Pallor

Neuroglycopaenic
Faintness
Loss of concentration
Drowsiness
Visual disturbances
Abnormal behaviour (agitation, aggressiveness)
Confusion
Coma

Other
Hunger
Headache
Perioral tingling/numbness

body response to hypoglycaemia is production of counterregulatory hormones (e.g. glucagon and adrenaline), which increase glucose levels through glycogenolysis and gluconeogensis. However, when patients have taken insulin or oral hypoglycaemic agents, the drug effects may outlast the counterregulatory hormone effects, causing hypoglycaemia. This must be corrected by consuming carbohydrates or by administration of glucose or glucagon.

Causes of hypoglycaemia

The most common causes of hypoglycaemia are either a decrease in carbohydrate consumption, excess carbohydrate utilization or increase in circulating insulin (Table 44.4).

Hypoglycaemic unawareness

This is when a patient loses the sensation associated with the autonomic symptoms of hypoglycaemia and is therefore not alerted to correct the hypoglycaemia. Hypoglycaemia unawareness is a problem especially for those who are on insulin, and may necessitate more frequent blood glucose monitoring. It is estimated that about 25% of people with type 1 diabetes are affected. There may be a number of reasons why hypoglycaemia unawareness occurs. These include recurrent hypoglycaemia, long duration of diabetes, autonomic neuropathy, excessive alcohol consumption and other concurrent medication. Some patients treated with β-blocking agents may lose the adrenergic warning signs, with the exception of sweating, which may increase. β-Blockers are not contraindicated in diabetes but if hypoglycaemia unawareness becomes a problem, then an alternative should be sought.

Nocturnal hypoglycaemia

Sometimes hypoglycaemia occurs throughout the night. Symptoms may include restlessness although this may not be identified unless observed by another person. When nocturnal hypoglycaemia occurs the person often wakes feeling unrested, unwell or with a headache. Contrary to what might be expected, morning blood glucose readings may be high because a sustained hypoglycaemic episode leads counterregulatory hormones to raise blood glucose levels. This could present a confusing picture as the obvious solution to a raised blood glucose level in the morning would be to increase the evening/night-time dose of insulin. However, in the case of nocturnal hypoglycaemia this would make the problem worse. If nocturnal hypoglycaemia is suspected then blood glucose should be measured at night (e.g. 2.00 to 3.00 am). If confirmed, the patient should either have a snack before bedtime or reduce the evening/night-time dose of insulin.

Treatment of hypoglycaemia

If the patient is able to swallow safely without the risk of aspiration, then glucose should be taken orally. However, if unable to swallow or if there is a risk that aspiration might occur, parenteral treatment should be given, either intravenous glucose or glucagon.

The most effective oral treatments are pure sources of glucose, e.g. glucose tablets, glucose powder, and glucose drinks such as Lucozade®. In an emergency hot drinks should be avoided as they might burn and drinks containing milk are not suitable as the fat in milk slows down sugar absorption. Blood glucose levels should be measured about 10–15 minutes after treating hypoglycaemia. If below 3.5 mmol/L, more glucose should be consumed. If above 3.5 mmol/L and the next meal will be over 1 hour, then a long-acting carbohydrate is also required, e.g. bread or biscuits. However, if the person is taking an α-glucosidase inhibitor, e.g. acarbose, then monosaccharide carbohydrates must be given because disaccharides and polysaccharides will not be absorbed due to inhibition of the enzymes cleaving carbohydrate into absorbable monosaccharide units.

Should parenteral treatment be required, intravenous glucose or glucagon is recommended, especially if the patient is

Table 44.4 Causes of hypoglycaemia

Cause	Comment
Missed meals or delays in eating	Reduced carbohydrate intake, therefore reduction in glucose levels
Not eating the usual amount of carbohydrates	Reduced carbohydrate intake, therefore reduction in glucose levels
Increased doses of insulin	Increased uptake of glucose into cells and increased storage of glucose as glycogen
Increased doses of oral insulin secretagogues	Increased levels of insulin therefore increased uptake of glucose into cells and increased storage of glucose as glycogen
Introduction of other blood glucose-lowering agents to oral insulin secretagogues	Enhanced hypoglycaemic effects
Increase in exercise	Increased uptake of glucose into cells
Excessive alcohol consumption	Impaired gluconeogenesis
Liver disease	Impaired gluconeogenesis and glycogenolysis

restless. Glucagon takes approximately 15–20 minutes to work but if the person has liver disease (cirrhosis) or is malnourished then glucagon may not work. In such cases intravenous glucose must be given. A number of serious extravasation injuries, some necessitating amputation of the affected limb, have been caused by 50% glucose. As a consequence many hospitals now use 20% glucose.

Diabetic ketoacidosis

Diabetic ketoacidosis is serious and in developed countries it has a mortality rate of 5–10%. It occurs because absence of insulin causes extreme hyperglycaemia. At the same time the normal restraining effect of insulin on lipolysis is removed. Non-esterified fatty acids are released into the circulation and taken up by the liver, which produces acetyl coenzyme A (acetyl CoA). The capacity of the tricarboxylic acid cycle to metabolize acetyl CoA is rapidly exceeded. Ketone bodies, acetoacetate and hydroxybutyrate are formed in increased amounts and released into the circulation. Furthermore, osmotic diuresis, caused by hyperglycaemia, lowers plasma volume, causing dizziness and weakness due to postural hypotension. Weakness is increased by potassium loss, caused by urinary excretion and vomiting due to stimulation of the vomiting centre by ketones, and catabolism of muscle protein. When insulin deficiency is severe and of acute onset, all of these symptoms are accelerated. Ketoacidosis exacerbates the dehydration and hyperosmolarity by producing anorexia, nausea and vomiting. As plasma osmolarity rises, impaired consciousness ensues with coma developing in approximately 10% of cases. Metabolic acidosis causes stimulation of the medullary respiratory centre, giving rise to Kussmaul respiration (deep and rapid breathing) in an attempt to correct the acidosis. The patient's breath may have the fruity odour of acetone (ketones) commonly described as smelling like pear drops or nail varnish remover.

Precipitating factors for diabetic ketoacidosis in type 1 disease are usually omission of insulin dose, acute infection, trauma or myocardial infarction. Although diabetic ketoacidosis is normally associated with type 1 diabetes, it may rarely occur in people with type 2.

Diagnosis of diabetic ketoacidosis

Diagnosis requires demonstration of hyperglycaemia and metabolic acidosis with the presence of ketones. The biochemical diagnosis of ketoacidosis is usually made at the bedside and confirmed in the laboratory. Urinalysis will show marked glycosuria and ketones. A blood glucose test strip usually shows a blood glucose level of more than 22 mmol/L. Formal laboratory measurement of glucose, urea, creatinine, electrolytes, bicarbonate and arterial pH, P_aO_2 and P_aCO_2 (to determine the extent of the acidosis) should be carried out. Two potentially misleading laboratory results are the white blood cell count and plasma sodium. The former will always be raised but correlates with the ketone body level and is not therefore a guide to infection. The plasma sodium level will often be low due to the osmotic effect of glucose draining water from the cells and diluting the sodium. The sodium concentration will also be spuriously low if there is marked dyslipidaemia.

Treatment of diabetic ketoacidosis

Treatment comprises fluid volume expansion (initially with 0.9% sodium chloride), correction of hyperglycaemia and the presence of ketones (by infusion of insulin), prevention of hypokalaemia, and identification and treatment of any associated infection.

Hyperosmolar non-ketotic hyperglycaemia

Hyperosmolar non-ketotic hyperglycaemia is associated with type 2 disease and has a higher mortality rate (5%) than diabetic ketoacidosis. Hyperosmolar non-ketotic hyperglycaemia usually occurs in middle-aged or elderly people, about 25% of whom have previously undiagnosed type 2 diabetes.

In hyperosmolar non-ketotic hyperglycaemia, unlike diabetic ketoacidosis, there is no significant ketone production and therefore no severe acidosis. Hyperglycaemia occurs gradually over a sustained period of time, leading to dehydration due to osmotic diuresis which, if severe, results in hyperosmolarity. Hyperosmolarity may increase blood viscosity and the risk of thromboembolism. Factors precipitating hyperosmolar non-ketotic hyperglycaemia are infection, myocardial infarction, poor concordance with medication regimens or medicines which cause diuresis or impair glucose tolerance, e.g. glucocorticoids.

Diagnosis of hyperosmolar non-ketotic hyperglycaemia

The diagnostic features of hyperosmolar non-ketotic hyperglycaemia are hyperglycaemia (often in the region of 55.5 mmol/L, which is generally much higher than for diabetic ketoacidosis), dehydration and hyperosmolarity. There may be a mild metabolic acidosis but without marked ketone production. Consciousness levels on presentation range from slight confusion to coma. In some cases seizures occur. Plasma sodium and potassium levels are usually normal but creatinine is high. The average fluid deficit is 10 L so circulatory collapse is common.

Treatment of hyperosmolar non-ketotic hyperglycaemia

Treatment requires fluid replacement to stabilize blood pressure and improve circulation and urine output. Sodium chloride 0.9% or 0.45% (if plasma sodium is greater than 150 mmol/L) is given and monitoring of blood pressure and cardiovascular status undertaken. Potassium may be added if required. Insulin treatment is started via intravenous infusion but is not aggressive, since fluid replacement also lowers plasma glucose levels. Prophylaxis or treatment for thromboembolism may also be required.

Long-term diabetic complications

Diabetes and its long-term complications cost the NHS substantial amounts of money – approximately 5% of the total budget (£10 million per day). This spend is estimated to rise to 10% by 2011.

Although all long-term complications may occur in each type of diabetes, the spectrum of incidence is different. Many patients with type 2 diabetes have had their disease a long time before the diagnosis, by which time many have developed diabetic complications (Figs 44.1, 44.2). However, diabetic complications can

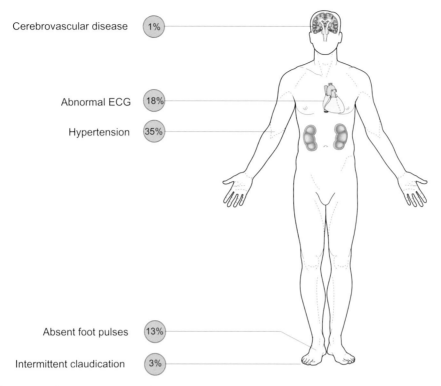

Figure 44.1 Incidence of macrovascular complications at diagnosis in type 2 diabetes.

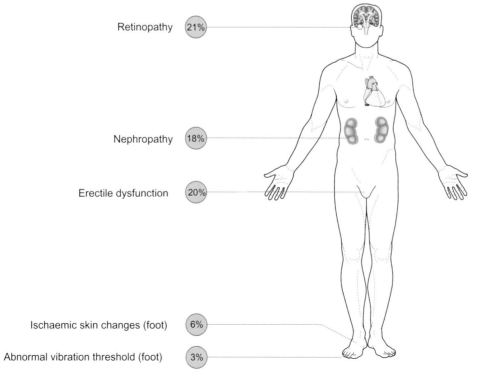

Figure 44.2 Incidence of microvascular complications at diagnosis in type 2 diabetes.

be limited and sometimes prevented altogether if good management occurs from an early stage. Hyperglycaemia and hypertension are the two major controllable factors that influence the development of diabetic complications.

Patients with diabetes should undergo regular review of their disease management for early signs of associated complications. Diabetic complications are frequently divided into macrovascular and microvascular complications. Macrovascular complications arise from damage to large blood vessels and microvascular complications occur from damage to smaller vessels. The general aetiology of macro- and microvascular complications is the same and results from atherosclerosis of the vessels, which may lead to occlusion. The main aims of treatment are first, to prevent the immediate symptoms associated with diabetes (polyuria, polydipsia, etc.) and second, to prevent development, or slow the progression of the long-term disease complications.

Macrovascular disease

The risk of macrovascular complications, including cardiovascular disease (coronary heart disease and stroke) and peripheral vascular disease, is 2–4 times higher for people with diabetes.

Cardiovascular disease

The most common cause of death in patients with type 2 diabetes is cardiovascular disease (CVD) (estimated 80% of deaths). The risk of a person with diabetes having a myocardial infarction (MI) is the same as someone without diabetes having a second myocardial infarction. The risk of cardiovascular disease is increased further if nephropathy is present. Other cardiovascular disease risk factors are the same as in the non-diabetic population and include smoking and dyslipidaemia. However, these risk factors are enhanced in the presence of diabetes and therefore smokers are encouraged to stop, and individuals with hypertension and lipid disorders are actively reviewed and treated. Silent myocardial infarction (and infarction with no symptoms) is more common in those with diabetes and may be due to cardiac autonomic neuropathy. Cerebrovascular disease is also more commonly associated with diabetes, and patients have a greater mortality and morbidity compared to the general population.

Hypertension Hypertension is twice as common amongst the diabetic population compared to the general population. It affects over 80% of those with type 2 diabetes. The treatment target ranges for people with diabetes are generally lower than for people without diabetes, as hypertension is associated with the development of macro- and microvascular complications. For people with type 2 diabetes, hypertension is a feature of the metabolic syndrome and is associated with insulin resistance. For those with type 1 disease, it is closely associated with retinopathy and renal disease.

Peripheral vascular disease

Peripheral vascular disease (PVD) affects the blood vessels outside the heart. In people with diabetes it often affects the arteries of the legs and may give rise to intermittent claudication, a cramping pain experienced on walking, due to reversible

muscle ischaemia secondary to atherosclerosis. The iliac vessels can be affected, causing buttock pain and also erectile dysfunction. If peripheral vascular disease is present, the risk of cardiovascular disease increases. About 20% of people with peripheral vascular disease die from myocardial infarction, within 2 years of symptom onset.

Peripheral vascular disease is also responsible for much of the morbidity associated with diabetic foot problems.

Microvascular disease

Microvascular complications include retinopathy, nephropathy and neuropathy.

Retinopathy

Diabetic retinopathy is the leading cause of blindness in people under the age of 60 in industrialized countries. After 20 years from the onset of diabetes over 90% of people with type 1, and over 60% of people with type 2, will have diabetic retinopathy. The main problem with diagnosing retinopathy is that it is symptomless until the disease is far advanced. Therefore if regular screening is not undertaken diagnosis may not be made early enough for successful treatment intervention. Tight glycaemic control has been shown to prevent and delay the progression of mild or moderate retinopathy in patients with type 1 disease. Likewise, for patients with type 2 diabetes, both tight glycaemic control and tight blood pressure control reduce the risk of developing retinopathy. When retinopathy is detected early, sight may be saved by laser photocoagulation. In advanced cases surgery may be required.

Pregnancy may worsen moderate-to-severe retinopathy, particularly if there is poor or sudden improvement in glycaemic control. However, tight glycaemic control during pregnancy reduces the long-term risks of retinopathy.

Nephropathy

In diabetic renal disease, the kidneys become enlarged and the glomerular filtration rate (GFR) initially increases. However, if the nephropathy progresses, the GFR starts to decline. Serum creatinine used alone to estimate renal function has limitations. The GFR can be estimated (eGFR). The most popular method is the modified Modification of Diet in Renal Disease (MDRD) formula, which requires serum creatinine, age, sex and ethnicity:

$$eGFR = 175 \times [\text{serum creatinine (umol/L)} \times 0.011312\,]^{-1.154}$$
$$\times\,[\text{age in years}]^{-0.203} \times [1.212 \text{ if patient is black}]$$
$$\times\,[0.742 \text{ if female}]$$

$eGFR$ = glomerular filtration rate (mL/min per 1.73 m^2)

The presence of nephropathy is indicated by the detection of microalbuminuria (small amounts of albumin present in urine). If higher amounts of albumin are detected, this is termed proteinuria (or macroalbuminuria) and signifies more severe renal damage. Microalbuminuria is defined as an albumin: creatinine ratio (ACR) greater or equal to 2.5 mg/mmol (men) and 3.5 mg/mmol (women). Proteinuria may be defined as an albumin:creatinine ratio greater than 30 mg/mmol or albumin concentration greater than 200 mg/L. Proteinuria may progress to end-stage renal disease and require dialysis. Albumin in the urine increases the risk of cardiovascular disease, with microalbuminuria associated with 2–4 times the risk, proteinuria with nine times the risk and end-stage renal disease increasing risk by 50 times.

Tight control of both glycaemic levels and blood pressure reduces the risk of developing nephropathy. Angiotensin converting enzyme (ACE) inhibitors and/or angiotensin receptor blockers (ARBs) are the treatments of choice, since both have been demonstrated to provide renal protective effects additional to their antihypertensive effects. ACE inhibitors and ARBs have been shown to delay the progression to proteinuria in patients with microalbuminuria. Although not proven for all individual drugs in these classes, it is considered to be a class effect. However, these drugs should be used with care if there is a risk of renovascular disease.

Peripheral neuropathy

Peripheral neuropathy is the progressive loss of peripheral nerve fibres resulting in nerve dysfunction. Diabetic neuropathies can lead to a wide variety of sensory, motor and autonomic symptoms. The most common is the distal sensory type, which is particularly evident in the feet. It often manifests as the loss of the sensation of vibration and may progress to a complete loss of feeling. It is most prevalent in elderly patients with type 2 but may be found with any type of diabetes, at any age beyond childhood. Painful diabetic neuropathy is another manifestation of sensory neuropathy; it can be extremely disabling and may cause considerable morbidity. Diabetic proximal motor neuropathy is rapid in onset and involves weakness and wasting, principally of the thigh muscles. Muscle pain is common and may require opiate analgesia. Distal motor neuropathy can lead to symptoms of impaired fine co-ordination of the hands and/or foot slapping.

Autonomic neuropathy may affect any part of the sympathetic or parasympathetic nervous systems. The most common manifestation is diabetic impotence. Bladder dysfunction usually manifests as loss of bladder tone with a large increase in volume. Diabetic diarrhoea is uncommon, but can be troublesome as it tends to occur at night. Gastroparesis may cause vomiting and delayed gastrointestinal transit and variable food absorption, causing difficulty in the insulin-treated patient. Postural hypotension due to autonomic neuropathy is uncommon but can be severe and disabling. Disorders of the efferent and afferent nerves controlling cardiac and respiratory function are more common, but rarely symptomatic. Autonomic neuropathy may also cause dry skin and lack of sweating, both of which may contribute to diabetic foot problems.

Macro- and microvascular disease combined

Diabetic foot problems

Infected diabetic foot ulcers account for the largest number of diabetes-related hospital bed-days and are the most common non-trauma cause of amputations. The rate of lower limb amputation in people with diabetes is 15 times higher than in the general population. Diabetic foot ulcers are a costly problem and are associated with considerable morbidity. Foot problems often develop as a result of a combination of specific problems associated with having diabetes, i.e. sensory and autonomic neuropathy, peripheral vascular disease and hyperglycaemia. Poor foot care and poorly controlled diabetes are also contributory factors. Development of foot ulcers may be partly preventable by patient education. People with diabetes learn that their feet are particularly vulnerable and if problems arise, they must seek immediate professional advice.

There are three main types of foot ulcers: neuropathic, ischaemic and neuroischaemic. Neuropathic ulcers occur when peripheral neuropathy causes loss of pain sensation. The ulcers can be deep but are usually painless and are caused by trauma to the foot which is not noticed until after significant damage has occurred. Ischaemic ulcers result from peripheral vascular disease and poor blood supply causing a reduction in available nutrients and oxygen required for healing. Ischaemic ulcers are painful and usually occur on the distal ends of the toes. Most ulcers have elements of both neuropathy and ischaemia and are termed neuroischaemic.

Diabetic foot ulcers are prone to infection, the most common pathogens being staphylococci and streptococci. Wounds with an ischaemic component are commonly infected with anaerobic organisms.

Charcot arthropathy This is a rare foot complication caused by severe neuropathy. It results in chronic, progressive destruction of joints with marked inflammation. Reduced bone density leads to bone fractures, altered foot shape and gross deformity.

Treatment

Treatment for people with diabetes includes advice on nutrition, physical activity, weight loss and smoking cessation if appropriate. Drug therapy is prescribed where necessary.

Diet

Dietary control is the mainstay of treatment for type 2 diabetes and plays an integral part in the management of type 1. Dietary recommendations have undergone extensive review in recent years and considerable changes have been made. Generally speaking, healthy eating advice for people with diabetes is the same as for the general population. Some of the general dietary advice that patients should be given is shown in Table 44.5.

Carbohydrates and sweeteners

The blood glucose level is closely affected by carbohydrate intake. Previous guidance for people with diabetes recommended eating about the same amount of carbohydrate at approximately the same time each day and generally advised restriction of carbohydrates. As a consequence of this advice, a number of people tended to eat more fat. Current guidance for carbohydrate consumption still emphasizes the importance of total carbohydrate intake but it focuses on selecting carbohydrates with a lower glycaemic index, i.e. carbohydrates which give sustained release of sugars over time, as opposed to carbohydrates with a high glycaemic index that give high peaks in blood glucose

Table 44.5 General dietary advice for people with diabetes

- Eat regular meals based on starchy foods such as bread, pasta, potatoes, rice and cereals. Whenever possible, choose high-fibre varieties of these foods, e.g. wholemeal bread and wholemeal cereals which have a lower glycaemic index.

- Try to cut down on fat, particularly saturated (animal) fats. Monounsaturated fats such as olive oil are preferred. Use less butter, margarine, cheese and eat fewer fatty meals. Choose low-fat dairy foods, e.g. skimmed milk and low-fat yoghurt. Grill, steam or oven bake instead of frying or cooking with oil or other fats.

- Try to eat at least five portions of fruit and vegetables every day. This provides vitamins and fibre as well as helping to balance the overall diet.

- Cut down on sugar and sugary foods. Sugar can still be used as an ingredient in foods and baking as part of a healthy diet. Use sugar-free, low-sugar or diet squashes and fizzy drinks, as sugary drinks cause blood glucose levels to rise quickly.

- Use less salt as high intake can raise blood pressure. Food can be flavoured with herbs and spices instead of salt.

- Drink alcohol in moderation. Two units per day for a woman and three for a man. A small glass of wine or half a pint of normal strength beer is one unit. Never drink on an empty stomach as alcohol can exacerbate hypoglycaemia.

concentration. Examples of carbohydrates with a low glycaemic index include beans, pulses and starchy foods like wholemeal pasta and wholegrain bread. Total carbohydrate consumption should not exceed 45–60% of energy intake, with monounsaturated fat and carbohydrate combined making up 60–70% of energy intake.

Sucrose or 'sugar' may be included in the diet, according to the new guidance, but sucrose should account for no more than 10% of total energy and should be spaced throughout the day, rather than being consumed all in one go. Sugar alcohols (sorbitol, maltitol and xylitol), often used as sugar substitutes in diabetic foods, are expensive and may cause diarrhoea. They are therefore considered to confer little advantage over sucrose. Non-nutritive or intense sweeteners (aspartame, saccharin, acesulfame K, cyclamate and sucralose) may be useful, especially for those who are overweight.

Alcohol Alcohol contains carbohydrates and, if consumed in excess, may cause hyperglycaemia. However, more dangerously, it is also associated with later onset (up to 16 hours post alcohol) hypoglycaemia and hypoglycaemia unawareness. Alcohol must be restricted to the same maximum weekly quantities as for the general population, i.e. 14 units (women) and 21 units (men), with 1–2 alcohol-free days per week. In these quantities, alcohol has cardioprotective effects.

Dose adjustment training for normal eating A clinical trial comparing outcomes in type 1 patients demonstrated benefits in glycaemic control and quality of life for those who had undertaken an intensive insulin dose adjustment training and were able to eat more 'normally' by adjusting their insulin

doses in conjunction with their carbohydrate consumption. Many diabetes centres now offer this type of intensive training programme for selected, motivated patients with type 1 diabetes.

Fats

Since obesity is a major problem in type 2 diabetes and fats contain more than twice the energy content per unit weight than either carbohydrate or protein, consumption of fats should be limited. Monounsaturated fats have a lower atherogenic potential and are therefore recommended as the main source of dietary fat. Intake of fat should be less than 35% of total energy consumption, with saturated and trans unsaturated fats accounting for less than 10% of energy intake and monounsaturated fats providing 10–20%.

Examples of monounsaturated fats are olive oil and rapeseed (also known as canola) oil. Saturated fats are chiefly of animal origin (beef, pork, lamb, whole milk products) with some found in plants (cocoa butter, coconut oil and palm oil). Trans unsaturated fats are found in hydrogenated vegetable oils and hard margarines. N-6 polyunsaturated fats (cornflower, sunflower, safflower, soyabean oil and seed oils) should account for less than 10% of energy intake and n-3 polyunsaturated fats (fish oils) should be eaten as fish (as opposed to fish oil supplements) once or twice a week.

Protein

For adults without nephropathy, protein intake is recommended as less than 1 g per kg of body weight, equivalent to about 10–20% of total energy intake. For those with nephropathy, protein intake may need to be further restricted but this requires expert dietetic advice and supervision.

Fibre

There is no quantitative dietary recommendation for fibre intake. Dietary fibre has useful properties in that it is physically bulky and it delays the digestion and absorption of complex carbohydrates, thereby minimizing hyperglycaemia. For the average person with type 2 diabetes, 15 g of soluble fibre (from fruit, vegetables and pulses) is likely to produce a 10% improvement in fasting blood glucose, glycated haemoglobin and low-density lipoprotein cholesterol (LDL-C). Insoluble fibre from cereals, wholemeal bread, rice and pasta has no direct effect on glycaemia or dyslipidaemia but it has an overall benefit on gastrointestinal health and may help in weight loss by promoting satiety.

Salt

Sodium chloride should be limited to a maximum of 6 g per day. A reduction in salt intake from 12 g to 6 g per day has been shown to produce a reduction in systolic blood pressure of 5 mmHg and a reduction of 2–3 mmHg in diastolic pressure.

Insulin therapy in type 1 diabetes

All patients with type 1 diabetes require treatment with insulin in order to survive. Exogenous insulin is used to mimic the normal physiological pattern of insulin secretion as closely as possible, for each individual patient. However, a balance is required between tight glycaemic control and hypoglycaemia risk. If the risk of hypoglycaemia is high, then it may be necessary to aim for less tight glycaemic control. There is a wide variety of insulin preparations available which differ in species of origin, onset of action, time to peak effect and duration of action (Table 44.6).

Table 44.6 Insulin preparations

Preparation	Origin	Onset (h)	Peak (h)	Duration (h)
Soluble insulin				
Human Actrapid (pyr)	H	0.5	2–5	8
Human Velosulin (pyr)	H	0.5	1–3	8
Humulin S (prb)	H	0.5	1–3	5–7
Hypurin Bovine Neutral	B	0.5/1	2–5	6–8
Pork Actrapid	P	0.5	1–3	8
Apidra (insulin glulisine)	H	0.25	1	3–4
Humalog (insulin lispro)	H	0.25	1–1.5	2–5
Novorapid (insulin aspart)	H	0.25	1–3	3–5
Hypurin Porcine Neutral	P	0.5/1	2–5	6–8
Insuman Rapid (crb)	H	0.5	1–3	7–9
Biphasic insulin				
Human Mixtard 10 (pyr)	H	0.5	2–12	24
Human Mixtard 20 (pyr)	H	0.5	2–12	24
Human Mixtard 30 (pyr)	H	0.5	2–12	24
Human Mixtard 40 (pyr)	H	0.5	2–12	24
Human Mixtard 50 (pyr)	H	0.5	2–12	24
Humulin M3 (prb)	H	0.5	1–8.5	14–15
NovoMix 30	H	0.25	1–4	Up to 24 hrs
Humalog Mix 25	H	0.25	1–2	22
Humalog Mix 50	H	0.25	1–2	22
Pork Mixtard 30	P	0.5	4–8	24
Hypurin Porcine 30/70	P	0.5	4–12	24
Insuman Comb 15 (prb)	H	0.5	2–4	12–20
Insuman Comb 25 (prb)	H	0.5	2–4	12–19
Insuman Comb 50 (prb)	H	0.5	1–4	12–16
Isophane insulin				
Hypurin Porcine Isophane	P	2	6–12	24
Insuman Basal (crb)	H	1	3–4	12–20
Human Insulatard (pyr)	H	2	4–12	24
Humulin I (prb)	H	0.5	2–8	18–20
Hypurin Bovine Isophane	B	2	6–12	24
Pork Insulatard	P	2	4–12	24
Insulin zinc suspension (mixed)				
Human Monotard (pyr)	H	3	7–15	24
Hypurin Bovine Lente	B	2	8–12	30
Insulin zinc suspension (crystalline)				
Human Ultratard (pyr)	H	4	8–24	28
Protamine zinc				
Hypurin Bovine PZI	B	4	10–20	36
Long-acting analogues				
Lantus (insulin glargine)	H	2–4	No peak	20–24
Levemir (insulin detemir)	H	2–4	6–14	16–20

Insulin preparations classified as being of human (H), beef (B) or pork (P) origin; prb, proinsulin recombinant bacteria; crb, chain recombinant bacteria; pyr, precursor yeast recombinant.

Species of origin

Until the 1980s insulin was obtained and purified from the pancreas of pigs and cows. Human sequence insulins have subsequently been developed using recombinant DNA technology and are now the most common insulins in use. Many of the animal-derived products have been withdrawn but some animal insulin continue to be available, mainly from pork sources. Porcine insulin only differs from human insulin in one amino acid at the end of the B chain (position B30). Human insulin may be produced semisynthetically by enzymatic modification of porcine insulin (emp). However, most human insulin is manufactured using genetic engineering and recombinant DNA technology. This is done by inserting either synthetic genes for the insulin A chain and B chain, or the proinsulin gene, or a proinsulin-like precursor into *Escherichia coli* (crb, prb) or yeast cells (pyr). The cells are fermented, resulting in large amounts of the recombinant protein, which is then converted into insulin and purified. More recently human insulin analogues have been developed through genetic and protein engineering, to produce insulin molecules with differing pharmacokinetic properties.

It is now standard practice to commence all patients requiring insulin on human insulin. In those who have been changed from porcine to human insulin, there has been concern that human insulin may be associated with an increase risk of hypoglycaemic unawareness although current evidence suggests that this is unlikely if the switch is done appropriately. Human insulin may be more potent dose for dose than porcine insulin due to the formation of anti-porcine insulin antibodies. Conventionally, doses are reduced by 25% or more when changing from porcine to either human or analogue insulin.

Insulin preparations

The onset of action, peak effect and duration of action are determined by the insulin type and by the physical and chemical form of the insulin.

Fast-acting insulins Conventional fast-acting insulins are soluble insulins (also known as neutral insulins). After subcutaneous injection, soluble insulin appears in the circulation within 10 minutes. The concentration rises to a peak after about 2 hours and then declines over a further 4–8 hours. This absorption curve can be contrasted with the physiological insulin concentration curve, where peak concentrations are reached 30–40 minutes after a meal and decline rapidly to 10–20% of peak levels after about 2 hours.

The fast-acting recombinant insulin analogues (insulin lispro, insulin aspart and insulin glulisine) are more rapidly absorbed than the non-analogue soluble insulins and have a shorter duration of action. The analogues therefore offer more flexibility. They are more convenient for some patients as they can be given immediately before a meal rather than the 30 minutes before recommended for human soluble insulin. Another benefit is a reduced risk of hypoglycaemia because of the shorter duration of action. These pharmacokinetic differences arise as the short-acting analogues remain as monomers (single units) unlike regular soluble human insulins which self-associate into a hexameric (6-unit) form. Hexamers need to dissociate into dimers and monomers to be readily absorbed from subcutaneous tissue, which causes delayed absorption.

Intermediate-acting insulins Conventional intermediate-acting insulins are insoluble, cloudy suspensions of insulin complexed with either protamine (also known as isophane or NPH insulin) or zinc (lente insulin).

Over time, insulin dissociates from the protamine, which gives the preparation its extended activity. The onset of action is usually 1–2 hours with the peak effect being seen at 4–8 hours. There is considerable inter-patient variation in the duration of action, but it usually requires twice-daily administration to adequately cover a 24-hour period. Protamine insulin and soluble insulin do not interact when mixed together. As a result there is a wide range of ready-mixed (biphasic) preparations available containing varying proportions of isophane and soluble insulin.

Lente insulin is formed by producing a 30:70 mixture of an amorphous insulin and a crystalline zinc–insulin complex in suspension. It has a slower onset of action than isophane insulin and a longer duration of effect at the same dose. In order to maintain the integrity of the insulin crystals, all insulin zinc suspensions contain significant amounts of free zinc in solution. If mixed with soluble insulin, some of the latter may be precipitated into a loose complex if they remain in contact. Therefore, if these two insulins are mixed, they should be injected immediately.

Long-acting insulins More recently, long-acting insulin analogues such as insulin glargine and insulin detemir have been developed using recombinant DNA technology. They both have a duration of action of about 24 hours, a more predictable, flat profile of action with no pronounced peaks and less inter- and intra-subject dosing variability.

Insulin glargine differs from human insulin as two arginine molecules have been added to the B chain at the C-terminal end. This alters the isoelectric point from pH 5.4 to 6.7. Also, the neutral amino acid glycine replaces the asparagine residue at position A21. The changes mean that insulin glargine remains soluble at a slightly acidic pH. The product is buffered at a pH of 4. Once it is injected into subcutaneous tissue, it forms a microprecipitate in the more neutral surrounding pH. This allows slow absorption from the injection site .

Insulin detemir has a long duration of action and is formulated at neutral pH. It differs from human insulin by omission of the amino acid threonine at position B30 and the attachment of a fatty acid chain (myristic acid) to lysine at position B29. The modification allows the insulin molecule to reversibly bind to albumin, via the fatty acid chain, following absorption from subcutaneous injection. This reduces the amount of free, active insulin detemir (bound insulin is inactive). The long duration of action is produced by dissociation of the insulin molecule from albumin.

Insulin delivery

The majority of licensed products are only available by injection, although a new inhaled insulin is available. Currently the subcutaneous route is used for maintenance therapy. Insulin can be injected into the thigh, abdominal wall, buttocks or upper arm. Its main advantages are accessibility, which allows most patients to administer their own insulin. However, this route cannot be regarded as physiological as it delivers insulin to the systemic rather than portal circulation.

A small number of patients still use disposable plastic syringes with insulin from a vial as their means of insulin administration, although the vast majority now use pen injection devices. Insulin pens may either be refillable or disposable. Although not in themselves improving diabetic control, they are popular amongst users since they are compact and more convenient as they remove the need to draw up insulin from a vial. Intravenous delivery should be used in the management of ketoacidosis and hyperosmolar states. The intravenous route is also preferable for diabetic patients due to have major surgery and who may be 'nil by mouth' after surgery. The short half-life of insulin means that changes in infusion rate have a rapid effect on insulin action and glycaemic control. This type of intravenous insulin delivery is commonly referred to as a 'sliding scale' insulin regimen, whereby the rate of infusion is adjusted according to frequent blood glucose readings. A 'sliding scale' insulin regimen is not recommended for patients who are eating and drinking.

Insulin regimens

Standard insulin regimens for managing type 1 disease vary between two to five injections daily. They must be tailored to the individual patient and will depend on lifestyle, willingness to achieve the best control and ability to cope with both injecting insulin and subsequent monitoring of blood glucose. Starting doses of insulin and the ratio of short- to intermediate-acting insulin are very variable. In patients who are very active, such as manual workers and those who exercise regularly, the starting dose should be kept low to reduce the risk of significant hypoglycaemia.

Mealtime plus basal regimens The best control for type 1 diabetes may be attained using a mealtime plus basal regimen, also referred to as a basal-bolus regimen. This mimics normal physiological insulin release more closely than other regimens. A mealtime plus basal regimen requires mealtime injections of insulin with a fast-acting preparation, preferably with an analogue, plus one or two injections of a basal (intermediate- or long-acting) insulin. This may require up to five injections a day. As a general rule, with this regimen the soluble insulin injections given before each meal usually comprise 40–60% of the total daily dosage. Both basal and mealtime insulin may be administered as a continuous subcutaneous infusion delivered by an insulin pump.

These regimens offer the most flexibility of dosing and eating habits, and often better blood glucose control. A number of patients have been taught to count mealtime carbohydrates and calculate their own insulin dose on the basis of the preprandial blood glucose concentration, which allows greater scope for 'normal eating'. An example is the DAFNE (dose adjusted for normal eating) programme (DAFNE Study Group 2002), in which patients are required to attend structured, group education on 5 consecutive days.

The disadvantage of mealtime plus basal regimens is that they require multiple injections, unless a pump is in situ, and require regular blood glucose monitoring. For some people this is too difficult.

Twice-daily regimens The mealtime plus basal regimen may be too hard for some, e.g. school-age children, to manage. In this type of situation a twice-daily regimen may be more suitable. The simplest and most effective twice-daily regimens use premixed insulin, comprising a short- or rapid-acting plus an intermediate-acting insulin. Regular human insulin mixes and analogue mixes are available. The regular human insulin mixes should be given 30 minutes before breakfast and 30 minutes before the evening meal, whereas analogue mixes may be given immediately before these meals. The longer acting component of the insulin mix given at breakfast time must span the lunchtime meal and the evening dose must bridge the night time. Twice-daily regimens using intermediate- or long-acting insulins alone are not sufficient for maintenance control of type 1 diabetes. Occasionally they are used in newly diagnosed patients who are not acutely ill, adding the short-acting preparation if and when indicated by self-monitoring.

Adjusting the insulin dose

The information on which insulin dosage adjustment is based is derived from blood glucose self-monitoring and the incidence and timing of hypoglycaemia. On twice-daily fast- and intermediate-acting insulin regimens, the soluble insulin may be considered as acting up to the next meal or to bedtime, while the extended-acting insulins act up to the next injection. The glucose concentration at the end of the period can be taken as a measure of the appropriateness of the relevant dose.

Adjustments to a dose of insulin should depend on the degree of insulin resistance present. In order to determine a suitable adjustment dose, the effect of other dosage adjustments in the same patient should be taken into consideration, as should the total insulin dose. For example, a 2-unit dose increase in someone taking 6 units of insulin would be a 33% dosage increase; however, a 2-unit dose increase in someone taking 60 units of insulin would be proportionately much less and make less impact.

Storage of insulin

Insulin formulations are stable if kept out of light, and they are not subject to freezing or extremes of heat. Loss of potency of 5–10% occurs in vials kept at high ambient room temperatures for 2–3 months. Insulin should therefore be stored in a domestic refrigerator except for the vial(s) and/or cartridge(s) in current use which, depending on the individual preparation, may be stable for 4–6 weeks (see manufacturers' recommendations). When pen injector devices are in use, they should never be stored in a refrigerator. Injecting cold or refrigerated insulin is undesirable because it is more painful and the absorption profile is altered.

Adverse effects of insulin

Hypoglycaemia is a common physiological complication of insulin therapy and is often a source of great anxiety to patients and carers. The symptoms (see Table 44.3) may occur at different blood glucose levels in different individuals.

Thickening of subcutaneous tissues can occur at injection sites because of recurrent injection in the same area, known as lipohypertrophy. As well as looking unsightly, it can result in impaired and erratic insulin absorption, leading to poor glycaemic control. The solution is to rotate injection sites. Bruising is usually a sign of superficial injections. Localized skin reactions occasionally occur but resolve even with continued use of the same insulin preparation.

Systemic allergic reactions rarely occur with the current universal use of highly purified insulins. Though not usually species specific, it is worthwhile trying insulin of a different species if allergy occurs.

Management of type 2 diabetes

About 80% of patients with type 2 diabetes are overweight at diagnosis, and this is known to cause insulin resistance. This means that higher doses of medication may be required to control blood glucose levels. Advice on weight loss by increased physical exercise and calorie restriction, in addition to education about general healthy eating, is required. Targets for weight reduction should be to achieve a normal body mass index of between 20 and 25 kg/m^2 or a waist circumference of less than 100 cm which lowers the risk of developing insulin resistance (Wahrenberg et al 2005).

Some people normalize their glycaemic control by weight loss and attention to diet (diet controlled). Nevertheless, such individuals still have diabetes and are at risk of developing diabetic complications. Hyperglycaemia may occur, especially in times of stress or if dietary control is lost, and consequently they should be monitored regularly.

For over 75% of people with type 2 diabetes, dietary measures and exercise alone do not produce adequate glycaemic control and oral hypoglycaemic therapy is required. Within 3 years of diagnosis, a large majority of patients will require oral drug therapy. In the UK, there are five classes of agents currently available: a biguanide (metformin), sulfonylureas, meglitinides (repaglinide and nateglinide), thiazolidinediones (rosiglitazone and pioglitazone) and an α-glucosidase inhibitor (acarbose).

Acarbose has beeen poorly tolerated in trials, with only 39% of those receiving the drug still taking it after 3 years. The main reason for non-compliance appears to be flatulence. Acarbose is rarely prescribed in the UK but is popular in other countries such as Germany. Metformin remains the cornerstone of oral treatment for type 2 diabetes. The sulfonylureas and meglitinides are known as insulin secretagogues, since they both enhance secretion of insulin from the pancreatic β-cells.

The progressive decline in β-cell function in type 2 diabetes with time and increasing insulin resistance means people with type 2 diabetes show a progressive loss of glycaemic control and usually require two or three drugs to maintain control before ultimately requiring insulin.

The factors used to select a particular treatment include the patient's clinical characteristics, such as their degree of hyperglycaemia, weight and renal function (Fig. 44.3). In acutely ill people with significant hyperglycaemia, insulin therapy may well be required, albeit transiently.

Biguanides

Metformin is the only biguanide available in the UK. The mechanism of action of biguanides is still not completely understood. However, the principal mode of action is via potentiation of insulin action at an unknown intracellular locus, resulting in decreased hepatic glucose production by both gluconeogenesis and glycogenolysis. Metformin also stimulates tissue uptake of glucose, particularly in muscle, and is thought to reduce gastrointestinal absorption of carbohydrate. The action of metformin does not involve stimulation of pancreatic insulin secretion and therefore it is still a beneficial agent when β-cell function has declined. Another advantage of metformin over insulin secretagogues, and sulfonylureas in particular, is that it does not usually cause hypoglycaemia and weight gain. Metformin has a short duration of action, with a half-life of between 1.3 and 4.5 hours, and does not bind to plasma proteins. It is not metabolized and is totally renally eliminated.

It has been shown that diabetes-related death was reduced by 42% in overweight subjects who took metformin for 10 years, compared to those who took conventional therapies such as a sulfonylurea or insulin. Myocardial infarction was also reduced by 39% over the 10-year follow-up period. Consequently metformin has become the first-line therapy for glycaemic control when oral agents are indicated in overweight patients.

Adverse effects   The most common adverse effects of metformin, affecting about a third of patients, result from gastrointestinal disturbances including anorexia, nausea, abdominal discomfort and diarrhoea. In some patients diarrhoea can be extreme and can preclude metformin use. However, the gastrointestinal side effects are usually transient and can be minimized by starting with a low dose, increasing the dose slowly and administering the drug with or after food. A suggested regimen is to start with 500 mg daily for 1 week, then 500 mg twice daily for 1 week, increasing the dosage at weekly intervals until the desired glycaemic response is achieved or intolerance occurs. The maximum licensed dose is 3 g per day but doses of more than 2 g per day often cause intolerance. If the initial dose of 500 mg daily causes side effects then some prescribers reduce the starting dose to 250 mg daily for a week. This may be difficult for some patients as the 500 mg strength tablets are not scored and are not easy to halve.

Recently a modified-release preparation of metformin has become available that permits once-daily dosing. Clinical evidence suggests that this formulation causes fewer problems with gastrointestinal side effects. The maximum licensed dose of the modified-release preparation (2 g daily) differs from the standard preparation.

The two previously available biguanides, phenformin and buformin, were withdrawn due to deaths associated with lactic acidosis. Lactic acidosis is a rare complication with metformin, with an estimated incidence of five cases per 100 000 patient-years. However, it is potentially life threatening. Patients at most risk are those with renal insufficiency in whom the drug accumulates, individuals with co-existing conditions where lactate accumulates, and those who are unable to metabolize lactate. In practice, metformin should not be prescribed for patients who have renal impairment (eGFR <50 μmL/min or serum creatinine

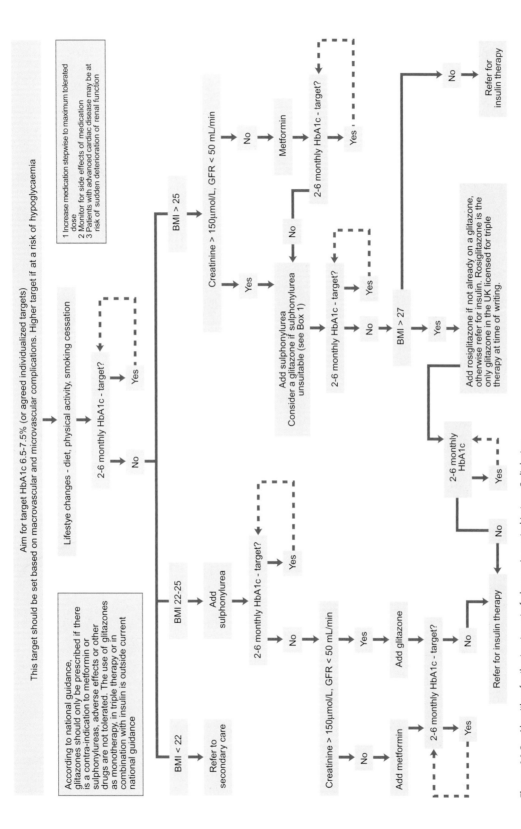

Figure 44.3 Algorithm for the treatment of glycaemic control in type 2 diabetes.

Agent		Recommended dose range	Comments
BIGUANIDE	Metformin	500 mg to 3 g daily in divided doses. Start at 500 mg daily and titrate dose weekly. Maximum 3 g daily	• Contraindicated in renal impairment • Doses in company literature may differ to other sources • Doses are normally taken with meals (breakfast, lunch, dinner) • Most physicians limit maximum dose to 2.5 g daily
SULPHONYLUREAS			
	Gliclazide	Initially 40-80 mg daily, titrate according to response. Maximum 320 mg daily	• Avoid suphonylureas where possible in severe hepatic and renal impairment and in porphyria • Up to 160 mg daily can be taken as a single dose with breakfast • Doses higher than this should be taken as divided
	Glipizide	Initially 2.5-5 mg daily, titrate dose according to response. Maximum 20 mg daily	• Doses are taken just before breakfast or lunch • Up to 15 mg daily can be taken as a single dose Doses higher than this should be taken as divided doses
GLITAZONES			

• The glitazones are contraindicated in hepatic impairment, patients with a history of heart failure, in combination with insulin (due to risk of heart failure)
• Monitor liver function before treatment, then every 2 months for 12 months and periodically thereafter
• Advise patients to seek medical advice if symptoms such as nausea, vomiting, abdominal pain, fatigue and dark urine develop

	Pioglitazone	15-30 mg once daily, increased to a maximum of 45 mg daily according to response	• Not licensed for triple therapy
	Rosiglitazone	Initially 4 mg daily, when used in combination with metformin, the dose can be increased to 8 mg daily (in 1 or 2 divided doses) after 8 weeks according to response	• There is currently no experience with doses of rosiglitazone above 4 mg/day in combination with sulphonylureas • Licensed for triple therapy

When to refer patients:

1 Acutely unwell patients (these patients may require insulin urgently, refer to specialist service)
  • Severe hyperglycaemia or
  • Urinary ketones or
  • Rapid weight loss or
  • Dehydration
2 Patients with advanced cardiac disease or hepatic impairment
3 Referral for insulin start in those with sub optimal control on maximal tolerated oral agents
4 Pregnant women, urgent referral to diabetes antenatal clinic

Figure 44.3 continued

>150 μmol/L), severe liver disease, uncontrolled cardiac failure or severe pulmonary insufficiency. It should be withdrawn in patients with severe intercurrent illness, for example acute myocardial infarction or septicaemia, or those undergoing major surgery or requiring investigation using radiographic contrast media.

Role of metformin   Metformin is useful in obese patients with diabetes as it does not cause weight gain. If there are no contraindications it can be used in conjunction with diet as second-line therapy in patients not adequately controlled on diet alone. As it has a different mode of action to the sulfonylureas, meglitinides, thiazolidinediones and α-glucosidase inhibitors, it can be valuable when prescribed in combination.

Sulfonylureas

Mode of action   The major actions of this class of drug rely on the ability of the pancreas to secrete insulin and hence require functioning β-cells to exert a beneficial effect. Sulfonylureas lower blood sugar by increasing pancreatic β-cell sensitivity to glucose, allowing more insulin to be released from storage granules for a given glucose load. Sulfonylurea therapy is also associated with increased tissue sensitivity to insulin, resulting in improved insulin action. Studies also suggest that sulfonylureas may promote an increased systemic bioavailability of insulin due to reduced hepatic extraction of the insulin secreted from the pancreas.

Pharmacokinetics   The pharmacokinetic parameters of oral hypoglycaemic agents are shown in Table 44.7. Chlorpropamide is the slowest and longest acting agent but it is now very rarely used. Although glibenclamide has been shown to have a short elimination half-life, it has a prolonged biological effect, which may be explained by slower distribution and the existence of a deep compartment, possibly the islet cells. All sulfonylureas are metabolized by the liver to some degree and some may have active metabolites.

Choice of drug   There are many factors which influence the choice of sulfonylurea. These may relate to the drug itself, the patient or the prescriber. There are few well-controlled long-term clinical comparisons between sulfonylureas. It would appear that when dosage is individualized and governed by the effect on fasting blood glucose, there is little or no difference in clinical efficacy between different agents. In general, if a patient is not well controlled on the maximum dosage of one sulfonylurea, it is not worthwhile changing to another one, except possibly for tolbutamide.

Adverse effects   The frequency of adverse effects from sulfonylureas is low. They are usually mild and reversible on drug withdrawal (Table 44.8). The most common adverse effect is hypoglycaemia, which may be profound and long lasting. Hypoglycaemia due to sulfonylureas is often misdiagnosed, particularly in the elderly. The major risk factors for the development of hypoglycaemia include: use of a long-acting agent, increasing age, renal or hepatic dysfunction and inadequate carbohydrate intake. The major side effect is, however, weight gain.

Other adverse effects are rare; blood dyscrasias occur in 0.1% of patients and rashes in up to 3%. Chlorpropamide can produce troublesome flushing after ingestion of alcohol, and about 5% of patients develop hyponatraemia due to its effect on increasing renal sensitivity to antidiuretic hormone (ADH). Most patients are asymptomatic with this problem but occasionally severe hyponatraemia is observed.

Table 44.7   Pharmacokinetic properties of oral hypoglycaemic agents

Drug	Main route of elimination	Elimination half-life (h)	Duration of action (h)	Daily dose range	Doses per day
Sulfonylureas					
First generation					
Tolbutamide	Hepatic	4–24	6–10	0.5–2 g	1–3
Chlorpropamide	Hepatic (80%) Renal (20%)	24–48	24–72	100–500 mg	1
Second generation					
Glibenclamide	Hepatic (40%) Biliary (60%)	2–4	16–24	2.5–15 mg	1–2
Glipizide	Hepatic	2–4	6–24	2.5–40 mg	1–3
Gliquidone	Hepatic	1–2	6–24	15–180 mg	2–3
Gliclazide	Hepatic	10–12	10–24	40–320 mg	1–2
Glimepiride	Renal (60%) Biliary (40%)	5–8	12–24	1–6 mg	1
Biguanides					
Metformin	Renal	1–5	5–8	1–3 g	2–3
Non-sulfonylurea insulinotropic					
Repaglinide	Hepatic	1	4–6	1–16 mg	With each main meal
Nateglinide	Hepatic	1	3–4	180–540 mg	3 (before each main meal)
Thiazolidinediones					
Rosiglitazone	Hepatic	3–4	6–24	4–8 mg	1–2
Pioglitazone	Hepatic	5–6	16–24	15–30 mg	1

Table 44.8 Adverse effects of sulfonylureas

Adverse effect	Comments
Gastrointestinal	Affects approximately 2% Most commonly nausea and vomiting Dose related Advise patient to take with or after food
Dermatological	Affects 1–3% Usually occur within the first 2–6 weeks Most commonly: generalized photosensitivity, pruritus, maculopapular rash May require discontinuation of drug Cross-sensitivity between sulfonylureas is common Rare cases of severe allergic reactions, e.g. erythema multiforme Stevens–Johnson syndrome
Haematological	Rare cases of fatal agranulocytosis or pancytopenia Other haematological effects usually reversible on discontinuing drug Some reports of reversible haemolytic anaemia
Hepatic	Mild, reversible elevation of liver function tests Cholestatic jaundice Usually a hypersensitivity reaction associated with fever, rash and eosinophilia
Cardiovascular	Possible excess of cardiovascular mortality in patients treated with tolbutamide (not proven)
Hypothyroidism	Association not proven May be rare cases
Alcohol flush	Rarely seen with sulfonylureas other than chlorpropamide Change to another agent
Syndrome of inappropriate antidiuretic hormone (SIADH)	Chlorpropamide and, to a lesser extent, tolbutamide enhance the effect of ADH on the kidney Results in hyponatraemia Risk factors are: increasing age, congestive cardiac failure and diuretic therapy
Hypoglycaemia	The most common adverse effect and may be severe and prolonged Highest incidence with chlorpropamide and glibenclamide All sulfonylureas and meglitinides have been implicated Risk factors include increasing age, impaired renal or hepatic function, reduced food intake, weight loss Decrease dose, change to a shorter-acting agent or discontinue sulfonylurea therapy

Sulfonylurea dosage The dosage should be individualized for each patient. The lowest possible dose required to attain the desired levels of blood glucose, without producing hypoglycaemia, should be used. Treatment should start with a low dose and be increased if necessary approximately every 2 weeks. For many agents the maximum effect is seen if the dose is taken half an hour before a meal, rather than with or after food. The number of daily doses required will depend on the agent used and the total daily dose. For several drugs it becomes necessary to administer the drug two or three times daily when the dose is increased.

Recently a modified-release preparation of gliclazide has become available. A dose of 30 mg of the modified-release product is equivalent to 80 mg of the standard-release preparation.

Drug interactions Several drugs can interfere with the efficacy of sulfonylureas by influencing either their pharmacokinetics or pharmacodynamics, or both. Despite much literature about displacement interactions with sulfonylureas, the clinical significance is doubtful. Many reported cases involve first-generation agents, which have a different protein-binding site from the second-generation agents, which bind in a non-ionic fashion and

are not readily displaced. Ingestion of alcohol can cause hypoglycaemia in itself and can also prolong the hypoglycaemic effect of sulfonylureas.

Meglitinides

The meglitinides are insulin-releasing agents (insulin secretagogues), also called 'postprandial glucose regulators'. They are characterized by a more rapid onset and shorter duration of action than sulfonylureas. Their site of action is pharmacologically distinct from that of the sulfonylureas. Repaglinide, a benzoic acid derivative, was the first member of the class. It is licensed for use as a single agent when diet control, weight reduction and exercise have failed to regulate glucose levels, or in combination with metformin. Nateglinide was introduced later and is a derivative of the amino acid D-phenylalanine. Nateglinide is only licensed for combination therapy with metformin when metformin alone is inadequate.

Mode of action Like the sulfonylureas, the meglitinides stimulate first-phase insulin secretion by inhibiting ATP-sensitive potassium channels in the membrane of the pancreatic β-cells. This causes depolarization and gating of the calcium channels (which are voltage sensitive), increasing the intracellular concentration of calcium and stimulating insulin release. The release of insulin only occurs in the presence of glucose. As glucose levels drop, less insulin is secreted. Conversely, if carbohydrates are consumed and glucose levels rise, insulin secretion is enhanced.

Pharmacokinetics The pharmacokinetic properties of the meglitinides confer a rapid onset and a short duration of action. The individual parameters are shown in Table 44.7. The meglitinides are extensively metabolized in the liver, repaglinide by oxidative biotransformation and direct conjugation with glucuronic acid. The cytochrome P450 enzymes CYP2C8 and CYP3A4 have been shown in vitro to be involved its metabolism. Nateglinide is metabolized predominantly by cytochrome P450 enzyme CYP2C9, and to a lesser extent by CYP3A4. Repaglinide has no active metabolites but nateglinide has partially active metabolites, one-third to one-sixth the potency of the parent compound. The meglitinides should be taken immediately before main meals although the time can vary up to 30 minutes before a meal. The pharmacokinetic profile of meglitinides offers some advantages in patients with poor renal function or irregular eating habits.

Adverse effects The meglitinides may cause a range of side effects, most commonly hypoglycaemia, visual disturbances, abdominal pain, diarrhoea, constipation, nausea and vomiting. More rarely, hypersensitivity reactions can occur as well as elevation of liver enzymes. The meglitinides may also cause weight gain.

Dosage The recommended starting dose for repaglinide is 500 μg before or with each meal, increasing as necessary (depending on blood glucose measurements) every 1–2 weeks to a maximum single dose of 4 mg and a maximum daily dose of 16 mg. When patients are transferred from other therapies the recommended starting dose is 1 mg preprandially. The recommended starting dose of nateglinide is 60 mg three times a day before meals, which may be subsequently increased to 120 mg three times a day. The maximum single dose is 180 mg, which may be given with the three main meals of the day.

Drug interactions Drugs which induce or inhibit the cytochrome P450 enzymes CYP2C8 and CYP3A4 interact with repaglinide. Examples of drugs which enhance or prolong the hypoglycaemic effect include gemfibrozil, clarithromycin, ketoconazole, itraconazole, trimethoprim, other hypoglycaemic drugs, monoamine oxidase inhibitors, non-selective β-blockers, ACE inhibitors, salicylates, NSAIDs, octreotide, alcohol and anabolic steroids. Drugs which induce cytochrome P450 enzymes may also interact, e.g. rifampicin and phenytoin, and may decrease repaglinide plasma levels. Drugs that inhibit CYP2C9 may interact with nateglinide. Drugs that may enhance or prolong the hypoglycaemic effect include ACE inhibitors, gemfibrozil and fluconazole. The hypoglycaemic effects of nateglinide may be reduced by diuretics, corticosteroids and β-blockers.

Role of meglitinides The meglitinides are an effective hypoglycaemic therapy in type 2 diabetes. They may be most beneficial in patients who experience problems with postprandial glucose elevation and as single therapy in patients who eat at unpredictable times or have a tendency to miss meals.

However, no outcome studies have been undertaken and so their long-term use has not been proven to be more effective than the less expensive sulfonylureas. Therefore their exact place in therapy is currently unclear.

Thiazolidinediones

Recent research into the action of the thiazolidinediones, also known as glitazones, has lead to greater understanding of the development of type 2 diabetes. Two glitazones are currently available, rosiglitazone and pioglitazone. Pioglitazone has been shown to have a significant benefit on macrovascular morbidity and mortality, demonstrating the benefit of a glucose-lowering agent on macrovascular disease (Dormandy et al 2005).

Mode of action The glitazones act as agonists of the nuclear peroxisome proliferator-activated receptor-γ (PPAR-γ). PPAR-γ is mostly expressed in adipose tissue, but is also found in pancreatic β-cells, vascular endothelium and macrophages. It is also expressed weakly in those tissues that express predominantly PPAR-α, e.g. skeletal muscle, liver and heart. The thiazolidinediones lower fasting and postprandial glucose levels in addition to lowering free fatty acid and insulin concentrations. They enhance insulin sensitivity and promote glucose uptake and utilization in peripheral tissues. They also suppress gluconeogenesis in the liver and, by increasing insulin sensitivity in adipose tissue, suppress free fatty acid concentrations. In addition, patients with impaired glucose tolerance have shown increased insulin secretory responses. However, they do not have a direct effect on insulin secretion. The indirect effects of glitazones on adipose tissue are due to alterations in the regulation of gene expression. This is not identical for both glitazones. Various adipokines (adiponectin, tumour necrosis factor-α, resistin and 11β-hydroxysteroid dehydrogenase 1) are regulated by PPAR-γ agonists in animal studies. Other effects of glitazones on the vasculature include antiatherogenic effects thought to be caused by a reduction in the inflammatory response, decrease in vasoconstriction and an increase in plaque stability.

Pharmacokinetics Rosiglitazone is metabolized in the liver by N-demethylation and hydroxylation followed by conjugation with sulfate and glucuronic acid to form inactive compounds. These are excreted mainly by the kidney but also by the liver. Pioglitazone is also metabolized extensively in the liver to both active and inactive metabolites. The pharmacokinetic parameters of both agents are shown in Table 44.7.

Adverse effects The primary side effect of both rosiglitazone and pioglitazone is oedema, particularly in patients with hypertension and congestive cardiac failure. As combination therapy with insulin and thiazolidinediones results in a higher incidence of oedema, use with insulin is contraindicated in the UK. Anaemia also occurs in about 1% of patients and is seen as a small decrease in the haemoglobin concentration during the first 4–12 weeks of therapy. However, it is suggested this decrease is due to dilutional effects caused by an increase in plasma volume. Both agents caused weight gain of up to 3.5 kg during trials. Some patients also experience headache, abdominal pain, myalgia and upper respiratory infection. Both drugs cause elevated liver transaminases. Another thiazolidinedione, troglitazone, was withdrawn from the UK market in 1997 because of liver failure, and therefore liver function is checked before initiating therapy and monitored every 2 months for the first year, and periodically thereafter. However, liver failure caused by thiazolidinediones is not a class effect but was due to a metabolic idiosyncrasy product of a toxic troglitazone metabolite from a specific side chain.

Dosage Rosiglitazone is usually started at a dose of 4 mg daily. If used alone or in combination with metformin, the dose may be increased to 8 mg daily after 8 weeks, should glycaemic control be inadequate. It may be given as one or two daily doses. Pioglitazone is started at a dose of 15 mg or 30 mg which may be increased to 45 mg once daily. In combination with metformin or a sulfonylurea, the current dose of these drugs can be continued. Administration of glitazones may be either with or without food. Dosage adjustment is not necessary in patients with mild or moderate renal impairment or in the elderly. However, neither agent should be used in patients with severe renal impairment or in those with hepatic impairment.

Drug interactions Rosiglitazone is metabolized by CYP2C8 and 2C9. As these are not major P450 pathways, there have been no clinically relevant interactions reported with other agents. Concurrent administration of NSAIDs may increase the risk of oedema. Pioglitazone is metabolized by cytochrome P450 CYP3A4. Therefore drugs which induce or inhibit this enzyme interact with pioglitazone. Ketoconazole, itraconazole, erythromycin and fluconazole increase plasma concentrations, while rifampicin and phenytoin decrease plasma levels of pioglitazone.

Role of thiazolidinediones Thiazolidinediones improve glycaemic control in patients, especially in those with insulin resistance, by reducing HbA_{1c} levels up to 1.5% compared to sulfonylurea or metformin alone. National guidance (NICE 2002a) recommends rosiglitazone or pioglitazone in combination with metformin or a sulfonylurea should a combination of metformin and a sulfonylurea be unsuitable. However, since this guidance was issued, both glitazones have been licensed for use as monotherapy. Rosiglitazone is also licensed for triple therapy (sulfonylurea, metformin and glitazone). Combining a thiazolidinedione with metformin is preferred rather than in combination with a sulfonylurea, especially in obese patients. However, thiazolidinediones in combination with sulfonylureas may be useful in patients in whom metformin is contraindicated. Monotherapy may be a valuable treatment option for patients who are known to be insulin resistant. Triple therapy can be an alternative to transferring a patient to insulin but the modest reduction in HbA_{1c} usually means that many patients will eventually require insulin.

α-Glucosidase inhibitors

Acarbose reduces carbohydrate digestion by interfering with gastrointestinal glucosidase activity. Although overall carbohydrate absorption is not significantly altered, the postprandial hyperglycaemic peaks are markedly reduced. Acarbose is minimally absorbed in unchanged form from the gastrointestinal tract.

Adverse effects The most common adverse effect of acarbose is abdominal discomfort associated with flatulence and diarrhoea. These symptoms usually improve with continued treatment but can be minimized by starting with a low dose and titrating slowly. Systemic adverse effects are rare but high doses have been associated with idiosyncratic elevations of plasma hepatic

transaminase levels. Patients titrated to the maximum dose of 200 mg three times daily should be closely monitored, preferably at monthly intervals for the first 6 months. If elevated transaminase levels are observed, reduction in dose or withdrawal of therapy should be considered.

Role of acarbose Acarbose is a therapeutic option in type 2 patients inadequately controlled on diet alone, or on diet and other oral hypoglycaemic agents. However, the gastrointestinal side effects do limit the use of acarbose in clinical practice.

Insulin therapy in type 2 diabetes

The younger age of onset of type 2 diabetes and tighter glycaemic targets mean that the majority of patients with type 2 diabetes progress to insulin therapy. Evidence indicates that overweight patients who are not acutely unwell should be initiated on once-daily basal insulin (usually at night) with continuation of metformin. The basal insulin is titrated to achieve normal fasting glucose levels and the patient may be taught this self-titration protocol (Davies et al 2005). Use of a basal analogue in this regimen, as compared with a conventional intermediate-acting insulin, does not seem to offer better HbA_{1c} outcome but may result in less hypoglycaemia. The starting dose of insulin does not appear to be crucial but titration against fasting glucose is more important. If daytime hyperglycaemia persists despite normalization of fasting glucose (<6 mmol/L) then a fast-acting insulin may be added preprandially, typically with the largest meal of the day. However, sometimes patients are switched to a premixed twice-a-day regimen.

In a lean patient (BMI <25 kg/m²), significant insulin deficiency is more likely and therefore from the outset of insulin treatment either a basal-bolus or twice-daily regimen may be preferred.

In type 2 patients who require temporary insulin during intercurrent illness, a soluble preparation such as Humulin S or Human Actrapid can be given two or three times daily with a small dose of isophane insulin at bedtime to control blood glucose quickly and eliminate symptoms. The dose is selected initially according to the patient's previous insulin requirements, if any, and adjusted according to four times daily blood glucose measurements.

Treating hypertension

The co-existence of hypertension and diabetes dramatically increases the risk of microvascular and macrovascular complications. Most important is the increased risk of cardiovascular disease. Tight control of blood pressure may be a more effective method of preventing complications in patients with type 2 diabetes than tight glycaemic control. Current guidelines (Joint British Societies 2005) recommend a target of <130/80 mmHg for individuals with diabetes.

Patients with evidence of nephropathy, whether or not they have an increased cardiovascular event risk, should include an ACE inhibitor or angiotensin receptor blocker, if tolerated, in their treatment (NICE 2002b). A treatment algorithm is shown in Figure 44.4.

In young patients with type 1 diabetes, hypertension is usually a consequence of renal disease and should be treated aggressively

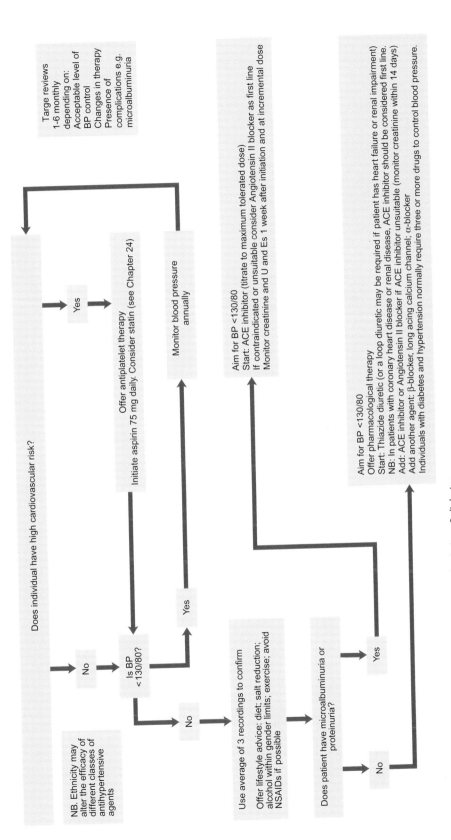

Figure 44.4 Algorithm for the treatment of hypertension in type 2 diabetes.

(to a target of <125/75 mmHg) with maximal doses of either an ACE inhibitor or angiotensin receptor blocker.

Treating obesity

Obesity is a significant risk factor in the development of type 2 diabetes. Evidence suggests that for each kilogram increase in body weight, the risk of diabetes increases by 4.5%. It is estimated that almost one-fifth of the population has a BMI of over $30 \, kg/m^2$ and is therefore obese.

Treatment of obesity may require modification of lifestyle (diet and exercise regimens) to reduce calorie intake and increase calorie utilization, pharmacological intervention and/or surgery. There are currently two drugs available for treating obesity, orlistat and sibutramine, with a third drug, rimonabant, a selective cannabinoid-1 (CB_1) receptor blocker, to be launched.

Orlistat is licensed for use with a 'mildly hypocalorific diet' to treat obese people (BMI >30 kg/m^2) or overweight patients with a BMI >28 kg/m^2 and associated risk factors. It should be discontinued after 12 weeks if a 5% weight reduction since the start of treatment has not been achieved. Orlistat increases the amount of faecal fat excretion but is associated with a number of gastrointestinal side effects such as oily leakage from the rectum, flatulence, faecal urgency and incontinence.

A greater reduction in the incidence of type 2 diabetes has been observed in patients treated with both orlistat and lifestyle modification (Torgerson et al 2004). Sibutramine is also licensed for use as part of a weight reduction programme for those with a BMI >30 kg/m^2 or above and those with a BMI of 27 kg/m^2 or higher if other risks such as diabetes or dyslipidaemia are present. Treatment is started at 10 mg daily and increased to 15 mg daily if an inadequate response is seen. Treatment should be discontinued if at least 2 kg body weight has not been lost after 4 weeks of treatment. Treatment should also be discontinued if weight stabilizes at less than 5% of initial body weight or if the patient has not lost 5% of initial body weight after 3 months. For patients with co-morbidities such as diabetes, it is recommended that treatment with sibutramine is only continued if weight loss is associated with other clinical benefits such as improvement in lipid profile or glycaemic control.

Patient care

Patient education

Patient involvement is paramount for the successful care of diabetes. This is highlighted in national service standards for diabetes (DH 2002) which state that all patients, and carers, where appropriate, will be encouraged to develop a partnership with their clinicians to enable them to manage their diabetes and maintain a healthy lifestyle, often through shared care plans.

Education will depend upon the individual patient and the availability of local resources. Individual tuition is preferable in the early stages after diagnosis and is usually delivered by a diabetes specialist nurse. The educational aspect of care is a gradual and ongoing process. At a later stage, group education can be effective and many patients appreciate and find support in meeting others who have the same disease. Many such

programmes are multidisciplinary and involve doctors, nurses, dieticians, pharmacists and chiropodists. It is also essential to involve the patient's family and carers in the educational process. Patients can also obtain support and information from specialist organizations such as Diabetes UK (available at www.diabetes.org.uk/home.htm).

Patients require education and information about many subjects, ranging from general lifestyle advice through to knowledge about the medicines they are prescribed (Table 44.9). Advice about the use of over-the-counter medications, diet, foot care products and diabetic food products is frequently requested.

Table 44.9 Patient education in diabetes

1. **The disease**
   Signs and symptoms

2. **Hyperglycaemia**
   Signs, symptoms and treatments

3. **Hypoglycaemia**
   Signs, symptoms and treatments

4. **Exercise**
   Benefits and effect on blood glucose control

5. **Diet**

6. **Insulin therapy**
   - Injection technique
   - Types of insulin
   - Onset and peak actions
   - Storage
   - Stability

7. **Urine testing**
   - Glucose
   - Ketones

8. **Home blood glucose testing**
   - Technique
   - Interpretation

9. **Oral hypoglycaemic agents**
   - Mode of action
   - Dosing
   - Need for multiple therapies

10. **Foot care**

11. **Management during illness**

12. **Cardiovascular risk factors**
    - Smoking
    - Hypertension
    - Obesity
    - Hyperlipidaemia

13. **Regular medical and ophthalmological examinations**

Annual review

People with diabetes should attend their clinic for an annual review to screen for diabetic complications. Monitoring and optimizing glycaemic control is also undertaken although this should be done on a more regular basis, as should review of patients with known complications. The annual review is increasingly taking place in primary care, with referral to secondary care if required. The typical assessments undertaken at an annual review are described in Table 44.10.

Glycaemic management targets

The theoretical ideal for all patients with diabetes is to achieve normoglycaemia. As this is not always possible, the aim is to achieve the best possible control compatible with an acceptable lifestyle for the patient. In some patients this may mean only symptomatic control, in others this may be tight control. In making this decision, the following factors should be considered: the patient's age, motivation, intelligence, understanding, likely compliance, co-existing diseases, ability to recognize hypoglycaemia, duration of their diabetes and the presence/absence/severity of diabetic complications.

Targets for pre-meal blood glucose of between 4 and 7 mmol/L and post-meal values of <10 mmol/L may be set for most patients provided there is no significant hypoglycaemia. In special cases such as diabetes in pregnancy, postprandial targets may be tighter. National guidelines (NICE 2002a) have set a target range for HbA_{1c} of between 6.5% and 7.5%, based on the risk of macrovascular and microvascular complications. Those at risk of macrovascular disease have lower targets unless this would put them at risk of hypoglycaemia.

The diabetes treatment goals in older people may be different and more conservative than in younger adults. For example, some elderly patients may have poor vision and limited manual dexterity, which may or may not be linked to a degree of cognitive impairment. Others may have multiple pathology and take a number of other medications. Therefore the goals of therapy need to be both individual and realistic. In some people they will involve only the optimization of body weight, control of symptoms and avoidance of hypoglycaemia (which has an increased risk of severe brain damage and may occur without the usual warning signs in the elderly). In others, reasonably tight control may be appropriate. There is, therefore, a difficult balance between the use of aggressive treatment with its associated risk of hypoglycaemia and the benefits of reducing complications to maintain an acceptable quality of life. Table 44.11 sets out some of the common therapeutic problems in diabetes.

Monitoring glycaemic control

Clinic monitoring

There are several ways in which glycaemic control can be monitored in primary and secondary care. Estimates of average control are often useful. Glycation of minor haemoglobin components occurs in the blood, with the extent depending on both the amount of glucose present and the duration of exposure of the haemoglobin to glucose. Estimates of glycated haemoglobin (HbA_{1c}) provide an index of average diabetes control over the preceding 2–3 months, i.e. the lifespan of a red blood cell. HbA_{1c} can be measured at any time, the patient does not need to be fasted, and levels are not normally affected by acute changes in therapy, diet or exercise. However, they may be lower in those with reduced red cell lifespan, e.g. pregnancy or advanced renal failure. Plasma fructosamine represents the glycation of all plasma proteins and gives information about control over the preceding 3 weeks. As albumin is the major plasma protein, hypoalbuminaemia may affect fructosamine levels. However, HbA_{1c} is the preferred marker for average glycaemic control.

Home monitoring

Type 1 diabetes All patients treated with insulin should be offered home blood glucose monitoring (HBGM). Capillary blood is applied to a reagent strip which has been

---

Table 44.10 Annual review for diabetes

Routine assessment
Capillary blood glucose level
Weight, body mass index and waist circumference
Blood pressure
Urinalysis for glucose, protein and ketones
Foot assessment

Laboratory investigations
Fasting lipid profile
HbA_{1c}
U&E, creatinine
Liver function tests
Urine specimen for albumin:creatinine ratio (ACR)

Referral, if appropriate
Retinopathy screening (should be done annually)
Dietician
Podiatry
Exercise programme
Smoking cessation programme

Table 44.11 Common therapeutic problems in diabetes

- Achieving normoglycaemia or HbA_{1c} targets

- Achieving an acceptable balance between improving glycaemic control and minimizing episodes of hypoglycaemia

- Achieving adequate control in type 2 diabetes with diet alone, especially in patients who are overweight

- Drug-related weight gain, notably with insulin and sulfonylureas

- Achieving blood pressure targets in patients with co-existing hypertension

- Ensuring adherence as drug regimens become complex, requiring multiple drug therapies

- Making insulin therapy acceptable to patients with type 2 diabetes, inadequately controlled with oral therapies

impregnated with enzymes, e.g. glucose oxidase. Some HBGM methods require visual comparison of colour changes which correspond to various blood glucose concentrations. More commonly, meters may be used to give readings and are more convenient for people who are colour blind or who have poor eyesight. HBGM enables patients and carers to make a direct assessment of the effect of changes in medicines, dietary habits, exercise and patterns of illness. It has the additional benefit that it can detect hypoglycaemia and, unlike urine testing in which glycosuria may only be detected some time after changes in blood glucose have occurred, it enables more accurate calculations of insulin doses.

Patients with type 1, who are by definition ketosis prone, should also know how and when to test their urine for ketones. This test need not be carried out as part of routine monitoring, but is essential at times of intercurrent illness, especially when the blood glucose is ≥17mmol/L.

Type 2 diabetes Most people with type 2 diabetes are treated with diet alone or with oral hypoglycaemic agents, and urine glucose monitoring is adequate. This is a simple non-invasive test that can detect hyperglycaemia but not hypoglycaemia. Home blood glucose monitoring is used by some patients with type 2, particularly if control is poor, if they are being treated with insulin or if the patient wishes to use this method.

CASE STUDIES

Case 44.1

Mrs PH is a 62-year-old lady who has hypertension, for which she takes bendroflumethiazide 2.5 mg daily. She has smoked for over 40 years and is overweight. This morning she had a 'funny turn' and fell to the floor. Her husband called an ambulance and she was taken to hospital. She said that she felt generally unwell but could not specify any particular symptoms other than nausea. In the Accident and Emergency department of the hospital an ECG showed acute ST elevation. Blood tests showed that she had raised creatinine kinase-MB and troponins. A venous blood glucose level of 23.6 mmol/L was reported and confirmed.

Questions

1. What is her diagnosis?
2. What are her risk factors for cardiac disease?
3. How should she be treated acutely?
4. What important lifestyle changes should she make?
5. What targets for glycaemic control would be appropriate?

Answers

1. Mrs PH has ST elevation on her ECG and raised cardiac isoenzymes, which indicate that she has had an acute myocardial infarction (MI). Her raised blood glucose level suggests that she has type 2 diabetes (previously undiagnosed) and the presentation of MI is likely to be associated with this. Her presentation is atypical in that she does not complain of any pain, but in people with diabetes there is a greater incidence of MI where pain is absent. This is often referred to as a silent MI where all symptoms are absent. A pain-free MI can often delay a diagnosis and sometimes means that a diagnosis is not made, since the patient may not realize that something is wrong.

2. Her risk factors are hyperglycaemia, obesity, hypertension and smoking. Hyperglycaemia is associated with a substantially increased risk of developing cardiovascular disease. Additionally, she is a long-term smoker which increases the risk of macrovascular and microvascular complications of diabetes. Cardiovascular disease and death are more common in people with diabetes who smoke, the risk being greater than in people who do not have diabetes.

3. This lady requires thrombolysis, aspirin, intravenous insulin and glucose treatment, β-blocker, ACE inhibitor and an antiemetic. Analgesia should also be considered. Thrombolysis should be given promptly on confirmation of the diagnosis of acute MI, even if the diabetic patient has proliferative retinopathy, since the risk of vitreous haemorrhage is small and outweighed by the benefits of thrombolysis. The benefits of thrombolysis appear to be greater for diabetic patients than in the non-diabetic population. Aspirin taken as soon after the infarct as possible has been shown to reduce mortality even if thrombolysis is given. Intravenous insulin and glucose were used acutely in the DIGAMI (Diabetes mellitus, Insulin, Glucose infusion Acute Myocardial Infarction) Study, after which a multiple injection regimen was used for 3 months post MI. Results showed a relative reduction in mortality of 29% at 12 months (Malmberg et al 1999). The early administration of β-blockers has been shown to limit infarct size and reduce mortality from early cardiac events, potentially more so in those with diabetes. Contrary to common belief, β-blockers are not contraindicated in diabetes. ACE inhibitors have also been shown to reduce the incidence of heart failure and mortality and should be prescribed. However, there is a risk of the presence of bilateral renal artery stenosis in this lady, especially since she has cardiovascular disease. Careful observation of her creatinine levels after starting the ACE inhibitor is advised.

4. Mrs PH needs to stop smoking and try to reduce her weight. Macroalbuminuria, proteinuria and neuropathy are 2–3 times more likely in those who smoke. Smoking cessation services are offered in some hospitals and also in primary care. Nicotine replacement therapy is available on prescription and may be used if required. Access to a support network may also be of considerable benefit to many patients. Mrs PH should also be advised that losing weight may greatly improve her condition and access to dietetic services should be provided.

5. Future management targets for glycaemic control should be set to reflect the individual patient. Since this lady is not particularly old and already has macrovascular disease, a target for HbA$_{1c}$ of below 6.5% would be ideal. However, if this puts her at risk of hypoglycaemia in the future then the target may be raised to a level that does not pose such a risk.

Case 44.2

Mr FM is a 67-year-old man with type 2 diabetes, diagnosed 18 years ago. He normally takes Mixtard 30 insulin 24 units with breakfast and 16 units with his evening meal, which, combined with careful attention to diet, maintains his blood sugar levels between 5 and 11 mmol/L. His HbA$_{1c}$ 2 months ago was 6.3%. Just over a week ago he had a severe headache, jaw pain and temporary loss of vision in one eye, leading to a diagnosis of temporal arteritis for which he was prescribed prednisolone 60 mg daily. Mr FM now reports that his blood sugars have become chronically elevated, sometimes giving readings of above 20 mmol/L, which is most unusual for him. He also reports polyuria and polydipsia and is feeling tired and lethargic.

Questions

1. What is the likely cause of Mr FM's symptoms and elevated blood glucose levels?
2. How should his symptoms be managed?

3. What advice should he be given regarding long-term management of his blood glucose levels?

Answers

1. Mr FM is normally well controlled, indicated by his recent HbA$_{1c}$ of 6.3%, so compliance is unlikely to be problem. It is highly likely that Mr FM is experiencing elevated blood glucose levels and the symptoms of hyperglycaemia due to taking high-dose steroids. Glucocorticoids lead to the production of glucose via hepatic gluconeogenesis and inhibition of glucose uptake into muscle, and cause insulin resistance, all potentially giving rise to hyperglycaemia. When steroids are taken there may be postprandial hyperglycaemia and a blood glucose peak that may occur 8–12 hours following a once-daily dose of glucocorticoids.

2. There are very few studies examining how best to treat steroid-induced hyperglycaemia. Mr FM will need to increase his dose of insulin; however, since there is no formula to predict his new insulin requirements, he will have to carefully increase his dose in order to lower his blood glucose to satisfactory levels. He must therefore increase the frequency of home blood glucose monitoring.

3. With respect to the treatment of his temporal arteritis, Mr FM will be advised to reduce his prednisolone dose after the initial high treatment dose. As his steroid dose is reduced, his insulin dose will also need to be reduced otherwise he is likely to experience hypoglycaemia. Mr FM should be advised, with each reduction in steroid dose, to monitor his blood glucose levels diligently and to reduce his insulin dose. This is important because as his blood glucose levels fall he will be at risk of hypoglycaemia. If, during his reducing steroid regimen, he needs to take an alternate-day dose of steroid, then he may need to counteract hyperglycaemia by alternate-day increases in his insulin dose.

Case 44.3

Mrs DB is a 55-year-old lady with type 2 diabetes, which she has had for 4 years. She presented to her primary care clinician complaining of tiredness and lethargy. Her normal medication includes metformin 500 mg three times a day, Mixtard 30 insulin (18 units in the morning and 12 in the evening), aspirin 75 mg daily, simvastatin 40 mg daily and lisinopril 5 mg daily. Her primary care clinician did blood tests and discovered a serum creatinine of 207 μmol/L, eGRF of 24 mL/min, haemoglobin (Hb) of 8.4 g/dL. Her HbA$_{1c}$ was 9.2% and a random blood glucose test was 14.2 mmol/L. Her blood pressure was 170/95 mmHg and a urine dipstick was positive for protein.

Questions

1. What might be the cause of her tiredness and lethargy?
2. What immediate interventions should be made by her primary care clinician?
3. How might the rate of renal decline be further slowed?

Answers

1. Tiredness and lethargy may be symptoms of poorly controlled diabetes, which cannot be ruled out as her HbA$_{1c}$ and random blood glucose levels are high. However, tiredness and lethargy can also be symptoms of anaemia, which may be diagnosed from the low Hb of 8.4 g/dL (normal range for females 11.5–16 g/dL). Anaemia may occur with diabetic nephropathy because as well as glomerular damage, the endocrine function of the kidneys is impaired. (The kidneys produce erythropoietin, required for synthesis of haemoglobin.) Untreated anaemia is an additional risk factor for developing cardiovascular disease.

2. Mrs DB's primary care clinician should stop her metformin immediately since there is an increased risk that she may develop life-threatening lactic acidosis. She needs referral to a specialist nephrologist. Her blood pressure and blood glucose levels should be optimized. Blood pressure should be reduced to a target of less than 130/80. She is already taking lisinopril 5 mg daily and the dose should be increased, in a minimum of two stages, to at least 20 mg daily. ACE inhibitors slow the progression of nephropathy. If the ACE inhibitor dose is increased, then serum creatinine must be checked soon after each dose increase, since a marked rise >30% above baseline or out of the normal range might indicate bilateral renal artery stenosis. Most hypertensive people require more than one antihypertensive agent to bring their blood pressure down to acceptable limits, so additional antihypertensive agents should be commenced. Since her metformin must be stopped, her insulin dose may need to be increased although one should consider the increased risk of hypoglycaemia. In patients with renal disease this is due to reduced renal clearance of insulin and failure of renal gluconeogenesis.

3. The rate of decline of renal function in people with diabetic nephropathy may be as high as 12 mL/min/year but with effective control of hypertension and glycaemic control, this may be reduced to about 5 mL/min/year. Dietary protein restriction to approximately 1 g/kg body weight per day may be considered although the benefits are unclear and poor nutrition with failing appetite is also a risk. Administration of exogenous erythropoietin with parenteral iron therapy may be required. Eventually renal replacement may be necessary, e.g. CAPD, haemodialysis or renal transplant.

Case 44.4

Miss RH is a 16-year-old girl with type 1 diabetes who is brought to the Accident and Emergency department at 10.30 am by her mother. She is acutely unwell, slurring her words and unable to maintain concentration for more than a few seconds. She has been vomiting since waking that morning, is clutching her abdomen and groaning in pain. Her mother is very distressed as her daughter's condition has deteriorated rapidly over a short period of time. She says that she thought her daughter smelt of ketones the previous evening although at the time Miss RH told her mother that her blood glucose readings were fine, although her mother now thinks that her daughter's response was evasive. Six months ago Miss RH's care was transferred from paediatric to adult diabetic services and a month ago she was switched from a long-standing twice-daily insulin mix regimen to a basal-bolus regimen with insulin aspart and glargine. Since her insulin regimen has been altered Miss RH has already been admitted twice with ketoacidosis. Prior to this her blood glucose levels sometimes ran high but she had never been diagnosed with ketoacidosis.

Questions

1. How should the diagnosis be confirmed?
2. What are the likely explanations for Miss RH experiencing ketoacidosis?
3. How should she be managed acutely?
4. What future changes would you recommend with regard to her insulin treatment?

Answers

1. Diabetic ketoacidosis is a medical emergency and requires prompt treatment, therefore it is imperative to make a speedy diagnosis. The clinical presentation and history of two previous recent admissions with diabetic ketoacidosis and the mother's report of smelling ketones on her daughter the night before indicate another episode of diabetic ketoacidosis. The suspected diagnosis should be confirmed by physical examination and bedside testing of blood (and/or urine if possible). A physical examination for dehydration, hypotension, ketosis (by smelling the breath; however, up to 30% of the population cannot detect the smell of ketones) and Kussmaul breathing should be undertaken. The diagnosis should be further confirmed by laboratory testing of venous blood (glucose, Na+, K+, Cl−, HCO_3^-, urea, creatinine, anion gap, lactate) and arterial blood (pH, HCO_3^- base excess, P_aO_2, P_aCO_2). Further tests including ECG, cardiac enzymes, FBC, chest x-ray and blood/urine/sputum for culture may also be performed if necessary and to elucidate any precipitating factors.

2. Precipitating factors (e.g. the presence of infection) should be investigated. Glycaemic control is notoriously difficult in adolescents. This may be due to a number of reasons, some due to changes associated with puberty, e.g. hormonal changes, and some due to psychosocial factors. Psychosocial factors may include a desire to be independent from parental help in controlling blood sugar levels, to be 'normal' like other adolescent peers who do not need to conform to strict diet and insulin regimens and a desire to 'not conform' with medical recommendations. Many adolescents become more body and image conscious and resent the weight gain often associated with insulin use and for this reason have been known to skip insulin injections. The change to a basal-bolus regimen requiring more injections which was intended to improve control and offer more flexibility in eating habits may be another reason for non-compliance.

3. Immediate treatment should include fluid and electrolyte replacement and an infusion of intravenous soluble insulin. Fluid replacement should be undertaken with 0.9% sodium chloride and with added potassium if required (see below) until blood glucose levels fall below 15 mmol/L, at which point it should be switched to 5% dextrose. Soluble insulin should be infused at a rate of 5–10 units per hour until blood glucose levels fall below 15 mmol/L, then the insulin infusion rate should be reduced to 1–4 units per hour. Blood glucose should be maintained at between 4 and 10 mmol/L using the insulin infusion until Miss RH is eating again. Potassium is required as there is likely to have been potassium loss because of diuresis and vomiting. In addition, the insulin infusion and subsequent rise in pH will cause extracellular potassium to enter into the cells, causing hypokalaemia. Regular potassium monitoring is required; however, generally potassium should not be given with the first litre of 0.9% sodium chloride unless a level of less than 3.5 mmol/L is measured. With subsequent rehydration fluids, to achieve a potassium level of less than 3.5 mmol/L, 40 mmol/L potassium is added; for a potassium level of 3.5–5.5 mmol/L then 20 mmol/L is added. However, if a potassium level is above 5.5 mmol/L then potassium is omitted from the infusion fluid.

4. Since Miss RH was admitted in such a serious condition, and it is suspected that she may have omitted or reduced her insulin doses, the situation needs to be handled sensitively, yet frankly. Whether or not her mother should be present during any such discussions should be established with Miss RH who may have a strong desire to be independent from parental control of her diabetes. Basic education should be given about the need to rotate injection sites and her sites should be checked for the presence of lipohypertrophy as this may explain erratic absorption. She should also be educated about the correct storage of insulin, in case the insulin she is using has been incorrectly stored and hence become less active. Miss RH needs to be fully informed of the risks associated with diabetic ketoacidosis, especially as this is the third time in a month that she has been admitted with this condition. If the basal-bolus regimen is too complex and contributing to the non-adherence then the twice-daily regimen can be readopted.

ACKNOWLEDGEMENTS

The authors would like to acknowledge the contribution of the previous authors, J A Cantrill and J Wood.

REFERENCES

DAFNE Study Group 2002 Training in flexible, intensive insulin management to enable dietary freedom in people with type 1 diabetes: dose adjustment for normal eating (DAFNE) randomised controlled trial. British Medical Journal 325: 746-749

Davies M, Storms F, Shutler S et al 2005 Improvement of glycaemic control in subjects with poorly controlled type 2 diabetes. Diabetes Care 28: 1282-1288

Department of Health 2002 National Service Framework for Diabetes: Standards. Department of Health, London

Dormandy J A, Charbonnel B, Eckland D J A et al 2005 Secondary prevention of macrovascular events in patients with type 2 diabetes in the PROactive Study (PROspective pioglitAzone Clinical Trial In macroVascular Events): a randomised controlled trial. Lancet 366: 1279-1289

Joint British Societies 2005 JBS 2: Joint British Societies' guidelines on prevention of cardiovascular disease in clinical practice. Heart 91: v1-v52

Khan R, Buse J, Ferrannini E et al 2005 The metabolic syndrome: time for a critical appraisal. Joint statement from the American Diabetes Association and the European Association for the Study of Diabetes. Diabetes Care 28(9): 2289-2304

Malmberg K, Norhammar A, Wedel H et al 1999 Glycometabolic state at admission: important risk marker of mortality in conventionally treated patients with diabetes mellitus and acute myocardial infarction: long-term results from the Diabetes and Insulin-Glucose Infusion in Acute Myocardial Infarction (DIGAMI) study. Circulation 99(20): 2662-2632

National Institute for Clinical Excellence 2002a Management of type 2 diabetes: management of blood glucose. Clinical Guideline G. National Institute for Clinical Excellence, London. Available online at: http://www.nice.org.uk/page.aspx?o=GuidelineG&c=endocrine

National Institute for Clinical Excellence 2002b Management of type 2 diabetes: management of blood pressure and blood lipids. Clinical Guideline H. National Institute for Clinical Excellence, London. Available online at: http://www.nice.org.uk/page.aspx?o=GuidelineH&c=endocrine

Torgerson J S, Hauptman J, Boldrin M N et al 2004 XENical in the Prevention of Diabetes in Obese Subjects (XENDOS) Study. Diabetes Care 27: 155-161

Wahrenberg H, Hertel K, Leijonhufvud B-M et al 2005 Use of waist circumference to predict insulin resistance: retrospective study. British Medical Journal 330: 1363-1364

World Health Organization 1999 Definition, diagnosis and classification of diabetes mellitus and its complications, part 1: Diagnosis and classification of diabetes mellitus. World Health Organization, Geneva

FURTHER READING

Aldhahi W, Hamdy O 2003 Adipokines, inflammation, and the endothelium in diabetes. Current Diabetes Reports 3: 293-298

Herald K C, Hagopian W, Auger J A et al 2002 Anti-CD3 monoclonal antibody in new-onset type 1 diabetes mellitus. New England Journal of Medicine 346: 1692-1698

Keymeulen B, Vandemeulebroucke E, Ziegler A G et al Insulin needs after CD3-antibody therapy in new-onset type 1 diabetes. New England Journal of Medicine 352: 2598-2608

Lipsky B A, Berendt A R, Gunner Deery H et al 2004 Infectious Disease Society of America (IDSA) guidelines – diagnosis and treatment of diabetic foot infections. Clinical Infectious Diseases 39: 885-910

Royal Pharmaceutical Society of Great Britain Diabetes Task Force in conjunction with Diabetes UK 2004 Practice guidance on the care of people with diabetes. Royal Pharmaceutical Society of Great Britain, London. Available online at: www.rpsgb.org/pdfs/diabguid3. pdf#xml=http://www.rpsgb. org/search/pdfhi.php?all=1&filepath=../pdfs/diabguid3.pdf&search=diabetes%202004

45 Menstrual cycle disorders

K. Marshall   S. Calvert

KEY POINTS

- Girls can begin experiencing menstrual disorders once ovulatory cycles are established.
- Up to 95% of women experience some changes premenstrually, but severe premenstrual syndrome is more common in the 30–40 year age group.
- The aetiology of premenstrual syndrome is multifactorial, the symptomatology complex and treatment options diverse.
- It has been estimated that 50–80% of women of child-bearing age will suffer from dysmenorrhoea at some time.
- Treatment options vary according to the type of dysmenorrhoea (primary or secondary) but include: non-steroidal anti-inflammatory drugs; combined oral contraceptive pills; and progestogen-only preparations.
- Menorrhagia (excessive menstrual blood loss) affects up to 30% of menstruating women. The management of the condition depends upon the cause and can be either surgical or medical.
- Endometriosis (the presence of extrauterine endometrial tissue) can give rise to an array of symptoms including subfertility. Treatment may be designed to improve fertility and manage symptoms. Medical and surgical treatments are available.

Once a girl reaches puberty, various physiological events occur, leading to the onset of menstruation, or the menarche. The average age of the menarche has decreased to around 12.5 years and a halt in this trend towards earlier menarche is not evident. This decline has been attributed to an improvement in nutrition and overall health. Body weight is linked to menarchal age and it is possible that as body fat increases so does serum leptin (hormone which influences calorie intake) which in turn may increase the pulsatile release of gonadotrophin-releasing hormone (GnRH).

Menstruation is an event that occurs relatively late in puberty and 95% of girls reach the menarche between the ages of 11 and 15 years. One UK study has shown that one girl in eight begins to menstruate whilst still at primary school. Even before the first ovulatory cycle has taken place, childhood ovarian activity will have gradually increased the production of oestrogen, leading to the development of the secondary sexual characteristics. These events are probably initiated by the central nervous system which ultimately triggers the necessary gonadal changes that will eventually lead to the establishment of the menstrual cycle. It may take up to 2 years for the hypothalamic pituitary gonadal axis to mature and for regular ovulation to take place. In girls who only start to menstruate when they are older, it may take even longer. This should be considered when taking a patient's medical history.

Menstruation itself occurs as a result of cyclic hormonal variations (Fig. 45.1). During the first half or follicular phase of the menstrual cycle, the endometrium thickens under the influence of increasing levels of oestrogen (most notably estradiol, which at the peak of its preovulatory surge reaches around 2000 pmol/L) secreted from the developing ovarian follicles. Once the serum oestrogen level has surpassed a critical point it triggers, by positive feedback, the anterior pituitary to release, about 24 hours later, a surge of luteinizing hormone (up to 50 iu/L) and after 30–36 hours, ovulation follows.

After ovulation, which occurs around day 14 of a 28-day menstrual cycle, and as the luteal phase progresses, the endometrium begins to respond to increasing levels of progesterone. Both progesterone and oestrogen are secreted from the corpus luteum which is formed from the remains of the ovarian follicle after ovulation. The lifespan of the corpus luteum is remarkably constant and lasts between 12 and 14 days; hence the length of the second half or the luteal phase of the menstrual cycle is between 12 and 14 days. Between days 18 and 22 of a 28-day cycle, both sex steroids peak, with levels of progesterone reaching around 30 nmol/L. As progesterone has a thermogenic effect upon the hypothalamus, basal body temperature increases by about 1°C in the second half of an ovulatory cycle (Fig. 45.2). Most ovulatory cycles range from 21 to 34 days.

These synchronized changes mean that about a week after ovulation, the endometrium is prepared for implantation, providing fertilization has taken place. If conception does not occur then

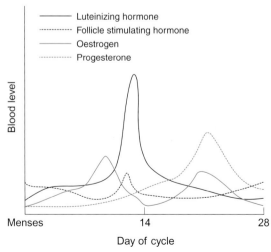

Figure 45.1 The hormonal events that occur during the menstrual cycle in women.

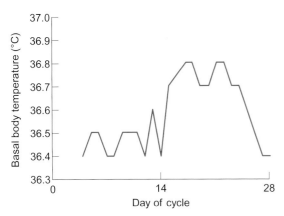

Figure 45.2 Typical temperature chart from a 28-day ovulatory menstrual cycle.

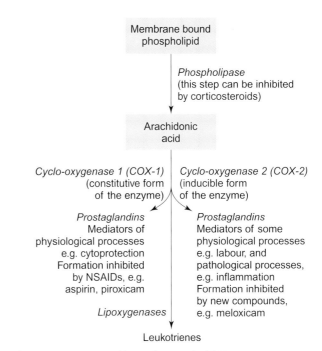

Figure 45.3 Eicosanoid biosynthesis and inhibition.

luteolysis begins and steroid levels fall. This means that the endometrium cannot be maintained, there is a loss of stromal fluid, leucocyte infiltration begins, and there is intraglandular extravasation of blood. Finally, endometrial blood flow is reduced and this leads to necrosis and sloughing, i.e. menstruation. Initially the blood vessels that remain intact after sloughing are sealed by fibrin and platelet plugs; subsequent haemostasis is probably achieved as a result of vasoconstriction of the remaining basal arteries. Nitric oxide may be involved in the initiation and maintenance of menstrual bleeding by promoting vasodilation and inhibiting platelet aggregation. The myometrium is the muscular layers of the uterus that contract spontaneously throughout the menstrual cycle, the frequency of these contractions being influenced by the hormonal milieu. The myometrium is also more active during menstruation. The average blood loss per period is between 30 and 40 mL.

There is evidence which suggests a physiological and pathological role for the local hormones, known as prostaglandins, in the process of menstruation. Prostaglandins are 20-carbon oxygenated, polyunsaturated bioactive lipids, which are cyclo-oxygenase derived products of arachidonic acid. Indeed, both the myometrium and the endometrium are capable of synthesizing and responding to prostaglandins. A potential role for another family of autocoids, the leukotrienes, in the regulation of uterine function remains uncertain although it is known that leukotrienes can also be synthesized from arachidonic acid by lipoxygenase enzymes (Fig. 45.3).

Disorders associated with menstruation are a major medical and social problem for women which also impact upon their families.

Premenstrual syndrome

Premenstrual syndrome (PMS) encompasses both mood changes and physical symptoms. Symptoms may start up to 14 days before menstruation, although more usually they begin just a few days before and disappear at the onset of, or shortly after, menstruation. However, for some women the beginning of menstruation may not signal the complete resolution of symptoms. Numerous studies have demonstrated that this condition can cause substantial impairment of normal daily activity, including reduced

occupational activity and significant levels of work absenteeism. Severity varies from cycle to cycle, and may be influenced by other life factors such as stress and tiredness. The most severe form of PMS may be referred to as premenstrual dysphoric disorder (PMDD) as defined by the Modified Diagnostic and Statistical Manual of Mental Disorders appendix IV, or DSM-IV (APA 2000) and for which the criteria are set out in Table 45.1. Other bodies (ACOG 2000) have published diagnostic criteria

Table 45.1 Summary of DSM-IV diagnostic criteria for premenstrual dysphoric disorder (PMDD)

One year duration of symptoms which are present for the majority of cycles (occur luteal/remit follicular)

Five of the following symptoms (with at least 1 of these*) must occur during the week before menses and remit within days of menses.

- Irritability*
- Depressed mood or hopelessness*
- Affective lability* (sudden mood swings)
- Tension or anxiety*
- Decreased interest in activities
- Change in sleep patterns
- Difficulty concentrating
- Feeling out of control or overwhelmed
- Lack of energy
- Other physical symptoms, e.g. breast tenderness, bloating
- Change in appetite, e.g. food cravings

Seriously interferes with work, social activities, relationships

Not an exacerbation of another disorder

Confirmed by prospective daily ratings during at least 2 consecutive symptomatic cycles

for PMS (Table 45.2). There is considerable overlap between PMS and PMDD.

Epidemiology

Up to 95% of menstruating women experience some changes premenstrually. PMS occurs in about 5% of these women and PMDD has an estimated incidence of 3–9%. PMS affects young and older women alike and does not appear to be influenced by parity. Severe PMS is more common in the 30–40 year age range, and married women with young children commonly seek help. Certain events may be linked with the onset of PMS, including childbirth, cessation of oral contraceptive use (incidence of reported PMS is lower in pill users), sterilization, hysterectomy or even increasing age. PMS may be exacerbated by other stresses, typically those associated with family life. Women with a body mass index over 30 are more likely to suffer from PMS. There is also some evidence that crimes, accidents, examination failure, absenteeism and marital disturbances may be more common premenstrually.

Aetiology

PMS is not seen before puberty, during pregnancy or in post-menopausal women and therefore, the ovarian hormones have been implicated. The mineralocorticoids, prolactin, androgens, prostaglandins, endorphins, nutritional factors (for example, pyridoxine, calcium and essential fatty acids) and hypoglycaemia may be involved. In addition, changes in central nervous system function have been implicated as cerebral blood flow in the temporal lobes is decreased premenstrually in PMS sufferers, and noradrenergic cyclicity is disrupted. As symptoms vary so much from cycle to cycle, and from individual to individual, it is likely that different aetiological factors apply to different

women, all of which may be affected by extenuating emotional circumstances.

Hormones

The cyclicity of PMS suggests an ovarian involvement. This is substantiated by the fact that it is still experienced after hysterectomy if the ovaries are left intact and that it disappears during pregnancy and after the menopause. One theory attributes PMS to luteal phase progesterone deficiency leading to a progesterone/estradiol imbalance, but there is no direct clinical evidence to support this in terms of serum progesterone levels. However, the problem could lie at the cellular level, i.e. a paucity of functional steroid receptors leading to differential sensitivity to hormones. Alternatively it could be a central control defect, as ovarian suppression by GnRH analogues can alleviate symptoms in some women; however, the use of these drugs is generally not recommended because of their unwanted effects associated with production of a hypo-oestrogenic state.

The central actions of the sex steroids or their neuroactive metabolites could also be significant. Estradiol increases neuronal excitability possibly via increasing the activity of glutamate (an important excitatory neurotransmitter). Progesterone, and its metabolites, can bind to the γ-aminobutyric acid A (GABA$_A$) receptor and this interaction would induce an effect similar to that evoked by benzodiazepines. The mineralocorticoid aldosterone may be associated with the increase in fluid retention as serum levels of this hormone are elevated in the luteal phase. However, no significant difference in blood levels of this mineralocorticoid has been found between PMS sufferers and non-sufferers. In contrast, one study has found that baseline levels of cortisol were elevated during the luteal phase in PMS sufferers.

Prolactin is secreted from the decidual cells at the end of the luteal phase of the menstrual cycle as well as from the anterior pituitary. This hormone has a direct effect upon breast tissue and hence may be associated with breast tenderness. Prolactin is also associated with stress, and has an indirect relationship with dopamine metabolism and release in the central nervous system. It promotes sodium, potassium and water retention. However, there are no consistent differences in hormone blood levels of prolactin between PMS sufferers and non-sufferers. Again, the differences could lie at the receptor level. Local hormones such as the prostaglandins may also be implicated in the aetiology of PMS as synthesis of these autocoids can be affected by the sex hormones as well as substrate availability. Prostaglandin imbalance is implicated in PMS as increased synthesis of certain prostaglandins, e.g. PGE$_2$, have antidiuretic and central sedative effects as well as promoting capillary permeability and vasodilation. Deficiencies of others, e.g. PGE$_1$, which can attenuate some of the actions of prolactin, may also contribute to the syndrome.

Vitamins and minerals

Pyridoxine phosphate is a co-factor in a number of enzyme reactions, particularly those leading to production of dopamine and serotonin (5-hydroxytryptamine). It has been suggested that disturbances of the oestrogen/progesterone balance could cause a relative deficiency of pyridoxine, and supplementation with this vitamin appears to ease the depression sometimes associated

---

Table 45.2 Diagnostic criteria for premenstrual syndrome (PMS)

Patient reports ≥1 of the following affective and somatic symptoms during the 5 days before menses in each of three prior menstrual cycles:

Affective	Somatic
Depression	Breast tenderness
Angry outbursts	Abdominal bloating
Irritability	Headache
Anxiety	Swelling of extremities
Confusion	
Social withdrawal	

Symptoms relieved within 4 days of menses onset without recurrence until at least cycle day 13

Symptoms present in absence of any pharmacological therapy, hormone ingestion, or drug or alcohol abuse

Symptoms occur reproducibly during two cycles of prospective recording

Patient suffers from identifiable dysfunction in social or economic performance

with the oral contraceptive pill. Decreased dopamine levels would tend to increase serum prolactin, and decreased serotonin levels could be a factor in emotional disturbances, particularly depression. There is now some evidence that premenstrual mood changes are linked to cycle-related alterations in serotonergic activity within the central nervous system and, therefore, serotonin may be important in the pathogenesis of PMS.

There are also data to suggest that a variety of nutrients may play a role in the aetiology of PMS, specifically calcium and vitamin D. Oestrogen influences calcium metabolism by affecting intestinal absorption, and parathyroid gene expression and secretion, so triggering fluctuations throughout the menstrual cycle. Disruption of calcium homeostasis has been associated with affective disorders.

Essential fatty acids

Essential fatty acids, such as GLA (γ-linolenic or gamolenic acid), provide a substrate for prostaglandin synthesis. GLA is converted into dihomo-γ-linolenic acid, which forms the starting point for the synthesis of prostaglandins of the 1 series (e.g. PGE_1). It has been suggested that women with PMS are abnormally sensitive to normal levels of prolactin and that PGE_1 is able to attenuate the biological effects of this hormone. Hence, if there is a GLA deficiency then there is less substrate for PGE_1 synthesis. Therefore, the effect of prolactin with respect to breast tenderness, fluid retention and mood disturbances may be exaggerated. Numerous other dietary factors may also be involved, including excess saturated fats and cholesterol, moderate-to-high alcohol consumption, zinc and magnesium deficiencies, diabetes, ageing and viral infections, all of which hinder the conversion of cis-linolenic acid to GLA. Pyridoxine, ascorbic acid and niacin also increase conversion of GLA to PGE_1, while there is some evidence to suggest that linolenic acid metabolite levels are reduced in women with PMS.

Psychological factors

PMS may not be wholly explicable in pathophysiological terms but it should not be regarded as a psychosomatic disorder as there is no simple relationship between its existence and severity and personality. It is not strictly confined to particular types of women, although there is no doubt that PMS interacts with many aspects of life, especially difficult or stressful times. The latter has been termed the 'vulnerability factor' which, although not a function of the menstrual cycle, can affect the way a woman reacts.

Symptoms

Symptoms occur 1–14 days before menstruation begins and disappear at the onset or shortly after menstruation begins. For the rest of the cycle the woman feels well. Symptoms are cyclical, although they may not be experienced every cycle, and can be either physical and/or psychological (see Tables 45.1 and 45.2 for more detailed symptomatology). The lives of the 5% or so of women who are severely affected may be completely disrupted in the second half of the menstrual cycle. The symptoms of PMS tend to decrease as a woman gets closer to the menopause as her ovulatory cycles become less frequent.

Management

The first step in the management of PMS is recognition of the problem and realization that many other women also suffer. Keeping a menstrual diary is useful and will establish any link between symptoms and menstruation, and this will provide a cornerstone for diagnosis. After a few months it will allow the patient to make predictions and help her deal with changes when they arrive. The effectiveness of medical intervention depends upon which symptoms are being experienced, underlining the importance of a menstrual diary and experimentation. In terms of treatment, self-help and perseverance will be required in the management of PMS. The wide variety of symptoms may require exploring a number of treatment options before optimal relief can be achieved.

Non-pharmacological strategies

Maintenance of good general health is important, especially with respect to diet and possible deficiencies. Dietary modifications that may be helpful include restricting caffeine and alcohol intake. Smoking can also exacerbate symptoms. Exercise may help, as may learning simple relaxation techniques. If fluid retention is a problem, then reducing fluid and salt intake may be of value. Increasing the intake of natural diuretics such as prunes, figs, celery, cucumber, parsley and foods high in potassium such as bananas, oranges, dried fruits, nuts, soya beans and tomatoes may all be useful. Hypoglycaemia may also be involved in premenstrual tiredness so eating small protein-rich meals more frequently may help.

Results from clinical trials involving pyridoxine (vitamin B_6) have shown conflicting results. However, some women do respond to pyridoxine and show improvement, particularly with respect to mood change, breast discomfort and headache. A typical dosage regimen would be 50 mg twice daily after meals or 100 mg after breakfast. The dose should not exceed 100 mg a day. Gastric upset and headaches have been reported at doses greater than 200 mg. High doses over long periods have also been associated with peripheral neuropathies. Pyridoxine should be commenced 3 days before symptom onset and continued for 2 days after menstruation has started.

A double-blind placebo-controlled study of over 450 women with PMS reported that calcium supplementation was effective in reducing emotional, behavioural and physical symptoms.

Some women find that supplementation with γ-linolenic acid (GLA), found in evening primrose oil, gives relief from physical symptoms, especially breast tenderness. However, this has not been substantiated by trial data.

Pharmacological management

Progestogens Synthetic progestogens, in preparations such as Cyclogest and Duphaston, have been used in the past. However, because of the lack of convincing trial evidence and the risk of side effects, the use of progestogens is no longer recommended. Possible side effects include weight gain, nausea, breast discomfort, breakthrough bleeding and changes in cycle length. Problems usually arose because some synthetic progestogens, especially 19-nor compounds such as norethisterone and levonorgestrel, also display some affinity for glucocorticoid, mineralocorticoid and androgen receptors. The specificity of these synthetic agents is influenced by the substituents present on the steroid nucleus, particularly at C13. For example, the third-generation progestogens that have an ethyl group at C13 (gestodene, desogestrel and norgestimate) have the least androgenic activity of all the 19-nor compounds but are still orally active.

Combined oral contraceptives Some women are helped by the combined oral contraceptive pill (COC) because it prevents ovulation from taking place. However, the use of exogenous oestrogen may be contraindicated because it can increase the risk of venous thromboembolism (VTE). This occurs because oestrogen decreases blood levels of the potent natural anticoagulant antithrombin III and at the same time increases serum levels of some clotting factors. Women with other risk factors for thromboembolic disease should also avoid this form of therapy. The incidence of VTE in healthy, non-pregnant women who are not taking an oral contraceptive is about five cases per 100 000 women per year. For those using combined oral contraceptives containing second-generation progestogens, e.g. levonorgestrel, this incidence is about 15 per 100 000 women per year of use. Some studies have reported a greater risk of VTE in women using preparations containing the third-generation progestogens desogestrel and gestodene. The incidence in these women is about 25 per 100 000 women per year of use. However, it should be noted that the absolute risk of VTE in women using combined oral contraceptives containing these third-generation progestogens remains very small and well below the VTE risk associated with pregnancy.

It is thought that use of third-generation progestogens is associated with increased resistance to the anticoagulant action of activated protein C. Oral contraceptive treatment diminishes the efficacy with which activated protein C downregulates in vitro thrombin formation. This is known as activated protein C resistance and is more pronounced in women using COCs containing desogestrel than in women using those containing levonorgestrel. However, it has also been recognized that women who do react to third-generation progestogens with VTE may be revealing a latent thrombophilia. There are several conditions, congenital or acquired, that can cause thrombophilic alterations. A genetic factor known as factor V Leiden mutation is the most common inherited cause of thrombophilia and this mutation results in resistance to the effects of activated protein C. Carriers of this mutation have more than a 30-fold increase in risk of thrombotic complications during oral contraceptive use, although this has been disputed (Farmer et al 2000) because no increase in risk of VTE was found with the third-generation progestogens. In conclusion, if there is a history of thromboembolic disease at a young age in the immediate family then disturbances of the coagulation system must be ruled out.

The combination of ethinylestradiol with drospirenone is also available as an oral contraceptive and appears to be useful in the management of PMS. Drospirenone is a derivative of spironolactone, with affinity for progesterone receptors, but it also acts as a mineralocorticoid antagonist. This progestogen, therefore, alleviates some of the salt-retaining effects of the ethinylestradiol.

Bromocriptine Bromocriptine stimulates central dopamine receptors and thus inhibits the release of prolactin. It may be useful for breast tenderness and occasionally has beneficial effects upon fluid retention and mood changes. It should be used in small doses, for example 1–1.25 mg at bedtime with food, to avoid the side effects of nausea and faintness due to hypotension. The dose can be slowly increased to 2.5 mg twice a day if required. It is advised that ergot-derived dopamine receptor agonists, such as bromocriptine, have been associated with pulmonary, retroperitoneal and pericardial fibrotic reactions (Anon 2002). Excessive daytime sleepiness and sudden onset of sleep can also occur with dopaminergic drugs.

Danazol Danazol is a synthetic steroid derived from ethisterone. It is weakly androgenic and has been described as an attenuated androgen. Danazol interacts with androgen receptors but it also has some affinity for the progesterone receptor. It inhibits the pulsatile release of gonadotrophins from the anterior pituitary and so abolishes cyclical ovarian activity, leading to amenorrhoea in the majority of women and a subsequent fall in serum oestrogen levels. However, because of the high incidence of side effects it tends to be used as a last resort for relief of severe mastalgia and mood changes. These side effects relate to the androgenicity of the compound and include nausea, giddiness, muscular pain, weight gain, acne and virilization. These can be minimized by using low doses of 200 mg a day.

Gonadotrophin-releasing hormone analogues GnRH analogues, sometimes referred to as gonadorelin analogues, are useful for managing the physical symptoms, but are less effective with respect to emotional symptoms. These agents inhibit the hypothalamic–pituitary–gonadal axis. However, they can only be used for short periods of time, no more than 6 months, because they induce a hypo-oestrogenic state and therefore bone loss becomes significant after 6 months' treatment. Should a patient respond well to GnRH analogues for PMS following hysterectomy because of underlying pelvic pathology then bilateral oophorectomy may also be of benefit.

Prostaglandin synthesis inhibitors Improvements in tension, irritability, depression, headache and general aches and pains can be seen in some women who take prostaglandin synthesis inhibitors. Most of the information available centres upon the use of mefenamic acid at doses of 250 mg three times a day 12 days before a period is due, increasing to 500 mg three times a day 9 days before the period and continuing until the third day of menstruation. Other inhibitors of prostaglandin synthesis are likely to be just as effective and may be associated with fewer side effects. Some experimental evidence, however, suggests that, in addition to being a cyclo-oxygenase inhibitor, mefenamic acid also has activity as an antagonist at prostaglandin E receptors and therefore this may be useful if heavy menstrual bleeding is also a problem. For optimum effectiveness this form of therapy should be started 24 hours before the onset of symptoms. However, this starting point may be difficult to predict for women with irregular cycles.

Antidepressants The serotonin reuptake inhibitors (SSRIs) are becoming more popular in the treatment of PMS-related depression because they are effective and well tolerated (Dimmock et al 2000). Several randomized controlled trials using fluoxetine, sertraline, citalopram, fluvoxamine or paroxetine concluded that SSRIs are an effective first-line therapy for severe PMS and the side effects at low doses are generally acceptable. Two studies also found that not only do SSRIs improve behavioural symptoms, but some improvement in physical symptoms was also noted. Common side effects experienced include headache, nervousness, drowsiness and fatigue, sexual dysfunction and gastrointestinal disturbances. Other agents such as tricyclic antidepressants and anxiolytics such as buspirone have been used. However, they appear to improve fewer PMS symptoms than the SSRIs.

A small study using St John's Wort indicated that this may reduce the severity of PMS and that there is scope for larger randomized trials.

Dysmenorrhoea

Dysmenorrhoea is usually subdivided into primary and secondary dysmenorrhoea. The former may also be referred to as spasmodic dysmenorrhoea, which is a uterine problem and is predominantly a complaint of young women. Secondary dysmenorrhoea is so called because it occurs secondary to some underlying pelvic pathology such as endometriosis or pelvic inflammatory disease.

Epidemiology

The estimates vary but epidemiological studies suggest that between 50% and 80% of women will suffer from dysmenorrhoea at some time during their reproductive life, and up to 15% of these women will be seriously debilitated by the condition, with social and economic consequences.

Primary dysmenorrhoea

Aetiology and symptoms

The incidence of primary dysmenorrhoea peaks in women in their late teens and early 20s, the pain coinciding with establishment of ovulatory cycles. A typical sufferer will usually complain of lower abdominal pain (cramping), which may radiate down into the thighs, and backache. Some women also suffer gastrointestinal symptoms (nausea, vomiting, diarrhoea), headaches and faintness. Symptoms are intense on the first day of menses but rarely continue beyond day 1 or 2 of the cycle. Factors that appear to increase the severity include young age at menarche, extended duration of menstrual flow (pain can be most severe when the flow is lighter), smoking and parity (the prevalence and severity of dysmenorrhoea is decreased in parous women). Other factors such as weight, length of menstrual cycle or frequency of physical exercise do not influence the condition.

In terms of the aetiology of this condition, work carried out in the 1950s and 1960s first drew attention to the possible role of the prostaglandins. Following on from this, many in vivo studies have shown that women suffering from primary dysmenorrhoea do have greater concentrations of prostaglandins, predominantly $PGF_{2\alpha}$, and to some extent PGE_2, in their menstrual fluid compared with matched control subjects. Such a prostaglandin imbalance would favour increased myometrial contractility. The effects of the prostaglandins on human myometrium are now well documented, and increased biosynthesis of prostaglandins may also account for the gastrointestinal problems encountered by some sufferers. A role for the prostaglandins is further substantiated by the fact that women whose diet contains

more omega-3 fatty acids tend to suffer less. When eicosapentaenoic acid (EPA) is the substrate for prostaglandin biosynthesis, prostaglandins of the three series are produced (e.g. PGE_3 and TXA_3). Such local hormones are less potent stimulators of the myometrium and less effective vasoconstrictors. Other potential mediators are the endothelins, vasoactive peptides produced in the endometrium that may play a role in the local regulation of prostaglandin synthesis, and vasopressin, a posterior pituitary hormone that stimulates uterine activity and decreases uterine blood flow. The smaller branches of the uterine arteries are very sensitive to the vasoconstrictor actions of these mediators and it is these resistance vessels that are important in the control of uterine blood flow. The interrelationship between blood flow and myometrial activity is summarized in Figure 45.4.

Measurements of intrauterine pressure and myometrial activity have been made for research purposes, but there are no simple objective measurements for dysmenorrhoea.

Secondary dysmenorrhoea

Aetiology and symptoms

Secondary dysmenorrhoea tends to afflict women in their 30s and 40s, and usually occurs as a consequence of some other pelvic pathology such as endometriosis or pelvic inflammation. In terms of symptoms, it differs from primary dysmenorrhoea in that the pain may actually start before menstruation begins, continue for the duration of menses and be associated with abdominal bloating and backache and a general feeling of 'heaviness' in the pelvic area. The intrauterine contraceptive device may also exacerbate menstrual pain, since it causes localized inflammation that triggers the release of prostaglandins. The prostaglandins may also be implicated in the chain of events that lead to the pain associated with secondary dysmenorrhoea. For example, if the cause is endometriosis, in which endometrial tissue is found outside the uterine cavity, then this extrauterine tissue can also synthesize prostaglandins, which may in turn disrupt normal uterine function.

Treatment

In terms of analgesia, the most rational choice would be a non-steroidal anti-inflammatory drug (NSAID), as these compounds decrease prostaglandin biosynthesis by inhibiting cyclooxygenase. Differences in anti-inflammatory activity between different NSAIDs are small. However, there is considerable

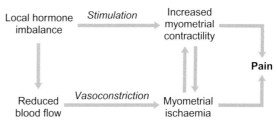

Figure 45.4 The interactive role of myometrial stimulants and vasoconstrictive agents in the pathway leading to pain in dysmenorrhoea.

variation in individual patient tolerance and response, and a lack of response to one particular agent does not mean that a patient would not respond to a different NSAID.

Mefenamic acid is frequently used to manage pain due to dysmenorrhoea. As stated previously, this compound not only inhibits prostaglandin production but also appears to possess some prostaglandin E receptor blocking activity which may serve to augment its effect. However, these preparations are not suitable for all women and some, about 30% of women, will not respond.

The lack of an effect with an NSAID may be explained by pathway diversion, since the arachidonic acid that was to be converted to a prostaglandin via the action of cyclo-oxygenase can be utilized by an alternative biosynthetic route, leading to increased formation of leukotrienes. Alternatively the second cyclo-oxygenase enzyme (COX-2), which is generally induced under pathological conditions, may be involved. Many of the currently available NSAIDs are relatively poor inhibitors of COX-2, and if some of the prostaglandins in these uterine disorders are produced via the action of this form of cyclo-oxygenase, then it is not surprising that the NSAIDs are not 100% effective. The availability of selective COX-2 inhibitors may be useful in the treatment of dysmenorrhoeic pain and at the same time spare the patient from the potential problem of gastric irritation that appears to occur as a result of COX-1 inhibition. Celecoxib, etoricoxib and rofecoxib are effective against this type of pain and show a lower incidence of gastrotoxicity although none is currently licensed for use in dysmenorrhoea. In 2004 rofecoxib was withdrawn because of adverse effects on the cardiovascular system.

It has been estimated that approximately 50% of primary dysmenorrhoea sufferers will gain relief from taking the oral contraceptive pill although, as this is a condition afflicting young girls, there may be attitudinal problems to the use of these products either in the patient or her parents. The oral contraceptive pill inhibits ovulation and thereby prevents increased luteal phase prostaglandin synthesis and so decreases uterine contractility. However, not all women are suitable candidates for COC use because of the potential problems associated with exogenous oestrogen. Contraindications include high blood pressure, obesity and a significant personal or family history of VTE. Progestogenic preparations (for example, dydrogesterone 10 mg twice daily from day 5 to 25 of cycle, norethisterone 5 mg three times daily from day 5 to 24 of the cycle) or progestogen-only pills may be useful if they inhibit ovulation. Antispasmodics such as hyoscine butylbromide and propantheline bromide have a very limited role in the treatment of dysmenorrhoea, not least because of their poor oral bioavailability. Related compounds such as atropine also have negligible effects upon the human uterus. A summary of the treatment options for dysmenorrhoea is presented in Table 45.3. Future therapy may involve use of vasopressin antagonists. Clinical trials have shown these compounds to be effective and well tolerated and they do not affect bleeding patterns.

For secondary dysmenorrhoea the best treatment lies in finding the underlying cause and then taking an appropriate therapeutic route. For example, if some form of pelvic inflammatory disease (PID) is diagnosed that can be attributed to a causative organism, then antimicrobial therapy is appropriate. PID is most commonly caused by the presence of a sexually transmitted infection. The most frequent causative organisms are *Chlamydia trachomatis* and *Neisseria gonorrhoeae*. In addition, any procedure that may compromise the mucus barrier of the cervix, for example insertion of an intrauterine device, may also increase the risk of contracting PID. Treatment of endometriosis will often reduce symptoms of dysmenorrhoea. Surgical treatment for secondary dysmenorrhoea such as hysterectomy is also possible for those woman who do not want to become pregnant.

Non-pharmacological management options have recently been reviewed and include high-frequency transcutaneous nerve stimulation (TENS) and acupuncture (Proctor et al 2006).

Table 45.3 Summary of treatment options for dysmenorrhoea

Drug	Side effects
NSAIDs	Gastric irritation, which can be minimized by taking with or after food or selecting an agent with less gastrotoxicity, e.g. ibuprofen. Hypersensitivity reactions, particularly bronchospasm. Headache, dizziness, vertigo, hearing problems (e.g. tinnitus) and haematuria. NSAIDs may adversely affect renal function and provoke acute renal failure
Combined oral contraceptives	Many side effects are dose related and so the development of the ultra-low dose preparations (i.e. those containing 20 µg ethinylestradiol) is beneficial. An alternative to the oral preparations is the low-dose transdermal combined contraceptive which releases 20 µg ethinylestradiol and 150 µg of norelgestromin (active metabolite of the third-generation progestogen, norgestimate). The most serious potential adverse effect is the increased risk of thromboembolism due to a decrease in circulating levels of antithrombin III while increasing serum levels of some clotting factors. This risk increases with age and smoking. Analysis of current data suggests that the risk of breast cancer is not increased for most women who use the combined oral contraceptive for the major portion of their reproductive years. Use of the combined oral contraceptive also conveys several health benefits besides being an effective contraceptive. The progestogenic side effects are discussed below
Progestogen-only preparations	Use of these agents may cause menstrual disturbances, e.g. breakthrough bleeding. Other adverse effects relate to the selectivity of the synthetic hormone, e.g. norethisterone is a first-generation progestogen and has some affinity for steroid receptors other than progesterone and so possesses androgenic, oestrogenic and anti-oestrogenic activity. The third-generation progestogens (gestodene, norgestimate and desogestrel) have the least androgenic activity. This should be advantageous as it is the androgenicity of the compounds that correlates with the decrease in high-density lipoproteins

Both of these therapies showed some potential benfit. Some Chinese herbal medicines are also under study. There is limited evidence to support the use of uterine nerve ablation and presacral neurectomy, to interrupt the sensory nerve fibres near the cervix blocking the pain pathway.

Menorrhagia

Blood loss is considered to be excessive if it exceeds 80 mL per period, although both women themselves and clinicians find it difficult to objectively quantify the blood loss. In practice, it is defined by the woman's subjective assessment of blood loss. Any change in menstruation, whether real or perceived, may be disturbing with respect to social, occupational or sexual activities and can lead to other problems including depression and concern about an undiagnosed problem such as cancer. Physically excessive blood loss will precipitate iron deficiency anaemia (haemoglobin <12 g/dL) which, if left undiagnosed and untreated, will only compound the problems outlined above.

If a patient has any intermenstrual or postcoital bleeding, then referral to a gynaecologist for endometrial biopsy is essential to exclude intrauterine pathology. Up-to-date cervical cytology is also required.

Epidemiology

In the UK about 30% of women complain of heavy menstrual bleeding, and about 1 in 20 women aged 25–44 years consults their primary care doctor about this problem. Historically, once referred to a gynaecologist, 60% of women could expect to have a hysterectomy within 5 years. Recent changes in the management of women with menorrhagia and new treatment options, particularly endometrial ablations and the levonorgestrel intrauterine contraceptive devices (LNG-IUS), have significantly reduced hysterectomy rates for menorrhagia to a third of the number 10 years ago.

Aetiology and investigation

With respect to aetiology, menorrhagia can be divided into three categories: underlying pelvic pathology, systemic disease and dysfunctional uterine bleeding (Table 45.4). The typical symptoms suggestive of underlying pelvic pathology are presented in Table 45.5. Pelvic pathologies associated with menorrhagia include: myomas (fibroids, common benign tumours of the myometrium); endometriosis; adenomyosis (penetration of endometrial tissue into the myometrium); endometrial polyps; polycystic ovarian disease; and endometrial carcinoma. Although endometrial cancer is more typically seen in postmenopausal women, approximately 50% of those patients diagnosed with it premenopausally will have associated menorrhagia. Systemic diseases from which menorrhagia may stem include hypothyroidism, disorders involving the coagulation system such as elevated endometrial levels of plasminogen activator, and systemic lupus erythematosus. Very few women fall into this group. About 60% of menorrhagia sufferers have no underlying systemic or pelvic pathology and have ovulatory cycles. These patients are said to have dysfunctional uterine bleeding and local uterine

Table 45.4 Causes of menorrhagia (percentage frequency)

Dysfunctional uterine bleeding (60%), i.e. cause is unknown

Other gynaecological causes (30%):
 Uterine or ovarian tumours
 Endometriosis
 Pelvic inflammatory disease
 Intrauterine contraceptive devices
 Early pregnancy complications

Endocrine and haematological causes (<5%)
 Thyroid disorders, e.g. hypothyroidism
 Platelet problems and clotting abnormalities

Table 45.5 Symptoms suggestive of underlying pelvic pathology

Irregular bleeding

Sudden change in blood loss

Intermenstrual bleeding

Postcoital bleeding

Dyspareunia

Pelvic pain

Premenstrual pain

mechanisms appear to be important in the control of menstrual blood loss. Occasionally cycles may be anovulatory, with heavy blood losses because the endometrium has become hyperplastic under the influence of oestrogen. It should also be mentioned that use of an intrauterine contraceptive device may also increase menstrual blood loss.

The prostaglandins appear to play a role in the aforementioned local mechanisms, and have been implicated in menorrhagia. Studies have suggested an association between the type and quantity of endometrial prostaglandin synthesis and the degree of menstrual blood loss. In the mid 1970s it was discovered that women with heavy periods had raised endometrial levels of $PGF_{2\alpha}$ and PGE_2 and that blood loss could be reduced by the use of drugs inhibiting prostaglandin formation. More studies suggested that in menorrhagic women there is a shift towards increased biosynthesis of PGE_2, which is known to dilate uterine vasculature, and/or increased numbers of membrane receptors for this prostanoid. The availability of arachidonic acid, a substrate for prostaglandin synthesis, is also greater in women with menorrhagia. Levels of the vasodilators or their metabolites, PGI_2 and nitric oxide (NO), are also increased in the menstrual blood collected from women with excessive blood loss. Recent studies suggest that menorrhagia is an angiogenesis-related disease associated with changes in the pattern of vascular fragility involving the upregulation of various vascular endothelial growth factors.

Excessive menstrual blood loss is the most common cause of iron deficiency anaemia in women of reproductive age. In an otherwise healthy, well-nourished woman it has been estimated that menstrual blood loss would have to exceed 120 mL to precipitate iron deficiency anaemia. Objective measurement of menstrual blood loss is difficult so measurement of full blood count (including red blood cell indices and serum ferritin levels), and in particular haemoglobin concentration, gives some indication of blood loss. Thyroid function should also be assessed. If fibroids are suspected, then pelvic ultrasound may be required. Endometrial biopsy is needed if there is an associated irregularity of menstruation or if intermenstrual or postcoital bleeding is present. In the case of regular menses, however, investigation of the uterine cavity would usually only be required in women over the age of 35 years or if medical treatment had failed to alleviate symptoms. Young women presenting with dysfunctional uterine bleeding may have underlying coagulopathies such as von Willebrand's disease or Christmas disease, which should be excluded.

Treatment

The management of menorrhagia depends upon the cause of the condition. Treatment can be either surgical or medical (Table 45.6). The effectiveness of drug therapy is obviously influenced by the accuracy of the diagnosis. Drug treatment is also influenced by a woman's contraceptive needs; for example, combined oral contraceptives can reduce menstrual blood loss by up to 50%, but in women over 35 years of age who smoke, this form of therapy would need careful consideration. Low-dose luteal phase progestogens are no longer recommended for treatment of heavy but regular periods as they increase menstrual blood loss in this situation. However, they may be of value in women with an irregular cycle. Long-term, long-acting progestogens, however, may render a woman amenorrhoeic. Other hormonally based therapies include the GnRH analogues, although their propensity to induce a hypo-oestrogenic state with long-term use may be problematic (a 6-month course would reduce trabecular bone density by 5–6%). Danazol can reduce

Table 45.6 Summary of drug treatment options for menorrhagia

Drug	Comments
Combined oral contraceptive	See Table 45.3. These preparations are taken for 21 days with a 7-day pill-free (or placebo) period to allow for a withdrawal bleed
Progestogen-only preparations	See Table 45.3. Compounds such as norethisterone can be used, e.g. 5 mg three times daily or 10 mg twice daily for the latter half of the cycle. Ten days of therapy should be sufficient from day 15 of the cycle in ovulatory cycles. However, if the cycles are anovulatory then a minimum of 12 days' therapy is more appropriate. Progestogens for 12 days are also required to prevent endometrial hyperplasia in peri- and postmenopausal women taking oestrogen. When progestogens such as norethisterone are used, the dosage required is higher than that used in the combined oral contraceptive pill, and the adverse effects associated with the synthetic progestogens, particularly the 19-nortestosterone derivatives, may be more pronounced
Intrauterine progestogen-only contraceptive	The levonorgestrel-releasing intrauterine device (LNG-IUS) typically releases 20 μg of levonorgestrel/24 hours. Unlike non-medicated IUCDs, which may increase menstrual blood loss, this device appears to reduce it, as a result of the local endometrial actions of the progestogen. The device also offers contraceptive cover without many of the side effects associated with the non-medicated IUCDs. Progestogen-related side effects should be minimized because of the low dose of levonorgestrel employed. Initially bleeding patterns may be disrupted, but menstrual blood loss should become lighter within three menstrual cycles
Danazol and gestrinone	These agents suppress the pituitary–ovarian axis. Side effects include amenorrhoea, hot flushes, sweating, changes in libido, vaginitis and emotional lability. Danazol also causes androgenic side effects such as acne, oily skin and hair, hirsutism, oedema, weight gain, voice deepening and decreasing breast size. Gestrinone appears to be better tolerated, and only needs to be taken twice a week, while danazol has to be taken daily
GnRH analogues (gonadorelin)	After an initial period of stimulation these agents suppress the pituitary–ovarian axis. As result of inducing a hypo-oestrogenic state, these compounds should only be used for 6 months because they may decrease trabecular bone density
NSAIDs	These agents only need to be taken for the first 3–4 days of menses
Tranexamic acid	This drug appears well tolerated, but can produce dose-related gastrointestinal disturbances. Patients who may be predisposed to thrombosis are at risk if given antifibrinolytic therapy. This compound is usually only taken for the first 3 days of menses

IUCDs, intrauterine contraceptive devices
GnRH, gonadotrophin-releasing hormone

menstrual blood loss but its use is generally prohibited by its side effect profile. Prostaglandins have been implicated in the aetiology of several forms of menorrhagia. Therefore NSAIDs may be of use in some patients, especially if there is pain associated with menstruation. The NSAIDs appear to be most effective in women with the heaviest blood loss, for example mefenamic acid 500 mg three times daily from day 1 until heavy flow ceases.

Women with menorrhagia have greater endometrial fibrinolytic activity, hence the use of antifibrinolytic drugs, such as tranexamic acid, which are plasminogen activator inhibitors. Tranexamic acid reduces menstrual blood loss by up to 50% (Lethaby et al 2000). It is considered the treatment of first choice for the management of menorrhagia (RCOG 1998), the recommended dose being 1 g three times daily starting on the first day of menses. Agents such as tranexamic acid carry a risk of unwanted thrombogenesis but this does not appear to be translated into practice as increased numbers of deep vein thromboses. A Cochrane review found that this class of drugs decreases menstrual blood loss better than NSAIDs and oral luteal phase progestogen (Lethaby et al 2000).

The levonorgestrel intrauterine contraceptive devices (also known as intrauterine systems or LNG-IUS) can be left in place for up to 5 years following insertion. They reduce menstrual blood loss by up to 90% after 12 months of use. The levonorgestrel-releasing intrauterine system provides relief from dysmenorrhoea, effective contraception and long-term control of menorrhagia. A Cochrane review stated that the LNG-IUS improved quality of life of women with menorrhagia as effectively as surgical treatments (Marjoribanks et al 2003). In addition, other slow-release progestogenic devices such as nesterone implants and vaginal rings also reduce menstrual blood loss and promote amenorrhoea.

Hysterectomy has been the traditional surgical treatment for menorrhagia, with either an abdominal or vaginal approach used. Newer alternatives to hysterectomy include endometrial ablation, which can be done by electrosurgical, laser, microwave or thermal techniques. Endometrial ablation is less invasive than hysterectomy but recurrence of menorrhagia can occur and amenorrhoea cannot be guaranteed. There is evidence that pretreatment with a single dose of a GnRH agonist before the ablation procedure gives a better result. These preparations cause an initial stimulation of gonadotrophin release which then suppresses the hypothalamic–pituitary axis, producing a hypo-oestrogenic state. If circulating levels of oestrogen are low, then endometrial growth will not be stimulated; thus it will be thinner, making the surgical endometrial destruction more effective. With GnRH pretreatment, modern techniques such as microwave ablation have achieved amenorrhoea rates of about 50% and patient satisfaction rates of 90%.

Endometriosis

Endometriosis is a condition in which endometrial tissue is found outside the uterus. These so-called ectopic endometrial foci have been found outside the reproductive tract in the gastrointestinal tract, the urinary tract and even the lung.

Aetiology

Aetiology remains unclear, although retrograde menstruation, when shed endometrial cells migrate up through the fallopian tubes, would appear to be involved. This may occur because abnormalities in uterine innervation cause disruption in the usual patterns of myometrial contractility with consequent loss of the usual fundocervical polarity. Endometriosis is found in women in whom the normal route for the menstrual flow is disrupted, such as when there is some genital tract abnormality. Women who have frequent and heavier periods also seem to be more likely to suffer from endometriosis. Familial predisposition may also be a factor.

Studies suggest that endometrium from endometriosis sufferers tends to be more invasive. This may reflect either biological or genetic differences in the peritoneal milieu and may be explained by the upregulation of certain types of metalloproteinase responsible for the degradation of basement membrane. Endometrial tissue from women with endometriosis has aromatase activity which can be stimulated by PGE_2. Therefore ostensibly the endometriotic lesions have their own oestrogen supply as aromatase converts androgenic precursors into oestrogen and oestrogen stimulates biosynthesis of PGE_2; thus the cycle is self-perpetuating. Pilot studies using aromatase inhibitors, such as anastrozole, look promising.

Epidemiology

Endometriosis was previously considered to be a disease affecting women in their 30s onwards, but increasing use of laparoscopy has revealed that it can occur at any time throughout a woman's reproductive life. The condition is dependent upon oestrogen stimulation and, as such, it does not occur before the menarche or after the menopause. The exact incidence of the disease is unknown but it is believed to be about 10% in the general female population of reproductive age. One study has found a positive correlation between a menarche before 13 years and increased risk of developing endometriosis.

Symptoms

Although not all women with endometriosis are symptomatic, the pelvis is the most commonly affected site. Consequently, most of the symptoms of endometriosis relate to this region. Symptoms take the form of dysmenorrhoea and pelvic pain. However, the severity of the pain does not necessarily reflect the extent of the disease because women with severe pain may have few lesions, and vice versa. Dyspareunia (often with postcoital discomfort) is also common. There may also be menstrual irregularities.

The link between endometriosis and infertility is recognized but the mechanisms involved have not been established. If the ovaries or fallopian tubes themselves are directly affected by the endometriotic lesions then fertility may be compromised by purely mechanical means. However, the situation is less clear when the endometriosis does not cause any anatomical distortions. In this case some of the postulated causes of infertility associated with endometriosis include: ovulation disorders such as luteinized unruptured follicle syndrome, anovulation, premature ovulation; hyperprolactinaemia; and changes in the peritoneal environment such as extrauterine endometrial material which, like normal endometrium, is subject to control by the ovarian steroids and like its uterine counterpart is also capable of producing prostaglandins. Prostaglandin levels, along with macrophage concentrations, are raised in the peritoneal fluid of women with endometriotic explants, and these may alter tubular and uterine motility within the abdomen.

Outside the reproductive tract, endometrial deposits can be found along the urinary and gastrointestinal tracts. If the former is involved then the patient may suffer from cyclical haematuria, dysuria or even ureteric obstruction. If there is gastrointestinal tract involvement, then symptoms could include dyschezia, cyclical tenesmus and rectal bleeding or even obstruction. Very occasionally the lesions are found at more distant sites such as the lungs, where they could cause cyclical haemoptysis. A reduction in bone mass in women with endometriosis has also been reported.

Treatment

The aims of treatment in endometriosis are to relieve symptoms and improve fertility if pregnancy is desired. Treatment can be either surgical or medical. Surgery is increasingly performed laparoscopically, and can be employed to restore normal pelvic anatomy, divide adhesions or ablate endometriotic tissue using either laser treatment or electrodiathermy. Medical treatment utilizes the fact that endometriotic tissue is oestrogen dependent, and any drug therapy that will oppose the effects of oestrogen should, among other things, inhibit the growth of the endometriotic tissue. Hence the choices of drug treatment are as follows.

- GnRH analogues such as buserelin, goserelin, leuprorelin and nafarelin. These initially stimulate the hypothalamic–pituitary–ovarian axis but thereafter induce a hypo-oestrogenic state by paradoxically inhibiting follicle-stimulating hormone (FSH) and luteinizing hormone (LH) release.
- Low-dose COC (20–30 μg of ethinylestradiol) monophasic preparations have been found to be as effective as GnRH analogues and they may slow down disease progression in young women and preserve future fertility.
- Compounds with androgenic activity such as danazol and gestrinone also inhibit pituitary gonadotrophin release by interfering with the negative feedback, and cause atrophy of endometrial tissue.
- Progestogens such as dydrogesterone, medroxyprogesterone acetate and norethisterone initially cause decidualization of the endometrial tissue followed by glandular atrophy.

None of the above drug therapies is free from side effects. Use of the GnRH analogues may evoke menopausal symptoms such as hot flushes, decreased libido, vaginal dryness (topical vaginal lubricants may be helpful), mood changes, headache, etc. The problems associated with the hypo-oestrogenic state limit the long-term use of GnRH analogues. Although lipoprotein levels are not affected adversely, bone mass is, and this loss of bone density may not be entirely reversible after cessation

of therapy. Various 'add-back' hormone replacement therapies have been successfully used to minimize bone demineralization, for example low-dose oestrogen/progestogen combinations used continuously. Such regimens protect against osteoporosis and other hypo-oestrogenic side effects without apparently affecting clinical efficacy.

The androgenic compounds, because of their very nature, are associated with hirsutism, weight gain and acne. Side effects associated with synthetic progestogens relate again to androgenicity, although dydrogesterone is free from virilization. However, using LNG-IUS ensures the low dose of levonorgestrel is delivered locally and the more direct pelvic distribution may be useful in the management of endometriosis. Recent results suggest this device causes the downregulation of endometrial cell proliferation and increased apoptotic activity. More longer term studies (over 5 years) need to be undertaken to determine how long this effect is maintained and also effectiveness on symptoms such as dyspareunia and dyschezia.

Researchers have also found that certain dietary changes may be beneficial and reduce symptoms. A decreased intake of glycaemic carbohydrates such as sugar, rice and potatoes in addition to reducing/eliminating caffeine and increasing the intake of omega-3 oils such as flax seed oil may also be helpful. In addition, one study found that women with endometriosis tended to have a lower body mass index than those without the condition.

Total pelvic clearance, including the removal of the ovaries, is practical in women who have completed their family. This tends to be a last resort treatment but it is usually effective. However, surgery may be difficult if multiple lesions are present. There is no evidence that hormonal suppression improves surgical outcome.

Neither surgical nor medical management is effective in all cases. Studies suggest that pain associated with endometriosis responds well to both surgical and medical treatment but symptoms of recurrence occur in about 50% of patients within 5 years of stopping treatment. Fertility may be increased by the use of surgery to remove endometriotic foci causing anatomical distortion. The same benefit is not associated with medical treatment.

CASE STUDIES

Case 45.1

TM is a 46-year-old woman who is concerned about her constant tiredness. Her primary care clinician has attributed this to her heavy periods. While discussing possible management strategies her primary care doctor mentions the possibility of her having an IUD (intrauterine device) fitted. TM is alarmed by this. She has used an IUD in the past and it did not suit her because it made her bleed more frequently.

Questions

1. What sort of IUD will the clinician be considering in this case?
2. How should this patient be counselled?

Answers

1. In this case the doctor will be referring to the possible use of the intrauterine system (LNG-IUS). In the UK there is currently only one such device, namely Mirena. This device releases 20 μg of the second-generation progestogen levonorgestrel every 24 hours into the uterine cavity. In terms of potential progestogenic side effects it should be noted that this is a relatively low dose of hormone compared with that used in oral contraceptive pills.

2. TM should be reassured that although the medicated intrauterine system is indeed an intrauterine device, and it will offer her excellent contraceptive cover, it will eventually decrease her menstrual blood loss. The locally delivered progestogen will effectively prevent proliferation of the endometrium, reduce menstrual blood loss, and may even precipitate amenorrhoea. However, TM should be warned that initially she may suffer some irregular or breakthrough bleeding, but this is a tolerance effect and usually disappears within the first 3 months after device insertion. One study has estimated that levonorgestrel-releasing IUD treatment could replace approximately 75% of endometrial ablations. This also helps to contextualize the cost of devices such as Mirena (net price of about £90 for 5 years) compared with the cost of an ablation (about £1200–1300). Use of the intrauterine system will also provide contraceptive cover at a time when the oestrogen in the combined contraceptive may be contraindicated.

Case 45.2

YS is a 16-year-old girl who presents with her mother at a pharmacy with a prescription for: Loestrin-20, 3 × 21. Mother and daughter are concerned that the doctor has prescribed a contraceptive pill when YS went about her period pains. YS suffers from severe cramping pains which begin just before she starts to bleed and continue for the first 3–4 hours of her period. She also seems to be more irritable and prone to tears just before her periods, which are rather irregular.

Questions

1. What is YS likely to be suffering from?
2. Why has she been prescribed a combined oral contraceptive pill?

Answers

1. In this case it seems as if YS is suffering from primary dysmenorrhoea, a diagnosis suggested by her age, timing of symptoms (pain) just before menses which abate once the menstrual flow is established and her description of symptoms. She is also exhibiting some symptoms of premenstrual syndrome.

2. Hormonal contraceptives that work by inhibiting ovulation such as the combined oral contraceptives may be useful in alleviating dysmenorrhoea and premenstrual syndrome in many women. Both of these conditions can begin with the commencement of ovulatory cycles, hence the ovarian steroids have been implicated, either directly or indirectly, in their aetiology. However, these drugs may be contraindicated for some women, and there may be an attitudinal problem from either the patient or her parents because they are contraceptives and parents may fear contraceptive use could lead to promiscuity. In this case it might be helpful if the

pharmacist emphasized some of the non-contraceptive benefits of oral contraceptive usage such as decreased blood loss, reduced risk of developing iron deficiency anaemia, cycles regularized, and a reduced risk of developing certain cancers of the endometrium and ovary.

Case 45.3

AW is a 36-year-old woman who, 6 years ago, was treated for endometriosis with a 6-month course of danazol. She subsequently became pregnant and her child is now 3 years old. Her symptoms have returned and are increasing in severity; the most prominent of these is dysmenorrhoea. Her pain begins around day 24 of her 30-day cycle, progressively worsening until 3 days into her menstrual bleed. AW would prefer to avoid danazol treatment as she found it difficult to tolerate. She asks if there are any new treatments available. She has a BMI of 30 kg/m³ and is a smoker.

Questions

1. What alternative therapies would be suitable for AW?
2. Would over-the-counter analgesia be helpful for her?

Answers

1. Drug therapy (or pregnancy) rarely cures endometriosis and the condition recurs in about 50% of women within 5 years of stopping treatment. In terms of alternatives to attenuated androgens such as danazol, the combined oral contraceptives compare well with other hormonal treatments as they reduce dysmenorrhoic pain (and they are cheap). However, a combined oral contraceptive would not be suitable for AW because of her weight, age and smoking status. If she still requires contraception a progestogen-only contraceptive method may be an option.

   An alternative hormonal therapy would be a GnRH analogue usually given for 6 months. The hypo-oestrogenic side effects of these compounds are generally better tolerated than the androgenic side effects of agents such as danazol. Women should also be alerted to the possible vasomotor symptoms, similar to those suffered by perimenopausal women. Other potential side effects such as dyspareunia may be eased by using a vaginal lubricant. Troublesome vasomotor symptoms can be treated with add-back hormone replacement therapy by using a continuous combined preparation or tibolone. This will also help ameliorate the effects of GnRH agonists on bone loss. These add-back regimens do not appear to adversely affect clinical outcome but offer some protection against osteoporosis. The effects of GnRH analogues on bone density are reversed within 1 year after treatment is stopped. However, the use of add-back HRT treatment for longer than 6 months is not recommended

   Evidence also suggests that changes in diet can positively influence endometriosis symptom score. Reducing the intake of glycaemic carbohydrates such as those found in potatoes and rice while increasing omega-9 oils (e.g. olive oil) and eliminating caffeine can help some sufferers. Surgery is also an option for some women depending on the degree of endometriosis and their desire for fertility.

2. Some women can be managed by NSAIDs alone. One study has shown that substantial analgesia was achieved in 80% of women with endometriosis after taking naproxen. The most useful NSAID available over the counter would be ibuprofen.

REFERENCES

American College of Obstetricians and Gynecologists 2000 Premenstrual syndrome. ACOG Practice Bulletin No 15. American College of Obstetricians and Gynecologists, Washington, DC

American Psychiatric Association 2000 Diagnostic and statistical manual of mental disorders. American Psychiatric Publishing Inc., Arlington, VA

Anon 2002 Fibrotic reactions with pergolide and other ergot-derived dopamine receptor agonists. Current Problems in Pharmacovigilance 23: 3

Dimmock P W, Wyatt K M, Jones P W et al 2000 Efficacy of selective serotonin-reuptake inhibitors in premenstrual syndrome: a systematic review. Lancet 356: 1131-1136

Farmer R D T, Williams T J, Simpson E L et al 2000 Effect of 1995 pill scare on rates of venous thromboembolism among women taking combined oral contraceptives: analysis of General Practice Research Database. British Medical Journal 321: 477-479

Lethaby A, Farquhar C, Cooke I 2000 Antifibrinolytics for heavy menstrual bleeding. The Cochrane Database of Systematic Reviews 2000, Issue 4. John Wiley, Chichester

Marjoribanks J, Lethaby A, Farquhar C 2003 Surgery versus medical therapy for heavy menstrual bleeding. The Cochrane Database of Systematic Reviews 2003, Issue 2. John Wiley, Chichester

Proctor M L, Smith C A, Farquhar C M et al 2006 Transcutaneous electrical nerve stimulation and acupuncture for primary dysmenorrhoea. The Cochrane Database of Systematic Reviews, Issue 1. John Wiley, Chichester

Royal College of Obstetricians and Gynaecologists 1998 The initial management of menorrhagia. Evidence-Based Clinical Guidelines No 1. Royal College of Obstetricians and Gynaecologists, London

FURTHER READING

Adashi E Y 1995 Long term gonadotrophin-releasing hormone 'add-back' paradigms. Keio Journal of Medicine 44: 124-132

Barnhart K T, Freeman E W, Sondheimer S J 1995 A clinician's guide to the premenstrual syndrome. Medical Clinics of North America 79: 1457-1472

Brooks P M, Day R O 2000 COX-2 inhibitors. Medical Journal of Australia 173: 433-436

Ismail K M K, O'Brien S 2005 Premenstrual syndrome. Current Obstetrics and Gynaecology 15: 25-30

Lesley D, Acheson N (eds) 2004 Endometriosis. Royal College of Obstetricians and Gynaecologists, London

Oelkers W 2004 Drospirenone, a progestogen with antimineralocorticoid properties: a short review. Molecular and Cellular Endocrinology 217: 255-261

O'Flynn N, Britten N 2000 Menorrhagia in general practice – disease or illness? Social Science and Medicine 50: 651-661

Rapkin A 2003 A review of treatment of premenstrual syndrome and premenstrual dysphoric disorder. Psychoneuroendocrinology 28: 39-53

Romer T 2000 Prospective comparison study of levonorgestrel IUD versus roller-ball endometrial ablation in the management of refractory recurrent hypermenorrhoea. European Journal of Obstetrics and Gynaecology and Reproductive Biology 90: 27-29

Tapanainen J S 2004 Madical management of menstrual disorders. International Congress Series 1266: 63-68

Yu S L 2004 Mirena. International Congress Series 1266: 69-71

Menopause 46

K. Marshall   S. Calvert

Menopause

The UK, like many countries in the developed world, has an ageing population, life expectancy is increasing and women continue to live longer than men, whilst birth rates are declining. Currently a woman can expect to live about 35% of her life in a postmenopausal state.

The menopause is signalled by a woman's last menstrual period and is defined as the permanent cessation of menstruation resulting from loss of ovarian follicular activity. The occurrence of the last menstruation can only be diagnosed retrospectively, and is usually taken as being final if it is followed by a 12-month bleed-free interval; such women are defined as being postmenopausal. The mean age of the menopause in the UK is 51 years, and by the age of 54 years around 80% of women will be postmenopausal. If the menopause occurs before 40 years it would be classed as a premature menopause. Many women will experience erratic periods before the final cessation due to inadequate ovarian oestrogen secretion; these women are described as being perimenopausal. This transitional phase usually lasts around 4–5 years. The problems associated with the menopause result from oestrogen deprivation. Hormone replacement

therapy (HRT) reduces the effects of this deprivation and overcomes the associated symptoms.

The menopause is a natural event in the anatomical, physiological and psychological changes which form the female climacteric. Some women will go from the transition of being premenopausal to postmenopausal with no symptoms at all. Many will experience the symptoms associated with oestrogen lack, whether in the perimenopausal or postmenopausal phase, which include:

- vasomotor symptoms
- localized atrophy of urogenital tissues
- osteoporosis
- psychological problems
- coronary heart disease.

Initially the symptoms are more likely to include vasomotor symptoms such as hot flushes, night sweats and palpitations, and psychological problems such as mood changes, irritability, sleep disturbance, depression and decreased libido. Many women suffer from vaginal dryness and dyspareunia, which serve to enhance the loss of libido and this in turn can adversely affect psychological well-being. The urethral mucosa may become atrophied, leading to an increased incidence of urinary tract infections or urinary incontinence. In some women the urethra may eventually become fibrosed, leading to dysuria, frequency and urgency (urethral syndrome). The long-term consequences of oestrogen deprivation are often symptomless. There is a significant loss of calcium from the bones, which may give rise to frequent fractures, and there is a change in the blood lipid profile, which is associated with a rise in coronary heart disease.

Physiological changes

Ovarian

The approaching menopause is associated with loss of ovarian follicular activity. Human ovaries contain approximately 700 000 follicles at birth but these cells have a high mortality rate and fewer than 500 of them will be ovulated. This number falls progressively with increasing age so that by the time the woman approaches 50 years of age, the number of follicles has fallen to zero or very few. The rate of follicle loss is highest during the decade between 40 and 50 years of age, possibly due to an increase in the rate of degeneration (atresia) of the earliest follicles. Women over the age of 45 years who are menstruating regularly have been shown to have 10 times as many follicles as those with irregular cycles; those who have not had a period for 12 months have few follicles remaining. Thus, the size of the follicular pool is an important determinant in ovarian function.

Ovarian function includes two major roles: the production of eggs (gametogenesis) and the synthesis and secretion of hormones (hormonogenesis). Both of these functions undergo subtle changes with ageing so that fewer ova are produced and they are less readily fertilized, and the hormone levels become irregular. It is the granulosa cells in the developing follicle that normally secrete estradiol, and lack of this follicular activity results in diminishing oestrogen secretion. The diminution in the number of active follicles is followed by an increase in follicle-stimulating hormone (FSH) secretion from the anterior pituitary gland as the normal feedback mechanisms between ovarian estradiol secretion and the hypothalamus–pituitary axis become disrupted. It may be that there is an age-related decrease in sensitivity to feedback inhibition that exacerbates this increase in FSH levels. In women who are still bleeding, a FSH level exceeding 10–12 iu/L on day 2 or 3 of the bleed is indicative of a diminished ovarian response. A high FSH level (above 30 iu/L) and a low estradiol level (below 100 pmol/L) in the plasma characterize the menopause. The low oestrogen level fails to stimulate growth of the uterine endometrium. As endometrial growth has not occurred there can be no menstruation (shedding of the endometrium) and the menopause has arrived. Since ova are not being released, the production of progesterone from the ovary also ceases, and the levels of luteinizing hormone (LH) eventually rise. Thus, perimenopausal and menopausal women are subjected to an increasing ovarian hormone deficiency, as shown in Table 46.1.

When the ovaries are conserved after hysterectomy they will usually continue to produce some estradiol, but the levels of this hormone will decline up to the age of the natural menopause. Postmenopausally, in all women, androstenedione (secreted from the adrenal cortex) is converted in adipose tissue and muscle (peripheral conversion) to estrone, which becomes the major circulating oestrogen (but estrone is about 10 times less potent than estradiol). The levels of FSH and LH remain elevated for many years if no HRT is given, but these elevated levels have no effect on the ovary since the follicles are atretic.

The cessation of reproductive function in the woman and declining oestrogen production from the ovary are not the only physiological events associated with the menopause. For many years oestrogen was considered to be associated only with the genitourinary system, but its effects are more wide-ranging and the major tissues affected include blood vessels, bones and the brain.

Table 46.1 Ovarian hormone secretion after the onset of the normal menstrual cycle

	Premenopausal (normal cyclic)	Perimenopausal (irregular cycles)	Postmenopausal (cessation of cycle)
Oestrogens	+++	++	+ → −
Progesterone	+++	+	−
Androgens	+	+	+ → −

Urogenital system

With the failure in ovarian oestrogen production the number of uterine endometrial oestrogen receptors occupied falls and endometrial growth is not sustained. Thus in the postmenopausal woman the endometrium becomes thin and atrophic. Likewise, in the other target tissues containing oestrogen receptors, the basal layers of the vaginal epithelium are no longer stimulated to maintain the vaginal epithelium and produce natural lubricants from the vaginal glands. The result is vaginal atrophy and a thin, dry vagina may result in dyspareunia. Because the lower urinary tract and the lower genital tract share common embryological origin, deprivation of oestrogen can result in urethral and bladder problems. Often perimenopausal and postmenopausal women report an increase in urinary frequency, nocturia and urge incontinence. For some women these changes may become manifest as long as 10 years after the menopause.

Bone

Risk factors for osteoporosis include low body mass index ($<19 \, kg/m^2$), smoking, early menopause, family history of maternal hip fracture, long-term systemic corticosteroids use and conditions affecting bone metabolism, especially those causing prolonged immobility. Osteoporosis is most common in white women. People with osteoporosis are at risk of fragility fractures, which occur as a result of mechanical forces that would not ordinarily cause fracture. The clinically relevant outcome in evaluating treatments for osteoporosis is the incidence of fragility of fracture as otherwise this condition is asymptomatic and therefore undiagnosed. The most common sites for these fractures are the hip, vertebrae and wrist. In 2000, it was estimated that the total cost of treating osteoporotic fractures in postmenopausal woman was between £1.5 and £1.8 billion. This is expected to increase to £2.1 billion by 2010.

Cardiovascular system

Young adult women are protected against the development of hypertension and its deleterious consequences in the cardiovascular system. Levels of low-density lipoprotein cholesterol (LDL-C) and very low-density lipoprotein cholesterol (VLDL-C) are decreased by oestrogen, and the levels of high-density lipoprotein cholesterol (HDL-C) are increased, thereby giving protection against atherosclerosis. HDL-C is known to promote cholesterol efflux from macrophages in the arterial wall, thereby reducing atheromatous plaque and conferring a protective effect against heart disease. However, after the menopause this protection is lost and the incidence of high blood pressure and associated cardiovascular disease increases to levels similar to those found in age-matched men.

Oestrogen has direct beneficial effects in the control of blood pressure, possibly via regulating endothelium-mediated control of arteriolar tone. In women deprived of oestrogen, endothelium-dependent vasodilation is impaired. This dysfunction is largely associated with a reduction in nitric oxide availability. Oestrogen increases nitric oxide availability by stimulating endothelial nitric oxide synthase (eNOS). Oestrogen also stimulates the production of other endothelium-derived relaxing factors such as prostacyclin (prostaglandin I$_2$). Research suggests that the oestrogen receptor (ER)α is important in mediating the vascular effects of oestrogen. Studies using selective ERα agonists are being undertaken. However, many pathways are stimulated by oestrogen receptor activation and the relative importance of these different pathways varies from tissue to tissue.

Miscellaneous

Thinning of the skin, brittle nails, hair loss and generalized aches and pains are also associated with reduced oestrogen levels (Hall & Phillips 2005). The skin is the largest non-reproductive target on which oestrogen acts. Oestrogen receptors, predominantly of the ERβ type, are widely distributed within the skin. Both types of oestrogen receptor (ERα and ERβ) are expressed within the hair follicle and associated structures. Thus epidermal thinning, declining terminal collagen content, diminished skin moisture, decreased laxity and impaired wound healing (selective ERα ligands are being investigated for their wound-healing properties) have been reported in postmenopausal women.

In addition, women also show increasing body weight associated with ageing. This weight gain tends to increase or begin near the menopause. Body fat redistribution to the abdomen also occurs independent of weight gain. This type of centralized abdominal fat distribution is widely recognized as an independent risk factor for cardiovascular disease in women.

Psychological changes

Depression is twice as common in women as in men and may increase during times of changing hormonal levels such as the menopause. Some aspects of decreased central nervous system function have been related to falling oestrogen levels. Preclinical studies have shown oestrogen to have several positive effects on central nervous system function. Perhaps the most important is promotion of acetylcholine synthesis and increased synaptogenesis in the hippocampus. ERβ is expressed in this area of the brain as well as the entorhinal cortex and thalamus, areas crucially involved in explicit memory. Human neuroimaging studies have also indicated that oestrogen influences regional cerebral blood flow in women.

Management

Hormone replacement therapy

HRT is a complicated clinical issue requiring an in-depth risk/benefit assessment. The vast amount of study data are often conflicting and careful analysis is required. Many factors need to be reviewed before it is prescribed. One important factor is age, as data have shown that if a woman aged less than 35 has a hysterectomy and a bilateral oophorectomy, her risk of non-fatal myocardial infarction is nearly eight times that of her age-matched counterpart who has retained her ovaries. Age at time of HRT prescription in relation to menopausal age, i.e. number of years of oestrogen deprivation before replacement, is also of importance when considering outcomes. Individual differences in hormone metabolism (both endogenous and exogenous) are also likely to be important as several different cytochrome

enzymes metabolize oestrogen and may be affected by inherited polymorphisms. Therefore some women may produce oestrogenic metabolites possessing considerable oestrogenic activity, whilst others produce metabolites which are relatively non-oestrogenic. Body mass index (BMI) also influences response to HRT, with increased plasma estradiol levels observed in women with higher BMIs.

HRT is effective for symptomatic relief of menopausal symptoms and its use is justified when symptoms adversely affect quality of life. Current advice is that the lowest effective dose for a particular woman should be used for the shortest period of time. Local oestrogen replacement may be used to reverse the symptoms of urogenital atrophy as it appears to be more effective than systemic therapy. There is no evidence to suggest that local oestrogen treatment is associated with significant risks.

Treatment with HRT should be reviewed at least annually, with alternative therapies considered for the management of osteoporosis. In the treatment of menopausal symptoms, the benefits of short-term HRT outweigh the risks in the majority of women but in healthy women without symptoms the risks outweigh the benefits.

Contraindications to the use of HRT include undiagnosed vaginal bleeding in postmenopausal women, the presence of an oestrogen-dependent tumour, liver disease (where liver function tests have failed to return to normal), active thrombophlebitis, and active or recent arterial thromboembolic disease (e.g. angina or myocardial infarction). A history of deep vein thrombosis and pulmonary embolism requires careful evaluation before the use of oestrogen therapy. Use in patients with Dubin–Johnson and Rotor syndromes may also be contraindicated.

Oestrogen therapy

Since the symptoms and long-term effects of the menopause are due to oestrogen deprivation, the mainstay of HRT is oestrogen. This may be administered orally or parenterally but, in either case, the oestrogens used are naturally occurring and include:

- estradiol
- estriol
- estrone
- estropipate
- conjugated equine oestrogen (estrone sulphate 40%, equilin sulphate 60%)
- estradiol valerate.

The use of 'natural' oestrogens reduces the risk of the potentially dangerous oestrogenic effects such as raised blood pressure, alteration in coagulation factors and an undesirable lipid profile, which sometimes occur with the more potent synthetic oestrogens used in the oral contraceptive agents. A 'natural' oestrogen is defined as one that is normally found in the human female and has a physiological effect. Natural oestrogens are less potent (up to 200 times) than synthetic oestrogens. Because they are naturally occurring compounds, the plasma half-life of these oestrogens is similar to that of the ovarian-secreted oestrogens and the duration of action is shorter than the synthetic oestrogens, such as ethinylestradiol, used in many formulations of the contraceptive pill. The plasma ratio of estradiol to estrone is normally about 1:1 to 2:1, and the aim of HRT should be to preserve this ratio.

There are five routes of administration for oestrogens in HRT:

- oral
- transdermal (patches/gels/cream)
- intranasal
- subcutaneous (implants)
- vaginal (creams and medicated rings).

The use of oral oestrogen therapy, while convenient for the patient, does mean that the oestrogen will be subjected to conversion to estrone by the liver and gut, thereby altering the estradiol:estrone ratio in favour of the less active oestrogen, estrone. The oral preparations have different metabolic effects due to first-pass hepatic metabolism. Smoking stimulates metabolism of oestrogens by cytochrome P450 and decreases plasma oestrogen levels by 40–70% in oral oestrogen users. Smoking has no significant effect on plasma oestrogen levels in users of transdermal preparations. Oral delivery compared to transdermal delivery also has different effects on lipid levels (Table 46.2). In addition, orally administered oestrogens undergo first-pass hepatic metabolism, which may result in some reduction in antithrombin III, a potent inhibitor of coagulation. Implants and patches show smaller changes in coagulation, platelet function or fibrinolysis.

More constant levels of oestrogen result from the use of transdermal patches containing estradiol, and these have the added advantage of a more physiological estradiol:estrone ratio. However, the adhesive used in these transdermal patches and the alcohol base can cause skin irritation. The patch is applied to the non-hairy skin of the lower body, and care should be taken to ensure that it is placed away from breast tissue. The patch is changed either once or twice a week, thus providing a constant reservoir of estradiol to provide a controlled release into the circulation. Estradiol is also available in a gel formulation that is applied daily to the skin over the area of a template (to ensure correct dosage), but this formulation may give erratic absorption. The intranasal preparation, administered as a nasal spray, also avoids hepatic first-pass metabolism.

The oestrogen implant gives a constant level of oestrogen from a few days after insertion for up to 6 months. This formulation maintains the best estradiol:estrone ratio and is a convenient method of administration, requiring repeat implants only every 6 months. However, because the levels of oestrogen are constantly raised there will be some increase in oestrogen receptor numbers, and this can lead to a recurrence of symptoms of oestrogen deficiency due to the presence of unoccupied oestrogen receptors, even in the presence of normal or even high oestrogen levels. This phenomenon, called tachyphylaxis, results in patients becoming symptomatic and requesting repeat implants earlier and earlier. In such cases it is unwise to treat with additional oestrogen; the patient should receive counselling and perhaps a change of preparation. The disadvantage of the implant is that, once inserted, it cannot be removed readily and even if it is removed, the oestrogen level will take at least a month to fall. There is also evidence that the uterine endometrium, if present, remains stimulated for some time after removal of the implant.

Both the transdermal and implant preparations avoid the first-pass hepatic effects of oral oestrogens and are less likely to affect liver enzyme systems and clotting factors. Some studies show an increase in the incidence of venous thromboembolism (VTE) in women taking HRT. Therefore patients who have a history of deep vein thrombosis or pulmonary embolism will need careful guidance, with each woman being considered individually, and the relative risks evaluated. Other risk factors include severe varicose veins, obesity or a family history of deep vein thrombosis (DVT). If HRT is justified in such patients, transdermal preparations are a better alternative than oral preparations.

Vaginal creams containing oestrogen are available but generally fail to produce the reliable plasma levels required to protect against the long-term effects of oestrogen deprivation. They provide short-term relief from menopausal symptoms, in particular atrophic vaginitis. A vaginal ring which releases estradiol at a controlled rate in physiological levels for up to 3 months is an alternative for women who cannot tolerate transdermal patches.

The dose of oestrogen used in HRT sufficient to preserve bone density is usually higher than that necessary to alleviate vasomotor symptoms. The doses suggested to protect bone density are estradiol 2 mg per day orally, 50 µg per day transdermally, and 50 mg every 6 months by implant. If the conjugated equine oestrogens are used, the oral dose should be 0.625 mg per day. The lower doses found in vaginal creams may alleviate the vasomotor symptoms but will not protect against osteoporosis. Current guidelines advise the use of the lowest possible dose of HRT to relieve vasomotor symptoms and recommend alternative treatment to prevent and treat osteoporosis.

Oestrogens should be used alone only in women who have undergone a hysterectomy; if the uterus is present the endometrium will be stimulated and this increase in endometrial growth may be a precursor to development of a malignant condition. Current practice is to administer progestogens with oestrogen. In the early 1970s, when oestrogen was used alone, HRT received a bad press because in women who had not undergone hysterectomy, there was an increased incidence of endometrial carcinoma. In women who have undergone hysterectomy, oestrogens are usually administered continuously.

Progestogen therapy

The only proven reason for adding a progestogen to oestrogen therapy for HRT in women with an intact uterus is to protect the endometrium from hyperplasia and possible neoplasia. There are many preparations which contain progestogens added to oestrogen for a number of days per month. However, to effectively prevent endometrial hyperplasia, the progestogen must be taken

Table 46.2   Effect of HRT adminstration route on lipid profile

Oral	Transdermal
↓ Low-density lipoprotein	↓ Low-density lipoprotein
↓ Total cholesterol	↓ Total cholesterol
↑ High-density lipoprotein	↔ High-density lipoprotein
↑ Triglycerides	↓ Triglycerides
↑ Bile cholesterol	↔ Bile cholesterol

for a minimum of 12 days. The minimum dose of progestogen required to protect against hyperplasia depends on the potency of the compound used.

The progestogens commonly available in HRT preparations are either derivatives of progesterone, such as medroxyprogesterone and dydrogesterone, or 19-nortestosterone substitutes such as norethisterone or levonorgestrel. All these synthetic progestogens are active following oral administration and provide adequate protection of the endometrium against oestrogen stimulation. Some transdermal preparations also incorporate a progestogenic compound in the regimen. As with all semi-synthetic or synthetic hormones, these compounds may act on receptors other than the progesterone receptor, and the long-term consequence of this is not predictable.

Progesterone is the only progestogen to act solely on the progesterone receptor, but it has poor oral bioavailability and so it is difficult to achieve satisfactory plasma concentrations. However, the micronized preparations are better absorbed. Progesterone may also be administered at night in the form of a pessary or suppository, or by injection in the form of a long-lasting subdermal implant. The progestogen in HRT is most commonly administered orally or transdermally and usually one of the synthetic progestogens is used.

Oestrogen and progestogen regimens

The monthly withdrawal bleed is perceived by some postmenopausal patients to be an unacceptable side effect of HRT and this has resulted in the development of a number of regimens (Table 46.3) in an effort to minimize this effect. Formulations have been produced with which bleeding only occurs every 3 months instead of every 4 weeks, or it does not occur at all.

The use of the 70-day oestrogen preparation, while being more popular with women because bleeding only occurs every 3 months, needs further evaluation as regards endometrial protection. Bleeding can be avoided altogether if a combination of oestrogen and progestogen is given continuously throughout the treatment (continuous combined HRT). Such a preparation should only be given to women who are at least 12 months postmenopausal and have an atrophied endometrium, otherwise breakthrough bleeding may occur. Bleeding in the first 6 months (usually just spotting) is not uncommon but bleeding after this time should be investigated, although the incidence of endometrial hyperplasia is low with this continuous regimen.

Table 46.3 Regimens of combined oestrogen and progestogen therapy for use in HRT

- Oestrogen 28 days + progestogen 12 or 14 days then repeat without interval (bleed every 4 weeks)

- Oestrogen 70 days + progestogen 14 days followed by 7 days placebo tablets (bleed every 3 months)

- Oestrogen + progesterone continuously (no bleed)

- Oestrogen continuously + Mirena IUS

Others recommend a 28-day interval between courses of treatment to allow the endometrium to become atrophic in patients who are changing from the cyclical therapy to the continuous combined therapy. Patients who commence cyclical HRT prior to ceasing menstruation should change to a continuous combined preparation only after the age of 54 (when there is a 80% chance that they will be post- rather than perimenopausal) to reduce the risk of breakthrough bleeding. An alternative option is to use the levonorgestrol-loaded intrauterine device (IUS or Mirena) in conjunction with oral oestrogen. This option can be particularly useful for women intolerant of progestogenic side effects.

Not all progestogens have the same pharmacological profile and these differences have implications for their usage. Two of the most widely used synthetic progestogens are medroxyprogesterone acetate and norethisterone. These are used as the progestogenic component of an HRT regimen in combination with oestrogen but have been shown to increase the risk of breast cancer in long-term HRT users (Million Women Study 2003, Women's Health Initiative 2002). Structurally, medroxyprogesterone acetate is more similar to natural progesterone than norethisterone. The metabolism of these two compounds is also different, as medroxyprogesterone acetate is the major progestogenic compound rather than its metabolites. In contrast, the metabolites of norethisterone exhibit significant activity in addition to a wide range of non-progestogenic actions. Norethisterone also binds to sex hormone-binding globulin whereas medroxyprogesterone acetate does not.

The most notable difference in steroid receptor-binding affinity between the two synthetic progestogens and endogenous progesterone is that although all the compounds have affinity for the mineralocorticoid receptor, only the natural compound has antagonist activity. As a consequence, the synthetic compounds may be unable to counteract the sodium-retaining and blood pressure-raising effects of the oestrogens used in HRT. Endogenous progesterone affinity for the glucocorticoid receptor is also different, with medroxyprogesterone acetate a more potent antagonist than norethisterone. This may influence their side effect profiles and impact on inflammation, immune response, adrenal function and bone metabolism.

Tibolone

Tibolone is a synthetic steroid that has oestrogenic, progestogenic and androgenic effects that alleviate menopausal symptoms without a monthly bleed. The oestrogenic effects are weak and should not promote endometrial hyperplasia, but 10–15% of women on this treatment experience breakthrough bleeding. The drug is given continuously but is not suitable for women within 1 year of the menopause or immediately after oestrogen therapy because in such cases breakthrough bleeding is most likely to occur. The evidence suggests that this drug is protective against osteoporosis but the long-term cardioprotective effects remain unclear as there is some evidence of a lowering of HDL-C. It should also be withdrawn if signs of thromboembolic disease occur. The androgenic action of tibolone tends to increase libido. It has been reported that tibolone does have fewer breast-related adverse effects than oestrogenic or oestrogenic–progestogenic HRT regimens.

Raloxifene

Raloxifene is a non-steroidal benzothiophene that binds to some oestrogen receptors and belongs to a class of drugs referred to as selective oestrogen receptor modulators (SERMs). These compounds act selectively on some oestrogen receptors to increase bone mineral density and antagonize oestrogen-dependent effects on breast and endometrial tissues in postmenopausal women. However, there is a reported increased risk of thromboembolism, particularly in the first 4 months of use. Raloxifene cannot be used to treat vasomotor symptoms in perimenopausal women. In fact, it is reported to induce hot flushes. It has little or no stimulatory effect on the uterine endometrium and is not associated with uterine bleeding.

In summary, raloxifene is a compound that selectively stimulates one group of oestrogen receptors and may be considered a curative treatment for osteoporosis and a preventive agent in the development of oestrogen-dependent breast tumours.

Clinical monitoring

Before initiating HRT, a detailed patient history and physical examination are essential to eliminate medical disorders and genital malignancy. Bone mineral densitometry can also be helpful to establish a baseline for subsequent measurements. Blood tests should include serum electrolytes and creatinine, liver function tests, haemoglobin and lipids and a full blood count. Urine analysis should also be performed. The history and findings from the physical examination may indicate other tests. The patient should have undergone routine cervical smear examination and, preferably, mammography. In women with an intact uterus, any irregular vaginal bleeding should be investigated to exclude endometrial pathology.

After starting therapy, the woman should be seen within 3 months in the first instance and then at intervals between 6 and 12 months so that symptoms may be assessed and any side effects of therapy can be reported. Blood pressure measurements are undertaken on these routine visits; HRT is usually associated with a fall in blood pressure due to a vasodilator action of oestrogen. Hypertension is not a contraindication to treatment with HRT but does need treatment before starting on oestrogen therapy. Some women may have an elevated blood pressure on oral oestrogen but show no such effect with the non-oral route. Weight gain may occur some months after treatment has been initiated, and the patient should be advised to reduce calorie intake accordingly.

Stopping HRT

Current guidelines indicate that there are a number of signs and symptoms which suggest that women should be advised to immediately stop taking HRT and these include:

- sudden severe chest pain
- sudden breathlessness or cough with blood-stained sputum
- unexplained severe pain in calf of one leg
- severe stomach pain
- serious neurological effects
- hepatitis, jaundice, liver enlargement

- blood pressure above systolic 160 mmHg and diastolic 100 mmHg
- detection of a risk factor, e.g. prolonged immobility after surgery or leg injury.

Once HRT has been stopped investigation and treatment should be undertaken as appropriate.

Examples of serious neurological effects include unusual severe, prolonged headache. This is especially important if the headache occurs for the first time or it becomes progressively worse. Marked numbness, especially if it suddenly affects one side or part of the body, is important. Other neurological effects are sudden partial or complete loss of vision or disturbance of hearing or other perceptual disorders. HRT should also be stopped if the following occur: dysphasia, bad fainting attack or collapse, a first unexplained epileptic seizure/weakness and motor disturbances.

Alternatives to HRT

HRT remains the most effective treatment for vasomotor symptoms, resulting in 80–90% reduction in hot flushes. Of the non-hormonal agents, selective serotonin reuptake inhibitors such as venlafaxine appear to be the next most useful treatments; gabapentin may be equally effective, whilst clonidine is only modestly effective in reducing hot flushes. Generally, there is a lack of safety information and trial data regarding alternative therapies. Trials with black cohosh, red clover and soy foods, all of which contain phytoestrogens, have yielded conflicting results and have raised concerns about hepatoxicity (black cohosh) and interactions with anticoagulants (red clover).

Bisphosphonates (e.g. alendronate, etidronate and risedronate) are inhibitors of bone resorption and increase bone mineral density by altering osteoclast activation and function. Bisphosphonates are used with care in women with upper gastrointestinal problems and their posology is complex. They are contraindicated in patients with hypocalcaemia. Etidronate is also contraindicated in patients with severe renal impairment.

Teriparatide, a recombinant human parathyroid hormone, is licensed to treat osteoporosis in postmenopausal women. It stimulates new formation of bone and may increase resistance to fracture. However, it has several contraindications including hypercalcaemia, severe renal impairment, metabolic bone diseases and unexplained elevations of alkaline phosphatase.

Treatment with HRT

Vasomotor symptoms

Vasomotor symptoms include hot flushes, headaches, insomnia, giddiness and faintness. They occur in about 70–80% of women and result in physical distress in about 50%, lasting for up to 5 years in around one-quarter of the women. Flushes and sweats, particularly night sweats, indicate vasomotor instability and probably result from unoccupied oestrogen receptors on blood vessels. Oestrogens cause a rapid rise in blood flow through the blood vessels, and lack of oestrogen will render the oestrogen receptors in these vessels supersensitive to any subsequent rise in oestrogen level. During the perimenopause and menopause, oestrogen levels tend to fluctuate and it is suggested that it is these fluctuations that result in vasomotor symptoms. The extreme sensitivity of blood vessel oestrogen receptors tends to mean that a clinical response to vasomotor symptoms is achieved with low doses of oestrogen. General advice regarding diet, for example avoiding certain foods and drinks that cause vaso-dilation such as hot spicy foods and alcohol, may be helpful to some women. There is some evidence that regular exercise, which stimulates the production of hypothalamic β-endorphins, may reduce the risk of hot flushes.

Urogenital tract

These symptoms include:

- vaginal dryness and dyspareunia (painful sexual intercourse)
- vaginal discharge and bleeding
- urinary incontinence, urgency of micturition, recurrent symptoms of cystitis.

Symptoms result from oestrogen deficiency in menopausal woman and may be treated either with systemic HRT prepara-tions or with topical applications of oestrogen incorporated into vaginal creams, pessaries and silicone vaginal rings. Such topi-cal routes of administration do result in some systemic absorption of oestrogen through the vaginal mucosa and since this may be erratic, vasomotor symptoms may ensue. Absorption of oestro-gen from these topical applications may also stimulate uterine endometrial development, if present. Consequently, it is recom-mended that these treatments should not be used for more than 6 months. The dose of oestrogen required to stimulate the oestrogen receptors in the vagina and the lower urethra is about 10 μg per day, and the efficiency of such low doses has been demonstrated in a number of clinical trials. The effect of oestrogen on vagi-nal symptoms is more marked than its effect on urinary symp-toms, but the incidence of urinary sensory dysfunction may be improved. Menopausal atrophic vaginitis may respond to a short course of a topical vaginal oestrogen preparation used for a few weeks and repeated if necessary. Current guidance is that the minimum effective dose should be used for the shortest duration.

Initial treatment with local oestrogen may result in a reaction to the presence of oestrogen in tissues containing oestrogen receptors, such as the breast and vagina. The longer the time between starting HRT and the menopause, the greater these effects. During initial treatment other effects observed include headache, appetite increase and calf muscle cramps, but these side effects usually resolve without intervention. HRT with small doses of an oestrogen (together with a progestogen in women with an intact uterus) is appropriate for alleviating menopausal symptoms such as vaginal atrophy or vasomotor instability.

Bone

Osteoporosis is defined as a reduced bone mass per unit volume of bone; that is, a reduction in bone density. In a woman not treated with HRT, approximately 15% of bone mass is lost within 10 years of the menopause, resulting in an increased incidence of fracture, typically of the hip. Such fractures take up at least 10% of orthopaedic beds and the total cost in terms of morbidity

and mortality is high. The effect of oestrogen lack is to increase osteoclastic bone resorption. There is an overall increase in bone turnover, more bone is resorbed than replaced and there is an associated increase in the rate of bone loss which may continue for 5–10 years. Oestrogens may exert effects on bone through the calcium-regulating hormones such as calcitonin and para-thyroid-regulating hormones. Evidence also exists for the effect of oestrogens on the local production of bone growth factors, cytokines and prostaglandin E_2.

The greatest effect of oestrogen on bone is seen with implants, where an approximately 8% increase in vertebral bone density is seen within 1 year of treatment. Estradiol patches are the next most effective route of administration (Fig. 46.1), while oral therapy only achieves an increase in bone density of about 2% per annum. However, 5 years of oral oestrogen therapy will still achieve a lifetime reduction in femoral neck fracture of as much as 50%.

Oestrogen improves the quality and quantity of bone in the postmenopausal woman. It may be started at any time after the menopause and the benefit will continue for the duration of treat-ment. Bone loss will continue after treatment ceases, which leads into the difficult area of how long treatment should con-tinue. It was previously recommended that to obtain maximum benefit from treatment with oestrogen, the duration of the course should be at least 10 years. However, studies have identified some potential adverse effects of HRT (Million Women Study 2003, Women's Health Initiative 2002). Therefore this recommen-dation is controversial, particularly in women with an intact uterus, where a combined HRT preparation is required as there is probably a greater risk of adverse outcome. Oestrogen given systemically in the perimenopausal and postmenopausal period or tibolone given in the postmenopausal period also diminish postmenopausal osteoporosis but other drugs are preferred.

Raloxifene is now licensed for the prevention and treatment of osteoporosis as an alternative to HRT. Raloxifene reduces bone loss and increases bone density at the spine and hip in postmenopausal women. With its oestrogen antagonist effect on breast and endometrium, raloxifene may prove to be an advance over oestrogen treatment in osteoporosis prevention and

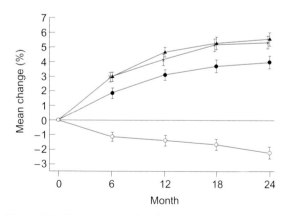

Figure 46.1 Percent change from baseline (mean ± SEM) in lumbar spine bone mineral density in patients receiving placebo (open circles) or transdermal 17β-estradiol 50 μg/day (filled circles), 75 μg/day (asterisks) or 100 μg/day (filled triangles) (from Delmas et al 1999).

treatment in postmenopausal women. It does, however, cause hot flushes which may be unacceptable for some.

Cardiovascular system

Coronary heart disease

Women at 45 years are significantly less likely than men to die of coronary heart disease, but by the age of 60 years the death rate from the disease is similar in both sexes. Oestrogen is probably central to this gender difference as women who experience early loss of endogenous estradiol have an accelerated risk of developing coronary heart disease. Intuitively it would appear logical that postmenopausal women would gain benefit from receiving exogenous oestrogen. However, there are conflicting views as to whether this is, or is not, the case. A 4-year study of women with coronary heart disease in the USA (Heart and Estrogen-progestin Replacement Study [HERS]) who were also receiving HRT (conjugated equine oestrogen and medroxyprogesterone acetate) demonstrated no significant reduction in stroke (Simon et al 2001). This was in contrast to the increased risk of myocardial infarction in the first year of starting HRT in the original HERS report (Hulley et al 1998). The Women's Health Initiative (2002), another USA-based study, also reported an increase in coronary events in the first year of receiving HRT.

The relevance of both studies to UK practice has been challenged as both involved use of conjugated equine oestrogen/medroxyprogesterone acetate regimens. In the UK natural progesterone is preferred and this differs from medroxyprogesterone acetate in that it does not attenuate the beneficial effects of oestrogen in reducing the development of coronary artery atherosclerosis and protecting against coronary vasospasm. A recent study (De Vries et al 2006) using the UK General Practice Research Database found HRT was associated with a decrease in risk of acute myocardial infarction and there was no difference between the different oestrogen–progestogen combinations. The current situation is probably best summed up by the guidelines of the International Menopause Society (2004) which state that there is no clear reason to commence HRT treatment solely or primarily to confer cardiovascular benefit.

Venous thromboembolism

It is known that the oestrogen in the combined oral contraceptive pill contributes to thromboembolic disorders. Whether the same applies to the oestrogen in HRT is unclear as the dose of oestrogen found in HRT is much lower and more physiological than that in the oral contraceptive pill. Analysis of the results from the Women's Health Initiative (2002) has confirmed that there is an increased risk of pulmonary embolism with HRT and the risk is greater with oral HRT than transdermal oestrogen.

Oral oestrogen, in contrast to the transdermal route, undergoes extensive first-pass metabolism. This increases the production of prothrombotic factors in the liver and is associated with a reduction in fibrinogen and factor VII activation, such as von Willebrand's factor and antithrombin, and enhanced fibrinolysis (RCOG 2004). HRT is also associated with increased resistance to activated protein C.

Whilst oestrogen exposure and age increase the risk of VTE, they do not explain the increased risk seen in the first year of HRT use. An underlying thrombophilia, a known risk in hyperoestrogenic situations, is thought to be the additional factor that makes certain women susceptible to VTE. Guidelines (RCOG 2004) to manage the risk of VTE have been produced for women starting or continuing HRT (Table 46.4). The selective oestrogen receptor modulators (SERMS) such as raloxifene are considered to carry the same risk of thrombosis as oestrogen-containing HRT.

Overall, minimizing cardiovascular risk whilst obtaining the benefits of HRT is influenced by the age of the women treated,

---

Table 46.4 Summary of guidelines for dealing with the risk of venous thromboembolism (VTE) in women receiving HRT (adapted from RCOG 2004)

Women starting or continuing HRT
- Women starting or continuing HRT should be counselled with regard to perceived benefits and possible risks for their individual situations, including consideration of alternative therapies
- All women commencing HRT should be counselled about the risk of VTE, should be aware of the signs and symptoms of VTE and should be able to access medical help rapidly if they suspect that they have developed a thrombus
- Universal screening of women for thrombophilic defects prior to or continuing the prescription of HRT is inappropriate
- Prior to commencing HRT, a personal history and a family history assessing the presence of VTE in a first- or second-degree relative should be obtained
- HRT should be avoided in women with multiple pre-existing risk factors for VTE

Women with a personal or family history of VTE
- Testing for thrombophilia should be discussed with, and available for, women with a personal or family history of VTE
- In women with a previous VTE, with or without underlying heritable thrombophilia, oral HRT should be usually avoided in view of the relatively high risk of recurrent VTE
- In women with a personal history of VTE but with an underlying thrombophilic trait identified through screening, HRT is not recommended in high-risk situations such as antithrombin deficiency or with combinations of defects
- In women over 50 years with a history of VTE within the previous year, a full clinical history and examination with appropriate investigations is warranted for underlying disease
- If a woman who is on HRT develops VTE, HRT should be discontinued
- If a woman wants to continue on HRT after VTE, long-term anticoagulation should be considered

their body mass index, cardiovascular health and menopausal history, the timing of initiation of HRT, the formulation of the product used, and polymorphism.

Cancer

Colorectal cancer

Colorectal cancers tend to occur in women over 50 and several studies have indicated that HRT can reduce the risk by around 35%. The exact mechanism for this protective effect on the colon is unclear, although it has been suggested that oestrogen may decrease the formation of potentially carcinogenic bile acids.

Ovarian cancer

The risk of ovarian cancer risk is known to be affected by exogenous hormones, with a reduced incidence consistently reported in users of oral contraceptives. The relationship between the hormones used in HRT and ovarian cancer is, however, less clear. Women who use oestrogen plus a progestogen do not appear to be at increased risk of ovarian cancer, perhaps because the progestogenic component has an apoptotic effect on the ovarian epithelium. This has been supported by studies in small goups of women with a mutation in either the *BRCA1* or *BRCA2* gene (point mutations associated with breast and ovarian cancer) which demonstrated that HRT did not adversely influence the risk of developing ovarian cancer. In contrast, other large HRT trials have suggested a possible increase in risk of ovarian cancer, particularly in women who have had a hysterectomy and are receiving long-term oestrogen-only HRT.

Endometrial cancer

Unopposed oestrogen therapy at least doubles the risk of endometrial cancer but the addition of a progestogen, either in continuous combined or sequential regimens, reduces this risk. Of the two regimens, continuous combined administration is more effective than sequential therapy in reducing the risk of endometrial hyperplasia.

Breast cancer

Breast cancer is the most common cause of disease and death in middle-aged women, affecting around one in 11 women before the age of 75 in developed countries. Over the past 20 years there has been a growing body of evidence to suggest that progesterone contributes to the development of breast cancer. Evidence to support this came from trials in which use of combined regimens increased breast cancer risk more than oestrogen alone. This is thought to have occurred because the synthetic progestogens possessed some non-progesterone like effects that potentiated the proliferating action of oestrogen. In the USA, the most commonly used progestogen in HRT is medroxyprogesterone acetate combined with conjugated equine oestrogen and administered orally. In contrast, in central and southern Europe, a wider range of progestogens is used, particularly the 19-nortestosterone derivatives. Studies investigating the use of natural micronized progesterone to improve bioavailability in HRT regimens have

demonstrated no increased risk of breast cancer. In vitro studies with medroxyprogesterone have found it promotes the reproductive transformation of estrone into estradiol by influencing the activity of 17β-hydroxysteroid dehydrogenase. The properties of the synthetic progestogens are outlined in Table 46.5.

The oestrogen-only arm of the Women's Health Initiative study (2002) found no increase in the relative risk of breast cancer during 6.8 years of therapy.

Overall, there is only a small increased risk of breast cancer for women receiving short-term treatment, typically 1–3 years. HRT may also modify the pathological presentation of breast cancer. Users of HRT have more lobular carcinomas although the implications of this for prognosis are unclear. It is also recognized that women who use HRT have a slight increase in mammographic density and this may affect diagnosis.

Psychological symptoms

These symptoms include:

- depression
- mood changes and irritability, which may also be associated with other life changes occurring at this time
- exhaustion
- poor concentration and memory
- panic attacks
- lowered libido, which may be exacerbated by the above symptoms together with dyspareunia linked to lack of oestrogen and falling androgen levels.

The role of HRT in this area has not been clearly defined although in several studies surgical menopause has been associated with depression, indicating a correlation with oestrogen lack. Many women experience psychological symptoms around the menopause and although these may be associated with oestrogen lack, they may also result from the changes in family

Table 46.5 Properties of progestogens and their link to breast cancer (adapted from Campagnoli et al 2005)

Progestogen	Action
19-Nortestosterone derivatives	Oestrogenic activity
Medroxyprogesterone acetate	Influence on 17β-hydroxysteroid dehydrogenase
19-Nortestosterone derivatives Medroxyprogesterone acetate	Metabolic effects, opposing those of oestrogen, on insulin sensitivity Hepatic effects, opposing those of oestrogen, i.e. increasing IGF-1 (insulin-like growth factor), decrease in sex hormone-binding globulin
19-Nortestosterone derivatives	Binding to sex hormone-binding globulin with consequent reduction in capacity to bind oestrogen

life that often occur around this time. Disturbance of sleep pattern and sleep deprivation, associated with the menopause, are likely to contribute to the psychological symptoms. Many women find treatment with estradiol restores normal sleep and psychological problems are then reduced. Some of the mood changes will respond to counselling and psychotropic drugs. Treatment with oestrogens at high doses (patches $100\,\mu g$ or implants $50\,mg$) has also been shown to improve depression scores. If a progestogen is added into the regimen then the results are less predictable since progestogen use is related to mood changes, particularly in women who have previously suffered from the premenstrual syndrome. Age negatively influences almost all sexual function domains in a significant manner.

HRT improves some aspects of sexual function during menopause but it does not appear to improve the domains of desire and arousal. The lowered libido experienced during the menopause is associated with reduced levels of circulating androgen resulting from ovarian failure. It has been demonstrated that subcutaneous implants of testosterone, $100\,mg$ every 6 months, will increase the libido in a high proportion of patients.

Central nervous system

The relationship between oestrogen and neurodegenerative conditions, in particular Alzheimer's disease, has received attention in the light of an observation that there is an increased incidence of the disease in older women. The development of plaques of amyloid-β, a protein that disrupts nerve cell connections in the brain, occurs more rapidly in the absence of oestrogen. This effect of amyloid-β production results in the symptoms of short-term memory loss and disorientation which occur in Alzheimer's disease. Hope that oestrogen administration would halt the progression of Alzheimer's disease has not been vindicated (Mulnard et al 2000). Further studies are essential to clarify the relationship between HRT and Alzheimer's disease. A trial of raloxifene over 3 years revealed no significant effect upon cognitive scores (Yaffe et al 2001) although there was a trend toward a smaller decline in verbal memory and attention scores. However, it is premature to conclude that oestrogen replacement therapy or use of a SERM such as raloxifene has no role in preserving cognitive function. It is possible that HRT may have a neuroprotective effect under certain circumstances in some women and neuroimaging may reveal effects not detectable using cognitive testing.

CASE STUDIES

Case 46.1

Elizabeth is a 54-year-old woman who has been on HRT in the form of oestrogen–progestogen patches for the past 5 years. Before treatment with HRT, she had been suffering from irregular and frequent heavy menstrual bleeding, irritability and lack of concentration. Full gynaecological and general investigation (including endometrial biopsy) at the time indicated no detectable pathology but her FSH levels were raised above normal to 35 iu/L. She is now complaining about still having monthly bleeds, although apart from this she is symptom free.

Questions

1. What was the likely cause of Elizabeth's symptoms 5 years ago?
2. What is available to her as an alternative to the monthly bleeds?

Answers

1. As the menopause approaches, ovarian function becomes irregular and at 49 years of age, Elizabeth was showing classic signs of ovarian changes. Since this patient had no regular cycles it was unlikely that she was still ovulating; thus she was not producing ovarian progesterone. Peripheral levels of ovarian steroids fluctuate and are difficult to measure; FSH levels are a more reliable indication of ovarian activity. This patient showed moderately high levels of FSH, indicating some failure of the normal FSH/oestrogen feedback mechanisms 5 years ago. The ovary was still producing oestrogen sufficient to stimulate endometrial development but when the oestrogen level was not sustained, the endometrium was shed, accounting for the heavy and irregular periods. Now, after 5 years of HRT, using a combined oestrogen–progesterone regimen to regularize the uterine endometrium and alleviate symptoms, it is time to review her treatment. As there was a possibility of some ovarian activity being present at the initial diagnosis, a high dose of oestrogen was required to override any remaining activity of the pituitary–ovarian pathway. The progestogen component of the treatment was included to protect the uterine endometrium from overstimulation by the oestrogen. In patients such as Elizabeth, in whom the uterus is still present, the progestogen should be used for at least 12 days in each month.
2. Now that the patient is questioning the need for the monthly bleeds which she has experienced with the HRT over the past 5 years, treatment must be reviewed. It is possible that HRT to alleviate the menopausal symptoms will no longer be needed and the patient may decide to try and manage without HRT. If she wishes to continue HRT or expresses concern about osteoporosis developing in later life then the possibility of using tibolone (oestrogenic, progestogenic and weak androgenic activity) or a continuous combined preparation could be discussed. These preparations will not cause her to have a monthly bleed although spotting is common in the first few months. The patient should be made aware of the recent concerns about the safety of long-term HRT so she can make a fully informed decision.

Case 46.2

Sally is a 49-year-old obese woman (BMI $31\,kg/m^2$) with a family history of coronary heart disease. She underwent a total hysterectomy 10 years ago when suffering from endometriosis and has since been treated with HRT in the form of oestrogen implants. Her primary care clinician is concerned about a raised blood pressure that is reasonably controlled with lisinopril $20\,mg$ daily. She has raised serum cholesterol and her LDL cholesterol is greater than $3\,mmol/L$. Her doctor suggests stopping the oestrogen implants but the patient has read that HRT is useful in older women with heart disease.

Questions

1. Sally has hypercholesterolaemia. Should she continue with the HRT?
2. What advice should be given to Sally about her lifestyle?

Answers

1. HRT should not be used as a means of trying to reduce the risk of cardiovascular disease, as recent evidence suggests there may be an increase in the risk of stroke and cardiovascular disease in HRT users. However, the findings are controversial. If this patient is still

symptomatic after stopping HRT it would be reasonable to use the lowest dose of HRT that relieves her vasomotor symptoms and to review the decision to continue HRT annually. She should continue to take lisinopril but she will also need a statin to control her raised LDL and serum cholesterol level.

2. If Sally stops HRT she will no longer have any exogenous oestrogen and may lose a little weight spontaneously as patients on oestrogen treatment tend to have a feeling of well-being and an increase in appetite. She will need to have counselling about her diet to reduce her weight and her risk of cardiac disease. She should also be encouraged to take weight-bearing exercise to reduce her long-term risk of osteoporosis. Sally should also be told that the 10 years of treatment with oestrogen she has already received would be protective against the future development of osteoporosis.

Case 46.3

Geraldine is a 54-year-old solicitor with three children and a busy lifestyle. She is 1.6 m tall and weighs 53 kg, has never smoked or drunk alcohol, but she tends to have a small appetite and to take meals when she can. She spends much of her working day sitting at her desk and does not take regular exercise. Her periods ceased 2 years ago and she has not suffered from any menopausal symptoms. At a recent routine cervical smear examination she raised the question of using HRT to prevent osteoporosis as her mother had suffered from recurrent fractures in later life. She was referred for investigation and all her investigations and tests were normal except for her bone densitometry, which was 2 standard deviation units below normal, and her FSH level, which was above 50 iu/L.

Questions

1. What risk factors does Geraldine have for osteoporosis and how could these be minimized?
2. What would be a suitable preparation for starting HRT in this patient and how long should her duration of treatment be?

Answers

1. Geraldine has the following risk factors for osteoporosis:

- female gender
- perimenopausal oestrogen deficiency
- low bone density
- family history of osteoporosis
- takes little exercise
- haphazard dietary intake.

She probably has an inadequate calcium intake in her diet, and three pregnancies will have reduced her calcium stores. However, on the positive side she does not smoke or take alcohol. She should be advised to ensure she receives at least 1000 mg of calcium daily either from her diet or by the addition of calcium supplements. If she does not take HRT she will need 1500 mg of calcium daily. The richest sources of dietary calcium can be found in dairy products:

- 0.5 L of skimmed milk contains 750 mg calcium
- 60 g of cheddar cheese contains 420 mg calcium
- a small pot of yogurt contains 250 mg calcium.

Calcium supplements are available either as over-the-counter medicines or on prescription. Geraldine should also be recommended to take regular meals and undertake some form of weight-bearing exercise.

2. Geraldine is clearly postmenopausal since her FSH level is high and this suggests that no viable follicles are remaining in the ovary. HRT is no longer recommended as first-line therapy for the prevention or treatment of osteoporosis but in a woman who is taking HRT for vasomotor symptoms, it may help preserve bone density if continued for 10 years. An alternative drug is raloxifene which shows oestrogenic activity in bone but antagonistic activity in the breast and endometrium as well as favourable lipid profiles. The risks of thromboembolism are similar to those with oestrogen. Raloxifene can also cause hot flushes and this may limit its use in some women. Non-hormonal treatment for osteoporosis is available, with the bisphosphonate drugs being the treatment of choice.

REFERENCES

Campagnoli C, Abbà C, Ambroggio S et al 2005 Pregnancy, progesterone and progestins in relation to breast cancer risk. Journal of Steroid Biochemistry and Molecular Biology 97: 441-450

Delmas P D Pornel B, Felsenberg D et al 1999 A dose-ranging trial of a matrix transdermal 17β-estradiol for the prevention of bone loss in early postmenopausal women. Bone 24: 517-523

De Vries C S, Bromley S E, Farmer R D T 2006 Myocardial infarction risk and hormone replacement: differences between products. Maturitas 53: 343-350

Hall G, Phillips T J 2005 Oestrogen and skin: the effects of estrogen, menopause, and hormone replacement therapy on the skin. Journal of the American Academy of Dermatology 53: 555-568

Hulley S, Grady D, Bush T et al 1998 Randomised trial of oestrogen plus progestin for secondary prevention of coronary heart disease in postmenopausal women. Journal of the American Medical Association 280: 605-613

International Menopause Society 2004 Guidelines for hormone treatment of women in the menopausal transition and beyond. Climacteric 7: 333-337. Available online at: www.imsociety.org

Million Women Study Collaborators 2003 Breast cancer and hormone-replacement therapy in the Million Women Study. Lancet 362: 419-427

Mulnard R A, Cotman C W, Kawas C et al 2000 Oestrogen replacement therapy for treatment of mild to moderate Alzheimer disease. Journal of the American Medical Association 283: 1007-1015

Royal College of Obstetricians and Gynaecologists 2004 Hormone replacement therapy and venous thromboembolism. Guideline 19. Royal College of Obstetricians and Gynaecologists, London. Available online at: www.rcog.org.uk/resources/public/pdf/hrt_venous_thromboembolism_no19.pdf

Simon J A, Hsia J, Cauley J A et al 2001 Postmenopausal hormone and risk of stroke. Heart and Estrogen-progestin Replacement Study (HERS). Circulation 103: 638-642

Women's Health Initiative 2002 Risks and benefits of oestrogen plus progestin in healthy postmenopausal women: principal results from the Women's Health Initiative randomized controlled trial. Journal of the American Medical Association 288: 321-333

Yaffe K, Krueger K, Sarkar S et al 2001 Cognitive function in postmenopausal women treated with raloxifene. New England Journal of Medicine 344: 1207-1213

FURTHER READING

Brockie J 2005 Alternative approaches to the menopause. Reviews in Gynaecological Practice 5: 1-7

Dantas A P V, Sandberg K 2005 Challenges and opportunities associated with targeting oestrogen receptors in treating hypertension and cardiovascular disease. Drug Discovery Today: Therapeutic Strategies 2(3): 245-251

Dubey R K, Imthurn B, Barton M, Jackson E K 2005 Vascular consequences of menopause and hormone therapy: importance of timing of treatment and type of estrogen. Cardiovascular Research 66: 295-306

Panay N, Rees M 2005 Alternatives to hormone replacement therapy for management of menopausal symptoms. Current Obstetrics and Gynaecology 15: 259-266

Warren M P, Halpert S 2004 Hormonal replacement therapy: controversies, pros and cons. Best Practice and Research in Clinical Endocrinology and Metabolism 18: 317-332

Drugs in pregnancy and lactation 47

Sharon J. Gardiner   David J. Woods

Drug use in pregnancy

In 1961 thalidomide was withdrawn from the UK market following numerous reports of severe anatomical birth defects after mothers took the drug in early pregnancy. Subsequently, it was realized that drugs have the potential to traverse the placenta and harm the developing fetus. There is now a greater appreciation of the risks of drug use in pregnancy, and it is generally accepted that maternal pharmacotherapy should be avoided or minimized where possible. Nevertheless, it has been estimated that over 90% of expectant mothers take three or four drugs at some stage of pregnancy. Indications for drug use range from chronic illnesses such as epilepsy and depression to those commonly associated with pregnancy such as hypertension, urinary tract infections and gastrointestinal complaints. Further, a significant number of women are taking medication at the time when their pregnancy is detected.

Pregnancy stages

The human gestation period is approximately 40 weeks from the last menstrual period (38 weeks post conception) and is conventionally divided into the first, second and third trimesters, each lasting 3 calendar months. Another method for classifying the stage of pregnancy is according to the stage of fetal development. This is a more useful approach when assessing drug safety in pregnancy. The pre-embryonic stage is the first 17 days post conception and involves implantation of the fertilized ovum. The embryonic stage (days 18–56) is when the major organ systems are formed. The fetal stage (weeks 8–38) involves maturation, development and growth. It is common practice to describe drug exposure at any stage during pregnancy as fetal exposure, and for simplicity this convention is followed in this chapter.

Placental drug transfer

Most drugs diffuse easily across the placenta and thus enter the fetal circulation to some extent. In fact, sometimes drugs are administered to pregnant women in order to treat fetal disorders; for example, flecainide has been used to resolve fetal tachycardia. Drugs with very large molecular weights such as insulin and heparin have negligible transfer. Lipophilic, un-ionized drugs cross the placenta more easily than polar drugs, and weakly basic drugs may become 'trapped' in the fetal circulation due to the slightly lower pH compared with maternal plasma. Some other factors such as enzymes or transporters in the placenta may facilitate or restrict the transfer of a drug to the fetus. However, the extent of placental drug transfer is seldom employed to evaluate the safety of a drug when given during pregnancy. Knowledge of the pharmacology and toxicity and experience of use of the drug in pregnancy are much more important.

Considerations in pregnancy

There are two major considerations regarding drug use in pregnant women: the effect of the drug on the pregnancy, fetus or neonate (teratogenicity and pharmacological effects), and the effect of the pregnancy on drug handling (pharmacokinetics).

Teratogenicity

A teratogen is an agent, e.g. drug, chemical or infectious disease, that interferes with the normal growth and development of the fetus. Approximately 2–3% of all live births are associated with a congenital anomaly. However, the cause of the malformation cannot be identified in most cases, and exogenous factors such as drugs may account for only 1–5% of these (affecting <0.2% of all live births). As drug-associated malformations are largely preventable, they remain an important consideration.

Congenital anomalies such as spina bifida and hydrocephalus are obvious at birth, but some defects may take many years to develop or be identified. Examples of delayed anomalies are behavioural and intellectual disorders associated with in utero alcohol exposure and the development of vaginal cancer in young women following maternal intake of diethylstilbestrol for the prevention of miscarriage. Examples of drugs that are known to be human teratogens are shown in Table 47.1.

Drug use during the first trimester (especially during the embryonic stage) carries the greatest risk of malformations, as this is when the fetal organs are being formed. Ideally, all unnecessary drug therapy should cease prior to conception. However, inadvertent drug exposure frequently occurs, as approximately half of all pregnancies are unplanned. Thus, it is important to make careful drug choices when prescribing for women of reproductive potential.

Teratogenicity is often regarded as unpredictable (idiosyncratic) and seemingly unrelated to dose. However, it is likely that there is an unknown threshold dose above which drug-induced malformations are more likely to occur. Clearly, complex mechanisms are involved such as fetal genetic predisposition. The possibility of a dose relationship justifies the use of the lowest effective dose in pregnancy.

Pharmacological effects

Pharmacological effects on the fetus are by far the most common drug effects during pregnancy, and the consequences are often minor and reversible compared to the idiosyncratic effects that often lead to major irreversible anomalies. Pharmacological effects are usually dose related and to some extent predictable. Drugs may cross the placenta and exert a direct pharmacological effect on the fetus, or they may adversely affect the fetus via effects on the maternal circulation. For example, high doses of corticosteroids (>10 mg prednisone daily) may cause fetal adrenal suppression. Antihypertensive drugs can cause fetal hypoxia secondary to maternal hypotension (Table 47.2).

Table 47.1 Examples of drugs considered to be human teratogens

ACE inhibitors	Misoprostol
Androgens	Penicillamine
Carbamazepine	Phenytoin
Carbimazole	Tetracyclines
Cytotoxics (some)	Thalidomide
Danazol	Valproic acid
Diethylstilbestrol	Vitamin A and derivatives, e.g. isotretinoin
Ethanol	Warfarin
Lithium	

Table 47.2 Examples of drugs with pharmacological effects on the fetus or neonate

Drug	Adverse effect
ACE inhibitors	Renal dysfunction, oligohydramnios, intrauterine growth retardation
Antidepressants	Withdrawal reactions/pharmacological effects
Antihypertensives	Fetal hypoxia if excessively treated
Benzodiazepines	Withdrawal reactions/pharmacological effects, e.g. 'floppy infant syndrome'
Corticosteroids	Adrenal suppression
NSAIDs	Premature closure of the ductus arteriosus, renal impairment
Opioids	Withdrawal reactions/pharmacological effects

Drugs may also have significant effects on maintenance of the pregnancy. For example, β_2-agonists such as salbutamol inhibit labour and have been used therapeutically to delay delivery.

The neonate can also be adversely affected by maternal drug therapy. It is generally only at birth that signs of fetal distress are observed due to in utero drug exposure or the effects of abrupt discontinuation of the maternal drug supply. The capacity of the neonate to eliminate drugs is reduced and this can result in significant accumulation of some drugs, leading to toxicity. Neonatal withdrawal effects can also be very distressing and symptoms may require treatment with sedatives or drug replacement. Morphine oral solution is used to wean babies off methadone and its use can often be planned before birth. Other classes of drugs associated with adverse effects in neonates include antidepressants and antipsychotics (see Table 47.2). Idiosyncratic drug effects in the fetus and neonate are possible but occur rarely compared with pharmacological effects.

Timing of drug exposure

The stage of pregnancy at which a drug is administered can help determine the likelihood, severity or nature of any adverse effect on the fetus. Drug effects on the fetus are usually described in terms of the trimester of risk, and some drugs can present a different risk according to the trimester of exposure. An example is phenobarbital, which can cause congenital anomalies if given in the first trimester and neonatal bleeding if given in the third trimester. In addition, there may be variable risk within a trimester. For example, folic acid antagonists, e.g. trimethoprim, would not be expected to cause neural tube defects if exposure occurred after neural tube closure, between the third and fourth week post conception. Thalidomide is estimated to cause malformations in 20–30% of cases when exposure occurs between the 20th and 36th days post conception

Drug exposure during the pre-embryonic stage is understood to elicit an 'all-or-nothing' response, leading to either death of the embryo or complete recovery and normal development.

Malformations are thought to be unlikely unless the half-life of the drug is sufficient to extend exposure into the embryonic stage.

Organogenesis occurs predominantly during the embryonic stage and with the exception of the central nervous system, eyes, teeth, external genitalia and ears, formation is complete by the end of the 10th week of pregnancy. Exposure to drugs during this period represents the greatest risk of major birth defects by interfering with organ formation. The general principle is to avoid or minimize all drug use in the first trimester, whenever possible.

In the fetal stage, the fetus continues to develop and mature and there is susceptibility to some drug effects. This is especially the case with the central nervous system, which can be damaged by exposure to some drugs, e.g. ethanol, if given at any stage of pregnancy. The external genitalia continue to form from the seventh week until term and consequently danazol, which has weak androgenic properties, can cause virilization of a female fetus if given in any trimester. Conversely, because of their anti-androgenic properties, spironolactone and cyproterone have the potential to cause feminization of the male fetus. The pharmacological effects of angiotensin-converting enzyme (ACE) inhibitors given in the second and third trimesters can result in fetal renal dysfunction and oligohydramnios (small amount or absence of amniotic fluid), and sulfonamides can cause neonatal haemolysis when given at the end of the third trimester. Another important group of drugs that can cause problems specifically in the third trimester is the NSAIDs. These drugs inhibit prostaglandin synthesis in a dose-related fashion and when given late in pregnancy, can cause closure of the fetal ductus arteriosus, fetal renal impairment, bleeding disorders and delay in labour and birth. NSAIDs should therefore be avoided during the third trimester.

Pharmacokinetic changes

Volume of distribution The weight gain of pregnancy is significant as a result of the fetus and an increase in total body water and fat. These factors increase the volume of distribution of drugs such that increased loading doses may be required. This may be important if a rapid drug effect is required or if the magnitude of the effect is proportional to peak plasma concentration.

Protein binding Albumin is the main plasma protein responsible for binding acidic drugs such as phenytoin and salicylates, and α_1-acid glycoprotein predominantly binds basic drugs, including β-blockers and opioid analgesics. Plasma albumin concentrations fall significantly in pregnancy and this leads to an increase in the *fraction* of unbound drug. Clinical effect is related to the *concentration* of unbound drug, which usually remains unchanged even though the total (bound plus unbound) plasma concentration is decreased. Thus, a fall in the total plasma concentration does not usually require an increase in dose. Phenytoin is bound to albumin and exhibits these effects but the situation is further complicated by increased hepatic metabolism that may necessitate a dose increase. Consequently, therapy can only be reliably guided by clinical assessment or measurement of unbound rather than total plasma concentration. Generally speaking, management of epilepsy in

pregnancy is so complicated that it should be undertaken by specialists in the area.

Clearance Within the first few weeks of pregnancy the glomerular filtration rate increases by approximately 50% and remains raised until after delivery. Consequently, the clearance of drugs that are excreted unchanged mainly by the kidneys, e.g. lithium and some β-lactam antibiotics, is increased and higher maintenance doses may be required. The hepatic metabolism of many drugs is also increased during pregnancy, in part due to enzyme induction, but the effects on individual drugs are inconsistent and difficult to predict. The metabolism of methadone and phenytoin is often significantly increased in the third trimester, requiring higher maintenance doses. Conversely, in some women, metabolism of theophylline is reduced and a decrease in the maintenance dose is required.

Drug dosing in pregnancy

As a general principle, the dose of a drug given at any stage of pregnancy should be as low as possible to minimize toxic effects to the fetus. Drug therapy that is considered essential can be tapered to the lowest effective dose either before conception (ideally) or at the time the pregnancy is diagnosed. The doses of antidepressants and antipsychotics could be slowly reduced close to parturition to minimize neurological disturbances due to direct toxicity in the neonate and to minimize withdrawal reactions, e.g. jitteriness, altered muscle tone. However, this may not be appropriate in many cases, particularly given the increased risk of psychiatric problems in the immediate postpartum period. In addition, pharmacokinetic changes are common in pregnancy and these may dictate a dose increase to maintain symptom/disease control. Pregnancy itself can cause a temporary worsening or amelioration of some diseases and thus influence drug dosages.

Drug selection

There are few, if any, drugs for which safe use in pregnancy can be absolutely assured but only a handful of drugs in current clinical use have been conclusively shown to be teratogenic. Animal studies are not necessarily predictive of drug safety in human pregnancy, and there are species differences in the sensitivity to dysmorphogenic effects. In general, drugs that have been used extensively in pregnant women without apparent problems should be selected in preference to new drugs for which there is less experience of use. For example, methyldopa is used rarely to treat hypertension in the non-pregnant state but is frequently used to treat chronic hypertension in pregnancy because of a long history of safe use.

A frequent recommendation is that the benefits of drug treatment should outweigh any possible risk to the fetus, but this analysis is sometimes difficult to perform with certainty. Some countries use pregnancy risk categories which can be helpful in summarizing the available information on a particular drug. The best established system is that created by the FDA which classifies a drug from category 'A' (no demonstrable risk, e.g. replacement doses of thyroid hormones) to 'D' (implies risk, e.g. ACE inhibitors). An additional category, 'X', is used to describe teratogenic agents that are considered to be completely contraindicated in pregnancy, e.g. thalidomide, retinoids. These categories can be helpful but are very simplified and often difficult to interpret. In general, they should not be relied upon as the sole means of assessing the safety of a drug in pregnancy.

It is worth noting that standard literature sources often contain unhelpful information such as 'do not use in pregnancy unless the benefits outweigh the risks'. This is understandable from a medicolegal point of view but offers little in terms of risk assessment. The primary literature is frequently inadequate because ethical, legal and emotional reasons mean that randomized controlled trials are rarely undertaken in pregnant women. Often, the only information that is available is confined to retrospective studies, voluntary reporting schemes and/or animal studies. The rate of anomalies in retrospective studies and voluntary reporting databases may be erroneously elevated as normal outcomes may be under-reported. Individual case reports are also difficult to interpret as the denominator of drug exposure is unknown. More recently, prospective controlled trials have been utilized where the pregnancy outcomes of a defined cohort of women exposed to the drug are compared with outcomes of a matched control group. Complete follow-up of each pregnancy and postnatal monitoring is an essential feature of this type of investigation.

For some new drugs, pregnancy registries have been initiated that record all reported drug exposures and follow up the outcome of the pregnancy. These registries are cumulative and work on the basis that specific anomalies would be identified relatively quickly and that there will eventually be sufficient statistical power to detect the magnitude of any increased risk relative to the general population. The safety data for aciclovir have largely been derived from a pregnancy registry. All studies have inherent methodological problems and require critical review but in general, the most recent investigations provide the most reliable data.

Preconception advice

All women planning pregnancy should be offered advice to minimize the risk of congenital anomalies. General advice includes avoidance of all drugs, alcohol, smoking and vitamin A products (teratogenic) minimization of caffeine consumption, and beginning daily supplementation with at least 400 μg of folic acid to reduce the risk of neural tube defects. The daily dose of folic acid should be increased to around 4–5 mg daily in women who have epilepsy or who have had a previous child with a neural tube defect. Some infectious diseases may carry important fetal consequences if contracted during pregnancy. For example, rubella infection in the first 20 weeks of pregnancy is associated with an increased risk of miscarriage and a syndrome comprising problems such as deafness, cardiac defects and mental retardation in more than 20% of pregnancies. Women who lack immunity to rubella should be immunized prior to conception.

Women with chronic illnesses requiring drug treatment should be offered specialist counselling before conception, and the options explored to reduce or change drug therapy to a safer agent. Epilepsy is an example, in which, if continued drug treatment is necessary, attempts are made to stabilize treatment with a single drug at the lowest effective dose. It is also important to note that many pregnant women become less compliant with

their drug therapy out of concern about possible harm to their infant. In many cases, e.g. asthma, inflammatory bowel disease, epilepsy, inadequate treatment of the underlying disease may be more detrimental to the mother–fetus pair than the drugs used to treat the condition. Therefore, it is essential that mothers are advised of this so that unrealistic fears about the risks to their baby do not result in undesirable outcomes such as unnecessary pregnancy termination or disease relapse.

Drug use in lactation

Human milk provides the optimal form of infant nutrition. Other important health benefits include reduced maternal postpartum blood loss and protection for the infant against infectious disease. Breast feeding also facilitates establishment of the mother–infant bond and is cheaper than alternative food sources such as formula milk. These benefits have lead groups such as the World Health Organization to advocate exclusive breast feeding for the first 6 months of life. As contraindications to breast feeding are few, e.g. HIV infection in developed countries, this advice should be achievable for most women. Unfortunately, the percentage of women exclusively breast feeding their infants at 6 months of age is generally low in developed countries, at less than 20%. This is likely to be due to a number of issues such as the requirement for the mother to return to work or the perception of inadequate milk supply. Drug therapy is a frequent cause for concern and may result in unnecessary avoidance, interruption or cessation of breast feeding. As most women ingest at least one drug during the lactation period, it is essential that health professionals understand the principles of drug safety in breast feeding to facilitate informed decisions during this time.

All drugs distribute into breast milk to a greater or lesser extent and could therefore pose risk to the suckling infant. The only exceptions are drug molecules such as insulin and heparin that are very large and do not readily cross biological membranes. The important factors to consider are the amount of drug that passes into the milk and the likely effect of this 'dose' on the suckling infant. In most cases, it is possible to select a drug that adequately treats maternal disease while posing negligible risk to the baby (Table 47.3). In other cases, the therapeutic options available to the mother may result in unacceptable risk to the infant by virtue of the amount present in milk and/or the toxicity of the drug. In addition, maternal concern about the effects of the drug on the baby may result in other issues such as noncompliance with maternal drug therapy.

Transfer of drugs into milk

The transfer of drugs into milk is almost always by passive diffusion, although drug transporters, e.g. organic cation/anion transporters, are increasingly recognized as playing a role. Several factors affect the rate and extent of passive diffusion; these include maternal pharmacokinetics, the physiological nature of blood versus milk and the physicochemical properties of the drug. Maternal pharmacokinetics determine the amount of drug that is available for transfer. The physiological composition of blood versus milk determines which physicochemical characteristics influence diffusion. Milk differs from blood in that it has a lower

Table 47.3 Drugs regarded as 'safe' when breast feeding full-term healthy babies[a]

Classes	Individual drugs
ACE inhibitors	Aciclovir
Antihistamines	Aminosalicyclic acid
Benzodiazepines	Carbamazepine
β-Lactam antibiotics	Citalopram
Calcium channel blockers	Clarithromycin
NSAIDs (except piroxicam)	Codeine
Phenothiazines	Co-trimoxazole
Tricyclic antidepressants	Digoxin
	Domperidone
	Erythromycin
	Famotidine
	Heparin
	Insulin
	Labetalol
	Mebendazole
	Methadone
	Methyldopa
	Metoprolol
	Morphine
	Nefopam
	Nitrofurantoin
	Paracetamol
	Paroxetine
	Phenytoin
	Prednisone
	Propranolol
	Trimethoprim
	Valproic acid
	Warfarin (monitor infant's bleeding time)

[a] This table is to be used as a guide only. 'Safe' is defined as an infant dose less than 10% of the maternal dose on a mg/kg basis, and a low likelihood of toxicity, remembering that the infant is an innocent bystander. Some drugs within a particular class have more data confirming safety than others and should be the preferred choice. Expert advice is required when the maternal dose is high, or the infant is premature, has renal or hepatic disease or G6PD deficiency.

Table 47.4 Composition of blood and breast milk

	Blood	Milk[a]
Protein	19%	2.5%
Lipid	1%	4.5%
pH	7.4	7.2 (range: 6.8–7.7)

[a] Milk composition varies considerably, both within and between feeds.

pH and less buffering capacity, lower protein-binding capacity and higher fat content (Table 47.4). Therefore, the following drug characteristics affect the extent of transfer.

- *pKa*. This is a measure of the fraction of drug that is ionized at a given pH, e.g. physiological pH. For basic drugs a greater fraction will be ionized at an acidic pH so the milk phase will tend to 'trap' weak bases. In contrast, acidic drugs are more ionized at higher pH values and will tend to be 'trapped' in the maternal plasma.
- *Protein binding*. Drugs that are highly bound to plasma proteins are likely to be relatively retained in maternal plasma because there is a lower total protein content in the milk. Milk concentrations of these drugs are usually low.
- *Lipophilicity*. Drugs that are highly lipophilic will dissolve into the lipid content of the milk, potentially increasing the extent of transfer from maternal plasma.

The profile of a drug that passes minimally into milk would therefore be an acidic drug that is highly protein bound and

has low to moderate lipophilicity, e.g. a NSAID. In contrast, a weakly basic drug that has low plasma protein binding and is relatively lipophilic will achieve higher concentrations in the milk phase, e.g. sotalol.

It should be noted that the composition of milk varies between mothers and within the same mother. For example, milk produced in the first few weeks post partum is termed colostrum and contains more protein and less fat than mature milk. Milk at the end of a feed (hind milk) contains up to five times more fat and about 50% more protein than milk from the beginning of a feed (fore milk). These changes in milk composition are quantitatively less important than the physicochemical properties of the drug.

Milk to plasma concentration ratio

The milk to plasma (M/P) ratio is often used as a measure of the extent of drug transfer into breast milk. It is usually obtained from case reports or small clinical studies and may be based on paired concentrations or full area under the concentration-time curve (AUC) analysis. M/P ratios that are based on a pair of milk and plasma samples collected simultaneously may be inaccurate as they assume that the concentrations of drug in milk and plasma are in parallel, which may not be the case. It is better to collect multiple samples of plasma and milk across a dosing interval, or until the drug is cleared from both phases after a single dose, for determination of an M/P ratio based on the respective AUCs (M/P_{AUC}). Figure 47.1 demonstrates the markedly different estimates of M/P ratio that can be obtained via both sampling methods.

If human-derived M/P ratios are lacking for a particular drug, it may be possible to predict the extent of transfer using known physicochemical properties, e.g. pKa, and a published predictive model (Atkinson & Begg 1990, Begg et al 1992). M/P ratios obtained from animal studies should not be used for clinical decision making, as they may not correlate well with human M/P ratios.

Studies in humans demonstrate that most drugs have an M/P ratio less than 1.0, with the range of reported ratios being from around 0.1 to 5.0. It is often thought that drugs with high M/P ratios (e.g. 5.0) are unsafe because the concentration in milk exceeds that in plasma while those with low ratios (<1.0) are believed to be safe. This is not always the case as the M/P ratio often fails to correlate with the 'dose' of drug the infant ingests via milk. Therefore, the M/P ratio must never be used

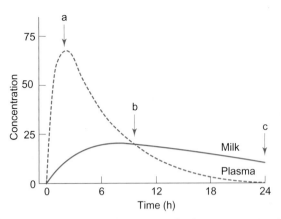

Figure 47.1 Diagrammatic representation of a drug concentration–time profile in the maternal plasma and milk phases after a single oral dose. The points a, b and c illustrate simultaneous sampling times from both phases. Sampling at 'a' would yield an estimated M/P value of 0.2, at 'b' a value of 1.0, and at 'c' a value of 9.3. All can be misleading. The true M/P ratio calculated by the AUC method is 1.2 when extrapolated to infinity.

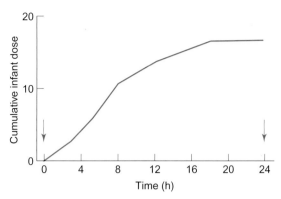

Figure 47.2 The cumulative dose received by the infant is plotted against time. The arrows represent the maternal dose times. This type of study is undertaken by the mother expressing all the milk, from both breasts, at usual feeding times. An aliquot of milk is taken and assayed for the drug. The volume of milk is measured and the total amount of drug at each time is calculated as the product of concentration and volume. This type of study must be undertaken at steady state.

as the sole measure of drug safety in breast feeding. However, it can be used to estimate the 'dose' ingested via milk, which is a better predictor of safety (see below).

Estimating risk to the infant

The risk to the infant depends on the 'dose' ingested through milk, and the concentration and potential toxicity of the drug in the infant.

The most accurate estimation of the infant 'dose' is from studies in which the milk is collected over a complete dose interval at steady state and the total dose is calculated (Fig. 47.2). Unfortunately, these studies are seldom performed. Therefore, information must be obtained from less than ideal conditions.

If the M/P ratio is known from published studies, the likely infant dose (D_{inf}) can be calculated as follows, with some assumptions:

$$D_{inf} = Cp_{mat} \times M/P \times V_{milk}$$

where Cp_{mat} is the average maternal plasma concentration and the M/P_{AUC} is used in preference to a ratio based on paired concentrations when available. The volume of milk (V_{milk}) is not known but is generally assumed to be around 150 mL of milk per kilogram of body weight per day. The above equation simplifies if the actual milk concentration data are available:

$$D_{inf} = C_{milk} \times V_{milk}$$

The likely infant plasma drug concentration (Cp_{inf}) can be calculated by:

$$Cp_{inf} = \frac{F \times D_{inf}}{Cl_{inf}}$$

where F is oral availability and Cl_{inf} is the infant clearance. Unfortunately, neither F nor Cl_{inf} is known accurately for infants so estimation of the likely steady-state average plasma drug concentration will be very approximate. Weight-adjusted Cl_{inf} values (i.e. L/h/kg) are often significantly less than adult values in the

early stages of life (Table 47.5). It is worth remembering that drugs that are not appreciably absorbed orally in adults are also not likely to be absorbed by the infant. Therefore, drugs such as aminoglycosides, vancomycin and proton pump inhibitors are in most circumstances safe to use in breast-feeding mothers.

Given the difficulty in estimating infant plasma drug concentrations, the relative infant dose, e.g. compared with a therapeutic infant dose, is often used as a surrogate of exposure. To give some basis for comparison, the likely infant dose from milk can be compared with an infant therapeutic dose. This is reasonable for drugs such as paracetamol that are usually administered to infants but is unsuitable for drugs such as antidepressants that are not. In the absence of a clearly defined range of infant doses, it is common to compare the dose to the maternal dose (D_{mat}):

$$\% \text{ dose} = \frac{D_{inf} \text{ (mg / kg / day)}}{D_{mat} \text{ (mg / kg / day)}} \times 100$$

For the great majority of drugs this calculation yields infant doses in the order of 0.1–5.0% of the weight-adjusted maternal dose expressed as a percentage (% dose).

Table 47.5 Approximate clearance by age

Age	Percentage of adult clearance[a]
2–3 months preterm	10%
Term	33%
1–2 months	50%
3–6 months	66%
>6 months	100%

[a]Expressed as an approximate fraction of the typical adult clearance values on a weight-adjusted basis.

What is a safe level of exposure?

While there is no simple way of determining a safe level of infant exposure, it is possible to devise guidelines that account for differing possibilities. What needs to be considered are the possible effects that the dose of the drug might have on the infant. For drugs with a low order of toxicity, e.g. amoxicillin, a significant '% dose' would be tolerated, while any exposure to cytotoxic agents is usually considered unacceptable. Clearly, each case needs to be considered on its own merits. As a guideline, for drugs of low-to-moderate toxicity (most drugs), an exposure of less than 10% of the weight-adjusted maternal dose is considered acceptable. This figure is arbitrary and may require modification if the infant is expected to clear the drug slowly. Thus, for a premature neonate whose weight-adjusted clearance might be a tenth of an adult's, a maximum exposure of only 1% might be appropriate as plasma concentrations will be higher for any given dose due to the reduced clearance (dose = $Cp \times Cl$). Assuming the arbitrary cut-off of 10% and ignoring intrinsic toxicity, there are only a small number of drugs that should be avoided during lactation (Table 47.6).

The disparity in the information provided by the M/P ratio and the '% dose' can be demonstrated by considering sumatriptan and lithium. Sumatriptan has a high M/P ratio (4.9) but a relatively low weight-adjusted maternal dose (0.3–6.7%), while lithium has a low M/P ratio (<1.0) and a high relative infant dose (up to 80%).

If there is no information on the extent of transfer and the drug is given as a single dose it might not be too inconvenient for the mother to avoid breast feeding for a short time after the dose until the drug is largely eliminated, about five elimination half-lives. However, if the drug is being used to treat a chronic condition such as epilepsy, then the risk of ongoing infant exposure must be considered. In addition, if the drug has been used regularly throughout pregnancy then the relative exposure of the infant to the drug via milk must be considered with respect to the probable exposure in utero. In general, fetal exposure to

the drug during pregnancy will be substantially greater than the infant exposure from breast feeding.

Variability

To complicate matters further, there will be significant variability between and within individuals in the values used to estimate infant exposure (i.e. D_{inf}, F, Cl_{inf}, where D_{inf} is itself a function of the estimated parameters Cp_{mat}, M/P, volume of milk). Some of this variability will systemically change over time due to developing organ function in the maturing baby and part will be unexplained variability. In addition to this pharmacokinetic variability, there will be variability in response of the infant to any given concentration of the drug. It is fortunate that most drugs seem to fall readily into safe (<10%) and not safe (>10%) categories based on expected exposure. However, care should be taken for drugs that fall between these two extremes, when variability in the estimates of the parameters used may impact on the prediction of their safety. This is especially true for those circumstances when initial estimates of these parameters are less precise, for example in neonates.

Reducing infant exposure

A technique that is often recommended for reducing infant exposure is to give the maternal dose immediately after the infant has been fed in an attempt to avoid feeding at the maximum milk concentration. This assumes that peak milk concentrations occur at a similar time to peak concentrations in plasma. Unfortunately, dosing after a feed is often impractical and may not avoid peak milk concentrations when infants feed up to 2 hourly. Thus, it is better to use this recommendation selectively. For example, it is most likely to be helpful if the mother is feeding less frequently, e.g. 4 hourly, and the drug has a short half-life.

Other methods of helping to reduce infant exposure may be more readily achievable. These include using topical treatments for local effect, e.g. short-term use of a corticosteroid cream for a minor skin complaint rather than oral antihistamines or steroids, and avoiding large immediate oral/parenteral doses in favour of a longer course of a lower dose.

Special situations

Allergy

The theoretical possibility exists of an allergic reaction in an infant exposed to a drug in breast milk, such as a rash from antibiotics. Allergic reactions are by nature unpredictable and a clear dose–response relationship is often not observed. Even minimal exposure of the infant to a drug through milk may confer a significant underlying risk. Only isolated cases have been reported that document an allergic reaction in an infant subsequent to the ingestion of a drug in milk, although adverse effects such as this are generally underreported. However, it is thought that the incidence of this type of reaction must be very low and need not be considered in normal practice. However, if an infant has already experienced an allergic reaction to a given drug in a therapeutic setting, subsequent maternal use should be discouraged or breast feeding avoided.

Table 47.6 Examples of drugs that give high infant exposure during lactation

Amiodarone
Carbimazole
Ethosuximide
Isoniazid
Lithium
Metronidazole
Phenobarbital
Theophylline
Propylthiouracil

Glucose-6-phosphate dehydrogenase deficiency

The other main circumstance when adverse reactions may occur in response to small amounts of drug present in milk is in infants with glucose-6-phosphate dehydrogenase (G6PD) deficiency G6PD is an enzyme present in erythrocytes that is responsible for maintaining the antioxidant compound glutathione in its active form. Deficiency of this enzyme makes the erythrocyte more susceptible to oxidative stress, resulting in haemolysis. Typically only small amounts of drug are needed to precipitate such reaction. Breast feeding should be avoided if the infant has a known or suspected G6PD deficiency and the mother is taking drugs that have been reported to cause oxidative stress, e.g. nitrofurantoin.

Recreational drug use

Recreational drug use is widespread, variable and probably underreported. Many drugs may be taken at any one time, and doses used vary widely between individuals and within the same individual. Information from studies of recreational drug use is difficult to interpret as a result of the questionable accuracy of dosing history or the measurement of the M/P ratio, and the confounding of residual effects due to in utero exposure. It is not appropriate to use the 10% cut-off rule in these circumstances since the doses used are not standardized and therapeutic benefit is lacking. However, the '% dose' remains useful as a guide to the level of infant exposure.

In general, it appears that infant exposure to caffeine, ethanol and nicotine is approximately 10–20%. All these drugs are best avoided in breast feeding. However, the occasional consumption of a small alcoholic beverage, e.g. celebratory, is acceptable provided the mother avoids breast feeding for about 2 hours (per drink) to enable the ethanol to be eliminated. Breast milk does not need to be expressed and discarded during this time unless the mother feels more comfortable to do this or it is needed to maintain milk supply, since milk and blood concentrations decline in parallel and the principles of passive diffusion apply.

Opioid agonists are poorly distributed into milk and the '% dose' found in milk is less than 5%. The data on the active components of marijuana, Δ9-tetrahydrocannabinol, and cocaine are incomplete and assessment of infant exposure is not possible. Erring on the side of caution is advised.

Drug effects on lactation

Hormonal agents such as oestrogens and those that affect dopamine activity are the main drugs shown to have effects on milk production, mainly mediated via effects on prolactin. Oestrogens distribute minimally into milk but are best avoided in the early stages of lactation when progestogen-only contraceptives are preferred. Drugs that are agonists at dopamine receptors, such as cabergoline, decrease milk production while dopamine antagonists, such as domperidone, increase milk production. Both cabergoline and domperidone are occasionally used therapeutically for their effects on milk production. Thiazide diuretics, pseudoephedrine and serotonin antagonists such as cyproheptadine may also inhibit lactation.

CASE STUDIES

Case 47.1

A woman is 6 weeks' pregnant and has been diagnosed with depression that warrants pharmacological intervention. She wishes to recommence venlafaxine, which has been helpful in the past. She is also anxious that the ethanol she consumed around the time of conception may have harmed her baby.

Questions

1. What are the safest antidepressants in the first trimester of pregnancy?
2. Is it reasonable for her to commence venlafaxine?
3. Is there any risk from the ethanol ingestion?

Answers

1. Tricyclic antidepressants have been extensively used in pregnancy and are generally regarded as safe. Within this class, amitriptyline and imipramine have the best evidence supporting safety; therefore these drugs or their metabolites, nortriptyline and desipramine respectively, should be used preferentially. Of the SSRIs, fluoxetine is best studied and does not appear to increase the risk of malformations. However, recent data suggests that this class may increase the risk of persistent pulmonary hypertension of the newborn. Further, new studies on paroxetine suggest a small increased risk of defects, especially cardiac defects, compared with other antidepressants. This information is difficult to interpret, in part because it contradicts earlier studies with paroxetine. Until further information is available it may be prudent to avoid the use of paroxetine where possible.
2. Experience with the use of venlafaxine and many other antidepressants, e.g. moclobemide, in pregnancy is very limited. The use of these agents is best avoided until more data are available. However, in some instances it may be necessary to use an agent such as venlafaxine which has little supportive data. For example, if the mother had a history of severe depression that did not respond to multiple trials of other antidepressants then it may be necessary to use venlafaxine. In this case, the unknown risks associated with venlafaxine are likely to be less than those associated with inadequately treated depression.
3. Ethanol is a human teratogen. The fetal alcohol syndrome includes low birth weight, facial dysmorphogenesis and retarded mental development. The safe limit has not been defined, and it is possible that very low amounts of alcohol may produce subtle effects on the fetus. Therefore, the best practice is to avoid all alcohol exposure in pregnancy. In this case, the mother ingested ethanol at the time of conception. She should be reassured that this is regarded as a relatively safe period and is not expected to adversely affect the fetus. However, further ethanol ingestion should be avoided.

Case 47.2

A 30-year-old woman with epilepsy is currently taking valproic acid 1500 mg daily. She wishes to conceive but is concerned about the possibility of birth defects due to valproate exposure in pregnancy. Her seizures have been difficult to control with alternative anticonvulsants.

Questions

1. What are the risks associated with valproate treatment in pregnancy?
2. How can these risks be minimized?

Answers

1. Valproate is a human teratogen, with early first-trimester exposure associated with a 1–2% risk of neural tube defects, as well as other malformations such as orofacial clefts. Valproate has also been associated with neonatal complications such as seizures. It is generally advised that valproate is avoided in pregnancy. Ideally, the valproate dose should be gradually tapered and discontinued prior to conception. However, this is not a realistic option for many women with epilepsy. In fact, seizures may lead to greater problems such as maternal–fetal injury, miscarriage or hypoxia.

2. The patient should be reassured that most pregnancies in women with epilepsy end with a healthy baby without malformations. Concern about the risk of fetal abnormalities may result in reduced compliance, which may have greater maternal–fetal risk than the drug itself. There is some evidence to suggest that higher doses/concentrations of valproate are associated with greater risk of malformations. Therefore, the lowest effective dose should be used throughout pregnancy. Monitoring free valproate concentrations may be useful in pregnancy, perhaps with the view to maintaining those concentrations shown to be effective in the non-pregnant stage. However, doses should be adjusted based on clinical need and not concentrations alone. Women with epilepsy should be commenced on folic acid 4–5 mg daily. They should also receive prenatal diagnostic techniques such as ultrasound and serum α-fetoprotein.

Case 47.3

A 3-day-old term baby has excessive shrill crying, is feeding poorly and seems jittery. The medical team cannot find any cause for these effects. The mother is worried they may be due to paroxetine exposure via breast milk and wonders whether St John's wort is a safer alternative. She has taken paroxetine 20 mg daily throughout pregnancy.

You note from a specialist textbook that the likely infant exposure is around 1% of the maternal dose, corrected for weight.

Questions

1. What is the most likely drug-related explanation?
2. Is it safe for the mother to continue to take paroxetine during breast feeding?
3. Is St John's wort a reasonable alternative?

Answers

1. The most likely drug-related cause is paroxetine exposure during pregnancy and not breast feeding. The half-life of paroxetine in adults is about 24 hours and is likely to be longer in a neonate. There will be a gradual decline in paroxetine plasma concentrations in the neonate after delivery. As a general rule, drug exposure in pregnancy is much greater than exposure through breast milk. Paroxetine is one of the preferred antidepressants in breast feeding as studies have shown that the likely infant exposure is low and typically less than 3% of the weight-adjusted maternal dose. Further, in these studies the concentration of drug in infant plasma was below the limit of detection in almost all cases.

2. The mother should be reassured that the effects are not likely to be due to the transfer of excessive amounts of paroxetine into milk. They are most likely to be a carry-over effect from taking the drug in pregnancy. These effects should resolve naturally within the week as the baby eliminates the remaining drug. If they persist, further medical advice should be sought.

3. Herbal remedies are often perceived as safe because they are natural. However, data on the extent of transfer of the active constituent(s) are lacking. As a general rule it is better to avoid treatment with herbal remedies in favour of non-pharmacological treatment (if appropriate) or the use of a pharmaceutical option (such as paroxetine in this case), with known safety.

Case 47.4

A woman developed stomach cramps, bloating and diarrhoea following a visit to a farm. Her doctor suggests this is likely to be giardiasis and decides to initiate treatment while waiting for the faecal specimen test results. The mother is prescribed metronidazole 200 mg three times daily for 5 days and given general advice such as ensuring adequate hydration. She is exclusively breast feeding a healthy 2-month-old infant and has been told that metronidazole 'passes into breast milk' and 'caution' is required in breast feeding.

Data

- The mother weighs 60 kg.
- The average steady-state plasma metronidazole concentration on this dosage schedule is 10 mg/L.
- Metronidazole concentrations in milk are comparable to those in plasma.

Questions

1. What is the calculated '% dose' exposure for this infant?
2. Would it be safe for the mother to breast feed her child during this course?
3. What if the dose was 400 mg three times daily? Would this change your recommendation?

Answers

1. The '% dose' is 15%. The mother is 60 kg and is prescribed 600 mg/day so her dose is 10 mg/kg/day. The average milk concentration is 10 mg/L and infant milk ingestion rate is assumed to be 0.15 L/kg/day. The infant dose is therefore ~1.5 mg/kg/day (10 mg/L × 0.15 L/kg/day). As a percent of the weight-adjusted maternal dose, it is (1.5 mg/kg/day ÷ 10 mg/kg/day) × 100 = 15%.

2. The infant exposure is greater than the generally recommended cut-off of 10% (in fact, it may vary from 7% to 36%, according to the published data). Metronidazole is not a particularly toxic drug, although it causes gastrointestinal side effects in approximately 12% of patients and has been associated rarely with neuropathies. As the mother is on a relatively low dose and the infant is healthy and born at term, it is probably reasonable to breast feed while on metronidazole. The mother should be advised to monitor the infant for excessive vomiting or diarrhoea or poor suckling (metronidazole may make the milk taste bitter) during the course. The statement that caution is required in breast feeding is unhelpful and is unfortunately consistent with information found in many of the readily available reference sources.

3. The relative infant dose will remain the same (15%) while the absolute infant dose will double. Therefore, methods of reducing infant exposure should probably be considered. These might include alternating breast feeding with bottle feeding, or abstaining from breast feeding for the duration of the treatment course. These techniques must be tailored to the individual as they may not be easy to achieve for many women, especially if they are unwell, and might lead to undesirable outcomes such as cessation of breast feeding. Mothers who might be the best candidates for this sort of approach include those who have a supply of previously expressed breast milk and whose babies are used to taking some of this milk via a bottle. In some cases, an alternative antimicrobial may be safer. For example, paromomycin is a non-absorbable aminoglycoside that is safe in breast feeding, although somewhat less effective than metronidazole for giardiasis.

ACKNOWLEDGEMENTS

We gratefully acknowledge the work of Dr Stephen B. Duffull on the previous versions of this chapter.

REFERENCES

Atkinson H C, Begg E J 1990 Prediction of drug distribution into human milk from physicochemical characteristics. Clinical Pharmacokinetics 18: 151-167

Begg E J, Atkinson E J, Duffull S B 1992 Prospective evaluation of a model for the prediction of milk:plasma drug concentrations from physicochemical characteristics. British Journal of Clinical Pharmacology 33: 501-505

FURTHER READING

American Academy of Pediatrics 2005 Breast feeding and the use of human milk. Paediatrics 115: 496-506

Barclay M, Begg E, Doogue M, Gefken T 2005 Interactive clinical pharmacology. Department of Clinical Pharmacology, Christchurch Hospital/School of Medicine, New Zealand. Available online at: www.icp.org.nz

Bennett P N (ed) 1988 Drugs and human lactation. Elsevier, Amsterdam

Briggs G G, Freeman R K, Yaffe M D 2005 Drugs in pregnancy and lactation, 7th edn. Lippincott, Williams and Wilkins, Philadelphia

Hale T W, Ilett K F 2002 Drug therapy and breast feeding: from theory to clinical practice. Parthenon Publishing, New York

Benign prostatic hyperplasia 48

R. L. Gower

KEY POINTS

- Benign prostatic hyperplasia (BPH) is a common condition which becomes increasingly prevalent with age.
- The enlarging prostate compresses the urethra and produces lower urinary tract symptoms (LUTS) and bladder outflow obstruction (BOO).
- Surgical treatments such as transurethral resection of the prostate (TURP) are effective, but less invasive procedures such as thermotherapy and laser therapy are commonly used.
- α-Adrenoceptor blocking drugs are effective in reducing symptoms within 6 weeks.
- Drugs which block α_{1A}-adrenoceptors are believed to have more specific activity on the prostate and produce fewer systemic adverse effects.
- 5α-Reductase inhibitors such as finasteride reduce prostate size, improve symptoms and urinary flow rates over a period of about 6 months and are most effective in men with larger size prostates.

Benign prostatic hyperplasia (BPH) is the most common benign tumour in men and is responsible for urinary symptoms in the majority of males over the age of 50 years

Epidemiology

Autopsy studies have revealed the histological presence of benign prostatic hyperplasia in 50% of males aged 51–60 years, increasing to 90% in those over 85. By the age of 80 years virtually all men exhibit one or more of the symptoms associated with benign prostatic hyperplasia.

From puberty to the third decade of life there is considerable expansion in the size of the prostate gland. It has been estimated that the time for it to double in size between the ages of 31 and 50 years is 4.5 years, and between 51 and 70 years it is 10 years. Theoretically there is very little increase in size of the male prostate after 70 years.

Benign prostatic hyperplasia is seen in all races although the overall size of the prostate varies from race to race.

Pathophysiology

The prostate is a part glandular, part fibromuscular structure about 3.5 × 2.5 cm in size surrounding the first part of the male urethra at the base of the bladder (Fig. 48.1). It develops at the 12th week of embryonic life, under the influence of androgenic fetal hormone from outpouchings of the urethra.

Simplistically, the prostate can be divided into an inner and an outer zone. The inner zone is generally the site of benign hypertrophic changes, and the outer zone the site of malignant change.

The aetiology of benign prostatic hyperplasia is multifactorial but it is well recognized that prostatic hypertrophy is directly related to the ageing process and to hormone activity. Within the prostate, testosterone is converted by 5α-reductase to dihydrotestosterone (DHT), an androgen with five times the potency of testosterone. Dihydrotestosterone is responsible for stimulating growth factors that influence cell division and lead to enlargement and hyperplasia of the prostate.

Histologically the hypertrophied prostate can vary, depending on the predominance of the type of prostatic tissue present, from stromal, fibromuscular or muscular to fibroadenomatous and fibromyoadenomatous enlargement.

The enlarging prostate does not produce any constitutional change in its own right, other than that mediated by its effect on the urethra of the lower urinary tract (Fig. 48.2). As the prostate enlarges, it tends to elongate and compress the urethra and this, together with increased adrenergic tone, leads to outlet obstruction. Benign prostatic hyperplasia therefore comprises benign clinical enlargement (BPE), bladder outflow obstruction (BOO) and lower urinary tract symptoms (LUTS).

Symptoms

Lower urinary tract symptoms can be divided into symptoms of failure of urine storage (irritative) and those caused by failure to empty the bladder (obstructive or voiding).

Irritative

- Frequency
- Nocturia
- Urgency and urge incontinence

Obstructive

- Poor flow
- Hesitancy in initiation of micturition
- Postmicturition dribble
- Sensation of incomplete emptying
- Occasional acute retention of urine requiring emergency treatment

Lower urinary tract symptoms can be quantified by various scoring systems such as the international prostate symptom score

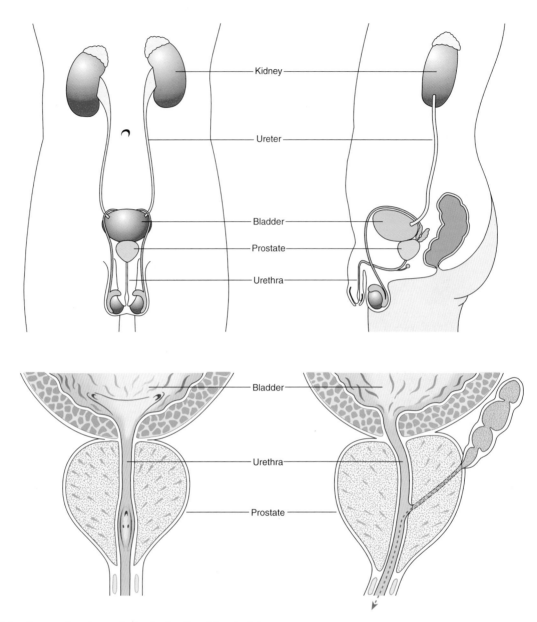

Figure 48.1 Male urinary system demonstrating the location of the prostate.

(IPSS), though each system has its limitations. Other scores measure flow rate, residual volume, prostate size and quality of life.

A digital rectal examination (DRE) is essential to reveal the presence of a tumour. The measurement of prostate-specific antigen (PSA) is controversial but may be offered if the diagnosis of cancer would change the treatment plan (see Chapter 6, Laboratory data).

Benign prostatic hyperplasia can produce haematuria, but the presence of a large bladder that does not empty and leads to chronic renal failure is potentially the most serious sequela.

This often happens in relatively young patients without any other prostatic symptoms. Fortunately, the vast majority of cases can be easily reversed by catheterization and decompressing the bladder.

Examination and investigations

All patients who present with suspected benign prostatic hyperplasia should undergo a digital rectal examination. An enlarged bladder can be palpated and the size of the prostate

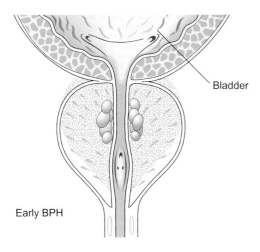

Bladder

Early BPH

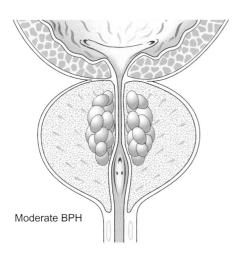

Moderate BPH

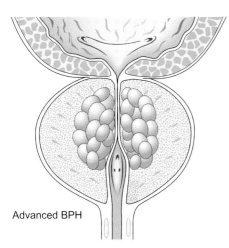

Advanced BPH

Figure 48.2 Diagrammatic representation of the impact of prostate hyperplasia on the urethra demonstrating overgrowth of cells in the inner zone of the prostate.

determined although size has no direct relationship to the severity of symptoms. The most important reason for doing a rectal examination is to detect prostate cancer.

Further investigations include simple urinalysis, urine for culture if infection is considered, serum assessment of renal function to ascertain upper tract damage and the measurement of levels of prostate-specific antigen to detect the presence of a carcinoma of the prostate.

Urodynamic assessment

Urodynamic measurements may range from simple measurement of urinary flow through to cystometry and pressure flow studies. In most cases a urinary flow is enough, where the peak flow and average flows of urine are recorded. Most young men should void at a peak flow of 25 mL/s, while a flow of less than 12 mL/s strongly suggests outflow obstruction.

Imaging

Simple digital ultrasound scanning of the bladder is sufficient to detect and measure a residual volume. Upper tract imaging by means of an ultrasound scan and intravenous urography is no longer routinely done unless indicated by the presence of haematuria, impaired renal function or infection.

Flexible cystoscopy

An evaluation of the bladder using a fibre-optic telescope inserted into the urethra and advanced into the bladder under topical anaesthetic is invaluable in the assessment of the type of prostatic obstruction. If the prostate has grown in such a way that there is intravesical extension where the prostatic tissue can be imagined to hinge at the bladder neck, then each time the patient tries to void, the internal urethral meatus is obstructed by this ball valve effect. This type of tissue requires surgical removal, whereas simple lateral lobe enlargement may well respond to non-surgical measures.

Prostatic ultrasound scan

This is invaluable in accurately documenting the size of the prostate and detecting malignant change. In institutions where it is freely available, it gives the confidence of diagnosis and the ability to more accurately predict the outcome of various treatment options.

Treatment

Most men over the age of 50 years exhibit some of the symptoms of benign prostatic hyperplasia. The problem, therefore, is deciding who should be treated and when. With improved anaesthetic techniques the majority of surgical procedures on the prostate can be done under regional anaesthesia, considerably reducing operative risks and complications. This, together with the development of less invasive surgical procedures and the refinement of medical treatments, offers a range of management options for the individual with benign prostatic hyperplasia.

Surgery

Transurethral resection of the prostate

Transurethral resection of the prostate (TURP) is a common and effective procedure which achieves a high level of improvement in symptoms and flow rate and only requires a short hospital stay. Sections of prostate are removed using electrical loops attached to a resectoscope, a tube-like telescope inserted into the urethra. The electrical wire loop enables the surgeon to gradually remove small amounts of tissue, which is collected for histological assessment.

There is a small incidence of perioperative mortality associated with transurethral resection along with complications such as bleeding, urinary tract infections and epididymitis. Long-term complications include stress incontinence, urethral and bladder neck strictures and erectile dysfunction.

Open prostatectomy

Open prostatectomy involves the surgical removal of an enlarged prostate and is done under general or spinal anaesthesia. Typically, an incision is made through the lower abdomen although sometimes the incision is between the rectum and the base of the penis. This procedure is now performed infrequently and restricted to very enlarged prostate glands, individuals with bladder diverticula or stones or where transurethral resection is not possible (Stoevelaar & McDonnell 2001). Open prostatectomy requires a longer hospital stay than transurethral resection and is associated with a higher incidence of bleeding and other complications.

Minimally invasive techniques

Various treatment modalities have been tried as alternatives to TURP to reduce the risks associated with resection. Thermotherapy and laser technology are the most commonly used.

Thermotherapy

Thermotherapy uses techniques such as electrovaporization, which heats the prostate using bipolar diathermy to cause vaporization of the tissue, and transurethral microwave thermotherapy which uses radiative heating.

Laser therapy

Various types of laser energy can be used to destroy prostatic tissue and it has the advantage of desiccating the tissue so that it is less likely to bleed.

Although alternative measures for surgical intervention give the surgeon a choice in management, transurethral resection still gives the best result for the patient and provides samples for histological assessment.

Non-invasive treatment

In some men, benign prostatic hyperplasia does not progress significantly and one management option is that of so-called 'watchful waiting'. Guidelines for the treatment of benign prostatic hyperplasia in primary care have been published (Speakman et al 2004) and focus on when urological referral is required and when non-invasive treatment can be initiated (Fig. 48.3). Where medical treatment is indicated, the principal options are α-adrenoceptor blocking drugs or inhibition of 5α-reductase.

α-Adrenoceptor blocking drugs

The prostate gland is very responsive to adrenergic stimulation and it has been found that about half of the prostatic outlet obstruction in BPH arises from an increase in adrenergic tone, the other half being due to the hypertrophied bulk of the gland. This increase in sympathetic tone is potentially reversible by drugs. In the prostate, α_1-receptors predominate and mediate the contraction of the gland's smooth muscle. At least three subtypes of this receptor exist (α_{1A}, α_{1B} and α_{1D}) and it is believed that α_{1A} is the dominant receptor in the prostate, although its role clinically has still to be confirmed. The search for drugs which selectively inhibit this receptor subtype has led to the introduction of several new agents in recent years.

Patients with benign prostatic hyperplasia frequently experience problems with erectile and ejaculatory function. The treatment of benign prostatic hyperplasia should therefore aim to restore sexual function. However, the effect of α_1-adrenoceptor antagonists on male sexual function is variable and influenced by the drug chosen and patient characteristics (Van Dijk et al 2006).

The antihypertensive drug prazosin was the first α_1-blocking drug used to relieve the symptoms of benign prostatic hyperplasia but it lacks relative selectivity for α_{1A} receptors and has been associated with many adverse affects such as drowsiness, weakness, headache and postural hypotension (especially after the first dose). It has been replaced by other drugs.

Tamsulosin This drug is a selective inhibitor at the α_{1A}- and α_{1B}-adrenoceptor. It increases urinary flow rates and reduces lower urinary tract symptoms in men with benign prostatic hyperplasia within 8 hours and 1 week respectively, as well as improving quality of life scores (O'Leary 2001). Tamsulosin has an elimination half-life of about 10 hours which allows once-daily dosing and there is no requirement to titrate the dose upward when initiating treatment. It is well tolerated but can cause dizziness, headache, asthenia and syncope. Arthralgia, back pain and myalgia are common adverse effects, each affecting up to 11% of patients treated.

Tamsulosin interacts with cimetidine, which reduces its clearance and thereby increases plasma levels, whilst furosemide can produce a fall in plasma level. In both cases dose adjustment is not normally required as levels remain within the therapeutic range. In common with all α-adrenoceptor blocking agents, there is a risk of enhanced hypotension when administered with other drugs which reduce blood pressure.

A systematic review (Wilt et al 2006) of tamsulosin concluded that it provides a small-to-moderate improvement in urinary symptoms and flow compared to placebo. Effectiveness was similar to other α_1-adrenoceptor antagonists and only increased slightly at higher doses. Adverse effects were noted to increase with use of higher doses

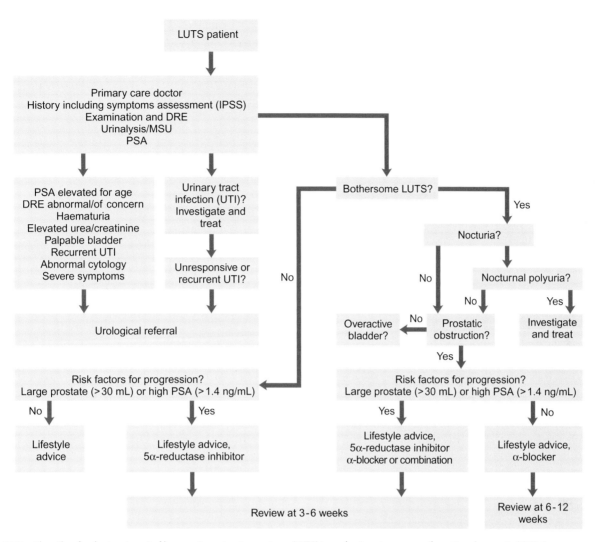

Figure 48.3 Algorithm for the treatment of lower urinary tract symptoms (LUTS) in males in primary care (from Speakman et al 2004). (DRE, digital redial examination; MSU, mid sliream urine sample; PSA, prostate-specific antigen)

Alfuzosin In isolated human tissue, alfuzosin displays a higher selectivity for the prostate over vascular tissue compared with tamsulosin and doxazosin. It has a half-life of 5 hours but is available as a once-daily formulation. It has a rapid onset of action and good tolerability in short-term studies (MacDonald & Wilt 2005). It reduces the overall clinical progression of benign prostatic hyperplasia, does not reduce the primary occurrence of acute urinary retention but appears to have a sustained beneficial effect on quality of life (Roehrborn 2006).

Alfuzosin should not be co-administered with potent inhibitors of cytochrome P450 3A4 such as erythromycin, clarithromycin, itraconazole and ketoconazole.

Indoramin Indoramin is readily absorbed from the gastrointestinal tract and undergoes extensive first-pass hepatic metabolism. Its hypotensive effect may be increased by diuretics and other antihypertensive agents. Alcohol has been reported to increase the bioavailability and sedative effects of indoramin. Randomized clinical trials have generally been small and of short duration and demonstrated no consistent benefit over other α_1-adrenoceptor antagonists.

Doxazosin Doxazosin has a long half-life of about 20 hours which allows for once-daily dosing. As with many other α_1-adrenoceptor antagonists, the dose requires titrating to limit postural hypotension. It has been found to improve symptoms and peak flow rates when compared to placebo, but it has demonstrated no consistent benefit over other α_1-adrenoceptor antagonists. There would also appear to be no significant difference in symptom score regardless of whether the standard or controlled-release preparation is used (Kirby et al 2001).

Terazosin Like doxazosin, terazosin is an α_1-adrenoceptor antagonist that is administered once daily and requires dose titration. It improves the symptoms and flow rates associated with benign prostatic hyperplasia, is more effective than placebo or finasteride, and similar to other α_1-adrenoceptor antagonists. Adverse effects are generally mild but occur more frequently than with other α_1-adrenoceptor antagonists and result in up to a fourfold increase in treatment discontinuation.

5α-Reductase inhibitors

Finasteride The primary androgen responsible for the development and progression of benign prostatic hyperplasia is dihydrotestosterone. There are two isoenzymes of 5α-reductase: type 1 is found in most 5α-reductase producing tissues such as

Table 48.1   Common therapeutic problems in benign prostatic hyperplasia

Problem	Solution
Patient taking α-blocker still symptomatic after 2 weeks' treatment	Patients should be advised that it may take 2–6 weeks before symptomatic relief is seen
Patient taking an α-adrenoceptor blocker complains of cardiovascular adverse effects such as dizziness, syncope, palpitations, tachycardia or angina	These side effects are more likely in elderly patients. They are most common after the first dose and reflect the hypotensive effects of the drugs. They can be reduced by titrating the dose or using more uroselective drugs such as tamsulosin
Sexual dysfunction	Decreased libido or impotence can occur in patients taking finasteride and dutasteride. Abnormal ejaculation can be caused by α-blockers. Tamsulosin in particular can cause a dry climax (retrograde ejaculation). Patients should be forewarned when discussing treatment options
Patient taking finasteride notices breast enlargement	Unilateral or bilateral gynaecomastia is a frequently reported side effect with finasteride and patients need to be counselled accordingly when discussing treatment options
Patient taking finasteride or dutasteride has a sexual partner who is pregnant	Exposure to semen should be avoided as both drugs can cause abnormalities to genitalia in a male fetus. The patient should be advised to use a condom

the liver, skin and hair; type 2 is predominant in genital tissue, including the prostate. Finasteride is a type 2 5α-reductase inhibitor and can thereby downregulate prostate growth. It has been shown to reduce prostate size by about 30%, improve symptom scores and increase urinary flow rates. Meta-analysis has shown that changes in symptoms and peak urinary flow rates were greatest in men with prostate volumes greater than 40 mL. It may take 6 months before symptomatic benefit is felt by the patient but once attained, it may continue for several years with continued treatment. Finasteride has been shown to reduce the number of men who go on to develop acute urinary retention and require surgical intervention (Roehrborn et al 2000).

Side effects include decreased libido, impotence, reduced ejaculatory volume and reversal of male pattern baldness. Plasma concentrations of PSA may be reduced by 50% in the first year of treatment with finasteride, a fact which must be taken into account if a patient has or is suspected of having prostate cancer.

Dutasteride   Like finasteride, dutasteride suppresses the activity of 5α-reductase and thereby reduces levels of dihydrotestosterone and the stimulus for prostate growth. A decrease in volume of the prostate by up to 26% after 4 years of treatment has been reported. Urinary symptoms improve after 6 months of treatment and progression to serious complications is reduced (Thomson 2005). Dutasteride is well tolerated although side effects, which include reduced libido, impotence and gynaecomastia, are troublesome and occur with similar frequency to finasteride. Dutasteride inhibits both type 1 and type 2 isoenzymes of 5α-reductase although the clinical significance of this is unclear.

Combination therapy

It is widely accepted that α-adrenoceptor antagonists are best for managing acute symptoms and delaying symptomatic progression of benign prostatic hypertrophy but have no impact on the rates of acute urinary retention or prostate surgery. In contrast, the 5α-reducatase inhibitors have little impact on short-term acute symptoms but demonstrate improvements in urinary flow rates and symptoms after 1–2 months. Continued treatment with the 5α-reducatase inhibitors decreases the risk of acute urinary retention and prostate-related surgery. It therefore appears logical to use a combination of an α-adrenoceptor antagonist and 5α-reductase inhibitor to manage symptoms and decrease progression of benign prostatic hypertrophy and avoid surgical intervention. A study of over 3000 men for 5 years (McConnell et al 2003) in the Medical Therapy of Prostate Symptoms (MTOPS) trial confirmed the additional benefits of using a combination of doxazin and finasteride and this approach has now been adopted into routine practice.

Phytotherapy

A number of plant extracts are reputed to be effective in the management of symptoms of benign prostatic hypertrophy. They include saw palmetto berry (*Serenoa repens*), African plum tree (*Pygeum africanum*), stinging nettle (*Urtica dioica*) and rye grass pollen. Many of the trials are uncontrolled, short term and use different preparations that may not be equivalent, and few use a validated symptom score to measure outcome. As a consequence it is difficult to assess efficacy meaningfully. The proposed mechanisms of action include an anti-inflammatory effect (by inhibition of prostanoid formation), and inhibition of 5α-reductase.

Patient care

The patient generally seeks treatment for benign prostatic hyperplasia because of the impact of symptoms on quality of life. Most men tolerate a high degree of symptoms and impact on daily activities before they seek help. In patients with troublesome bladder-filling symptoms such as frequency, urgency and urge incontinence, formal bladder training may be appropriate, using a frequency–volume chart that records intake and output over several days. This bladder training may involve asking the patient to go longer between voiding and increasing the volume voided. Keeping a chart may also help the patient better regulate fluid intake, particularly before going to bed, and raise awareness of the need to minimize the intake of drinks containing caffeine or alcohol to reduce symptoms.

Bladder training may be undertaken as part of a 'watch and wait' approach or concurrently with drug therapy. For those patients in whom drug therapy is appropriate, the choice lies between an α_1- or α_{1A}-adrenoceptor antagoniste and a 5α-reductase inhibitor, and each, in turn, requires its own specific information to be given to the patient.

Table 48.1 lists some common therapeutic problems in the management of benign prostatic hyperplasia. There are also two websites which produce valuable resource material: the Men's Health Forum at www.menshealthforum.co.uk, and the Prostate Research Campaign UK at www.prostate-research.org.uk.

CASE STUDIES

Case 48.1

A 64-year-old man presents with complaints of poor urinary flow and having to visit the toilet at least twice during the night to pass urine. There is no family history of prostate disease and he is taking no medication.

Question

What investigations are appropriate and how should this patient be managed?

Answer

This patient should be asked to present a frequency–volume chart of voided urine and undergo a full clinical examination, including measurement of PSA. A post void residual volume of urine within the bladder should be measured after micturition.

If the PSA is within the normal range and the residual volume is less than 100 mL, the patient can be reassured about his condition and a 'watch and wait' policy adopted. If the patient finds this unacceptable then he should be offered treatment with an α-adrenoceptor antagonist. If he is not hypertensive a uroselective drug such as tamsulosin can be considered. This should have few systemic side effects and requires no initial titration of dose. If he is hypertensive, a less specific α-blocker may be more appropriate which will serve the dual purpose of an antihypertensive agent as well as treating his urinary symptoms. Careful dose titration may be necessary initially to counter any potential postural hypotension.

Following publication of the MTOPS trial (McConnell et al 2003), combination of an α-adrenoceptor antagonist and 5α-reductase inhibitor may be considered the treatment of choice for this patient.

Case 48.2

A 50-year-old man requests treatment from his primary care doctor for a 'bladder infection'. On questioning, he describes symptoms of urinary frequency, urgency and urge incontinence, but fever is absent.

Question

How should this patient be treated?

Answer

The lay person may interpret the symptoms of frequency and urgency as representing a urinary tract infection, but in the absence of dysuria this is unlikely. The patient should be referred for a full clinical assessment which should include urodynamic studies, filling and voiding cystometry, an ultrasound scan of the upper urinary tract and measurement of PSA and assessment of renal function. It is likely the patient has an outflow obstruction which has given rise to secondary instability of the detrusor muscle in the bladder, causing involuntary contractions of the bladder and resulting in incontinence. The obstruction may be due either to prostate enlargement or a dysfunctional bladder neck. In either case, treatment with an α-adrenoceptor antagonist is appropriate to reduce the outflow resistance. Should the flow be adequate but symptoms of incontinence persist, then concurrent treatment with an antimuscarinic drug may be necessary to inhibit the cholinergic-mediated contractions of the detrusor. Examples include oxybutynin, tolterodine and propiverine.

There is emerging evidence that phosphodiesterase-5 inhibitors may also be useful in the management of lower urinary tract symptoms. It is known there is an abundance of the phosphodiesterase-5 isoenzyme in the prostate and it is thought this is involved in the regulation of smooth muscle tone. A number of small-scale studies have shown the benefit of agents such as sildenafil and tadalafil, although both are currently licensed only for the treatment of erectile dysfunction. It may therefore be appropriate to prescribe one of these agents for the patient in question.

Case 48.3

An 80-year-old man presents with severe symptoms of outflow tract obstruction with dribbling and initial haematuria. A rectal examination reveals a large prostate.

Question

What is the optimal treatment for this man?

Answer

A full clinical assessment is necessary to eliminate a diagnosis of cancer. If the diagnosis is benign prostatic hypertrophy, then surgery may be considered necessary. If it is decided that surgery is not an option because of the patient's age or preference, then treatment with finasteride would be appropriate to reduce bleeding over 3–6 months, as well as to reduce the size of the prostate and improve outflow symptoms. If successful, treatment may be continued indefinitely with finasteride. If finasteride does not provide satisfactory remission, consideration should be given to carrying out a transurethral resection of the prostate with concurrent finasteride to reduce excessive surgical bleeding.

Case 48.4

A 50-year-old man presents complaining of lower abdominal swelling and feeling tired. On questioning, he admits to poor urinary flow and bedwetting.

Question

What is the optimal treatment for this man?

Answer

Full clinical examination and renal function tests should be arranged urgently. If the abdominal swelling is thought to be caused by a large bladder and laboratory tests show the renal function is deranged then urgent urethral catheterization should take place to drain the bladder.

The catheter should be left in place to allow the renal function to recover before proceeding to surgical prostatectomy.

Outflow tract obstruction with renal impairment requires urgent management. This alone may not relieve the situation as chronic overstretching may cause bladder atony and the patient may well have to continue with intermittent self-catheterization.

REFERENCES

Kirby R S, Andersen M, Gratzke P et al 2001 A combined analysis of double blind trials of the efficacy and tolerability of doxazosin-gastrointestinal therapeutic system, doxazosin standard and placebo in patients with benign prostatic hyperplasia. BJU International 87: 192-200

MacDonald R, Wilt T J 2005 Alfuzosin for treatment of lower urinary tract symptoms compatible with benign prostatic hyperplasia: a systematic review of efficacy and advers effects. Urology 66: 780-788

McConnell J D, Roehrborn C G, Bautista A M et al 2003 The long-term effect of doxazosin, finasteride, and combination therapy on the clinical progression of benign prostatic hyperplasia. New England Journal of Medicine 349: 2387-2398

O'Leary M P 2001 Tamsulosin: current clinical experience. Urology 58: 42-48

Roehrborn C G, Bruskewitz R, Nickel G C et al 2000 Urinary retention in patients with BPH treated with finasteride or placebo over four years. European Urology 37: 528-536

Roehrborn C G for the ALTESS Study Group 2006 Alfuzosin 10 mg once daily prevents overall clinical progression of benign prostatic hyperplasia but not acute urinary retention: results of a 2-year placebo-controlled study. BJU International 97: 734-741

Speakman M J, Kirby R S, Joyce A et al 2004 Guidelines for the primary care management of male lower urinary tract symptoms. BJU International 93: 985-990

Stoevelaar H J, McDonnell J 2001 Changing therapeutic regimens in benign prostatic hyperplasia. Pharmacoeconomics 19: 131-153

Thomson A 2005 Dutasteride: an evidence-based review of its clinical impact in the treatment of benign prostatic hyperplasia. Core Evidence 1: 143-156

Van Dijk M M, de la Rosette J, Michel M C 2006 Effects of α_1-adrenoceptor antagonists on male sexual function. Drugs 66: 287-301

Wilt T, MacDonald R, Rutks I 2006 Tamsulosin for benign prostatic hyperplasia. Cochrane Database of Systematic Reviews, Issue 3. John Wiley, Chichester

FURTHER READING

Batista-Miranda J E, de la Cruz Diez M, Bertran P A et al 2001 Quality of life assessment in patients with benign prostatic hyperplasia. Pharmacoeconomics 19: 1079-1090

Disantostefano R L, Biddle A K, Lavelle J P 2006 An evaluation of the economic costs and patient-related consequences of treatments for benign prostatic hyperplasia. BJU International 97: 1007-1016

Loughlin K R 2004 Clinical guide to prostate specific antigen. Bladon Medical Press, Chipping Norton

McVary K T 2004 Management of benign prostatic hypertrophy. Humana Press, New Jersey

Milani S, Djavan B 2005 Lower urinary tract symptoms suggestive of benign prostatic hyperplasia: latest update on alpha-adrenoceptor antagonists. BJU International 95: 29-36

Nandipati K C, Raina R, Agarwal A et al 2006 Erectile dysfunction following radical retropubic prostatectomy: epidemiology, pathophysiology and pharmacological management. Drugs and Aging 23: 101-117

Nicholson T A, Kirby M, Miles A (eds) 2000 The effective management of benign prostatic disease and lower urinary tract symptoms. Aesculapius Medical Press, London

Sandhu J S, Vaughan E D 2005 Combination therapy for the pharmacological management of benign prostatic hyperplasia Drugs and Aging 22: 901-912

Anaemia 49

C. Acomb   J. Holden

KEY POINTS

- Anaemia is a common condition which is caused by a number of different pathologies.
- Iron deficiency causes a microcytic, hypochromic anaemia. Once the primary cause has been corrected, ferrous iron is the standard treatment.
- Folate deficiency results in a macrocytic anaemia and is treated with replacement therapy.
- Lack of intrinsic factor prevents absorption of vitamin B_{12} and leads to a macrocytic anaemia. Treatment with parenteral B_{12} reverses the blood picture but does not always alleviate the accompanying neuropathy.
- Haemolytic anaemias include the genetic disorders of sickle cell anaemia, thalassaemia and glucose-6-phosphate dehydrogenase deficiency. In these diseases, abnormal forms of haemoglobin cause damage to the structure of the red cells and haemolysis.
- Sideroblastic anaemia is a rare anaemia in which haem synthesis is impaired owing to an enzyme deficiency.

Table 49.1 Examples of conditions that cause reduced haemoglobin synthesis

Reduced proliferation of precursors	Defective maturation of precursors
Iron deficiency	Vitamin B_{12} deficiency
Anaemia of chronic disease	Folate deficiency
Anaemia of renal failure	Iron deficiency
Aplastic anaemia (primary)	Disorders of:
Aplastic anaemia (secondary to drugs, etc.)	globin synthesis (thalassaemias)
Infiltration of the bone marrow: leukaemia or lymphoma myelofibrosis metastases	iron metabolism (e.g. sideroblastic) Myelodysplastic syndrome

Anaemia is not one disease but a condition that results from a number of different pathologies. It can be defined as a reduction from normal of the quantity of haemaglobin in the blood. The World Health Organization defines anaemia in adults as haemoglobin levels less than 13 g/dL for males and less than 12 g/dL for females. However, there are apparently normal individuals with levels less than this. The low haemaglobin level results in a corresponding decrease in the oxygen-carrying capacity of the blood.

Epidemiology

Anaemia is possibly one of the most common conditions in the world and results in significant morbidity and mortality, particularly in the developing world. Worldwide, over 50% of pregnant women and over 40% of infants are anaemic. In the UK, 14% of women aged 55–64 and 3% of men aged 35–64 have been found to be anaemic.

Aetiology

Anaemia results from two different mechanisms:

- reduced haemoglobin synthesis, which may be due to lack of nutrient or bone marrow failure. This leads to either reduced proliferation of precursors or defective maturation of precursors or both (see Table 49.1)

- increased haemoglobin loss due to haemorrhage (red cell loss) or haemolysis (red cell destruction).

It is not unusual to find more than one cause in a patient.

This chapter will cover some of the more common anaemias that involve drug therapy.

Microcytic anaemias	– iron deficiency anaemia
	– anaemia of chronic disease
	– sideroblastic anaemia
Megaloblastic anaemias	– folate deficiency
	– vitamin B_{12} deficiency
Haemolytic anaemias	– autoimmune haemolytic anaemia
	– sickle cell disease
	– thalassaemia
	– glucose-6-phosphate dehydrogenase deficiency

Normal erythropoiesis

It is thought that white cells, red cells and platelets are all derived from a common cell known as the pluripotent stem cell found in the bone marrow. As these cells mature, they become committed to a specific cell line (Fig. 49.1). The red cells mature through the various stages, during which time they synthesize haemoglobin, DNA and RNA. Reticulocytes are found in the peripheral circulation for 24 hours before maturing into erythrocytes. Reticulocytes are released into the peripheral circulation prematurely during times of increased erythropoiesis.

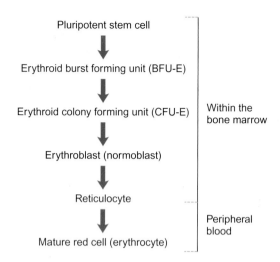

Figure 49.1 Simplified diagram of some of the stages within erythropoiesis.

Table 49.2   Non-specific signs and symptoms associated with anaemia

Tiredness
Pallor
Fainting
Exertional dyspnoea
Tachycardia
Palpitations
Worsening angina
Worsening cardiac failure
Exacerbation of intermittent claudication

Erythropoietin is a hormone produced by the cells of the renal cortex. The kidney responds to hypoxia and anaemia by increasing the production of erythropoietin. The red cell progenitors BFU-E and CFU-E have receptors on their surface. When erythropoietin binds to these receptors, it promotes differentiation and division, and consequently increased erythropoiesis. Patients with end-stage renal disease fail to produce appropriate amounts of erthropoietin and so develop anaemia. Erythropoietin production is also impaired in other conditions such as rheumatoid arthritis, cancer and sickle cell disease, though the impairment is not as great as in renal disease. Also of interest is the fact that theophylline decreases erythropoietin production, though the clinical relevance of this is uncertain.

Each day approximately 2×10^{11} erythrocytes enter the circulation. Normal erythrocytes survive in the peripheral circulation for about 120 days. Abnormal erythrocytes have a shortened lifespan. At the end of their life the red cells are destroyed by the cells of the reticuloendothelial system found in the spleen and bone marrow. Iron is removed from the haem component of haemoglobin and transported back to the bone marrow for re-use. The pyrole ring from globin is excreted as conjugated bilirubin by the liver and the polypeptide portion enters the body's protein pool.

Clinical manifestations

In its mildest form anaemia results in tiredness and lethargy (Table 49.2); at its most severe it results in death, unless treated. There is some suggestion that even mild anaemia may inhibit physical exercise and result in reduced mental performance. The reduced oxygen-carrying capacity of the blood leads to reduced tissue oxygenation and widespread organ dysfunction.

A rapid blood loss, e.g. haemorrhage, produces shock, with collapse, dyspnoea and tachycardia. Anaemia that develops over a period of time allows the body to partially compensate. As the anaemia becomes worse, so more and more signs and symptoms may develop.

Even though in anaemia the amount of haemoglobin is reduced, all the blood that passes through the lungs is fully oxygenated.

Increasing the respiratory rate or increasing the FiO_2 (fraction of inspired oxygen) will not improve tissue oxygenation. When the haemoglobin falls below 7 or 8 g/dL there is almost always a compensatory increase in cardiac output.

Investigations

It is essential to find the cause of the anaemia; there is no place for 'blind' treatment. In most patients the anaemia is a consequence of a reduced concentration of haemoglobin in each red cell and/or a reduced number of red cells in the peripheral circulation. Blood volumes may be increased in pregnancy and heart failure and haemoglobin concentration appear falsely low. Splenomegaly and signs of heart failure are sure signs of an increased blood volume. A blood transfusion in such a patient would precipitate left ventricular failure.

The most important parameter to assess in anaemia is the haemoglobin concentration of the blood. It is also usual to count the number of red cells. In addition, the size, shape and colour all contribute to the investigation (Table 49.3). The mean corpuscular volume (MCV) is a useful parameter that helps determine the type of the anaemia. However, care must be taken

Table 49.3   Anaemia classified by size and colour of red cells

Hypochromic microcytic
  Iron deficiency
  Sideroblastic
  Anaemia of chronic disease

Normochromic macrocytic
  Folate deficiency
  Vitamin B_{12} deficiency

Polychromatophilic macrocytic
  Haemolysis

since the MCV indicates the *average* size of the cells. If there are two pathologies, where one causes large cells and one causes small cells, the MCV may appear normal or be misleading. Following on from this baseline, other investigations may be required. Bone marrow examinations by either aspiration or trephine may be needed to make a diagnosis.

Iron deficiency anaemia

Epidemiology

Worldwide, iron deficiency anaemia is the most common form of anaemia and may be present in up to 20% of the world's population. A diet deficient in iron, parasitic infestations, e.g. hookworm (causing blood loss), and multiple pregnancies contribute to its high prevalence in underdeveloped countries. Even in Western societies it has been reported that as many as 20% of menstruating women show a rise in haemoglobin levels on iron therapy.

Aetiology

In Western societies the most common cause of iron deficiency is blood loss. In women of child-bearing age, this is most commonly due to menstrual loss. Amongst adult males the most likely cause is gastrointestinal bleeding. Other causes of blood loss associated with iron deficiency anaemia include haemorrhoids, nosebleeds or postpartum haemorrhage. A loss of 100 mL of blood represents the amount of iron normally absorbed from a Western diet over 40 days. The major causes of iron deficiency anaemia are listed in Table 49.4.

Pathophysiology

The elimination of iron is not controlled physiologically so the homeostasis is maintained by controlling iron absorption. Iron is absorbed mainly from the duodenum and jejunum. Absorption itself is inefficient; iron bound to haem (found in red meat) is better absorbed than iron found in green vegetables. The presence of phosphates and phytates in some vegetables leads to the formation of unabsorbable iron complexes, whilst ascorbic acid increases the absorption of iron. In a healthy adult, approximately 10% of the dietary iron intake will be absorbed.

Anaemia may result from a mismatch between the body's iron requirements and iron absorption. The demand for iron varies with age (Table 49.5). Diets deficient in animal protein or ascorbic acid may not provide sufficient available iron to meet the demand. Poor nutrition in children in inner cities in the UK frequently leads to anaemia. Milk fortified with iron given to inner-city infants up to the age of 18 months has been shown to increase haemoglobin levels and improves developmental performance compared to unmodified cow's milk (Williams et al 1999).

Malabsorption of iron has been reported in patients with coeliac disease and in 50% of patients following partial gastrectomy. Tetracyclines, penicillamine and fluoroquinolines bind iron in the gastrointestinal tract and reduce the absorption of iron from supplements. They probably do not affect the absorption of dietary iron.

Table 49.4 Major causes of iron deficiency anaemia

Inadequate iron absorption
  Dietary deficiency
  Malabsorption

Increased physiological demand

Loss through bleeding

Table 49.5 Typical daily requirements for iron

Infant (0–4 months)	0.5 mg
Adolescent male	1.8 mg
Adolescent female	2.4 mg
Adult male	0.9 mg
Menstruating female	2.0 mg
Pregnancy	3–5 mg
Postmenopausal female	0.9 mg

During pregnancy there is an increase in red cell mass but there is also a proportionally bigger increase in plasma volume, which results in a physiological dilutional anaemia. It is thought that the gut increases its ability to absorb iron during pregnancy to meet the additional demands of fetal red cell production. Some of the increased demand is met by the stopping of menstruation. If, however, there is inadequate iron absorption, then anaemia may result.

Clinical manifestations

In addition to the general symptoms of anaemia, various other features may be present (Table 49.6). The colour of the skin is very subjective and often unreliable. Patients at risk of heart failure may present with breathlessness when anaemic. Koilonychia, dysphagia and pica are found only after chronic iron deficiency and are relatively rare.

Table 49.6 Features of iron deficiency anaemia

Pale skin and mucous membranes

Painless glossitis

Angular stomatitis

Koilonychia (spoon-shaped nails)

Dysphagia (due to pharyngeal web)

Pica (unusual cravings)

Atrophic gastritis

A full blood count is an essential screening test. The cells of the peripheral blood are microcytic and hypochromic with poikilocytes (often pencil shaped) and occasional target cells (abnormal thin erythrocytes which when stained show a dark centre and peripheral ring).

Three parameters help establish the iron status of the patient: the plasma iron, the total iron binding capacity (TIBC) and the plasma ferritin. The plasma iron exhibits diurnal variation, being higher in the morning. Iron is transported around the body bound to a plasma protein called transferrin. Normally this protein is only one-third saturated with iron. The TIBC is the sum of the plasma iron and the unsaturated iron-binding capacity (UBIC) of the iron transport proteins in the blood. The plasma iron and TIBC vary with iron status (Fig. 49.2). The plasma ferritin level is low in iron deficiency anaemia and markedly raised in iron overload.

Investigations

The aim of treatment is to correct the anaemia and to replenish iron stores. Although the treatment of iron deficiency anaemia is relatively simple, it should not be embarked upon lightly. It is important to resolve the underlying cause as far as possible. Since gastrointestinal blood loss is the most common cause in men and postmenopausal women, examination of the upper and lower tract is an important investigation. If necessary, this may include upper gastrointestinal tract endoscopy, colonoscopy, barium enema and small bowel biopsy.

Over-the-counter sales of iron should be discouraged except in those patients who have been fully investigated. It is not unknown for patients to be given iron unnecessarily, resulting in iron overload. Also, giving iron therapy to a patient who is continuing to bleed from their gastrointestinal tract is not helping to resolve the underlying problem.

Treatment

Prophylaxis of iron deficiency anaemia was widely used in pregnancy (together with folic acid); however; it is now only used for women who have additional risk factors for iron deficiency such as poor diet. Prophylaxis may also be used in menorrhagia, after partial gastrectomy and in some low birth weight infants, e.g. premature twins.

If gastrointestinal investigation has been performed and any underlying cause treated, all patients should receive iron supplementation to correct their anaemia and replenish stores. Oral iron in the ferrous form is cheap, safe and effective in most patients. Depending on the state of the body's iron stores, it may be necessary to continue treatment for up to 6 months to both correct the anaemia and replenish body stores. The standard treatment is ferrous sulphate 200 mg 2–3 times a day. It typically takes between 1 and 2 weeks for the haemoglobin level to rise 1 g/dL. An earlier indication of the patient's response can be seen by looking at the reticulocyte count, which should start to rise 2–3 days after starting effective treatment.

Nausea or abdominal pain troubles some patients and this tends to be related to the dose of elemental iron. Giving the iron with food makes it better tolerated but tends to reduce the amount absorbed. Alternative salts of iron are sometimes tried; these cause fewer side effects simply because they contain less elemental iron (Table 49.7). Taking fewer ferrous sulphate tablets each day would have the same effect. A change in bowel habit (either constipation or diarrhoea) is sometimes reported and this is probably not dose related. During the early stages of treatment the body absorbs oral doses of iron better. Absorption is commonly around 15% of intake for the first 2–3 weeks but falls off to an average of 5% thereafter. It has been shown that for some patients, eradication of *Helicobacter pylori* aids recovery from iron deficiency anaemia (Annibale et al 1999).

There are a number of modified-release oral preparations available. They have no clear therapeutic advantage over ferrous sulphate and are not recommended. Indeed, the modified-release characteristic may cause the oral iron to be carried into the lower gut, which is much poorer at absorbing iron than the duodenum. Modified-release preparations may be more likely to exacerbate diarrhoea in patients with inflammatory bowel disease or diverticulae.

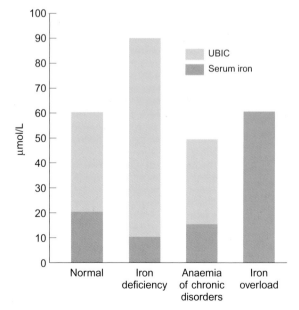

Figure 49.2 Typical examples of plasma iron and unsaturated iron binding capacity (UBIC).

Table 49.7 Elemental iron content of common oral preparations

Preparation	Approximate iron content
Tablets	
Ferrous sulphate 200 mg	65 mg
Ferrous gluconate 300 mg	35 mg
Ferrous fumarate 200 mg	65 mg
Oral liquids	
Ferrous fumarate 140 mg in 5 mL	45 mg
Ferrous glycine sulphate 141 mg in 5 mL	25 mg
Sodium feredetate 190 mg in 5 mL	27.5 mg

There is a limited place for parenteral iron in iron deficiency anaemia; it should be reserved for patients who fail on oral therapy, usually because of poor co-operation and intolerable gastrointestinal side effects. For most patients, when equivalent doses of oral and parenteral iron are used there is no difference in the rate at which the haemoglobin level rises. Patients who have lost blood acutely may require blood transfusions. The need for a rapid rise in haemoglobin is not an indication for parenteral iron. However, some patients with chronic renal failure appear to have a functional iron deficiency that responds to intravenous iron. These patients, despite receiving oral iron and epoetin (recombinant human erythropoietin), do respond with a rise in haemoglobin when given regular intravenous iron (Silverberg et al 1996).

There is a risk of anaphylactoid reactions with intravenous iron but the incidence appears to be lower with current products than with those previously on the market. Patients given the newer licensed products, iron dextran (CosmoFer) or iron sucrose (Venofer), should have a test dose and facilities for cardiopulmonary resuscitation must be available. The dose for both products is calculated from the body weight and iron deficit. Both preparations are given by slow intravenous injection or intravenous infusion. Iron dextran may also be given by deep intramuscular injection or by total dose infusion (though an increased incidence of adverse reactions is reported with this method). In renal patients a regular weekly dose is often given and the patient's plasma ferritin monitored to check for iron overload. Concerns have been expressed (Cavill 2003) about the possible long-term complications of intravenous iron such as atherosclerosis and increased risk of infection, but current direct evidence remains inconclusive.

Patient care

It is usual practice to advise patients to take iron products with or after meals as this probably reduces the incidence of nausea. Patients should be told that their faeces may become darker and that this is nothing to worry about. This is important in patients who have had melaena since they may associate their dark stools with the bleed and worry that they are still bleeding from the gastrointestinal tract. The length of treatment and compliance should be discussed and an explanation given that iron stores need to be replenished and that this takes time.

Anaemia of chronic disease

Epidemiology

Anaemia of chronic disease is a common disorder associated with a wide variety of inflammatory diseases including; arthritis, malignancies and inflammatory bowel disease.

Aetiology

In some cases there appears to be impaired response to erythropoietin. However, there is also a shift of iron from the circulation into the reticuloendothelial system leading to iron-restricted erythropoiesis despite normal iron stores.

Pathophysiology

Hepcidin, a peptide produced by hepatocytes, is now thought to play a key role in the regulation of iron. During infections, inflammation and in cancer, there is an upregulation of interleukin-6 which leads to an increased production of hepcidin. Hepcidin reduces intestinal iron absorption and 'locks' iron within hepatocytes and macrophages. The reduction of circulating iron is thought to limit this essential nutrient's availability to invading microbes and tumour cells, blocking their proliferation.

Clinical manifestations

Patients have the general symptoms of anaemia in addition to their symptoms of the chronic inflammatory condition. This frequently leads to a reduced quality of life for these patients.

Investigation

Patients have a hypochromic microcytic anaemia with low plasma iron but normal or raised plasma ferritin.

Treatment

Blood transfusions are rarely needed. Oral iron therapy is not usually indicated despite the apparent reduced iron availability since these patients have a functional iron deficiency rather than an actual iron deficiency. Some patients respond to erythropoietin. Treating the underlying inflammatory condition is important. It has been suggested that drugs which down regulate interleukin-6 may have some benefit (Altschuler & Kast 2005). Olanzepine and quetiapine (potent H_1 antagonists) are known to be regulators of interleukin-6 though not used clinically for this purpose. Furthermore, it is not known what other effects modifying interleukin-6 or hepcidin would have on the chronic inflammatory condition.

Patient care

Some patients hearing that they have anaemia may be tempted to go and purchase iron or other supplements. Careful explanation will help them make an informed decision.

Sideroblastic anaemias

Epidemiology

Sideroblastic anaemias are a group of conditions that are diagnosed by finding ring sideroblasts in the bone marrow. There are both hereditary and acquired forms. The hereditary forms are rare, whilst some of the acquired forms are relatively common, with as many as 30% of alcoholics admitted to hospital having sideroblastic anaemia.

Aetiology

In the majority of hereditary forms there is an X chromosome-linked pattern of inheritance. Both autosomal dominant and autosomal recessive families have been described. The main defect is a reduced activity of the enzyme 5-aminolaevulinate synthase (ALAS) which is involved in haem synthesis.

The acquired disorders include idiopathic forms, those associated with myeloproliferative disorders and forms secondary to the ingestion of drugs (Table 49.8). Regardless of the cause, there is impaired haem synthesis.

Pathophysiology

An examination of the bone marrow typically shows a number of erythroblasts that have iron granules surrounding the cell nucleus. These cells are known as ring sideroblasts. In the hereditary forms there are low levels of ALAS. This mitochondrial enzyme is involved in the first step in the synthesis of haem and requires pyridoxal phosphate as a co-factor. Pyridoxine is a precursor for pyridoxal.

Drugs and toxins

Alcohol can lead to the formation of ring sideroblasts. Ethanol is metabolized to acetaldehyde and it is the acetaldehyde that lowers the levels of ALAS and pyridoxal. Isoniazid is a known cause of sideroblasts. In slow acetylators of isoniazid, the drug reacts with pyridoxal and the resulting product is then rapidly excreted. Pyridoxine prophylaxis is usually given to all patients on isoniazid. Doses of chloramphenicol over 2 g a day invariably lead to sideroblasts. This is thought to be due to the inhibition of mitochondrial protein synthesis. Sideroblastic anaemia is also associated with copper deficiency which can be caused by an overdose of the chelators penicillamine and triethylene tetramine dihydrochloride (used in the treatment of Wilson's disease).

Clinical manifestations

The hereditary forms typically develop in infancy or childhood. The anaemia can be severe or mild (Hb 4–10 g/dL). There may be splenomegaly, which can lead to mild thrombocytopenia. The idiopathic acquired forms tend to develop insidiously, usually in

middle age or later. Many patients may be asymptomatic for long periods. In the forms associated with other disorders, the clinical picture tends to be dominated by the underlying disease.

Investigations

In the hereditary form the red cells in the peripheral blood are hypochromic and microcytic. Despite this, there are frequently increased iron stores in the bone marrow. The plasma iron and ferritin may also be high. In the acquired forms the peripheral blood has hypochromic cells, which may be either normocytic or macrocytic. The common finding is the presence of sideroblasts in the bone marrow.

Treatment

In patients with the hereditary forms, large doses of pyridoxine (typically 100–200 mg daily or even up to 400 mg) may reduce the severity of the anaemia. Long-term high-dose pyridoxine has been associated with peripheral neuropathy and so lower maintenance doses are sometimes tried. There have been case reports of patients responding to parenteral pyridoxal-5-phosphate after failing to respond to pyridoxine. Patients with an acquired form occasionally respond to high-dose pyridoxine, and a 2–3 month trial may be helpful in symptomatic patients. The response tends to be slow and only partial. The investigational agent haem arginate has been shown to increase the red cell count and decrease the number of ring sideroblasts in some patients with acquired sideroblastic anaemia. In common with other conditions where an increased turnover of cells in the bone marrow is a feature, folate supplements are often necessary.

Although the peripheral blood cells are frequently hypochromic and microcytic, the condition is associated with increased iron stores so iron supplements should be avoided. The drugs and toxins (see Table 49.8) tend to cause a reversible anaemia. Removing the offending agent usually resolves the anaemia.

Iron overload

Inevitably some patients fail to respond to these treatments and frequent blood transfusions are required. This leads to the complications of iron overload and sensitization and the risk of blood-borne virus transmission.

The chelating agent desferrioxamine is given by either intravenous or subcutaneous infusion. It binds free iron and iron bound to ferritin. Therapy should be considered when the plasma ferritin level reaches 1000 μg/L. Patients with very high ferritin levels may need daily infusions. Daily subcutaneous infusions using a disposable infusor or small infusion pump are suitable for home use. In the UK a number of commercial healthcare companies provide a desferrioxamine home care service. Published evidence suggests that for an equivalent dose, a longer infusion time results in increased iron excretion. Intravenous infusions can be given whenever the patient goes into hospital for a blood transfusion. Small doses (<200 mg) of vitamin C increase the effectiveness of desferrioxamine, probably by facilitating iron release from the reticuloendothelial system. Higher doses of vitamin C are reported to increase the cardiotoxicity of iron overload. Patients with cardiac failure should

Table 49.8 Acquired sideroblastic anaemia
Associated with other disorders
Myelodysplastic syndromes
Myeloid leukaemia
Myeloma
Collagen diseases
Associated with drugs and toxins
Alcohol
Isoniazid
Chloramphenicol
Penicillamine
Pyrazinamide
Cycloserine
Progesterone (single case report)
Copper deficiency (associated with penicillamine and triethylene tetramine dihydrochloride)

not be given vitamin C with desferrioxamine. Desferrioxamine should not be given concurrently with prochlorperazine as prolonged unconsciousness may result.

An oral agent, deferiprone, has been shown to be beneficial (Al-Refaie et al 1997). Unfortunately, it is reported to cause reversible neutropenia in some patients. It is licensed for patients intolerant of desferrioxamine and weekly neutrophil counts are required. There are few reports of trials using a combination of deferiprone and desferrioxamine. A new, orally active, N-substituted bis-hydroxyphenyl-triazole (Exjade) has completed phase I and phase II clinical trials and is showing promise. Early studies suggest that it is at least as effective as deferrioxamine, with a tolerability and safety profile suitable for chronic, once-daily administration.

Patient care

Few patients with hereditary or idiopathic acquired forms have completely reversible anaemia. Patients need to be aware that pyridoxine may take several months before there is any improvement. They should be advised not to purchase over-the-counter iron or vitamin supplements, particularly ascorbic acid or pyridoxine, without discussing it with their consultant.

Megaloblastic anaemias

The megaloblastic anaemias are macrocytic anaemias (raised MCV) associated with an abnormality in the maturation of haematopoietic cells in the bone marrow. In addition to abnormal red cells, the white cells and platelets may be affected. The two major causes are folate deficiency and vitamin B_{12} deficiency. Pernicious anaemia is a specific autoimmune disease that causes malabsorption of vitamin B_{12} due to a lack of intrinsic factor.

Epidemiology

Folate deficiency anaemia

Much of the world's population has a marginal dietary intake of folate. Body stores are low and as soon as there is a decrease in dietary intake or there is increased folate demand, deficiency readily occurs.

Vitamin B_{12} deficiency anaemia

Strict vegans (e.g. Hindus) commonly have low vitamin B_{12} levels due to their dietary deficiency though actual anaemia is rarer. All patients who have had a total gastrectomy and up to 15% of those with a partial gastrectomy will develop vitamin B_{12} deficiency anaemia.

Pernicious anaemia

Pernicious anaemia is found most commonly in people of northern European descent. In the UK, the incidence is about 120 per 100000 and is higher in Scotland than in the south of England. Pernicious anaemia is usually a disease of the elderly, the average patient presenting at 60 years of age.

Aetiology

Folate deficiency anaemia

Folate is readily available in a normal diet. Fruit, green vegetables and yeast all contain relatively large amounts of folate. Despite this relative abundance of folate in many foods, dietary deficiency is common, either as the sole cause of the folic acid deficiency anaemia or in conjunction with increased folate utilization.

Vitamin B_{12} deficiency anaemia

Deficiency occurs from inadequate intake or malabsorption. The only dietary source of vitamin B_{12} (cyanocobalamin) is from food of animal origin. It is present in meat, fish, eggs, cheese and milk. Cooking does not usually destroy vitamin B_{12}. Daily requirements are between 1 and $3\,\mu g$. Deficiency arises either from inadequate intake over a prolonged period or, more commonly in the West, from impaired absorption due to lack of intrinsic factor.

Malabsorption occurs if the distal ileum is removed; it may also occur with certain intestinal pathologies, particularly stagnant loop syndrome, tropical sprue and fish tapeworm infestation. Passive absorption does take place in the jejunum but this is very inefficient and usually accounts for less than 1% of an oral dose.

Pathophysiology

The common biochemical defect in all megaloblastic anaemias is the inhibition of DNA synthesis in maturing cells.

Folate deficiency anaemia

The folate found in food is mainly conjugated to polyglutamic acid. Enzymes found in the gut convert the polyglutamate form to monoglutamate, which is readily absorbed. During absorption the folate is methylated and reduced to methyltetrahydrofolate monoglutamate. This travels through the plasma and is transported into cells via a carrier specific for the tetrahydrofolate form. Within the cell the methyl group is removed (in a reaction requiring vitamin B_{12}) and the folate is reconverted back to a polyglutamate form (Fig. 49.3). It has been suggested that the polyglutamate form prevents the folate leaking out of cells. The folate eventually acts as a co-enzyme involved in a number of reactions, including DNA and RNA synthesis.

Defective DNA synthesis mainly affects cells with a rapid turnover, e.g. gastrointestinal cells and red blood cells, hence the sore tongue and anaemia seen in folate deficiency. During DNA synthesis the folate co-enzyme is oxidized to the dihydrofolate form, which is inactive and has to be reactivated by the enzyme dihydrofolate reductase. This is the enzyme inhibited by methotrexate and to a lesser extent by trimethoprim and pyrimethamine. Co-trimoxazole, although much less used now than in the past, has been shown to increase the severity of megaloblastic anaemia.

Vitamin B_{12} deficiency

Absorption of vitamin B_{12} is mainly by an active process. Enzymes in the stomach release vitamin B_{12} from protein complexes. One

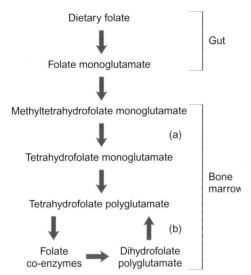

Dietary folate

Folate monoglutamate

Gut

Methyltetrahydrofolate monoglutamate

(a)

Tetrahydrofolate monoglutamate

Tetrahydrofolate polyglutamate

Bone marrow

Folate co-enzymes → Dihydrofolate polyglutamate

(b)

Figure 49.3 Simplified pathway of folate metabolism. **(a)** Vitamin B$_{12}$ is required as a co-enzyme for this reaction; **(b)** the enzyme dihydrofolate reductase converts inactive dihydrofolate back to the active tetrahydrofolate.

Table 49.9 Features of megaloblastic anaemia

Glossitis (sore, pale, smooth tongue)
Angular stomatitis
Altered bowel habit (diarrhoea or constipation)
Anorexia
Mild jaundice
Insidious onset
Sterility
Bilateral peripheral neuropathy (mainly vitamin B$_{12}$ deficiency)
Melanin skin pigmentation (rare)
Fever (mainly vitamin B$_{12}$ deficiency)

molecule of vitamin B$_{12}$ then combines with one molecule of a glycoprotein called intrinsic factor. The intrinsic factor protects the vitamin B$_{12}$ from breakdown by micro-organisms. There are specific receptors in the distal ileum for the intrinsic factor–vitamin B$_{12}$ complex. The vitamin B$_{12}$ enters the ileal cell and is then transported through the blood attached to transport proteins. Intrinsic factor does not appear in the blood.

Since intrinsic factor is only produced by the gastric parietal cells, a total gastrectomy always leads to vitamin B$_{12}$ deficiency. Approximately 10–15% of patients who have had a partial gastrectomy also develop deficiency. The onset of anaemia is usually delayed because the body typically has stores of 2–3 mg, which is sufficient for 2–3 years. Vitamin B$_{12}$ is a co-enzyme for the removal of a methyl group from methyltetrahydrofolate. Lack of vitamin B$_{12}$ traps the folate as methyltetrahydrofolate, and prevents DNA synthesis (see Fig. 49.3). The exact mechanism by which vitamin B$_{12}$ deficiency causes neuropathy is not clear but it may be due to a defect in the methylation reactions needed for myelin formation.

Pernicious anaemia

Pernicious anaemia is probably autoimmune in origin. Patients typically have a gastric atrophy and no (or virtually no) intrinsic factor secretion. Although not present in all patients, two different antibodies have been found in the plasma of some patients with pernicious anaemia.

Clinical manifestations

In addition to the general features of anaemia, megaloblastic anaemia, of which folic acid deficiency and B$_{12}$ deficiency anaemia are the two most common examples, has certain specific characteristics (Table 49.9).

Folate deficiency anaemia

Alcoholics and the elderly are particularly prone to nutritional deficiency. Elderly people living alone on tea and toast are typical examples of at-risk patients. Many alcoholics develop deficiency due to their poor diet; although some beers contain small amounts of folate, spirits contain none. A number of drugs have been implicated in causing folate deficiency (Table 49.10). Actual megaloblastic anaemia from drug therapy is uncommon and the exact mechanism(s) has not always been established. Serious malabsorption can occur in tropical sprue and coeliac disease. Reduced absorption is seen in Crohn's disease and following partial gastrectomy or jejunal resection.

There is a physiological increase in folate utilization during pregnancy. There may also be an increased utilization in various pathological conditions in association with inflammation or in a number of chronic haemolytic anaemias, particularly thalassaemia major, sickle cell disease and autoimmune haemolytic anaemia. Chronic folate deficiency probably predisposes patients to thrombosis, depression and neoplasia.

Table 49.10 Drugs implicated in causing folate deficiency anaemia

Malabsorption
Phenytoin
Barbiturates
Sulfasalazine
Colestyramine
Oral contraceptives

Impaired metabolism
Methotrexate
Pyrimethamine
Triamterene
Pentamidine
Trimethoprim

Vitamin B$_{12}$ deficiency anaemia

The megaloblastic anaemia caused by vitamin B$_{12}$ deficiency has similar features to folate deficiency (see Table 49.9). In addition to the macrocytosis, anisocytosis and poikilocytosis, there is often mild thrombocytopenia. The spleen may be slightly enlarged and there may be a slight fever. Mild jaundice may be present due to the increased breakdown of haemoglobin found in the abnormal red cells. The onset is slow and insidious so patients often present late or are diagnosed during other investigations. The feature that separates vitamin B$_{12}$ deficiency from the other megaloblastic anaemias is progressive neuropathy. It is symmetrical and affects the legs rather than the arms. Patients notice a tingling in their feet and a loss of vibration sense. Occasionally patients have muscle weakness or difficulty in walking or experience frequent falls.

Investigations

Folic acid deficiency anaemia

Many patients are symptomless initially, and the diagnosis is often made following a full blood count carried out for another reason. The peripheral blood reveals large oval red cells. Anisocytosis and poikilocytosis are common. Some of the neutrophils are hypersegmented, and thrombocytopenia may be present. The red cell folate concentration accurately reflects folate stores and is a preferable parameter than the plasma folate concentration, which is subject to changes in diet and does not correlate as closely with anaemia.

Vitamin B$_{12}$ deficiency anaemia

Following the detection of macrocytes in the full blood count, one of the first investigations will be the determination of the plasma vitamin B$_{12}$ level. This level is low in mild anaemia and may be very low if there is marked megaloblastic anaemia or neuropathy. If there is no concurrent folate deficiency the folate level tends to be raised whilst the red cell folate level falls, possibly due to a failure of folate polyglutamate synthesis in cells. False positives (low vitamin B$_{12}$ level without true deficiency) may be seen in multiple myeloma, excessive ascorbic acid intake and pregnancy. In contrast, liver disease, lymphoma, autoimmune disease and myeloproliferative disorders may lead to a false-negative result (normal levels in the presence of true deficiency).

The detection of autoantibodies is helpful in distinguishing pernicious anaemia from other forms (Table 49.11). The presence of intrinsic factor antibodies is virtually diagnostic of pernicious anaemia because it is rarely found in any other condition. However, it is not a very sensitive test since only half the patients with pernicious anaemia have these antibodies. Gastric parietal cell antibodies are found in 85% of patients with pernicious anaemia (a more sensitive test) but unfortunately also found in up to 10% of people without pernicious anaemia (less specific).

Oral vitamin B$_{12}$ absorption can be measured using the Schilling test though this is now rarely used in practice as most vitamin B$_{12}$ deficiencies are treated in the same way. The test is based on giving a radiolabelled oral dose of vitamin B$_{12}$ and an unlabelled parenteral dose that saturates the vitamin B$_{12}$-binding proteins. The amount of labelled vitamin in the urine gives a measure of oral absorption. The test can be repeated by giving the radiolabelled oral dose with intrinsic factor. The absorption should now be approaching normal if the patient has intrinsic factor deficiency but remains low if there is ileal disease.

Treatment

It is necessary to establish whether the patient with megaloblastic anaemia has vitamin B$_{12}$ deficiency or folic acid deficiency or both. Treatment of vitamin B$_{12}$ deficiency with folic acid may lead to the resolution of the haematological abnormalities but does not correct the neuropathy, which continues to deteriorate. If it is not possible to delay treatment until a definitive diagnosis is made, both folic acid and vitamin B$_{12}$ may be given.

Folate deficiency anaemia

Folate deficiency is usually managed by replacement therapy. The duration of the treatment depends on the cause of the deficiency. Changes in dietary habits or removal of any precipitating factor should also be considered.

The normal daily requirement of folic acid is approximately 100 μg a day; despite this, the usual treatment doses given are 5–15 mg a day. Even in malabsorption states, because of these large doses, sufficient folate is usually absorbed. Therefore parenteral folic acid treatment is not normally required. Treatment for 4 months will normally be sufficient to ensure that folate-deficient red cells are replaced.

Large doses of folic acid can produce a partial haematological response in patients with vitamin B$_{12}$ deficiency. The blood picture appears nearly normal but the neurological damage due to the vitamin B$_{12}$ deficiency continues. Folic acid therapy should not be started until vitamin B$_{12}$ deficiency has been excluded. It has also been suggested that patients on long-term folic acid therapy should have their vitamin B$_{12}$ levels checked at regular intervals, e.g. yearly.

Pregnancy The folate requirement increases in pregnancy and is higher in twin pregnancies. Folate deficiency regularly occurs in patients with a poor diet who do not take supplements. Prophylaxis with folate (350–500 μg daily) is now frequently given in pregnancy, often in combination with iron, starting before conception and during the first 12 weeks of pregnancy. It is important that products with low doses of folate are not used to treat megaloblastic anaemia. Although this low-dose folate should be started before conception to prevent a first occurrence of neural tube defect, higher doses (5 mg daily) are required for

Table 49.11 Autoantibodies in pernicious anaemia		
	Intrinsic factor antibodies	Parietal cell antibodies
Patients with pernicious anaemia	Detected in 50% of patients	Detected in 85% of patients
People who do not have pernicious anaemia	Rarely detected	Detected in up to 10%

the first 12 weeks of pregnancy in women with a history of neural tube defects.

Vitamin B$_{12}$ deficiency anaemia

The majority of patients with vitamin B$_{12}$ deficiency require life-long replacement therapy. Occasionally specific therapy related to the underlying disorder may be all that is necessary, e.g. treatment of fish tapeworm.

Since the anaemia has developed slowly the cardiovascular system does not tolerate blood transfusions very well and can be easily overloaded. Transfusions should not normally be given. In severe cases where emergency transfusion is deemed necessary, packed cells may be given slowly whilst blood (mainly plasma) is removed from the other arm. Diuretics may also need to be given, especially if the patient has congestive heart failure and poorly tolerates fluid overload.

For most patients a definite diagnosis is made before treatment is started. The standard treatment is hydroxocobalamin 1 mg intramuscularly three times a week for 2 weeks, then 1 mg every 3 months. Where there is neurological involvement a slightly higher dose regimen is recommended of 1 mg on alternate days until no further improvement then 1 mg every 2 months. There is no evidence that larger doses provide any additional benefit in neuropathy. In the UK, hydroxocobalamin is the treatment of choice. It is retained in the body longer than cyanocobalamin, and reactions to it are very rare. US texts recommend cyanocobalamin rather than hydroxocobalamin because of the fear that some patients appear to develop antibodies to the vitamin B$_{12}$ transport protein complex in the serum. The haematological response to both is probably identical. A small amount of passive absorption of vitamin B$_{12}$ does take place from the gastrointestinal tract. An oral dose of 1 mg every day is worth trying in patients who are unable to have injections. In the UK cyanocobalamin tablets are not available on the NHS except to treat or prevent vitamin B$_{12}$ deficiency in a patient who is a vegan or who has proven vitamin B$_{12}$ deficiency of dietary origin.

Hypokalaemia develops in some patients during the initial haematological response because potassium is an intracellular ion and is used in the production of new cells. Potassium supplements may be needed in the elderly and patients receiving diuretics or digoxin. The plasma iron level also falls as it is incorporated into haemoglobin. The more severe the anaemia, the more likely it is to see a fall in the potassium or iron level.

Not only is it gratifying to follow the response to treatment, it is also important to monitor the response to ensure the patient returns to normal without any attendant problems. There is often a subjective improvement before an objective one. Typically the patient feels better within 24–48 hours and yet there may be no discernible haematological response. The first haematological change in the peripheral blood is a rise in the reticulocyte count starting around day 3 or 4 and peaking after 7–8 days. The more severe the anaemia, the higher the peak reticulocyte count. The reticulocyte count should remain raised whilst the haematocrit is less than 35%. Failure to remain raised during this time indicates the need for further evaluation. The arrest or slowing down of erythropoiesis may be due to inadequate stores of other essential factors, e.g. iron, or may be due to co-existing disease such as hypothyroidism or infection.

The red cells return to normal and the platelet count rises to normal (or even higher) after 7–10 days. The haemoglobin takes much longer to return to normal. It should rise by approximately 2–3 g/dL each fortnight. Neurological damage may be irreversible. Peripheral neuropathy of recent onset often partially improves but any spinal cord damage is irreversible, even with optimum therapy.

Patient care

Folic acid deficiency anaemia

In patients who have a dietary component to their deficiency, appropriate nutritional advice should go alongside their folic acid therapy. If the cause of the deficiency has been eliminated patients can expect to receive folic acid for approximately 4–6 months. In patients with a continuing requirement (e.g. haemolytic anaemia), treatment will be lifelong. Those starting out on folic acid therapy can anticipate feeling better after a few days but should be informed that their blood count will take much longer to return to normal.

Vitamin B$_{12}$ deficiency anaemia

Patients feel subjectively better very shortly after their first hydroxocobalamin injection. They can be told that their sore tongue will start to improve within 2 days and be back to normal after 2–4 weeks. Patients need to be informed that they need regular injections, usually every 3 months. Surprisingly, some patients say they feel ready for the injection as they approach their appointment time and feel better after the injection. Compliance is not usually a problem.

Haemolytic anaemias

In the haemolytic anaemias there is a reduced lifespan of the erythrocytes. If the rate of destruction of the erythrocytes exceeds the rate of production then anaemia results. There is a wide range of haemolytic anaemias with both genetic and acquired disorders (Table 49.12). Only autoimmune haemolytic anaemia, sickle cell anaemia, thalassaemia and glucose-6-phosphate dehydrogenase deficiency will be briefly discussed. Haemolytic anaemias account for approximately 5% of all anaemias.

General clinical manifestations

Patients with acute haemolytic anaemia commonly complain of malaise, fever, abdominal pain, dark urine and jaundice. They have haemoglobulinaemia, hyperbilirubinaemia, reticulocytosis and increased urobilinogen levels in the urine. Patients with chronic haemolytic anaemia also usually have splenomegaly. Their anaemia is usually normochromic and normocytic.

General treatment

Many patients with chronic haemolytic anaemia will have an overactive bone marrow to compensate for the chronic haemolysis. This increases demand for folate and folic acid

Table 49.12 Examples of haemolytic anaemia

	Examples
Genetic disorder of	
Membrane	Hereditary spherocytosis
	Hereditary ovalcytosis
Haemoglobin	Sickle cell anaemias
	Thalassaemias
Energy pathways	Glucose-6-phosphate deficiency
Acquired disorders	
Immune	Rh or ABO incompatibility
	Autoimmune
Non-immune	Infections (parasitic, bacterial)
	Drugs and chemicals
	Hypersplenism

Table 49.13 Drugs associated with autoimmune haemolytic anaemia

Ciclosporin
Fludarabin
Interferon A
Levodopa
Mefenamic acid
Methyldopa
Penicillin
Quinine
Quinidine

supplements are therefore often required, particularly for patients with a poor diet.

Autoimmune haemolytic anaemia

Epidemiology

This is a range of conditions consisting of warm autoimmune haemolytic anaemia (WAIHA) and cold autoimmune haemolytic anaemia, also known as cold agglutinin disease (CAD). Both forms can be subdivided into idiopathic and acquired forms and are found in all races. The most common form is idiopathic WAIHA which occurs in approximately 40% of all cases with an incidence of between 1 in 40000 and 1 in 80000. Idiopathic CAD tends to present in middle age.

Aetiology

WAIHA is frequently associated with other diseases which have an immunological component, e.g. chronic lymphocytic leukaemia, systemic lupus erythematosus, hepatitis B. Acquired CAD is sometimes associated with viral or bacterial infections; cold agglutinins develop in more than 60% of patients following infectious mononucleosis but haemolytic anaemia is rare. A number of drugs have been implicated as leading to immune haemolysis (Table 49.13).

Pathophysiology

The anaemia results from the presence of autoantibodies which agglutinate or lyse the patient's own erythrocytes. In WAIHA the haemolysis is usually extravascular and mediated by IgG. These antibodies react best at body temperature. CAD is usually mediated by IgM and is capable of fixing complement. The IgM antibody attaches to the erythrocytes and causes them to agglutinate at temperatures below 37°C, resulting in impaired blood flow to fingers, toes, nose and ears when exposed to cold.

Clinical manifestations

The symptoms in WAIHA depend on the severity of the haemolysis. In CAD, severity of the clinical manifestations ranges from an inconsequential laboratory finding in the benign variety to acute haemolytic crises and Raynaud-type phenomena. A common complaint is painful fingers and toes with purplish discoloration associated with cold exposure. In chronic CAD, the patient is more symptomatic during the colder months.

Investigations

A positive direct Coombs test indicates the presence of antibodies to red blood cells. Further laboratory serological testing helps determine the exact nature of the reaction. Drug-induced haemolytic anaemia may be difficult to distinguish from other forms of autoimmune haemolytic anaemia and a clear medication history will help. The antibodies produced may react with the red cells only in the presence of the drug or one of its metabolites, or may also react without the drug being present.

Treatment

Treatment is dependent on the specific cause (Pruss et al 2003). In WAIHA the standard treatment is high-dose corticosteroids. Patients who do not respond can be managed with azathioprine or cyclophosphamide. Blood transfusions are necessary in severe cases, though providing blood free from underlying alloantibodies is difficult. Rituximab has been shown to be beneficial in some patients who fail to respond to corticosteroids. Patients with CAD need to be kept warm and provided with supportive measures as well as treatment for any underlying disorder.

Patient care

Patients requiring rituximab will need careful explanation of its unlicensed use and the necessary pretreatment with paracetamol and chlorphenamine.

Sickle cell anaemia

Epidemiology

Sickle cell disease is a hereditary condition and several different variants exist. It is found in a number of ethnic groups, mainly in populations that originate from tropical regions. In the UK approximately 5000 people, largely from the Afro-Caribbean population, have sickle cell disease.

Aetiology

Patients with sickle cell disease have a different form of haemoglobin. Patients with the most common variant of sickle cell disease have haemoglobin S (Hb S) whereas normal haemoglobin is usually designated Hb A. Haemoglobin S has valine substituted for glutamic acid as the sixth amino acid in the β-polypeptide compared with normal haemoglobin. Patients with homozygous Hb S develop many problems, including anaemia.

Sickle cell trait is where a person is a carrier of the gene (heterozygous for the sickle cell gene) and is usually asymptomatic. The offspring from a father with trait (AS) and a mother with trait (AS) has a 1 in 4 chance of having sickle cell disease (see Fig. 49.4).

Pathophysiology

The membrane of red cells containing Hb S is damaged, which leads to intracellular dehydration. In addition, when the patient's blood is deoxygenated, polymerization of Hb S occurs, forming a semisolid gel. These two processes lead to the formation of crescent-shaped cells known as sickle cells. Sickle cells are less flexible than normal cells (flexibility allows normal cells to pass through the microcirculation) and this leads to impaired blood flow through the microcirculation, resulting in local tissue hypoxia. Anaemia results from an increased destruction of red cells. Some red cells in patients with sickle cell disease contain fetal haemoglobin (Hb F). These cells do not sickle, i.e. sickle cells do not form as described above.

Clinical manifestations

Patients with severe variants of the disease have chronic anaemia, arthralgia, anorexia, fatigue and splenomegaly. They have crises more frequently than patients with other variants of the disease. A crisis can be precipitated by infection and fever, dehydration, hypoxia or acidosis. A combination of these factors is sometimes present. The clinical manifestation of a crisis can vary, with the most common being an infarct crisis. Infarction of the long bones and larger joints or an infarction of a large organ, e.g. liver, lungs or brain, may occur. Severe pain is a common feature, depending on the site of the infarction. Destructive bone and joint problems are frequently seen.

Investigations

The common form usually presents in the first year of life. From then on patients have a chronic haemolytic anaemia interspersed with crises. Abnormal haemoglobin can be detected using electrophoresis. The proportion of Hb S is a useful monitoring parameter. Regular plasma ferritin determinations identify the need for desferrioxamine therapy and are used to monitor progress.

Treatment

Patients with sickle cell disease have a high incidence of pneumococcal infections and a number of studies have shown the benefit of prophylactic antibiotics. Penicillin V 250 mg twice a day is usual for adults (erythromycin for patients allergic to penicillin). Administration of pneumococcal vaccine and *Haemophilus influenzae* vaccine is now common.

Attempts have been made to increase the proportion of Hb F and reduce the proportion of Hb S in the circulation. Several drugs (Table 49.14) have been shown (some only in animal models) to stimulate fetal haemoglobin production (Charache et al 1995).

Hydroxycarbamide is effective and may reduce the frequency of crises but is limited by its cytotoxicity. Erythropoietin has been shown to increase Hb F in some animal models, but this

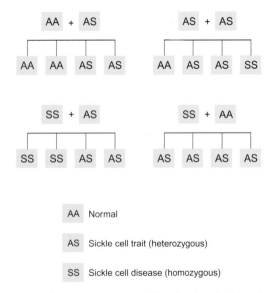

AA	Normal
AS	Sickle cell trait (heterozygous)
SS	Sickle cell disease (homozygous)

Figure 49.4 Inheritance patterns in sickle cell trait and sickle cell disease.

Table 49.14 Drugs that may increase fetal haemoglobin production (Hb F)
5-azacytidine
Cytarabine
Vinblastine
Hydroxycarbamide
Erythropoietin
Short chain fatty acids (butyrates, valproate)

has yet to be fully demonstrated in humans. Transfusions and exchange transfusions have also been used to decrease the proportion of Hb S. This is limited by the usual complications of chronic infusions: iron overload, the risk of blood-borne virus transmission and sensitization.

Sickle cell crises require prompt and effective treatment. Removal of the trigger factor, hydration and effective pain relief are the mainstays of treatment. Appropriate antibiotic therapy should be started at the first sign of infection and strong opioids are required for pain relief. Traditionally many patients have been given frequent intramuscular injections of pethidine. Pethidine is not ideal since it is short-acting, not very potent and repeated injections lead to the accumulation of metabolites that have been associated with seizures. Morphine is a more logical choice of opioid. Some centres are having success with morphine in a patient-controlled analgesia system (PCAS).

Patient care

Patients need to be encouraged to take their prophylactic penicillin and folic acid therapy regularly between crises. During a crisis some health professionals worry about the patient developing opioid addiction. While this may happen, it is also important to recognize that crises are extremely painful and the patient requires effective analgesia.

Thalassaemias

Epidemiology

The β thalassaemias occur mainly in populations from around the Mediterranean, North and West Africa, Middle East and Indian subcontinent. More than 100 β thalassaemia mutations have been identified and they tend to produce severe anaemia. The α thalassaemias are more common, of which the milder variants do not cause severe anaemia whilst the severe homozygotes lead to death in utero or infancy.

Aetiology

In α thalassaemia there is either no α chain production (α^0 thalassaemia) or reduced production of a chain (α^+ thalassaemia). Similarly for α thalassaemia. Heterozygotes are usually symptomless whilst homozygotes are more severely affected, as are compound heterozygotes in which there is a thalassaemia gene and a gene from another haemoglobin variant (e.g. Hb S).

Pathophysiology

In β thalassaemias there is reduced or absent production of the globin β chain. This leads to a relative excess of α chain which, when unpaired, becomes unstable and precipitates in the red cell precursors. There is ineffective erythropoiesis and those mature cells that reach the circulation have a shortened lifespan.

In α thalassaemias the pathology is slightly different. The deficiency of α chains leads to an excess of γ or β chains. This time erythropoiesis is less affected but the haemoglobin produced (haemoglobin Bart's or haemoglobin H) is unstable when the cells are in the circulation and precipitates as the cells grow older.

This leads to a shortened lifespan with the spleen trapping many of the cells. Haemoglobin Bart's and haemoglobin H are also physiologically useless.

Clinical manifestations

The anaemia causes erythropoietin production to increase and results in expansion of the bone marrow. In severe disease this causes bone deformity and growth retardation. The spleen is actively involved in removing the abnormal mature cells from the circulation and becomes enlarged.

Investigations

For β thalassaemia the diagnosis is relatively straightforward: haemolytic anaemia from infancy and racial background. Haemoglobin electrophoresis is used to determine the amounts of abnormal haemoglobin.

Treatment

There is currently no effective treatment. Many patients with severe forms are transfusion dependent from an early age and this inevitably leads to iron overload. Desferrioxamine and deferiprone are routinely used. Splenectomy helps some patients. Prevention is actively explored, with genetic counselling programmes in Italy and Greece and antenatal screening in a number of countries.

As in sickle cell disease, much attention is being placed on the idea of switching the bone marrow to the production of fetal haemoglobin rather than the defective adult haemoglobin of β thalassaemia. These therapies are still in the early stages of development. It is likely that a combination of drugs (hydroxycarbamide and erythropoietin) will provide some clinical improvement.

Patient care

Currently drug therapy does not play a large part in treatment.

Glucose-6-phosphate dehydrogenase deficiency

Epidemiology

Approximately 400 million people in the world are affected by glucose-6-phosphate dehydrogenase (G6PD) deficiency. There are more than 300 different forms of G6PD deficiency, only some of which cause anaemia. The most common form of G6PD deficiency is found in 15% of black Americans. It causes anaemia when the individual is exposed to a trigger factor. A more severe form is the Mediterranean variant of G6PD deficiency. Some of these individuals may have chronic haemolytic anaemia even in the apparent absence of exposure to a precipitating factor.

Aetiology

There are many variants of G6PD activity found in different populations and ethnic groups. G6PD is an erythrocyte enzyme that is indirectly involved in the production of reduced glutathione.

Glutathione is produced in response to, and protects red cells from, oxidizing reagents.

Pathophysiology

G6PD is essential for the production of nicotinamide adenine dinucleotide phosphate (NADPH) in erythrocytes. If there is a deficiency in G6PD this decreases the production of NADPH which is needed to keep glutathione in a reduced form. Reduced glutathione helps erythrocytes deal with oxidative stress. Hence in G6PD deficiency, if the erythrocytes are exposed to an oxidizing agent, the cell membrane becomes damaged, the haemoglobin becomes oxidized and forms Heinz bodies. Some of the red cells haemolyse and others have their Heinz bodies removed by the spleen to form 'bite cells'.

Clinical manifestations

Clinically the two most important types of G6PD deficiency occur in the black population and in people originating from the Mediterranean. The black population has a milder form that results in an acute self-limiting haemolytic anaemia following exposure to an oxidizing agent, e.g. infection, acute illness, fava beans or drugs (Table 49.15). The haemolytic anaemia is self-limiting because the young cells produced by the bone marrow have higher levels of G6PD activity than old cells. Following exposure to the oxidizing agent, the old cells are haemolysed but the new cells produced in response are more capable of tolerating the insult until they grow old. In the Mediterranean form of the disorder, the enzyme activity is very low, haemolysis is not usually self-limiting and, indeed, some patients have a chronic haemolytic anaemia despite the absence of an obvious causative factor.

Investigations

The history and the clinical findings steer the diagnosis, which is then confirmed by measuring G6PD activity. Care must be taken during the acute phase since there are increased numbers of young cells with higher levels of activity that may be misleading. The increased numbers of young cells result from the selective destruction of older cells and the increased production of reticulocytes.

Treatment

In cases of acute haemolytic anaemia, the causative oxidizing agent should be stopped and general supportive measures adopted. In chronic haemolytic anaemia most patients become reasonably well adjusted to their anaemia. They need to avoid known precipitating factors to prevent acute episodes occurring on top of their chronic haemolytic anaemia.

There is no specific drug treatment. During acute episodes the patient should be kept well hydrated to ensure good urine output to prevent haemoglobin damaging the kidney. Blood transfusions may be necessary. Vitamin E (an antioxidant) appears to have little clinical benefit in preventing haemolysis.

Table 49.15 Common drugs implicated in causing haemolysis in G6PD deficiency

Drugs to be avoided in all variants
Ciprofloxacin (and probably other quinolones)
Dapsone
Methylene blue
Primaquine (reduced dose may be used in milder variants)
Nalidixic acid
Sulfonamides (including co-trimoxazole)

Drugs to be avoided in more severe variants
Aspirin (low dose used under supervision)
Chloramphenicol
Chloroquine (may be acceptable in acute malaria)
Menadione
Probenicid
Quinidine
Quinine (acceptable in acute malaria)

Patient care

Drug therapy does not play a large part in the management of these patients. Patients can be given a list of drugs to avoid but since most of these drugs are prescription-only medicines it is important that patients remind healthcare professionals of their condition.

CASE STUDIES

Case 49.1

Mr HA, a 62-year-old single, unemployed man, was admitted to hospital for investigation of anaemia. He presented with a 6-month history of lethargy, chest pain, dizziness and falls, and a past history of having a partial gastrectomy 16 years ago. The drug history taken by the junior doctor showed that Mr HA was taking diazepam and a GTN spray on admission.

Review of systems revealed no vomiting and no melaena. He complained of some indigestion after meals and reported his appetite as 'fine if someone else cooks'. On examination he was pale, with a blood pressure of 140/80, a pulse of 90 and a haemoglobin level of 2.5 g/dL (normal range 13.5–18.0 g/dL). A gastroscopy was normal and a biopsy showed no evidence of coeliac disease. A barium enema was normal and faecal occult bloods (FOBs) negative.

Over the first 3 days he was transfused with 8 units of blood and was given furosemide (frusemide) 40 mg with alternate bags. On day 7 he was started on ferrous sulphate 200 mg three times a day, folic acid 5 mg twice daily and ascorbic acid 200 mg three times daily.

Questions

1. How might a full drug history taken by a pharmacist help this patient?
2. Comment on the use of vitamin C in Mr HA.
3. How long should Mr HA remain on ferrous sulphate?

Answers

1. Although all Mr HA's prescribed drugs were documented, it is possible that he was taking purchased medication. On admission he complained of indigestion over the last 3 months, and on questioning revealed that he was self-medicating with aluminium hydroxide mixture. From a theoretical point of view, antacids may reduce the amount of iron absorbed by increasing the pH of the stomach and by reducing the solubility of ferrous salts. It is unlikely that this contributed significantly to the development of his anaemia, but if he intends to continue using an antacid after discharge, it would be better not to take a dose of antacid within 1–2 hours of his ferrous sulphate. It would also be worth checking to see if he has been self-medicating with a purchased aspirin- or ibuprofen-based product; both drugs have been implicated in causing gastrointestinal blood loss, though in this case his gastroscopy was normal and the FOBs negative.

2. Ascorbic acid slightly increases the absorption of iron in some patients. It probably keeps iron in solution either in the ferrous form or by forming a soluble chelate with the ferric form. In most patients this is of little clinical benefit. It may have an advantage in Mr HA since he appears to have had a poor diet and may be vitamin C deficient. He may also benefit from a short course of multivitamins.

3. Mr HA needs to continue iron therapy until he has at least replenished his iron stores. This may take up to 6 months, after which time he should be reassessed, taking into account whether he is now having a suitable diet. In practice, since his haemoglobin was dangerously low on admission it may be quite reasonable to leave him on iron for the rest of his life.

Case 49.2

Mr WK, a 46-year-old mechanic, was referred to hospital by his primary care doctor. He gave a history of diarrhoea and vomiting a week ago and now was complaining of headaches and feeling 'lousy'. His doctor had given him metoclopramide and ferrous sulphate. Mr WK did not appear jaundiced although he said he had noticed his urine was unusually dark a few days ago. On examination he was obese, with a blood pressure of 120/80 mmHg and a pulse of 80. Rectal examination revealed black stools. He had a normal gastroscopy and three negative FOBs. His serum biochemistry showed a normal level of alanine transaminase and a slightly raised total bilirubin level. Mr WK's reticulocyte count was 13.5% (normal range 0.5–1.5%). He was diagnosed as having G6PD deficiency, probably triggered by an infection.

Questions

1. How do you explain Mr WK's dark urine and dark stools?
2. Would Mr WK benefit from any medication following his admission?
3. Why would it be necessary to repeat his red cell G6PD after 2 months?

Answers

1. Mr WK's dark urine was a consequence of his haemolytic anaemia. Bilirubin is a breakdown product of haemoglobin that is transported to the liver and conjugated before being excreted in the bile. Bacteria in the intestine convert this to urobilinogen, most of which is excreted in the stool. Small amounts of urobilinogen are reabsorbed and some of this appears in the urine. Urobilinogen is oxidized to urobilin, which is coloured. During episodes of haemolysis, erythrocytes are destroyed faster than normal and hence there is an increase in the formation of bilirubin and increased excretion of urobilinogen in the urine. Also during haemolysis, free haemoglobin may be released into the blood. If the haemolysis is severe enough the normal mechanism

for removing haemoglobin from the circulation is overcome and haemoglobin may appear in the urine.

Dark stools may indicate melaena and upper gastrointestinal bleeding. In Mr WK's case his gastroscopy was normal and he had three negative FOBs. His dark stools were due to the ferrous sulphate prescribed by his primary care doctor prior to admission.

2. His raised reticulocyte count indicates he is rapidly replacing his lost red cells. Erythropoiesis consumes folate and iron and since his folate is towards the lower end of the reference range it may be worth giving him a short course of folate supplements.

3. Young red cells tend to have higher levels of enzyme activity than more mature cells. Determining G6PD levels during the acute phase may be misleading since there is a relatively high proportion of young cells. Mr WK's result 2 months later would more accurately represent his normal state.

Case 49.3

Miss PR, a grey-haired, 58-year-old lady, was admitted from casualty. She had fallen over and bruised herself but had not broken any bones. The casualty officer thought Miss PR appeared pale with possibly a lemon-yellow tinge to her skin, she was slightly confused and had paraesthesiae of the feet and fingers. She had a past history of heart failure and was taking furosemide and enalapril. She was admitted for investigation and discovered to have a macrocytic anaemia. Pernicious anaemia was suspected. Folate levels, vitamin B$_{12}$ levels and a Schilling test were carried out before commencing treatment.

Questions

1. What are the features that may lead you to consider pernicious anaemia as a diagnosis?
2. Can Miss PR have a blood transfusion after samples have been taken for folate and vitamin B$_{12}$ levels?
3. The red cell folate is reported as 150 mg/L (reference range 160–640 mg/L). Would Miss PR benefit from folate therapy?

Answers

1. Macrocytic anaemia and paraesthesiae are typical features (though not diagnostic) of pernicious anaemia. Patients may be mildly jaundiced, which is often described as lemon-yellow in colour. Interestingly, pernicious anaemia is more common in women than men and is associated with blue eyes and early greying of the hair. Miss PR may have other features of pernicious anaemia, which include glossitis, angular stomatitis and altered bowel habit.

2. Patients with pernicious anaemia develop their anaemia over a long period of time and tend not to tolerate increases in blood volume very well. A transfusion may result in fluid overload and precipitate heart failure. Miss PR already has heart failure so, unless she becomes severely compromised by the anaemia, a transfusion should not be given. In patients who have such a pronounced anaemia that an urgent transfusion is required, an exchange transfusion of a small volume of packed cells may be appropriate.

3. In vitamin B$_{12}$ deficiency, folate tends to leak from cells and the red cell folate is often low (serum folate is sometimes raised). Many patients initially require both folate and vitamin B$_{12}$ although the folate can usually be stopped after a short course. Folate therapy must never be given to patients who have not been fully investigated for vitamin B$_{12}$ deficiency. If vitamin B$_{12}$-deficient patients are given large doses of folate without hydroxocobalamin, the full blood count can appear to improve but the peripheral neuropathy from the vitamin B$_{12}$ deficiency progresses.

Case 49.4

Mrs GN, a 76-year-old retired textile factory worker, was seen by her primary care doctor, complaining of tiredness. She had been seen 2 months earlier and started on ferrous sulfate for a microcytic anaemia. Initially she had felt better but the tiredness soon returned. A bone marrow aspiration revealed increased erythropoiesis, iron stores and red cell precursors.

A diagnosis of sideroblastic anaemia was made and it was decided to give her monthly transfusions. She was also started on pyridoxine 50 mg three times a day in addition to the ferrous sulphate.

Questions

1. What are the potential problems of Mrs GN's treatment?
2. After 3 months there appeared to be little benefit to show from the pyridoxine. How might the management be improved?

Answers

1. Mrs GN's bone marrow aspiration and serum ferritin level showed that she had high levels of stored iron. Repeated monthly transfusions will also contribute to further iron accumulation. In sideroblastic anaemia the bone marrow appears to be inefficient at incorporating iron into haem. The administration of iron leads to iron overload which may result in damage to the heart, liver and endocrine organs. The ferrous sulphate must be stopped. If iron accumulation remains a problem, desferrioxamine therapy may be tried.
2. Pyridoxine does not always improve the blood picture in patients with sideroblastic anaemia. Doses up to 400 mg a day have been used. In the case of Mrs GN an increase in dose should be tried. Patients with sideroblastic anaemia often do not realize that pyridoxine is not just a simple vitamin but a specific treatment for anaemia. Counselling the patient may improve compliance. Some patients also benefit from folate and this should be tried especially if Mrs GN's serum folate level was found to be low.

Case 49.5

Mrs RO, a 70-year-old retired teacher, presented with a history of increasing tiredness over the last 6 weeks. She had a past history of a partial gastrectomy 4 years ago. On questioning, her relevant symptoms included 'pins and needles' in her toes and loose bowels. She said that she had never been a good eater but ate red meat twice a week.

Questions

1. Why was it 4 years after her gastrectomy before Mrs RO developed vitamin B_{12} deficiency?
2. How long will it take for Mrs RO to respond to treatment?
3. What long-term therapy will Mrs RO require?

Answers

1. Vitamin B_{12} requires intrinsic factor produced by the stomach for absorption. Patients who have had a total gastrectomy, and some with a partial gastrectomy, malabsorb vitamin B_{12}. Most patients have good body stores and even with no new vitamin B_{12} entering the body (e.g. following a total gastrectomy), it takes at least 2 years to deplete the stores.
2. Many patients feel better within days of starting hydroxocobalamin and before a change in their haemoglobin concentration can be detected. Mrs RO's blood picture may take a number of weeks to return to normal, but the 'pins and needles' may be a sign of peripheral neuropathy, which is frequently irreversible and may not respond to the hydroxocobalamin treatment.
3. Mrs RO will need lifelong replacement therapy with hydroxocobalamin. This is usually given at a dose of 1 mg i.m. every 3 months.

REFERENCES

Al-Refaie F N, Hershko C, Hoffbrand A V et al 1997 Results of long term deferiprone (L1) therapy: a report of the International Study Group on Oral Chelators. British Journal of Haematology 91: 224-229

Altschuler E L, Kast R E 2005 Using histamine (H1) antagonists in particular atypical antipsychotics to treat anaemia of chronic disease via interleukin-6 suppression. Medical Hypotheses 65: 65-67

Annibale B, Marignani M, Monarca B et al 1999 Reversal of iron deficiency anaemia after Helicobacter pylori eradication in patients with asymptomatic gastritis. Annals of Internal Medicine 131: 668-672

Cavill I 2003 Intravenous iron as adjuvant therapy: a two edged sword? Nephrology Dialysis and Transplantation 18 (suppl 8): viii24-viii28

Charache S, Terrin M L, Moore R D et al 1995 Effect of hydroxyurea on the frequency of painful crises in sickle cell anemia. New England Journal of Medicine 332: 1317-1322

Pruss A, Salama N, Ahrens A et al 2003 Immune hemolysis – serological and clinical aspects. Clinical and Experimental Medicine 3: 55-64

Silverberg D S, Blum M, Peer G et al 1996 Intravenous ferric saccharate as an iron supplement in dialysis patients. Nephron 72: 413-417

Williams J, Wolff A, Daly A et al 1999 Iron supplemented formula milk related to reduction in psychomotor decline in infants from inner city areas: randomised study. British Medical Journal 318: 693-698

Leukaemia 50

G. Jackson   G. Jones

KEY POINTS

- Leukaemias are uncommon malignancies.
- Acute lymphoblastic leukemia (ALL) is the most common malignancy in childhood.
- With the exception of ALL, leukaemias are more common in the elderly.
- Age is one of the most important prognostic factors in the treatment of leukaemia. With the exception of neonates, older patients are less likely to be cured than younger patients.
- The treatment of leukaemia is continually improving with the introduction of more focused therapy and improvements in supportive care.
- The use of bone marrow transplantation in the treatment of all forms of leukaemia is increasing. Some of the results are exciting but the short- and long-term problems of this type of intensive treatment need to be considered.

Table 50.1   Incidence of leukaemia in the UK (Leukaemia Research Fund 2005)

	New cases/year	Incidence per 100 000 of the population
CLL	2750	4.58
CML	750	1.25
ALL	650	1.00
AML	1950	3.25

Leukaemias, together with lymphoma, are the main haematological malignancies. Although rare, they are of particular interest in that dramatic improvements in the prognosis for patients with these cancers have been achieved through the use of chemotherapy, and cure is now a possibility for many patients.

Many forms of leukaemia exist but they are all characterized by the production of excessive numbers of abnormal white blood cells. The leukaemias can be broadly divided into four groups:

- acute myeloblastic leukaemias (AMLs)
- acute lymphoblastic leukaemias (ALLs)
- chronic myelocytic leukaemias (CMLs)
- chronic lymphocytic leukaemias (CLLs).

The leukaemias were formerly defined as either acute or chronic on the basis of the patient's life expectancy and on how quickly they initially become unwell. They are now classified on the basis of cell morphology, maturity, surface antigens and cytogenetics. The adjectives 'myeloid' and 'lymphoid' refer to the predominant cell involved, and the suffix -cytic and -blastic to mature and immature cells, respectively.

Epidemiology

Together the haematological malignancies account for only 5% of all cancers; of these, CLL is the most common form of leukaemia (UK incidence data are presented in Table 50.1). CLL mainly affects an older age group: 90% of patients are over the age of 50 and nearly two-thirds are over 60 years old at diagnosis. It rarely occurs in young people and is twice as common in men as in women. CML is primarily a disease of middle age with the median onset in the 40–50 year old age group, but it can occur in younger people.

Acute leukaemia is rare, with a total annual incidence of approximately 4 per 100 000 population. The more common form of the disease is AML, which accounts for 75% of cases of acute leukaemia. The incidence of AML rises steadily with age, occurring only rarely in young children. In contrast, ALL is predominantly a childhood disease, with the peak incidence in the 3–5 year age group, and is the most common childhood cancer.

Aetiology

In common with other cancers, the aetiology of leukaemia is not fully understood. Leukaemia is thought to result from a combination of factors that induce genetic mutations which allow mutated cells to proliferate faster than normal cells and/or to fail to die in response to normal apoptotic signals. Epidemiological studies have, however, identified a number of specific risk factors for the development of leukaemia, which are described below.

Radiation

The association between ionizing radiation and the development of leukaemia is evident from nuclear disasters such as Hiroshima and more recently Chernobyl. Long-term follow-up of survivors of Nagasaki and Hiroshima has shown an increase in all forms of leukaemia other than CLL. The link is also apparent for patients who received radiotherapy for the treatment of malignant and non-malignant conditions such as Hodgkin's disease or ankylosing spondylitis. The effect of chronic low-level exposure to radiation is less certain.

Exposure to chemicals and cytotoxic drugs

There is a small but definite risk of acute leukaemia occurring in patients successfully treated for other malignancies with cytotoxic and immunosuppressive agents. The combination of chemotherapy, especially alkylating agents such as cyclophosphamide, and radiotherapy presents the highest risk. This has practical implications as an increasing number of patients achieve a 'cure' as a result of combination therapy, while occupational exposure of health professionals to these agents is also an area of concern. Occupational exposures to paint, insecticides and solvents, in particular the aromatic solvent benzene, have all been associated with the development of leukaemia but it is difficult to be certain whether such exposures genuinely cause the disease.

Viruses

Human T-cell lymphotrophic virus, an RNA retrovirus endemic in Japan and the West Indies, has been linked to a rare T-cell leukaemia/lymphoma.

Genetic factors

Down's syndrome, constitutional trisomy of chromosome 21, is associated with an increased risk of leukaemia development. Disorders that predispose to chromosomal breaks such as Fanconi's anaemia and ataxia telangectasia are also associated with an increased risk of developing acute leukaemia. These alterations may permit the expression of oncogenes, which promote malignant transformation.

Haematological disorders

Many patients with other haematological disorders have a greatly increased risk of developing leukaemia, particularly AML. These disorders include the myelodysplastic syndromes, the non-leukaemic myeloproliferative disorders, aplastic anaemia and paroxysmal nocturnal haemoglobinuria.

Pathophysiology

In leukaemia the normal process of haemopoiesis is altered (Fig. 50.1). Transformation to malignancy appears to occur in a single cell, usually at the pluripotential stem cell level, but it may occur in a committed stem cell with capacity for more limited differentiation. Accumulation of malignant cells leads to progressive impairment of the normal bone marrow function and bone marrow failure.

Acute leukaemias

In acute leukaemia the normal bone marrow is replaced by a malignant clone of immature blast cells derived from the myeloid (AML) or lymphoid (ALL) series. More than 30% of the cellular elements of the bone marrow are replaced with blasts. This is usually associated with the appearance of blasts in the peripheral circulation accompanied by worsening pancytopenia as a result of the marrow's reduced ability to produce normal blood cells. In ALL the blasts may infiltrate lymph nodes and other tissues such as liver, spleen, testis and the meninges, in particular. In AML blasts tend to infiltrate skin, gums, liver and spleen.

Classification of acute myeloblastic leukaemia

AML has traditionally been classified on the basis of morphological features of the disease. Subtypes displaying granulocytic, monocytic, erythroid and megakaryocytic differentiation were defined using the French–American–British (FAB) system (Bennett et al 1976). Recently the World Health Organization (WHO) has updated this system (Table 50.2). AML is now classified using a combination of morphological,

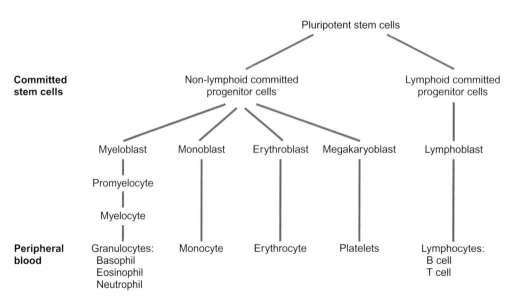

Figure 50.1 Haemopoiesis.

Table 50.2   WHO classification of AML

Subgroup	Examples
AML with recurrent genetic abnormalities	Inversion chromosome 16 (inv 16) t(15;17) t(8;21)
AML with multilineage dysplasia	
Therapy-related AML	
AML not otherwise classified	AML without maturation AML with granulocytic maturation AML with granulocytic and monocytic differentiation AML with monocytic differentiation AML with erythroid differentiation AML with megakaryocytic differentiation

genetic and immunological cell marker features in an attempt to define disease groups of greater prognostic significance (Jaffe et al 2001).

Classification of acute lymphoblastic leukaemia

A WHO classification scheme has now superseded the morphology-based FAB system (Jaffe et al 2001). As with AML, the WHO definitions now take account of morphological, genetic and immunological features. The disease is, however, mainly classified immunologically, based on the presence or absence of B- or T-cell markers (Table 50.3). Each subtype displays different clinical presentations, response to treatment and ultimately, prognosis, with pre-B having the best prognosis and B-ALL the worst. It is worth noting that B-ALL (Burkitt's type), which is associated with translocations of the *myc* gene normally located on chromosome 8, seems to be a morphologically and biologically distinct form of leukaemia.

Chronic leukaemias

In chronic leukaemia the normal bone marrow is replaced by a malignant clone of maturing haemopoietic cells.

Chronic lymphocytic leukaemia

CLL is characterized by a clonal expansion of morphologically mature lymphocytes, which are usually of B-cell origin. These

Table 50.3   Classification of ALL

Pre-B ALL	Possessing the common ALL antigen CD 10
B-cell type	B-ALL of Burkitt's type
T-cell type	T-ALL
Null	Non-B, non-T and lacking the common ALL antigen CD 10

cells accumulate in the peripheral blood and give rise to a lymphocytosis which may be very marked. Lymphocytes accumulate in lymph nodes and spread to the liver and spleen, which become enlarged. The bone marrow is progressively infiltrated. Although the cells appear morphologically normal they are functionally deficient.

Chronic myelocytic leukaemia

The characteristic feature of CML is the predominance of maturing myeloid cells in blood, bone marrow, liver, spleen and other organs. CML was the first cancer to be associated with a specific chromosomal abnormality: the Philadelphia chromosome translocation (Ph), seen in over 90% of cases. This is a translocation of genetic material between the long arms of chromosome 22 and chromosome 9. This results in the apposition of the BCR gene (chromosome 22) and the ABL gene (chromosome 9). This novel BCR-ABL gene encodes a fusion protein which has tyrosine kinase activity. This genetic event is believed to be crucial in the pathogenesis, or perhaps even to initiate the development of, CML since overactivity of the tyrosine kinase results in the uncontrolled growth characteristic of leukaemic cells (Faderl et al 1999).

Clinical manifestations

Acute leukaemia

Most of the clinical manifestations of acute leukaemia are related to bone marrow failure. The disease commonly presents with a short history and, left untreated, it is rapidly fatal. Symptoms of infection, anaemia and bleeding are common and life-threatening presenting problems. Bleeding may be particularly severe in one subtype of AML, acute promyelocytic leukaemia. This condition is associated with a translocation of genetic material between chromosomes 15 and 17, t(15;17). Disseminated intravascular coagulation (DIC) is commonly the presenting feature of this disease. Some patients with AML develop symptoms and signs due to infiltration of major organs by leukaemic cells.

The involvement of other tissues such as spleen, liver, lymph nodes and meninges is more common in ALL than AML. Involvement of the central nervous system (CNS) may give rise to headaches, vomiting and irritable behaviour. CNS disease is rare at presentation, but develops in up to 75% of children with ALL unless specific prophylactic treatment is given. Less commonly, patients present with features of hypermetabolism, hyperuricaemia or generalized aches and pains.

Chronic leukaemia

Chronic myelocytic leukaemia

Patients with CML commonly present with non-specific symptoms, such as malaise, weight loss and night sweats. The main physical sign is an enlarged spleen that may give rise to abdominal discomfort. Hepatomegaly is also detected in approximately 40% of newly diagnosed patients. Neutropenia and thrombocytopenia are uncommon at presentation. Thus, unlike the acute leukaemias, patients with CML rarely present with symptoms of infection or haemorrhage. In up to 30% of cases, patients are asymptomatic and the disease is detected as a result of a routine blood test performed for other reasons.

CML is a triphasic disease. The initial chronic phase may last from several months to 20 years; the median is around 5 years. During this time treatment can alleviate symptoms and reduce the white blood count (WBC) and spleen size, allowing patients to lead near-normal lives. An accelerated phase eventually occurs where the disease becomes more aggressive with progressively worsening symptoms: unexplained fevers, bone pain, anaemia, thrombocytopenia or thrombocytosis. Finally, after a period of weeks or months a blast crisis occurs, resembling fulminating acute leukaemia. In a small percentage of patients this occurs abruptly.

Chronic lymphocytic leukaemia

An increasing number of patients are diagnosed as having CLL by chance, when a full blood count is performed for an unrelated reason. Symptomatic patients often suffer with B symptoms; these are night sweats, unexplained fever and weight loss. At diagnosis, findings may include generalized lymphadenopathy and some enlargement of the liver and spleen. The course of CLL is variable; in some patients the disease may remain indolent for many years while others experience a steady deterioration in their health. Survival varies from 2 to 20 years depending on the extent of disease. Patients are immunocompromised with a reduction in serum γ-globulin and are at increased risk of bacterial and viral infections. There is an increased susceptibility to autoimmune disease, particularly immune haemolytic anaemias and thrombocytopenia. With progressive disease bone marrow failure becomes apparent, resulting in fatigue, infection and bleeding, and the disease becomes less responsive to treatment. Patients with CLL also have an increased risk of developing a more aggressive malignancy such as high-grade non-Hodgkin's lymphoma or prolymphocytic leukaemia.

Investigations

Examinations of peripheral blood and bone marrow are the key laboratory investigations carried out in cases of suspected leukaemia. However, some additional investigations can help in the diagnosis and classification of this group of diseases. Some of the main findings at diagnosis are presented in Table 50.4.

In acute leukaemia, leukaemic blast cells are usually seen on the peripheral blood film. The blasts of ALL and AML are distinguished using morphology, cytochemical stains, cytogenetics and cell surface antigen analysis. In CML the principal feature is a leucocytosis with WBC ranging from 30×10^9 to 250×10^9/L comprising the complete spectrum of myeloid cells. In CLL it is lymphocytes in particular which are increased, with levels exceeding 10×10^9/L. Non-random chromosome abnormalities are increasingly being identified in patients with leukaemia. The information obtained from cytogenetic analysis of bone marrow or peripheral blood cells can be used to confirm

Table 50.4 Findings at diagnosis in leukaemia

	AML	ALL	CML	CLL
WBC	↑ in 60% may be N or ↓	↑ in 50% may be N or ↓↓	↑↑ commonly 100×10^9–250×10^9/L	Commonly ↑
Differential WBC	Mainly myeloblasts	Mainly lymphoblasts	Granulocytes ↑↑, especially neutrophils, myelocytes, basophils and eosinophils <10% blasts present	Lymphocytes >10×10^9/L
RBC	Severe anaemia	Severe anaemia	Anaemia common	Anaemia in 50% of patients, generally mild
Platelets	↓↓	↓↓	Usually ↑, may be N or ↓	↓ in 20–30%
Bone marrow aspiration and trephine	Predominantly blasts	Predominantly blasts	Hypercellular blasts <15%	Lymphocytic infiltration
Cytogenetic analysis	Important abnormalities detected	Important abnormalities detected	Presence of Ph chromosome	
Lymphadenopathy	Rare	Common	Rare	Common
Splenomegaly	50%	60%	Usual and severe	Usual and moderate
Other features	DIC, high urate	High urate, CNS involvement	↑ serum uric acid	Immunoparesis

N, normal; ↓, reduced; ↑, increased
Ph, Philadelphia; DIC, disseminalid intravascular coagulation

the diagnosis and classification of leukaemia and may provide a guide to the likely response to treatment and prognosis.

Treatment

Although significant progress has been made in the treatment of leukaemia, work continues to further improve prognosis. As leukaemias are rare malignancies the most important studies are undertaken on a national or international basis and in the UK many of these are co-ordinated by the Medical Research Council (MRC).

In addition to the specific anti-leukaemia treatment, general supportive therapy is vital, to manage both the disease and the complications of therapy.

Acute leukaemia

At the outset, intensive combination chemotherapy is given in the hope of achieving a complete remission (CR). This initial phase of treatment is termed induction or remission induction chemotherapy. A CR can only be achieved by virtual ablation of the bone marrow, followed by recovery of normal haemopoiesis. If two cycles of therapy fail to induce CR an alternative drug regimen can be used. If this is unsuccessful it is unlikely that CR will be achieved. The subsequent duration of the first remission is closely linked to survival.

Remission is defined as the absence of all clinical and microscopic signs of leukaemia, less than 5% blast forms in the bone marrow and return of normal cellularity and haemopoietic elements. Despite achieving CR, occult residual disease

(also termed minimal residual disease or MRD) will persist and further intensive therapy is given in an attempt to sustain the remission. This postremission consolidation therapy may be chemotherapy or a combination of chemotherapy, radiotherapy and bone marrow transplantation.

Acute lymphoblastic leukaemia

Treatment of ALL in childhood has been one of the success stories of the last three decades. Over 80% of children will achieve a remission lasting more than 5 years (Pui et al 2004). Unfortunately the results in adults are not so impressive. The combination of vincristine, prednisolone, anthracyclines and asparaginase induces complete remission in about 90% of children with ALL and 80% of adults, though sadly relapse is far more common in adults (Table 50.5). Other active drugs in the treatment of ALL include methotrexate, 6-mercaptopurine, cyclophosphamide and mitoxantrone.

Patients with ALL are at a high risk of developing central nervous system infiltration. Cytotoxic drugs penetrate poorly into the central nervous system which thus acts as a sanctuary site for leukaemic cells. For this reason all patients with ALL receive central nervous system prophylaxis. Cranial irradiation plus intrathecal methotrexate or high-dose systemic methotrexate can be used.

Maintenance treatment is important to sustain a complete remission. It is usually milder than induction or consolidation chemotherapy, but is carried on for at least 18 months. Treatment usually consists of weekly methotrexate and daily 6-mercaptopurine with intermittent vincristine and prednisolone.

The treatment of relapsed disease varies with the site of relapse. Isolated central nervous system or testicular relapse may be

Table 50.5 Treatment of ALL (adapted from MRC protocol)

	Dose	Route	Regimen
Induction (4 weeks)			
Vincristine	1.5 mg/m^2	i.v.	Weekly for 4 weeks
Prednisolone	40 mg/m^2	oral	Daily for 4 weeks
L-Asparaginase	6000 u/m^2	i.m.	3 × weekly for 3 weeks
Daunorubicin	45 mg/m^2	i.v.	Daily for 2 days
Intensification (1 week)			
Vincristine	1.5 mg/m^2	i.v.	1 dose
Daunorubicin	45 mg/m^2	i.v.	Daily for 2 days
Prednisolone	40 mg/m^2	oral	Daily for 5 days
Etoposide	100 mg/m^2	i.v.	Daily for 5 days
Cytarabine	100 mg/m^2	i.v.	2 × daily for 5 days
Thioguanine	80 mg/m^2	oral	Daily for 5 days
CNS prophylaxis (3 weeks)			
Cranial irradiation	24 Gy		
Methotrexate	i.t. weekly for 3 weeks also given during induction and intensification		
Maintenance therapy (2 years)			
Methotrexate	20 mg/m^2	oral	Weekly
6-Mercaptopurine	75 mg/m^2	oral	Daily
Prednisolone	40 mg/m^2	oral	5 days/month
Vincristine	1.5 mg/m^2	i.v.	Monthly

i.m., intramuscular; i.v., intravenous; i.t., intrathecal; MRC, Medical Research Council; ALL, acute lymphoblastic leukaemia

successfully treated with radiation and reinduction therapy. Cure can still be achieved for some patients. Bone marrow relapse is much more difficult to cure, especially if it occurs early.

A small proportion of paediatric patients and a larger proportion of adult patients have the Philadelphia chromosome translocation within their ALL blasts. Such patients have a relatively poor prognosis and therefore require more intensive therapy. There is some evidence that drug combinations including imatinib may enhance the response of these leukaemias to therapy.

Acute myeloblastic leukaemia

As for ALL, the treatment of AML involves induction and consolidation chemotherapy. In AML therapy, however, the chemotherapy regimens used to achieve remission are much more myelotoxic, and patients require intensive supportive care to survive periods of bone marrow aplasia (Fig. 50.2). The pyrimidine analogue cytarabine has formed the basis of treatment for AML for 20 years. The addition of daunorubicin and oral thioguanine has achieved a CR rate of 75% in patients under the age of 60 years and about 50% in those over 60 years (Löwenberg et al 1999). The precise dose and scheduling of these agents is continually being refined in order to improve the response rates. Despite the numbers of patients who achieve CR following induction therapy, the majority relapse, with only about 25% becoming long-term disease-free survivors (Stone et al 2004). Thus, in common with ALL, additional postremission therapy is required. Intensive consolidation chemotherapy with high-dose cytarabine and daunorubicin or amsacrine appears to improve survival rates to approximately 50% after 3 years, with even more encouraging results being obtained in patients under 25 years of age (Löwenberg et al 1999). There is generally no

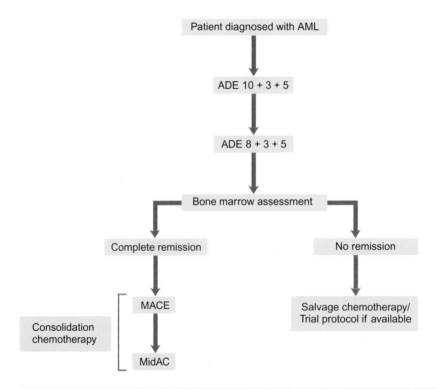

List of abbreviations

ADE 10+3+5   Cytosine arabinoside 100mg/m^2 iv twice daily days 1 to 10
Daunorubium 50mg/m^2 iv once daily days 1,3,5
Etoposide 100mg/m^2 iv once daily days 1 to 5

ADE 8+3+5   Cytosine arabinside 100mg/m^2 iv twice daily days 1 to 8
Daunorubium 50mg/m^2 iv once daily days 1,3,5
Etoposide 100mg/m^2 iv once daily days 1 to 5

MACE   Amsacrine 100mg/m^2 iv once daily days 1 to 5
Cytosine arabinoside 200mg/m^2 iv by continuous infusion days 1 to 5
Etoposide 100mg/m^2 once daily days 1 to 5

MidAC   Mitoxantrone 10mg/m^2 iv once daily days 1 to 5
Cytosine arabinside 1g/m^2 iv once daily days 1 to 3

Figure 50.2 One example of a possible treatment regimen for AML. The figure demonstrates that patients are treated with initial induction therapy then remission is consolidated with at least two courses of chemotherapy. This figure provides a summary only and should not be used as a guide to prescribing or dispensing therapy.

role for maintenance therapy in AML. Similarly, central nervous system prophylaxis is not routinely indicated though patients thought to be at particularly high risk of CNS disease, such as those with testicular or sinus involvement, should receive prophylactic therapy.

It has been shown that acute promyelocytic leukaemia, AML associated with t(15;17), is sensitive to all-trans retinoic acid (ATRA), which induces blast maturation and remission when used as a single agent (Soignet & Maslak 2004, Tallman et al 1997). In combination with standard chemotherapy, remission rates are significantly better than those seen when chemotherapy is used alone. In contrast to other subtypes of AML, studies have also shown that inclusion of ATRA as part of a maintenance strategy significantly increases the long-term survival of patients with this subtype of AML.

An alternative approach to postremission therapy is stem cell transplantation. In patients under 40 years of age, allogeneic bone marrow transplantation has resulted in disease-free survival of 45–65% at 5 years post transplant. These patients are considered cured of their disease. Only about 10% of patients are suitable for allogeneic bone marrow transplants and there is little evidence to suggest that autologous stem cell transplantation improves the outcome for patients with AML in first complete remission. It is always worth remembering that AML is most common in the elderly, and intensive intravenous chemotherapy regimens are not always appropriate for this population of patients.

Treatment of AML in relapse is difficult and the prognosis is generally poor. Encouraging results have been seen using a combination of fludarabine, cytosine arabinoside and granulocyte colony stimulating factor (GCSF). Novel approaches in AML therapy are often piloted in this group of poor-risk patients. A combination of anti-CD33 antibody, which targets myeloid blasts, with calicheamicin, an anthracycline antibiotic, is a promising and effective approach (Stone et al 2004), but appears most effective when given in combination with conventional chemotherapy. Arsenic trioxide has potent and specific activity against AML M3 blasts and is useful for patients who have relapsed. A newly developed purine analogue, clofarabine, has also been shown to have activity against AML. This drug is a promising agent, particularly in the treatment of older patients, as pilot studies suggest that its toxic effects may be less severe than those associated with other chemotherapy regimens (Faderl et al 2005).

Chronic leukaemia

Chronic myelocytic leukaemia

Until recently the treatment of CML has been essentially palliative, producing modest increases in survival, but with the main aim of keeping patients asymptomatic by normalizing the WBC. Hydroxycarbamide was the most widely used drug in the management of CML in chronic phase. Treatment with hydroxycarbamide (hydroxyurea) is initiated at a dose of 1.5–2 g/day, and usually brings the WBC under control within 1–2 weeks. The dose can then be reduced to a maintenance dose of 0.5–2 g/day. Withdrawing or reducing the dose abruptly can cause a rebound increase in WBC. The side effects of hydroxycarbamide are generally mild but include rashes and gut disturbances.

Interferon can control symptoms of CML but also was the first agent shown to modify the disease process. It promotes the expression of suppressed normal haemopoiesis at the expense of the malignant clone. Studies have shown that interferon-α therapy prolongs the chronic phase and improves the median survival of patients with CML and its effects seem to be enhanced by the addition of low-dose cytarabine (Sawyers 1999).

Another approach is the use of allogeneic stem cell transplantation in selected patients under 50 years of age for whom a suitable donor can be found. There is a high risk of mortality with this procedure (10%) and 5–10% of patients relapse within the first 3 years, but there are now long-term survivors who can be considered cured. Patients who relapse following allogeneic bone marrow transplantation may go into remission after an infusion of lymphocytes from the donor. To date, allogeneic transplantation is the only proven curative therapy in CML.

Therapeutic options for patients with CML have changed dramatically in the last 5 years due to the development of imatinib mesylate. This drug was specifically designed to target the abnormal tyrosine kinase product of the BCR-ABL fusion gene (Fig. 50.3). Initial results with this agent are exciting. In

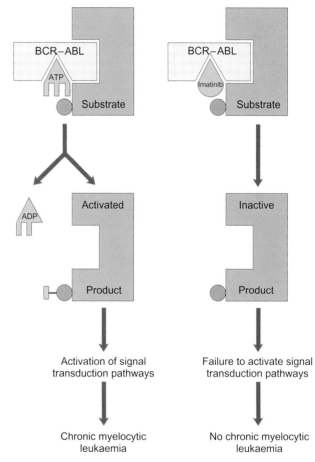

Figure 50.3 Inhibition of BCR-ABL protein by imatinib. The protein product of the BCR-ABL fusion gene (BCR-ABL protein) acts as a constitutively active tyrosine kinase and uses ATP, bound within a kinase pocket in the molecule, to phosphorylate tyrosine (o) in a variety of substrates. In doing so ATP (adenosine triphosphate) is reduced to ADP (adenosine diphosphate) which falls out of the kinase pocket to be replaced by further ATP. Imatinib prevents the action of the BCR-ABL protein by blocking ATP entry into the kinase pocket.

a large randomized controlled trial, patients were randomized to receive imatinib or a combination of interferon-α and cytarabine. Many patients were intolerant of the interferon and cytarabine combination and crossed over to receive imatinib after trial commencement. Despite this problem, progression-free survival at 1 year was 97% in the imatinib arm and 80% in the interferon and cytarabine arm in an intention-to-treat analysis (O'Brien et al 2003). The Philadelphia chromosome became undetectable in 68% of imatinib recipients compared to 7% of those in the alternative arm (Hughes et al 2003). However, more sensitive testing methods, such as real-time polymerase chain reaction (PCR), have now shown that many patients who are Philadelphia chromosome negative still possess very low levels of the abnormal BCR-ABL gene produced by the Philadelphia translocation.

Thus, whilst results with imatinib are encouraging, allogeneic transplantation is still considered the only curative therapy in CML and the primary therapy for many young patients. For older patients, at higher risk of transplant-related morbidity and mortality, a trial of imatinib is often considered the best option. Clinical trials are under way to study the effect of changes in dose and addition of other chemotherapeutic agents such as interferon-α on the efficacy of this agent.

Transformation of CML into acute leukaemia can be treated in the same manner as de novo acute leukaemia, in an effort to achieve a second chronic phase. Treatment is slightly more successful if transformation is lymphoid rather than myeloid. Imatinib, typically at higher doses than are used in chronic phase disease, can also be used to attempt to return patients to chronic phase disease. In general remissions are rare and the median survival is less than 6 months.

Chronic lymphocytic leukaemia

Currently there is no cure for CLL. All treatment is, therefore, considered palliative. There is no evidence that early treatment of asymptomatic patients improves outcome. Indications for treatment are:

- rapidly increasing WBC
- increasing or troublesome lymphadenopathy
- systemic symptoms
- marrow failure
- autoimmune complications.

The alkylating agents chlorambucil and cyclophosphamide are commonly used. Prednisolone can reduce the lymphocyte count without contributing to myelosuppression and is used to treat autoimmune phenomena such as haemolytic anaemia and immune thrombocytopenia. The use of purine analogues, particularly fludarabine, has been an exciting development in the treatment of CLL. Although complete remissions are unusual, good responses are seen even in patients whose leukaemia is resistant to alkylating agents. With regard to initial therapy of CLL, fludarabine-treated patients show a higher response rate than patients treated with chlorambucil. However, no survival advantage for the use of fludarabine has been demonstrated (Rai et al 2000). Splenic complications may necessitate splenectomy or splenic irradiation. Radiotherapy can also be used to control localized

painful lymphadenopathy. Combination chemotherapy, such as CHOP (see Chapter 51) used in lymphoma, may be beneficial in advanced disease.

Campath-1H is a humanized monoclonal anti-CD52 antibody. CD52 is present on most lymphocytes including malignant lymphocytes in CLL. Binding of this antibody induces both antibody-mediated and complement-mediated T-cell cytotoxicity against malignant B-cells. In relapsed patients, the duration of response to Campath-1H is relatively short. However, the agent is currently being studied, both in combination with other drugs and as a possible means of purging the bone marrow of residual cells prior to autologous stem cell harvest and transplantation.

Patients with CLL are very susceptible to infection. Herpes viruses, in particular herpes zoster, can cause significant problems. This susceptibility is increased because many treatments, such as campath-1H and fludarabine, have generalized antilymphocyte action and are not absolutely specific for malignant lymphocytes.

Stem cell transplantation

The potential role of stem cell transplantation is increasingly being explored in the management of all types of leukaemia.

The basic principle

This technique provides a means of rescuing the patient from the potentially lethal effects on the bone marrow of ablative therapy given in an attempt to eradicate all traces of disease (Fig. 50.4). The conditioning regimen most commonly used is a combination of high-dose cyclophosphamide and total body irradiation. Other conditioning regimens include high-dose melphalan, etoposide, busulphan or cytarabine.

Following administration of conditioning therapy, 2–3 days elapse to allow its elimination from the body and then previously harvested stem cells are reinfused peripherally. The stem cells will return to and repopulate the marrow, restoring normal haemopoiesis. Peripheral blood counts recover in 2–4 weeks. Throughout this time patients require intensive supportive care and the procedure, particularly allogeneic stem cell transplantation, causes significant morbidity and has a mortality rate of 5–30%.

The source of stem cells

During allogeneic stem cell transplantation (allograft), stem cells are obtained from a human leucocyte antigen (HLA)-matched donor. These stem cells can be removed directly from the bone marrow, under general anaesthetic, or harvested from the peripheral blood. Under certain circumstances, in the absence of a matched donor, an autologous bone marrow or peripheral blood stem cell transplant (autograft) can be performed. Following conditioning, the patients receive their own cryopreserved marrow or peripheral blood stem cells, previously harvested from them while in complete remission. There is a potential risk, however, that stem cells obtained in this way may contain undetected, residual disease. Attempts have been made to purge the bone marrow of disease in vitro but these have generally been unsuccessful.

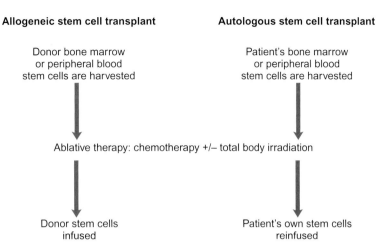

Allogeneic stem cell transplant

Donor bone marrow
or peripheral blood
stem cells are harvested

Autologous stem cell transplant

Patient's bone marrow
or peripheral blood
stem cells are harvested

Ablative therapy: chemotherapy +/– total body irradiation

Donor stem cells
infused

Patient's own stem cells
reinfused

Figure 50.4 Stem cell transplantation.

Peripheral blood stem cell transplantation

This technique for rescuing bone marrow following ablative conditioning therapy is increasingly used to restore haemopoiesis (Russell 1998). Patients receive the haematopoetic growth factor GCSF, either alone or following an infusion of high-dose chemotherapy such as high-dose cyclophosphamide. Patients receive GCSF for a period of about 7 days. This stimulates the release of stem cells into the peripheral circulation. Stem cells are then harvested from the peripheral circulation by a process of cell pheresis. The harvested cells can then be reinfused, fresh, into the patient following conditioning therapy or frozen and stored for later use.

Peripheral stem cell transplantation offers some advantages over conventional bone marrow transplant techniques; collection of peripheral stem cells negates the need for general anaesthesia and it has been found that the haemopoietic recovery period following transplantation is shortened by 5–10 days. This technique can also be used to harvest stem cells from allogeneic donors. In this case GCSF is used alone to stimulate stem cell release into the peripheral circulation.

Complications

Infection is almost inevitable in patients undergoing bone marrow transplantation. Other significant complications of allografts include interstitial pneumonitis and hepatic veno-occlusive disease, but the major life-threatening complication is acute graft-versus-host disease (GVHD). The likelihood of GVHD occurring increases with age and for this reason allografts are largely restricted to patients under 45 years of age. GVHD is caused by T-lymphocytes in the donated marrow reacting to host tissues. The severity of the reaction ranges from a mild maculopapular rash to multisystem organ failure with a high mortality rate. Acute GVHD typically occurs within 100 days of the bone marrow transplantation and typically presents with fever, rash, diarrhoea and liver dysfunction. Prophylactic therapy is routinely given with methotrexate or ciclosporin, alone or in combination, for 6–12 months post transplant. Should acute GVHD develop, high-dose methylprednisolone,

ciclosporin, antithymocyte globulin and more recently, anticytokine monoclonal antibodies, e.g. anti-TNF (tumour necrosis factor) antibodies, have been used to treat the condition.

Chronic GVHD can occur after 3 months following bone marrow transplantation. It is a multisystem disorder associated with chronic hepatitis, severe skin inflammation and profound immunosuppression. Treatment is successful in approximately 50% of patients and consists of immunosuppression with azathioprine and prednisolone together with prophylactic antibiotics. Ciclosporin and thalidomide have also been used successfully in the treatment of chronic steroid-refractory GVHD. The main cause of death amongst patients with chronic GVHD is infection.

Reduced intensity allografting

Allogeneic transplantation is a very intensive procedure associated with significant morbidity and mortality, hence its restriction to younger patients. Recently attempts have been made to reduce the intensity of transplant conditioning regimens whilst using increased immunosuppression to facilitate marrow engraftment. Although such an approach reduces the intensity of therapy delivered to any residual tumour, the possible downside of this reduction is offset by an immunological graft-versus-tumour effect and by reduced early post-transplant mortality. This form of transplant is often offered to older patients who are considered unfit to receive a standard allograft. However, the long-term outcomes of this approach are under continual review.

The place of stem cell transplantation

The place of stem cell transplantation in the management of a particular form of leukaemia depends very much on the prognosis of patients treated with conventional chemotherapy (Table 50.6). For example, the results of intensive chemotherapy in children with ALL are good and bone marrow transplantation is generally only considered for children who have relapsed and in whom a second remission can be achieved. However, conventional treatment of adults is less successful and allogeneic bone marrow transplantation may be offered to adults in first remission.

Table 50.6   Indications for allogeneic stem cell transplantation in leukaemia

AML	First remission with the exception of patients with good risk genetic abnormalities: t(15;17), t(8;21) and inversion of chromosome 16
	Second remission
CML	Chronic phase
ALL	First remission in adults
	Second remission in children
CLL	Not generally appropriate as part of standard therapy but under investigation within several clinical studies

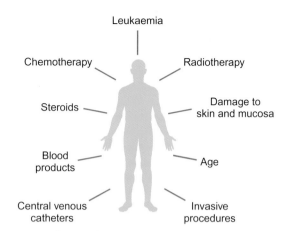

Figure 50.5   Infection risk in immunocompromised patients.

Patient care

Supportive care

The treatment of CLL and CML is largely carried out on a hospital outpatient basis, with patients taking oral medication at home or attending outpatient clinics on a weekly or monthly basis for injections of chemotherapy. Patients are routinely monitored to follow the progress of disease and to observe treatment-related side effects. Supportive therapy such as blood transfusions can also be given on an outpatient basis. In contrast, the intensity of induction and consolidation regimens used in the management of patients with acute leukaemia renders them pancytopenic. Therapy is usually given as a hospital inpatient with patients often remaining in hospital following treatment for 3–4 weeks until their bone marrow recovers sufficiently. This is in contrast to therapy for most solid tumours where, following administration of treatment, patients are often well enough to remain at home until their next cycle of chemotherapy is due.

Advanced leukaemia, bone marrow transplantation and aggressive chemotherapy for acute leukaemia all result in pancytopenia. Red cell transfusions are given to patients to maintain their haemoglobin above 9–10 g/dL. Evidence of bleeding includes petechial haemorrhages in skin and mucous membranes, and patients receiving aggressive treatment must be examined daily for any of the above signs. Platelet concentrates are given to thrombocytopenic patients who have signs of bleeding and are given prophylactically should platelets fall below 10×10^9/L. The probability of infection developing rises as the WBC, specifically the neutrophil count, falls. With an absolute neutrophil count of below 0.5×10^9/L, patients are at high risk of infection, with the risks being even greater if the period of neutropenia is prolonged.

Chapters 51 and 52 examine many of the non-haematological toxicities which result from the use of cytotoxic drugs and these are clearly pertinent to haematology patients. The major contributors to morbidity and mortality in patients with leukaemia are relapsed disease and infection.

Infection in the immunocompromised patient

A number of intrinsic and extrinsic factors all contribute to the risk of infection in this vulnerable group of patients (Fig. 50.5).

While cross-infection can occur via staff, other patients or contaminated objects, the main sources of infection in this group of patients are endogenous, arising from commensal gut and skin organisms. The normal host defences to infection are broken down; damage to mucous membranes, particularly in the gastrointestinal tract, occurs with chemotherapy and radiotherapy, allowing infecting organisms to enter the bloodstream. Most infections in neutropenic patients arise from three main sites: the gastrointestinal and respiratory tracts, and the skin. Table 50.7 lists the main pathogens responsible for infection in this group of patients.

Table 50.7   Pathogens commonly causing infection in neutropenic patients

Gram-negative bacteria	*Pseudomonas* spp.
	Escherichia coli
	Klebsiella spp.
	Enterobacter spp.
	Proteus spp.
	Serratia spp.
	Legionella pneumophila
Gram-positive bacteria	*Streptococcus* spp.
	Staphylococcus epidermidis
	Staphylococcus aureus
Anaerobes	*Clostridium difficile*
	Clostridium perfringens
	Bacteroides spp.
Fungi	*Candida* spp.
	Aspergillus spp.
Viruses	Herpes simplex
	Herpes zoster
	Cytomegalovirus
	Hepatitis
Protozoa	*Pneumocystis jiroveci*

Preventive measures

Oral hygiene Mouth care is important in all patients receiving chemotherapy but particularly neutropenic patients. Patients are generally asked to use mouthwashes regularly and prophylactic antifungal therapy may also be given. Although it is important to avoid any sort of trauma to the oral mucosa, teeth should be cleaned regularly using a soft toothbrush. Attention must also be paid to the care of dentures. Patients require careful counselling on mouth care, stressing the importance of oral hygiene.

Prophylactic anti-infectives In general, prophylactic antibiotics are avoided because of the possible development of resistant organisms, but they may have a place in the management of periods of prolonged myelosuppression following chemotherapy and bone marrow transplantation. Prophylactic antifungal agents are often given and patients undergoing bone marrow transplantation and therapy for ALL require prophylaxis against herpes virus and *Pneumocystis jiroveci* (Table 50.8).

Gut decontamination Gut decontamination using a combination of non-absorbable oral antibiotics and antifungal agents reduces the population of potentially pathogenic organisms in the intestine. One such combination includes neomycin sulfate, colistin sulfate, nystatin and amphotericin. However, opinions are divided over this practice, as gut decontamination can lead to the overgrowth of resistant organisms.

Growth factors An exciting development in the care of patients with leukaemia has been the production of haemopoietic growth factors using recombinant DNA technology. The first of these, GCSF, given daily by subcutaneous injection or intravenous infusion after completion of chemotherapy, stimulates neutrophil production and may reduce the duration of neutropenia by up to 7 days. The cost of these compounds is a major issue and results of studies investigating the effects of GCSF on morbidity and mortality, following chemotherapy, have been disappointing (Pagliuca et al 2003). Newer pegylated growth factors have recently been introduced. These have a longer half-life than standard agents and thus fewer injections are required. The impact of these agents on morbidity and mortality post chemotherapy, however, remains controversial.

Aseptic technique Careful attention should be paid to the care of intravenous cannulae, particularly central venous catheters. The increased incidence of staphylococcal infection in immunocompromised patients can largely be attributed to their use. Invasive procedures, such as venepuncture, must be carried out using strict aseptic technique. Similarly, urinary catheters are a major source of infection and their use should be avoided if at all possible.

Protective isolation Reverse barrier isolation during periods of neutropenia, nursing in strict sterile environments and high-efficiency particulate air (HEPA) filtration have been used in an attempt to reduce infection rates. This is extremely demanding for staff and patients alike and is generally only appropriate following bone marrow transplantation.

Treatment of infection

Commonly, neutropenic patients show no signs of focal infection; they are unable to form pus. The only clinical manifestations of septicaemia might be general malaise, fever or hypotension. A patient's condition can deteriorate very rapidly, with collapse occurring within hours of the first signs of infection. Treatment should be instigated as soon as infection is suspected. Following a clinically serious febrile episode (temperature 37.5°C for more than 1 hour or 38°C or more on a single reading) samples are taken for culture; these may include blood, urine, sputum and stool cultures along with line and throat swabs. Intravenous antibiotics must be started empirically, without delay (Sipsas et al 2005). Standard empirical therapy varies from unit to unit but may involve the combination of an aminoglycoside with an antipseudomonal penicillin such as piperacillin to provide broad-spectrum bactericidal cover. In penicillin-allergic patients ceftazidime or cefotaxime may be substituted, but local resistance patterns are of paramount importance. Antibiotics with a broad spectrum of activity, such as ciprofloxacin, have been used as single agents.

Vancomycin or teicoplanin are often prescribed if an infected central venous catheter is suspected, to provide additional cover against Gram-positive organisms. Microbiological advice should be sought in cases of methicillin-resistant *Staphylococcus aureus* (MRSA) infection. Metronidazole may be added to the antibiotic regimen to cover anaerobes if the clinical presentation suggests that the source of the infection may be oral, perineal or gut. Anti-infective therapy should subsequently be modified on the basis of cultures but in the majority of neutropenic patients a causative organism is never identified.

If the pyrexia persists for more than 3 days in spite of broad-spectrum antibiotics, or if the patient's condition is deteriorating, systemic fungal infection should be suspected. Empirical antifungal therapy for neutropenic patients with antibiotic-resistant fever reduces mortality and is considered a standard of care. A number of broad-spectrum agents are now available for use in this setting, including standard amphotericin, lipid formulation of amphotericin, caspofungin and voriconazole. Intravenous amphotericin is often the first choice to ensure that *Aspergillus* and *Candida* are covered. The main limitation of amphotericin is its toxicity, in particular nephrotoxicity. Lipid formulation of amphotericin may be appropriate in patients with pre-existing renal impairment or in cases where conventional amphotericin has induced nephrotoxicity. Voriconazole is a useful agent with a similarly broad spectrum of activity. Hepatotoxicity, visual disturbances and prolonged QT interval are the most common side effects of voriconazole. This agent has the advantage of being available as both intravenous and oral preparations so the conversion from parenteral to oral therapy is straightforward.

Table 50.8	Prophylactic anti-infectives
Gram-negative bacteria	Ciprofloxacin
Candidiasis	Nystatin
	Fluconazole
	Itraconazole
Herpes simplex	Aciclovir
Pneumocystis jiroveci	Co-trimoxazole

Table 50.9 Common therapeutic problems in the leukaemias

Problem	Cause	Solutions
Mucositis and oral ulceration	Chemotherapeutic agents directly toxic to mucosal epithelium	Regular mouth toilet including use of antibacterial mouthwash
	Radiotherapy is directly toxic to the mucosa and also reduces saliva production by salivary glands	Prophylactic use of antiviral and antifungal agents for patients in whom myelosuppression is likely to be prolonged
	Vulnerable mucosa is likely to be attacked by infective agents, e.g. herpes simplex, *Candida*	
Fever in neutropenic patients	Infection predominantly caused by bacteria and/ or fungi	Broad-spectrum antibiotics must be commenced as soon as blood cultures have been taken. A strategy of planned progressive therapy, including use of an antifungal agent in non-responsive fever, is appropriate
Graft-versus-host disease (GVHD)	T-lymphocytes from the donor react against host tissues	Use a sibling donor if possible
		Use the donor most closely HLA matched to the patient
		Consider T-cell depletion of graft (though this may increase the risk of disease relapse)
		Prophylactic therapy with methotrexate and ciclosporin
		Treat GVHD with corticosteroids, ciclosporin, antithymocyte, globulin, FK 506, anticytokine monoclonal antibodies
		Irradiate all blood products
Late complications of treatment	Risks of haemopoietic malignancy and non-haemopoietic malignancy are increased post chemotherapy	Aim to tailor therapy to the underlying disease, i.e. do not overtreat and do not undertreat
	Late cardiotoxicity secondary to anthracyclines	Do not exceed maximum cumulative doses of anthracyclines
		Liposomal anthracyclines may be useful in the future

Although the antifungal activity of the echinocandin caspofungin is more limited than that of amphoteracin or voriconazole, it has been shown to be effective for empirical therapy as it has good efficacy against *Candida* and *Aspergillus* spp. It has the advantage of reduced toxicity in comparison with other available agents. The most common side effect is hepatotoxicity. Since this agent has a relatively limited spectrum of activity it is probably best avoided in the setting of presumed fungal sinus or central nervous system infection, which are often caused by fungi other than *Aspergillus* or *Candida* spp.

Table 50.9 lists some of the common problems encountered in the treatment of the leukaemias.

The practice points listed below should be used to control infection in immunocompromised patients.

- Measures to prevent infection are important.
- Particular attention should be paid to scrupulous hand washing, mouth care and the use of antifungal, antiviral and anti-*pneumocystis* prophylaxis for patients at high risk.
- Preventive measures do not eliminate the risk of infection.
- Treatment of fever in a neutropenic patient is a medical emergency.

- Empirical antifungal therapy should be used to treat neutropenic patients with antibiotic-resistant fever, at high risk of fungal infection.

CASE STUDIES

Case 50.1

A 30-year-old woman recently diagnosed with CML attends the haematology clinic to discuss the options for treatment.

Questions

1. Which treatment options are available?
2. Which treatment is likely to be the best choice for this patient?

Answers

1. There are clearly a number of potential treatment options but it is often very difficult, in these circumstances, to determine the optimal treatment for an individual patient. It is vitally important to fully inform

patients regarding their condition and its prognosis, and about treatment options and their potential advantages and disadvantages. Only if this patient has all the necessary information can she decide on the treatment option that is most appropriate/acceptable to her individual circumstances.

The various treatment options are:

- palliative therapy with hydroxycarbamide to control cell counts
- interferon-α
- interferon-α and cytosine
- imatinib
- allogeneic matched sibling transplant
- matched unrelated donor (MUD) transplantation if a matched sibling is not available
- treatment as part of a clinical trial which is likely to involve imatinib in varying doses or in combination with other effective agent such as interferon-α.

2. A purely palliative approach is unlikely to be acceptable to a young patient but hydroxycarbamide can still be used acutely to control high cell counts. There is no doubt that use of interferon-α alone results in cytogenetic remission in a small percentage of patients and this effect is enhanced by the addition of cytosine. The side effects of interferon-α include flu-like and affective symptoms. The addition of cytosine increases myelosuppression and risk of mucositis. Although these treatments can induce cytogenetic remission, the duration of such responses is unclear and only a minority of patients respond completely. The high risk of side-effects and low chance of complete cytogenetic response to interferon-α, with or without cytosine, are likely to make these therapeutic modalities unattractive to this patient.

It remains true that allogeneic stem cell transplantation is the only proven curative therapy for patients with CML. The difficulty with this approach is that the mortality rate for transplant recipients remains high. The 1-year mortality rate for a 30-year-old patient transplanted using a sibling donor is approximately 15–20% and this may rise to 25–30% if a MUD has to be used. The major causes of death in this group are acute GVHD and infection. In addition to this high risk of mortality in the short term, there is also a risk of long-term morbidity post allograft. Chronic GVHD can have a significant impact on quality of life for many patients and requires long-term medical follow-up. Ironically, patients with a degree of chronic GVHD are at reduced risk of disease relapse since a graft-versus-host response is also associated with a graft-versus-leukaemia effect; hence some disparity between the immune systems of the transplant donor and recipient is helpful. In addition to these problems, all transplanted patients are at increased risk of a second malignancy developing later in life as a consequence of the conditioning therapy received before transplant and probably also as a consequence of deficiencies within the transplanted immune system.

Given the problems associated with the various therapeutic strategies discussed above, it is not surprising that there has been great excitement surrounding the development of a new targeted tyrosine kinase inhibitor, imatinib. The initial results with this agent, particularly for patients with newly diagnosed chronic phase disease, are very encouraging. Complete cytogenetic responses have been seen although very sensitive quantitative PCR techniques can still detect the abnormal BCR-ABL gene in the vast majority of CML patients in whom the Philadelphia chromosome itself is undetectable. In addition, the drug has been shown to delay progression to accelerated phase disease or blast crisis. Imatinib use has not yet, however, been shown to associate with improved overall survival as compared with standard therapies such as interferon-α with or without cytosine or in the long term with allogeneic transplantation. Although no randomized study has been undertaken, it is clear from historical data that in the short term the mortality associated with allogeneic stem cell transplantation far exceeds that associated with imatinib. In addition to these very encouraging data which pertain to the effect of the drug on the disease, the side effects of imatinib are generally mild and patients report this agent far easier to tolerate than

interferon-α. The main side effects are rash, cytopenias, fluid retention and abnormalities of liver function tests.

There is clearly a dilemma here; imatinib appears to be a well-tolerated and effective agent but it is too early to say whether it represents a cure for CML and in addition, its potential long-term toxicities are unknown since it has only been in use since 1998. In contrast, allogeneic transplantation does represent a curative therapy for CML and the acute and chronic toxicities of this therapy are well documented and are high. The patients themselves may have strong views about the risks they are prepared to accept and clearly they need to be fully involved at all stages of the decision-making process. In view of the encouraging results seen with imatinib, many patients and their treating physicians choose to begin therapy with a trial of this drug. The patient is then monitored closely both haematologically and molecularly to determine whether they have a good response to imatinib. In the event of a good response to imatinib, the patient continues to take the drug. If at a later stage the molecular response to the agent begins to diminish then transplantation is reconsidered. Amongst patients who fail to respond or respond poorly to imatinib, transplantation options are likely to be considered at an earlier stage. It is worth pointing out that historical data show that patients initially treated using interferon-α did better post transplant if that transplant was undertaken during the first year after diagnosis. Ongoing studies will determine whether the same effect is seen amongst patients initially treated with imatinib. However, given the problems associated with transplantation, even when undertaken early, it seems reasonable at this time to take transplant decisions on basis of responses to imatinib.

Case 50.2

A patient with AML is currently in first complete remission and has a fully HLA-matched brother who is medically fit. You have been asked to counsel the potential transplant donor about stem cell collection.

Questions

1. What methods are available for the collection of stem cells for haemopoietic stem cell transplantation?
2. What are the advantages and disadvantages of each of these stem cell collection methods for the transplant donor?
3. What are the advantages and disadvantages of each of these stem cell collection methods for the transplant recipient?

Answers

1. There are two main methods of collection of haemopoietic stem cells from a sibling donor. These are:

- direct harvesting of cells from the bone marrow in the pelvis
- collection of circulating peripheral blood stem cells using an apheresis technique after stimulation of the stem cell compartment using (GCSF).

2. Direct harvesting of marrow stem cell from the bone marrow is an operative procedure and is performed under general anaesthetic. Clearly there are risks associated with the use of general anaesthesia but the risk of death associated with this approach is less than 1 in 10 000 procedures. There are no known long-term complications of such anaesthetics. Marrow harvesting involves a hospital stay, usually for one night postoperatively, but some units also require donors to be admitted the night before surgery. Donors are likely to experience pain around the pelvis and there is a risk of mechanical back pain in the short to medium term due to pressure applied to the pelvis during repeated needle insertions. This risk is increased in those with a history of back problems prior to the procedure. Indeed, such potential donors may prefer a peripheral blood stem cell harvesting approach. Donors must be warned about bruising and potential infection at the site of their wounds.

One of the other potential problems associated with marrow harvesting is that it is impossible to select the type of blood cell harvested and a large component of the volume of fluid collected comprises red blood cells. This can lead to a degree of anaemia in the donor who may take several weeks to normalize their haemoglobin. It is usually possible to avoid blood transfusion in this situation as it is unusual for donors to be significantly symptomatic. Nonetheless, donors must be warned that the need for allogeneic blood transfusion is a possibility with this procedure.

Peripheral blood stem cell harvesting has several advantages over direct marrow harvesting from the iliac crests. The procedure can be undertaken during hospital outpatient visits and does not require the use of a general anaesthetic. As the stem cell harvesting procedure allows selective collection of mononuclear cells, significant anaemia is very unlikely after this procedure. Clearly red cells do circulate within the apheresis circuit and if the circuit clots off and has to be disconnected from the donor then red cells will be lost. This is unlikely to be of clinical significance unless the donor is a child and hence has a relatively low blood volume.

Disadvantages of this approach include the need for stimulation of donor haemopoiesis by the GCSF. Marrow stimulation can result in significant pain especially around the shoulders, back and pelvic girdle. Most donors can manage this pain at home with simple analgesia but very occasionally hospital admission is required for pain control. Very occasional patients develop splenic pain and there have been a couple of reports of splenic rupture in normal donors after GCSF stimulation but this is very rare. One difficulty with the use of GCSF is that it has only been in routine use for the last 10 years. This makes it impossible to categorically reassure potential stem cell donors that use of GCSF in this way is absolutely safe in the long term. There is, however, currently no evidence that acting as a peripheral blood stem cell donor increases one's risk of leukaemia development later in life. Some potential donors find this element of uncertainty difficult and prefer to undertake a marrow harvest in which the risks, although present, are better quantified.

The apheresis procedure itself involves the donor lying relatively still with a needle in one or both arms (depending upon the type of apheresis kit used) for approximately 4–5 hours. Some collections can be done in one procedure but some donors will need to be harvested in two procedures, over 2 days. One prerequisite for peripheral blood stem cell donation is that the potential donor has good enough peripheral veins to allow reliable venous access. If this is not the case and the donor prefers to donate using this method, a temporary central venous line has to be inserted.

Most donors tolerate the apheresis procedure with few problems. One of the most common complications of the procedure is hypocalcaemia which results from calcium binding by the citrate anticoagulant used to prevent clotting within the apheresis circuit. Donors may notice perioral tingling or paraesthesia in other areas and are asked to report this immediately. The problem is easily treated by reducing the concentration of anticoagulant in the circuit and by asking the donor to drink a small amount of milk. If this problem is not picked up early the consequences can be more severe, with the development of tetany which would clearly require intravenous calcium replacement.

In summary, peripheral blood stem cell donation is generally a less invasive and better tolerated procedure than direct stem cell harvest from the marrow space. However, the associated procedural risks are more easily quantifiable for the latter procedure.

3. There are some potential advantages, to the transplant recipient, in the use of peripheral blood stem cells as opposed to bone marrow stem cells. Engraftment is quicker so the recipient spends less time in the neutropenic phase and hence the risk of infection is reduced. Similarly there is evidence that duration of hospital stay is

reduced when peripheral blood stem cells are used. One potential disadvantage of this approach is that the graft includes a larger dose of T-lymphocytes than a graft of stem cells derived directly from the marrow (approximately a 10-fold increase). There is some evidence that rates of chronic GVHD are increased amongst recipients of peripheral blood stem cells but this observation has not been borne out in all studies. This potential disadvantage of peripheral blood stem cells is negated if a T-cell depleted approach is used, as is the case for most matched unrelated procedures.

Case 50.3

Mrs RY is a 40-year-old woman undergoing an allogeneic bone marrow transplant for chronic myelocytic leukaemia. Post transplant she experienced severe mucositis and gastrointestinal toxicity. She was unable to eat and so take in adequate nutrition and in view of this was commenced on total parenteral nutrition. On day 16 she had a temperature and antibiotic therapy was initiated with gentamicin and piperacillin. The fever had not resolved 72 hours later and blood cultures remained negative. Daily blood counts taken to monitor the fall and recovery of her peripheral blood count revealed she was still pancytopenic.

Questions

1. Would you advise commencement of an antifungal agent at this stage?
2. Which agents are available for therapy and what advantages and disadvantages are associated with each?

Answers

1. The commencement of empiric antifungal therapy is considered the standard of care in the management of neutropenic patients. The use of empirical intravenous amphotericin B has been shown to reduce mortality in the setting of a fever which is non-responsive to antibacterial agents in severely neutropenic patients.
2. There is a range of agents available for use in this setting. Firstly, the azoles; fluconazole has a limited spectrum of activity, with no efficacy against *Aspergillus* which is one of the most frequently seen fungal infections in this setting. Fluconazole is therefore not a suitable choice for empirical therapy. Itraconazole has a broader spectrum of activity and has anti-*Aspergillus* activity. The absorption of the agent when given orally is variable and thus to be sure of attaining good tissue levels, if this agent were chosen it should be given via the intravenous route. Voriconazole is a new agent with a broad spectrum of activity. This agent was recently compared with ambisome in a randomized trial. Although the results with voriconazole did not reach the criteria for non-inferiority when compared with ambisome, the rate of breakthrough fungal infections was lower in the voriconazole arm. Voriconazole could be considered for use in this setting, particularly if there were specific reasons why alternative agents would cause problems, for instance amongst patients with renal impairment who may experience worsening of their renal function using an amphotericin-based product. One major advantage of voriconazole is that it is available as both an oral and intravenous preparation; conversion of patients to oral therapy for home treatment is straightforward if their infection has been controlled with voriconazole.

Amphotericin-based drugs have a broad spectrum of activity against fungal infections and would be an excellent choice in this setting. The only agent that has been proven to be associated with a reduction in mortality in the empiric therapy of potential fungal infections in neutropenic patients is standard amphotericin B. Unfortunately this agent is associated with significant renal toxicity, which limits dose intensity and necessitates the cessation of use in many cases. Lipid-formulated amphotericin drugs are now available which are efficacious and reduce renal toxicity.

Caspofungin is a relatively new antifungal agent. Its use is not associated with significant renal toxicity but elevations in liver enzymes can occur and may necessitate withdrawal of the drug. It is easier to give to patients than amphotericin-based agents as patients experience fewer infusional toxicities. It does not have such a broad spectrum of activity as amphotericin-based agents or voriconazole and in particular, *Mucor* tends to be resistant to this drug. In a large randomized controlled trial caspofungin was not found to be inferior to ambisome, a lipid-formulated amphotericin-derived product.

Case 50.4

A 24-year-old patient with ALL is undergoing chemotherapy and needs intrathecal chemotherapy to prevent relapse in the meninges. Giving drugs by this route is EXTREMELY DANGEROUS. Several patients have died as a result of the inadvertent administration of vinca alkaloids into the CSF.

Question

What steps have been taken nationally to try to prevent the inadvertent intrathecal injection of vincristine and other agents not suitable for intrathecal use?

Answer

In the UK there are now strict guidelines for administration of intrathecal chemotherapy. They can only be performed in hospital units which have passed a rigorous peer review process. The procedure must be undertaken in a specially designated area. Intravenous drugs must not be given in this area. The intrathecal drugs must only be prescribed by a consultant or specialist registrar who has been trained to prescribe or give intrathecal chemotherapy and whose name appears on a locally held register. Drugs for intrathecal administration must only be prescribed on a specially designated prescription sheet. Once the prescription has arrived in pharmacy the drugs must be made up and checked by pharmacists trained in the manufacture and checking of intrathecal prescriptions. The drugs must be positively labelled 'for intrathecal use only' and must be dispensed by a trained pharmacist. They can only be dispensed once the patient has been given any intravenous drugs that are due that day. The doctor collecting the drugs must sign to confirm that the i.v. drugs, if due, have been given before the drugs are dispensed. The drugs must only be dispensed to a doctor trained and on the register for giving intrathecal drugs. The intrathecal drugs must be transported in a specially designated container and if they need to be stored then it must be in a separate, specially designated fridge, i.e. separate from any intravenous chemotherapy. Once the procedure is under way the intrathecal drugs must be checked by the registered doctor and by a nurse who has been trained and appears on a register of nurses trained to check intrathecal drugs. The drugs should also be checked by the patient or a patient's representative. Intrathecal drugs must not be given in hospitals not approved for the procedure, in non-designated areas, outside office hours or at the weekend unless there are exceptional circumstances. All staff working on oncology or haematology units should be taught about the rules for giving intrathecal therapy. Hospitals giving intrathecal chemotherapy should follow special rules for labelling vinca alkaloid prescriptions and vinca alkaloids should be made up in a minimum volume of 20 mL.

Case 50.5

A 37-year-old dental technician presented with acute promyelocytic leukaemia (APML). He had a number of bleeding problems at presentation. He was commenced on oral all-trans retinoic acid (ATRA) followed by chemotherapy with daunorubicin, cytosine arabinoside and tioguanine. Within 4 weeks he had achieved a complete remission. He went on to receive a further two courses of intensive chemotherapy followed by maintenance therapy with 6-mercaptopurine, methotrexate and ATRA.

Question

Why is ATRA used in this circumstance and what are its side effects?

Answer

APML is a variant of AML which presents with coagulation defects, low platelet counts and severe bleeding. Patients are at risk of severe haemorrhage at presentation but have a relatively good prognosis with chemotherapy. ATRA can rapidly correct the coagulopathy found at presentation. This agent also increases the likelihood of the patient entering remission, when combined with standard high-dose chemotherapy. It is also used as a maintenance agent and when used with 6-mercaptopurine and methotrexate, it increases the number of patients who remain in long-term remission. The side effects of ATRA include dry eyes and a dry mouth. In addition, ATRA can cause a severe and life-threatening sterile pneumonitis. It is important to recognize this syndrome quickly as it often responds to high-dose dexametason and if left untreated leads to respiratory failure and death.

Case 50.6

A 57-year-old man with a 6-year history of CLL presented with a rising white cell count, worsening lymphadenopathy and hepatosplenomegaly. He had previously been treated with six courses of chlorambucil. Treatment was commenced with fludarabine 25 mg/m² daily for 5 days.

Question

What additional precautions would you advise the physician to take and why?

Answer

Fludarabine is a new agent available for the treatment of CLL. It is usually used as a second-line therapy although many haematologists are now considering its use as a first-line therapy. It can be given either orally or intravenously. It is very immunosuppressive, with particular activity against T-cells, and patients treated with this drug are at high risk of developing *Pneumocystis* pneumonia. It is important that patients are given prophylaxis against this severe infection.

As patients are immunosuppressed they are also at risk of developing transfusion-related GVHD. This is a complication of blood product transfusion, caused by engraftment of lymphocytes from the transfused product, which is frequently fatal. This complication can be prevented by irradiation of blood products prior to transfusion.

REFERENCES

Bennett J M, Catovsky D, Daniel M T et al 1976 Proposals for the classification of the acute leukaemias (FAB cooperative group). British Journal of Haematology 33: 451-458

Faderl S, Talpaz M, Estrov Z et al 1999 The biology of chronic myeloid leukaemia. New England Journal of Medicine 341(3): 164-172

Faderl S, Gandhi V, Keating M J et al 2005 The role of clofarabine in hematologic and solid malignancies – development of a next-generation nucleoside analogue. Cancer 103: 1985-1995

Hughes T P, Kaed J, Branford S et al 2003 Frequency of major molecular responses to imatinib or interferon-alfa plus cytarabine in newly diagnosed chronic myeloid leukaemia. New England Journal of Medicine 349: 1423-1432

Jaffe E S, Harris N L, Stein H et al 2001 World Health Organization classification of tumours. Pathology and genetics: tumours of haematopoietic and lymphoid tumours. IARC Press, Lyon

Leukaemia Research Fund 2005 Facts and statistics. Available online at: www.Lrf.org.uk

Löwenberg B, Downing J R, Burnett A 1999 Acute myeloid leukaemia. New England Journal of Medicine 341(14): 1051-1062

O'Brien S, Guilhot F, Larson R A et al 2003 Imatinib compared with interferon and low-dose cytarabine for newly diagnosed chronic-phase chronic myeloid leukaemia. New England Journal of Medicine 348: 994-1004

Pagliuca A, Carrington P A, Pettengell R et al 2003 Guidelines on the use of colony-stimulating factors in haematological malignancies. British Journal of Haematology 123: 22-33

Pui C H, Relling M V, Downing J R 2004 Mechanisms of disease: acute lymphoblastic leukaemia. New England Journal of Medicine 350: 1535-1548

Rai K R, Peterson B L, Appelbaum F R et al 2000 Fludarabine compared with chlorambucil as primary therapy for chronic lymphocytic leukaemia. New England Journal of Medicine 343: 1750-1757

Russell N H 1998 Developments in allogeneic peripheral blood progenitor cell transplantation. British Journal of Haematology 103: 594-600

Sawyers C L 1999 Medical progress: chronic myeloid leukaemia. New England Journal of Medicine 340: 1330-1340

Sipsas N V, Bodey G P, Kontoyiannis D P 2005 Perspective for the management of febrile neutropenic patients with cancer in the 21st century. Cancer 103: 1103-1113

Soignet S, Maslak P 2004 Therapy of acute promyelocytic leukaemia. Advances in Pharmacology 51: 35-58

Stone R M, O'Donnell M R, Sekeres M A 2004 Acute myeloid leukaemia. Hematology 2004: 98-117

Tallman M S, Andersen J W, Schiffer C et al 1997 All-trans-retinoic acid in acute promyelocytic leukaemia. New England Journal of Medicine 337(15): 1021-1028

FURTHER READING

Hoffbrand A V, Pettit J E 2001 Essential haematology, 4th edn. Blackwell Publishing, Oxford

Howard M R, Hamilton P J 2002 Haematology: an illustrated colour text, 2nd edn. Churchill Livingstone, Edinburgh

Negrin R S, Blume K G 2001 Allogeneic and autologous hematopoietic stem cell transplantation. In: Beutler E, Lichtman M A, Coller B S, Kipps T J, Seligsohn U (eds) Williams' hematology, 6th edn. McGraw-Hill Medical Publishing Division, New York

Provan D, Gribben J G 2005 Molecular hematology, 2nd edn. Blackwell Publishing, Oxford

Provan D, Henson A 2002 ABC of clinical haematology, 2nd edn. BMJ Books, London

Lymphomas 51

L. Cameron   C. Loughran

KEY POINTS

- Hodgkin's lymphoma (HL) and non-Hodgkin's lymphoma (NHL) are aggressive diseases that are fatal if untreated.
- Early-stage Hodgkin's lymphoma patients are treated with combined modality treatment usually consisting of 2–4 cycles of ABVD (adriamycin (doxorubicin), bleomycin, vinblastine, dacarbazine) and involved field radiotherapy (20–30 Gy); a relapse-free survival rate of 80% at 5–10 years is achieved.
- ABVD chemotherapy is the current gold standard regimen for advanced Hodgkin's lymphoma, and overall survival at 5 years is 70%.
- Low-grade non-Hodgkin's lymphoma may be treated using either a 'watch and wait' policy or a single alkylating agent such as chlorambucil or combination chemotherapy.
- CHOP-R (cyclophosphamide, hydroxydaunorubicin (doxorubicin), Oncovin (vincristine), prednisolone, rituximab) chemotherapy is the standard for the treatment of aggressive (intermediate and high-grade) non-Hodgkin's lymphoma, curing 60% of patients.
- Relapsed Hodgkin's lymphoma and non-Hodgkin's lymphoma may be treated with further chemotherapy followed by high-dose chemotherapy with bone marrow or peripheral stem cell transplantation.
- Patients receiving chemotherapy for Hodgkin's lymphoma and non-Hodgkin's lymphoma should have full blood count and blood biochemistry monitored at frequent intervals.
- Complications such as nausea and vomiting, tumour lysis syndrome, mucositis and bone marrow suppression may occur as a result of chemotherapy and are significant factors in morbidity.
- Supportive care of the patient undergoing chemotherapy includes appropriate drug therapy to minimize the adverse effects of the treatment.

Lymphoma is cancer of the lymphatic system and accounts for approximately 3% of new cases of cancer reported in the UK each year. The primary cancerous cell of origin is the lymphocyte; as a result there is often considerable overlap between lymphomas and lymphoid leukaemias. Lymphomas are subdivided into two main categories: Hodgkin's lymphoma and non-Hodgkin's lymphoma. Both Hodgkin's lymphoma (HL) and non-Hodgkin's lymphoma (NHL) can be further classified based on histology.

The site of malignancy is usually a lymph node. Extranodal disease, most frequently of the stomach, skin, oral cavity and pharynx, small intestine and CNS, can occur and is more common in non-Hodgkin's lymphoma than Hodgkin's lymphoma .

Hodgkin's lymphoma

Hodgkin's disease, now known as Hodgkin's lymphoma, was first described by Thomas Hodgkin in 1832. Hodgkin's lymphoma accounts for 30% of all lymphomas and has an incidence in the UK of 2.2 per 100 000 for women and 3.3 per 100 000 for men. It is predominantly a disease of young adults, having a peak incidence between the ages of 15 and 35 years.

Aetiology

The cause of HL is unknown but a number of risk factors have been identified. Epstein–Barr (glandular fever) virus has been identified in 50% of HL cases and is likely to be associated with an increase in risk of developing Hodgkin's lymphoma. Certain associations have been identified which suggest a genetic link with Hodgkin's lymphoma; for example, same-sex siblings of patients with Hodgkin's lymphoma have a 10 times higher risk of developing the disease. Patients with reduced immunity, e.g. AIDS or those taking immunosupressants, may have an increased risk of developing Hodgkin's lymphoma.

Pathology

The diagnosis is made by histological examination of an excised lymph node biopsy. The characteristic pathological finding in Hodgkin's lymphoma is the identification of a large, abnormal binucleate lymphocyte called a Reed-Sternberg cell. Hodgkin's lymphoma is classified as two distinct entities: classic Hodgkin's lymphoma and nodular lymphocyte-predominant Hodgkin's lymphoma (NLPHL). Classic Hodgkin's is further subdivided into four histological types:

- nodular sclerosis: this is the most common type in the UK, predominating in young adults and females, and has an excellent prognosis
- mixed cellularity: this is second most common type of classic Hodgkin's lymphoma and more common in males (70% male)
- lymphocyte depleted: this carries a poor prognosis and is more common in HIV-positive individuals
- lymphocyte rich: this is a rare type of classic Hodgkin's lymphoma.

NLPHL accounts for 5% of Hodgkin's lymphoma cases and is more common in men.

Signs and symptoms

Hodgkin's lymphoma usually presents with painless enlargement of lymph nodes, often in the neck. About 40% of patients will present with fever, night sweats and/or weight loss. These have prognostic significance and are designated B symptoms; others include malaise, itching (25%) or pain at the site of enlarged nodes after drinking alcohol. Bone pain may result from skeletal involvement. Primary involvement of the gut, central nervous system or bone marrow is rare.

If lymph nodes in the chest are involved patients may present with breathlessness. There is often a disturbance of immune function due to a progressive loss of immunologically competent T-lymphocytes, with patients becoming particularly prone to viral and fungal infections.

Laboratory findings

Laboratory findings include normochromic, normocytic anaemia, a raised erythrocyte sedimentation rate and eosinophilia. One-third of patients have a leucocytosis due to an increase in neutrophils. Advanced disease is associated with lymphopenia (lymphocytes $<0.6 \times 10^9$/L). Plasma lactate dehydrogenase (LDH) is raised in 30–40% of patients at diagnosis and has been associated with a poor prognosis.

Investigations and staging

Once the diagnosis has been made on biopsy, further investigations are needed to assess disease activity and the extent of its spread through the lymphoid system or other body sites. This is called staging and is essential for assessing prognosis, with cure rates for localized tumours (stage I or II) being much higher than those for widespread disease (stage IV). The staging of Hodgkin's lymphoma is assessed by the Cotswolds modification of the Ann Arbor classification system (Table 51.1). Information about prognostic factors such as mediastinal mass and bulky disease is included in the classification system. The tests required to establish the stage include a complete history, physical examination, full blood count (FBC), urea and electrolytes (U & Es), chest x-ray and computed tomography (CT). Other useful tests include erythrocyte sedimentation rate (ESR), plasma lactate dehydrogenase (LDH) and liver function tests (LFTs). PET (positron emission tomography) can be used to detect active residual disease.

Management

Hodgkin's lymphoma is potentially curable and, in general, sensitive to both chemotherapy and radiotherapy; therefore the two main goals of treatment are to maximize the likelihood of cure whilst minimizing the risk of late toxicity such as infertility. Stage of disease is the biggest factor in treatment choice and outcome. The management of classic Hodgkin's lymphoma is determined by the stage of the disease and this is summarized in Figure 51.1. Localized NLPHL frequently involves one isolated lymph node and tends to be indolent (slow growing). If there are no risk factors it can be treated with involved field radiotherapy

Table 51.1 Cotswolds modification of the Ann Arbor classification system for Hodgkin's lymphoma

Stage	Defining features
I	Involvement of a single lymph node region or lymphoid structure
II	Involvement of two or more lymph node regions on the same side of the diaphragm
III	Involvement of lymph node regions or structures on both sides of the diaphragm: III$_1$ – with or without involvement of splenic, hilar, coeliac or portal nodes III$_2$ – with involvement of para-aortic, iliac or mesenteric nodes
IV	Involvement of extranodal site(s) beyond that designated E

Modifying characteristics
- A: no symptoms
- B: fever, drenching sweats, weight loss
- X: bulky disease
  > one-third width of the mediastinum
  >10 cm maximal dimension of nodal mass
- E: involvement of a single extranodal site, contiguous or proximal to known nodal site
- CS: clinical stage
- PS: pathological stage

alone (30 Gy); all other types are treated as advanced (stage III or IV) classic Hodgkin's lymphoma.

In Europe the treatment of classic Hodgkin's lymphoma is determined by whether the disease is staged as early favourable disease, early unfavourable disease, advanced disease or relapsed.

Early-stage (favourable) disease

The cure rate for patients with stage I and IIA disease is greater than 90%. Patients with stage I and IIA disease may be cured with radiotherapy alone (wide or extended field irradiation). However, due to radiation-related late effects, cardiac toxicity and secondary malignancy and the incidence of relapse (25–30%), most receive combined modality treatment (chemotherapy and radiotherapy). This usually consists of 2–4 cycles of ABVD chemotherapy followed by involved field radiotherapy (IFRT) of 20–30 Gy (Diehl et al 2004). The aim of chemotherapy is to destroy subclinical disease outside the field of radiotherapy.

Where disease is confined to above the diaphragm, the mantle field is used (Fig. 51.2). The inverted Y is employed when the disease is confined below the diaphragm. This group of patients have a relapse-free survival rate of 80% at 5–10 years. However, a recent study suggests that radiotherapy with ABVD, compared to ABVD alone, increases progression-free survival but not overall survival. It would appear that any advantage of radiotherapy plus ABVD is offset by deaths due to causes other than Hodgkin's lymphoma (Meyer et al 2005).

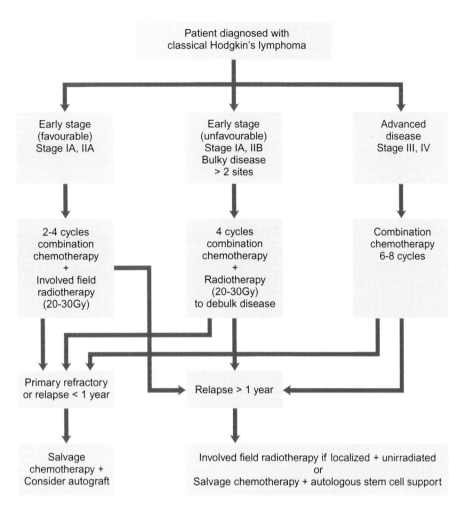

Figure 51.1 Treatment algorithm for classic Hodgkin's lymphoma.

Early-stage (unfavourable) disease

Patients with stage I or II presenting with bulky disease, B symptoms or with more than two sites of disease are considered to be poor risk if treated with radiotherapy alone. These patients are treated with four cycles of combination chemotherapy, e.g. ABVD, and radiotherapy (20–30 Gy) to sites of bulky disease.

Advanced disease

Patients with advanced disease (stages III and IV) are treated with combination chemotherapy. The first widely used combination chemotherapy regimen was MOPP (mechlorethamine, vincristine (Oncovin), procarbazine and prednisolone) which produced a response rate of 80% and long-term disease-free survival of approximately 50%. ABVD has replaced MOPP chemotherapy as the regimen of choice as it is as effective but less toxic in terms of fertility, haematological toxicity, and the development of acute leukemia and myelodysplasia. Six to eight cycles of ABVD is considered the current standard treatment for advanced disease. The role of consolidative radiotherapy in advanced disease is unclear. Patients with partial remission after chemotherapy may benefit from IFRT, whereas those in complete remission may not receive any further benefit. The decision

whether to give radiotherapy needs to be made on an individual basis (Connors 2005).

Despite advances in Hodgkin's lymphoma, 30–40% of patients progress or relapse and respond poorly to salvage chemotherapy. A number of regimens have been investigated over the past decade; two regimens that have shown promise are Stanford V (mustine, adriamycin (doxorubicin), vinblastine, prednisolone, vincristine, bleomycin, etoposide) and BEACOPP (bleomycin, etoposide, adriamycin (doxorubicin), cyclophosphamide, vincristine (Oncovin), procarbazine, prednisolone) (Table 51.2) In a trial comparing dose-increased BEACOPP, standard-dose BEACOPP and COPP-ABVD, dose-increased BEACOPP demonstrated increased overall survival compared with the other two treatment arms. BEACOPP is associated with a higher rate of haematological toxicity and secondary acute myeloid leukaemia (AML). Of men treated with BEACOPP, 80% will suffer sterility, whereas those treated with ABVD are unlikely to have problems (Pfreundschuh et al 2004). It is because of this toxicity that ABVD remains the standard treatment but trials are ongoing to investigate the role of dose-intensified chemotherapy in advanced Hodgkin's lymphoma. The International Prognostic Index (IPI) for advanced Hodgkin's lymphoma was developed to identify high-risk patients who may benefit from dose-intensified

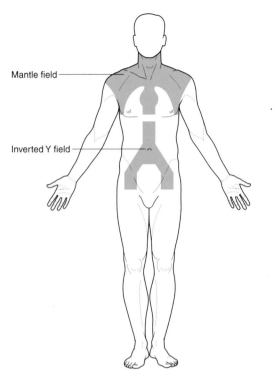

Figure 51.2   The mantle and inverted Y fields commonly employed in the treatment of Hodgkin's lymphoma with radiotherapy (from Souhami & Tobias 1998, p. 437, with permission from Blackwell Science).

Mantle field

Inverted Y field

chemotherapy. However, stratification and treatment based on this index are still experimental.

Salvage therapy for relapsed disease

Relapsed disease refers to disease progression after completion of primary treatment which resulted in a complete remission. Dependent on previous treatment, options include salvage radiotherapy, salvage chemotherapy or high-dose chemotherapy with autologous stem cell support. In this procedure stem cells are collected from the patient and returned following high-dose chemotherapy. Patients who relapse after initial radiotherapy alone have a good chance of cure with combination chemotherapy, at least equal to that of patients initially treated with chemotherapy for advanced disease. Occasionally radiotherapy is used if the disease is localized and previously non-irradiated. Those who relapse after combination chemotherapy have a worse prognosis, although durable remissions can be obtained with further conventional therapy.

Length of remission following first-line chemotherapy influences the success of subsequent salvage therapy and so failure of chemotherapy can be used to classify disease and determine appropriate therapy. If the duration of remission was greater than 12 months (late relapse) then the patient can be retreated with their initial chemotherapy, salvage regimen or considered for high-dose chemotherapy with autologous transplantation. Commonly used chemotherapy salvage regimens are listed in

Table 51.2   Combination chemotherapy regimens effective in the treatment of Hodgkin's lymphoma

Regimen	Dose and route	Frequency
ABVD (28-day cycle)		
Doxorubicin	25 mg/m² i.v.	Days 1 and 15
Bleomycin	10 000 iu/m² i.v.	Days 1 and 15
Vinblastine	6 mg/m² i.v.	Days 1 and 15
Dacarbazine	375 mg/m² i.v.	Days 1 and 15
BEACOPP 14 (14-day cycle)*		
Bleomycin	10 000 iu/m² i.v.	Days 8
Etoposide	100 mg/m² i.v.	Days 1–3
Adriamycin (doxorubicin)	25 mg/m² i.v.	Day 1
Cyclophosphamide	650 mg/m² i.v.	Day 1
Vincristine	1.4 mg/m² i.v. (max. 2 mg)	Day 8
Procarbazine	100 mg/m² orally	Days 1–7
Prednisolone	40 mg/m² orally	Days 1–14
GCSF is used to maintain a 14-day cycle		
Stanford V (28-day cycle)*		
Mustine	6 mg/m² i.v.	Weeks 1,5,9
Doxorubicin	25 mg/m² i.v.	Weeks 1,3,5,7,9,11
Vinblastine	6 mg/m² i.v.	Weeks 1,3,5,7,9,11
Prednisolone	40 mg/m² alternate days orally	Days 1–63, taper over days 64–84
Vincristine	1.4 mg/m² i.v. (max. 2 mg)	Weeks 2,4,6,8,10,12
Bleomycin	5000 iu/m² i.v.	Weeks 2,4,6,8,10,12
Etoposide	60 mg/m² i.v. for 2 consecutive days	Weeks 3,7,11

*Stanford V and BEACOPP-14 are chemotherapy regimens that have shown activity in Hodgkin's lymphoma, but their usage is not common in the UK.

Table 51.3. If relapse occurs less than a year after treatment (early relapse) then high-dose chemotherapy with autologous stem cell support should be considered. A patient who has never achieved complete remission (primary refractory disease) should receive high-dose chemotherapy with autologous stem cell support.

High-dose chemotherapy plus autologous stem cell support is associated with a 40–50% 5-year survival rate. However, the significant toxicity of autologous stem cell transplantation means that it should be reserved for patients in whom there is a clear increase in chance of cure.

The role of allogeneic transplantation is controversial. Early results indicate a high transplant-related mortality (up to 50%) and disappointing survival. Allogeneic transplantation for Hodgkin's lymphoma should be restricted to prospective trials (Bartlett 2005).

New agents

The anti-CD20 antibody rituximab has shown remission in 80% of cases of (NLPHL but due to short follow-up its use is still considered experimental. Other monoclonal antibodies targeting CD30, which is expressed in the majority of classic Hodgkin's lymphoma cases, are being investigated. Gemcitabine has shown activity in relapsed classic Hodgkin's lymphoma with response rates up to 79% in a small series of heavily pretreated patients (Ng et al 2005). Bortezomib, a proteosome inhibitor licensed for myeloma, is also being investigated in those who have relapsed Hodgkin's lymphoma.

Non-Hodgkin's lymphoma

The non-Hodgkin's lymphomas are a heterogeneous group of lymphoid malignancies ranging from indolent, slow-growing

Table 51.3 Salvage chemotherapy regimens effective in the treatment of lymphoma

Regimen	Dose and route	Frequency
DHAP		
Cisplatin	100 mg/m² i.v.	Days 1
Cytarabine	2000 mg/m² i.v. 12 hourly	Day 2
Dexametasone	40 mg orally	Days 1–4
ESHAP		
Etoposide	40 mg/m² i.v	Days 1–4
Methylprednisolone	500 mg/m² i.v	Days 1–5
Cytarabine	2000 mg/m² i.v	Day 1
Cisplatin	25 mg/m² i.v	Days 1–4
ICE		
Ifosfamide	5000 mg/m² i.v	Day 2
Carboplatin[a]	AUC 5 i.v.	Day 2
Etoposide	100 mg/m² i.v	Days 1–3

[a]Carboplatin dose (mg) = target AUC (mg/mL × min) × (GFR (mL/min) + 25)
AUC: area under the curve
GFR: glomerular filtration rate

tumours to aggressive, rapidly fatal disease. Paradoxically, the more aggressive non-Hodgkin's lymphomas are more susceptible to anticancer therapy. The overall incidence of non-Hodgkin's lymphoma in the UK is 11 per 100 000 per year and accounts for approximately 3% of all cancers in the UK. The disease is rare in subjects under 30 years of age and the incidence steadily increases with increasing age; the median age at presentation is about 60. Non-Hodgkin's lymphoma is slightly more common in men than in women (1.5:1).

Aetiology

The aetiology is unclear although immunosuppression, for example following organ transplantation, may predispose to the development of lymphoma. Several viruses have been implicated in the pathogenesis of non-Hodgkin's lymphoma; for example, there is some evidence that Burkitt's lymphoma, an aggressive B-cell lymphoma observed in West African children, is linked to malaria. Burkitt's lymphoma is also one of the most common neoplasms to develop in HIV-related immunosuppressed patients. The human T-lymphotrophic virus type 1 (HTLV-1) is associated with a rare type of T-cell lymphoma. Exposure to certain chemicals such as pesticides and solvents can increase the risk of developing non-Hodgkin's lymphoma. There is an increased incidence of gastrointestinal lymphomas in patients with Crohn's disease.

Signs and symptoms

The most common presentation of non-Hodgkin's lymphoma is painless lymphadenopathy, frequently in the neck area in the supraclavicular and cervical regions. Spread of disease is haematogenously (via the blood) and so extranodal sites may be involved. Signs and symptoms of infection, anaemia or thrombocytopenia may be present in patients with bone marrow involvement. Hepatospenomegaly may also be present. Patients may also present with any of the following symptoms: unexplained loss of weight, unexplained fever, drenching night sweats. These symptoms are described as B symptoms and patients without these symptoms are classified as category A. B symptoms are more commonly seen in advanced or aggressive non-Hodgkin's lymphoma but may be present in all stages and histological subtypes.

Laboratory findings

Laboratory examinations may reveal anaemia, a raised erythrocyte sedimentation rate and a raised plasma lactate dehydrogenase level. There may be a reduction in circulating immunoglobulins and a monoclonal paraprotein may be seen in a small number of cases. The immune disruption caused by the disease may also result in an increased susceptibility to viral infection or autoimmune haemolytic anaemia or thrombocytopenia.

Histopathology and classification

There have been many attempts to classify the non-Hodgkin's lymphomas into histological categories that have clinical significance. Despite this, many problems and areas of confusion remain.

Approximately 85% of non-Hodgkin's lymphomas are of B-cell origin, while 15% are of T-cell origin or are unclassifiable.

There are two classification systems in common use. The Working formulation, developed in 1982, divides the lymphomas into low, intermediate and high grade. More recently, the revised European–American lymphoma (REAL) classification system has been developed (Table 51.4) and adopted by the World Health Organization (Table 51.5) to classify the grade of lymphoma. The REAL/WHO classification incorporates some diagnoses not included in the Working formulation and is a list of lymphomas using morphology, immunophenotype, genotype and clinical behaviour. It recognizes the three major categories of lymphoid malignancies: B-cell neoplasms, T-cell/natural killer cell neoplasms and Hodgkin's lymphoma. However, in practice, the clinical behaviour of lymphomas informs the treatment strategies employed as these are based on the initial classification into indolent (low grade) or aggressive (intermediate and high grade) non-Hodgkin's lymphoma. A more biologically relevant classification of lymphoma using the REAL/WHO classification and immunological and molecular characteristics increases the diagnostic specificity and improves selection and targeting of therapy.

Diagnosis

Diagnosis is based on a thorough history, physical examination and investigation of a lymph node. A definitive diagnosis of non-Hodgkin's lymphoma can only be made by biopsy of pathological lymph nodes or tumour tissue. An expert histopathologist may need to utilize sophisticated techniques such as immunophenotyping or genotyping to obtain an accurate subclassification.

Chromosomal abnormalities are of diagnostic importance. The most commonly associated chromosomal abnormality in non-Hodgkin's lymphoma is the t(14;18)(q32;q21) translocation. This is found in 85% of follicular lymphomas and 28% of more aggressive lymphomas.

Additional investigations should also be performed to accurately stage the disease and exclude other disease. Full blood count from peripheral blood should be performed. Peripheral blood lymphocytosis (increased lymphocytes) with circulating malignant cells is common in low-grade and mantle cell lymphomas. A bone marrow aspirate and trephine is required to exclude leukaemia and will detect bone marrow involvement, which is more common than in Hodgkin's lymphoma. CT scans of the chest, abdomen and pelvis are required to assess the extent of the disease. The use of positron emission tomography (PET) scans, capable of locating sites not thought to be affected from CT scan images, is increasing. Lumbar punctures should be performed for patients at high risk of CNS involvement, e.g. Burkitt's lymphoma. Erythrocyte sedimentation rate, plasma

Table 51.4 Clinical grade and frequency of lymphomas in the REAL classification

Diagnosis	% of all cases
Indolent lymphomas	
Follicular lymphoma	22
Marginal zone B-cell, mucosa-associated lymphoid tissue	8
Chronic lymphocytic leukaemia/small lymphocytic lymphoma	7
Marginal zone B-cell nodal	2
Lymphoplasmacytic lymphoma	1
Aggressive lymphoma	
Diffuse large B-cell lymphoma	31
Mature (peripheral) T-cell lymphomas	8
Mantle cell lymphoma	7
Mediastinal large B-cell lymphoma	2
Anaplastic large cell lymphoma	2
Very aggressive lymphomas	
Burkitt's lymphoma	2
Precursor T-lymphoblastic	2
Other lymphomas	7

Table 51.5 Revised European–American lymphoma classification as adopted by the WHO (REAL/WHO classification)

Precursor B-cell neoplasm
Precursor B-cell acute lymphoblastic leukaemia or lymphoma

Mature (peripheral) B-cell neoplasm
B-cell chronic lymphocytic leukaemia or small lymphocytic lymphoma
B-cell prolymphocytic leukaemia
Lymphoplasmacytoid lymphoma
Splenic marginal zone B-cell lymphoma (with or without villous lymphocytes)
Hairy cell leukaemia
Plasma cell myeloma or plasmacytoma
Extranodal marginal zone B-cell lymphoma (with or without monocytoid B-cells)
Follicular lymphoma
Mantle cell lymphoma
Diffuse large B-cell lymphoma
Mediastinal large B-cell lymphoma
Primary effusion lymphoma
Burkitt's lymphoma or Burkitt's cell leukaemia

Precursor T-cell neoplasm
Prescursor T-cell acute lymphoblastic leukaemia or lymphoma

Mature (peripheral) T-cell and natural killer neoplasms
T-cell prolymphocytic leukaemia
T-cell granular lymphocytic leukaemia
Aggressive natural killer cell leukaemia
Adult T-cell lymphoma or leukaemia
Extranodal natural killer/T-cell lymphoma
Enteropathy type T-cell lymphoma
Hepatosplenic T-cell lymphoma
Subcutaneous panniculitis-like T-cell lymphoma
Mycosis fungoides/Sezary syndrome
Primary cutaneous anaplastic large cell lymphoma
Peripheral T-cell lymphoma
Angio-immunoblastic T-cell lymphoma
Primary systemic anaplastic large cell lymphoma

lactate dehydrogenase and plasma β_2-microglobulin levels may indicate disease activity and can be of prognostic importance.

Staging

Determining the extent of disease in patients with non-Hodgkin's lymphoma provides prognostic information and is useful in treatment planning. Patients with extensive disease usually require different therapy from those with limited disease. The non-Hodgkin's lymphomas can be staged according to the Ann Arbor classification (see Table 51.1). In this system, non-Hodgkin's lymphoma is defined as stage I, II, III or IV, stage I being disease limited to a single lymph node and stage IV being advanced disease, with involvement of extralymphatic sites. The International Prognostic Index (Table 51.6) uses the following factors as predictors of poor prognosis: elevated lactate dehydrogenase (LDH), stage III or IV disease, greater than 60 years of age, the higher the number of extranodal sites involved and the Eastern Co-operative Oncology Group (ECOG) performance status of two or higher. Other prognostic factors include bulky disease, presence of B symptoms and transformation from low- to high-grade disease. Prognostic indicators are important because they inform the treatment plan to avoid overtreating those with good prognosis and undertreating those with poor prognosis.

Treatment

When designing a treatment plan for an individual patient, various factors must be taken into account. These include the patient's age and general health, the extent or stage of the lymphoma and the particular histological subtype. Indolent (low-grade) lymphoma tends to run a slow course and although it is not curable, patients survive for prolonged periods with minimal symptoms. Aggressive (high-grade) lymphomas result in death within weeks or months if untreated. These lymphomas, however, are very responsive to chemotherapy and up to 50–60% may be cured with combination chemotherapy. Figure 51.3 summarizes the management of non-Hodgkin's lymphoma.

Indolent non-Hodgkin's lymphoma

The median age at which patients present with indolent non-Hodgkin's lymphomas is 50–60 years and generally patients have a good performance status. If left untreated, indolent non-Hodgkin's lymphoma has a comparatively long survival (median 9 years). Follicular lymphoma is the most common of the indolent lymphomas. For the minority of patients presenting with limited stage disease (stage I), radiotherapy to the involved field is generally used. However, the majority (80%) of patients present with advanced disease (stage II–IV) and the aim of treatment is to reduce disease bulk and offer symptom relief. Advanced-stage low-grade non-Hodgkin's lymphoma is responsive to both chemotherapy and radiotherapy but patients usually relapse over time, even those who achieve a complete response. Cure is unusual for the majority of patients. Patients who are asymptomatic at diagnosis can be followed with a 'watch and wait' policy and treated when symptomatic or until disease progression. The median time until chemotherapy is required is around 3 years.

Systemic treatment consists of oral alkylating agents, e.g. chlorambucil, cyclophosphamide, with or without steroid, purine analogues (fludarabine) or combination chemotherapy. Chlorambucil is commonly used as a first-line agent. Repeated courses of chlorambucil may be given for recurrences occurring at intervals over a prolonged period of time. Combination chemotherapy, e.g. CVP (cyclophosphamide, vincristine, prednisolone) or CHOP, tends to be used as first-line treatment for young patients with aggressive disease and is an option in relapsed disease (Table 51.7). It is not clear which chemotherapy agents or combination of agents provide the best treatment outcome. Recent studies have shown that the addition of rituximab to CVP chemotherapy (R-CVP) as first-line therapy for advanced (stage III or IV) follicular lymphoma compared to CVP alone improves clinical outcome (Marcus et al 2005). This approach has been incorporated into national guidance (NICE 2006). Fludarabine as a single agent or in combination with mitoxantrone and dexamethasone (FMD) is the treatment of choice for second-line therapy. Although treatment is often associated with symptomatic and clinical improvement, there is little proof that it affects survival. The use of rituximab alone in newly diagnosed, asymptomatic patients is being investigated and it is hoped this may delay the time to initiation of chemotherapy.

Relapsed indolent non-Hodgkin's lymphoma

Rituximab, a monoclonal antibody with specificity for CD20, has shown benefit in patients with relapsed or chemoresistant follicular lymphoma. CD20 is essential for cell cycle regulation and cell differentiation and is expressed on normal B-cells and the majority of malignant B-cell lymphomas. The mechanism of action of rituximab is not fully understood but is thought to involve complement-mediated lysis of B-cells and antibody-dependent cellular cytotoxicity. Other potential mechanisms include induction of apoptosis and inhibition of cell cycle progression. In practice, therefore, it is used for patients who have failed to respond or relapsed after receiving chlorambucil or fludarabine. There are several ongoing clinical trials to determine the best strategy for rituximab treatment for varying subtypes and stages of non-Hodgkin's lymphoma.

Some resistant or relapsing patients, particularly if elderly, will be in too poor a condition to merit further radical chemotherapy and palliation will be appropriate. There are a number of agents which may be useful in this field. Yttrium-90 labelled

Table 51.6 International Prognostic Index	
Factor	Adverse prognosis
Age	≥60 years
Ann Arbor stage	III or IV
Plasma lactate dehydrogenase level	Above normal
Number of extranodal sites of involvement	≥2
Performance status	≥ECOG 2 or equivalent

ECOG, Eastern Co-operative Oncology Group

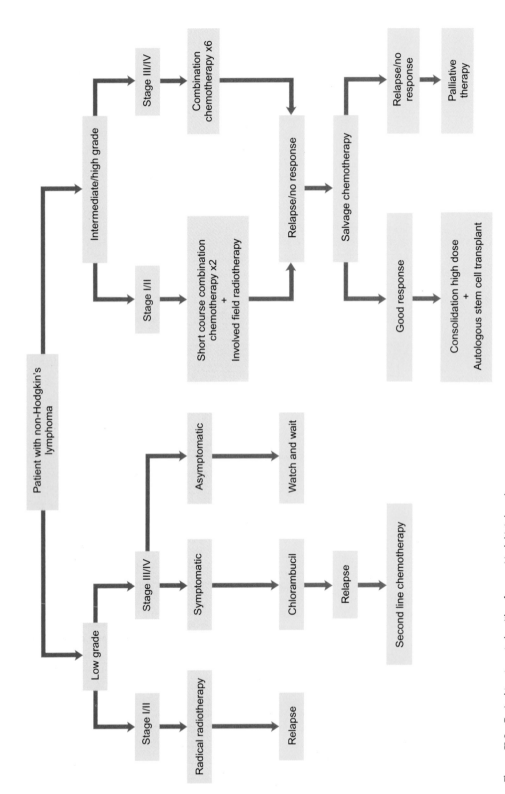

Figure 51.3 Typical treatment algorithm for non-Hodgkin's lymphoma.

Table 51.7 Chemotherapy regimens effective in the treatment of non-Hodgkin's lymphoma

Drug	Dose and route	Day of administration
CHOP-R (21-day cycle)		
Cyclophosphamide	750 mg/m^2 i.v.	Day 1
Doxorubicin (hydroxydaunorubicin)	50 mg/m^2 i.v.	Day 1
Vincristine (Oncovin)	1.4 mg/m^2 (max. 2 mg) i.v	Day 1
Prednisolone	100 mg orally	Days 1–5
Rituximab	375 mg/m^2 i.v.	Day 1
CVP (21-day cycle)		
Cyclophosphamide	750 mg/m^2 i.v.	Day 1
Vincristine (Oncovin)	1.4 mg/m^2 (max. 2 mg) i.v	Day 1
Prednisolone	100 mg orally	Days 1–5
FMD (28-day cycle)		
Fludarabine	40 mg/m^2 orally	Days 1–3
Mitoxantrone	10 mg/m^2 i.v.	Day 1
Dexametasone	20 mg daily	Days 1–5
FC (28-day cycle)		
Fludarabine	40 mg/m^2 orally	Days 1–3
Cyclophosphamide	250 mg/m^2 daily orally	Days 1–3
CHOP (21-day cycle)		
Cyclophosphamide	750 mg/m^2 i.v.	Day 1
Doxorubicin (hydroxydaunorubicin)	50 mg/m^2 i.v.	Day 1
Vincristine (Oncovin)	1.4 mg/m^2 (max. 2 mg) i.v	Day 1
Prednisolone	100 mg orally	Days 1–5
CHOP-14 (14-day cycle)		
Cyclophosphamide	750 mg/m^2 i.v.	Day 1
Doxorubicin (hydroxydaunorubicin)	50 mg/m^2 i.v.	Day 1
Vincristine (Oncovin)	1.4 mg/m^2 (max. 2 mg) i.v	Day 1
Prednisolone	100 mg orally	Days 1–5

GCSF is used to maintain a 14-day cycle

ibritumomab tiuxetan (Zevalin) and iodine-131 tositumomab (Bexxar) are therapeutic developments that utilize monoclonal antibodies as tumour-specific vehicles to deliver systemic radiation therapy concurrent with immunotherapy to the targeted tumour. There are also ongoing clinical trials investigating the value of newer agents such as bortezomib, a proteosome inhibitor.

Aggressive non-Hodgkin's lymphoma

The median age of presentation of aggressive non-Hodgkin's lymphoma is 60–70 years when 50–60% of patients will present with an advanced stage of the disease. The most common presentation is diffuse large B-cell lymphoma (DLBCL), and therefore the treatment strategies described below refer to this alone. Other aggressive lymphomas, e.g. mantle cell, are managed differently. The most important strategy when treating this group of patients is to maintain the dose intensity of chemotherapy and minimize any delay in chemotherapy administration. Treatment is given with curative intent.

Stage I disease These lymphomas are treated with a combination chemotherapy regimen and IFRT. Radiotherapy alone can achieve long-term disease control in approximately 90% of patients with a disease-free survival of 60–70% at 5 years However, a better outcome can be obtained with the combination of CHOP and radiation therapy. Rituximab is not generally indicated for this patient group.

Stage II–IV disease The treatment for advanced-stage aggressive non-Hodgkin's lymphoma is the combination of CHOP and rituximab (CHOP-R). Elderly patients have a lower response rate to CHOP compared with younger patients. The poor outcome seems to be related to a poor initial response and an increase in treatment-related toxicity and a decrease in dose because of age.

A number of clinical trials are under way to determine whether an improvement in survival can be achieved by increasing the dose intensity of chemotherapy using granulocyte colony stimulating factor (GCSF).

Relapsed aggressive non-Hodgkin's lymphoma

Combination chemotherapy with CHOP probably cures 40–50% of patients with aggressive lymphoma and the addition of rituximab may increase this by a further 10% (Burton & Linch

2005). This, therefore, implies that over half of all patients have refractory disease or relapse after first treatment.

In younger patients with aggressive non-Hodgkin's lymphoma, the aim will be to introduce remission with further chemotherapy, using an alternative, salvage regimen, and then to consolidate remission with high-dose therapy (HDT). HDT is usually supported by mobilized peripheral blood stem cells and an autologous peripheral blood stem cell transplantation (auto PBSCT). Lymphoma is the most frequent indication for HDT and autologous peripheral blood stem cell transplantation in Europe. The European Group for Blood and Marrow Transplantation (EBMT) suggests that the upper age limit for autologous transplantation is 65 years. HDT, with autologous stem cell support, is also used as part of primary treatment for younger patients with indolent lymphoma. Patients who receive HDT after their initial treatment can have progression-free survival rates of around 50% at 5 years.

To induce a remission in patients with aggressive lymphoma and relapsed disease, it may be reasonable to use the same or similar regimen used for front-line chemotherapy. However, in most cases the regimen chosen introduces new agents that are potentially not cross-resistant with those used in the initial treatment regimen. There are several salvage regimens in use and they generally have response rates of between 40% and 70%. Examples of salvage regimens are ICE (ifosfamide, carboplatin, etoposide), ESHAP (etoposide, methylprednisolone, cytarabine, cisplatin) and DHAP (cisplatin, cytarabine, dexametasone) (see Table 51.3). Gemcitabine, a pyrimidine analogue, may be of benefit for patients with relapsed or refractory disease after two lines of treatment. Gemcitabine is used in combination with other agents, such as cisplatin and methylprednisolone. Rituximab can also be added to these salvage regimens. Peripheral blood stem cells (PBSC) are usually harvested after the third course of the salvage regimen. Patients then receive a high-dose regimen such as BEAM (carmustine, etoposide, cytarabine, melphalan) (Table 51.8) conditioning prior to stem cell infusion. It is not clear if patients should first receive salvage chemotherapy, with high-dose therapy and autologous peripheral blood stem cell transplantation reserved for those patients who do not respond to chemotherapy, or alternatively if all patients should be offered HDT regardless of the success of the salvage chemotherapy. In addition, whether patients should undergo HDT without previous salvage chemotherapy has also yet to be determined.

Table 51.8 Conditioning chemotherapy for autologous transplantation

Drug	Dose and route	Day of administration
BEAM		
Carmustine	300 mg/m² i.v.	6 days before reinfusion
Etoposide	200 mg/m² i.v.	5 to 2 days before reinfusion
Cytarabine	200 mg/m² 12 hourly i.v.	5 to 2 days before reinfusion
Melphalan	140 mg/m² i.v.	1 day before reinfusion
Reinfusion of stem cells		Day 0

CNS prophylaxis for diffuse large B-cell lymphoma
Approximately 5% of patients with DLBCL develop CNS disease. The optimum approach to CNS prophylaxis is uncertain and it usually involves a course of intrathecal chemotherapy. The updated national guidance for the safe administration of intrathecal chemotherapy (DH 2003) sets out the minimum requirements of a hospital providing an intrathecal chemotherapy service.

Very aggressive lymphoma

Burkitt's lymphoma is a rare form of B-cell non-Hodgkin's lymphoma which occurs most commonly in children and young adults. The median age of adult patients is 30 years. Untreated, survival is measurable in days or weeks and it is widely accepted that combination chemotherapy should be urgently commenced. Intensive chemotherapy is necessary, together with CNS prophylaxis, and cure is possible in a high proportion of cases.

Multi-agent chemotherapy regimens including high-dose methotrexate, high-dose cytarabine, etoposide and ifosfamide are used and a schedule such as CODOX-M (cyclophosphamide, vincristine, doxorubicin, high-dose methotrexate)/IVAC (ifosfamide, etoposide, high-dose cytarabine) is common.

Lymphoblastic lymphomas/leukaemia

Lymphoblastic lymphomas comprise about 2% of adult non-Hodgkin's lymphomas. Patients are often treated with the same regimens used in acute lymphoblastic leukaemia (ALL). Despite a very high rate of complete responders, long-term survival remains poor. Patients who fail after first-line chemotherapy have a long-term disease-free survival of less than 10%. These cases are subsequently treated as leukaemias (see Chapter 50).

Patient care

The chemotherapy regimens used to treat Hodgkin's lymphoma and non-Hodgkin's lymphoma (see Tables 51.2 and 51.7) are usually administered on a hospital outpatient basis with the patient visiting the clinic regularly for assessment and treatment. The patient is monitored by full blood counts carried out before each cycle of chemotherapy and at the 'nadir' between cycles. The nadir is when the blood count is at its lowest point, usually 10–14 days after the first day of chemotherapy. The interval between each cycle of chemotherapy enables normal body cells to recover before the patient receives further treatment. Disease response to treatment is monitored by repeating some of the diagnostic investigations, such as CT, at suitable intervals and the use of PET. If there is little or no response to treatment a different chemotherapy regimen will be used or a decision made to withdraw from active therapy and provide optimum supportive care.

Counselling and support

Counselling is an essential part of the care of the cancer patient and involves not only the explanation of drug therapy and investigations but also the provision of psychological support for the patient and family. Prior to treatment with chemotherapy, the patient will be counselled by the doctor, chemotherapy nurse and, increasingly, by oncology pharmacists. It is necessary to explain how the chemotherapy is to be given and discuss both potential and inevitable side effects. The probability of successful treatment must be weighed against the prospect of serious and life-threatening adverse effects. Patients must be made aware of the long-term complications of chemotherapy and radiotherapy, such as secondary malignancy.

The support available to the cancer patient, to help cope with both the illness and its treatment, has improved dramatically in recent years. Multidisciplinary teams working within specialized units have become skilled in anticipating the problems of lymphomas and their treatment. In addition, many charities provide care, support and advice – for example, BACUP (British Association of Cancer United Patients; www.cancerbackup.org.uk), Macmillan Cancer Relief (www.macmillan.org.uk) and the Lymphoma Association (www.lymphoma.org.uk).

Patient-specific treatment modifications

The selection of appropriate therapy must also take into consideration the individual patient. Factors include the patient's age, renal and hepatic function and underlying medical conditions, such as heart disease, diabetes or chronic pulmonary disease. The patient's tolerance of side effects and complications of therapy may then be predicted. The decision is based on an understanding of the pharmacodynamics and pharmacokinetics of the drugs being used as well as the clinical condition of the patient.

Supportive care

During a course of chemotherapy the patient requires supportive care to minimize the adverse effects of treatment. The common adverse effects of the chemotherapy regimens discussed in this chapter are outlined in Table 51.9. These will occur to varying

Table 51.9 Adverse effects associated with chemotherapy regimens used in the lymphomas with supportive measures and counselling points

Adverse effect	Cytotoxics implicated	Supportive measures	Counselling points
Bone marrow suppression	Chlorambucil Cyclophosphamide Dacarbazine Etoposide Vinblastine Prednisolone	Blood transfusion Platelet transfusions Mouth care Antibiotic therapy for febrile episodes Granulocyte-colony stimulating factor (G-CSF)	Expect tiredness Report bleeding or unusual bruises Importance of good personal hygiene Adhere to mouth care regimen Avoid people with infections Monitor temperature Report febrile episodes or signs of infection immediately
Nausea and vomiting	Cyclophosphamide Doxorubicin Procarbazine Dacarbazine	Antiemetic therapy	Emphasize regular use. A short course is more effective than 'as required' treatment Take tablets before meals Report episodes of vomiting (especially if taking oral cytotoxics) For dexametasone, emphasize short course not to be continued to ensure the patient does not receive repeat prescriptions from primary care doctor
Mucositis	Doxorubicin	Mouth care regimen	Importance of good oral hygiene, instruct how mouthwashes are used, stress importance of regular use
Tumour lysis syndrome	High tumour load sensitive to chemotherapy	Hydration Allopurinol Rasburicase	Stress importance of regular allopurinol until appropriate to stop Drink plenty of fluids
Alopecia	Cyclophosphamide Doxorubicin Etoposide	Provision of wig if wanted	Hair usually regrows on completion of therapy
Impaired gonadal function	Alkylating agents Procarbazine Doxorubicin (to a lesser degree)	Sperm storage	Refer to doctor, depends on regimen, reversible some cases

continued

Table 51.9 (continued)

Adverse effect	Cytotoxics implicated	Supportive measures	Counselling points
Neuropathy	Vincristine	Discontinue use or substitute vinblastine	Report tingling sensations or difficulty with buttons, jaw pain or stiffness, constipation. Do not self-treat but refer to doctor
Cardiomyopathy	Doxorubicin		Report breathlessness, tiredness
Lung fibrosis	Bleomycin		Report breathlessness

degrees depending on the combination of drugs and the doses used as well as individual patient factors.

Nausea and vomiting

Nausea and vomiting is the most distressing and most feared adverse effect of chemotherapy. Its effect on the patient should not be underestimated and its treatment is an important part of supportive care. The severity will depend on the combination of drugs used. For example, oral chlorambucil is generally well tolerated by almost all patients and requires no antiemetic cover. Regimens such as FMD (fludarabine, mitoxantrone, dexametasone) and ABVD, which are moderately and highly emetic respectively, will make most patients vomit if no antiemetics are given. The patient should be counselled on the appropriate use of prescribed antiemetics (see Table 51.9).

Tumour lysis syndrome

The lymphomas are, in general, highly sensitive to chemotherapy. The resulting lysis of cells which occurs following initiation of chemotherapy may lead to hyperuricaemia, hyperkalaemia and hypercalcaemia in patients with bulky disease, and result in urate nephropathy. There is a high incidence of tumour lysis syndrome (TLS) in tumours with high proliferation rates and tumour burden such as Burkitt's lymphoma and T-lymphoblastic lymphoma. The mainstay of tumour lysis syndrome prevention is hydration with the patient encouraged to maintain a high fluid intake. Hyperuricaemia is controlled with allopurinol and close monitoring of renal function, plasma urate levels and electrolytes. Allopurinol must be commenced before chemotherapy and continued until the tumour load has reduced and plasma urate levels are normal. In aggressive forms of non-Hodgkin's lymphoma, rasburicase, a recombinant urate oxidase, may be indicated as prophylaxis. Allopurinol should not be prescribed concurrently with rasburicase because it will inhibit the production of uric acid, the substrate for rasburicase.

Rasburicase can also be used to treat tumour lysis syndrome but will only correct hyperuricaemia. Treatment of tumour lysis syndrome should include vigorous hydration and diuresis. Historically alkaline diuresis has been recommended but overzealous alkalinization can lead to problems such as metabolic acidosis (Cairo & Bishop 2004). Hypocalcaemia should be corrected if the patient is symptomatic but this may increase calcium phosphate deposition. Hyperkalaemia and hyperphosphataemia should be corrected; patients may require haemofiltration or dialysis.

Mucositis

Chemotherapy may cause mucositis, which is inflammation of or damage to the surface of the gastrointestinal tract. In the mouth this may lead to painful ulceration, local infection and difficulty in swallowing. Dependent on the severity of mucositis, patients may require analgesia from benzydamine mouthwash to systemic opiates. Disruption of the mucosal barrier will give bacteria and fungi easier systemic access. A mouth care regimen should therefore be instituted with myelosuppressive therapy. This involves good oral hygiene, e.g. gentle brushing with a toothbrush to remove plaque or rinsing with saline to remove debris. An antiseptic mouthwash such as chlorhexidine 0.2% should also be used regularly to prevent infection.

Bone marrow suppression

Myelosuppression is usually the dose-limiting factor with these regimens and it is necessary to carry out full blood counts before treatment to confirm that recovery has occurred. Each chemotherapy protocol should be referred to so as to ensure appropriate management. Generally, if the platelet count is below $100 \times 10^9/L$ and/or the absolute neutrophil count is less than $1 \times 10^9/L$, the subsequent dose may be reduced or treatment delayed by a week.

Anaemia is treated with blood transfusions and thrombocytopenia with platelet transfusions as necessary. Erythropoietin administration reduces blood transfusion requirements and can improve quality of life. However, the evidence suggesting improvement in patient survival is inconclusive.

Neutropenia is the most life-threatening acute toxicity; the neutropenic patient is at constant risk from infections. Seemingly minor infections such as cold sores can spread rapidly, and infections not seen in the normal population, such as systemic fungal infections, can occur. Supportive measures involve reducing the risks and the aggressive treatment of any infectious episodes. The patient is counselled to avoid contact with people with infection or those who may be carriers. Most infections, however, are from an endogenous source such as the gut or skin. The patient is educated on the importance of good personal hygiene, mouth care, how to monitor body temperature and to report any febrile episodes immediately. Co-trimoxazole 960 mg may be prescribed as prophylaxis against *Pneumocystis* pneumonia in patients receiving chemotherapy for lymphomas, particularly in those receiving a regimen containing fludarabine. Thorough and frequent hand washing helps to prevent the transmission of opportunistic infection to the neutropenic patient.

Febrile neutropenia

A febrile episode in the neutropenic patient is an indication for immediate treatment with broad-spectrum intravenous antibiotics. Susceptibility to infection is likely when the neutrophil count is less than 1×10^9/L with increasing risk at levels less than 0.5×10^9/L and 0.01×10^9/L. Fever, usually defined as a temperature above 38°C maintained for 1 hour or 38.3°C on one occasion, may be the only sign of infection. The patient should be assessed to determine the site of infection, if possible. Blood cultures from all venous access ports and any other appropriate cultures, e.g. midstream urine sample and stool sample, are taken and then antibiotic therapy commenced. Blood cultures are taken prior to starting antibiotics to increase the likelihood of obtaining a positive culture. Infection with Gram-negative bacilli, e.g. *Escherichia coli, Klebsiella pneumoniae* and *Pseudomonas aeruginosa,* and Gram-positive cocci, e.g. coagulase-negative staphylococci, β-haemolytic streptococci, enterococci, and *Staphylococcus aureus* is probable in this situation. Therefore first-line therapy is usually a third-generation cephalosporin or antipseudomonal penicillin with gentamicin. If the patient does not respond to this combination within 24–48 hours, then second-line therapy, which includes a glycopeptide for Gram-positive cover, is commenced.

Gram-positive infections are becoming more common with the use of indwelling intravenous catheters. If positive microbiological cultures are found, the appropriate antibiotic can be prescribed on the basis of sensitivities; however, if the patient is responding to empiric therapy the antibiotics should not be changed. Only one-third of suspected infections are ever confirmed, and the pathogen may not be isolated. The febrile episode may not be due to infection; non-infectious causes include blood transfusion and underlying disease.

Growth factor support

Patients with persistent neutropenia or those who have repeated admissions for neutropenic sepsis may be supported with GCSF. There is evidence that patients with lymphomas receiving a reduced dose of chemotherapy as a consequence of myelosuppression have a worse prognosis when compared with patients who receive full doses. GCSF is indicated as primary prophylaxis, before any episode of febrile neutropenia, for regimens where there is a high (>40%) incidence of febrile neutropenia. GCSF has been investigated as a prophylactic measure to increase the dose intensity of chemotherapy in regimens such as CHOP-14 (cyclophosphamide, hydroxydaunorubicin (doxorubicin), Oncovin (vincristine), prednisolone at 14 day intervals) and BEACOPP-14 (bleomycin, etoposide, Adriamycin (doxorubicin) cyclophosphamide, vincristine, procarbazine, prednisolone at 14 day intervals).

CASE STUDIES

Case 51.1

Mr RB is a 50-year-old man receiving a course of fludarabine and cyclophosphamide (see Table 51.7) for mantle cell lymphoma. He has no other medical problems and has normal renal and hepatic function.

Questions

1. What are the key counselling points for the oral chemotherapy drug fludarabine?
2. What antibacterial agent would you expect to see prescribed with fludarabine?
3. What antiemetic regimen would you recommend with the fludarabine and cyclophosphamide?

Answers

1. Immunocompromised patients, e.g. those receiving purine analogues, fludarabine, cladribine and pentostatin, are at risk of developing transfusion-associated graft versus host disease (TAGVHD), a rare but usually fatal complication of transfusion. Viable T-lymphocytes in donated blood can recognize the recipient as 'foreign', leading to fever, skin rash, hepatitis and bone marrow involvement. Death occurs in 90% of cases, predominantly due to infection.

   γ-Irradiation of cellular blood components is the mainstay of TAGVHD prevention. Patients should be given an appropriate patient information leaflet and an alert card. The risk of TAGVHD is minimized by informing transfusion staff and the patient of their need for irradiated blood products.
2. Mr RB should be prescribed co-trimoxazole prophylactically to prevent *Pneumocystis jiroveci* infection.
3. Chemotherapy drugs are grouped by how likely they are to cause emesis if antiemetics are not given, called emetogenic potential. Antiemetic regimens are then prescribed to prevent the degree of vomiting expected for each group.

   Fludarabine is rarely emetogenic and oral cyclophosphamide is moderately emetogenic. Therefore the regimen should be classified and treated as moderately emetogenic. Dexametasone, granisetron and metoclopramide are frequently employed for moderately emetogenic regimens. Guidelines for antiemetic use in oncology are available (American Society of Clinical Oncology 2006). As corticosteroids are associated with immunosupression, some clinicians prefer not to use them for emesis prevention with FC chemotherapy.

Case 51.2

Mrs BC is a 72-year-old widow who has been newly diagnosed with low-grade non-Hodgkin's lymphoma. She has been seen in the hospital outpatient haematology clinic and has brought a prescription to the pharmacy for chlorambucil 10 mg daily for 14 days. When she hands in her prescription she expresses concern about the side effects of the tablets. The doctor who saw her had spent a lot of time talking to her about her treatment but she feels confused with all the information given.

Questions

1. What are the side effects of chlorambucil?
2. How would you counsel this patient?

Answers

1. Chlorambucil, an alkylating agent, is generally well tolerated. The major side effect is bone marrow suppression. Other side effects are uncommon, and include nausea and vomiting, rash, mucositis and diarrhoea. Hepatotoxicity and jaundice have been reported. Mrs BC is an elderly patient and is thus more likely to experience toxicity because of deteriorating renal and hepatic function and underlying medical conditions.

2. Mrs BC may be distressed by her diagnosis and may not have been able to absorb all the information she was given in the clinic. She may also be seeking confirmation of information.

    Mrs BC should be counselled to complete the course of tablets as prescribed. She should be told that she will probably feel tired and be more prone to infection because the tablets lower the blood count and resistance to infection. She should be advised to inform the haematologist if she feels unwell. Chlorambucil is unlikely to make her feel nauseous, but if this occurs she should inform the doctor, who will be able to prescribe an antiemetic.

Case 51.3

Mr F is 56 years old and was diagnosed with stage III high-grade non-Hodgkin's lymphoma over 10 weeks ago. Since then he has received three cycles of CHOP-R and has come to the hospital for his nadir blood count. He complains of painful mouth ulcers and a sore throat. On examination he has mucositis and oropharyngeal candidiasis. He has a white blood cell count (WCC) of 3.2 (normal range 3.5–11 × 10⁹/L) with 25% neutrophils (normal range 30–75%).

Questions

1. How would you treat Mr F's *Candida* infection?
2. How would you counsel this patient?

Answers

1. Mr F has an absolute neutrophil count (ANC) of 0.8×10^9/L (25% of WCC) and is therefore neutropenic (ANC $<1.0 \times 10^9$/L). Localized candidal infections can spread rapidly in the immunosuppressed patient, so local therapy with an antifungal mouthwash will be inadequate therapy. A course of fluconazole, 100 mg daily for at least 7 days, should be prescribed. Therapy should continue for a further 7 days if Mr F is still neutropenic or if the thrush has not completely resolved.

    An antibacterial mouthwash, such as chlorhexidine 0.2% 10 mL four times daily, should be used. As Mr F is complaining of pain, an analgesic should be added. Benzydamine mouthwash, a locally acting analgesic, could be prescribed initially. If this does not give adequate pain relief, then systemic analgesics such as dihydrocodeine should be given.

3. Regular mouth care reduces the risk of infection but does not entirely remove it. It is not necessarily a reflection of how well the patient has adhered to his mouth care regimen. Chlorhexidine mouthwash should be used first, held in the mouth as long as possible, ensuring the entire mucosa is covered before spitting out. The mouthwash should be used after meals and at bedtime. He should not eat or drink for at least half an hour after using the mouthwash.

    The benzydamine mouthwash should be used before meals as Mr F will probably find eating painful. He should be advised to use a soft toothbrush, to eat soft foods and to avoid hot and spicy dishes. He may be reassured that once his blood count recovers his mouth ulcers should resolve and that the fluconazole should relieve his sore throat.

Case 51.4

Mr D, 38 years old with advanced Hodgkin's lymphoma, is admitted to the haematology ward at the local hospital as an emergency. He had a temperature of 39°C on the morning of admission, feels generally unwell but has no specific symptoms. It is 12 days since he started his third cycle of ABVD. On admission he is taking the following medication:

- **co-trimoxazole 960 mg twice daily on 3 days a week**
- **chlorhexidine 0.2% mouthwash 10 mL four times daily.**

Blood cultures are taken and piperacillin 4.5 g i.v. three times daily and gentamicin 480 mg i.v. once daily are prescribed, to be commenced immediately. Blood biochemistry results are normal; his full blood count was Hb 10.8 (normal range 13.5–18.0 g/dL for men), WCC 2.5 (normal range 3.5–11 × 10⁹/L), neutrophil count 0.6 (normal range 1.5–7.5 × 10⁹/L) and platelets 150 (normal range 150–400 × 10⁹/L). Mr D weighs 86 kg and is 186 cm tall.

Questions

1. Comment on the rationale for the antibiotic therapy prescribed.
2. How would you monitor this patient?
3. What would be an appropriate second-line regimen if he remains pyrexial?
4. What modifications would need to be made to subsequent cycles of chemotherapy?

Answers

1. Mr D's full blood count is probably at its nadir following his last course of chemotherapy. He is neutropenic and febrile; fever is often the only sign of infection in neutropenic patients. Immunosuppression is also a feature of Hodgkin's lymphoma and contributes to susceptibility to infection. Treatment should commence immediately after cultures have been taken, as infection can be rapidly fatal in these patients. The antibiotics selected should provide broad-spectrum cover and follow local policy as there are institutional variations in predominant pathogens and antimicrobial sensitivities. The organisms responsible for infectious episodes are constantly changing: in the 1970s, Gram-negative infections predominated but now Gram-positive organisms account for 65% of positive cultures. As Gram-negative infections are more rapidly fatal, first-line therapy should be biased towards these infections. Piperacillin, an antipseudomonal pencillin, and gentamicin are therefore an appropriate combination to use in this patient.

    The dose of piperacillin is appropriate. Infection is considered to be severe in these patients as signs and symptoms are often muted. Single daily dose gentamicin is at least as effective as multiple dosing and less nephrotoxic; it is more convenient and cost-effective and overcomes deficiencies of the traditional method such as subtherapeutic dosing and inadequate monitoring. The dose is 5–7 mg/kg and has been calculated correctly for Mr D. He has normal renal function, so no dose modifications are necessary.

2. Monitor temperature, pulse and blood pressure and any patient symptoms for signs of improvement or deterioration. Blood biochemistry should be checked daily to detect any deterioration in renal function. Microbiology reports should be checked and antibiotics reviewed if any micro-organisms have been cultured. However, no change should be made to antibiotics if the patient is showing signs of improvement. The administration of gentamicin should be monitored, checking both administration and sampling time for drug levels. The results should be checked and recommendations for dose modification made where appropriate, using a method such as the Hartford monogram.

3. If the patient remains pyrexial 24–48 hours after the first-line antibiotics have been commenced, they should be replaced with second-line therapy, again following local policy. This should be a combination of a glycopeptide (vancomycin or teicoplanin) and a second broad-spectrum antibiotic to provide Gram-negative cover, e.g. ceftazidime. If blood cultures show growth, found in only 30–40% of neutropenic patients, the choice of antibiotics should be on the basis of sensitivities. It is important to note that febrile episodes lasting several days may involve more than one infecting organism.

The patient's full blood count should start to recover from day 14 but may be delayed by this infection. It is unusual for patients on conventional chemotherapy for Hodgkin's lymphoma to require more than one change to antibiotic therapy, and clinical improvement is often seen with recovery of neutrophil count. If Mr D is still pyrexial at 96 hours then the likelihood of fungal infection must be considered and an intravenous amphotericin-based product or caspofungin commenced if appropriate. The incidence of fungal infection is increasing in patients with prolonged neutropenia. As Mr D's neutropenia is short-lived, he is more likely to have a bacterial infection.

4. A dose reduction for subsequent cycles of chemotherapy may be considered. However, as this patient is being treated with curative intent, it may be more appropriate to give GCSF and maintain the dose intensity.

ACKNOWLEDGEMENTS

The authors thank Denise Blake and Mary Maclean for permission to use material originally included in their chapter that appeared in the third edition of this book.

REFERENCES

American Society of Clinical Oncology 2006 Guideline for antiemetics in oncology: update 2006. Journal of Clinical Oncology 24: 2932-2947

Bartlett N L 2005 Therapies for relapsed Hodgkin lymphoma: transplant and non-transplant approaches including immunotherapy. Hematology (Am Soc Hematol Educ Program) 245-251

Burton C, Linch D 2005 Management of relapsed histologically aggressive non-Hodgkin's lymphoma. British Journal of Cancer Management 2: 4-7

Cairo M S, Bishop M 2004 Tumour lysis syndrome: new therapeutic strategies and classification. British Journal of Haematology 127: 3-11

Connors J 2005 State-of-the-art therapeutics: Hodgkin's lymphoma. Journal of Clinical Oncology 23: 6400-6408

Department of Health 2003 Updated national guidance on the safe administration of intrathecal chemotherapy. Available online at: www. doh.gov.uk/publications/coinh.html

Diehl V, Thomas R K, Re D 2004 Part II: Hodgkin's lymphoma – diagnosis and treatment. Lancet Oncology 5: 19-26

Marcus R, Imrie K, Belch A et al 2005 CVP chemotherapy plus rituximab compared with CVP as first-line treatment for advanced follicular lymphoma. Blood 105: 1417-1423

Meyer R M, Gospodarowicz M K, Connors J M et al 2005 Randomized comparison of ABVD chemotherapy with strategy that includes radiation therapy in patients with limited-stage Hodgkin's lymphoma: National Cancer Institute of Canada clinical trials group and the Eastern Co-operative Oncology Group. Journal of Clinical Oncology 23: 4634-4642

National Institute for Health and Clinical Excellence 2006 Non-Hodgkin's lymphoma – rituximab. National Institute for Health and Clinical Excellence, London. Available online at: www.nice.org.uk

Ng M, Waters J, Chau I et al 2005 Gemcitabine, cisplatin and methylprednisolone (GEM-P) is an effective salvage regimen in patients with relapsed and refractory lymphoma. British Journal of Cancer 92: 1352-1357

Pfreundschuh M, Trümper L, Kloess M et al 2004 Two-weekly or 3-weekly CHOP chemotherapy with or without etoposide for the treatment of elderly patients with aggressive lymphomas: results of the NHL-B2 trial of the DSHNHL. Blood 104: 634-641

Souhami R, Tobias J (eds) 1998 Cancer and its management. Blackwell Science, Oxford

FURTHER READING

Dearden C, Matutes E 2000 Non-Hodgkin's lymphoma. Medicine 28: 71-77

Laport G F, Williams S F 1998 The role of high-dose chemotherapy in patients with Hodgkin's disease and non-Hodgkin's lymphoma. Seminars in Oncology 25: 503-517

Leonard J P, Coleman M (eds) 2006 Hodgkin's and non-hodgkin's lymphoma. Springer-Verlag, New York

Molina A, Al-Kadhimi Z, Nicolaou N 2005 Non-Hodgkin's lymphoma. In: Pazdur R, Coia L R, Hoskins W J, Wagman L D (eds) Cancer management: a multidisciplinary approach. PRR Melville, New York, pp 697-748. Available online at: www.cancernetwork.com/handbook/contents.htm

Pettengell R 2000 Hodgkin's disease. Medicine 28: 68-71

Provan D, Singer C R J, Baglin T et al 2004 Oxford handbook of clinical haematology. Oxford University Press, Oxford

52 Solid tumours

J. So

KEY POINTS

- Although cancer is a disease which predominantly affects the elderly, it is the leading cause of death in adults aged under 65.
- Superior outcomes are seen when treatment is supervised by, or given at, a specialized cancer centre.
- Before treatment, patients must be carefully staged to establish the type and extent of disease.
- Dependent on the stage of the disease, treatment goals may be cure, prolongation of survival or palliative symptom control.
- Cytotoxic chemotherapy is the main treatment for disseminated disease.
- Optimum patient management relies on tailoring treatment to the individual, anticipating adverse effects and taking into account patient preferences.
- New approaches include the use of targeted treatments which have more tolerable side effect profiles and may be given on a more long-term basis compared to conventional chemotherapy.

The term 'cancer' is used to describe more than 200 different diseases, including the haematological malignancies as well as those affecting discrete organs, i.e. solid tumours. Although some solid tumours are benign and mainly harmless this chapter will focus on the management of patients with solid malignancies which require some form of treatment. Treatment is best carried out in specialized cancer centres (or units closely linked with cancer centres) and therapy may include surgery, radiotherapy, chemotherapy or a combination of these. Care of the cancer patient demands a broad range of services involving multidisciplinary team working across the hospital, community and hospice network.

Epidemiology

Cancer is a common disease, affecting about one in three of the UK population, and one in four will die from it. Mortality statistics for 2003 show that in the UK, 154 547 people were registered as dying from a malignancy. Although male lung cancer death rates continue to fall, it is still the most common cause of male cancer death (25%), followed by prostate (13%) and colorectal (11%) cancer together accounting for half of male cancer deaths (Fig. 52.1). For women (Fig. 52.2) the decline in breast cancer deaths has seen lung cancer (18%) overtake breast cancer (17%) as the leading cause of female cancer death followed by colorectal (10%) and ovary (6%).

Although more than a quarter of a million people develop cancer each year in the UK, it is predominantly a disease of the elderly, with 64% of new cases diagnosed in people aged over 65 years. However, in adults under 65 years, 54% female deaths are due to cancer compared with 35% in men.

Over the decade from 1994 to 2003, mortality from cancer fell despite the growing incidence of the disease. Reducing mortalities in lung, breast and colorectal cancer have more than counteracted an upward trend in deaths from oesophageal cancer and melanoma.

Aetiology

The causes of cancer may be categorized as either environmental or genetic, although these may be interrelated and the causes of some cancers are multifactorial.

Environmental factors

Increasingly, lifestyle factors play a large part in the development of many cancers. Cigarette smoking has been identified as the single most important cause of preventable disease and premature death in the UK. About one-third of all cancer deaths are linked to tobacco use, which causes about 80% of lung cancer deaths as well as other cancers including bladder and oesophagus. The most important lifestyle factor for bowel cancer is likely to be diet. Table 52.1 lists a number of factors which have been associated with cancer development.

Genetic factors

A number of rare tumours are known to be associated with an inherited predisposition. Examples include the paediatric malignancies Wilms' tumour of the kidney and bilateral retinoblastoma, a rare cancer of the eye. Some common cancers such as breast, ovary, colon and melanoma may also show a tendency to occur in families but these are rare (5% common cancers). A woman's risk of developing breast cancer is increased if her mother, sister or daughter has had premenopausal or bilateral breast cancer and referral to a breast family history clinic is advisable.

Screening and prevention

Screening

Screening (secondary prevention) programmes aim to detect pre-clinical cancer in asymptomatic individuals in the general population to provide earlier, and thus more effective, treatment. Any

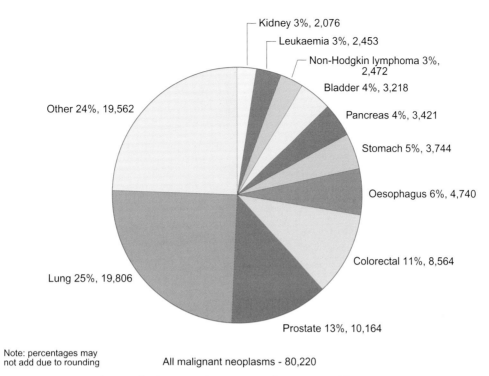

Figure 52.1   The 10 most common causes of cancer death in UK males in 2003. (With permission of the Cancer Research UK 2005)

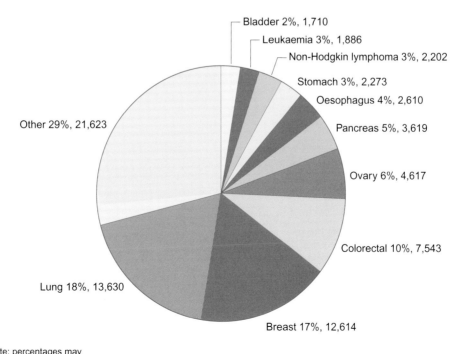

Figure 52.2   The 10 most common causes of cancer death in UK females in 2003. (With permission of the Cancer Research UK 2005).

Table 52.1 A–K of factors associated with specific cancer sites: an empirical basis for recommending life style changes (Jankowski & Boulton 2005)

Factor	Associated cancer
Alcohol consumption >3 units a day	Most squamous cancers, especially bladder and oesophagus
Body mass index >25 and certainly >30	All solid cancers
Cigarette smoking at any level (even passive smoking)	Bladder, lung, head and neck, oesophagus, and oropharyngeal cancers
Diet, especially one that is high in fat	All solid cancers
Exercising <30 minutes a day	All solid cancers
Family history of cancer (in at least one first-degree relative and at least three people in two or more generations)	Inherited cancer syndromes, including breast, colorectal, diffuse gastric, ovarian, prostate, and uterine cancers
Genital and sexual health (sexually transmitted infections)	Cervical cancer
Health-promoting drugs that may decrease global cancer risks (but need a careful risk/benefit analysis)	Colonic adenomas can be treated with low-dose aspirin but can have serious side effects. Hormone replacement therapy linked with breast cancer
Intense sunburn	Melanoma
Job-related factors	Lung cancer (exposure to asbestos and particulates), skin cancer (contact with arsenic)
Known disease associations	Colorectal cancer has predisposing mucosal pathology – adenomas, coeliac disease, ulcerative colitis

screening test must be simple, reliable, highly specific (to exclude healthy individuals) and highly sensitive (detection 90–95%). Screening is well established for cancers of the breast and cervix. From April 2006, screening in the form of a home testing kit (for faecal occult blood) will be introduced for bowel cancer. This will be phased in nationally over 3 years and offered to everyone aged 60–69 years. Population screening for prostate cancer using the prostate-specific antigen (PSA) blood test remains more controversial due to lack of specificity and sensitivity. It is currently not recommended for use in screening programmes in the UK.

Prevention

The strong association between cancer risk and lifestyle factors means there is great potential for the primary prevention of cancer through healthier eating, moderate drinking, limiting exposure to sunlight, avoiding cigarette smoke and encouraging physical exercise. Current public health campaigns such as the 5 (portions of fruit and vegetables) a day programme target the necessary lifestyle changes.

Chemoprevention

Chemoprevention (prevention of cancer by drug intervention) with the anti-oestrogen tamoxifen has been the subject of several trials to assess its value in preventing breast cancer. Although licensed for chemoprevention in the USA, on the basis of ongoing European studies, it is likely that tamoxifen will only be considered for younger women at high risk of breast cancer because of the associated increased risk and concerns of thrombosis. Continued follow-up of current trials will further inform UK practice.

Aspirin has been used in the primary prevention of colorectal cancer. Maximal effect was associated with high aspirin doses (more than 14 doses of 325 mg tablets per week) and only after 10 years of treatment (Chan et al 2005). More recently, individuals at high risk of colon cancer were targeted for participation in trials using cyclo-oxygenase 2 (COX-2) inhibitors until awareness of cardiovascular side effects associated with rofecoxib brought these to a halt.

Cancer at the cellular level

The normal cell and the role of p53

In the normal cell, there are genes associated with tumour suppression, notably the p53 gene which acts as a regulator of cell growth and proliferation. Agents which damage DNA cause p53 to accumulate. This switches off replication of abnormal cells, arresting them in the cell cycle and allowing them time to repair. If repair fails, p53 may trigger cell suicide by apoptosis. Thus p53 controls and halts the proliferation of abnormal cell growth.

Transformation of the normal cell

If a normal cell loses p53 function or the latter becomes impaired, then uncontrolled growth may result and this is more likely to produce malignant clones.

Alternatively, cells in which oncogenes (genes responsible for malignant transformation) are activated (such as c-myc) may also give rise to malignant clones. Cancer arises from the transformation of a single normal cell. Most cancers require a series of genetic mutations in a cell before an invasive tumour results.

The cancer cell

Cancer cells differ from normal cells in that they function differently. Inherently unstable, they may display different protein or enzyme content and chromosomal abnormalities (such as translocations or deletions) which may differ in their susceptibility to chemotherapy or radiotherapy. Also their changed appearance (visible under light microscopy) from normal cells allows them to be more easily detected.

Tumour growth

A solid tumour represents a population of dividing and non-dividing cells. The time it takes for a tumour mass to double in size is known as the doubling time. The latter will vary dependent on tumour type but for most solid tumours is about 2–3 months. In most solid tumours the growth rate is very rapid initially (exponential growth) and then slows as the tumour increases in size and age, a pattern described as Gompertzian growth. The growth fraction is the percentage of actively dividing cells in the tumour and this decreases with tumour size.

This pattern of tumour growth kinetics has implications for chemotherapy treatment. Generally, chemotherapy is most successful when the number of tumour cells is low and the growth fraction high, which is the situation in the very early stages of cancer.

Tumour spread

As a primary tumour grows and invades normal tissue, malignant cells often infiltrate blood vessels and the lymphatic system. Malignant cells are thereby transported to other organs of the body where they can subsequently form secondary cancers or metastases. The pattern of spread tends to be predictable for different tumour types. Breast cancer usually metastasizes to the lungs and central nervous system while prostate cancer tends to metastasize to bone, in particular to the lumbar spine. Generally, the larger the tumour mass, the more likely that it has metastasized to other sites.

Patient management

Clinical assessment

Presentation

The clinical features of cancer vary with tumour type. Table 52.2 depicts the frequency of presenting symptoms in small cell lung cancer. Generally, patients most commonly present with non-specific complaints which include weight loss, bleeding, malaise, pain or the presence of a painless lump. In general, solid tumours are clinically detectable when there are approximately 10^8–10^9 tumour cells present. The patient is usually in the terminal stages

Table 52.2 Frequency of presenting symptoms in small cell lung cancer (Jackman & Johnson 2005)

Symptom or sign	Frequency %
Local	
Cough	50
Dyspnoea	40
Chest pain	35
Haemoptysis	20
Hoarseness	10
General	
Weight loss	50
Weakness	40
Anorexia	30
Fever	10

of the disease when there are 10^{12} cells present. This means that unless a tumour is detected by chance during a routine physical examination or by screening, the disease at presentation is usually at an advanced stage.

Before treatment, each patient must undergo a thorough assessment to establish diagnosis, stage of disease and general fitness level. These factors will influence the choice of treatment and give a guide to prognosis.

Diagnosis

An accurate diagnosis is usually made from a tissue sample. This sample may be obtained invasively as a biopsy, for example during bronchoscopy when lung cancer is suspected, or, as in the case of a patient presenting with a breast lump, aspiration through a fine needle is possible.

Malignant tumours vary in their sensitivity to chemotherapy. For example, there are two major groups of lung cancer: small cell and non-small cell lung cancer. Each of these groups is treated with different combinations of chemotherapy drugs, so precise histopathology is important.

Tumour markers

Tumour markers are usually proteins associated with a malignancy and are clinically useful to diagnose a specific tumour, monitor response to treatment or detect recurrent disease. They may be detected in a solid tumour, in circulating tumour cells in peripheral blood, in lymph nodes, in bone marrow or in other body fluids. A number of the tumour markers used to help confirm the diagnosis of particular tumours are presented in Table 52.3.

Staging investigations

Since the cancer is often disseminated at the time of presentation, it is absolutely vital that patients undergo thorough staging investigations to establish the extent and nature of disease. This will determine the most appropriate treatment offered to the patient. Baseline investigations range from clinical examination, blood tests, liver function tests, diagnostic imaging such as chest and

Table 52.3 Examples of tumour markers used in detection and diagnosis

Tumour marker	Indicative cancer
α-Fetoprotein (AFP) β-Human chorionic gonadotrophin (β-HCG)	Testicular tumour
CA125	Ovarian cancer
5-Hydroxyindole acetic acid (5HIAA)	Carcinoid tumours
Thyroglobulin	Thyroid cancer

skeletal x-rays, ultrasound, computed tomography (CT), magnetic resonance imaging (MRI) and positron emission tomography (PET), depending on the disease type and likely pattern of spread.

Staging classification

Most tumours are classified into three or four stages, denoted I, II, III and IV. In general, the higher the stage, the more advanced the disease and the poorer the prognosis. For some diseases, including breast cancer, a more complex staging classification is used: the TNM (tumour–nodes–metastases) system where T (0–4) indicates the size of the primary tumour, N (0–4) the extent of

lymph node involvement and M (0–1) the presence or absence of distant metastases.

Performance status

The patient's general level of fitness (performance status) at the time of diagnosis is often a good indicator of prognosis and will help determine if they are likely to withstand intensive chemotherapy and therefore influences the choice of treatment. A number of physical rating scales have been devised to assess performance status, including the Karnofsky performance index and the World Health Organization (WHO) performance scale (Table 52.4).

Prognostic factors

These are factors that can predict outcome in individual patients. Table 52.5 lists favourable prognostic factors in patients with small cell lung cancer.

Treatment

Treatment goals

After the diagnosis of cancer has been confirmed and the extent of disease fully investigated, the goals of treatment have to be considered. The primary goal is to cure. Patients are said to be 'cured' of cancer when they are completely disease free and have a normal life expectancy. The smaller the tumour bulk when treatment is given, the greater the potential of achieving cure.

Table 52. 4 Performance status scales

Karnofsky performance index	WHO performance scale
100 Normal, no complaints, no evidence of disease	
90 Able to carry on normal activity, minor signs or symptoms of disease	0 Able to carry out all normal activity without restriction
80 Normal activity with effort, some signs or symptoms of disease	
70 Cares for self, unable to carry on normal activity or do active work	1 Restricted in physically strenuous activity but ambulatory and able to carry out light work
60 Requires occasional assistance but is able to care for most of own needs	
50 Requires considerable assistance and frequent medical care	2 Ambulatory and capable of all self-care but unable to carry out any work; up and about more than 50% of waking hours
40 Disabled, requires special care and assistance	
30 Severely disabled, hospitalization is indicated, although death is not imminent	3 Capable of only limited self-care; confined to bed more than 50% of waking hours
20 Very sick, hospitalization necessary, active supportive treatment is necessary	
10 Moribund, fatal processes progressing rapidly	4 Completely disabled; cannot carry on any self-care; totally confined to bed or chair

Table 52.5 Favourable prognostic factors in patients with small cell lung cancer (Jackman & Johnson 2005)

Limited stage disease
Good performance status
Female sex
Normal serum lactate dehydrogenase

If cure is not feasible, then the goal is to prolong survival while maintaining patient quality of life.

The third goal of cancer therapy is palliative care with relief of symptoms such as pain. Childhood malignancies, choriocarcinoma and testicular tumours in adults are most responsive to chemotherapy and these patients are regularly cured, even with advanced disease. However, for most patients treated with chemotherapy, cure is less likely and treatment will be given to prolong survival or be purely palliative.

The decision is influenced by factors such as the pace and extent of the disease as well as co-existing symptoms and concurrent medical conditions, performance status and, importantly, the patient's wishes.

The possibility of cure or long-term survival justifies aggressive treatment but with palliative therapy it is particularly important that the toxicity of treatment is carefully weighed against the potential benefits.

Treatment guidelines

Consensus on the best approach to managing each particular type of cancer is continually evolving, based on the evidence from clinical research (randomized controlled trials) conducted by cancer centres either nationally or internationally. National guidelines aim to promote equity for patients and ensure a consistent treatment approach. In the absence of clinical consensus, patients should be encouraged to participate in clinical trials.

Treatment methods

Three main options are available for the treatment of patients with solid tumours: surgery, radiotherapy and chemotherapy. Each treatment may play a number of roles, either alone or in combination, depending on the disease.

Role of surgery

Surgery can be curative when solid tumours are localized or confined to one primary anatomical site or region as in localized disease. It can also be used to remove isolated metastatic masses. Surgical techniques may be used to support chemotherapy administration when given by continuous infusion or by the intraperitoneal route. Surgery may also play a role in diagnosis through tissue biopsy or in staging to ascertain the extent of tumour involvement such as in ovarian cancer. In the latter it may also be used to debulk or reduce the size of the tumour to effect pain relief or to improve the effectiveness of subsequent radiation or chemotherapy. However, with more widespread disease, systemic treatment becomes necessary, with chemotherapy playing a major role.

Although cancer therapy encompasses cytotoxic drugs, endocrine (hormonal) therapy and cytokines (such as interferon), the remainder of this chapter will focus on cytotoxic drugs and the newer targeted therapies.

Cytotoxic chemotherapy

Chemotherapy regimen

Although chemotherapy is sometimes administered as a single agent it is more usual to combine two or more drugs to achieve additive or synergistic effects. Generally, drugs used in combination should have established efficacy as single agents, different mechanisms of action and differing toxicity profiles to allow their use at optimal doses.

Chemotherapy scheduling

Because chemotherapy does not specifically target malignant cells, any actively proliferating normal cell will be at potential risk of damage, in particular the cells of the bone marrow. This results in a fall in the white blood cell count and with many cytotoxic drugs, the white blood count is at its lowest level or nadir by around 10 days after treatment. Recovery generally occurs by day 20 post treatment and therefore chemotherapy treatment is repeated every 3–4 weeks. With agents such as mitomycin, haematological recovery may be delayed for 42–50 days following treatment, in which case the interval between treatment cycles needs to be increased. In most cases, a course of treatment will comprise a maximum of six cycles of chemotherapy.

Chemotherapy dose

The dose of most chemotherapy agents is calculated using the patient's body surface area (BSA) and is usually given in the form of milligrams per square metre. Body surface area may be calculated from the height and weight of the patient using a nomogram and may need to be recalculated for subsequent cycles of chemotherapy if the patient experiences significant weight changes. Table 52.6 gives an example of a chemotherapy regimen used in breast cancer.

Table 52.6 Example of a chemotherapy regimen E-CMF (epirubicin, cyclophosphamide, methotrexate, 5-fluorouracil) used in adjuvant breast cancer

Drug	Dose	Route
Epirubicin	$100\,mg/m^2$	Intravenous day 1
Repeated every 3 weeks for 4 cycles followed by:		
Cyclophosphamide	$100\,mg/m^2$	Oral days 1–14
Methotrexate	$40\,mg/m^2$	Intravenous days 1 and 8
5-fluorouracil	$600\,mg/m^2$	Intravenous days 1 and 8
Repeat every 28 days for 4 cycles		

Adjuvant chemotherapy

Historically, chemotherapy was used solely in the treatment of recurrent or advanced metastatic disease when it was not likely to yield cure. Increasingly chemotherapy is being used in the treatment of localized disease as adjuvant therapy postoperatively or following radiotherapy, in an attempt to eradicate any undetected metastatic disease and increase the likelihood of cure. Only patients whose cancers have a high or intermediate risk of recurrence are selected for adjuvant chemotherapy since it is not desirable to expose patients whose disease may already have been cured by surgery or radiotherapy to the toxicity of chemotherapy treatment.

In colorectal cancer, for example, the role of adjuvant chemotherapy is well established for stage III patients (lymph node positive) when it reduces the risk of relapse and improves 5-year survival by 10–15%. In patients with stage II or less advanced disease, the benefit of adjuvant chemotherapy is less well defined.

Similarly, in breast cancer, 5-year survival in women with node-positive cancer has risen from around 65% without adjuvant treatment to 85% with modern anthracycline-taxane chemotherapy.

Recent trials have also shown the benefit of adjuvant treatments in lung cancer (Pisters & Le Chevalier 2005).

Neo-adjuvant chemotherapy

In neo-adjuvant chemotherapy, chemotherapy is given before local therapy, often preoperatively, in order to reduce tumour size and facilitate surgical removal. Neo-adjuvant chemotherapy has been of particular value in cases of breast cancer, non-small cell lung cancer and Ewing's sarcoma, one of the most common bone tumours, when it allows limb-sparing surgery as an alternative to amputation.

Synchronous chemoradiation

The use of chemotherapy alongside radical radiotherapy has been investigated in several cancers, including those of the cervix, head and neck, lung and stomach. Studies to date have indicated superior results compared to either radiation alone or radiation followed by chemotherapy. It is thought that synchronous chemotherapy may act chiefly as a radiosensitizer and allow shortening of radiation therapy time. Further studies will be needed to inform and define its future role.

Adverse effects of cytotoxic drugs

Most cytotoxic drugs have been developed because of their effect on dividing cells. Consequently, and as previously mentioned under chemotherapy scheduling, proliferating normal tissue such as bone marrow is at risk. Myelosuppression is frequently the dose-limiting toxicity with these compounds. Neutropenia and thrombocytopenia place patients at risk of life-threatening infection and bleeding, respectively.

The other acute adverse effects occurring most frequently include nausea and vomiting, mucositis, anorexia and alopecia. Individual drugs will also give rise to specific adverse effects,

some of which may not be reversible on stopping treatment. Cardiotoxicity, nephrotoxicity and pulmonary toxicity, which are specific to the chemotherapeutic agent or class, may depend on cumulative drug exposure, the schedule of administration and previous therapy. Long-term side effects include infertility due to suppression of ovarian and testicular function and occasionally the induction of a second malignancy.

Chemotherapy-related toxicity is an important issue. Not only can it result in prolonged hospitalization and a reduction in patients' quality of life, but also successful treatment can be compromised. A reduction in dose intensity, i.e. the dose of cytotoxic delivered for unit time, because of dose reductions or treatment delays, can result in reduced response rates and survival.

Chemotherapy-specific adjunctive treatments

Both ifosfamide and cyclophosphamide are metabolized to the inactive acrolein which is responsible for bladder toxicity. The co-administration of mesna, a sulphydryl-containing compound which binds to acrolein, has reduced the incidence of haemorrhagic cystitis associated with intravenous regimens of ifosfamide and high-dose cyclophosphamide.

Calcium leucovorin or folinic acid is a reduced form of folic acid. Competing directly with methotrexate for transport into cells, folinic acid is effectively used as a form of rescue when high doses of intravenous methotrexate are used.

Targeted therapies

In recent years there has been an increased understanding of biochemical signalling pathways involved in the growth and progression of tumours. This has allowed the development of therapies targeted specifically at the cell receptors involved. A number of these are described. Because they are targeted at tumour cells, they suppress disease without inflicting the non-selective toxic effects of cytotoxic chemotherapy on the patient. Benefits in terms of overall survival and potential cure are anticipated when these agents are given together with, or following, conventional chemotherapy.

Epidermal growth factor receptor

The epidermal growth factor receptor (EGFR) is a transmembrane protein with an intracellular tyrosine kinase domain. Extracellular binding of the epidermal growth factor receptor induces tyrosine phosphorylation which activates signal cascade pathways. These ultimately lead to cellular proliferation and metastasis. EGFR expression is low in normal tissues and overexpression is associated with a variety of tumours including non-small cell lung cancer, colon, and head and neck.

Inhibitors of EGFR (also known as human epidermal growth factor receptor type 1 [HER1]) include:

- small molecules such as the orally administered erlotinib used in the treatment of non-small cell lung cancer and imatinib used in the treatment of gastrointestinal stromal tumours (GIST) which specifically inhibit tyrosine kinase
- monoclonal antibodies such as cetuximab which binds to the EGFR. Cetuximab has demonstrated synergy when

given in combination with irinotecan chemotherapy, offering prolonged survival in selected patients with metastatic colorectal cancer.

Vascular endothelial growth factor receptor

Angiogenesis is the formation of new blood vessels on which tumour growth depends. Vascular endothelial growth factor (VEGF) is key in angiogenesis and its overexpression has been associated with increased vasculature, aggressive disease and poor prognosis. The monoclonal antibody bevacizumab inhibits VEGF, thereby reducing new blood vessel growth and interstitial pressure within the tumour, allowing improved chemotherapy access. Studies have demonstrated meaningful survival benefits when bevacizumab is administered in conjunction with chemotherapy in patients with advanced or metastatic colorectal cancer (Hurwitz et al 2004).

Human epidermal growth factor receptor type 2

Overexpression of human epidermal growth factor receptor 2 (HER2) is associated with a particularly aggressive form of breast cancer (about 20% cases are HER2 positive) linked with a poor prognosis. Trastuzumab, a humanized monoclonal antibody, specifically targets HER2 and is only effective in patients with elevated levels. Used widely in the treatment of metastatic breast cancer, trastuzumab is likely to have broader application in the adjuvant setting.

Capecitabine

Although capecitabine does not target a particular receptor, it is probably worth a mention under this section, as it preferentially targets tumour cells.

Capecitabine is a fluoropyrimidine carbamate precursor of 5-fluorouracil (5FU). Given orally, it is converted via enzyme pathways to 5-fluorouracil. As these enzymes are found in higher concentrations in tumour cells, treatment is targeted. Proven to be at least as effective as intravenous 5-fluorouracil, it is anticipated that capecitabine will substantially replace traditional 5-fluorouracil in regimens commonly used in colorectal and breast cancer.

Management of patients receiving cytotoxic chemotherapy

Prescription verification

Table 52.7 summarizes the key factors which need to be taken into consideration to ensure safe, appropriate and optimal patient treatment. Although each cytotoxic drug varies in its particular spectrum of toxicity, some general precautions can be taken to minimize the risk of predictable adverse effects occurring.

Cumulative dosing

The use of doxorubicin is limited by a dose-dependent cardiomyopathy. A number of other factors have been implicated,

Table 52.7 Patient care: monitoring chemotherapy

Diagnosis	• Is prescription in accordance with treatment protocol/established regimen?
Protocol	• Is the selected treatment protocol appropriate?
Regimen	• Is the prescribed regimen appropriate?
Weight/height	• Check body surface area calculation • Verify dose • Calculate total exposure to drugs with cumulative toxicity

Clinical factors:
  Age
  Haematological status
  Renal/hepatic function
  Concurrent disease
  Allergy
  Toxicity from previous cycle
	• Is dose adjustment required?
	• Are there any contraindications to planned therapy?

Administration	• Is the route appropriate? • Does the patient have suitable venous access? • Has treatment been scheduled correctly?
Interactions	• What are the concurrent medications? • Has the potential for interactions being checked? • Are there incompatibilities with intravenous drugs or infusion fluids?
Supportive care (e.g. antiemetics, analgesia, laxatives, growth factors, etc.)	• Has appropriate supportive therapy been prescribed? • Has appropriate monitoring been undertaken?
Documentation	• Has treatment been accurately documented in the patient's records, including discussions of the different treatment options and patient preference? • If care is managed jointly with a supplementary prescriber, is there a clear clinical management plan?

including treatment schedule, patient age and pre-existing cardiac disease, but dose is the most important. The maximum recommended cumulative dose is $550\,mg/m^2$ or $400\,mg/m^2$ for patients who have received radiotherapy to the mediastinum, so treatment should be monitored closely to make sure the cumulative dose is not exceeded throughout the patient's lifetime.

Dose modification or delay

Appropriate investigations must be carried out before treatment to ensure that patients are fit for chemotherapy; in particular, the patient's haematological, renal and hepatic function should be investigated. For some cytotoxic drugs it may be necessary to adjust the dose, or even stop treatment, in the presence of renal or hepatic impairment to ensure that delayed excretion or reduced metabolism does not result in toxicity (Table 52.8).

If the bone marrow does not recover sufficiently between cycles of treatment then a dose reduction or a delay in treatment may be necessary. In general, patients with a white cell count below 3×10^9/L or a platelet count below 100×10^9/L should not be given myelosuppressive cytotoxics.

Table 52.8 Cytotoxic drugs requiring monitoring or dose adjustment depending on organ dysfunction

| | Monitoring or dose adjustment required | |
	Renal	Hepatic
Bleomycin	√	
Capecitabine	√	√
Carboplatin	√	
Cisplatin	√	
Cyclophosphamide	√	
Dacarbazine		√
Dactinomycin		√
Docetaxel		√
Doxorubicin		√
Epirubicin		√
Etoposide	√	
Gemcitabine	√	√
Ifosfamide	√	
Irinotecan	√	√
Methotrexate	√	
Mitomycin		√
Mitoxantrone		√
Nitrosoureas	√	
Paclitaxel		√
Raltitrexed	√	√
Vinca alkaloids		√
Vinorelbine		√

Drug interactions

Prescriptions for cancer chemotherapy are often complex, sometimes involving combinations of both parenteral and oral cytotoxic drugs, intravenous fluids and other supportive therapies. The potential for drug interactions to arise is considerable. However, care is required when assessing the clinical significance of potential drug interactions. A documented interaction does not necessarily imply that drugs should not be used together but will necessitate close monitoring of the patient.

Patient information and counselling

All patients must be provided with information about their treatment, including any anticipated side effects. Patients should be encouraged by health professionals to ask questions about their treatment. A report on the cancer 'information maze' (ABPI 2005) suggests that health professionals develop 'information prescriptions' for patients which signpost them to the most appropriate sources of information.

Patients must understand the different medications, specific use and duration of treatment. The last point is particularly important in order to prevent highly potent medicines from being inadvertently continued beyond their intended course.

Symptom control

Nausea and vomiting

Nausea and vomiting are considered by most patients to be the most distressing side effects of chemotherapy, and in extreme cases poor symptom control can result in patients refusing further treatment. In selecting an appropriate antiemetic regimen, relevant factors include the emetogenic potential of the chemotherapy drugs prescribed (see Chapter 34, Table 34.3), the putative mechanism(s) of inducing emesis, and the likely onset and duration of symptoms. Individual patient characteristics also have to be taken into consideration. For example, sickness in pregnancy and travel sickness are well-recognized predisposing factors which increase a patient's susceptibility to emesis following chemotherapy treatment. Differences in the severity of emesis can also occur between patients receiving the same type of chemotherapy and even between treatment cycles in the same patient.

The 5-hydroxytryptamine type 3 ($5HT_3$) receptor antagonists which include dolasetron, granisetron, ondansetron, palonosetron and tropisetron, have become the gold standard in the management of acute chemotherapy-induced nausea and vomiting when treating patients with highly or moderately emetogenic chemotherapy regimens such as those including cisplatinum. They are most effective in dealing with acute emesis (less than 24 hours duration) when combined with dexametasone. It is important to achieve optimal control of nausea and vomiting at the outset to avoid subsequent anticipatory symptoms which can prove very difficult to treat.

The route of administration for antiemetics is an important consideration. With intravenous chemotherapy it may be simpler to administer all treatments by the intravenous route. Alternatives to the oral route may be useful when vomiting occurs and include the rectal and buccal route.

Pain control

Drug therapy remains the cornerstone of effective pain management but it is often undertreated, thus highlighting the importance of regular patient assessment and appropriate dose or drug treatment changes. For example, patients experiencing intolerable side effects to morphine may be transferred to transdermal fentanyl skin patches. Analgesia should be prescribed both regularly and for breakthrough pain, and laxatives should be prescribed to prevent constipation.

The route of administration is also important. When patients are unable to manage oral medication, it is important to assess the use of alternative routes such as the rectal, subcutaneous, epidural and transdermal routes.

Bone marrow suppression

Myelosuppression following chemotherapy is common, and for some patients profound. The risk of systemic infection can be reduced by good oral hygiene and mouth care using antiseptic mouthwashes and antifungal prophylaxis. Patients must be advised to immediately report symptoms of infection and bruising. Platelets may be required, but fever or other evidence of infection occurring in a neutropenic patient when the neutrophil count is less than $0.8 \times 10^9/L$ must be aggressively treated with broad-spectrum intravenous antibiotics to prevent overwhelming infection developing.

The duration and depth of neutropenia can be dramatically reduced by the administration of haemopoietic growth factors which stimulate neutrophil production and, in cases of severe neutropenia, effectively rescue the patient. Once the patient's neutrophil count has recovered sufficiently, their use may be safely discontinued. These agents may also be used prophylactically in patients with a high risk of febrile neutropenia before receiving chemotherapy.

Blood transfusions are commonly required by patients at some stage of their treatment due to anaemia. Alternatively, erythropoietin may be useful in some patients receiving chemotherapy to shorten the period of anaemia and improve the patient's quality of life.

Extravasation

Extreme care must be taken when administering cytotoxic drugs parenterally because of the dangers of extravasation. Extravasation, which is the accidental leakage of an intravenous drug into the surrounding tissue, can cause pain, erythema and severe local necrosis, resulting in permanent tissue damage. The patient must be asked to immediately report any pain or a stinging sensation at the injection site since the degree of damage is determined by the amount of drug extravasated and the speed at which it is detected. If extravasation is suspected, the administration of further chemotherapy must stop and remedial treatment must commence as soon as possible. Drugs most likely to cause problems on extravasation are listed in Table 52.9.

Inpatient or outpatient treatment

The majority of patients receive chemotherapy in the outpatient clinic or day-care setting, where cytotoxics are administered mainly by short intravenous infusion at 3- or 4-week intervals. Initiation of monoclonal antibody treatment usually requires close monitoring of the patient for several hours in case of anaphylactic reactions. More complex treatment, such as cisplatinum-containing regimens, require prehydration with intravenous fluids and aggressive use of antiemetics, so necessitating inpatient treatment.

Domiciliary treatment

Oral cytotoxic drugs can safely be taken at home so long as the patient is fully informed to monitor side effects. Availability of a 24-hour helpline is essential for those patients who encounter problems whilst on treatment. Administration of intravenous treatments such as the monoclonal antibody trastuzumab may subsequently be maintained in a home setting and it seems likely that this area of treatment delivery will expand in future years to cope with the growing demand for these treatments.

Monitoring anticancer therapy

As well as desirable outcomes, treatment with chemotherapy may result in a variety of undesirable outcomes; both require careful monitoring.

Toxicity

The toxicity resulting from treatment is routinely assessed following each cycle of chemotherapy, and may result in therapy being modified on subsequent cycles, for example a dose reduction, a delay in treatment or, in some cases, an alternative treatment. A number of international rating scales are available for rating predictable acute reactions arising from chemotherapy, including that of the WHO (Table 52.10). Standardizing the assessment of treatment-related toxicity in this way allows comparison to be made between published reports of clinical trials.

Table 52.9 Cytotoxic drugs with the highest potential for tissue damage if extravasated

Actinomycin D	Mechlorethamine (mustine)
Amsacrine	Mitomycin C
Carmustine	Paclitaxel
Dacarbazine	Streptozocin
Daunorubicin	Treosulphan
Doxorubicin	Vinca alkaloids (vinblastine, vincristine, vindesine)
Epirubicin	Vinorelbine
Idarubicin	

For more information visit: www.extravasation.org.uk

Table 52.10   WHO grading of acute and subacute toxicity

	Grade 0	Grade 1	Grade 2	Grade 3	Grade 4
Nausea/vomiting	None	Nausea	Transient	Vomiting requiring vomiting therapy	Intractable vomiting
Diarrhoea	None	Transient <2 days	Tolerable, but >2 days	Intolerable, requiring therapy	Haemorrhagic dehydration
Constipation	None	Mild	Moderate	Abdominal distension	Distension and vomiting
Oral	No change	Soreness/erythema	Erythema, ulcers; can eat solids	Ulcers; requires liquid diet only	Alimentation not possible
White blood cells (× 10^9/L)	>4.0	3.0–3.9	2.0–2.9	1.0–1.9	<1.0
Platelets (× 10^9/L)	>100	75–99	50–74	25–49	<25
Haemoglobin (g/dL)	>11.0	9.5–10.9	8.0–9.4	6.5–7.9	<6.5
Hair	No change	Minimal hair loss	Moderate patchy alopecia	Complete alopecia, but reversible	Non-reversible alopecia

Response to treatment

Throughout treatment, the response to therapy is closely monitored, noting changes in performance status, symptoms and objective measurements of the tumour. This may necessitate repeating some or all of the initial staging investigations. Should the initial treatment prove ineffective, an alternative can then be considered without delay. Assessment of response should be formally documented before proceeding to further therapy.

Definitions of response   These have been standardized by the WHO.

- *Complete response or remission (CR).* Disappearance of all recognizable tumour masses and/or biochemical changes directly related to the tumour and resolution of symptoms determined by two observations at least a month apart.
- *Partial response (PR).* Decrease by 50% or more in all tumour masses, measured by the product of the longest × the widest perpendicular diameters for at least a month.
- *Stable disease (SD) or no change (NC).* Changes smaller than those described above for PR or less than for PD for at least a month.
- *Progressive disease (PD).* Occurrence of any new lesion or increase in the longest × widest perpendicular diameters of measurable disease by at least 25%.

Again, this allows comparison of results between different reported studies. An update of the WHO guidelines has been published (Therasse et al 2000) called RECIST or Response Evaluation Criteria in Solid Tumours. To avoid confusion, it is important to stipulate in trial protocols which system is to be used. Although clinical response indicates tumour sensitivity, it may not necessarily predict long-term survival nor does it measure other benefits such as quality of life.

CASE STUDIES

Case 52.1

Mrs BH, a 53-year-old postmenopausal mother of two teenage children, has recently completed six cycles of epi-CMF (epirubicin, cyclophosphamide, methotrexate and 5-fluorouracil) as adjuvant chemotherapy for her node-positive early breast cancer. She tolerated her chemotherapy well and did not require any dose reductions or delays.

Her receptor status at diagnosis was oestrogen receptor positive and progestogen receptor negative (ER +/ PR–); she was also HER2 positive.

Her oncologist has recommended that she commences treatment with trastuzumab.

Questions

1. What treatment regimen should be followed for this patient?
2. What side effects should Mrs BH be informed about when giving consent for treatment?
3. What other treatments should be considered for this patient?

Answers

1. Trastuzumab targets the EGFR and is indicated for the treatment of early breast cancer overexpressing HER2 following surgery, chemotherapy (neo-adjuvant or adjuvant) and radiotherapy if applicable. The product licence for trastuzumab recommends the dosing schedule used in the HERA study (Piccart-Gebhart et al 2005), i.e. loading dose of 8 mg/kg body weight, followed by 6 mg/kg body weight 3 weeks later and then 6 mg/kg repeated at 3-weekly intervals administered as infusions over approximately 90 minutes. This is continued for 12 months, stopping sooner if disease recurs.

2. The most common side effects experienced by patients are infusion related, such as fever and chills, usually following the first or second treatment. Patients should be closely monitored for at least 6 hours after the start of the first infusion and if the treatment has been well tolerated, for 2 hours after the start of subsequent infusions. If a reaction occurs the infusion should be stopped, appropriate symptomatic treatment administered and treatment recommenced at a slower rate only when the symptoms have subsided. Trastuzumab has been associated with cardiotoxicity and patients who have previously received anthracyclines are at increased risk. All patients should have their cardiac function closely monitored at baseline and during the period that they are being treated with trastuzumab. There was an approximate 5% increase in the number of patients with a significant change in cardiac function in the HERA study (Piccart-Gebhart et al 2005).

3. In view of her receptor status this patient should be offered hormonal treatment. Depending on the perceived level of risk of recurrence as estimated using a model such as the Nottingham Prognostic Index (Galea et al 1992), she should be offered either 5 years' treatment with an aromatase inhibitor or planned sequential treatment with tamoxifen switching to an aromatase inhibitor after 2–3 years' therapy. The long-term effect on cardiovascular health (tamoxifen) or bone health (aromatase inhibitors) together with the expected level of benefits should be used to guide choice of treatment. Further information can be found in national guidance for the early management of breast cancer with hormonal treatments (NICE 2006a).

Case 52.2

Mr BS, a 67-year-old man with a history of localized prostate cancer, is reviewed by his oncologist. Mr BS was previously treated with radical radiotherapy and more recently several lines of hormonal therapy.

His PSA has risen over the last 6 months and is now 80 ng/mL. It was 0.1 ng/mL on completion of radical x-ray radiation therapy. He also complains that his back pain that was previously controlled has now returned.

Questions

1. What is the most likely cause of Mr BS's back pain and raised PSA?
2. What treatment options should be discussed with the patient?
3. Why should he be referred for a dental examination before commencing any further treatment?

Answers

1. The fact that the PSA is markedly raised demonstrates a recurrence of prostate cancer; moderate rises in the PSA would have warranted a change in hormonal therapy. The elevated PSA together with the increased back pain suggest metastatic bone disease as a result of distant recurrence of his prostate cancer. This can be confirmed with a bone scan. The risk of both local and distant recurrence depends on the stage at presentation:

   • stage I   less than 10% at 10 years
   • stage II   15–25% at 10 years
   • stage III   20–30% at 5 years.

2. Treatment options for recurrent prostate cancer include second-line hormonal therapy, chemotherapy with or without corticosteroids, and best supportive care. The choice of therapy depends on the symptoms, the site of relapse, the performance status of the patient and the presence of other co-morbidities. Best supportive care can be provided with radiotherapy, bisphosphonates, steroids and analgesics, and

is the only option for patients who are too ill to tolerate further active intervention. Tolerability of chemotherapy is of concern, particularly because most patients with prostate cancer are elderly and many have other medical problems. Mr BS has already received more than one line of hormonal therapy; his tumour is unlikely to respond to further hormonal manipulation. Localized radiotherapy to specific bone lesions could improve his back pain; this would depend on the number of treatable lesions identified. An alternative strategy that is becoming available is the use of radioactive isotopes for systemic treatment of multiple bone metastases. The use of chemotherapy in the treatment of hormone-refractory prostate cancer should be considered in patients with a Karnofsky performance status of 60% or greater. Further information on the use of docetaxel for the treatment of hormone-refractory metastatic prostate cancer is available (NICE 2006b).

3. Future treatment options for this patient may include use of bisphosphonates to stabilize his bone lesions and reduce his pain. Long-term use of bisphosphonates has been associated with osteonecrosis of the jaw; the risk is exacerbated by poor dental hygiene, concurrent dental procedures, chemotherapy, corticosteroids and malignant disease. Examination and preventive dental treatment should be considered for patients prior to commencing therapy with bisphosphonates in order to avoid any invasive procedures, for instance dental extraction, during bisphosphonate therapy.

Case 52.3

Mr SG, a 46-year-old patient, was diagnosed with Dukes' C colon cancer several months ago. Since then he has undergone a left hemicolectomy. He is currently receiving capecitabine monotherapy as adjuvant treatment. He telephones the pharmacy department for advice on how to cope with the side effects he is currently experiencing.

Questions

1. What side effects are commonly associated with capecitabine?
2. How do these differ from those associated with intravenous 5-fluorouracil?
3. What advice should he be given?

Answers

1. Side effects most commonly associated with capecitabine treatment are mainly related to the skin and the gastrointestinal tract.

• Palmar–plantar erythema (hand–foot syndrome)	57%
• Diarrhoea	47%
• Nausea	35%
• Stomatitis	23%
• Vomiting	18%
• Fatigue	16%

2. Although capecitabine is converted enzymatically to 5-fluorouracil, there is a difference in the frequency with which specific side effects are experienced, making it more akin to continuous infusions of 5-flourouracil. Patients receiving intermittent bolus therapy with 5-fluorouracil are more likely to experience the gastrointestinal side effects, particularly diarrhoea or stomatitis, rather than the cutaneous reactions. Myelosuppression may also infrequently be a problem encountered by these patients.

3. Mr SG should be instructed to stop taking his course of capecitabine with immediate effect if he is experiencing any of the following side effects.

   • **Diarrhoea**: an increase of 4 or more bowel movements each day compared to normal or any diarrhoea at night.

- **Vomiting**: vomiting more than once in a 24-hour time period.
- **Nausea:** loss of appetite resulting in the amount of food eaten each day being much less than usual.
- **Stomatitis**: pain, redness, swelling or sores in the mouth.
- **Palmar–plantar erythema (hand–foot syndrome):** pain, swelling and redness of hands and/or feet.
- **Fever or infection:** temperature of 38°C or greater, or other signs of infection.
- **Chest pain:** pain localized to the centre of the chest, especially if it occurs during exercise.

If caught early, these side effects usually improve within 2–3 days. Treatment may be reinstated at the same dose if side effects are moderate (WHO grade 2) or at a reduced dose if more severe (WHO 3 or recurrent). Subsequent courses should be commenced at the new dose level. Symptomatic relief for palmar–plantar erythema may be provided by the use of emollients. There is little evidence to support the use of specific antidotes.

ACKNOWLEDGEMENTS

I gratefully acknowledge the contribution of Geoff Saunders, Macmillan Cancer Network pharmacist, Greater Manchester and Cheshire Cancer Network, for producing the case studies and answers.

REFERENCES

ABPI 2005 The cancer information maze: report investigating information access for people with cancer. Association of the British Pharmaceutical Industry in partnership with Cancer BACUP and Ask About Medicines. Available online at: www.askaboutmedicines.org

Chan A, Giovannucci E, Meyerhardt J et al 2005 Long-term use of aspirin and nonsteroidal anti-inflammatory drugs and risk of colorectal cancer. Journal of the American Medical Association 294: 914-923

Galea M H, Blamey R W, Elston C E et al 1992 The Nottingham prognostic index in primary breast cancer. Breast Cancer Research and Treatment 22: 207-219

Hurwitz H, Fehrenhacher L, Novotny W et al 2004 Bevacizumab plus irinotecan, fluorouracil and leucovorin for metastatic colorectal cancer. New England Journal of Medicine 350: 2335-2342

Jackman D, Johnson B 2005 Small cell lung cancer. Lancet 366: 1385-1396

Jankowski J, Boulton E 2005 Cancer prevention. British Medical Journal 331: 618

National Institute for Health and Clinical Excellence 2006a Breast cancer (early) – hormonal treatment. Hormonal therapies for the adjuvant treatment of early breast cancer. National Institute for Health and Clinical Excellence, London. Available online at: www.nice.org.uk

National Institute for Health and Clinical Excellence 2006b Breast cancer (early) – docetaxel. Docetaxel for the treatment of early breast cancer. National Institute for Health and Clinical Excellence, London. Available online at: www.nice.org.uk

Piccart-Gebhart M J, Procter M, Leyland-Jones B et al 2005 Trastuzumab after adjuvant chemotherapy in HER2-positive breast cancer (HERA Study). New England Journal of Medicine 353: 1659-1672

Pisters K, Le Chevalier T 2005 Adjuvant chemotherapy in completely resected non-small cell lung cancer. Journal of Clinical Oncology 23: 3270-3278

Therasse P, Arbuck S G, Eisenhauer E A et al 2000 New guidelines to evaluate the response to treatment in solid tumours. Journal of the National Cancer Institute 92: 205-216

FURTHER READING

Allwood M, Stanley A, Wright P 2004 The cytotoxics handbook, 4th edn. Radcliffe Medical Press, Oxford

Devita V T, Hellman S, Rosenberg S A 2005 Cancer – principles and practice of oncology, 7th edn. Lippincott, Williams and Wilkins, Philadelphia

Smith I, Chua S 2006 ABC of breast diseases. Medical treatment of early breast cancer: adjuvant treatment. British Medical Journal 332: 34-37

USEFUL WEBSITE

National Extravasation Information Service website, available online at: www.extravasation.org.uk

Rheumatoid arthritis and osteoarthritis

53

D. M. Bryant   A. Alldred

KEY POINTS

Rheumatoid arthritis

- About 2% of men and 5% of women over the age of 55 years have rheumatoid arthritis (RA).
- The cause of rheumatoid arthritis is unclear.
- The aims of treatment are to relieve pain and inflammation, prevent joint destruction and preserve functional ability.
- Non-steroidal anti-inflammatory drugs (NSAIDs) are the major group of drugs used for the relief of pain and inflammation in rheumatoid arthritis. They vary in their ability to inhibit different types of cyclo-oxygenase.
- Patients with rheumatoid arthritis should be treated early and aggressively with disease-modifying antirheumatic drugs (DMARDs).
- Cytokine inhibitors (biologic agents) are a major advance in the management of rheumatoid arthritis. They are particularly useful in patients with resistant disease and are being used earlier in the disease process.
- Patients with rheumatoid arthritis must be educated and counselled appropriately.

Osteoarthritis

- Osteoarthritis (OA) is uncommon in people aged less than 45 years, but prevalence increases up to the age of 65 years when at least 50% of the population have radiographic evidence in at least one joint.
- A wide variety of factors predispose patients to osteoarthritis, including genetic factors, age and joint loading.
- Lifestyle changes such as maintaining optimal weight and undertaking regular exercises are an essential part of treatment.
- Regular simple analgesics are effective. Oral NSAIDs may be of value in some patients.
- Intra-articular corticosteroids and hyaluronic acid derivatives may be useful in patients with osteoarthritis of the knee

RHEUMATOID ARTHRITIS

Rheumatoid arthritis (RA) is one of the most common chronic inflammatory conditions, affecting the population worldwide. It is a systemic inflammatory disease of unknown aetiology affecting both articular tissues and extra-articular organs. There is a wide range of extra-articular features (Table 53.1). The disease is progressive and results in pain, stiffness and swelling of joints which can lead to significant morbidity and increased mortality.

Table 53.1   Extra-articular features of rheumatoid arthritis

Common	Uncommon
Anaemia	Pleural and pericardial effusions
Nodules (subcutaneous)	Fibrosing alveolitis
Muscle wasting	Pericarditis
Dry eyes (Sjögren's syndrome)	Scleritis
Depression	Systemic vasculitis
Osteoporosis	Mitral valve and conduction defects
Episcleritis	Nodules (lungs, eyes, heart)
Carpal tunnel syndrome	Felty's syndrome (seropositive
Leg ulcers	rheumatoid arthritis, splenomegaly
Lymphadenopathy	and neutropenia, incidence <1%)
Nailfold vasculitis	

Epidemiology

Approximately 1% of the adult population worldwide is affected by rheumatoid arthritis with the gender ratio varying from 2:1 to 3:1 in favour of females (Alamanosa & Drosos 2005). The prevalence of rheumatoid arthritis increases with age in both sexes with nearly 5% of women and 2% of men over 55 years of age affected. The peak age of incidence is around 55–64 years in women and 65–75 years in men. The relative incidence in women compared to men falls with age from around 4:1 at age 15–24 to around 2:1 at age 65–74. Some ethnic variation has also been observed in the prevalence of rheumatoid arthritis. Among rural black Africans the prevalence is low, at about 0.1% of the population compared to 3% in caucasians. Comparative studies among urban and rural populations suggest that environmental factors associated with modern urban life may also be important.

Socio-economic impact

Rheumatoid arthritis is a disease that is associated with major socio-economic implications for the population it affects. The articular and extra-articular progressive nature of rheumatoid arthritis leads to both significant patient morbidity and mortality. Patients with rheumatoid arthritis have six times the probability of severe limitation of activity, four times as many restricted days and 10 times the work disability rate of the general population. Over a period of 6 years the average earnings of a patient with rheumatoid arthritis will be reduced by approximately 60% and after 10 years of disease duration more than 50% of patients are unable to work at all. Survival rates among patients with rheumatoid arthritis are lower than those in the general population. Median life expectancy is reduced by 7 years for men and 3 years for women. These reduced survival rates are similar to those observed for Hodgkin's disease, diabetes and stroke. The increased mortality in rheumatoid arthritis patients is mostly associated with cardiovascular disease.

Aetiology

The cause of rheumatoid arthritis remains unclear. It is postulated that a genetically susceptible host is exposed to an unknown pathogen (antigen) and this interaction gives rise to a persistent immunological response. It is possible that many different stimuli activate the immune response in the susceptible host. Whether the initiating agent is an infection, a self-antigen or an environmental factor remains unproven.

One proposed hypothetical disease model integrates the improved understanding of genetic risk factors and the inflammatory response (Weyand & Goronzy 1997). This model makes the assumption that the host's immune response is not involved in the initial disease process. The various immune human leucocyte antigen (HLA) response genes, immunoglobulin genes and T-cell receptor genes have an impact later in the chain of pathological events during stage II of the disease. The initial stage I, in this complex model, involves synovial tissue injury. This may result from a possible infection, with exposure to a wide spectrum of antigens, including many autoantigens generated by tissue injury.

Epidemiological data support the case for both environmental and genetic factors causing rheumatoid arthritis. There is a 30% concordance in monozygotic twins, compared to 5% in fraternal twins and first-degree relatives. Environmental factors must be related to rheumatoid arthritis development otherwise monozygotic twins would have 100% concordance. First-degree relatives of patients with rheumatoid arthritis develop rheumatoid arthritis at 4–6 times the standard population rate. Research in twins and other genetic studies suggest the genetic component is at best 30%. The most definite genetic association with rheumatoid arthritis is with HLA alleles. The HLA-DR4 allele is associated with development and severity of rheumatoid arthritis. The relative risk for an individual with HLA-DR4 to develop the disease is between 2 and 6. In American whites, 60–70% of rheumatoid arthritis patients are positive for HLA-DR4. This seems to be particularly important in severe forms of the disease. The frequency of HLA-DR4 among Dutch patients with severe extra-articular disease is greater than 90%.

The similarity of rheumatoid arthritis to other arthritides such as Lyme disease, for which an infectious agent has been identified, has prompted the search for similar candidates. Epstein–Barr virus has been linked to rheumatoid arthritis for many years. Of patients with rheumatoid arthritis, 80% have a circulating antibody directed against antigens specific for Epstein–Barr virus, and the autoantibody response in rheumatoid arthritis enhances the response to these antigens. Parvoviruses (small DNA viruses that cause disease in many species), particularly B19, have been linked to rheumatoid arthritis. Mycobacteria have also been linked to rheumatoid arthritis because these bacteria express heat shock proteins (HSPs). A potential hypothesis is that antibodies and T-cells exist that recognize epitopes shared by the HSPs of both the infectious agent and host cells. This would facilitate cross-reactivity of lymphocytes with host cells, triggering an immunological reaction.

Pathophysiology

Rheumatoid arthritis is characterized by the infiltration of a variety of inflammatory cells into the joint. The synovial membrane becomes highly vascularized, synovial fibroblasts proliferate and inflammatory cells release numerous cytokines and growth factors into the joint. These agents subsequently cause synovial cells to release proteolytic enzymes, resulting in destruction of bone and cartilage.

Normal synovial tissue consists of an intimal lining and the synovial sublining which merges with the joint capsule. The synovial sublining is relatively acellular, containing scattered blood vessels, fat cells and fibroblasts. In the early stages of the disease there is tissue oedema, which manifests clinically as joint swelling and pain. Vessel proliferation and new vessel formation are also observed, and synovial lining hyperplasia begins to develop.

In the chronic phase of the disease the synovial lining hyperplasia becomes more pronounced. The cells in the lining consist of type A (macrophage-like) and also type B (fibroblast-like) synoviocytes. The sublining also evolves and there is an infiltration with mononuclear cells comprising T-cells (predominantly CD4+ helper cells), B-cells, macrophages and plasma cells. New blood vessel formation continues and both the degree and content of the cellular infiltrate change. The hypertrophied synovium becomes locally invasive at the synovial interface with cartilage and bone. This results in the formation of a 'pannus'. It is this tissue that serves as the origin of joint erosions. The cells in the pannus express large amounts of messenger RNA encoding for destructive proteins called matrix metalloproteinases.

There is substantial evidence that T-cells, particularly CD4+ helper cells, are crucial in the early immunological response. However, it is likely that other cells and their products drive rheumatoid arthritis synovitis. Cytokines are soluble proteins that serve as chemical messengers between cells. It is clear that deregulation of the immune system and an excess production of proinflammatory cytokines, for example interleukin-1 (IL-1), IL-6, tumour necrosis factor-α (TNF-α), IL-18 and granulocyte macrophage colony stimulating factor (GM-CSF), play a crucial role. In particular, TNF-α appears to be a critical factor in the inflammatory cascade. Both TNF-α and IL-1 are considered to exert pivotal influence in the pathogenesis of rheumatoid arthritis. They stimulate the development of a proinflammatory phenotype on responding cells. This gives rise to positive effects on chemotaxis, angiogenesis, vessel permeability, matrix metalloproteinase production, which is responsible for matrix degradation, and T- and B-cell recruitment and activation.

Clinical manifestations

The diagnosis of rheumatoid arthritis is based on criteria developed by the American Rheumatism Association (Table 53.2).

Table 53.2   Criteria for diagnosis of rheumatoid arthritis

Criteria	Comment
1. Morning stiffness	Duration lasting >1 h for >6 weeks
2. Arthritis of at least three joint areas	Soft tissue swelling or exudation for >6 weeks
3. Arthritis of hand joints	Swelling in wrist, metacarpophalangeal joints or proximal interphalangeal joints lasting >6 weeks
4. Symmetrical arthritis	Symmetrical involvement of same joint areas on both sides of body lasting >6 weeks
5. Rheumatoid nodules	Subcutaneous nodules as observed by physician
6. Serum rheumatoid factor	Abnormal levels of serum rheumatoid factor assessed by a method positive in less than 5% of control subjects
7. Radiographic changes	Typical changes seen on anteroposterior films of wrists and hands

Presence of four or more of the above criteria indicates that the patient has rheumatoid arthritis.

These criteria were principally designed for disease classification in patients with established disease so they are not sensitive for patients in the early stages of disease (Aletaha et al 2005). The criteria do not necessarily need to be used for diagnosis as clinical history, physical examination and laboratory tests can also be used.

The course of rheumatoid arthritis is highly variable and although it is primarily a disease of the synovial joints, it can affect many organ systems. The disease is characterized by flares and remissions. Approximately 20% of patients achieve remission after a short illness with no further disease activity, 25% obtain remission with mild residual disease, 45% have persistent activity with variable progressive deformity, and 10% progress to complete disability.

The initial symptoms of rheumatoid arthritis typically present in one of two ways: with a slow insidious onset or an explosive sudden onset. Rheumatoid arthritis begins insidiously in 55–56% of cases over weeks to months, whilst 8–15% of patients have an acute onset of symptoms that peak within days (Khurana & Berney 2005). Early symptoms of rheumatoid arthritis are non-specific and consist of fatigue, malaise, diffuse musculoskeletal pain and stiffness. Joint pain and loss of function are the most obvious symptoms of rheumatoid arthritis. The peripheral joints of the hands and feet are usually involved first. Presentation is usually symmetrical. However, an asymmetrical presentation, with symmetry developing later in the course of the disease, has been observed. The metacarpophalangeal and proximal interphalangeal joints of the hands and the metatarsophalangeal joints of the feet are affected, but the distal interphalangeal joint is usually spared. Ultimately, any of the diarthrodial joints

can be affected. Larger joints generally become symptomatic after smaller joints. Synovial hypertrophy and effusion cause swelling, and the affected joints are warm and tender. Affected joints cannot be fully extended or fully flexed due to tenosynovitis. Erosive changes give rise to joint instability and subluxation. Characteristic deformities include ulnar deviation, swan neck and boutonnière deformities (Fig. 53.1). The most serious long-term disability is associated with damage to the larger weight-bearing joints. Patients usually experience prolonged morning stiffness, due in part to redistribution of interstitial fluid while sleeping, which improves during the day and often returns at night.

The extra-articular features of rheumatoid arthritis (see Table 53.1) occur in approximately 75% of seropositive patients and are often associated with a poor prognosis. A number of factors have been shown to be associated with a poor prognosis in rheumatoid arthritis (Table 53.3).

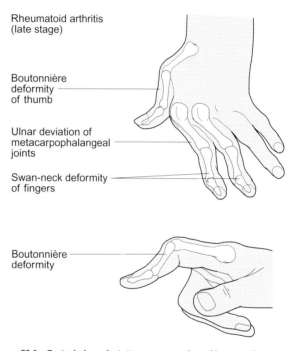

Figure 53.1   Typical ulnar deviation, swan neck and boutonnière deformities.

Table 53.3   Predictors of poor prognosis in rheumatoid arthritis

- Male with disease onset before age 50
- Disease duration >5 years before treatment
- Number of affected joints >20
- Lack of formal education
- Lower socio-economic status
- Functional disability within 1 year of onset
- Extra-articular involvement
- Several co-morbidities
- Seropositive disease (presence of rheumatoid factor)
- HLA-DR4 positive

Investigations

The diagnosis of rheumatoid arthritis is made on presenting signs, symptoms and some biochemical investigations. The most useful of these are the inflammatory markers, for example erythrocyte sedimentation rate (ESR), C-reactive protein (CRP) and plasma viscosity (PV), rheumatoid factor (RF) and antinuclear antibodies (ANA). A raised inflammatory marker simply confirms the presence of an inflammatory condition and occurs in many disease states. A normal inflammatory marker, however, does not preclude active disease. Although these markers are not specific to rheumatoid arthritis they may be used to assess response to drug treatment as they are usually raised when the disease is active.

Rheumatoid factors are autoantibodies directed against the host immunoglobulin. Routinely performed tests only detect IgM RF which is present in 75–80% of patients with rheumatoid arthritis (seropositive disease) and 5% of normal subjects. Extra-articular features of rheumatoid arthritis are much more common in patients with a high titre for RF. Antinuclear antibodies are investigated to rule out the possibility of other connective tissue disorders such as systemic lupus erythematosus (SLE). Antinuclear antibodies are raised in 80% of patients with SLE, and about 20% of patients with rheumatoid arthritis. Neither RF nor antinuclear antibodies are universal diagnostic tools, but they assist with the overall diagnostic picture. Other abnormal laboratory tests include an elevated alkaline phosphatase, an elevated platelet count, a decreased serum albumin level and a normochromic, normocytic anaemia.

Radiographs, mainly of the hands and feet, have been used to establish the diagnosis of rheumatoid arthritis and to follow its progression. Erosions can be seen at the joint margins and loss of joint space due to erosion of cartilage and bone may be identified. In severe long-standing disease the dominant features include subluxation and deformity. Modern imaging technology such as magnetic resonance imaging (MRI) and ultrasound (US) is being increasingly used to detect inflammatory activity. Erosions traditionally detected on x-ray will not be apparent in the early stages of the disease. Early diagnosis and treatment of inflammation are important to limit joint damage and so MRI and US are used to detect early changes in rheumatoid arthritis patients (Keen & Emery 2005).

Treatment

Goals for the management of a patient with rheumatoid arthritis include:

- decrease pain and inflammation
- prevent joint destruction
- preserve or improve functional ability
- maintain normal lifestyle.

Treatment of rheumatoid arthritis should begin as soon as possible as there is evidence that most patients develop joint destruction within the first 2 years of their disease. Early treatment is best achieved by having special arthritis clinics in which patients are often seen within 2 weeks of referral from their primary care doctor.

The multidisciplinary approach to treating rheumatoid arthritis patients is also important. Physiotherapists, occupational therapists, clinical nurse specialists, podiatrists, social workers and pharmacists all have a crucial role. Education of patients is an important aspect of treatment. The patient should gain knowledge of the disease process and understand the likely prognosis and treatment strategies. Psychological aspects of the disease should also be covered. The education is best carried out by the multidisciplinary team and should reinforce the importance of adherence to all aspects of the treatment plan.

The treatment for each patient is individualized and based on factors such as age, occupation and family responsibilities. Other considerations include the degree of disease activity and joint function, and the patient's response to previous therapy. There are several ways to measure response to treatment, both clinically and in the trial setting. One way is to use the American College of Rheumatology (ACR) guidelines. Patients are scored using various criteria and scores are compared to obtain an improvement in their symptoms. This is referred to as the ACR response. In clinical trials the ACR response is usually used to describe how many patients have a 20%, 50% or 70% improvement in their overall scores which equate approximately to the patient's ability to carry out activities of daily living (Table 53.4). Another way in which the severity or activity of a rheumatoid arthritis patient's disease can be measured is by the Disease Activity Score (DAS 28). This score is calculated using an assessment of 28 joints for swelling and tenderness, erythrocyte sedimentation rate, and patient global assessment of disease activity (Fig. 53.2).

Table 53.4 Criteria for defining an ACR 20 response

Over 20% improvement in tender joint count
Over 20% improvement in swollen joint count

Over 20% improvement in more than three of the aspects listed below:
     Patient pain assessment (using a visual analogue scale)
     Patient global assessment
     Physician global assessment
     Patient self-assessment of disability (using a health assessment questionnaire)
     ESR or C-reactive protein (CRP) levels

$$Das\ 28 = (0.56 \times \sqrt{28T}) + (0.28 \times \sqrt{28S}) + (0.70 \times \ln ESR) + (0.014 \times GH)$$

Where:

28T = 28 tender joint count
28S = 28 swollen joint count
ESR = erythrocyte sedimentation rate (mm/hr)
GH = patient global assessment of general health VAS (0–100mm)
ln = natural log

Fig 53.2 How to calculate a DAS 28 score.

Non-drug treatment

Physiotherapy is a vital part of treating rheumatoid arthritis, both in acute flares and in the chronic state. Heat, cold and electrotherapy help to reduce pain and swelling, and a programme of exercise strengthens joints to prevent disuse atrophy, mobilize joints to minimize deformity and increase the range of movement and functions. Occupational therapy educates patients to protect joints with the use of appliances and splints. Surgical techniques ranging from carpal tunnel decompression to major joint replacement can be effective in relieving pain and restoring function.

Drug treatment

Traditionally, treatment for rheumatoid arthritis was introduced in a stepwise 'pyramidal' manner. First-line agents such as analgesics and non-steroidal anti-inflammatory drugs (NSAIDs) were used to relieve symptoms. Then second-line (e.g. sulfasalazine) and third-line (e.g. azathioprine) disease-modifying antirheumatic drugs (DMARDs) were added when symptoms were not adequately controlled. Used in this way, DMARDs suppressed markers of disease activity and improved function but their impact on long-term disability was disappointing. The ultimate aim of treatment is to induce disease remission. This, in conjunction with the evidence that joint destruction occurs in the first few years of the disease, has led to the much earlier use of single DMARDs and combinations of DMARDs.

The treatment of rheumatoid arthritis continues to change rapidly. The advent of cytokine inhibitors has been a major step forward in the treatment of the disease. These agents are increasingly being used after failure of an adequate response to DMARDs (NICE 2002) although evidence is accumulating to support their earlier use. There is increasing evidence that the degree and severity of joint damage are linked to corresponding levels of inflammation. Thus, treatment that suppresses underlying inflammation is expected to produce improvements in function and bone erosions, although complete disease remission is rarely achieved.

Simple analgesics

Paracetamol, paracetamol combinations and weak opioids are all useful for simple pain relief. Although they have no anti-inflammatory properties and do not affect the disease process, they do have a place in both early and late stages of the disease. They may help with referred pain associated with muscle weakness and the general soreness associated with rheumatoid arthritis. Simple analgesic use is guided by the WHO analgesic ladder. Adjuvant analgesia, with low-dose antidepressants and anticonvulsants, also has a role in the relief of chronic pain later in the disease.

Non-steroidal anti-inflammatory drugs (NSAIDs)

The major pharmacological agents for the relief of pain and inflammation in rheumatic diseases are the NSAIDs. Their pharmacokinetic profiles are presented in Table 53.5. Although the NSAIDs differ in chemical structure, they all have similar pharmacological properties in terms of antipyretic, anti-inflammatory and analgesic action and are involved in essentially similar drug interactions (Table 53.6).

Patient response to NSAIDs is highly variable and therapeutic trials with several NSAIDs may be necessary to determine the best agent. Despite numerous clinical trials, differences between NSAIDs in objective measures of efficacy have not emerged. It is estimated that 60% of patients will respond to any one NSAID. If a patient does not respond it may be necessary to try several other NSAIDs before the most appropriate agent is found. It is recommended that the drug should be changed after 1 week of non-response if an analgesic effect is the desired outcome or 3 weeks if an anti-inflammatory effect is required. Approximately 10% of patients will not find any NSAID beneficial. This variability in response may be partly explained by the differing individual effects on the inflammatory pathways, although other factors are clearly important. Patient preference and adherence are the best indicators of success. Factors that should be considered in choosing a specific NSAID are relative efficacy, toxicity, concomitant drugs, concurrent disease states, patient age, renal function, dosing frequency and cost.

There is no evidence of synergism or reduced toxicity with the use of more than one NSAID. In fact, there is evidence that two NSAIDs may increase the risk of gastrointestinal side effects. Only one agent should be prescribed at a time. The NSAIDs can broadly be divided into those with a long or short plasma half-life; these are shown in Table 53.5.

Mechanism of action The main mechanism of action of NSAIDs (Fig. 53.3) is the inhibition of the enzyme cyclo-oxygenase (COX). COX converts the fatty acid arachidonic acid into endoperoxides, prostaglandins and thromboxanes in a cell-specific manner. These prostanoids have a diverse variety of physiological functions, including protection of the gastrointestinal tract, renal homeostasis, platelet aggregation, contraction of uterine smooth muscle, etc., and are widely implicated in pathological states associated with inflammation.

Over the years it has been shown that there are two isoforms of COX: COX-1 and COX-2. COX-1 is thought to function mainly as a physiological enzyme producing the prostaglandins critical for maintaining normal renal function, gastric mucosal integrity and haemostasis. COX-2 is virtually undetectable in most tissues under physiological conditions. However, it is induced by certain inflammatory stimuli, including IL-1 and TNF-α. Marked increases in levels of COX-2 have been found at sites of inflammation in musculoskeletal disease such as rheumatoid arthritis.

NSAIDs act by direct inhibition of COX-1 and COX-2, via blockade of the COX enzyme site. The subsequent inhibition of prostaglandins reduces inflammation but also results in additional activities on platelet aggregation, renal homeostasis and gastric mucosal integrity. In addition, NSAIDs interfere with a variety of other processes which may contribute to their effects. These include leukotriene synthesis, superoxide generation, lysosomal enzyme release, neutrophil function, lymphocyte function and cartilage metabolism.

NSAIDs differ in the extent and manner in which they inhibit COX-1 and COX-2. This is often expressed as the COX-2: COX-1 selectivity ratio, which shows significant variation according to

Table 53.5 Pharmacokinetic parameters of NSAIDs

Drug	T_{max} (h)	V_d(L/kg)	$t_{1/2}$(h)	Renal excretion (%)
Short half-life				
Aspirin	1–2	0.15	0.25	<2
Diclofenac	1–3	0.12	1.1	>1
Aceclofenac	1.25–3	0.25	4	66
Etodolac	2		3	
Fenoprofen	1–2	0.10	2.5	2–5
Flurbiprofen	1–2	0.10	3–4	<15
Ibuprofen	0.5–1.5		2.1	1
Indometacin	1–2	0.12	4.6	<15
Ketorolac	1	0.11–0.33	4–6	50–60
Ketoprofen	0.5–2	0.11	1.8	<1
Dexketoprofen	0.25–1	0.24	2	
Long half-life				
Azapropazone	3–6	0.16	15	62
Diflunisal	1–2	0.10	5–20	<3
Fenbufen	1–2		11	4
Meloxicam	1–2	0.16	20	3
Nabumetone	3–6	0.11	26	1
Phenylbutazone	2	0.17	50–100	1
Piroxicam	2	0.12	28	10
Sulindac	1		7 (sulindac), 16 (active sulfide)	7
Tenoxicam	1–2	0.12	60	<1
Celecoxib	2–3	7.14	11	27
Etoricoxib	1		22	70

T_{max}, time to maximum plasma concentration; V_d, volume of distribution; $t_{1/2}$, elimination half-life.

Table 53.6 Examples of drug interactions with NSAIDs

Affected drug	Drug causing effect	Effect
Oral anticoagulants	NSAIDs	Aspirin enhances hypoprothrombinaemic effect
		All increase risk of gastrointestinal bleed, all have antiplatelet effects
Hypotensive agents	NSAIDs	Decreased hypotensive effect
Diuretics	NSAIDs	Decreased diuretic effect
Potassium-sparing drugs, e.g. ACE inhibitors, potassium-sparing diuretics	Indometacin	Hyperkalaemia
Lithium	Most NSAIDs	Increased lithium levels
Methotrexate	All NSAIDs	Increased methotrexate levels
Most NSAIDs	Probenecid	Increased NSAID concentration

the source enzyme/type of cells used for the assays. Valid comparisons cannot therefore be made between different assays. It is also unclear how these ratios translate into clinical practice. However, the older traditional NSAIDs inhibit COX-1 and COX-2 to a similar degree. In contrast, etodolac and meloxicam inhibit COX-2 up to 50 times more than COX-1, and newer agents celecoxib and etoricoxib are even more COX-2 selective.

Adverse effects NSAIDs are widely used for the treatment of inflammatory conditions. They are also the drugs most

often reported as being responsible for adverse effects and use can be associated with significant morbidity and mortality. Gastrointestinal complications are the most important adverse reactions, with other serious reactions including renal impairment, angio-oedema, urticaria, hepatic dysfunction, haematological abnormalities and bronchospasm.

Gastrointestinal adverse events Gastric damage appears to require a direct mucosal effect as well as inhibition of prostaglandin biosynthesis. Impairment of mucosal defensive factors

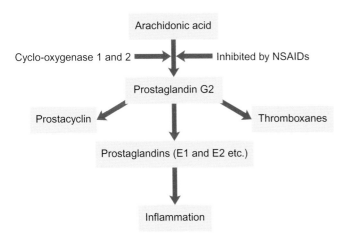

Fig 53.3 Mechanism of action of NSAIDs.

(mucus and bicarbonate secretion, mucosal blood flow) also plays a major role. Gastrointestinal adverse reactions range from superficial damage, with minor symptoms such as dyspepsia, abdominal pain and diarrhoea, to duodenal and gastric ulceration and potentially fatal complications. Patients generally complain of nausea and indigestion, but some of those presenting with bleeding or perforation will have no history of dyspepsia or peptic ulceration.

Finding the true incidence of gastrointestinal side effects due to NSAIDs is difficult. Short- and long-term treatment with aspirin and other NSAIDs is known to induce dyspeptic symptoms in up to 60% of cases and gastroduodenal lesions in 30–50% of patients. Others report the incidence of gastrointestinal side effects to be between 8% and 34%. The prevalence of symptomatic ulcers has been reported to be between 14% and 31%, with gastric ulcers most prevalent. Serious gastrointestinal haemorrhage or perforation can be expected in 1% and may be associated with a mortality rate in excess of 10%, especially in the elderly. Less than half these patients will experience dyspeptic symptoms before the serious event.

Other adverse events   Most NSAIDs can reduce creatinine clearance and produce a non-oliguric renal failure, possibly as a result of inhibition of prostaglandin synthesis in the kidney. This effect tends to be relatively minor, usually reversible and associated with long-term therapy. Those patients with impaired renal function, hepatic cirrhosis or circulatory volume depletion are most at risk. Indometacin is the most commonly reported cause of NSAID-induced renal failure. Fenoprofen is the NSAID most commonly associated with interstitial nephritis and nephrotic syndrome.

Asthmatic patients may develop wheezing following administration of NSAIDs. It is known that aspirin will provoke or worsen asthma in approximately 5% of patients.

Some NSAIDs have been shown to affect chondrocyte function in vitro in animal models. As a consequence, it has been suggested that NSAIDs may prevent regeneration of articular cartilage and hasten the development of osteoarthritis. Other possible adverse effects of NSAIDs involve the skin, liver and bone marrow. Indometacin, in particular, can cause headache, dizziness and psychiatric disturbances.

Strategies to reduce risk of NSAID-induced ulcers   A number of major risk factors that contribute to NSAID-induced

ulcers have been identified and classified according to whether they are related to the NSAID or to the patient (Table 53.7). The presence of one factor elevates the risk of gastrointestinal complications but the presence of more than one risk factor is even more deleterious. NICE (2001) further identified the following high risk factors for gastrointestinal toxicity:

- age over 65 years
- previous history of gastroduodenal ulcer, gastrointestinal bleed or gastroduodenal perforation
- concurrent treatment with corticosteroids and/or anticoagulation
- patients 'too frail to withstand a gastrointestinal emergency'
- serious co-morbidity, e.g. cardiovascular disease, diabetes, renal/hepatic impairment, hypertension and rheumatoid arthritis
- prolonged use of maximum doses of NSAIDs
- concurrent treatment with low-dose aspirin.

Patients treated with corticosteroids and NSAIDs are 15 times more likely to suffer from peptic ulcer disease than patients taking neither drug.

A number of strategies have been proposed to reduce the risk of ulcer development with NSAID treatment.

Choice of NSAID   A review of 12 controlled epidemiological studies examining 14 different NSAIDs demonstrated that there is a differential risk of gastrointestinal complications between drugs (Henry et al 1996). The work showed that ibuprofen (dose 1.2 g/day) has the lowest risk of gastrointestinal complications and azapropazone the highest. Diclofenac also ranks low, though higher than ibuprofen, with indometacin and piroxicam having intermediate risk (Table 53.8). The risk of gastrointestinal complications with NSAIDs is dose related and ibuprofen may be no safer than those NSAIDs defined as intermediate risk.

Preventive therapy   Preventive therapy cannot be recommended for all patients receiving NSAIDs on cost-effectiveness grounds. In patients at high risk of gastrointestinal toxicity, first-line choice of analgesic would be a simple agent such as paracetamol. If the anti-inflammatory effect of a NSAID is required, then either a standard low-risk NSAID such as ibuprofen or diclofenac can be used, in addition to a proton pump inhibitor (PPI), or misoprostol. Alternatively, a COX-2 selective

Table 53.7   Major risk factors that contribute to NSAID-induced ulcers

NSAID factor	Patient factor
Choice of NSAID	Age: older patients are at intrinsically increased risk of ulceration
High-dose NSAID	Previous history of gastrointestinal damage, e.g. perforation, ulceration
Concurrent low-dose aspirin plus NSAID	Other concurrent ulcerogenic medication, e.g. steroids
Concurrent NSAID plus anticoagulant	Presence of chronic disease, e.g. cardiovascular disease, rheumatoid arthritis

Table 53.8 Relative risk of major gastrointestinal complications with various NSAIDs (combined data from 12 controlled studies)

Drug	Mean rank (relative risk)
Ibuprofen	1.0
Diclofenac	2.3
Naproxen	7.0
Indometacin	8.0
Piroxicam	9.0
Azapropazone	11.7

inhibitor could be used by itself. However, a COX-2 selective inhibitor should not be used in patients taking low-dose aspirin, as the risk of gastrointestinal toxicity is not reduced. It should also be noted that there is currently no evidence to justify the use of a COX-2 inhibitor in combination with a PPI or misoprostol.

COX-2 selective inhibitors COX-2 selective inhibitors have a theoretical advantage over standard NSAIDs with respect to a reduction in gastrointestinal side effects. For example, meloxicam, a more preferential COX-2 selective inhibitor, has demonstrated a reduced incidence of symptomatic gastrointestinal adverse effects compared to non-selective NSAIDs when used at a dose of 7.5 mg per day. At a dose of 15 mg per day, meloxicam caused gastrointestinal mucosal injury intermediate between placebo and piroxicam 20 mg per day. The COX-2 selective inhibitors celecoxib and etoricoxib are more selective than the preferential COX inhibitors.

The COX-2 selective inhibitors are, however, not always appropriate as first-line therapy in patients with arthritis. They should not be administered concurrently with low-dose aspirin, as discussed above, and their use is contraindicated in patients with cardiovascular disease. All COX-2 selective inhibitors are contraindicated in patients with ischaemic heart disease, cerebrovascular disease, peripheral arterial disease and heart failure (NYHA class II–IV). Etoricoxib is also contraindicated in patients with uncontrolled hypertension. The traditional, nonselective NSAIDs, unlike the COX-2 selective inhibitors, are not known to cause increased cardiovascular toxicity.

Disease-modifying antirheumatic drugs

DMARDs have a major role in managing rheumatoid arthritis, and although they have very different chemical structures and different mechanisms of action, each shows activity in managing this disabling condition.

The DMARDs currently used in clinical practice include: methotrexate, sulfasalazine, injectable and oral gold, antimalarials, ciclosporin, penicillamine, azathioprine and leflunomide. The choice of DMARD depends upon the balance between adverse effects and efficacy. All the DMARDs possess a slow onset of action. Initial benefit can take 4–16 weeks, with response to treatment usually expected within 4–6 months.

The dose of a DMARD should generally be titrated upward as long as side effects allow. If the maximum recommended dose has been reached but the response is inadequate, an additional DMARD may be added or the initial DMARD stopped and switched to an alternative.

The developing knowledge and understanding of the pathophysiology of rheumatoid arthritis have radically altered the therapeutic approach to the use of DMARDs. Patients are no longer treated with NSAIDs first, with more toxic DMARDs being introduced at a later stage. This approach clearly failed to prevent the erosive changes and joint destruction associated with rheumatoid arthritis and has subsequently been replaced with a more aggressive approach (O'Dell 2002). The knowledge that disease progression is rapid within the first few years of onset has led to the much earlier use of DMARDs alone and in combination, although the evidence of benefit from using combination therapy is unclear.

In practice, initial treatment of rheumatoid arthritis is generally with a single agent. If a satisfactory response is not achieved after a 3–6 month trial with monotherapy, then combination treatment is usually given. This is most likely to be a combination of sulfasalazine and methotrexate. Some clinicians will prescribe triple therapy of methotrexate, sulfasalazine and hydroxychloroquine, added sequentially. A number of combinations have been shown to be beneficial and to carry no more toxicity than single DMARD therapy:

- methotrexate + sulfasalazine
- methotrexate + hydroxychloroquine
- methotrexate + sulfasalazine + hydroxychloroquine
- methotrexate + leflunomide
- ciclosporin + hydroxychloroquine
- ciclosporin + methotrexate.

Patients who fail to respond may be offered other therapeutic options such as a cytokine inhibitor (biologic agent).

Comparisons of the relative efficacy of DMARDs using a wide variety of disease symptoms and laboratory markers have been undertaken but the results are inconclusive. A more useful comparison is the continuation rates of the different DMARDs. Toxicity, loss of efficacy, or both, tend to limit continuation of therapy, frequently to less than 2 years. Methotrexate and sulfasalazine have the highest 5-year continuation rates of 50–60%. For parenteral gold and penicillamine, 5-year continuation rates are only about 20%, and the rate for oral gold is as low as 5%.

Sulfasalazine and methotrexate are generally regarded as firstline therapies because of their improved efficacy profile (approximately 40% response rates) and high continuation rates compared to the other DMARDs.

Mechanism of action The precise mechanism of action of these drugs is unclear. All DMARDs inhibit the release, or reduce the activity, of inflammatory cytokines. Activated T-lymphocytes appear to be particularly important in this process and it is known that methotrexate, leflunomide and ciclosporin all inhibit T-cells. Cytokines, which appear to be important in the inflammatory cascade, include TNF-α and the interleukins IL-1, IL-2 and IL-6. There is good evidence that DMARDs inhibit these cytokines in vitro and in vivo. Leflunomide has also been shown to inhibit the proliferation of B-cells with a subsequent inhibition of antibody production.

Use and monitoring The majority of DMARDs can cause bone marrow and hepatic toxicity and therefore require monitoring to ensure safe therapy. The monitoring requirements are set out in Table 53.9. Patient information leaflets and monitoring booklets are recommended for patients taking DMARDs.

Sulfasalazine has a high continuation rate, a low rate of serious adverse effects and has been shown to slow disease progression. It is often used in mild-to-moderate disease. The monitoring requirements are less arduous than most other DMARDs, conveying a significant benefit for patients. In order to reduce the problems of nausea, the dose is usually titrated from 500 mg daily, increasing at weekly intervals up to 1 g twice daily.

Methotrexate is first-line therapy in most centres in the UK. It is generally used in patients with moderate-to-severe disease, especially in those with poor prognosis (see Table 53.3). Methotrexate is probably the most effective DMARD. It has a high 5-year continuation rate and a low incidence of adverse effects at low weekly doses. It has a relatively rapid onset of action of 4–6 weeks and is easy to administer as a single weekly dose. It has a response rate of 40–50% and has been shown to improve quality of life and reduce joint destruction. Hepatic fibrosis and liver toxicity do, however, occur in a significant proportion of patients, and appear to be enhanced by a high alcohol intake. Patients should therefore be encouraged to either avoid alcohol while on methotrexate, or at the very least restrict it to special occasions. Liver function tests must be frequently monitored (see Table 53.9). Severe alveolitis can be a serious and sometimes fatal adverse event with methotrexate therapy, and requires urgent medical treatment. Any patient experiencing increasing dyspnoea should be advised to stop methotrexate and seek medical help immediately.

The dose range for methotrexate varies from 5 mg to 25 mg once a week. Nausea and stomatitis can be managed by the addition of folic acid although administration should be omitted on the day methotrexate is administered. Intramuscular or more frequently subcutaneous methotrexate (not licensed for use in rheumatoid arthritis) may be useful when side effects such as nausea and vomiting impede use of the oral route. The parenteral route may also be useful in patients with poor response despite high-dose oral therapy, especially in those with suspected poor oral absorption or compliance.

Perhaps one of the greatest concerns with methotrexate therapy is the potential for bone marrow suppression. This is of particular concern either in overdose or in patients on too high a maintenance dose. Bone marrow suppression includes neutropenia, thrombocytopenia and lymphopenia and can be fatal. This usually occurs in patients who inadvertently take methotrexate daily at the dose prescribed for weekly administration. Patients

Table 53.9 Dosage, side effects and monitoring guidelines for DMARDs

Drug	Dose schedule	Adverse effects	Monitoring
Sulfasalazine	Initially 500 mg once daily, increasing in weekly steps of 500 mg to 1 g twice daily	Nausea, reversible male, infertility, rashes, marrow suppressions hepatitis	FBC and LFTs fortnightly for 2 months then monthly for 4 months then 3 monthly
Methotrexate	5–25 mg once weekly	Rashes, nausea, stomatitis, marrow suppression, hepatitis, pneumonitis	FBC and LFTs fortnightly for 2 months then monthly for 4 months then 3 monthly
Sodium aurothiomalate (i.m. gold)	10 mg test dose, then 50 mg weekly until signs of remission, then reduce frequency to monthly	Rashes, stomatitis, marrow suppression, proteinuria	FBC and urinalysis weekly for first 16–20 injections then monthly. Urinalysis before each injection
Penicillamine	250–750 mg once daily (on empty stomach)	Rashes, taste disturbance, nausea, proteinuria, myasthenia, myositis, marrow suppression	FBC, U&E, urinalysis fortnightly for 2 months, monthly for 4 months then 3 monthly
Ciclosporin	2.5 mg/kg per day	Hirsutism, gingival hyperplasia, hypertension, renal impairment	U&E, LFT, FBC fortnightly until stable disease, then monthly for 4 months then 3 monthly. Check lipids and urate at 3-monthly intervals (optional). Use baseline creatinine to alter dose
Leflunomide	Maintenance dose of 10–20 mg per day (loading dose of 100 mg daily for 3 days rarely used and generally considered inadvisable)	Gastrointestinal disturbance, alopecia, liver abnormalities, hypertension, marrow suppression	FBC, U&E, LFTs and BP at week 1 then fortnightly for 2 months then monthly for 4 months then 3 monthly
Azathioprine	1.5–2.5 mg/kg day	Nausea, hepatitis, cholestatic jaundice, marrow suppression	FBC, U&E and LFTs fortnightly for 2 months then monthly for 4 months then 3 monthly

FBC, full blood count; LFT, liver function test; U&E, urea and electrolytes; i.m., intramuscular.

must be clear that they should take methotrexate only once per week, on the same day each week. Any sign of infection, such as unexplained fever or sore throat, etc., must be reported immediately and patients should avoid contact with people who may have chicken pox. Given the number of serious problems that may arise with patients receiving methotrexate, it is important that patients are counselled accordingly and receive appropriate written information.

Sodium aurothiomalate (gold injection) is a long-established DMARD and is a very effective agent in the treatment of rheumatoid arthritis. The use of injectable gold is, however, limited by its side effect profile. Important adverse events include rashes, stomatitis, proteinuria, leucopenia and thrombocytopenia. Injectable gold is usually reserved for use in patients who have a documented previous response or for those who demonstrate compliance problems.

Patients may be instructed to test their own urine for proteinuria. If significant protein is detected, the gold therapy should be withheld, urinary tract infection excluded and the proteinuria quantified by means of a 24-hour urine collection. Patients on gold injections should also be asked to report new side effects such as rashes or mouth ulcers.

Auranofin (oral gold) is a completely different drug entity to sodium aurothiomalate and although less toxic, it is generally less effective. It is now seldom used. Adverse effects are similar to injectable gold but are less frequent. The troublesome diarrhoea experienced with oral gold may be improved by a high-fibre diet.

Penicillamine (D-penicillamine) is now seldom used due to problems with toxicity and poor long-term efficacy. There is no evidence that penicillamine reduces joint erosions. It is initiated at a daily dose of 125 mg with monthly increases until a response is demonstrated. There is little benefit to increasing the dose above 750 mg as efficacy appears to have a ceiling effect. Penicillamine should be taken on an empty stomach as absorption is reduced by up to 50% when taken with food. The common side effects include thrombocytopenia, proteinuria, taste disturbances and rashes. Less common is neutropenia and, rarely, autoimmune side effects such as myositis and drug-induced lupus may occur. There have been reports of cutis laxa in infants born to mothers taking penicillamine.

Ciclosporin is an immunosuppressive agent that has proven efficacy in early and late disease but long-term data on reducing joint destruction are lacking. Ciclosporin is reserved for patients who have failed to respond to conventional therapies because of its potential for toxicity. It can cause nephrotoxicity and hypertension, which may have significant long-term consequences, and patients with a history of these are generally excluded from therapy. Treatment is initiated at a dose of 2.5 mg/kg/day and increased up to a maximum of 4.5 mg/kg dependent upon tolerance. There is no requirement to monitor ciclosporin blood levels in rheumatoid arthritis. Prior to commencing therapy, patients must have baseline blood pressure and creatinine measured, and both need to be carefully monitored. Other side effects include hirsutism, tremor and gum hyperplasia.

Hydroxychloroquine and other antimalarials are the least toxic of all the DMARDs. However, they are also the least effective and are generally reserved for less severe forms of the disease, or in combination regimens. Hydroxychloroquine requires little monitoring, with gastrointestinal toxicity the main adverse effect. Retinopathy is thought only to occur after high cumulative doses. The need for and frequency of eye tests are still debated. The typical dose is about 400 mg/day, although this has been increased up to 800 mg/day with the aim of achieving earlier efficacy.

Azathioprine is thought to have a steroid-sparing effect and is of particular use when treating rheumatoid arthritis refractory to other agents.

Cyclophosphamide is a potent cytotoxic agent that can be used either orally or as intravenous pulse therapy in the management of rheumatoid vasculitis.

Both azathioprine and cyclophosphamide have the potential to cause infertility and the development of malignancies. The risks must therefore be carefully balanced against intended clinical improvement.

Leflunomide is a novel isoxazole derivative, with both anti-inflammatory and immunomodulatory properties. It works by inhibiting the synthesis of DNA and RNA in immune response cells, particularly activated T-cells. It also inhibits the production of the proinflammatory cytokines TNF-α and IL-1. In short-term studies leflunomide appears to be equivalent to sulfasalazine and methotrexate. Patients have shown improvements in functional disability and quality of life and it has slowed radiographic progression of rheumatoid arthritis. It has a rapid onset of action, within 4 weeks, significantly faster than sulfasalazine, and is well tolerated. The most common side effects are gastrointestinal disturbances, reversible alopecia, rash, hypertension and abnormal liver function tests. Most of these are mild to moderate and resolve without any complications. Depending on the centre the patient attends, the clinician may sometimes omit the loading doses of leflunomide. Although the onset of action of the drug will take longer, it has been suggested that this approach avoids some of the side effects.

Corticosteroids

Systemic corticosteroids have long been used in the management of rheumatoid arthritis and were the first drugs to result in reversibility of the disease. Corticosteroids suppress cytokines and produce a rapid improvement in signs and symptoms of the disease. They have a potent anti-inflammatory effect and studies have suggested a slowing of radiological progression. However, side effects associated with long-term high-dose therapy, such as osteoporosis, diabetes mellitus and hypertension, have severely limited the long-term role of corticosteroids in rheumatoid arthritis.

Oral prednisolone may be used to provide temporary relief until a DMARD becomes effective, or in patients with aggressive disease who cannot be adequately controlled with a combination of DMARDs. Systemic corticosteroids can be difficult to withdraw once commenced, as the disease tends to flare with dose reductions. In order to minimize side effects, a daily maintenance dose of 7.5 mg of prednisolone or less should be used, given as a single dose in the morning. Prophylaxis against osteoporosis is recommended in patients likely to be on long-term therapy.

Intra-articular steroid administration (e.g. methylprednisolone or triamcinolone) can effectively relieve pain, increase mobility and reduce deformity in one or more joints. The duration of response to intra-articular steroids is variable. The dose used is dependent upon the joint size, with methylprednisolone acetate 40–80 mg or triamcinolone acetonide 20–40 mg appropriate for large joints such as knees. The frequency at which injections may be given is controversial, but repeated injections are usually given at intervals of 1–5 weeks or more, depending on the degree of relief obtained from the first injection. Joint injections should generally be limited to no more than three injections per year into an affected joint. They should never be used in prosthetic joints or if there is a possibility of sepsis. Intramuscular steroids may be useful in patients with an acute flare of disease, and intravenous pulses of methylprednisolone are particularly helpful in controlling rheumatoid vasculitis.

Cytokine inhibitors

Despite new approaches to the use of DMARDs, they have many limitations. The response to DMARD monotherapy or combination therapy is around 40–60% at best. This response rate and a high toxicity profile led to the search for new therapeutic strategies. Amongst the newer agents that have emerged are a group of drugs known as biologic therapies or cytokine inhibitors. These agents are expensive in comparison to traditional DMARDs, costing approximately £8000–9000 per patient per year.

The cytokine inhibitors target the inflammatory pathway which is modulated by various cytokines that act as local messengers and signalling molecules. The balance between proinflammatory and anti-inflammatory cytokines determines the signs, symptoms and degree of inflammation experienced by a patient. Proinflammatory cytokines include TNF-α, IL-1, IL-6 and other chemokines. TNF-α is the target of infliximab, etanercept and adalimumab and as a consequence these are often referred to as anti-TNF agents. Anakinra is a cytokine inhibitor that inhibits IL-1, and is referred to as an IL-1 receptor antagonist (IL-1 Ra).

Infliximab was the first of the biologic agents to be licensed. It is a human-murine chimeric monoclonal antibody that specifically and potently binds and neutralizes soluble TNF-α and its membrane-bound precursor. This high affinity binding prevents the interaction of TNF-α with its cellular receptors and attenuates the inflammatory response and other deleterious effects secondary to TNF-α overproduction.

Infliximab is licensed for concomitant use with methotrexate in patients who have failed to respond adequately to DMARDs and in patients with severe, active and progressive disease not previously treated with DMARDs. It is given by slow intravenous infusion typically at a dose of 3 mg/kg in adults at weeks 0, 2 and 6 and then every 8 weeks. The clinical response correlates with a positive radiological outcome in most patients although in some with a poor clinical response there may be a good radiological outcome. The infusion is generally well tolerated, with infusion-related events such as headache, diarrhoea, rash, fever, chills, uticaria and dyspnoea being the most common side effects.

Adalimumab is a recombinant human monoclonal antibody. It binds with high affinity and specificity to soluble and membrane-bound TNF. It is licensed for moderate-to-severe active arthritis when response to DMARDs has been inadequate and the treatment of severe, active and progressive rheumatoid arthritis in adults not previously treated with methotrexate. It is

administered subcutaneously, normally at a dose of 40 mg, once every 2 weeks.

Etanercept is a recombinant molecule that comprises part of the human TNF receptor plus the constant region of human immunoglobulin G$_1$. Etanercept binds to TNF-α before it can interact with the cell surface receptors. It can be used alone or in combination with methotrexate for the treatment of active rheumatoid arthritis in adults when the response to DMARDs has been inadequate. Etanercept is also indicated in the treatment of severe, active and progressive rheumatoid arthritis in adults not previously treated with methotrexate. In adults, etanercept is administered either twice a week at a dose of 25 mg or once a week at a dose of 50 mg.

Anakinra inhibits the activity of IL-1. In adults it is given daily as a 100 mg subcutaneous injection in combination with methotrexate. It is not recommended for the routine treatment of rheumatoid arthritis unless it is part of a long-term clinical study.

Guidelines for the use of etanercept and infliximab in rheumatoid arthritis have been published (NICE 2002) and were updated in 2006 to include adalimumab. The anti-TNF agents are effective drugs recommended for the treatment of rheumatoid arthritis in adults who continue to have active disease that has not responded adequately to at least two DMARDs, including methotrexate unless contraindicated. There is little to choose between the different anti-TNF therapies in the treatment of rheumatoid arthritis. One- and 2-year trials with infliximab, etanercept and adalimumab have consistently shown that joint progression has been slowed by 80–90%. The choice of drug, therefore, is often dictated by doctor and patient preference, route of administration, and the DMARDs previously prescribed. Where a patient is methotrexate intolerant, adalimumab or etanercept are favoured, whilst there is good evidence for etanercept in juvenile-onset inflammatory arthritis. When a patient fails on treatment with one anti-TNF agent there are emerging data to suggest benefit from switching to a different agent, perhaps reflecting the differences in molecular structures and mechanisms of action of the three compounds.

TNF blockade has significant advantages over existing DMARD treatments. The anti-TNF agents demonstrate a response rate of 60–70% compared to 40% for DMARDs. They also significantly reduce disease activity, prevent disease progression and improve quality of life. This, however, may come at a cost. Although side effects are generally minor, serious side effects have been reported. The serious side effects are all probably linked by the role of TNF as a key regulator of innate immunity. As a consequence, problems such as an increased risk of infection, malignancies, particularly of the breast and lung, and CNS demyelinating disorders such as multiple sclerosis have all been reported although causal links have not been confirmed.

There are reports of a range of infections including rhinitis, sinusitis, bronchitis, cystitis, skin infections and sepsis in patients treated with the cytokine inhibitors. Some have been fatal although these have mainly occurred in patients predisposed to infections. The cytokine inhibitors should not be used in patients with active infection, especially with *Mycobacterium tuberculosis* (TB). However, such patients may be eligible for treatment following successful completion of a course of anti-TB therapy.

There are many other safety concerns with the cytokine inhibitors in addition to those listed above. Nevertheless, these agents significantly improve symptoms and reduce long-term disease activity and joint inflammation. Short-term toxicity is relatively low and to clarify long-term toxicity, a national register for patients receiving treatment has been established.

Overall, the treatment of rheumatoid arthritis is evolving, from early treatment with DMARDs or an anti-TNF agent if the patients fails to respond to early treatment with aggressive DMARD therapy and/or an anti-TNF agent (Fig. 53.4).

Future therapies

There are several agents under development for the treatment of rheumatoid arthritis and these include rituximab, abatacept and tocilizumab.

Rituximab is a chimeric anti-CD20 monoclonal antibody currently licensed for non-Hodgkin's lymphoma. It targets the CD20 cell surface marker on B-cells which are thought to have a key role in the rheumatoid arthritis inflammatory cascade. Rituximab is given as two intravenous infusions of 1000 mg, 2 weeks apart, and this results in B-cell depletion lasting several months.

Abatacept is a genetically engineered fusion protein that interrupts the inflammatory process in rheumatoid arthritis by selectively blocking signals needed for T-cell proliferation. It is the first in a new class of selective co-stimulation modulators. T-cells are thought to play a significant role in activating synovial macrophages and fibroblast-like synoviocytes to produce proinflammatory cytokines and proteolytic enzymes that mediate joint inflammation and destruction. In addition, T-cells also affect the activation and proliferation of B-cells which in turn produce potentially pathogenic autoantibodies such as RF.

Tocilizumab is a humanized monoclonal antibody to IL-6, a proinflammatory cytokine. Early data from clinical trials show it is superior to DMARDs in preventing both erosion and joint space narrowing.

Other research is investigating intracellular signalling molecules involved in cell activation, adhesion molecules that facilitate cell migration into inflamed tissues, and blockage of enzyme (metalloproteinases) releases in inflammatory tissues.

Patient care

Education of the patient with rheumatoid arthritis is vital. The patient should have knowledge of the disease process, the likely prognosis and treatment strategies. Psychological aspects of the disease should also be covered.

Hospital inpatients may find self-medication particularly valuable. In general, NSAID preparations should be taken with or after food, and patients should be warned of potential adverse effects and what to do if these occur. Patients must be warned not to supplement their prescribed NSAIDs with purchased ibuprofen or aspirin and should be careful of consuming additional 'hidden' paracetamol.

Patient information sheets for DMARDs and biologic therapies are very useful. However, counselling must reinforce the need to comply with monitoring requirements and explain the time delay before a response is seen, potential toxicity and action to take in the event of adverse effects. Shared care agreements are beneficial for patients to avoid repeated hospital outpatient appointments, and also to aid in the monitoring of their treatments. A number of common therapeutic problems that may be encountered are presented in Table 53.10.

OSTEOARTHRITIS

Osteoarthritis (OA) is a chronic disease and the most common of all the rheumatological disorders. It is the most common joint problem in individuals over the age of 65 years and is the major cause of hip and knee replacements in developed countries. Osteoarthritis is painful and disabling and represents a major challenge to health resources. Until recently, it was generally considered to be an inevitable consequence of ageing. However, research in the last decade has led to the view that it is an active disease with potential for treatment.

Epidemiology

The prevalence of osteoarthritis increases with age. Generally, osteoarthritis is uncommon in people aged less than 45 years, with a prevalence of just 2%. This increases in people aged over 65 years to 68% of women and 58% of men. Osteoarthritis occurs in all populations irrespective of race, climate or geographical location. Most forms of the disease are more common and severe in women. Ethnic origin contributes to the pattern of the disease; for example, hip disease is less common in Chinese and Asians than in those of Western origin. Obesity has been shown to be associated with the development of osteoarthritis, especially in women and particularly with osteoarthritis of the knee. The proportion of osteoarthritis attributable to obesity is estimated to be 63%. A strong genetic component is thought to be present, particularly in women. Heberden's nodes are three times more common in sisters with osteoarthritis than in the general population. An inherited defect in type II collagen genes is linked to the development of early-onset polyarticular osteoarthritis.

Aetiology

Osteoarthritis is a complex disease involving both cartilage and bone and is generally believed to result from an imbalance in erosive and reparative processes. The disease process is not

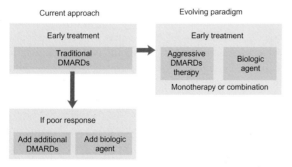

Fig 53.4 The evolving rheumatoid arthritis treatment paradigm.

Table 53.10 Common therapeutic problems in rheumatoid arthritis

Problem	Solution
Lack of efficacy of NSAID effect	Patient response at best around 60%; thus change after 2–3 weeks if lack of response. Consider adding simple/weak opioid analgesia
Intolerance to NSAID, e.g. dyspepsia	Consider changing NSAID If mild, treat with antacid If patient at high risk of gastrointestinal morbidity, consider gastroprotection Consider COX-2 selective NSAID If dyspepsia with COX-2 NSAID, treat with antacid
Need to reduce gastrointestinal morbidity with NSAID	Avoid NSAID if possible and use simple/weak opioid analgesia Consider lowest risk NSAID at lowest possible dose if NSAID required Use gastroprotection in high-risk patients Consider use of COX-2 NSAID with caution
Patient unwilling to commence DMARDs, especially in early disease	Counsel as to early irreversible joint destruction in first 2 years of disease Reassure as to adverse events with DMARDs
Lack of effect with DMARD	Ensure adequate trial of at least 12 weeks given Consider changing DMARD Consider combination DMARD therapy
Management of resistant rheumatoid arthritis	Consider addition of corticosteroids Consider triple DMARD therapy Consider TNF blockade therapy
Intolerance of DMARD	Titrate dose slowly Consider changing DMARD Treat mild side effects symptomatically Consider changing route of administration, e.g. parenteral methotrexate
Nausea and vomiting with methotrexate	Add folic acid Consider splitting the dose Consider changing to parenteral route Treat with antiemetics before and after administration

a simple wear-and-tear mechanism as inflammatory components may also be present. Osteoarthritis is multifactorial in aetiology and a wide variety of factors predispose an individual to this condition (Table 53.11). Other aetiological factors include mechanical overloading of joints, failure in the bone remodelling process, synovial and vascular changes, crystal deposition and catabolic enzyme secretion.

Pathogenesis

The pathogenesis of osteoarthritis has been classified into four stages:

1. initial repair
2. early-stage osteoarthritis
3. intermediate-stage osteoarthritis
4. late-stage osteoarthritis.

Table 53.11 Predisposing factors for the development of osteoarthritis

- Increasing age
- Race
- Genetic predisposition
- Gender: <45 years more common in males
  >55 years more common in females
  osteoarthritis knee more common in females
- Obesity
- Systemic disorders, e.g. hypertension
- Physical and occupational factors

Initial repair is characterized by proliferation of chondrocytes synthesizing the extracellular matrix of bone. Early-stage osteoarthritis results in degradation of the extracellular matrix as protease enzyme activity exceeds chondrocyte activity. There is net degradation and loss of articular cartilage. Intermediate osteoarthritis is associated with a failure of extracellular matrix synthesis and increased protease activity, further increasing cartilage loss. Finally, late-stage osteoarthritis will result in extreme or complete loss of cartilage with joint space narrowing. Bony outgrowths (osteophytes) appear at joint margins and there is general bone sclerosis. Clinically this stage manifests with pain and reduced joint movement.

Clinical manifestations

Osteoarthritis is characterized by joint pain, reduced joint movement, stiffness and joint swelling. The signs and symptoms are dependent upon the affected joints. The most commonly affected are the distal interphalangeal, proximal interphalangeal and first metacarpophalangeal joints, the knees, hips and the cervical and lumbar spine. Muscle weakness or wasting is usual. Pain, worsened by loading and movement but eased by rest, is the primary symptom. Pain is usually localized to the affected joint although it may be referred away from its origin (e.g. hip pain may be felt at the knee). Pain is often worse at the end of the day. Stiffness and reduced joint movement generally become worse as the day progresses, and are particularly troublesome after a long period of rest. Swelling, caused either by synovitis or osteophyte formation, and joint deformity restrict the range of joint movement and may lead to loss of function. The degree of disability depends on the site involved. Hip and knee disease are the most significant causes of morbidity associated with osteoarthritis. Crepitus may be heard in affected joints upon passive or active movement.

Investigations

Osteoarthritis is primarily diagnosed on the clinical presentation. Confirmation and evaluation of progression can be achieved using radiography. The presence of bone sclerosis, osteophyte formation and joint space narrowing is usually evident on radiography. There is, however, lack of association between symptoms and radiographic changes. On arthroscopy, normal cartilage is smooth, white and glistening, while osteoarthritis cartilage is yellowed, irregular and ulcerated. Synovial fluid analysis for crystals should be carried out to determine if pseudogout is present. In osteoarthritis the ESR/plasma viscosity and C-reactive protein levels are usually normal, and there is no extra-articular disease.

Treatment

The objectives in treating osteoarthritis are to:

- reduce pain
- increase mobility

- reduce disability
- minimize disease progression.

A variety of treatment options is available and includes both non-drug and drug strategies (Fig. 53.5).

Non-drug treatment

Non-drug treatment, particularly patient education, plays an important role in the management of osteoarthritis. Patients should be advised to protect joints through modification of daily living and reduction in weight. Physiotherapy may help patients regain muscle strength and improve the range of movement of affected joints. An exercise programme, heat, cold, ultrasound, diathermy and other aspects of physical therapy will support this strategy. Exercise regimens should encourage 'little and often' physical activity to improve muscle strength and resting tone. Occupational therapy may also help to protect joints and preserve function, especially with the use of physical aids and splints. Transcutaneous electrical nerve stimulation (TENS) and nerve blocks should be considered for severe pain and may also be assisted with orthopaedic surgery such as arthroplasty.

Depression and anxiety are common and should be treated to reduce the impact of pain and disability associated with osteoarthritis. Social support is essential for most patients.

Drug treatment

Most patients with osteoarthritis have pain as a result of the damage to bone and cartilage. In the absence of inflammation, simple analgesia and joint protection are often sufficient for the treatment of mild-to-moderate disease. The American College of Rheumatology (2000) has recommended simple analgesia as first-line therapy in patients with osteoarthritis of the hip and knee.

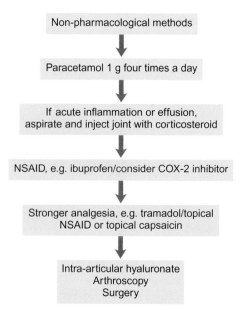

Non-pharmacological methods

↓

Paracetamol 1 g four times a day

↓

If acute inflammation or effusion, aspirate and inject joint with corticosteroid

↓

NSAID, e.g. ibuprofen/consider COX-2 inhibitor

↓

Stronger analgesia, e.g. tramadol/topical NSAID or topical capsaicin

↓

Intra-articular hyaluronate
Arthroscopy
Surgery

Fig 53.5 Algorithm for the management of osteoarthritis.

Paracetamol is safe and as effective as NSAID therapy in mild-to-moderate osteoarthritis. It is usually given at a dose of 1 g four times daily. This is often taken 'as required', although a regular regimen is frequently more successful. Addition of codeine to paracetamol may result in a slight increase in benefit although this must be assessed against an increased incidence of side effects (Eccles et al 1998). In the later stages of disease, other weak opioids and strong opioids may be used in line with chronic pain guidance.

There may be an associated inflammatory component to osteoarthritis. In these situations, NSAIDs may provide more effective pain control than simple analgesics. The evidence for the use of NSAIDs in the management of osteoarthritis is conflicting. Pooled data from trials indicate that NSAIDs have a greater effect in the symptomatic relief of people with osteoarthritis compared with paracetamol. However, the increased risk of adverse events with NSAIDs and the limited clinical significance of their greater effect means paracetamol is still the preferred first choice.

The choice of NSAID should be made after evaluation of risk factors for serious upper gastrointestinal and renal toxicity. Many osteoarthritis patients will be elderly and female and particularly susceptible to gastrointestinal side effects. A NSAID such as ibuprofen may be a suitable choice in such patients, and a 2-week trial should give an indication of its efficacy. The use of NSAIDs should be reviewed regularly and, if possible, restricted to short courses.

Gastroprotection with a PPI or misoprostol is recommended in patients at high risk of gastrointestinal events. These will include patients aged over 65 years, a history of peptic ulcer or gastrointestinal bleeding, concomitant steroids, concomitant anticoagulants or the presence of co-morbidity. COX-2 selective NSAIDs have been found to be more effective than placebo and comparable to standard NSAIDs in the management of osteoarthritis. These agents may provide an alternative NSAID strategy in patients at high risk of gastrointestinal events, although there is no evidence comparing these drugs to a standard non-selective NSAID with a gastroprotective agent.

Topical NSAIDs, topical capsaicin or simple rubefacients may be of use when pain is localized or if systemic therapy is not recommended. Topical NSAIDs can provide some pain relief and they are associated with fewer side effects than oral NSAIDs. However, they have been found to be no more effective than oral NSAIDs.

An alternative approach to the use of oral agents is the use of intra-articular injections. Intra-articular steroids may be of benefit in patients with acute inflammation or joint effusion. It has been recommended that repeat injections should not be given more often than every 3 months for a given joint. The duration of symptomatic improvement following intra-articular injection may range from a few days to 1 month or longer. Intra-articular hyaluronic acid derivatives (visco-supplementation) may prove useful in some patients. They are thought to supplement the natural hyaluronic acid in the synovial fluid in the joint space to return the elasticity and viscosity of the synovial fluid to normal. However, there is limited evidence to support this theory. These agents have been shown to be more effective than placebo and equivalent to intra-articular steroids and oral NSAIDs in reducing pain associated with osteoarthritis of the knee. Intra-articular hyaluronic acid derivatives are expensive and are indicated for patients who have failed non-drug treatment, simple analgesia, NSAIDs, strong analgesia and intra-articular corticosteroids (see Fig. 53.5).

New developments

Several chondroprotective agents or similar drugs have been proposed for the management of osteoarthritis. Chondroitin and glucosamine compounds are the most common. While some studies support the use of these agents in osteoarthritis, it is generally believed that there are insufficient data to support widespread use. A systematic review of 15 double blind RCTs of glucosamine and chondroitin in knee osteoarthritis reported significant short-term symptomatic benefits (Richy et al 2003). Glucosamine doses were mainly 1500 mg daily given for a duration between 6–8 weeks and 3 years. Chondroitin doses were 800–2000 mg daily with a duration of 3 months to 1 year.

CASE STUDIES

Case 53.1

Mr HP is a 52-year-old man who presents with increasing pain and stiffness in his hands and knees. He was diagnosed with rheumatoid arthritis 4 years ago, and his most recent medications include: methotrexate tablets 10 mg Sunday only, folic acid 5 mg once a day (except Sunday), calcium and vitamin D two tablets in the morning, ibuprofen 200 mg three times a day when required, and co-codamol 8/500 two tablets, three times a day when required. After a thorough examination the patient is diagnosed as having a flare of rheumatoid arthritis. It is decided to review his DMARD therapy in view of the current poor control of his disease.

Questions

1. What initial therapy would you advise to treat Mr HP's immediate flare symptoms, rather than his underlying disease?
2. What DMARD therapy(s) would you now recommend for the patient? List at least two side effects for each drug discussed.
3. What long-term monitoring is required to identify potential toxicity for the medication you have recommended?

Answers

1. Treatment is multimodal and this will include bed rest, physiotherapy, hydrotherapy and drug treatment. The patient's current analgesics and anti-inflammatories are suboptimal. In the acute flare phase of rheumatoid arthritis, a patient will need appropriate doses of their simple analgesia. As an example, this patient may be prescribed co-codamol 30/500, two to be taken four times a day. The dose of ibuprofen is also low for use in an acute flare. Either this dose should be increased or the therapy changed, for example, to diclofenac 50 mg three times a day or celecoxib 200 mg twice daily. However, it is not known whether a COX-2 selective drug is appropriate for this patient. Both drugs should be prescribed regularly, as opposed to the present 'when required' prescription. Corticosteroids may also be used depending on the severity of the flare, either a short course of oral steroids (20–30 mg prednisolone) or intra-articular injection into the worst affected joints. Depot intramuscular steroids are occasionally

used if the flare involves numerous joints, especially the small joints of the hands and feet.

2. Ideally triple therapy would be used: sulfasalazine, oral, intramuscular or subcutaneous methotrexate and hydroxychloroquine. The side effects for these DMARDs include:

- *sulfasalazine*: nausea, reversible male infertility, rashes, marrow suppression, hepatitis
- *methotrexate*: unusual bruising, rash, fever, cough, shortness of breath, nausea, alopecia, stomatitis, hepatic fibrosis, liver toxicity, severe alveolitis, pneumonitis, marrow suppression
- *hydroxychloroquine*: gastrointestinal toxicity, tinnitus, retinopathy, blurred vision.

Alternatively you could recommend increasing the dose of oral methotrexate. The patient has had a previous response to methotrexate, and doses of up to 25 mg a week are efficacious. Other possible alternatives would include leflunomide, azathioprine or cyclophosphamide. The side effects for these DMARDs include:

- *leflunomide*: gastrointestinal disturbances, reversible alopecia, rash, hypertension, hepatitis
- *azathioprine*: infertility, malignancy, gastrointestinal disturbance, marrow suppression
- *cyclophosphamide*: infertility, malignancy, bladder toxicity.

3. The monitoring for triple therapy is set out below.

- *Methotrexate*: baseline liver function tests (LFTs) and full blood count (FBC) and urea and electrolytes (U&E), then FBC and LFTs twice weekly for 2 months, then monthly for 4 months, then 3 monthly thereafter.
- *Sulfasalazine*: baseline LFTS and FBC and U&E, then FBC and LFTs twice weekly for 3 months, then monthly for 3 months, then 3 monthly thereafter.
- *Hydroxychloroquine*: ophthalmological screening dependant on the treatment centre.
- *Leflunomide*: baseline FBC, U&E, LFT and blood pressure twice weekly for 2 months then monthly for 4 months followed by 3 monthly thereafter.
- *Azathioprine*: baseline FBC, U&E, LFT, twice weekly for 2 months, then monthly for 4 months then 3 monthly thereafter.

Case 53. 2

Mrs VB is a 65-year-old woman with a 4-year history of rheumatoid arthritis, who presents to her primary care doctor with mouth ulcers, general lethargy, a sore throat, raised temperature and general bruising. Her current medication includes methotrexate 15 mg once each week, folic acid 5 mg three times per week, diclofenac SR 75 mg twice daily and a recent course of trimethoprim 100 mg tablets twice daily for a urinary tract infection.

Questions

1. What is the side effect profile of methotrexate?
2. What is the probable cause of the symptoms described by Mrs VB?
3. What treatment options are available for the management of Mrs VB's symptoms?

Answers

1. Methotrexate is a dihydrofolate reductase inhibitor, which is increasingly being used as the first-line DMARD for the management of rheumatoid arthritis. It is generally well tolerated, especially at the low weekly doses employed in rheumatoid arthritis. The main side effects with methotrexate include gastrointestinal toxicity, bone marrow toxicity, liver toxicity and pulmonary toxicity. Gastrointestinal side effects include nausea, vomiting and diarrhoea. Haematological side effects include bone marrow suppression, particularly thrombocytopenia and neutropenia. Regular full blood count monitoring is required and patients should be advised to report any signs of infection, especially sore throat, to their doctor. Methotrexate can cause liver toxicity, especially cirrhosis. Regular liver function test monitoring is required. Pulmonary toxicity includes dyspnoea and pulmonary fibrosis or alveolitis. Patients should be advised to report any sudden shortness of breath to their doctor. Mouth ulcers, stomatitis, alopecia, rash and bruising can also be troublesome adverse effects.

2. The probable cause of the signs and symptoms described by Mrs VB is methotrexate toxicity. She describes the classic symptoms of this syndrome. Methotrexate toxicity is a serious and potentially fatal event and should be managed accordingly. There are a number of risk factors for toxicity and these include age, reduced renal function, high-dose therapy, concomitant antifolate drugs, concurrent NSAIDs, etc. Mrs VB has recently had a course of trimethoprim for a urinary tract infection. Trimethoprim is also an antifolate agent and concomitant therapy can increase the risk of methotrexate toxicity. NSAIDs can reduce renal perfusion, thereby reducing methotrexate excretion and hence increasing toxicity. In clinical practice this is rarely significant and most patients are maintained on their NSAID plus methotrexate. However, in a patient with reduced renal function this combination should be avoided. A common cause of methotrexate toxicity is inadvertent daily rather than weekly administration. Patients must be counselled as to the weekly regimen. Careful risk analysis should be undertaken, especially in elderly patients with the potential for confusion. Mrs VB's methotrexate toxicity is probably due to a multitude of factors, principally the antifolate trimethoprim, concomitant diclofenac and possibly reduced renal function secondary to her age.

3. The most effective therapy for methotrexate toxicity is calcium folinate (calcium leucovorin). This is used to diminish the toxicity and counteract the folate antagonist action of methotrexate. The dosage depends on the severity of the leucopenia. In mild-to-moderate toxicity it is given in a dose of 15 mg every 6 hours for 48–72 hours. In more severe cases up to 120 mg is usually given in individual doses over 12–24 hours by intramuscular injection, intravenous bolus or infusion. Measures to ensure prompt excretion of methotrexate are also important, and include alkalinization of urine to a pH greater than 7.0 and maintenance of increased urine output. In cases where leucopenia is severe, treatment with GM-CSF may be required. It can induce marked increases in peripheral blood neutrophil counts within 24 hours of administration. A subcutaneous dose of 500 000 units/kg/day may be given and should be continued until the neutrophil count is greater than 1.5×10^9/L. Topical agents such as anti-inflammatory mouthwashes (benzydamine), analgesic gels (choline salicylate), protective agents (carmellose) or corticosteroids (hydrocortisone lozenges, triamcinolone in oral paste) may all be useful in managing mouth ulcers and stomatitis.

Case 53.3

A 68-year-old man with inflammatory osteoarthritis, particularly of the knees, presents at a hospital rheumatology clinic. He complains of worsening pain and mobility despite regular intra-articular corticosteroids, analgesia and NSAIDs. His current therapy includes tramadol MR 100 mg twice daily, celecoxib 200 mg twice daily, paracetamol 1 g four times daily and fluoxetine 20 mg once daily. The visco-supplementation agent Synvisc is also prescribed.

Questions

1. What is visco-supplementation?
2. What is the place of visco-supplementation in the management of osteoarthritis and in which patients would you advise therapy?
3. What are the contraindications and adverse reactions associated with visco-supplementation therapies?
4. How might you monitor the effectiveness of this therapy?

Answers

1. In joints affected by osteoarthritis the synovial fluid's capacity to lubricate and absorb shock is reduced. These changes are partly due to the reduction in the size and concentration of hyaluronic acid molecules in the synovium. A new approach in the management of osteoarthritis of the knee is to inject hyaluronic acid or its derivatives into the joint. Hyaluronan is a polysaccharide composed of repeating disaccharide units of glucuronic acid and N-acetyl glucosamine. When these molecules are very long they make a highly viscoelastic solution that is lubricant at low shear and shock absorbing at high shear. When injected into a joint, this is known as visco-supplementation.
2. The published evidence suggests that intra-articular hyaluronic acid derivatives are better than placebo and in some cases comparable to NSAIDs in the management of pain on movement associated with osteoarthritis of the knee. A summary of the relevant trials concludes that although these products are expensive, and available published data supporting their effectiveness are limited, there may be situations in which they have a role. This is likely to be in a small number of patients who meet the following criteria: osteoarthritis of the knee, daily pain, failure of adequate doses of stepwise analgesia, failure of tramadol and/or NSAIDs, failure of an adequate trial of physiotherapy and either failure of two separate intra-articular injections of corticosteroids or intolerance or contraindication to corticosteroids (failure in this context is when pain relief is not achieved after 4 weeks of treatment). They may also be indicated if surgery is either not appropriate or contraindicated, including patients too young for surgery and those who failed the above measures. In practice, this is a large number of resistant patients with osteoarthritis.
3. Intra-articular hyaluronic acid derivatives should not be injected if there is venous or lymphatic stasis or into severely inflamed or infected joints. Transient redness, pain, warmth and swelling of the injected joint may occur in about 10–40% of patients treated. There have been a small number of reports of severe synovitis following injection of hyaluronic acid requiring intra-articular corticosteroids. There have also been anecdotal reports of pseudogout following injection. Hyaluronic acid derivatives should not be used if there is a large intra-articular effusion whilst some preparations should not be used in patients who are hypersensitive to bird proteins because they contain small amounts of avian protein. Anaphylactic-like reactions have been reported following intra-articular Hyalgan injections.
4. It is unclear which patients will respond to visco-supplementation. All patients should receive close follow-up to evaluate this. The Western Ontario and McMasters Universities (WOMAC) index is a useful measure for determining response. It is a patient-completed questionnaire which evaluates pain, stiffness and functionality. WOMAC is the standard outcome measure used in osteoarthritis of the hip and knee. It is well validated and accepted worldwide. Patients can be monitored using the WOMAC prior to treatment and at 3 months. Response is defined as a 10–20% reduction in the pain subscale of WOMAC, with the use of supplemental analgesia and a physician assessment of response.

Case 53.4

Mrs AH is a 58-year-old woman with a long history of severe rheumatoid arthritis. She presents to the hospital rheumatology clinic with severe pain in her left foot. On examination, three toes are found to be discoloured and appear ischaemic. A large ulcer is also found on the heel of the same foot. She is diagnosed as having rheumatoid vasculitis.

Questions

1. What is rheumatoid vasculitis and what is its aetiology?
2. What is the role of cyclophosphamide and methylprednisolone in the management of this patient?
3. What precautions should be taken with cyclophosphamide use?
4. What other treatment options are available for Mrs AH?

Answers

1. Rheumatoid vasculitis is a severe, often life-threatening condition that may present as a complication of rheumatoid arthritis. Severe inflammation of blood vessels occurs, commonly producing pain and ulcers in the extremities. Many organs may be affected, particularly the kidneys. The primary aetiology is immune complex deposition in blood vessels.
2. Cyclophosphamide and methylprednisolone have been used effectively in rheumatoid vasculitis for their potent immunosuppressive actions. Regimens do vary, but intravenous pulses every 3–6 weeks are often used. Methylprednisolone at a dose of 500 mg to 1 g over an hour or more (to prevent cardiac arrhythmia or ischaemia) gives a rapid and intense anti-inflammatory action as well as immunosuppressive activity. Once the condition improves, oral steroids may be considered. Such an improvement may be seen by monitoring laboratory indices such as ESR, renal function and urine protein content. Patients usually tolerate cyclophosphamide although prophylactic antiemetics should be given and the possibility of fertility suppression should be discussed with patients.
3. Prior to administration of cyclophosphamide, patients should have a full blood count, urea and electrolytes, and creatinine measured. A full medical examination should also be carried out to exclude intercurrent illness or evidence of infection. A high fluid intake of at least 2.5 L on the infusion day should be maintained to reduce the risk of haemorrhagic cystitis, possibly with the addition of intravenous fluids. Mesna may also be given to reduce the risk of haemorrhagic cystitis although there is little clinical evidence that it is needed with such moderate doses of cyclophosphamide. Extravasation of cyclophosphamide is unlikely to be serious if infusion is promptly discontinued, and staff should be familiar with the extravasation management procedure.
4. Administration of iloprost has been used in rheumatoid vasculitis to improve vasculitic ulcers and reduce peripheral ischaemia although it is unlicensed for use in this condition. Iloprost is a prostacyclin analogue, which is a potent vasodilator and inhibitor of platelet aggregation. It is given either as an intravenous infusion over 6–8 hours for 3–6 days or, in severe peripheral ischaemia, as a continuous 24-hour infusion for up to 5 days. Infusion rates are titrated according to patient response and tolerance. Pulse and blood pressure should be monitored regularly as hypotension can occur and it is therefore usual practice to withhold any medication that might potentiate this, e.g. nifedipine. Doses of 2–10 μg/h are usually employed.

REFERENCES

Alamanosa Y, Drosos A A 2005 Epidemiology of adult rheumatoid arthritis. Autoimmunity Reviews 4: 130-136

Aletaha D, Breedveld F C, Simolen J S et al 2005 The need for new classification criteria for rheumatoid arthritis. Arthritis and Rheumatism 52: 3333-3336

American College of Rheumatology Subcommittee on Osteoarthritis Guidelines 2000 Recommendations for the medical management of osteoarthritis of the hip and knee. Arthritis and Rheumatism 43: 1905-1915

Eccles M, Freemantle N, Mason J 1998 North of England Evidence Based Guideline Development Project: summary guideline for non-steroidal anti-inflammatory drugs versus basic analgesia in treating the pain of degenerative arthritis. British Medical Journal 317: 526-530

Henry D, Lim L L-Y, Garcia Rodriguez L A et al 1996 Variability in risk of gastrointestinal complications with individual anti-inflammatory drugs: results of a collaborative meta-analysis. British Medical Journal 312: 1563-1566

Keen H I, Emery P 2005 How should we manage early rheumatoid arthritis? From imaging to intervention. Current Opinion in Rheumatology 17: 280-285

Khurana R, Berney S M 2005 Clinical aspects of rheumatoid arthritis. Pathophysiology 12: 153-165

National Institute for Clinical Excellence 2001 Guidance on the use of cyclo-oxygenase (COX) II selective inhibitors, celecoxib, rofecoxib, meloxicam and etodolac for osteoarthritis and rheumatoid arthritis. Appraisal 27. National Institute for Clinical Excellence, London

National Institute for Clinical Excellence 2002 Guidance on the use of etanercept and infliximab for the treatment of rheumatoid arthritis. Appraisal 36. National Institute for Clinical Excellence, London

O'Dell J R 2002 Treating rheumatoid arthritis early: a window of opportunity? Arthritis and Rheumatism 46: 283-285

Richy, F Bruyere O, Ethgen O et al 2003 Structural and symptomatic efficacy of glucosamine and chondroitin in knee osteoarthritis: a comprehensive meta-analysis. Archives of Internal Medicine 163(13): 1514-1522

Weyand C M, Goronzy J J 1997 Pathogenesis of rheumatoid arthritis. Medical Clinics of North America 81: 29-55

FURTHER READING

Khurana R, Berney S M 2005 Clinical aspects of rheumatoid arthritis. Pathophysiology 12: 153-165

Lipsky P E, Van Der Heijde D M, St Clair E W et al 2000 Infliximab and methotrexate in the treatment of rheumatoid arthritis. New England Journal of Medicine 343 (22): 1594-1602

Maini R, St Clair E W, Breedveld F et al 1999 Infliximab (chimeric anti-tumour necrosis factor alpha monoclonal antibody) versus placebo in rheumatoid arthritis patients receiving concomitant methotrexate: a randomised phase III trial. ATTRACT Study Group. Lancet 354: 1932-1939

Symmons D 2005 The British Rheumatoid Outcome Study Group (BROSG) randomised controlled trial to compare the effectiveness and cost-effectiveness of aggressive versus symptomatic therapy in established rheumatoid arthritis. NHS Health Technology Assessment Vol. 9 No. 34. Available online at: www.ncchta.org

Weinblatt M E, Keystone E C, Furst D E et al 2003 Adalimumab, a fully human anti-tumour necrosis factor a monoclonal antibody, for treatment of rheumatoid arthritis in patients taking concomitant methotrexate. The ARMADA trial. Arthritis and Rheumatism 48(1): 35-45

USEFUL WEBSITES

Oxford pain internet site: www.jr2.ox.ac.uk/bandolier/booth/painpag/index2

Prodigy guidance on osteoarthritis and rheumatoid arthritis: www.prodigy.nhs.uk

Gout and hyperuricaemia

54

A. Alldred   T. Capstick

'Gout' is a term that represents a heterogeneous group of diseases caused by an inflammatory response to the formation of monosodium urate crystals which develop secondary to hyperuricaemia. The hyperuricaemia may be due to an increased rate of synthesis of the purine precursors of uric acid or to a decreased elimination of uric acid by the kidney, or both.

Hyperuricaemia is a biochemical condition, while gout is a clinical diagnosis. Prolonged hyperuricaemia is necessary but not sufficient for the development of gout.

Gout is characterized by recurrent episodes of acute arthritis due to deposits of monosodium urate in joints and cartilage. Formation of uric acid calculi in the kidneys (nephrolithiasis) may occur.

Epidemiology

The prevalence of gout in the UK is approximately 2.6 cases per 1000. However, in some populations, such as adult male Maoris in New Zealand, it is as high as 10 cases per 1000. In the UK about 10% of cases of gout are a secondary manifestation, with diuretics being the most frequent causative factor. Figures for the incidence of gout vary between populations, and its prevalence is known to change with environmental and dietary factors in the same population over a short period of time.

Gout is a condition that most frequently affects middle-aged men, with only approximately 5% of cases occurring in women. Most women with gout have a family history of the disease, although studies in men have failed to detect a significant genetic component. However, evidence suggests the epidemiology of gout is changing because as the population ages there is an increasing prevalence amongst elderly females. This may reflect an increasing life expectancy with chronic diseases such as diabetes, atherosclerosis and the drugs used to treat these conditions. The risk of acute gout occurring secondary to hyperuricaemia is approximately equal for both sexes but hyperuricaemia is many times more common in men. Over half of the patients diagnosed with gout will admit to regular alcohol consumption.

The incidence and prevalence of gout increase in association with the level of serum uric acid. The risk of developing gout rises from about 0.5% per annum in men with serum urate of 420 µmol/L to 5.5% per annum at a serum urate of 540 µmol/L (Nuki 1998). The epidemiology of gout is summarized in Table 54.1.

Aetiology

Gout is a metabolic disorder of purine metabolism of which uric acid is the end-product. The development of gout is primarily related to the degree and duration of the elevated uric acid or

Table 54.1 Epidemiology of gout

Peak age (years)	Males: 40–50; females >60
Sex distribution (M:F)	2–7:1
Prevalence rate (/1000)	Males: 5–28; females: 1–6
Annual incidence (/1000)	Males: 1–3; females: 0.2
Geography	Worldwide; regional differences may reflect environmental factors as well as racial predisposition
Genetic associations	Inherited enzyme abnormalities Inherited urate excretion
Environmental associations	Diet, drugs, toxins (e.g. lead)

hyperuricaemia. Concentrations of urate in synovial fluid correlate closely with serum levels. A rigid definition of hyperuricaemia is not possible, but in general terms the upper limit of normal is 450 μmol/L for men and 380 μmol/L for women.

Overproduction of uric acid

Overproduction of uric acid may result from excessive turnover of nucleoproteins (as, for example, in type 1 glycogen storage disease, neoplastic diseases and myeloproliferative disorders), excessive dietary purines, or excessive synthesis of uric acid due to rare enzyme mutation defects (e.g. Lesch–Nyhan syndrome). Diet plays a minor role in this condition and thus dietary restrictions, with the exception of limiting alcohol intake, have a small part to play.

Two-thirds of the urate formed each day are excreted by the kidneys and one-third is eliminated via the gastrointestinal tract.

Patients who overproduce urate are identified as those with a 24-hour urinary urate excretion in excess of 4400 μmol.

Underexcretion of uric acid

Underexcretion of uric acid, defined as a 24-hour urinary urate excretion less than 1500 μmol, results from a defect in renal excretion. This occurs in approximately 75% of patients with primary (idiopathic) gout. Uric acid is filtered at the glomerulus, and almost completely reabsorbed in the proximal tubule. Of the reabsorbed uric acid, 50% is secreted distal to the proximal tubular reabsorption site and approximately 75% of this secreted urate is reabsorbed. In the hyperuricaemic state, large loads are filtered and urate reabsorption increases to avoid the dumping of poorly soluble urate into the urinary tract. Tubular urate secretion is not influenced by serum urate concentrations, and it is probably the impaired urate secretion which is responsible for the hyperuricaemia.

Another cause of gouty arthritic attacks can be physical stress. Factors such as tight shoes, hill walking and hiking have been reported to cause acute attacks in the great toe. A history of joint trauma may subsequently be associated with attacks of gout.

Clinical manifestations

The natural history of gout has five stages:

- asymptomatic hyperuricaemia which is 10 times more common than gout
- acute gouty arthritis
- chronic gout
- chronic tophaceous gout: aggregations of urate crystals affecting articular, periarticular and non-articular cartilage (e.g. ears)
- gouty nephropathy which can cause tubulo-interstitial disease due to parenchymal crystal deposition, acute intratubular precipitation, resulting in acute renal failure, or urate stone formation.

Acute gout is traditionally considered monoarticular, with only one joint affected in 90% of acute attacks. The great toe is most frequently affected, with approximately 80% of patients having the initial attack in the first metatarsophalangeal joint of the great toe (podagra). The majority of patients will have podagra at some time during the course of the disease. Other joints frequently affected are small joints of the feet or ankles, the hands (distal interphalangeal joints), elbows and knees. The initial presentation of the disease may be polyarticular and low-grade inflammation may be present in many joints.

The patient with acute gouty arthritis complains of severe pain with hot, red, swollen and extremely tender joints. The weight of the bedclothes or the jar of a person walking on the floor is said to be agony to the sufferer, and weight bearing is impossible. The affected joint has overlying erythema and signs of marked synovitis. The patient may be pyrexial with a leucocytosis (total white cell count in excess of 11×10^9/L), elevated erythrocyte sedimentation rate (in excess of 15 mm/h) and elderly patients may be confused. Untreated attacks last days or weeks before subsiding spontaneously, and resolution may be accompanied by pruritus and desquamation of the overlying skin.

Chronic tophaceous gout is associated with the presence of tophi (deposits of monosodium urate crystals, typically in subcutaneous and periarticular areas) and renal disease. The proportion of patients who go on to develop chronic gout is not known. It is thought to be dependent on the number whose hyperuricaemia is not controlled. Patients have usually suffered with gout for at least 10 years before tophi develop. In time, with treatment, the tophi disappear but renal function will probably remain static.

Premature atherosclerosis, cardiovascular disease and nephropathy are associated with gout but whether these are a consequence of hyperuricaemia remains unclear. In asymptomatic individuals gout, hypertension and coronary artery disease occur more commonly than in matched control groups. The half-lives of platelets in patients with gout are much shortened and thus platelet adhesiveness is increased. Studies have suggested that hyperuricaemia may be an independent risk factor for hypertension and atherosclerotic disease, while an association between hyperuricaemia and hypertriglyceridaemia has also been proposed. Obesity and alcohol excess are common factors rather than a direct causal mechanism for hyperuricaemia.

Gouty nephropathy is a form of chronic interstitial nephritis that occurs typically in patients who have had hyperuricaemia for many years. This is associated with hyperexcretion of urate and urine hyperacidity. Crystals are deposited around the renal tubules and incite an inflammatory response. The renal medulla becomes infiltrated with mononuclear cells and fibrosis occurs. Clinically this is manifested by proteinuria and/or renal impairment.

Events provoking acute gouty arthritis

Events provoking acute gouty arthritis are listed in Table 54.2. Diuretics are most frequently implicated.

These patients are characterized by the presence of tophi which often develop in Heberden's nodes (gelatinous cysts or bony outgrowths on the dorsal aspects of the distal interphalangeal joints). Patients affected rarely have acute attacks, and the condition usually responds to withdrawal of the diuretic. If the diuretic is essential, allopurinol may be used to lower uric acid levels.

Radiotherapy and chemotherapy in patients with leukaemias and lymphomas may lead to hyperuricaemia. Uric acid nephropathy may occur in association with acute increases in uric acid

Table 54.2 Events provoking acute gouty arthritis

- Trauma
- Unusual physical exercise
- Surgery
- Severe systemic illness
- Severe dieting
- Dietary excess
- Alcohol
- Drugs:
  Diuretics
  Initiation of uricosuric or allopurinol therapy
  Initiation of B$_{12}$ in pernicious anaemia
  Following drug allergy
  Cytotoxic drug therapy

production, and this is the most common cause of acute renal failure in patients with leukaemia. This can be treated prophylactically with allopurinol commencing 3 days before therapy and continuing for the duration of remission-inducing chemotherapy. Other measures adopted to prevent urate nephropathy in this situation include alkalinization of the urine and vigorous fluid intake.

Investigations

The diagnosis of acute gout can only be made through examination of synovial fluid aspirated from the inflamed joint. Monosodium urate crystals are needle shaped and are negatively birefringent under a polarizing microscope. Aspirated synovial fluid also contains large numbers of polymorphonuclear leucocytes.

Sudden onset of acute inflammatory monoarthritis, particularly in the foot or ankle, should always raise the suspicion of gout; however, in 10% of patients acute gouty arthritis is polyarticular.

Hyperuricaemia alone is not diagnostic of gout as many hyperuricaemic patients never develop symptomatic gout and some patients with acute gout have a normal serum uric acid concentration. Attacks of gout tend to be precipitated by changes in uric acid concentration, and the absolute level may have fallen back to normal during an attack. The diagnosis of gout is thus confirmed only by microscopic examination of synovial fluid aspirated from the affected joint.

Diagnosis

The differential diagnosis in acute gouty arthritis must include septic arthritis. Patients with gout commonly present with acute swelling and tenderness of the joint with a fever, raised plasma viscosity and leucocytosis, with no previous history of arthritis. Patients with joint sepsis are usually more ill and have other systemic signs of infection such as a swinging fever and severe

malaise. Large joints are most frequently infected, and the joint is hot, tender and swollen with effusion and marked limitation of movement.

Treatment

Patient education and an understanding of the basis for therapy are critical for successful management of gout. A fundamental part of the management strategy is avoidance of factors that may trigger an attack.

Gout is often associated with obesity, hypertriglyceridaemia, hypertension and high alcohol intake. A subgroup of patients, usually elderly women, taking diuretics has also been recognized.

The aims of treatment are to relieve the pain and inflammation of an acute attack; to terminate the attack as quickly as possible; to prevent the exacerbation of further attacks and so prevent long-term joint and associated organ damage (e.g. renal disease); and to consider long-term hypouricaemic therapy. The treatment goals are described in Table 54.3.

The management is often conveniently split into managing the acute attack (Table 54.4) and managing hyperuricaemia in patients with chronic gouty arthritis (Table 54.5). Therefore there are essentially three stages in the treatment of the disease:

- treating the acute attack
- reducing uric acid levels to prevent deposition of urate crystals into tissues, especially joints
- prophylactic treatment with hypouricaemic therapy.

Table 54.3 Treatment goals in the management of gout

Relieve pain and inflammation	Prevent joint damage
Terminate acute attack	Reduce the risk of uric acid calculi
Prevent exacerbation of further attacks	Prevent organ damage, e.g. renal involvement
Reduce serum urate levels in symptomatic patients	Reduce the formation of tophi

Table 54.4 Treatment of acute gout

Confirm diagnosis	If one or two joints affected, consider intra-articular steroids
Initial treatment with full-dose NSAIDs, early in the attack, unless contraindicated	If severe disease or NSAIDs/colchicine are not tolerated, consider systemic steroids
Consider oral colchicine if NSAIDs not appropriate. Use within 24–48 h of acute attack	Do not treat hyperuricaemia in an acute attack
Use colchicine cautiously because of toxicity and monitor response	

Table 54.5 Treatment of chronic gout

Start urate-lowering drugs in patients who have two or more attacks per year	Consider concomitant colchicine until serum urate levels have been lowered and no acute attacks have recurred (6–12 months)
Urate-lowering drugs should not be started during an acute attack	Monitor serum urate levels every 3–6 months and adjust therapy according to levels in symptomatic patients
Allopurinol is the urate-lowering drug of choice in the majority of patients	
Use uricosuric drugs in patients intolerant of/ allergic to allopurinol and in underexcreters with normal renal function	

Acute attacks

Rest and prompt treatment with full doses of non-steroidal anti-inflammatory drugs (NSAIDs) are first-line management in acute attacks. Aspirin and its derivative, choline salicylate benorilate, should be avoided as these agents compete with uric acid for excretion and can worsen an acute attack. NSAIDs will relieve pain and inflammation and they can abort an attack if commenced early. An alternative, but second choice, agent is colchicine. Deciding whether to choose an NSAID or colchicine in the management of acute gout depends on other patient factors. There are no controlled studies comparing colchicine with NSAIDs in the management of gout. Patients with cardiovascular disease including hypertension, those receiving diuretics in cardiac failure, those with gastrointestinal toxicity, bleeding diathesis or renal impairment should be treated with colchicine.

Agents that decrease the serum uric acid level, e.g. allopurinol, or uricosuric agents, e.g. probenecid and sulfinpyrazone, should not be used in an acute attack. Patients generally have been hyperuricaemic for several years, and there is no need to treat the hyperuricaemia immediately. In addition, agents that decrease serum uric acid concentrations may cause mobilization of uric acid stores as the serum level falls. This movement of uric acid may prolong the acute attack or precipitate another attack of gouty arthritis. However, if the patient is already stabilized on allopurinol at the onset of the acute attack, it should be continued.

Non-steroidal anti-inflammatory drugs

NSAIDs are effective first-line therapy for otherwise healthy patients presenting with acute gout. The most important factor determining therapeutic success is not the NSAID chosen but how soon NSAID therapy is initiated. NSAIDs should be administered in full doses for the first 24–48 hours or until the pain has settled. Lower doses should be continued until all symptoms and signs have resolved, usually after 7–10 days. NSAIDs usually take between 24 and 48 hours to work, although

complete relief of gouty signs and symptoms is usually seen after 5 days of treatment. Patients known to have gout should carry a supply of NSAIDs to treat the acute attack as soon as the first symptom appears. Indometacin is commonly prescribed for an acute attack of gouty arthritis, initially at a dose of 75–100 mg twice a day. This dose should be reduced after 5 days as the acute attack settles.

Adverse effects of indometacin include headaches, mental changes and gastrointestinal upset, although these resolve with decreasing dose. Other NSAIDs commonly used include: naproxen 750 mg to start followed by 250 mg three times a day; piroxicam 40 mg per day to start followed by 10–20 mg per day; and diclofenac 100 mg to start, then 50 mg three times a day for 48 hours, then 50 mg twice daily for 8 days.

COX-2 inhibitors

Etoricoxib is the only licensed coxib for the management of acute gout. It is an effective but comparatively expensive agent with a role in some patients, particularly those with gastrointestinal intolerance to other NSAIDs. COX-2 inhibitors have a lower risk of serious upper gastrointestinal side effects when compared to non-selective NSAIDs. However, similar risk is associated with symptomatic gastrointestinal events including uncomplicated gastric or duodenal ulcers, dyspepsia, abdominal pain, epigastric discomfort, nausea and heartburn. The COX-2 inhibitors have also been shown to increase the risk of thrombotic events, e.g. myocardial infarction and stroke, compared with placebo and some other NSAIDs. Therefore patients with established coronary heart disease, cerebrovascular disease or moderate-to-severe heart failure should not be prescribed these drugs, and they should be used with caution in patients with risk factors for heart disease. In addition, for all patients, the balance of gastrointestinal and cardiovascular risk should be considered before prescribing a COX-2 inhibitor. Evidence also indicates that etoricoxib, particularly at high doses, elevates blood pressure. As a consequence, it should not be prescribed in individuals with poorly controlled hypertension. In fact, blood pressure monitoring is advised for all patients taking etoricoxib.

Colchicine

Colchicine is an effective and specific treatment for gout, but less favoured than NSAIDs because of its slow onset of action and high incidence of side effects.

Oral colchicine has historically been first-line treatment for acute gout, but only one double-blind placebo-controlled trial of oral colchicine has been reported (Ahem et al 1987). This trial showed that two-thirds of patients treated with colchicine improved within 48 hours of commencement of therapy compared with only one-third of those receiving placebo.

For oral colchicine to be effective, it must be administered as quickly as possible after the onset of symptoms as it becomes less effective over time. Traditionally, an initial dose of 1 mg has been used followed by 0.5 mg every 2–3 hours during the acute attack until there is relief of joint pain, or the patient develops gastrointestinal symptoms or has received a maximum dose of 6 mg. However, a lower dose of 0.5 mg every 8 hours is suggested to reduce the risk of toxicity, especially in the elderly and patients with renal impairment (Morris et al 2003).

The titration of the dose between therapeutic response and gastrointestinal toxicity is difficult to achieve as the therapeutic and toxic doses are close. Deaths have occurred in patients who have received as little as 5 mg of colchicine. The therapeutic response to colchicine usually commences after about 6 hours, with pain relief after about 12 hours and resolution of pain, redness and swelling in 75% of patients after 48–72 hours. Colchicine thus has some diagnostic value. A course of colchicine should not be repeated within 3 days to prevent toxic reactions from occurring.

Adverse effects of colchicine include severe nausea and vomiting, diarrhoea and abdominal pain. These affect 80% of patients who have taken a therapeutic oral dose. Dehydration may be a major complication of therapy. Other side effects include seizure disorders, respiratory depression, hepatic and muscle necrosis, renal damage, fever, granulocytopenia, aplastic anaemia, disseminated intravascular coagulation and alopecia. Many of the serious side effects occur in patients with hepatic or renal dysfunction. The dose of colchicine should be reduced by 50% in patients with a creatinine clearance less than 10 mL/min.

Intravenous colchicine is no longer licensed for use because it has been associated with severe toxicity, such as bone marrow suppression, and was implicated in 20 deaths. However, a review of the published experience with intravenous colchicine suggested that the toxicity was caused by inappropriate use of the drug and usually involved dosage errors (Graham & Robert 1983, Wallace & Singer 1988).

Distribution of colchicine occurs rapidly, and after a single dose only 10% is excreted within the first 24 hours. Colchicine can still be detected in polymorphonuclear leucocytes 10 days after a single dose, implying a half-life of approximately 30 hours. The metabolism and excretion of colchicine are impaired in renal and hepatic disease.

It would be reasonable to give the patient one or two doses of opioid analgesic (e.g. morphine 10 mg) while awaiting the analgesic effect of NSAIDs or colchicine.

Steroids

An alternative strategy to NSAIDs or colchicine is to use intra-articular steroids. These can provide quick relief when only one or two joints are involved. However, the differential diagnosis between septic arthritis and acute gout must be certain as intra-articular steroids will exacerbate infection. Patients with a suboptimal response to NSAIDs may benefit from the administration of intra-articular steroid.

Systemic steroids can also be used to treat acute gout. In certain patients, such as those with severe or polyarticular attacks or those with renal disease or heart failure which may preclude NSAIDs or colchicine, prednisolone 20–40 mg per day initially may be useful. The recommended duration of therapy has been from 1 to 3 weeks. These agents usually take 12 hours to work (Gray et al 1981). Alternatively, intravenous methylprednisolone 50–150 mg daily or intramuscular triamcinolone 40–100 mg daily may be administered and reduced over 5 days.

Prophylactic control of symptomatic hyperuricaemia

Long-term control of hyperuricaemia is important to prevent acute attacks, chronic tophaceous gout, renal involvement and production of uric acid stones. However, the evidence to determine when urate-lowering drugs should be started is conflicting and controversial. Initial attacks of gout are usually infrequent and self-limiting and therefore long-term therapy is often not indicated. It has been advocated that treatment should only be started in patients who experience more than four episodes per year, whilst others suggest commencing patients who have only had one recurrent attack per year.

Expert consensus opinion suggests that long-term hypouricaemic agents should be considered for patients who suffer two or more gouty attacks per year and that urate-lowering drugs should not be started during an acute attack.

Allopurinol

Allopurinol is the hypouricaemic agent of choice in the management of chronic gout. This is effective for patients who overproduce or underexcrete urate. As well as controlling symptoms, it may protect renal function, especially in patients with familial disease. In patients under 30 years not taking diuretics, specialist advice should be sought to exclude metabolic defects before commencing treatment with allopurinol.

Patients with chronic tophaceous gout may benefit from resolution of tophi through prolonged treatment with allopurinol. Established tophi usually take approximately 6 months before they start to decline in size.

Allopurinol reduces uric acid production by inhibiting the enzyme xanthine oxidase. Allopurinol is not active but 60–70% undergoes hepatic conversion to an active metabolite, oxipurinol. The half-life of allopurinol is approximately 2 hours. Oxipurinol is excreted renally together with allopurinol. Oxipurinol undergoes net reabsorption in the renal tubule, as does urate itself. Therefore oxipurinol may accumulate in patients with renal failure. It will also accumulate in patients receiving thiazide diuretics where volume contraction and hypovolaemia may occur. Net reabsorption is also enhanced in states of volume contraction. In patients with normal renal function, the half-life of oxipurinol is 12–30 hours.

Allopurinol is generally well tolerated. However, many of the common adverse effects, especially pruritic maculopapular rash, affect up to 2% of patients and relate to inappropriate dosage in patients with renal impairment. Therefore renal function should be checked before allopurinol is started. Simple guidelines for allopurinol dosage in renal impairment have been published (Peterson et al 1990), and recommendations for dosing according to creatinine clearance have been made (Table 54.6).

A study of 66 patients taking allopurinol demonstrated that 35% were taking inappropriately high dosage with respect to recommendations on renal impairment (Singer & Wallace 1986).

In patients with normal renal function, the initial allopurinol dose should not exceed 300 mg in 24 hours. In practice, most patients are started on 100 mg daily with the dose increased every 3–4 weeks, if necessary, in order to produce a steady decrease in

Table 54.6 Sustained maintenance dose of allopurinol for patients with diminished renal function

Creatinine clearance (mL/min)	Allopurinol dose
0	100 mg thrice weekly
10	100 mg alternate days
20	100 mg daily
40	150 mg daily
60	200 mg daily
>100	300 mg daily

serum urate levels. The usual maintenance dose is 100–600 mg daily and a dose of 300 mg daily reduces serum urate to normal in approximately 85% of patients (Emmerson 1996). A decrease in serum urate levels between 274 and 393 μmol/L can produce a 30% reduction in the recurrence rate of acute gouty arthritis.

A response to allopurinol, reflected by a decrease in serum urate concentration, is seen about 2 days after starting therapy and is maximal after 7–10 days (Wood 1999). The serum urate concentration should be checked after 2–3 weeks to confirm a fall in levels.

In 3–5% of patients allopurinol causes a range of side effects which usually manifest as hypersensitivity reactions. Allopurinol hypersensitivity syndrome has been reported in 0.4% of patients and may present as symptoms of rash, fever, worsening renal insufficiency and vasculitis. There is a mortality rate of approximately 25% in patients with this syndrome. It is more common in elderly patients with renal insufficiency who are taking an inappropriately high daily dose with concomitant thiazide diuretic. This toxic syndrome most commonly occurs within the first 2 months of treatment although late reactions have been reported. Skin eruptions are the most common effects, but others include hepatotoxicity, acute interstitial nephritis and fever. These hypersensitivity reactions subside when treatment is discontinued. However, if treatment continues severe exfoliative dermatitis, various haematological abnormalities, hepatomegaly, jaundice, hepatic necrosis and renal impairment may occur.

Patients who have had minor hypersensitivity rashes may undergo an allopurinol desensitization regimen. The dose of allopurinol is gradually increased over a period of 3–4 weeks (Gillott et al 1999, McDonald et al 1988, Northridge & Almack 1986). This programme should not be used in patients who have had toxic epidermal necrolysis or drug-induced vasculitis (Emmerson 1996).

Allopurinol enhances the toxicity of cytotoxic drugs metabolized by xanthine oxidase. The doses of mercaptopurine and azathioprine should be reduced by 50% during concurrent allopurinol therapy. In addition, allopurinol enhances the bone marrow toxicity of cyclophosphamide.

As a sudden increase or decrease in serum uric acid levels may precipitate or prolong an acute gouty attack, allopurinol should not be commenced until an attack has subsided. The risk of

inducing an acute attack can be reduced by co-administration of an NSAID or colchicine (1.5 mg daily) for the first 3 months of chronic therapy. When prophylactic colchicine is used in patients with renal impairment (less than 50 mL/min), a full blood count and creatine kinase are checked at least once because of the risk of colchicine-related myopathy and myelosuppression.

Serum urate levels will fall within 2 days of the initiation of allopurinol, but maximal reduction will take 7–10 days.

Azapropazone

Although the exact mechanism of action is unknown, azapropazone, an NSAID, lowers serum urate levels. However, the use of azapropazone is restricted to acute gout only when other NSAIDs have been tried and failed. It is contraindicated in patients with a history of peptic ulceration, moderate-to-severe renal impairment, and the elderly with mild renal impairment. A maximum dose of 1.8 g in divided doses may be given until symptoms subside, followed by 1.2 g/day in divided doses until symptoms resolve. Adequate fluid intake must be ensured throughout treatment. In mild renal impairment or the elderly, 1.8 g in divided doses can be given for 24 hours, followed by 1.2 g daily then reduced as soon as possible to a maximum of 600 mg daily in divided doses.

Febuxostat

Febuxostat is a novel, oral, non-purine xanthine oxidase inhibitor currently being developed for hyperuricaemia associated with gout. A phase III 52-week randomized controlled trial comparing the safety and efficacy of febuxostat with allopurinol has demonstrated that more patients on febuxostat achieved a serum urate level below 360 μmol/L. However, there was no significant difference in the incidence of gout flares or reduction in tophus area between the two therapies. The incidence of adverse events was also similar (Becker et al 2005).

Uricosuric agents

Most patients with symptomatic hyperuricaemia underexcrete uric acid, and can be managed with uricosuric agents.

Uricosuric agents such as probenecid (500 mg to 1 g twice daily) and sulfinpyrazone (100 mg three or four times a day) offer an alternative to allopurinol. However, the availability of these drugs must be considered as probenecid has been discontinued in the UK and is only available on a named patient basis as an unlicensed product.

These agents should be avoided in patients with urate nephropathy and those who overproduce uric acid. They are ineffective in patients with poor renal function (creatinine clearance of less than 20–30 mL/min).

Probenecid is well absorbed orally with a serum half-life of 6–12 hours. Therapy should be initiated with a dose of 250 mg twice daily, increased to 500 mg twice daily after 2 weeks, with a further increase up to 2 g daily if required. In addition to prophylactic therapy against an acute attack using an NSAID or colchicine for 3 months, an initial low dose of uricosuric agent also prevents precipitation of an acute attack. Use of a uricosuric agent also decreases the risk of kidney stone formation. Patients should be advised to maintain a high fluid intake of at least 2 L per day to minimize the risk of stone formation.

Approximately 5–10% of patients receiving probenecid long term suffer nausea, heartburn, flatulence or constipation. A mild pruritic rash, drug fever and renal disturbances can also occur. Its major limiting factor is a lack of efficacy due to poor compliance, patients taking concurrent low-dose aspirin or renal insufficiency.

The serum level of probenecid is elevated by concomitant indometacin, whilst high-dose aspirin inhibits the uricosuric actions of probenecid and sulfinpyrazone. Other common drug interactions are listed in Table 54.7. The pharmacokinetic profiles of drugs used in the management of gout are presented in Table 54.8.

Benzbromarone

This unlicensed agent may be used at 100 mg daily, imported on a named patient basis, for patients with moderate renal impairment when other uricosuric agents are ineffective or allopurinol is precluded because of hypersensitivity. It is particularly useful as its uricosuric activity is maintained in patients with moderate renal impairment. However, as benzbromarone has been linked to severe hepatotoxicity its use is strictly monitored and controlled by the MHRA.

Table 54.7 Common drug interactions associated with therapy for gout and hyperuricaemia

Interacting drug	Affected drug	Effect
Allopurinol	Azathioprine	Increased levels of azathioprine
Allopurinol	Mercaptopurine	Increased levels of mercaptopurine
Allopurinol	Anticoagulants	Enhanced anticoagulant effect
Aspirin (high dose)	Uricosurics	Decreased hypouricaemic effect
Probenecid	Indometacin	Increased indometacin levels
Probenecid	Ketoprofen	Increased ketoprofen levels
Probenecid	Naproxen	Increased naproxen levels
Probenecid	Methotrexate	Increased methotrexate levels
Probenecid	Zidovudine	Increased zidovudine levels
Probenecid	Cephalosporins	Increased cephalosporin levels
Probenecid	Dapsone	Increased dapsone levels
Probenecid	Aspirin	Increased aspirin levels
Sulfinpyrazone	Anticoagulants	Enhanced anticoagulant effect

Table 54.8 Pharmacokinetic parameters for drugs used in the management of gout

Agent	$t_{1/2}$ (h)	t_{max} (h)	V_d (L/kg)	Protein binding	Clearance, hepatic (L/h)
Allopurinol	1–3[a]	2–6	–	0–4.5	46
Colchicine	20	2	1–2	31	36
Probenecid	4–12[b]	4	0.12–0.18	85–95	1.4
Sulfinpyrazone	1–2	3	0.06	98–99	1.4

[a] Active metabolite 12–30 h.
[b] 3–8 h (0.5 g); 6–12 h (2 g).

Prophylactic treatment of asymptomatic hyperuricaemia

It is unnecessary and excessive to treat all patients with hyperuricaemia with urate-lowering drugs although individuals with high serum uric acid levels are more likely to develop gout. The risk of hyperuricaemia causing renal disease is controversial although the consensus appears to be that hyperuricaemia alone does not have a deleterious effect on renal function. The presence of hyperuricaemia does seem to be a risk factor for development of cardiovascular disease although the evidence is not sufficiently strong at the moment for prophylactic therapy to be considered necessary. Obese patients (BMI greater than 28 kg/m^2) should lose weight gradually and their blood pressure and renal function should be monitored annually.

Drug-induced gout

Hyperuricaemia and gout occur with diuretics, especially thiazides. Where possible, an alternative agent should be used (e.g. vasodilator for hypertension) but where this is not possible, allopurinol should be used to lower urate levels. Other drugs that reduce renal urate excretion include low-dose aspirin and alcohol. Ciclosporin-induced hyperuricaemia and gout has been reported, especially in men, after an average of 24 months. The condition does not seem to be related to serum ciclosporin concentrations. Acute gout associated with omeprazole has also been reported.

Other drugs may interfere with renal excretion of uric acid, including ethambutol, pyrazinamide, niacin and didanosine (Agudelo & Wise 1998).

Radiotherapy and chemotherapy in patients with neoplastic disorders can cause hyperuricaemia. This can be treated prophylactically with allopurinol, commencing 3 days before therapy.

Patient care

Patients with gout should be advised about factors that may contribute to hyperuricaemia, such as fasting, obesity and alcohol excess. If these are avoided or corrected, drug treatment may not be needed. Asymptomatic hyperuricaemia need not be treated, but renal function can be checked to ensure that it is not deteriorating.

Patients at risk of recurrent gouty attacks should receive a supply of NSAIDs. They must be informed to start treatment at the first signs of an attack. In most patients this should abort the attack. Patients must be told the correct manner and dose in which NSAIDs should be used, the potential side effects and the action to take if side effects occur. Patients should be advised to avoid aspirin and use paracetamol for analgesia.

Patients treated with allopurinol should understand the need to continue single daily treatment in the absence of any symptomatic response. They must be warned of potential side effects and asked to report any adverse skin reactions.

The need to maintain a good fluid intake to reduce the risk of renal calculus formation should be explained to all patients receiving uricosuric agents. Urine flow of at least 2 L per day is required.

A therapeutic algorithm for the management of gout is presented in Figure 54.1. Common therapeutic problems are listed in Table 54.9.

Lifestyle choices

Gout has long been thought to be partly caused by different lifestyle choices including diet, alcohol intake and obesity. A 12-year, longitudinal study of 47 150 male healthcare professionals with no baseline history of gout has recently clarified a number of these issues. High levels of meat (beef, pork or lamb) and seafood consumption were associated with a 41% and 51% higher risk of gout, respectively. In contrast, high consumption of low-fat dairy products was associated with a 44% lower risk of gout (Choi et al 2004a). Alcohol intake was strongly associated with an increased risk of gout, with beer having a higher risk than spirits. Moderate wine drinking was not associated with an increased risk of gout (Choi et al 2004b).

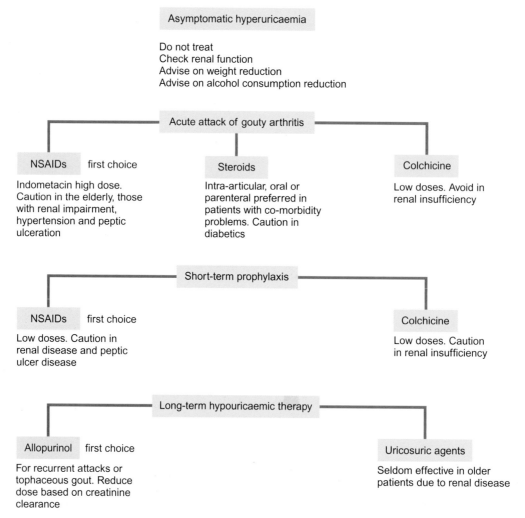

Figure 54.1 Algorithm for the management of gout.

Table 54.9 Common therapeutic problems in the treatment of gout

Problem	Possible solution
Treatment of acute attacks and short-term prophylaxis	
Elderly patients	These patients may not tolerate NSAIDs. Colchicine in low doses or corticosteroids are an option, but care with co-morbidity (see below)
Patients with renal failure	Avoid NSAIDs
Patients with heart failure	Use colchicine in low doses and with caution. Corticosteroids may be an option, but use with care in diabetic patients
Patients with a history of gastrointestinal problems	NSAID with a gastroprotective agent such as proton pump inhibitor or misoprostol. Consider colchicine
Long-term prophylaxis	
Elderly patients	Uricosuric agents are rarely effective in the elderly due to reduced renal function
Patients with renal failure	Uricosuric agents are not effective. Allopurinol dosage should be reduced
Recurrent attacks	Allopurinol dosage should be reduced if creatinine clearance is reduced

Obesity conferred an increased risk of gout and men with a BMI of 30–34.9 had three times the risk of gout than those with a BMI of 21–22.9. Hypertension and diuretic use both conferred an increased relative risk of gout of 2.31 and 1.77, respectively (Choi et al 2005).

CASE STUDIES

Case 54.1

Mr MG is 75 years old and weighs 95 kg. He presents with severe pain and swelling in his metacarpophalangeal joints. On examination he has hard nodules on his right elbow and right pinna. He has a past medical history of type 2 diabetes mellitus, hypertension, hyperlipidaemia and congestive heart failure. His current medication includes metformin 500 mg twice daily, perindopril 4 mg daily, amlodipine 10 mg daily, furosemide 40 mg daily, aspirin 75 mg daily and simvastatin 40 mg daily. He is a non-smoker and has an alcohol intake of 30 units per week. His blood pressure on admission is 160/95 mmHg, serum creatinine 190 μmol/L (62–133 μmol/L) and serum urate 675 μmol/L (140–380 μmol/L). A diagnosis of acute gout is made.

Questions

1. What factors predispose this patient to gout?
2. What options are available for the initial treatment of the acute gouty attack, and which would you recommend for this patient?
3. What advice would you give regarding the correction of hyperuricaemia?

Answers

1. Mr MG has gout which may be related to both overproduction and underexcretion of uric acid. He has hyperuricaemia and mild renal impairment (creatinine clearance 46 mL/min). The male:female incidence of gout is 2–7:1 and obesity is strongly associated with hyperuricaemia, reflecting excess dietary intake. Diuretic drugs, including both thiazides and loop diuretics, have been implicated in causing hyperuricaemia; furosemide causes hyperuricaemia in about 40% of men, and less frequently in women. Elderly women are, however, more likely to experience diuretic-induced tophaceous gout, but less likely to present with acute gout attacks than men. The mechanism is related to extracellular fluid contraction, whilst thiazides may also decrease uric acid excretion. Diuretic-induced hyperuricaemia is usually asymptomatic unless there is a family history of gout. Diuretic-induced gout may present as classic acute synovitis but sometimes appears as a generalized arthritis which can be misdiagnosed as osteoarthritis or rheumatoid arthritis. Mr MG also has a history of hypertension, hyperlipidaemia, diabetes and an excess alcohol intake, which can all predispose patients to gout.

2. The initial goal of treatment is to relieve the pain and inflammation of acute gout. Commonly used drugs include colchicine, NSAIDs and intra-articular steroids. Allopurinol or uricosuric agents should not be started at this stage. Lowering of urate levels is not urgent and the patient is likely to have been hyperuricaemic for some time. These agents cause mobilization of uric acid stores which may prolong or precipitate an acute attack. However, if the patient is already taking an antihyperuricaemic agent, it should be continued at the same dose.

    NSAIDs are effective in relieving symptoms and have a quicker onset of action than colchicine (2 hours compared to 6 hours). They are effective if used in high dosage for 1–3 days then reduced and continued for a further 7–10 days. However, NSAIDs may aggravate renal impairment and hypertension, and elderly patients are at a higher risk of gastrointestinal adverse drug reactions.

    Etoricoxib is the only COX-2 selective inhibitor licensed for the treatment of acute gout, with an efficacy similar to that of indometacin. However, etoricoxib may also aggravate renal impairment and elderly patients are at a higher risk of gastrointestinal adverse drug reactions. Etoricoxib is also contraindicated in patients with uncontrolled hypertension and so would not be suitable for Mr MG.

    Colchicine is effective for acute gout, commencing with 1 mg initially followed by 500 μg every 3 hours until pain is reduced or side effects occur or until a maximum dose of 6 mg is reached. The potential problems in this patient include gastrointestinal toxicity, as approximately 80% of patients are affected by vomiting, diarrhoea and abdominal pain. The dose should be reduced if renal function deteriorates to a creatinine clearance less than 10 mL/min.

    Intra-articular steroids are effective and work within 12–24 hours, but the differential diagnosis of joint infection must be made carefully. Intra-articular steroids are safe in renal impairment.

    Systemic steroids (e.g. prednisolone 20–40 mg daily for 1–3 weeks) may also be used in certain patients, such as those with severe polyarticular attacks or those with renal disease or heart failure which may preclude the use of NSAIDs or colchicine. These agents usually take 12 hours to work.

On balance, the most appropriate treatment would be to start colchicine: 1 mg initially, then 500 μg every 2–3 hours to a maximum cumulative dose of 6 mg.

3. Mr MG should be encouraged to reduce his alcohol intake. He should be encouraged to consider a low-fat diet, with less meat, in order to lose weight and reduce his risk of subsequent attacks of gout. These dietary modifications may also help reduce serum urate levels.

The administration of aspirin 300 mg, or more, can lead to elevation of serum urate levels, by inhibition of tubular secretion, and thus predispose patients to acute attacks of gout. In contrast, high-dose salicylate therapy acts in a similar manner to the uricosuric agents by inhibiting tubular reabsorption of urate, leading to an increased excretion and a fall in serum levels. Low-dose aspirin causes minimal interference with uric acid excretion and so treatment should continue.

The feasibility of discontinuing the diuretic or changing to bumetanide should be considered.

Treatment with antihyperuricaemic drugs is usually considered for recurrent gouty attacks, with radiological evidence of joint damage, tophaceous deposits or nephrolithiasis. This patient exhibits signs of chronic tophaceous gout, and so treatment with antihyperuricaemic drugs is justified but should not be commenced until the acute attack has settled completely. The treatment of choice in this patient is allopurinol. This will inhibit xanthine oxidase enzyme required for uric acid production and therefore is a logical choice for overproducers. Allopurinol will reduce serum urate levels after 2 days and the levels should be monitored after 2–3 weeks. In patients with renal impairment the dose should be reduced, and a suitable dose in this patient is 150 mg daily.

Since allopurinol may precipitate an acute attack of gout, the patient should continue on colchicine at a prophylactic dose of 500 μg twice daily to minimize the risk of acute attack. This should be continued for 1 month after correction of urate level. Mr MG is also taking simvastatin. Therefore he should be warned about the small number of case reports describing acute myopathy 10–20 days after starting colchicine in patients who have taken HMG CoA reductase inhibitors for several years (including simvastatin, pravastatin and fluvastatin). The mechanism of this interaction is not well understood and it appears to be rare, and so Mr MG should continue on both drugs and be asked to report any signs of myopathy.

Probenecid and sulfinpyrazone increase uric acid excretion, but are not suitable where overproduction is the major cause of hyperuricaemia. These agents are ineffective where the creatinine clearance is less than 50 mL/min and a high fluid intake is needed to reduce the risk of renal stone formation. In this patient these agents may be ineffective due to renal impairment. Sulfinpyrazone is also contraindicated since it may worsen heart failure by causing salt and water retention. High-dose aspirin (anti-inflammatory doses) may completely block the uricosuric action of probenecid and sulfinpyrazone, so concomitant therapy should be avoided. This interaction is negligible with low-dose aspirin, and therefore will not affect any treatment decision.

Case 54.2

Mr JD is 57 years old and is admitted to hospital with a deep vein thrombosis. He is known to have recurrent attacks of gout and takes a 300 mg allopurinol tablet each day as well as occasional analgesics.

Questions

1. It is decided to prescribe warfarin for Mr JD's deep vein thrombosis. What are the problems with using a standard loading dose of warfarin (day 1, 10 mg; day 2, 5 mg; day 3, 5 mg) to treat his deep vein thrombosis?
2. Explain why allopurinol is given once a day although it has a half-life of 2 hours.

Answers

1. Warfarin is highly protein bound and has a long plasma half-life. The administration of a 10 mg loading dose will reduce the time for the drug to reach a steady state, but in this patient the dose is excessive. Patients more than 60 years of age, or weighing less than 60 kg or with a serum albumin level less than 35 g/dL, all require a reduced loading dose. Although Mr JD does not fulfil any of these criteria, he is taking allopurinol. Allopurinol inhibits the metabolism of warfarin by inhibiting the oxidative metabolic pathway. The loading dose of warfarin should therefore be reduced by approximately 50%. The usual maintenance dose will also need to be reduced by approximately 50%. In the early stages of therapy the INR should be checked every few days until it has stabilized at twice normal.

2. Allopurinol has no activity on xanthine oxidase. Allopurinol undergoes hepatic conversion to its active metabolite, oxipurinol. The half-life of allopurinol is approximately 2 hours. Oxipurinol is excreted renally and undergoes net reabsorption in the renal tubule, as does urate itself. The half-life of oxipurinol is 13–18 hours in patients with normal renal function. Therefore, allopurinol may be successfully administered as a single daily dose.

Case 54.3

Mr KF is a 47-year-old factory worker who weighs 75 kg. He has a history of gout controlled with one 300 mg tablet of allopurinol each day. He was admitted to hospital after collapsing with chest pain while running to catch a bus. On admission he was diagnosed as having suffered a myocardial infarction and was treated with diamorphine, streptokinase, heparin and low-dose aspirin (150 mg).

Questions

1. What effect will the aspirin have on Mr KF's gout?
2. Should Mr KF's management be changed because of his history of gout?

Answers

1. Mr KF is already taking allopurinol as prophylaxis against further attacks of gout. In this situation the addition of aspirin to his drug regimen is probably of no consequence. His gout is already controlled with allopurinol.

   The administration of aspirin 300 mg or more can lead to elevation of serum urate levels, by inhibition of tubular secretion, and thus predispose patients to acute attacks of gout. In contrast, high-dose salicylate therapy acts in a similar manner to the uricosuric agents by inhibiting tubular reabsorption of urate, which leads to an increased excretion and a fall in serum levels.

   As a general principle, therefore, low-dose aspirin should be avoided in patients with gout. In the case of Mr KF, low-dose aspirin has been demonstrated in many studies to decrease mortality following myocardial infarction and for this reason treatment should continue, probably lifelong.

2. No changes in the management of Mr KF should be made because of his history of gout. It would be appropriate to counsel him over his risk factors for ischaemic heart disease and gout. He should be advised to stop smoking, reduce his alcohol intake and adopt a low-fat diet.

Case 54.4

Mrs AC is 87 years old and weighs 55 kg. She presents with a red, swollen and severely painful right first metatarsophalangeal joint, right elbow and right wrist. She has a past medical history of congestive heart failure, hypertension, chronic renal impairment and gout, with three previous gouty attacks this year. On admission, she was taking bumetanide 1 mg daily and ramipril 5 mg daily. She has previously been treated with allopurinol, but a hypersensitivity rash developed and treatment was discontinued. Colchicine 1 mg initially, followed by 500 μg was prescribed by the senior house officer. The results of her investigations include: temperature 38°C, serum creatinine 160 μmol/L (62–133 μmol/L), ESR 115 mm/h (1–15 mm/h), serum urate 745 μmol/L (140–380 μmol/L), synovial fluid analysis from the knee was positive for monosodium urate crystals. The diagnosis is a recurrent attack of acute gout.

Questions

1. Comment on the initial treatment of the acute gouty attack.
2. What are your recommendations for the long-term management of this patient?

Answers

1. Colchicine is an appropriate choice for the treatment of the acute attack. However, the recommended dose is 1 mg initially, followed by 500 μg every 2–3 hours until relief of pain is obtained or vomiting or diarrhoea occurs, or a total dose of 6 mg has been reached. If the patient's renal function deteriorates below 10 mL/min, the dose should be reduced by 50%. NSAIDs, such as indometacin, would be inappropriate because they may worsen Mrs AC's heart failure and hypertension. Intra-articular steroids are not suitable because of the number of joints affected, and the risk of infection. Oral steroids have a slow onset of action and can cause multiple side effects in the elderly.

2. Mrs AC has recurrent gouty arthritis secondary to hyperuricaemia and so prophylactic therapy is indicated, 2–3 weeks after resolution of the acute attack. The choice of prophylactic agents includes allopurinol, uricosuric agents or colchicine. Both probenecid and sulfinpyrazone are likely to be ineffective in patients with severe renal impairment (creatinine clearance less than 20–30 mL/min). Sulfinpyrazone is also contraindicated since it may worsen heart failure by causing salt and water retention. Colchicine does not reduce hyperuricaemia and therefore protect renal function, although it may prevent recurrent attacks of gout. Since Mrs AC has previously had a minor hypersensitivity rash when treated with allopurinol, a desensitization regimen can be employed to allow allopurinol to be reintroduced (Gillott et al 1999). Allopurinol should be introduced initially at 50 μg per day. If no reaction occurs after 3 days, then the dose can be increased gradually over 3–4 weeks to the required dose (Table 54.10).

Table 54.10 Allopurinol desensitization protocol

Day	Daily dose
1–3	50 μg
4–6	100 μg
7–9	200 μg
10–12	500 μg
13–15	1 mg
16–18	5 mg
19–21	10 mg
22–24	25 mg
25–27	50 mg
28+	100 mg

REFERENCES

Agudelo C A, Wise C M 1998 Crystal associated arthritis. Clinics in Geriatric Medicine 14: 495-513

Ahern M J, Reid C, Clardon T P et al 1987 Does colchicine work? Results of the first controlled study in gout. Australian and New Zealand Journal of Medicine 17: 301-304

Becker M A, Schumacher Jr H R, Wortman R L et al 2005 Febuxostat compared with allopurinol in patients with hyperuricaemia and gout. New England Journal of Medicine 353: 2450-2461

Choi H K, Atkinson K, Karlson E W et al 2004a Purine-rich foods, dairy and protein intake and the risk of gout in men. New England Journal of Medicine 350: 1093-1103

Choi H K, Atkinson K, Karlson E W et al 2004b Alcohol intake and risk of incident gout in men: a prospective study. Lancet 363: 1277-1281

Choi H K, Liu S, Curhan G 2005 Intake of purine-rich foods, protein, dairy products, and serum uric acid level: the third National Health and Nutrition Examination Survey. Arthritis and Rheumatism 52: 283-289

Emmerson B T 1996 The management of gout. New England Journal of Medicine 334: 445-450

Gillott T J, Whallett A, Zaphiropoulos G 1999 Oral desensitisation in patients with chronic tophaceous gout and allopurinol hypersensitivity. Rheumatology 38: 85-86

Graham W, Robert J B 1983 Intravenous colchicine in the management of gouty arthritis. Annals of the Rheumatic Diseases 12: 16-19

Gray R G, Tenenbaum J, Gottlieb N L 1981 Local corticosteroid injection treatment in rheumatic disorders. Seminars in Arthritis and Rheumatism 10: 231-254

McDonald J, Fam A G, Paton T et al 1988 Allopurinol hypersensitivity in a patient with coexistent systemic lupus erythematosus and tophaceous gout. Journal of Rheumatology 15: 865-868

Morris I, Varughese G, Mattingly P 2003 Colchicine in acute gout. British Medical Journal 327: 1275-1276

Northridge D B, Almack P M 1986 Allopurinol desensitisation. British Journal of Pharmacy Practice 8: 200

Nuki G 1998 Metabolic and endocrine arthropathies. Medicine 263: 54-59

Peterson G M, Boyle R R, Francis H W et al 1990 Dosage prescribing and plasma oxipurinol levels in patients receiving allopurinol therapy. European Journal of Clinical Pharmacology 39: 419-421

Singer J Z, Wallace S L 1986 The allopurinol hypersensitivity syndrome: unnecessary morbidity and mortality. Arthritis and Rheumatism 29: 82-87

Terkeltaub RA 2003 Gout. New England Journal of Medicine 349: 1647-1655

Wallace S L, Singer J Z 1988 Systemic toxicity associated with the intravenous administration of colchicine – guidelines for use. Journal of Rheumatology 15: 495-499

Wood J 1999 Gout and its management. Pharmaceutical Journal 262: 808-811

FURTHER READING

Choi H K, Mount D B, Reginato A M 2005 Pathogenesis of gout. Annals of Internal Medicine 143: 499-516

Katbamna R, Sutaria S, Underwood M R 2005 Diagnosing and treating gout. Practitioner 249: 773-777

Mikuls T R, MacLean C H, Olivieri J et al 2004 Quality care indicators for gout management. Arthritis and Rheumatism 50: 937-943

Nuki G 2002 Gout. Medicine 30: 71-79

Schlesinger N 2004 Management of acute and chronic gouty arthritis – present state of the art. Drugs 64(21): 2399-2416

Underwood M 2005 Gout. Clinical Evidence 13: 1435-1444

Glaucoma 55

L. C. Titcomb   S. D. Andrew

KEY POINTS

- Glaucoma is a large group of disorders with widely differing clinical features.
- Primary open-angle glaucoma (POAG) is a chronic progressive disease of insidious onset.
- The aim of treatment in POAG is to reduce the intraocular pressure (IOP) to a target pressure, specific to the patient, preventing further damage to the nerve fibres and the development of further visual field defects.
- A wide range of drugs is used to treat POAG. Surgery may be undertaken if the target pressure is not attained with medical therapy.
- POAG is a symptomless disease until well advanced. Concordance with therapy is an important issue.
- Acute primary angle-closure glaucoma (PACG) is a medical emergency that must be treated rapidly to prevent blindness.
- The aim of medical treatment in acute PACG is to reduce the IOP in preparation for surgery.
- A wide range of drugs can provoke an attack of PACG in susceptible individuals.

The term 'glaucoma' does not represent a single pathological entity. It consists of a large group of disorders with widely differing clinical features. It is therefore difficult to attempt a single definition of the term.

High intraocular pressure (IOP) was previously used as a diagnostic criterion for glaucoma but more recently it has been recognized purely as the most important risk factor for the disease. This is because glaucoma can occur even in patients with normal IOP (normal-pressure glaucoma or low-pressure POAG). The 'normal' IOP (10–21 mmHg), is a statistical description of the range of IOP in the population and is not applicable to an individual subject. It is thought to increase with age, at the rate of approximately 1 mmHg every decade after the age of 40 years in the Western population. There is a circadian cycle of IOP, with maximum levels often occurring between 8 a.m. and 11 a.m. and minimum levels between midnight and 2 a.m. This may affect IOP readings taken in outpatient clinics at different times of the day. The normal diurnal variation is between 3 and 5 mmHg and this is wider in untreated glaucoma. Although a raised IOP is not the only cause of glaucoma, it is the only parameter that can currently be changed by pharmacological intervention and therefore plays an important part in the evaluation of disease progression.

Current thinking is that once the rate of disease progression has been established, a 'target IOP' can be set. This is an estimate of the mean IOP obtained with treatment, to prevent further glaucomatous damage. However, it is extremely difficult to accurately assess in advance the IOP level at which further damage will occur for any one patient. As the correct target IOP is only discovered with hindsight, one limitation is that the chosen target IOP may not be low enough and a patient must get worse before it is realized that the target IOP was inadequate. There is no single safe IOP level for all patients, but in general the aim is to achieve at least a 20% reduction from the initial IOP at which damage occurred (Kass et al 2002). In advanced disease the aim is to achieve a IOP level below 18 mmHg at all times (AGIS Investigators 2000). This can be used as a good method to set an initial target IOP. However, it is essential that the patient receives regular periodic re-evaluation so that the target IOP can be adjusted according to disease progression and corresponding treatment adjusted accordingly.

Epidemiology

The diseases which make up the group known as glaucoma are usually classified according to the manner in which aqueous humour outflow is impaired.

Primary open-angle glaucoma

Primary open-angle glaucoma (POAG), also referred to as chronic simple glaucoma, is associated with a relative obstruction to aqueous outflow through the trabecular meshwork and is a chronic progressive disease of insidious onset, usually affecting both eyes. It is the most common type of glaucoma and affects approximately 1 in 200 of the population over the age of 40 years. POAG is responsible for about 20% of all cases of blindness in the UK, and affects both sexes equally. It is frequently an inherited condition, with approximately 10% of first-degree relatives of POAG sufferers eventually developing the disease (Pitts-Crick 1994). Two conditions similar to POAG are normal-tension glaucoma, where the IOP is not raised on initial screening although signs of damage are present, and ocular hypertension, where signs of damage do not accompany the raised IOP.

Primary angle-closure glaucoma

Primary angle-closure glaucoma (PACG), or closed-angle glaucoma, is a condition in which closure of the angle by the peripheral iris results in a reduction in aqueous outflow. It occurs in predisposed eyes and is frequently unilateral. There are ethnic variations as the disease affects approximately 1 in 1000 caucasian adults over the age of 40 years, about 1 in 100 Asians (especially mongoloids) and Hispanics, and 2–4 per 100 Inuits (Eskimos). It occurs in four times as many females as males.

Secondary glaucomas

Secondary glaucomas can arise for a number of reasons, including inflammation, intraocular tumour, raised episcleral venous pressure, or congenitally due to developmental abnormalities.

Aetiology

The factors that determine the level of IOP are the rate of aqueous humour production and the resistance encountered in the outflow channels. A fine balance between these is necessary to keep the pressure within the eye in the range of 16–21 mmHg.

Production of aqueous humour occurs in the ciliary epithelium by two mechanisms: secretion due to an active metabolic process, independent of the level of IOP, and ultrafiltration influenced by the level of blood pressure in the ciliary capillaries and the level of IOP.

Outflow of aqueous humour occurs by two routes. Approximately 80% of total outflow is through the trabecular meshwork into the canal of Schlemm and into the venous circulation via the aqueous veins. The uveoscleral pathway accounts for the remaining 20%: through the ciliary body into the suprachoroidal space, to be drained into the ciliary body, choroid and sclera via the venous circulation.

Pathophysiology

The primary site of damage is thought to be the optic nerve head, rather than any other point along the nerve axon. This most easily explains the progressive loss of visual field. Studies of axoplasmic flow show a vulnerability of the nerves to elevated IOP as they pass through the optic disc.

In POAG increased resistance within the drainage channels causes the rise in IOP. It is thought that the main route of resistance to aqueous outflow lies in the dense juxtacanalicular trabecular meshwork, or the endothelium lining the inner wall of Schlemm's canal.

In PACG the rise in IOP is caused by a decreased outflow of aqueous humour, due to closure of the chamber angle by the peripheral iris. It occurs in predisposed eyes, and the predisposing factors can be anatomical or physiological. The anatomical characteristics are lens size, corneal diameter and axial length of the globe. The lens continues to grow throughout life. This brings the anterior surface closer to the cornea. Slackening of the suspensory ligaments increases this movement. Both factors occur very gradually and lead to a progressive shallowing of the anterior chamber. The depth of the anterior chamber and width of the chamber angle are related to corneal diameter, and those eyes predisposed to PACG are observed to have a corneal diameter less than that seen in normal eyes. A short eye, which is frequently also hypermetropic, has a small corneal diameter and a thick and relatively anteriorly located lens.

The physiological precipitating factors of PACG in predisposed eyes are not fully understood. Two theories currently exist.

The dilator muscle theory suggests that contraction of the dilator muscle causes a posterior movement, which increases the apposition between the iris and anteriorly located lens and the degree of physiological pupillary block. The simultaneous dilation of the pupil renders the peripheral iris more flaccid, and causes the pressure in the posterior chamber to increase and the iris to bow anteriorly. Eventually the peripheral iris obstructs the angle and the IOP rises (Fig. 55.1).

The sphincter muscle theory postulates that the sphincter of the pupil precipitates angle closure. The pupillary blocking force of the sphincter is greatest when the diameter of the pupil is about 4 mm.

Clinical manifestations

POAG is typically characterized by the following: an IOP greater than 21 mmHg, an open angle, glaucomatous cupping and visual field loss. POAG, because of its insidious onset, is usually asymptomatic until it has caused a significant loss of visual field. In some eyes, subtle signs of glaucomatous retinal nerve damage can be detected prior to development of pathological cupping and detectable field loss. The earliest clinically significant field defect is a scotoma, which is an area of depressed vision within the visual field. Patients with POAG frequently show a wider swing in IOP than normal; therefore, a single pressure reading of 21 mmHg or less does not exclude the diagnosis. It may be necessary to measure IOP at different times of the day, or at periodic intervals.

Acute PACG is due to a sudden closure of the angle and a severe elevation in IOP. The symptoms include rapidly progressive visual impairment, periocular pain and congestion of the eye. In severe cases nausea and vomiting may occur. The signs include injection of the limbal and conjunctival vessels, giving a 'ciliary flush'. The IOP usually lies between 50 and 80 mmHg and causes corneal oedema with epithelial vesicles. The anterior chamber is shallow and iridocorneal contact can be observed. The pupil is vertically oval and fixed in a semidilated position. It is unreactive to light and accommodation. The fellow eye usually has a shallow anterior chamber and a narrow angle. The optic nerve head is oedematous and hyperaemic.

Investigations

Intraocular pressure may be measured by tonometry, such as indentation tonometry in which a plunger is applied to the cornea and the amount of indentation on the eye reflects the pressure within it. Tonography is a technique used to measure the outflow of aqueous humour from the eye, resulting from indentation of the eye, using a tonometer. Gonioscopy is used to estimate the width of the chamber angle, with the aid of a slit-lamp. Perimetry is important for both the diagnosis and management of glaucoma by detecting early scotomata and larger changes in visual field.

In patients with POAG, cupping of the optic disc becomes progressively apparent and is used in both diagnosis and assessment of the efficacy of treatment. The increased intraocular pressure appears to push the optic disc back into an excavation. This is known as glaucomatous cupping.

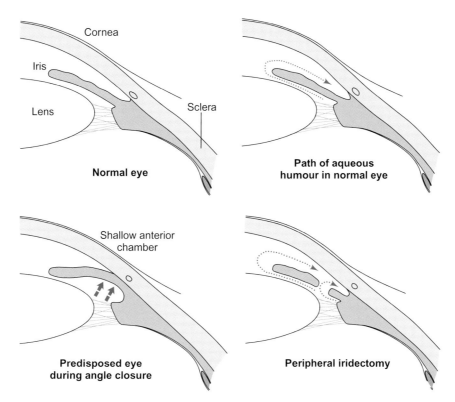

Figure 55.1 Changes to the eye seen during closed-angle glaucoma.

The colour of the optic disc will be observed to change from a creamy pink colour, due to the rich capillary network seen in the healthy eye, to increased pallor with advancing disease as the optic nerve tissue progressively atrophies.

Treatment

Primary open-angle glaucomas

The aim of treatment in POAG is to reduce the raised IOP to the target value, preventing further damage to the nerve fibres and the development of further visual field defects. The key to effective treatment is careful and regular follow-up, including measurement of visual acuity, tonometry, gonioscopy, evaluation of the optic disc and perimetry (of primary importance).

The actual safe level of IOP is unknown, the importance of disc and field assessment being underlined by evidence that IOP does not rise above the 'normal' range in up to 50% of glaucomas (normal-pressure glaucomas). However, in many cases maximal retardation of the disease process is achieved if the IOP is maintained in the lower teens. The effect on the visual field and the appearance of the optic disc are the only indications that IOP is being controlled at a safe level. A raised IOP without field or disc changes may not require treatment but will need regular review.

The initial treatment of POAG is usually medical. Topical administration is the preferred type of therapy and there is a wide range of preparations available (Table 55.1). The chosen drug should be administered at its lowest concentration and as infrequently as possible to obtain the desired effect over the whole 24-hour period as a high level of diurnal variation in intraocular pressure has been shown to be a more important factor in

Table 55.1 Drugs used in the treatment of primary open-angle glaucoma

Therapeutic category	Primary mechanisms of action
Topical β-blocking agents	Decrease aqueous formation
Topical miotics	Increase aqueous outflow
Topical adrenergic agonists	Increase aqueous outflow and decrease aqueous formation
Topical carbonic anhydrase inhibitors	Decrease aqueous formation
Oral carbonic anhydrase inhibitors	Decrease aqueous formation
Topical prostaglandins	Increase aqueous outflow
Topical prostamides	Increase aqueous outflow

visual field development than the average intraocular pressure. A drug with few potential side effects should be chosen, with oral therapy retained as the final option. The prostaglandin analogues latanoprost and travoprost and the prostamide bimatoprost are indicated for first-line use, as are the β-blockers as these produce the greatest fall in IOP (Table 55.2). Carbonic anhydrase inhibitors and sympathomimetics, which result in a smaller fall in IOP, are reserved for patients unresponsive to first-line drugs, in patients in whom the first-line agents are contraindicated or as adjunctive therapy.

Table 55.2 Comparison of reduction in IOP with a range of ocular hypotensive drugs (adapted from Van der Valk et al 2005)

Ocular hypotensive agent	Relative IOP reductions from baseline [mean (95% confidence interval)]			
	Peak	No of studies	Trough	No of studies
Betaxolol 0.5%	−23% (−25% to −22%)	5	−20% (−23% to −17%)	4
Timolol 0.5%	−27% (−29% to −25%)	15	−26% (−28% to −25%)	15
Dorzolamide 2%	−22% (−24% to −20%)	6	−17% (−19% to −15%)	6
Brinzolamide 1%	−17% (−19% to −15%)	1	−17% (−19% to −15%)	1
Brimonidine 0.2%	−25% (−28% to −22%)	4	−18% (−21% to −14%)	3
Latanoprost 0.005%	−31% (−33% to −29%)	12	−28% (−30% to −26%)	11
Travoprost 0.004%	−31% (−32% to −29%)	5	−29% (−32% to −25%)	4
Bimatoprost 0.03%	−33% (−35% to −31%)	6	−28% (−29% to −27%)	6
Placebo	−5% (−9% to −1%)	3	−5% (−10% to 0%)	3

In most cases the initial topical treatment is with a prostaglandin analogue or prostamide. If this is ineffective, another prostaglandin or prostamide may be substituted or a β-blocker used instead. Patients not reaching their target pressure on one first-line agent may be prescribed another concomitantly. Alternatively, a carbonic anhydrase inhibitor or a sympathomimetic may be added to one of the first-line drugs. Pilocarpine is usually reserved for those patients not controlled by a combination of the drugs listed above. Oral therapy with carbonic anhydrase inhibitors is usually reserved for use as the final stage of treatment in those complex glaucomas awaiting surgery (Fig. 55.2).

Strutton & Walt (2004) proposed that the improved control of IOP with newer therapies has led to a reduction in surgery for glaucoma. However, some patients will still require surgical intervention to reach their target pressure. Adding another anti-glaucoma medication to a regimen of two or three medications often fails to achieve the required fall of IOP, greater or equal to 20% of the original IOP (Neelakantan et al 2004).

The most frequently performed surgical procedures create a fistula to act as a new route for aqueous outflow. Occasionally argon laser trabeculoplasty (ALT) to promote increased aqueous humour outflow may be employed, but this tends to be reserved for elderly subjects with moderate glaucoma and an IOP of less than 30 mmHg. It is important to realize that the effect of laser trabeculoplasty may rapidly reverse, and therefore constant vigilance is necessary. Laser ciliary ablation to reduce aqueous humour production is used for some intractable glaucomas.

Primary angle-closure glaucoma

The medical management of acute PACG is essentially to prepare the eye for surgical treatment. The aim of treatment is to decrease the IOP and associated inflammation. Analgesics and antiemetics are sometimes needed, dependent on symptom severity, to make the patient comfortable. It is usual to treat the unaffected eye prophylactically with miotics (Fig. 55.3).

Paralysis of the iris sphincter usually occurs at an IOP of more than 60 mmHg, due to ischaemia. Therefore, intensive miotic therapy, previously the treatment of choice in many cases of PACG, is usually ineffective and the IOP needs to be lowered by drugs that reduce aqueous humour production rather than by trying to pull the peripheral iris away from the angle with miotics. An intravenous loading dose of acetazolamide followed by oral treatment, sometimes in combination with corneal indentation, to physically force aqueous humour to the peripheral anterior chamber and artificially open the angle, should allow the IOP to drop sufficiently to relieve iris ischaemia and allow the sphincter to respond to pilocarpine therapy.

If corneal indentation and acetazolamide fail to decrease IOP, hyperosmotic agents may be required. Once the IOP has been reduced medically, the condition is usually treated surgically, by either surgical peripheral iridectomy or laser iridotomy, to remove an area of the peripheral iris to allow flow of aqueous humour through an alternative pathway (see Fig. 55.1). Filtration surgery is indicated if a large proportion of the angle has been permanently closed by adhesions between the iris and the cornea.

Ocular hypotensive lipids: prostaglandins and prostamides

Prostaglandin analogues, such as latanoprost and travoprost, lower IOP with a once-daily application at night, primarily by increasing the uveoscleral outflow with no significant effect on other parameters of aqueous humour dynamics.

The prostamide bimatoprost is thought to increase outflow through both trabecular and uveoscleral outflow pathways.

All the drugs in this class are licensed for the reduction of elevated intraocular pressure in open-angle glaucoma and ocular hypertension, and administered once daily at night.

Details of drugs in this class are presented in Table 55.3. These drugs have some interesting local side effects (Table 55.4).

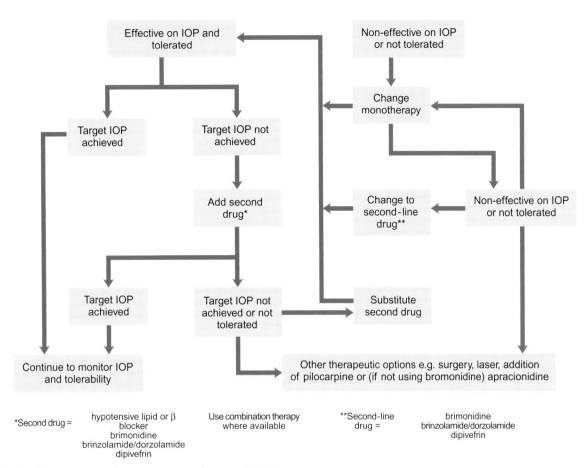

Figure 55.2 Topical therapy for primary open-angle glaucoma (POAG).

Pigmentation of the iris occurs in patients with mixed colour (green-brown or blue-brown) irides after 3–6 months of use and is a result of increased deposition of melanin in the melanocytes. An increase in the length and thickness of the eyelashes and pigmentation of the palpebral skin are side effects recognized during postmarketing surveillance. Bimatoprost, latanoprost and travoprost use may lead to disruption of the blood–aqueous barrier in patients with aphakia and pseudophakia (no or false lens respectively) and increase the risk of developing cystoid macular oedema; they should be used with caution in such patients.

Latanoprost

Latanoprost, which is converted to its active free acid on entering the eye, was the first of the hypotensive lipids to be launched and is the market leader. Like timolol amongst the β-blockers, latanoprost is the drug in this class against which new drugs or combinations are assessed. Travoprost and bimatoprost have been shown in studies to be superior in their ability to lower intraocular pressure. However, latanoprost is significantly more effective than β-blockers, carbonic anhydrase inhibitors and brimonidine (Van der Valk et al 2005). It is as effective and better tolerated than the dorzolamide-timolol fixed combination. Latanoprost is generally very well tolerated and patient persistence with latanoprost therapy is better than that with β-blockers or the other

hypotensive lipids (Day et al 2004, Reardon et al 2004). Latanoprost is not heat stable and requires refrigeration. It is stable enough to be stored at room temperature for the 4-week inuse period applied in the UK. The concentration of the preservative benzalkonium chloride in latanoprost eye drops may prevent its use in certain patients. The benzalkonium chloride concentration is 0.2%, which is 13 times the concentration in travoprost and 40 times that in bimatoprost.

Travoprost

Like latanoprost, travoprost is an ester pro-drug, converted to its active acid form by corneal hydrolytic enzymes as it is absorbed through the eye. Travoprost acid is a potent full agonist for prostaglandin $F_2\alpha$ receptors, producing 100% efficacy, whereas latanoprost has efficacy of 92%. It is highly selective, with no significant activity at non-prostanoid receptors and low affinity for the other prostanoid receptors responsible for pain, etc. It appears to be generally well tolerated by patients and is relatively free of systemic side effects although abdominal cramp has been reported. Travoprost has been found to be superior to timolol and equal or superior to latanoprost in lowering intraocular pressure in patients with POAG or ocular hypertension (OHT). It may be more beneficial in African American patients in whom the prevalence of POAG is four times greater than in

Time

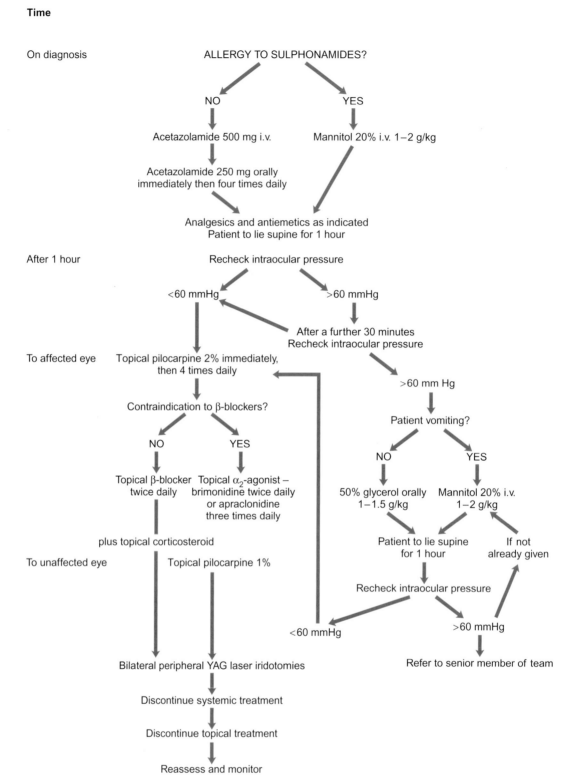

On diagnosis — ALLERGY TO SULPHONAMIDES?

NO → Acetazolamide 500 mg i.v. → Acetazolamide 250 mg orally immediately then four times daily

YES → Mannitol 20% i.v. 1–2 g/kg

Analgesics and antiemetics as indicated
Patient to lie supine for 1 hour

After 1 hour — Recheck intraocular pressure

<60 mmHg   >60 mmHg

After a further 30 minutes
Recheck intraocular pressure

>60 mm Hg

To affected eye — Topical pilocarpine 2% immediately, then 4 times daily

Contraindication to β-blockers?

NO → Topical β-blocker twice daily
YES → Topical α₂-agonist – brimonidine twice daily or apraclonidine three times daily

plus topical corticosteroid

To unaffected eye — Topical pilocarpine 1%

Patient vomiting?

NO → 50% glycerol orally 1–1.5 g/kg
YES → Mannitol 20% i.v. 1–2 g/kg

Patient to lie supine for 1 hour   If not already given

Recheck intraocular pressure

<60 mmHg   >60 mmHg

Bilateral peripheral YAG laser iridotomies

Discontinue systemic treatment

Discontinue topical treatment

Reassess and monitor

Refer to senior member of team

Figure 55.3 Algorithm for the treatment of primary angle-closure glaucoma (PACG). YAG, yttrium aluminium garnet.

other races because travoprost lowers IOP significantly more, and a higher percentage of such patients reach target pressure compared with latanoprost or timolol (Whitson 2002).

Patients treated with travoprost show good diurnal fluctuation control and an ocular hypotensive effect was shown to last for over 3 days (Dubiner et al 2004). Patients previously treated with β-blockers, α₂-agonists, carbonic anhydrase inhibitors, latanoprost and the dorzolamide-timolol fixed combination respond to travoprost. Within 1 month of starting therapy, the drug reduces the mean IOP to below 18 mmHg (Przydryga et

Table 55.3 Ocular hypotensive lipids

	Bimatoprost	Latanoprost	Travoprost
Strength	0.03%	0.005%	0.004%
Pharmacological class	Prostamide	Prostaglandin analogue	Prostaglandin analogue
Posology	Once daily in the evening	Once daily in the evening	Once daily in the evening
Preservative	BZC 0.005%	BZC 0.2%	BZC 0.015%
Storage requirements	≤25°C	2–8°C until opened then ≤25°C for period of use of 4 weeks	≤25°C

Table 55.4 Side effects of hypotensive lipids

Ocular		Systemic
Conjunctival hyperaemia	Cataract	Headache
Conjunctival oedema		Asthenia
Ocular pruritus	Corneal erosion	Infection (primarily URTIs)
Allergic conjunctivitis	Eye pain	Elevated liver function
Conjunctival follicles, papillae	Foreign body sensation	Abdominal cramp
	Punctate epithelial erosions	
Eyelash changes – increased number, length, thickness, pigmentation, misdirection, poliosis	Tearing	Dizziness
Increase in vellus hair on eyelids	Increased iris pigmentation	Hypertension
Distichiasis		Hypotension
	Ocular burning, dryness, irritation	Bradycardia
	Ocular fatigue	Peripheral oedema
		Hirsutism
Asthenopia		Asthma
Blepharospasm	Photophobia	Dyspnoea
Deepening of lid sulcus	Visual disturbance	Skin rash
Blepharitis	Cystoid macular oedema	
Eyelid and periocular skin darkening	Iritis, flare	
Localized skin reactions on the eyelids	Uveitis	
Lid margin crusting		
Eyelid oedema, eyelid retraction	Retinal haemorrhage	
Eye discharge	Browache	

al 2004). Travoprost is a stable compound throughout a range of temperatures and the commercially available product does not require refrigeration.

Bimatoprost

Bimatoprost, first marketed in 2002, is a fatty acid amide, pharmacologically similar to prostaglandin $F_{2\alpha}$1-ethanolamine (prostamide $F_{2\alpha}$). Administration of bimatoprost leads to an enhancement of both conventional or trabecular outflow and uveoscleral outflow without a significant effect on aqueous humour formation.

Several mechanisms of action have been proposed including activity of bimatoprost or its free acid, 17-phenyl $PGF_{2\alpha}$, at the prostaglandin $F_{2\alpha}$ receptor, prostamide mimetic activity, and inhibition of PGF synthase which leads to an increase in endogenous $PGF_{2\alpha}$. Although the free acid has been found in human eyes, its presence alone does not explain the 24-hour efficacy of bimatoprost or its hypotensive superiority over latanoprost. The pharmacology of bimatoprost itself is not explained wholly by its interaction with known prostaglandin $F_{2\alpha}$ receptors (Krauss & Woodward 2004). It is administered once daily in the evening; more frequent administration may lessen the intraocular pressure lowering effect.

Bimatoprost lowers the intraocular pressure to a greater extent than any other topical ocular hypotensive (see Table 55.2). It is superior to latanoprost in terms of response rate, fall in IOP and the percentage of patients reaching their target IOP (Simmons et al 2004). Bimatoprost is reported to be as effective as the fixed combination of latanoprost and timolol (Manni et al 2004). Many patients are non-responsive to latanoprost as they do not achieve a fall in IOP greater than 10%, although a large proportion of patients show a 20% or more fall in IOP with bimatoprost (Gandolfi & Cimino 2003).

Generally, bimatoprost causes similar ocular side effects to latanoprost and travoprost. Furthermore, while all the ocular hypotensive lipids cause subclinical ocular inflammation, bimatoprost and travoprost cause this to a lesser degree than latanoprost (Cellini et al 2004). However, bimatoprost causes hyperaemia more frequently than latanoprost, although this is described as mild. This may contribute to the higher discontinuation rate seen with bimatoprost therapy (Reardon et al 2004).

β-Adrenoceptor antagonists

The exact mechanism of action of β-adrenoceptor antagonists (β-blockers) in lowering IOP has not been fully established but is thought to result from the blockade of ciliary β-receptors, preventing the cyclic AMP-induced rise in aqueous secretion, as they have been shown to reduce aqueous humour formation rather than increase outflow. Although there are both β_1- and β_2-receptors in the eye, the latter predominate and even cardioselective β-blockers are thought to work by blockade of β_2-receptors. Five drugs are available in the UK for topical administration: betaxolol, carteolol, levobunolol, metipranolol and timolol (Table 55.5). β-Blockers have a number of important properties in addition to β-adrenoceptor blockade. These include intrinsic sympathomimetic activity (ISA), cardioselectivity and membrane-stabilizing activity, which are all of importance when considering the side effects seen with these agents (Table 55.6).

Table 55.5 Examples of ophthalmic β-blockers

Drug	Brand name	Strength (%)	Daily dosage frequency
Betaxolol	Betoptic solution	0.5	2
	Betoptic suspension[b]	0.25	2
Carteolol	Teoptic	1	2
		2	2
Levobunolol	Betagan[b] and generic form	0.5	1–2
Metipranolol[a]	Minims[c]	0.1	2
		0.3	2
Timolol	Timoptol[b] and generic form	0.25	2
		0.5	2
	Cosopt (with dorzolamide 2%)	0.5	2
	Xalacom (with latanoprost 0.005%)	0.5	1
	DuoTrav (with travoprost 0.004%)	0.5	1
	Ganfort (with bimatoprost 0.03%)	0.5	1
	Combigan (with brimonidine 0.2%)	0.5	2
	Timoptol-LA	0.25	1
		0.5	1

[a] Metipranolol multidose marketed as Glauline was withdrawn in 1990 due to the occurrence of granulomatous anterior uveitis.
[b] Available in unit dose and multidose forms.
[c] Available in unit dose form only.

Table 55.6 Pharmacological profile of ophthalmic β-blockers

	β-blocking potency[a]	ISA	Cardioselectivity	Membrane-stabilizing activity
Betaxolol	3–10	–	++	+
Carteolol	30	++	–	–
Levobunolol	6	–	–	–
Metipranolol	2	–	–	+
Timolol	5–10	–	–	+

[a] Propranolol = 1.

Ocular side effects of topically administered β-blockers are shown in Table 55.7.

It has been suggested that those β-blockers that show ISA are less likely to produce bronchospasm and peripheral vascular side effects. Carteolol is the only commercially available drug that shows ISA. The selectivity of cardioselective β-blockers diminishes with increasing dosage, even within the therapeutic range. Betaxolol is the only commercially available topical β-blocker that demonstrates cardioselectivity.

A degree of bradycardia and hypotension is commonly seen with all β-blockers, although it is more marked with non-selective agents. These may be of clinical significance and should be monitored, particularly if the patient is known to suffer cardiac disease or hypertension, for there may be a tendency to underestimate this particular problem.

The precipitation of bronchospasm in susceptible patients can occur with the administration of as little as one drop of timolol. Those β-blockers that show cardioselectivity or ISA are less likely to cause bronchoconstriction, although it has been demonstrated that respiratory function improved in patients whose treatment was changed from timolol to betaxolol or an adrenergic agonist, these same patients having previously been asymptomatic.

The property of membrane stabilization is relevant to the incidence of ocular side effects. The absence of anaesthetic properties reduces the number and severity of foreign body and dryness sensations, anaesthesia of the cornea and dry eye syndrome.

Table 55.7 Ocular and systemic side effects of topical β-blockers

Ocular	Systemic	
Allergic blepharoconjunctivitis	**Vascular**	**Endocrine**
Burning and itching	Hypotension	Hypoglycaemia (insulin induced)
Blurred vision	Arrhythmias	**Central nervous system**
Conjunctival hyperaemia	Reduced stroke volume	Anxiety
Corneal anaesthesia	Bradycardia	Depression
Dryness	Peripheral vasoconstriction	Irritability
Foreign body sensation	**Respiratory**	Fatigue
Macular oedema	Bronchoconstriction	Hallucinations
Pain	Dyspnoea	Sleep disturbances
Punctate keratitis	**Gastrointestinal**	
Uveitis[a]	Nausea	
	Diarrhoea	

[a] Granulomatous anterior uveitis has been reported with metipranolol.

All topical β-blockers have been reported to cause bronchospasm, hence 'at-risk' patients with a tendency to airway disease who require therapy for glaucoma should be treated with extreme caution.

Prescribers are advised that β-blockers, even those with apparent cardioselectivity, should not be used in patients with asthma or a history of obstructive airways disease unless no alternative treatment is available. In such cases the risk of inducing bronchospasm should be appreciated and appropriate precautions taken. Lacrimal occlusion with intracanalicular plugs may almost completely prevent the bronchoconstriction caused by topical timolol in asthmatics by inhibiting or decreasing systemic absorption of the medication (Hepsen et al 2004).

Ocular β-blockers are generally not contraindicated in diabetes although a cardioselective agent may be preferable. However, they are best avoided in patients who suffer frequent hypoglycaemic attacks as they do produce a slight impairment of glucose tolerance.

Systemic side effects of topically administered β-blockers are shown in Table 55.7.

The long-term benefits of β-blockers on visual function preservation have been shown to be less than would be expected. This may be due to adverse effects on the ocular microcirculation whereby the β-blockers interfere with endogenous vasodilation and cause optic nerve head arteriolar vasoconstriction. The various β-blockers demonstrate marked differences in their vasoconstrictive effect, with betaxolol possibly demonstrating the least vasoconstriction.

Betaxolol

In theory, because of its cardioselectivity, betaxolol should have fewer adverse effects on the pulmonary system. It should also have fewer adverse cardiovascular effects because of comparatively lower systemic β-receptor occupancy after ocular administration. Maximum occupancies for β_1 and β_2 receptors after ophthalmic administration were 52% and 88% for carteolol, 62% and 82% for timolol, and 44% and 3% for betaxolol, respectively. However, betaxolol is less effective than other β-blockers as an ocular hypotensive agent. On initiation of treatment, the fall in IOP is slower than with other topical β-blockers. The 0.25% suspension is as effective as the 0.5% solution and is better tolerated by the patient. Experimental studies showed the drug reaches the retina after topical administration and displays a voltage-dependent L-type calcium channel-blocking activity, which probably leads to improved retinal perfusion (Yarangumeli & Kural 2004). This effect may explain the significant improvement in visual field performance seen with betaxolol in a comparison study with timolol in open-angle glaucoma. The significant improvement with betaxolol occurred despite the more effective reductions in IOP with timolol (Araie et al 2003).

Carteolol

It has been suggested that because of the ISA of carteolol, attributable to its metabolite 8-hydroxycarteolol found in the plasma, smaller changes are seen in pulmonary and cardiovascular parameters than are seen with the non-cardioselective β-blockers without ISA. Carteolol appears to be neutral in its effect on serum lipid levels, whereas timolol adversely affects high-density lipoprotein cholesterol (HDL-C) and also the total cholesterol/HDL-C ratio. Carteolol is generally well tolerated and has been shown to be as effective as timolol at lowering IOP in the majority of patients. It has a greater vasodilator effect on the the retinal and choroidal vasculature than levobunolol but less than that of betaxolol. It is the least lipophilic of the topical β-blockers and consequently is likely to show a lower incidence of central nervous system side effects.

Levobunolol

Levobunolol is the potent L-isomer of bunolol. It is metabolized to dihydrolevobunolol in the eye, prolonging the drug's half-life and making it one of only two topical β-blockers licensed for once-daily use. It is as effective with once-daily dosing as the usual twice-daily regimen. It is not cardioselective, showing greater affinity for the β_2-receptor, and does not possess ISA. It is reported to be as effective as timolol 0.5% and metipranolol 0.6% in lowering IOP and more effective than betaxolol 0.5%. Levobunolol is better tolerated than betaxolol 0.5% and metipranolol 0.6%. Its tolerability is similar to that of timolol gel-forming solution and although its effect on tear volume and corneal epithelial barrier function is similar to that produced by timolol, it has less effect on non-invasive break-up time of the precorneal tear film. This may be attributable to its formulation which includes polyvinyl alcohol (Ishibashi et al 2003). Levobunolol appears to have no effect on the retinal and choroidal vasculature.

Metipranolol

This is a non-cardioselective β-blocker without ISA. The multidose form was discontinued following reports of anterior uveitis associated with its use. The remaining preservative-free, unit dose forms are indicated for treatment of patients who are hypersensitive to preservatives, to control postoperative increases of intraocular pressure and as an initial test for responsiveness to β-blocker therapy. Patient tolerability of the product is poor, stinging and dry skin around the eye being common complaints. The metipranolol unit dose presentation is considerably more expensive than those of the other topical β-blockers.

Timolol

This non-cardioselective β-blocker without ISA was the first to be introduced, and as such is the agent against which all newer β-blockers are compared. It is effective in the long-term treatment of glaucoma, often in conjunction with other antiglaucoma therapy in terms of IOP lowering. The Summary of Product Characteristics (SPC) for timolol indicates that many patients can be placed on once-a-day therapy provided the IOP is maintained at satisfactory levels. However, the presentation of timolol in a prolonged-release formulation (a polysaccharide-based, gel-forming solution) leads to a prolonged corneal contact time and increased penetration of timolol into the eye. This is the preferred form for once-daily administration. Both timolol eye gels, 0.1% and 0.5%, have been shown to be as effective as the 0.5% solution administered twice daily. The 0.1% gel has the advantage of a much lower drug load, giving rise to plasma levels of timolol 10 times lower than achieved after twice-daily dosage of timolol 0.5% eye drops (Rouland et al 2002). Timolol is available in combination products with the carbonic anhydrase inhibitor dorzolamide, the prostaglandin analogue latanoprost and the sympathomimetic brimonidine (see Table 55.5).

Sympathomimetic agents

The original sympathomimetic drug used in the treatment of ocular hypertension and open-angle glaucoma, adrenaline (epinephrine), has been discontinued. However, the more lipophilic pro-drug dipivefrine remains available. Adrenaline (epinephrine) is an α- and β-adrenoreceptor agonist. It decreases IOP by reducing aqueous inflow via an α-mediated vasoconstriction in the ciliary body and increased outflow due to a dilation of the aqueous and episcleral veins. Adrenaline (epinephrine) is a mydriatic and therefore its use is contraindicated in PACG and in patients who show a shallow anterior chamber, because of the risk of precipitating angle closure.

Dipivefrine

Enzymes in ocular tissues convert dipivefrine into its active form, adrenaline (epinephrine). Dipivefrine passes more rapidly through the cornea than adrenaline (epinephrine), and the effects of a 0.1% solution are comparable to a 1% solution of adrenaline (epinephrine). This lower concentration causes fewer local and systemic side effects although cystoid maculopathy may result in aphakic (i.e. without the lens) and perhaps pseudophakic eyes. Dipivefrine is rarely used today but it may have a place in patients intolerant of β-blockers who require adjunctive therapy to latanoprost, as it has been shown to be as efficacious as carbonic anhydrase inhibitors (Higginbotham et al 2002).

Ocular and systemic side effects of topical dipivefrine are detailed in Table 55.8.

Apraclonidine

Apraclonidine (a derivative of clonidine) was the first of the selective adrenergic agonists to be introduced. This drug, which acts predominantly on α_2 but also α_1-receptors, reduces the rate at which aqueous humour is produced due to ciliary vasoconstriction. Eye drops containing apraclonidine 1% are used to control or prevent postoperative elevation of IOP following anterior segment laser surgery. Eye drops containing a 0.5% solution are licensed for the short-term adjunctive treatment of patients with chronic glaucoma, not adequately controlled by other drugs, while awaiting surgery. Apraclonidine 0.5% is as effective in lowering IOP as brimonidine 0.2%, but has less effect on blood pressure and heart rate (Yuksel et al 2002). Although an off-licence use, apraclonidine is sometimes used in children in whom brimonidine is strictly contraindicated.

Topical and systemic side effects of α_2-agonists are shown in Table 55.9.

Brimonidine

More α_2 selectivity is seen with brimonidine, which results in miosis rather than mydriasis. Vasoconstriction of microvessels is

Table 55.8 Ocular and systemic side effects of topical dipivefrine

Ocular	Systemic
Allergic blepharoconjunctivitis	Contact dermatitis
Follicular conjunctivitis	Headache
Burning and stinging on instillation	Arrhythmias
Conjunctival hyperaemia	Tachycardia
Conjunctival adenochrome deposits	Hypertension
Macular oedema (aphakic eyes)	
Mydriasis	
Corneal vascularization and opacification	

Table 55.9 Ocular and systemic side effects of topical α2 agonists

Ocular	Systemic
Ocular pruritus	Dry mouth/nose
Discomfort	Headache
Tearing	Asthenia
Hyperaemia	Bradycardia
Conjunctival and lid oedema	Depression
Lid retraction, conjunctival blanching and mydriasis (reported after perioperative use of apraclonidine)	
Miosis (reported with brimonidine)	

also not seen. Brimonidine administered twice daily is almost as effective as timolol twice a day at peak. However, bromonidine is significantly less effective at trough and some researchers consider it to be more efficacious when administered three times a day, the frequency used in the United States. Brimonidine may be used as monotherapy to lower IOP in patients with open-angle glaucoma or ocular hypertension who are intolerant of β-blockers or in whom β-blockers are contraindicated, as there is no effect on pulmonary function and only minimal cardiovascular effect. It may also be used as an adjunctive therapy in those patients whose IOP is not adequately controlled with a topical β-blocker.

A 6-month study of 66 patients receiving glaucoma therapy showed that the agent most frequently associated with adverse drug reactions was brimonidine (73 ADRs) (Bhatt et al 2005). It has high allergenicity and may increase the likelihood of allergy to preparations subsequently used (Osborne et al 2005).

A new formulation of brimonidine, brimonidine-Purite 0.15%, given twice daily has been shown to be as effective as brimonidine 0.2% twice a day. However, it has a more favourable safety and tolerability profile, a reduced incidence of allergic conjunctivitis and better patient satisfaction and comfort rating (Katz 2002). Unfortunately, this product is not yet available in the UK.

Brimonidine is contraindicated in patients receiving MAOIs or antidepressants which affect noradrenergic transmission and there is the possibility of brimonidine potentiating or causing an additive effect with CNS depressants.

Commercially available preparations of sympathomimetic agents are shown in Table 55.10.

Table 55.10   Available ocular products containing sympathomimetic agents

Drug	Trade name	Strength	Daily dosage frequency
Dipivefrine	Propine	0.1%	2
Apraclonidine	Iopidine	1%	1 h prior to surgery and on completion
	Iopidine	0.5%	3
Brimonidine	Alphagan	0.2%	2

Table 55.11   Ocular side effects of topical pilocarpine

Allergic conjunctivitis	Pigment epithelial cysts
Blurred vision	Poor night vision
Ciliary/conjunctival injection	Posterior synechiae
Ciliary spasm	Pupillary block
Induced myopia	Retinal tear/detachments
Lens changes (chronic use)	Uveitis
Lid twitching	Vitreous haemorrhage
Pain	

Table 55.12   Systemic side effects of topical pilocarpine

Bradycardia	Lacrimation
Bronchial spasm	Nausea and vomiting
Browache, headache	Pulmonary oedema
Diarrhoea	Salivation
Hypotension	Sweating

Miotics

Miotics act to increase the outflow of aqueous humour by a stimulation of ciliary muscle and an opening of channels in the trabecular meshwork. Miotics are directly acting parasympathomimetic agents that act at muscarinic receptors. The only drug currently available commercially in the UK is pilocarpine.

The onset of action of pilocarpine is 20 minutes but its short duration of action necessitates four times daily dosing. Miosis is an unwanted incidental effect and can cause considerable difficulties to patients. Reduced visual acuity, especially in the presence of central lens opacities, spasm of accommodation, accompanied by severe frontal headache (browache) and diminished night vision may cause poor adherence in many patients.

Ocular side effects of pilocarpine are shown in Table 55.11. In eyes with narrow angles, PACG may be precipitated by an aggravation of pupillary block. Systemic side effects are due to parasympathetic stimulation and include anxiety, bradycardia, diarrhoea, nausea, vomiting and sweating (Table 55.12).

The frequency of instillation of pilocarpine eye drops is a major disadvantage and advances have been made to reduce the inconvenience of a four-times-daily dosage regimen. A slow-release gel preparation, Pilogel (Table 55.13), has been introduced. A single daily application, administered at bedtime, allows low IOP to be maintained for 24 hours, with the patient sleeping through the more troublesome ocular side effects, i.e. blurred vision.

Table 55.13   Commercially available forms of pilocarpine

Drug	Trade name	Strength	Daily dosage frequency
Pilocarpine	Pilocarpine	0.5–4%	4
	Minims	2 and 4%	4
	Pilogel	4%	1

Carbonic anhydrase inhibitors

There are many forms of the enzyme carbonic anhydrase, three of which (CA-I, CA-II and CA-IV) are present in ocular tissues. Inhibition of CA-II, the form of the enzyme involved in aqueous humour production in the ciliary body, results in a reduction in aqueous humour secretion. Inhibition of other forms of the enzyme results in many side effects.

Acetazolamide

This is the only systemic carbonic anhydrase inhibitor available in the UK. Although this agent is amongst the most potent ocular hypotensive agents available, it has limited use in the long-term management of glaucoma due to poor patient adherence following occurrence of side effects. The systemic side effects are shown in Table 55.14.

Paraesthesia occurs in almost all patients on commencement of therapy but usually disappears on continued therapy. The malaise complex can include fatigue, depression, weight loss and decreased libido.

Acetazolamide is also available in injection form, and given either intramuscularly or, preferably, intravenously. It is useful in the preoperative/emergency treatment of closed-angle glaucoma.

Topical carbonic anhydrase inhibitors

The topical carbonic anhydrase inhibitors dorzolamide and brinzolamide are useful alternatives to acetazolamide in glaucoma management. They are licensed as monotherapy for patients with ocular hypertension or open-angle glaucoma resistant to β-blockers or those in whom use of β-blockers is contraindicated. They are also licensed as adjunctive therapy to β-blockers.

Dorzolamide, which is also licensed for the treatment of pseudo exfoliative glaucoma, is used either alone three times a day or

Table 55.14 Side effects of systemic carbonic anhydrase inhibitors

Acidosis
Diarrhoea
Drowsiness
Elevated uric acid
Hypokalaemia
Nausea/vomiting
Malaise complex
Paraesthesia
Sulphonamide crystalluria
Sulphonamide sensitivity
Transient myopia

concurrently with a β-blocker twice daily. While the licence for brinzolamide states that the drug can be used twice a day as monotherapy, some patients may respond better to a thrice-daily dosage. Mean changes in intraocular pressure with brinzolamide administered twice daily and thrice daily and dorzolamide administered thrice daily are equivalent. However, these are less than those seen with timolol 0.5% twice daily. The lower fall in IOP with brinzolamide at peak reported in Table 55.2 was based on one study, while results for other drugs were based on between three and 15 studies.

Side effects similar to those of systemic sulfonamides may occur and should be watched for, but the most common side effects and the most frequent causes of patient discontinuation are local, as shown in Table 55.15. Of the two topical carbonic anhydrase inhibitors, brinzolamide appears to cause less burning and stinging on instillation (Stewart et al 2004a, Tsukamoto et al 2005).

Table 55.15 Side effects of topical carbonic anhydrase inhibitors

Ocular	Systemic
Blurred vision	Fatigue
Burning/stinging	Headache
Itching	Dry mouth
Tearing	Nausea
Conjunctivitis	Dyspnoea
Ocular discharge	Taste perversion
Eyelid pain/discomfort	

The likelihood of patients treated with dorzolamide changing therapy has been shown to be 1.28 times greater than that for those treated with brinzolamide. This has led Rouland and colleagues (2003) to examine the cost-effectiveness of various regimens for the treatment of ocular hypertension or primary open-angle glaucoma. They concluded that because brinzolamide can be prescribed twice daily in monotherapy, and because fewer patients treated with brinzolamide switch therapy due to local intolerance, brinzolamide is a cost-saving alternative to dorzolamide (Rouland et al 2003). This conclusion was confirmed following review of almost 50 000 patients in the UK General Practitioner Research Database (Deschaseaux-Voinet et al 2003).

Animal studies suggested that both topical carbonic anhydrase inhibitors may improve ocular blood flow independent of the IOP; however, only dorzolamide has been shown to have this effect in humans. It remains to be established whether this effect can help to reduce visual field loss in patients with glaucoma (Fuchsjager-Mayrl et al 2005, Zeitz et al 2005).

Combination products

A large number of patients require more than one medication to achieve target pressure. A need for the patient to use two products concomitantly may lead to confusion, with multiple instillation of one product and non-use of the other. Also, if the second drop is instilled too soon after the first, wash-out of the first product with the second drop, overflow of the precorneal tear film and a dilution of both products may occur. In addition, the patient receives a larger dose of preservative which can irritate the eye and is a common reason for non-tolerance of the regimen. The combination of two drugs in one topical ophthalmic preparation may improve compliance, results in a reduction in preservative load and also attracts only one co-payment charge, should this be applicable. The European Glaucoma Society recommends single rather than multi-drop combinations to improve compliance and maintain patients' quality of life.

For a combination of two drugs to be an acceptable alternative to the prescriber, the fixed combination must be more effective than either of the components used alone and at least as effective as the drugs administered separately (the loose combination), i.e. not demonstrate antagonism. In addition, adverse effects of the fixed combination must not be more numerous or more frequently encountered than with the components administered separately. There are five products in which timolol is combined with a second ocular hypotensive agent. Cosopt and Xalacom are indicated in the treatment of elevated IOP in patients with open-angle glaucoma or pseudoexfoliative glaucoma when topical β-blocker monotherapy is not sufficient, Combigan is indicated for the reduction of IOP in patients with chronic open-angle glaucoma or ocular hypertension who are insufficiently responsive to topical β-blockers, and Duotrav and Ganfort are indicated for the reduction of IOP in patients with open-angle glaucoma or ocular hypertension who are insufficiently responsive to topical β-blockers or prostaglandin analogues.

Fixed combination of timolol and dorzolamide

A combination of timolol 0.5% and dorzolamide 2% (Cosopt) was the first topical ocular hypotensive to be marketed. It is well tolerated, more effective than either timolol or dorzolamide alone, and as effective as its two components administered separately. Several studies have shown its efficacy with a response rate of over 80% in patients with initial IOPs over 30 mmHg (Henderer et al 2005).

Fixed combination of timolol and latanoprost

A combination of timolol 0.5% and latanoprost 0.005%, marketed as Xalacom, was first launched in the UK in 2001. Xalacom is indicated in the treatment of elevated IOP in patients with open-angle glaucoma or pseudoexfoliative glaucoma when topical β-blocker monotherapy is not sufficient. It is administered once a day in the morning.

Fixed combination of timolol and brimonidine

A combination of timolol 0.5% with brimonidine 0.2% is marketed as Combigan. and is indicated for the reduction of IOP in patients with chronic open-angle glaucoma or ocular hypertension who are insufficiently responsive to topical β-blockers. The fixed combination has been shown to be superior in reducing IOP than either brimonidine or timolol alone and is as safe and effective as concomitant treatment with the individual components.

Fixed combination of timolol and travoprost

A fixed combination of travoprost 0.004% and timolol 0.5% (DuoTrav) has been shown to be more effective than either of its components (Barnebey et al 2005) and as safe and efficacious as the components administered concomitantly (Hughes et al 2005). DuoTrav is indicated to decrease IOP in patients with open-angle glaucoma or ocular hypertension who are insufficiently responsive to topical β-blockers or prostaglandin analogues. The dose is one drop in the affected eye(s) once daily, in the morning or evening, but should be administered at the same time each day.

Fixed combination of timolol and bimatoprost

A fixed combination of bimatoprost 0.03% and timolol 0.5% (Ganfort) has also been shown to be more effective than either of its components used alone and as effective as the components used in their usual dosing regimen, i.e. bimatoprost once daily in the evening and timolol twice daily, used concomitantly.

Comparisons between combination products

A comparison of the effects of latanoprost/timolol against a dorzolamide/timolol combination on intraocular pressures between 8 a.m. and 8 p.m. in POAG and ocular hypertensive patients suggested that the daytime diurnal IOP was not different between these fixed combinations (Konstas et al 2004). Other studies comparing combinations are awaited. The fixed combinations have been compared with monotherapy and also with individual combinations of other drugs.

The dorzolamide/timolol combination has been compared with latanoprost 0.005% (Fechtner et al 2005), with bimatoprost 0.03% (Day et al 2005) and with concomitant brimonidine

0.2% and timolol 0.5% (Solish et al 2004) and found to be equally effective in lowering IOP in patients with ocular hypertension or glaucoma. Concomitant treatment with dorzolamide 2% and timolol 0.5% has been shown to be more effective in lowering IOP than concomitant treatment with dorzolamide 2% and brimonidine 0.2% (Ozturk et al 2005).

The fixed combination of latanoprost and timolol has been shown to produce similar diurnal IOP reduction, from an untreated baseline, to that achieved with concomitant therapy with latanoprost 0.005% and brimonidine 0.2% (Stewart et al 2004b). It was found to be more effective and better tolerated than the loose combination of brimonidine 0.2% and timolol 0.5% whether the latanoprost/timolol combination was given in the morning or in the evening (Garcia-Sanchez et al 2004, Stewart et al 2003).

Concomitant therapy with travoprost 0.004% and brinzolamide 1% showed greater efficacy, and also a greater percentage of responders, than seen with the fixed combination of latanoprost and timolol (Martinez-de-la-Casa et al 2004).

Hyperosmotic agents

Hyperosmotic agents are of great value during PACG emergencies due to their speed of action and effectiveness. The most commonly used agents are oral glycerol and intravenous mannitol, although isosorbide and urea have both been used in the past. Hyperosmotic agents act by drawing water out of the eye, and therefore lower IOP. The maximal effect of glycerol is seen within 1 hour and lasts for about 3 hours, while mannitol acts within 30 minutes with effects lasting for 4–6 hours.

Glycerol

Glycerol is given orally, usually as a 50% solution in water, the dose being 1–1.5 g/kg body weight given as a single dose. It is not a strong diuretic but may cause nausea and vomiting. Although it is metabolized to glucose in the body, it may be given to diabetics who are well controlled.

All practitioners should be aware of the difference in dose in mL required for a 50% solution of glycerol formulated as a 50% w/v solution and one formulated as a 50% v/v solution (Table 55.16).

Mannitol

Mannitol is given as a 20% solution in water for intravenous administration. The dose is 1–2 g/kg body weight up to a maximum of 500 mL given over 30–40 minutes at a rate not exceeding 60 drops per minute. It is a strong diuretic and as large volumes are required, it may cause problems due to cardiovascular overload, pulmonary oedema and stroke.

Patient care

Primary open-angle glaucoma

When the condition is first diagnosed, patients should be told that the disorder cannot be cured but only controlled by the regular use of the prescribed treatment. As POAG is, until far

Table 55.16 Doses of hyperosmotic agents in the treatment of POAG

Oral glycerol 50% at 1 g/kg				i.v. Mannitol 20% w/v[a]		
50% w/v solution		50% v/v solution				
Weight (kg)	Dose (mL)	Weight (kg)	Dose (mL)	Weight (kg)	Dose at 1 g/kg (mL)	Dose at 2 g/kg (mL)
40	80	44.5	70	40	200	400
50	100	50.8	80	50	250	500
60	120	57.2	90	60	300	–
		63.5	100	70	350	–
70	140	69.9	110	80	400	–
		76.2	120	90	450	–
80	160	82.6	130	100	500	–
90	180	88.9	140			
		95.3	150			
100	200	101.7	160			
For each additional 5 kg	Add 10 mL	For each additional 6.4 kg	Add 10 mL			

[a] Maximum dose 500 mL.

advanced, a symptomless disease, the result of non-adherence with treatment should be made clear and the importance of regular attendance at clinics stressed.

The existence of a patient self-help group, the International Glaucoma Association (www.glaucoma-association.com), should be brought to the patient's attention. They will be able to put the patient in contact with their nearest support group.

The patient's technique for instillation of eye drops should be checked and corrected if necessary. Emphasis should be on the dose (one drop), the position of instillation, into the temporal side of the lower conjunctival sac, and the importance of punctal occlusion to minimize systemic side effects.

The preferred times for administration of topical medication should be discussed with the patient. Prostaglandins, prostamides and the gel form of pilocarpine are best administered at bedtime; a 12-hourly regimen should be employed for twice-daily drugs; 8-hourly for drugs given three times a day; and as near a 6-hourly regimen as practical for the aqueous formulation of pilocarpine. β-Blockers given once daily should be administered in the morning. The importance of allowing a reasonable interval between drops should be emphasized. Sometimes the order of instillation of different types of eye drop is important for pharmacological or practical reasons. For example, the instillation of pilocarpine should always precede that of a sympathomimetic to prevent pain in the eye resulting from a strong miosis following a weak mydriasis. The instillation of aqueous eye drops, which remain in the conjunctival sac for a maximum of 10 minutes, should precede that of viscous eye drops, for example hypromellose eye drops, or suspensions (e.g dexametasone 0.1% eye drops) where the contact time is prolonged.

Eye drops containing benzalkonium chloride should not be instilled if soft contact lenses are in situ. The patient should be instructed to remove the lens immediately before instillation and replace it approximately 30 minutes later.

As POAG is a hereditary disorder, patients should be told to advise first-degree relatives to be screened. Such people over the age of 40 years are entitled to free eye tests by their optometrist.

Primary angle-closure glaucoma

Patients found to have shallow anterior chambers and narrow angles are normally promptly listed for peripheral iridectomies. However, if the procedure is delayed, they should be advised of the symptoms of an attack of acute PACG and details of the factors that are likely to precipitate an attack so that they can be avoided. They should be advised that there are a number of prescription and non-prescription drugs that they should not take. When visiting the doctor and purchasing medicines from a pharmacy, the patient should always remember to mention their condition, and the prescriber should ensure that the drug is appropriate for a patient prone to angle closure. Examples of drugs contraindicated in this condition are listed in Table 55.17. Note that the absence of a drug from this list does not imply safety.

Following an attack of angle closure and surgical treatment of the disorder, the patient should be told that the drugs previously contraindicated can be safely taken provided that iridectomy/iridotomy remains patent.

Patient adherence

The patient is more likely to comply with the prescribed treatment if the drug or drugs can be administered according to a

Table 55.17 Drugs contraindicated in narrow-angle glaucoma

Therapeutic class		Examples
Topical antimuscarinics		Atropine, cyclopentolate, homatropine, tropicamide
Topical sympathomimetics		Dipivefrine, cocaine, phenylephrine, naphazoline, xylometazoline
Systemic anticholinergics	Antiparkinsonian Antispasmodic Motion sickness	Trihexyphenidyl, benzatropine, biperiden, methixene, orphenadrine Atropine, dicycloverine, hyoscine, propantheline Hyoscine, promethazine, cyclizine
Antidepressants		Amitriptyline, amoxapine, clomipramine, dosulepin, doxepin, imipramine, lofepramine, nortriptyline, trimipramine (Maprotiline, mianserin – antimuscarinic effects may occur less frequently; citalpram – acute angle closure reported in case of overdose)
Antipsychotics		Chlorpromazine, fluphenazine, pericyazine, perphenazine, promazine, thioridazine, trifluoperazine
Antihistamines		Cyproheptadine, loratidine, terfenadine
Antiarrhythmics		Disopyramide
Antiepileptics		Topiramate
Systemic sympathomimetics		Ephedrine, isometheptene, pseudoephedrine, levodopa

simple, infrequent dosage regimen and cause no, or few, local or systemic side effects.

Thus, a patient treated with a once-daily prostaglandin analogue or prostamide or once- or twice-daily β-blocker would be expected to adhere to the regimen better than someone treated with pilocarpine, with its unfortunate side effects and inconvenient four-times-a-day dosage regimen. Common side effects of topical and systemic medication should be fully discussed with the patient so that the headache and the effects of miosis encountered with pilocarpine and the paraesthesia with acetazolamide are not unexpected, leading to premature discontinuation of therapy.

As glaucoma is predominantly a disease of elderly people, physical disability may prevent successful treatment, however conscientious the patient. For example, rheumatoid arthritis may reduce the patient's ability to squeeze the bottle of eye drops, while the tremor of Parkinson's disease can make correct positioning of instillation difficult. Various aids have been introduced to help with correct positioning and squeezing of eye drops and these should be made available to patients so disabled. Patients with poor visual acuity can be helped by colour coding of eye drop labels and supplying bottles labelled with large print. Some manufacturers have endeavoured to enhance adherence by including dose-reminder caps and facilitating instillation by supplying aids to open or position the bottle, e.g. timolol. Other manufacturers have made their eye drop containers easier to squeeze or supply aids to squeeze the bottle.

Where self-medication is impossible, a simple infrequent dosage regimen is more likely to be achieved when a relative,

Table 55.18 Common therapeutic problems in glaucoma

Problem	Comments
Lack of adherence	Treatment perceived to be worse than disease Complex multiple drug regimens Frequency of dosing Inability to differentiate between different types of medication Inability to instill medication
Contraindication to therapy	Pilocarpine in uveitis β-Blockers in asthma, bradycardia, heart block, uncontrolled heart failure Dipivefrine, prostaglandin analogues and prostamides in aphakia Dipivefrine and a wide range of other topical and systemic drugs in shallow anterior chamber α_2-Agonists in depression Carbonic anhydrase inhibitors in renal failure
Intolerance to drug	Miosis and ciliary spasm with pilocarpine Red eye with dipivefrine Bronchospasm with β-blockers Paraesthesia with acetazolamide
Use outside licensed indications	Paediatric patients Pregnant women Nursing mothers
Hypersensitivity	To active drug To preservative in multidose formulations

a neighbour or the district nursing service becomes responsible for administration of the medication. In these cases, a drug administered once daily, such as a long-acting timolol preparation or a prostaglandin analogue or bimatoprost, has an obvious advantage over one that should be administered at 12-hourly intervals. If pilocarpine is required and bedtime administration is possible, the prescribing of pilocarpine ophthalmic gel will be more practical than pilocarpine eye drops, the administration of which is totally impractical for anyone other than someone living with the patient.

Common therapeutic problems in glaucoma are listed in Table 55.18.

CASE STUDIES

Case 55.1

Mr DS is a 55-year-old accountant with POAG and a history of depression who has not reached the target pressure set by his ophthalmologist. His initial therapy was timolol 0.5% eye drops, one drop in each eye twice a day

Question

What choices are open to the prescriber and which would be the most appropriate choice for this patient?

Answer

There are several groups of ocular hypotensives which have been shown to lower IOP in patients on topical β-blockers. Sympathomimetics, parasympathomimetics, carbonic anhydrase inhibitors and the hypotensive lipids have all been used as adjunctive therapy.

The non-selective sympathomimetic dipivefrine is rarely used now because it has been superseded by the selective drug brimonidine. However, this is not a good choice for Mr DS who has a history of depression.

Due to its myriad local side effects and inconvenient four-times-a-day dosage, the parasympathomimetic pilocarpine is reserved for the treatment of patients who have not responded to other topical therapy so this would not be used as a second-line agent.

Either of the carbonic anhydrase inhibitors dorzolamide or brinzolamide would be suitable for Mr DS. Dorzolamide is administered three times a day when used as monotherapy, but can be used twice a day in conjunction with β-blockers so would not result in a great change to the patient's current regimen. Brinzolamide, which is always administered twice daily, is an alternative which is better tolerated than dorzolamide.

Finally, one of the hypotensive lipids, latanoprost, travoprost or bimatoprost, could be added to the β-blocker.

The ophthalmologist will need to monitor the response to, and the patient's tolerance of, the drugs prescribed before deciding on the best regimen. If the patient reaches target pressure following the addition of either dorzolamide or one of the hypotensive lipids to the existing regimen, the prescriber could consider use of a combination product, particularly where the patient pays an item-based co-payment charge.

Case 55.2

Miss VJ is a 35-year-old teacher with blue-brown eyes who wears soft contact lenses which she removes each night for cleaning.

Her mother has POAG. Her optometrist has referred her to one of the local ophthalmologists because her intraocular pressures are 27 mmHg left eye and 20 mmHg right eye, even though there are no signs of glaucomatous damage. The ophthalmologist diagnoses ocular hypertension and chooses to start topical ocular hypotensive therapy in the left eye.

Question

What factors should the ophthalmologist consider when choosing an ocular hypotensive for this lady?

Answer

The ophthalmologist has a choice of a hypotensive lipid or a β-blocker as first-line therapy but notes that the patient wears soft contact lenses which will affect the choice of therapy. Either of these groups of drugs would be suitable for Miss VJ as the hypotensive lipids should be instilled at night and could be used after the patient has removed her contact lenses. Four of the five β-blockers on the UK market are available in a preservative-free form so one of these could be used with the lenses in situ. However, betaxolol is only available in unit dose form as the 0.25% suspension. This is not the most suitable choice as the product's SPC states 'Contact lens wearers must remove their lenses prior to instillation and wait for 15 minutes after dosing before reinserting the contact lenses'.

The ophthalmologist discusses the side effects of both groups of drugs. Miss VJ, who is concerned that she will not be able to instill her drops efficiently without her lenses in and dislikes the idea of a change in iris colour which her students will notice, opts for a β-blocker. The ophthalmologist then has a choice of levobunolol, metipranolol and timolol and chooses the former drug because it can be used once daily.

Case 55.3

Mr JW is a 79-year-old POAG patient whose condition is very well controlled on travoprost at night and timolol 0.25% twice daily. His daughter comes in to see you as she is concerned that he is no longer able to administer his drops correctly due to the deterioration of his rheumatoid arthritis. He is now finding it very difficult to both position and squeeze the bottles correctly. He is a very independent person and does not want any help from outside agencies.

Question

What can you suggest?

Answer

There are several administration devices now available to assist in delivery of eye drops. Some devices are specific for particular products and some are universal. Devices are available specifically for both travoprost (Eyot) and latanoprost (Xal-ease). These are available from the manufacturers at no charge and can also usually be obtained from the glaucoma outpatient clinic.

As Mr JW is well controlled on his current treatment it would be appropriate to continue with both travoprost and timolol but with the aid of compliance devices.

The Eyot helps by positioning the bottle-tip relative to the patient's eye by gently pulling the lower eyelid downward, preparing the eye to receive the drop. The patient's head is positioned so that the drop falls directly into the eye. The device is easy for the physically impaired to use as a patient can self-administer the drops while sitting on a low-backed chair. It also requires minimal shoulder/arm mobility or hand strength.

Opticare and Opticare Arthro are two other devices which could be used in conjunction with the timolol bottle. These are available on prescription and both have a double-squeeze mechanism which lets the user dispense a single drop with only the lightest of squeezes. The dispensers can be used with either fingers or a grip squeeze. Both

models have an orbit-shaped, anatomically designed eye piece. This ensures that a single drop goes directly into the eye and not down the cheek. The design of the eye piece also ensures that the tip of the bottle cannot touch the eye. This prevents touch contamination and reduces the desire to blink.

REFERENCES

AGIS Investigators 2000 The Advanced Glaucoma Intervention Study (AGIS): 7. The relationship between control of intraocular pressure and visual field deterioration. American Journal of Ophthalmology 130: 429-440

Araie M, Azuma I, Kitazawa Y 2003 Influence of topical betaxolol and timolol on visual field in Japanese open-angle glaucoma patients. Japanese Journal of Ophthalmology 47: 199-207

Barnebey H S, Orengo-Nania S, Flowers B E et al 2005 The safety and efficacy of travoprost 0.004%/timolol 0.5% fixed combination ophthalmic solution. American Journal of Ophthalmology 140: 125-126

Bhatt R, Whittaker K W, Appaswamy S et al 2005 Prospective survey of adverse reactions to topical antiglaucoma medications in a hospital population. Eye 19: 392-395

Cellini M, Caramazza R, Bonsanto D et al 2004 Prostaglandin analogs and blood–aqueous barrier integrity: a flare cell meter study. Ophthalmologica 218: 312-317

Day D G, Schacknow P N, Sharpe E D et al 2004 A persistency and economic analysis of latanoprost, bimatoprost, or beta-blockers in patients with open-angle glaucoma or ocular hypertension. Ocular Pharmacology and Therapeutics 20: 383-392

Day D G, Sharpe E D, Beischel C J et al 2005 Safety and efficacy of bimatoprost 0.03% versus timolol maleate 0.5%/dorzolamide 2% fixed combination. European Journal of Ophthalmology 15: 336-342

Deschaseaux-Voinet C, Lafuma A, Berdeaux G 2003 Cost and effectiveness of brinzolamide versus dorzolamide in current practice: an analysis based on the UK-GPRD. Journal of Medical Economics 6: 69-78

Dubiner H B, Sircy M D, Landry T et al 2004 Comparison of the diurnal ocular hypotensive efficacy of travoprost and latanoprost over a 44-hour period in patients with elevated intraocular pressure. Clincal Therapeutics 26: 84-91

Fechtner R D, McCarroll K A, Lines C R et al 2005 Efficacy of the dorzolamide/timolol fixed combination versus latanoprost in the treatment of ocular hypertension or glaucoma: combined analysis of pooled data from two large randomized observer and patient-masked studies. Journal of Ocular Pharmacology and Therapeutics 21: 242-249

Fuchsjager-Mayrl G, Wally B, Rainer G et al 2005 Effect of dorzolamide and timolol on ocular blood flow in patients with primary open angle glaucoma and ocular hypertension. British Journal of Ophthalmology 89:1293-1297

Gandolfi S, Cimino L 2003 Effect of bimatoprost in patients with primary open angle glaucoma or ocular hypertension who are non-responders to latanoprost. Ophthalmology 110: 609-614

Garcia-Sanchez J, Rouland J F, Spiegel D et al 2004 A comparison of the fixed combination of latanoprost and timolol with the unfixed combination of brimonidine and timolol in patients with elevated intraocular pressure. A six month, evaluator masked, multicentre study in Europe. British Journal of Ophthalmology 88: 877-883

Henderer J D, Wilson R P, Moster M R et al 2005 Timolol/dorzolamide combination therapy as initial treatment for intraocular pressure over 30 mm Hg. Journal of Glaucoma 14: 267-270

Hepsen I F, Yildirim Z, Yilmaz H et al 2004 Preventive effect of lacrimal occlusion on topical timolol-induced bronchoconstriction in asthmatics. Clinical and Experimental Ophthalmology 32: 597-602

Higginbotham E J, Diestelhorst M, Pfeiffer N et al 2002 The efficacy and safety of unfixed and fixed combinations of latanoprost and other antiglaucoma medications. Survey of Ophthalmology 47: S133-140

Hughes B A, Bacharach J, Craven E R et al 2005 A three-month, multicenter, double-masked study of the safety and efficacy of travoprost 0.004%/timolol 0.5% ophthalmic solution compared to travoprost 0.004% ophthalmic solution and timolol 0.5% dosed concomitantly in subjects with open angle glaucoma or ocular hypertension. Journal of Glaucoma 14: 392-399

Ishibashi T, Yokoi N, Kinoshita S 2003 Comparison of the effects of topical levobunolol and timolol solution on the human ocular surface. Cornea 22: 709-715

Kass M A, Heuer D K, Higginbotham E J et al 2002 The Ocular Hypertension Treatment Study: a randomized trial determines that ocular hypotensive medication delays or prevents the onset of primary open-angle glaucoma. Archives of Ophthalmology 120: 701-713

Katz L J 2002 Twelve-month evaluation of brimonidine-purite versus brimonidine in patients with glaucoma or ocular hypertension. Journal of Glaucoma 11: 119-126

Konstas A G, Kozobolis V P, Lallos N et al 2004 Daytime diurnal curve comparison between the fixed combinations of latanoprost 0.005%/timolol maleate 0.5% and dorzolamide 2%/timolol maleate 0.5%. Eye 18: 1264-1269

Krauss A H, Woodward D F 2004 Update on the mechanism of action of bimatoprost: a review and discussion of new evidence. Survey of Ophthalmology 49: S5-S11

Manni G, Centofanti M, Parravano M et al 2004 A 6-month randomized clinical trial of bimatoprost 0.03% versus the association of timolol 0.5% and latanoprost 0.005% in glaucomatous patients. Graefe's Archive for Clinical and Experimental Ophthalmology 242: 767-770

Martinez-de-la-Casa J M, Castillo A, Garcia-Feijoo J et al 2004 Concomitant administration of travoprost and brinzolamide versus fixed latanoprost/timolol combined therapy: three-month comparison of efficacy and safety. Current Medical Research and Opinion 20: 1333-1339

Neelakantan A, Vaishnav H D, Iyer S A et al 2004 Is addition of a third or fourth antiglaucoma medication effective? Journal of Glaucoma 13: 130-136

Osborne S A, Montgomery D M, Morris D et al 2005 Alphagan allergy may increase the propensity for multiple eye-drop allergy. Eye 19:129-137

Ozturk F, Ermis S S, Inan U U et al 2005 Comparison of the efficacy and safety of dorzolamide 2% when added to brimonidine 0.2% or timolol maleate 0.5% in patients with primary open-angle glaucoma. Journal of Ocular Pharmacology and Therapeutics 21: 68-74

Pitts-Crick R 1994 Epidemiology and screening of open-angle glaucoma. Current Opinion in Ophthalmology 5: 3-9

Przydryga J T, Egloff C and the Swiss Start Study Group 2004 Intraocular pressure lowering efficacy of travoprost. European Journal of Ophthalmology 14: 416-422

Reardon G, Schwartz G F, Mozaffari E 2004 Patient persistency with topical ocular hypotensive therapy in a managed care population. American Journal of Ophthalmology 137: S3-12

Rouland J F, Morel-Mandrino P, Elena P P et al 2002 Timolol 0.1% gel (Nyogel 0.1%) once daily versus conventional timolol 0.5% solution twice daily: a comparison of efficacy and safety. Ophthalmologica 216: 449-454

Rouland J F, Le Pen C, Gouveia Pinto C et al 2003 Cost-minimisation study of dorzolamide versus brinzolamide in the treatment of ocular hypertension and primary open-angle glaucoma, in four European countries. Pharmacoeconomics 21: 201-213

Simmons S T, Dirks M S, Noecker R J 2004 Bimatoprost versus latanoprost in lowering intraocular pressure in glaucoma and ocular hypotension: results from parallel-group comparison trials. Advances in Therapy 21: 247-260

Solish A M, DeLucca P T, Cassel D A et al 2004 Dorzolamide/Timolol fixed combination versus concomitant administration of brimonidine and timolol in patients with elevated intraocular pressure: a 3-month comparison of efficacy, tolerability, and patient-reported measures. Journal of Glaucoma 13: 149-157

Stewart W C, Stewart J A, Day D et al 2003 Efficacy and safety of timolol maleate/latanoprost fixed combination versus timolol maleate and brimonidine given twice daily. Acta Ophthalmologica Scandinavica 81: 242-246

Stewart W C, Day D G, Stewart J A et al 2004a Short-term ocular tolerability of dorzolamide 2% and brinzolamide 1% vs placebo in primary open-angle glaucoma and ocular hypertension subjects. Eye 18: 905-910

Stewart W C, Stewart J A, Day D G et al 2004b Efficacy and safety of the latanoprost/timolol maleate fixed combination vs concomitant brimonidine and latanoprost therapy. Eye 18: 990-995

Strutton D R, Walt J G 2004 Trends in glaucoma surgery before and after the introduction of new topical glaucoma pharmacotherapies. Journal of Glaucoma 13: 221-226

Tsukamoto H, Noma H, Mukai S et al 2005 The efficacy and ocular discomfort of substituting brinzolamide for dorzolamide in combination therapy with latanoprost, timolol, and dorzolamide. Journal of Ocular Pharmacology and Therapeutics 21: 395-399

Van der Valk R, Webers C A, Schouten J S et al 2005 Intraocular pressure-lowering effects of all commonly used glaucoma drugs: a meta-analysis of randomized clinical trials. Ophthalmology 112: 1177-1785

Whitson J T 2002 Travoprost – a new prostaglandin analogue for the treatment of glaucoma. Expert Opinion on Pharmacotherapy 3: 965-977

Yarangumeli A, Kural G 2004 Are there any benefits of Betoptic S (betaxolol HCl ophthalmic suspension) over other beta-blockers in the treatment of glaucoma? Expert Opinion on Pharmacotherapy 5: 1071-1081

Yuksel N, Karabas L, Altintas O et al 2002 A comparison of the short-term hypotensive effects and side effects of unilateral brimonidine and apraclonidine in patients with elevated intraocular pressure. Ophthalmologica 216: 45-49

Zeitz O, Matthiessen E T, Reuss J et al 2005 Effects of glaucoma drugs on ocular hemodynamics in normal tension glaucoma: a randomized trial comparing bimatoprost and latanoprost with dorzolamide. BMC Ophthalmology 5: 6

FURTHER READING

Cordeiro F, Wells T (section curators) Glaucoma ophthalmology. eTextbook (online).www.eyetext.net/members/main/glaucoma/Glaucoma.html

European Glaucoma Society 2003 Terminology and guidelines for glaucoma, 2nd edn. European Glaucoma Society, London

Fraser S, Manvikar S 2005 Glaucoma – the pathophysiology and diagnosis. Hospital Pharmacist 12: 251-254

Goni FJ for the Brimonidine/Timolol Fixed Combination Study Group 2005 12-week study comparing the fixed combination of brimonidine and timolol with concomitant use of the individual components in patients with glaucoma and ocular hypertension. European Journal of Ophthalmology 15: 581-590

Royal College of Ophthalmologists 2004 Guidelines for the management of open angle glaucoma and ocular hypertension. Royal College of Ophthalmologists, London

Tripathi R C, Tripathi B J, Haggerty C 2003 Drug-induced glaucomas: mechanism and management. Drug Safety 26: 749-767

Drug-induced skin disorders 56

P. Magee

Adverse drug reactions are an inevitable consequence of modern drug therapy and important causes of iatrogenic illness in terms of morbidity and mortality. They bear serious medicolegal and economic consequences. Adverse cutaneous reactions to drugs are amongst the most frequent, affecting 2–3% of all hospitalized patients (Bigby 2001). Fortunately, only about 2% of all drug-induced skin reactions are severe and very few are fatal.

However, all drug-induced skin eruptions can cause considerable morbidity, affect the patient's confidence in the prescriber and future compliance with medication. It is important that all drug-associated rashes are carefully evaluated and documented in patient records so that recurrence can be avoided. It is especially important that allergic skin reactions are correctly identified as subsequent exposure to the drug may cause a more severe reaction.

The tendency for drugs to cause rashes is very variable; some drugs seldom if ever cause rashes, e.g. digoxin, potassium chloride and ferrous sulphate, while up to 5% of all patients given co-trimoxazole, ampicillin or carbamazepine develop rash. The evidence for these observations does not come from clinical trials designed to establish the incidence of adverse reactions as this would be unethical. Adverse drug reactions are identified from the systematic review of single case reports (Loke et al 2006) and information from clinical trials which are in fact looking at therapeutic efficacy.

Diagnosis

It is often difficult to determine the cause of a drug-induced eruption because:

- almost any drug can affect the skin
- unrelated drugs produce similar reactions
- the same drug may produce different reactions in different patients
- many reactions cannot be distinguished from naturally occurring eruptions.

Moreover, new drugs continue to be marketed and many drugs are prescribed as combined preparations. The possibility of a food additive or a pharmaceutical excipient causing a skin reaction must not be overlooked as re-exposure is likely and cross-reactivity can occur; for example, aspirin-sensitized patients may also be sensitized to tartrazine.

If a patient presents with a rash and is currently taking or has recently finished medication, it is important to:

- check that the rash is not due to a specific skin disease such as endogenous eczema or scabies
- take an accurate drug history, including over-the-counter medicines, herbal and homeopathic preparations and any injections. Record both generic and brand name of medicines
- ask if the patient has any history of sensitivity or allergy
- ascertain the time course of the eruption in relation to drug use
- note whether the appearance of the rash is typical of any classic drug-induced eruption.

It may then be possible to assess if a drug is the likely cause.

Rechallenge remains the most useful method of confirming a diagnosis. However, rechallenge is not possible for severe cutaneous reactions and even prick and patch testing methods are not without risk.

Treatment

Not all cutaneous reactions are serious but the implicated drug should usually be stopped, although in some cases a dosage reduction may be sufficient if alternative treatment is not appropriate. In a photosensitive reaction the drug may be continued if this is necessary, with the patient fully counselled on the use of sunscreen and sun avoidance.

In most cases the rash will disappear within a few days and the patient can be treated symptomatically with oral antihistamines.

In severe life-threatening disease, early diagnosis with early recognition and withdrawal of all potential causative drugs is essential to a favourable outcome. Symptomatic treatment will depend on the type and severity of the skin reaction. Patients may require intensive care and the use of immunomodulatory drugs.

Common drug-induced skin disorders

Erythematous (exanthematous) eruptions

An erythematous or exanthematous eruption is the most common type of drug-induced skin reaction (Table 56.1). The rash is characterized by erythema (abnormal flushing of the skin) and may be morbilliform (resembling measles) or maculopapular, consisting of macules (distinct flat areas) and papules (raised lesions conventionally less than 1 cm in diameter). The rash is usually

Table 56.1 Drugs causing erythematous eruptions
Allopurinol
Antituberculous drugs, especially rifampicin and second-line agents
Antidepressants, e.g. tricyclics, maprotiline
Barbiturates
Captopril
Carbamazepine
Cimetidine
Diuretics: thiazides, furosemide
Gold salts
Nalidixic acid
Nitrofurantoin
NSAIDs
Penicillin
Phenothiazines
Phenylbutazone, oxphenbutazone
Phenytoin
Oral retinoids
Ranitidine
Streptomycin (less common with other aminoglycosides)
Sulphonamides
Sulphonylureas
Ampicillin rashes do not necessarily indicate penicillin hypersensitivity.

bright red in colour and the skin may feel hot, burning or itchy. The whole of the skin surface can be involved, though the face is often spared. Sometimes the rash may disappear even though the drug is continued, but if itching is marked it is less likely that the rash will clear. In some severe cases erythroderma may follow an erythematous reaction. Here the erythema persists with continual scaling, which may be associated with lymphadenopathy, pyrexia, thirst and shivering with heat and fluid loss from the skin.

Most erythematous eruptions are probably allergic reactions but other mechanisms may sometimes be involved (Fitzpatrick et al 2001). Allergic reactions can occur early or late in therapy. Early reactions are more usual and start within 2–3 days of drug administration and occur in previously sensitized patients. In the late type of reaction the hypersensitivity develops during administration but the rash may not manifest itself until around the ninth day and can occur as late as 3 weeks after starting treatment and may also appear up to 2 weeks after cessation of therapy.

A distinct reddish coloured morbilliform rash may be caused by ampicillin, its derivative amoxicillin and its esters bacampicillin, pivampicillin and talampicillin. The reaction will occur in almost all patients with infective mononucleosis (glandular fever) and is not always an indicator of true penicillin allergy although patients often self-report penicillin sensitivity as a result of this reaction. A high incidence of this reaction also occurs in patients with cytomegalovirus. These are often transplant patients taking immunosuppressive drugs or patients with leukaemia.

Treatment of an erythematous eruption involves drug withdrawal and treatment for any associated itching. Measures should be taken to ensure that the patient is not re-exposed to the drug. A note of the suspected sensitivity should be made in medical records, and a personal card with the same information should be given to the patient.

A high incidence of erythematous rashes can be expected during or following treatment with penicillin or chemically related antibiotics, with gold salts and with non-steroidal anti-inflammatory drugs (NSAIDs). Sulphonamides are a frequent cause and more common in patients with AIDS (de Raevel et al 1988).

Erythroderma and exfoliative dermatitis

A widespread erythematous rash (erythroderma) with desquamation (exfoliative dermatitis) is a severe drug-induced skin reaction. There may be systemic symptoms and complications can include hypothermia, fluid and electrolyte loss, and infection. The sulphonamides, chloroquine, phenytoin, penicillin and isoniazid are the drugs most commonly implicated.

Pruritus

Pruritus (itching) can have many causes. Commonly these are systemic or psychological. However, drugs can induce pruritus either as a symptom of other cutaneous reactions or with itching as the only clinical manifestation. In either condition the itch can be so intense that the scratching this induces will cause lesions, so that it is not always possible to know if there was originally an underlying rash.

For most drugs the mechanism for inducing pruritus is not known but it is likely that both central and peripheral mechanisms are involved. Drug-induced pruritus is usually generalized but local anal pruritus can follow antibiotic-induced candidiasis. It can also be produced as a contact allergy following the local administration of ointments and suppositories when, for example, used to treat haemorrhoids. Drugs with autonomic activity may produce sweating and prickly heat followed by pruritus.

To treat pruritus, the itch-scratch-itch cycle must be broken once the drug cause has been eliminated. Topical steroids and occlusive dressings help to prevent scratching.

Urticaria and angio-oedema

Drug-induced urticaria is common and accounts for approximately 28% of all drug-induced skin disorders (Table 56.2).

The clinical appearance of drug-induced urticaria is indistinguishable from that of other causes but is often more severe and may be accompanied by hypotension, breathing difficulties, shock and even death.

An urticarial rash, often referred to as 'hives' or nettle rash, is an acute or chronic allergic reaction in which red weals develop. The weals itch intensely and may last for hours or days. Giant urticaria or angio-oedema is a severe form of urticaria involving swelling of the tongue, lips and eyelids, and requires urgent medical attention. Laryngeal oedema is the most serious complication.

Only acute urticaria is likely to be drug induced. It occurs immediately or shortly after the administration of the drug in a sensitized patient, and can be regarded as the cutaneous manifestation of anaphylaxis. Where urticaria or angio-oedema is a component of anaphylaxis or an anaphylactoid reaction,

resuscitation guidelines should be followed. When the reaction is less severe treatment with oral antihistamines is appropriate.

Chronic urticaria is rarely caused by a drug unless the patient is continually exposed, for example to trace amounts of penicillins in milk and dairy products. However, aspirin and codeine can exacerbate idiopathic chronic urticaria.

Fixed drug eruptions

Fixed drug eruptions are characterized by the fact that they tend to occur at the same site in a particular patient each time the drug is administered. Drugs causing fixed drug eruptions are listed in Table 56.3.

The lesions are flat and purplish brown in colour but may be raised in the acute stage. They take between 2 and 24 hours to develop following drug ingestion. On the first drug exposure there is usually only one lesion, but subsequent exposure can result in multiple lesions. The eruption usually involves the limbs rather than the trunk and often occurs on mucous membranes.

Once the drug has been stopped, the lesions heal with scaling followed by pigmentation, which may be the only physical sign at the time the patient presents.

Table 56.2 Drugs causing urticaria/angio-oedema

Aspirin/NSAIDs
ACE inhibitors
Barbiturates
Imipramine
Indometacin
Iodine
Monoclonal antibodies
Paracetamol
Penicillins (less often cephalosporins)
Ranitidine
Serum, toxoids, pollen vaccines
Sulphonamides
Tartrazine, aspartame, colourings, preservatives

Table 56.3 Drugs causing fixed drug eruptions

ACE inhibitors
Barbiturates
Calcium channel blockers
Chlordiazepoxide
Dapsone
Dichloralphenazone
Griseofulvin
Indometacin
Meprobamate
Paracetamol
Phenolphthalein
Phenylbutazone
Phenytoin
Proton pump inhibitors
Quinine
Salicylates
Sulphonamides
Tetracyclines

The fixed drug eruption is possibly the only case of a drug-induced cutaneous reaction where oral rechallenge can be safely used to confirm the diagnosis and patch testing at the site of the eruption, but not elsewhere, is often positive. Topical corticosteroids may reduce the intensity of the reaction.

Photosensitivity

Drug-induced photosensitivity can be either phototoxic or photoallergic and can result from systemic or topical therapy (Table 56.4). Up to 8% of cutaneous drug reactions are photosensitivity eruptions. A widespread eruption suggests exposure to a systemic photosensitizing agent, whereas a local eruption indicates a reaction to a locally applied topical photosensitizer.

Phototoxic reactions resemble severe sunburn and can progress to blistering. They are dose dependent for drugs and sunlight, occur within a few hours of taking the drug and subside quickly on drug withdrawal.

Photoallergic rashes are usually eczematous, lichenoid, urticarial, bullous or purpuric. They are not dose dependent and occur at usual doses of sunlight and can be delayed in onset. Recovery is slow following drug withdrawal. In some cases photoallergy can persist for years after the drug was taken.

Patients receiving photosensitizing drugs should be counselled to avoid strong sunlight and to use a total sun block that contains a reflective substance such as titanium oxide. This is because most sunscreens only provide protection against medium-wavelength radiation (UVB), while it is the long-wavelength radiation (UVA) that is responsible for photosensitive reactions.

Pigmentation

Hyperpigmentation, hypopigmentation or discoloration can all be drug induced (Table 56.5). Pigmentation can be widespread or localized and can occasionally occur in internal organs.

Table 56.4   Drugs causing light-induced eruptions

Topical preparations
   Antihistamines
   Antiseptics: bithionol, hexachlorophene
   Coal tar derivatives
   Sunscreens

Systemic drugs
   Amiodarone
   Antihistamines
   Cinoxacin
   Diuretics: thiazides, furosemide
   Griseofulvin
   Nalidixic acid
   NSAIDs
   Phenothiazines
   Psoralens used therapeutically
   Retinoids
   St John's wort
   Sulphonamides
   Sulphonylureas
   Tetracyclines
   Tricyclic antidepressants

Table 56.5   Drugs causing skin pigmentation

Drug	Pigmentation
Amiodarone	Blue grey
Anticonvulsants (hydantoin derivatives)	Brown
Antimalarials	Blue grey
β-Blockers	Brown
Imatinib	Hypo/hyperpigmentation
Imipramine	Blue grey
Methyldopa	Brown
Oral contraceptives	Brown spots/patches
Phenothiazines	Brown/blue grey
Psoralens	Brown
Tetracyclines	Blue black

The mechanism of drug induction is not always known. In some cases the drug itself may be responsible or it may induce a disturbance in melanin pigmentation.

Nail changes

Nail discoloration can be drug induced. Blue nails can result from therapy with mepacrine and blue-black nails from cytotoxic drugs and minocycline. Potassium permanganate solutions will dye nails brown, and white nails can result from therapy with antitumour agents.

Photo-onycholysis (separation of the nail from the nail plate associated with UVA radiation) can be exacerbated by oral contraceptives and tetracyclines. Cytotoxic agents may induce onycholysis by direct toxicity to the matrix whilst drug-induced psoriasis may cause nail pitting.

Hair disorders

Drug-induced alopecia

Drug-induced alopecia (Table 56.6) may be partial or complete and can involve sites other than the scalp, but the scalp is commonly affected. Hair loss may occur rapidly, as the drug affects the active 'anagen' growth. The most severe loss usually occurs with cytotoxic therapy; it begins shortly after administration of the drug and the effect is dose dependent and fortunately reversible, but a delay of several weeks is common before regrowth begins. The hair loss in patients receiving paclitaxel has unique characteristics. Hair loss is sudden and complete and many patients experience loss of all body hair, including axillary and pubic hair, eyelashes and eyebrows. The loss of body hair often occurs with cumulative therapy and is more severe after longer

Table 56.6 Drugs causing hair disorders

Alopecia

Acetretin
Anticoagulants
Anticonvulsants
Antithyroid drugs
β-Blockers
Withdrawal of oral contraceptives
Cytotoxic drugs
Etretinate
Gold salts
Interferons
Leflunomide
Lithium
Retinoids
Sodium valproate
Tacrolimus

Hirsutism/hypertrichosis

Acetazolamide
Anabolic steroids
Androgens
Corticosteroids (topical and systemic)
Ciclosporin
Danazol
Diazoxide
Dihydrotestosterone
Minoxidil
Nifedipine
Oral contraceptives
Penicillamine
Phenytoin
Tamoxifen
Verapamil

infusion times. Interferons have also been reported to produce hair loss.

Hair loss can occur 2–4 months after a drug is initiated, if it affects the 'telogen' phase of hair growth when hair is shed and new growth in the hair follicle begins. Alopecia of this type usually affects the scalp and may or may not be noticeable, depending on the proportion of follicles involved.

Drugs with androgen activity can induce male-pattern baldness and this can also occur with the oestrogen receptor antagonist tamoxifen.

Hirsutism and hypertrichosis

Hirsutism is excessive hairiness, especially in women, in the male pattern of hair growth, while hypertrichosis is the growth of hair at sites not normally hairy. Both conditions can be drug induced and in some cases the same drug can produce both patterns of hair growth (see Table 56.6). If it is not possible to withdraw the drug and there is no suitable alternative, then these patients should have this fully explained to them and be advised to use a depilatory cream if necessary. This particular side effect of minoxidil has been exploited in the treatment of male pattern baldness.

Some drugs can induce both alopecia and hirsutism. For example, the hydantoin anticonvulsants can cause alopecia of the scalp and hirsutism of the body. This occurs mainly in young women.

Severe and life-threatening drug-induced skin disorders

Erythema multiforme, Stevens–Johnson syndrome and toxic epidermal necrolysis

Erythema multiforme was initially described as an acute self-limited skin disease; when severe and life threatening, it was usually called Stevens–Johnson syndrome. Toxic epidermal necrolysis was considered to be a separate disorder. More recently, these drug-related severe diseases are considered to represent variants within a continuous spectrum of disease and some experts have proposed a new classification in which they separate Stevens–Johnson syndrome from erythema multiforme, adding it to toxic epidermal necrolysis.

Erythema multiforme

Erythema multiforme, as the name implies, can present in a variety of patterns. The usual erythematous lesions occur in crops on the hands and feet more often than on the trunk. Each maculopapular lesion increases in size, leaving a cyanotic centre that produces an 'iris' or 'target' lesion. The lesions appear over a few days, reaching a diameter of 1 or 2 cm within 48 hours. They may blister and can reach a size of up to 10 cm. They usually fade within 1 or 2 weeks of stopping the drug. Healing occurs without scarring although hyperpigmentation may persist for a long time. Involvement of the mucous membranes is common and the mouth, eyes and genitalia may be affected to varying degrees. Infections, for example herpes simplex, are a more common cause of erythema multiforme than drugs. When the condition is suspected all medicines, especially those introduced within the past month, should be stopped as there is a risk of progression to Stevens–Johnson syndrome or toxic epidermal necrolysis.

Stevens–Johnson syndrome

Stevens–Johnson syndrome comprises extensive erythema multiforme of the trunk and limbs with severe blistering and mucosal lesions. There is also systemic involvement, with fever, malaise, polyarthritis and diarrhoea. There have been case reports of haematuria and renal failure

Drugs are the most common cause of the Stevens–Johnson syndrome and all suspected drugs should be stopped as the disease has a mortality rate of approximately 5–15% without treatment. Rechallenge is never justifiable. Treatment with systemic steroids produces a rapid response in both erythema multiforme and the Stevens–Johnson syndrome (Table 56.7).

Toxic epidermal necrolysis

Toxic epidermal necrolysis (Lyell's syndrome) is a rare condition but with a mortality of approximately 33%. The main

Table 56.7 Drugs causing erythema multiforme and Stevens–Johnson syndrome

Barbiturates
Carbamazepine
Cimetidine
Dapsone
Ethosuximide
Gold salts
Isoniazid
Lamotrigine
Leflunomide
Macrolides
Mefloquine
NSAIDs
Penicillins
Phenytoin
Propranolol
Rifampicin
Nearly 200 other drugs have also been implicated.

Table 56.8 Drugs causing toxic epidermal necrolysis

Allopurinol
Barbiturates
Dapsone
Gold salts
Lamotrigine
Leflunomide
NSAIDs
Penicillins
Phenolphthalein
Phenylbutazone
Phenytoin
Sulphonamides
Tetracyclines

cause of toxic epidermal necrolysis in adults is drug therapy (Table 56.8). In children it is a phage type II staphylococcal infection, referred to as the staphylococcal scalded skin syndrome. A higher incidence of toxic epidermal necrolysis is reported in immunocompromised patients with systemic lupus erythematosus (SLE) and HIV.

The antiepileptic drug phenytoin is a known causative agent. More recently, lamotrigine has produced serious skin reactions including Stevens–Johnson syndrome and toxic epidermal necrolysis, with an increased risk in children and with the concomitant use of valproate.

Lyell's syndrome frequently has a prodromal phase of malaise sometimes accompanied by a sore throat and fever. The skin reaction starts with large areas of erythema involving most of the skin surface and is followed by a bullous (a large blister containing serous fluid) phase in which the epidermis peels off. This stage is complicated by fluid loss, septicaemia and bronchopneumonia. Mucous membrane involvement may precede the skin eruption by 10–14 days, giving a clinical appearance similar to the Stevens–Johnson syndrome.

Diagnosis is made clinically and from a skin biopsy. In drug-induced toxic epidermal necrolysis there is separation of the basal layer of the epidermis. In staphylococcal scalded skin syndrome, separation occurs in the granular layer without necrolysis. Drug rechallenge is never used to confirm a diagnosis. The patient with toxic epidermal necrolysis will require full intensive care support, preferably in a specialist burns unit, and antibiotic treatment at the first signs of sepsis. Corticosteroids are not indicated as these may increase mortality. The benefits of intravenous immunoglobulins and immunosuppressive agents such as cyclophosphamaide are still to be confirmed but appear promising.

Drug hypersensitivity syndrome

Drug eruption with eosinophilia and systemic symptoms (drug hypersensitivity syndrome) is a distinct severe and potentially fatal drug-induced skin disorder. It is almost exclusively associated with the anticonvulsants and sulfonamides but has been reported with other drugs.

It is characterized by eruption, fever, lymph node enlargement and internal organ involvement. It occurs in a delayed fashion, 3–8 weeks after starting the drug for the first time.

The mortality is estimated at near 10% but recovery can be total and the causative drug must be stopped as soon as possible to avoid progression of symptoms. In contrast to toxic epidermal necrolysis, corticosteroids may be useful.

Vasculitis

Vasculitis is inflammation in vessel walls. Several drugs can induce both systemic vasculitis with cutaneous manifestations, and cutaneous vasculitis without other organ involvement.

Drugs cause approximately 10% of vasculitic skin lesions and should be considered in any patient with small vesssel vasculitis (Table 56.9). Withdrawal of the causative drug is often sufficient to resolve the clinical manifestations without the need for treatment with systemic corticosteroids or more powerful immunosuppressants.

Table 56.9	Drugs that may cause cutaneous vasculitic reactions
Allopurinol
Aspirin
β-Lactam antibiotics
Carpamazepine
Carbimazole
Diltiazem
Erythromycin
Furosemide
Gold
Haematopoietic growth factors (G-CSF and GM-CSF)
Hydralazine
Interferons
Methotrexate
Minocycline
NSAIDs
Penicillamine
Propylthiouracil
Retinoids
Sulfasalazine
Sulphonamides
Thiazides
Thrombolytic agents

Table 56.10	Drugs causing systemic lupus erythematosus
Antiepileptics, e.g. phenytoin, primidone, ethosuximide
β-Adrenoceptor blockers
Chlorpromazine
Griseofulvin
Hydralazine
Isoniazid
Lithium
Methyldopa
Oral contraceptives
Penicillamine
Procainamide
Propylthiouracil
Sulfasalazine

The cutaneous manifestation of drug-induced systemic lupus erythematosus is the characteristic butterfly-shaped rash on the face. There may also be a rash on the neck and backs of the hands. Laboratory tests for antinuclear factor and lupus cells may be positive and the erythrocyte sedimentation rate may be elevated. Cerebral and renal involvement is rare. In some cases antinuclear antibodies occur without clinical manifestations.

Clinical manifestations of the systemic lupus erythematosus syndrome are predominant in women but the occurrence of antinuclear antibodies shows no preference for gender. The syndrome is usually reversible if the drug is withdrawn, although the antinuclear factor may persist for several months.

Skin necrosis

Necrosis can follow the extravasation of irritant drugs, particularly cytotoxic agents. Anticoagulants, both oral and heparin, can produce a severe haemorrhagic skin necrosis. Other causes of necrosis include the severe impairment of skin circulation which is occasionally produced by β-blockers, the synergistic effects of certain antitumour drugs with radiotherapy, and the topical application of gentian violet and brilliant green.

Skin malignancy

Skin malignancy is an increasing concern. Its growing prevalence is associated with exposure to sunlight, but also with increased immunocompromised populations, for example HIV patients.

Immunosuppressive drugs will facilitate the development of malignant and premalignant skin lesions. Azathioprine was believed to have a specific risk in organ transplantation because ultraviolet light leads to breakdown of the drug into mutagenic products. However, it has been shown that patients treated with

Erythema nodosum

Erythema nodosum is an acute inflammatory reaction with painful subcutaneous nodules, usually limited to the extremities. Transient erythema may precede the lesions.

Erythema nodosum is usually a complication of infection and is not commonly drug induced. However, it has been observed in women taking oral contraceptives and with other drugs such as sulfonamides, salicylates, penicillins and gold salts.

Systemic lupus erythematosus

Syndromes indistinguishable from systemic lupus erythematosus (SLE) may occur following drug administration (Table 56.10). It is not clear if drugs cause this by initiating the disease or by triggering it in predisposed patients.

ciclosporin but not azathioprine have a similar risk of skin malignancy. This suggests the skin cancer risk is mainly a result of reduced immune surveillance and human papilloma virus infection.

Malignancy shows significant latency, and caution has been expressed over the use of the very potent new generation of immunosuppressive agents such as the anti-TNF-α drugs. However, these drugs are proving to be very effective in otherwise highly disabling disease.

Immunosuppressive drugs are not directly photoallergenic. However, all patients receiving immunosuppressive therapies should be counselled on the risk of malignancy and advised to avoid exposure to sunlight, and those on long-term therapy should be monitored for skin lesions.

General conditions

Eczematous eruptions

An eczematous eruption may occur during systemic drug therapy, or it may develop as a result of allergy to a topical preparation (allergic contact dermatitis) or by direct contact with a primary irritant (contact dermatitis) (Table 56.11).

The skin lesions are characterized by redness with widespread exfoliation (peeling) and intense itching. Small blisters can develop, especially in contact dermatitis, that burst and weep exudate.

Primary irritant dermatitis is essentially a major public health problem although certain topical drugs, e.g. tar and dithranol, are primary irritants. However, allergic contact dermatitis is a common complication of topical therapy, for example persistent dermatitis from medication or dressings used to treat leg ulcers. It can be caused by the drug or any of the excipients of the preparation. Patch testing of all ingredients of a topical preparation is used to find the causative agent.

Cross-sensitivity reactions can occur when an eczematous eruption or anaphylaxis develops after administration of a systemic drug in a patient previously sensitized by topical application. Cross-sensitivity is one of the major reasons for not using topical antibiotics. Cases of cross-sensitivity have also been reported in patients and medical staff who handle systemic formulations of known sensitizers such as chlorpromazine.

Patch testing can be used to confirm a diagnosis of drug-induced dermatitis and treatment is the same as that used for idiopathic eczema and involves use of emollients and topical steroids.

Acneiform eruptions

Acne is a common complaint but is rarely drug induced. Drugs can, however, produce acne-like eruptions or aggravate existing acne (Table 56.12). The lesions are usually papular but no comedones (blackheads) are present.

Psoriasiform eruptions

Drugs can either exacerbate psoriasis in predisposed patients or induce psoriasiform rashes in previously unaffected patients (Table 56.13).

Table 56.11 Drugs causing eczematous eruptions

Local anaesthetics
Antibiotics, especially neomycin, streptomycin, chloramphenicol
Antihistamines
Antiseptics
Atropine
Captopril
Carbamazepine
Ethylenediamine (in aminophylline)
Gold salts
Imidazole antifungal drugs
Lanolin
Preservatives in creams and ointments
Methyldopa
Phenothiazines
Phenylbutazone
Phenytoin
Quinine, quinidine
Sulphonamides
Sulfonylureas
Thiazide diuretics

The psoriasiform eruptions mimic psoriasis and are characterized by itchy, scaly red patches on the elbows, forearms, knees, legs and scalp.

Vesicular and bullous eruptions

Vesiculobullous eruptions are termed 'pemphigoid' unless they are associated with specific skin conditions, e.g. erythema multiforme.

A vesicle is a blister filled with serum with a diameter up to 0.5 cm. If larger than this it is termed a bulla.

Pemphigoid reactions can be autoimmune or drug induced (Table 56.14). When drug induced, they can be part of a fixed drug eruption or generalized, as for example the large bullae that are seen in patients with barbiturate poisoning. The eruptions will resolve with drug withdrawal although they can persist for up to 2 years.

Table 56.12   Drugs causing acne
Androgens (in women)
Corticosteroids and ACTH (inlcuding inhaled preparations)
Ciclosporin
Ethambutol
Haloperidol
Isoniazid
Lithium
Oral contraceptives
Phenobarbital
Phenytoin
Propylthiouracil (resembling acne rosacea)
Topical corticosteroids (perioral dermatitis)
Quinine, quinidine (papular eruptions)

Table 56.14   Drugs causing vesicular and bullous eruptions
Azapropazone
Barbiturates (may be associated with drug-induced coma)
Captopril
Furosemide
Iodides
Nalidixic acid (phototoxic)
NSAIDs
Penicillamine
Phenylbutazone
Rifampicin
Salicylates
Sulfonamides

Table 56.13   Drugs causing psoriasiform eruptions
Aspirin
ACE inhibitors
β-Blockers (most frequently atenolol, oxprenolol and propranolol)
Chloroquine
G-CSF
Gold
Iodides
Lithium
NSAIDs
TNF-α antagonists
Withdrawal of topical steroids

Table 56.15   Drugs causing lichenoid eruptions
Aspirin
ACE inhibitors
β-Blockers
Carbamazepine
Chloroquine
Ethambutol
Gold salts
Interferon-α
Lithium
Mepacrine
Methyldopa
NSAIDs
Penicillamine
Phenothiazines
Quinidine
Quinine
Sulphonylureas

Lichenoid eruptions

Drug-induced lichenoid eruptions (Table 56.15) closely resemble lichen planus, occurring as flat mauve lesions, but they may be atypical, showing marked scaling. The lesions are found mainly on the forearms, neck and on the inner surface of the thighs. The mouth may be involved, and hair loss can occur.

The pathogenic mechanism is unknown. It is not allergic and is probably dose dependent.

The eruptions resolve with drug withdrawal, with or without topical steroids, but hyperpigmentation may remain. There is also a possibility of late malignancy.

Purpura

Purpura is a rash resulting from bleeding into the skin from capillaries. It can be caused by drug-induced thrombocytopenia or result from drugs that damage blood vessels (non-thrombocytopenic or vascular purpura). It can also occur with the hypocoagulation associated with reduced circulating clotting factors. In the latter case, drug interactions with the anticoagulants can be a cause.

Patient care

All adverse effects to drugs should be taken seriously. Rashes, even the less serious with no systemic involvement, are distressing, often irritant and disfiguring. Their presence can be indicative of drug allergy which can become more significant on drug rechallenge. It is therefore important to find the drug cause so patients are made aware and can report and avoid the sensitivity.

Treatment is symptomatic with oral antihistamines and corticosteroids (unless the patient is immunocompromised). In severe reactions intensive care support may be required but outcomes are usually favourable if the causative drug is promptly withdrawn. Patients should be reassured about the self-limiting nature of the disorder, and that disfigurement is unusual.

CASE STUDIES

Case 56.1

A female patient undergoing treatment for chronic hepatitis C presents with alopecia universalis – complete hair loss extending to the whole body. The patient is infected with genotype 1 and the alopecia occurred during the second half of an 8-week course of therapy.

Questions

1. What is the likely cause of the alopecia?
2. What treatment should be advised?

Answers

1. This lady will be receiving interferon and ribavarin therapy for her hepatitis C infection. Hair disorders have often been described during interferon therapy, which include reversible hair discoloration, hypertrichosis and alopecia. Ribavarin is reported to cause a photoallergic reaction.
2. Although alopecia universalis is very distressing, the patient should be counselled to complete her course of interferon if possible as the alopecia is reversible and hair regrowth is complete. Given the benign reversible nature of this side effect in patients who achieve a virological response, it is important to complete treatment with interferon to prevent disease relapse.

Case 56.2

A 69-year-old male patient with a history of erosive lichen planus on his feet and hands had been lesion free for 6 months. Two weeks following a myocardial infarction the erosive lesions on his palms and feet recurred.

He had been started on aspirin 75 mg once daily, atenolol 100 mg each morning, ramipril 2.5 mg each morning and simvastatin 40 mg at night.

Questions

1. What is the likely reason for the recurrence of the lichen planus?
2. How should this be treated?

Answers

1. The patient's lichen planus could have recurred spontaneously but is probably secondary to atenolol or ramipril.
2. Since lichen planus can be extensive and may be linked with or develop into an exfoliative dermatitis, the causative agent should be stopped. Atenolol is the likeliest cause and must be stopped. Ramipril could also be implicated, so stopping this and starting an angiotensin receptor blocker would be an appropriate plan. The lichen planus can be treated with topical tacrolimus.

Case 56.3

A 37-year-old man presents with swelling of his lips and face, noticeably his eyelids. He asks if this could be stress induced as he has had several previous episodes of localized swelling of the face over the last 6–12 months.

He has been taking bendroflumethazide and enalapril for hypertension for the last 3 years, but has not taken any other medications recently.

Questions

1. What condition do his symptoms suggest?
2. Could this be drug induced?
3. How should the condition be treated?

Answers

1. This pattern of non-pitting oedema of the face is characteristic of angio-oedema.
2. Angio-oedema is a known adverse effect of ACE inhibitors with an overall incidence of 0.5–1%. Although this commonly occurs in the first week of treatment, delayed-onset angio-oedema can occur even after many years of treatment. Predisposing factors for the development of angio-oedema include: complement C1 esterase inhibitor deficiency; African origin; a previous history of angio-oedema and possibly poor compliance.
3. Since angio-oedema can be life threatening any suspect drug should be stopped. There is a very low incidence of this occurring with an angiotensin 2 receptor blocker and this may be a suitable alternative for this patient. The acute presentation of angio-oedema is treated with antihistamine and corticosteroids. If the patient presents with respiratory symptoms subcutaneous epinephrine is indicated.

Case 56.4

Miss AF is a 15-year-old, 6 weeks post renal transplant patient. She is very distressed about the growth of facial hair and the worsening of acne.

Questions

1. What are the possible causes of Miss AF's skin complaints?
2. How might these conditions be treated?

Answers

1. It is likely that Miss AF is receiving transplant immunosuppression that includes ciclosporin and prednisolone. The ciclosporin is most likely to

have caused the growth of facial hair. The prednisolone could have worsened the acne, or this may be normal adolescent acne made worse by Miss AF's improved health. Ciclosporin could also be a causative agent for her acne.

2. Hirsutism was a side effect of ciclosporin that many young transplant patients had to cope with and depilatory creams had to be used. It is now possible that a switch to tacrolimus could be considered if the patient finds this side effect distressing. The prednisolone is low dose in transplantation. It will eventually be reduced to a maintenance dose, and could be stopped in most cases if acne were still a problem. Topical acne preparations and, if necessary, oral antibiotics can be used to treat the acne.

REFERENCES

Bigby M 2001 Rates of cutaneous reactions to drugs. Archives of Dermatology 137: 765-770

De Raevel L, Song M, Van Maldergen L 1988 Adverse cutaneous drug reactions in AIDS. British Journal of Dermatology 119: 521

Fitzpatrick T B, Johnson R A, Wolff K et al 2001 Color atlas and synopsis of clinical dermatology: common and serious disease, 4th edn. McGraw-Hill, New York

Loke Y K, Price D, Derry S, Aronson J K 2006 Case reports of suspected adverse drug reactions – systematic literature survey of follow up. British Medical Journal 332: 335-339

FURTHER READING

Aronson J K (ed) 2006 Meyler's side effects of drugs: the international encyclopedia of adverse drug reactions and interactions, 15th edn. Elsevier, Amsterdam

Breathnach S M, Hintner L 1992 Adverse drug reactions and the skin. Blackwell Scientific, Oxford

Ernst E 2000 Adverse effects of herbal drugs in dermatology. British Journal of Dermatology 143: 923-929

Wolf R, Orion E, Marcos B et al 2005 Life-threatening acute adverse cutaneous drug reactions. Clinics in Dermatology 23: 171-181

57 Eczema and psoriasis

M. M. Carr

Eczema and psoriasis are common inflammatory skin disorders that have some similarities and may sometimes be difficult to distinguish from each other in practice. Both may respond to some of the same treatments, and both can be functionally and socially disabling. However, they are distinct diseases with different causes, occurring in different groups of people.

ECZEMA

The terms 'eczema' and 'dermatitis' may be used interchangeably and describe the same clinical and histological entity. Both words are derived from the Greek: 'eczema', meaning 'to boil', describes the characteristic tiny bubble-like blisters of the condition, and 'dermatitis' means 'inflammation of the skin'. There are several patterns of the condition. A common convention is to describe as 'eczema' those that are endogenous or constitutional and as 'dermatitis' those that are exogenous or due to contact.

Pathophysiology and clinical features

The histological features of eczema/dermatitis are similar, regardless of cause, and differ in the acute and chronic phases. In the acute stage, fluid escapes from dilated dermal blood vessels to produce oedema, or swelling, in the epidermis. This collects into vesicles or tiny blisters, particularly where the skin is thick, as on the palms and soles. These vesicles may coalesce into larger blisters. Where the skin is thinner they tend to rupture onto the skin surface, causing exudation and crusting. The chronic stage

shows less oedema and vesiculation and more thickening of the epidermis and horny layers, produced by prolonged rubbing and scratching by the sufferer. Both stages are accompanied by a heavy inflammatory cell infiltration of the dermis and epidermis. These histological features are mirrored by the clinical picture; the different types of eczema/dermatitis have a number of features in common, although they vary in other ways according to their cause, site and severity.

Acute eczema/dermatitis

Acute eczema/dermatitis is characterized by a progression through a number of stages:

- red, hot, swollen and itchy skin
- papules and tiny blisters, sometimes coalescing to form large ones (called pompholyx on the palms and soles)
- exudation and crusting
- scaling.

Chronic eczema/dermatitis

In addition to the features listed above, chronic eczema/dermatitis may show:

- drier skin, becoming more scaly
- lichenification (dry, thickened, leathery skin with exaggerated skin markings, due to rubbing and scratching) (Fig. 57.1)
- painful fissures.

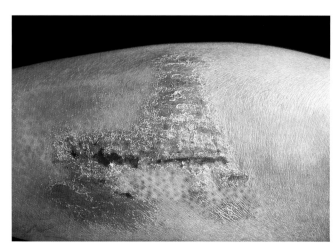

Figure 57.1 Dry, excoriated, lichenified chronic eczema.

Clinical types

Atopic eczema

Atopic eczema is a common condition affecting about 20% of children, the majority of whom recover before their teens, and 2–4% of adults. The tendency to this type of eczema is determined by a combination of genetic, environmental and immunological factors, with 70% of sufferers having a family history of atopy (one or more of eczema, asthma or hayfever). Between 30% and 50% of eczema patients will also develop asthma or hayfever.

At the cellular and molecular level, atopic eczema is characterized by activation of Langerhans cells in the epidermis by antigen/IgE complexes and presentation of the complexes to T-lymphocytes in the skin. A variety of inflammatory mediators are also produced by other cells in the skin, stimulated by a number of enzymes and intracellular processes. The inflammatory mediators cause the tissue reaction and destruction which produce the clinical features of atopic eczema.

Atopic eczema is typically symmetrical in distribution and affects particularly the face and flexures, such as the fronts of the elbows and wrists and backs of the knees (Fig. 57.2), although it may also affect the hands and feet or become generalized (erythroderma). The flexures tend to become lichenified as the child becomes older, and the skin is generally very dry and itchy. On the palms and soles, where the skin is naturally thick, an intensely itchy sago-like eruption known as pompholyx may occur, consisting of numerous tiny intact vesicles.

Atopic patients produce antigen-specific circulating IgE antibodies to allergens such as house dust mite, pollens, other inhalants, and foods such as dairy products. Scratch or prick testing to these allergens is unreliable; there is a high false-positive rate with this method, and it is becoming less popular. A more reliable method of detection is by radio-allergosorbent testing (RAST), although here too false-positive tests are common; the results may not necessarily be relevant to the state of an individual's eczema but may be a better reflection of allergies related to asthma or hayfever. For these reasons, allergy testing is not carried out routinely on atopics.

Provoking factors

A number of factors may aggravate atopic eczema, but none should be regarded as the sole cause of the problem.

- Dryness and extremes of temperature may increase itch, and so cause scratching.
- Inhalant and food allergens can produce similar effects.
- Irritants such as soap and water may have their effect, either by increasing dryness or by a direct effect on skin cells, having penetrated through fissures.
- Allergic contact dermatitis may complicate atopic eczema as loss of the natural lipid barrier function makes the entry of allergens into the skin easier.
- In older children, teenagers and adults, stress is a common exacerbating factor.

Probably the single most potent cause of a sudden deterioration in atopic eczema is infection, either bacterial or viral; atopics have impaired cell-mediated immunity, making them particularly prone to this problem. The most troublesome organisms are *Staphylococcus aureus,* herpes simplex virus and varicella. Milder viral infections such as warts and molluscum contagiosum are also very common (Figs 57.3, 57.4).

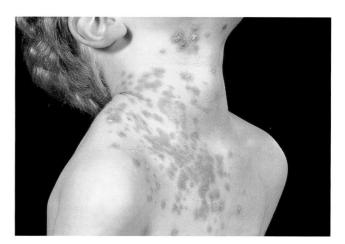

Figure 57.3 Impetigo complicating atopic eczema.

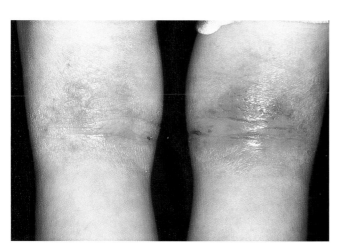

Figure 57.2 Flexural eczema in childhood.

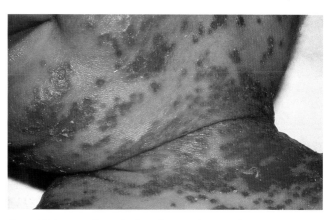

Figure 57.4 Typical 'punched-out' lesions of eczema herpeticum in an atopic baby.

Contact dermatitis

Two types of contact dermatitis exist: in the first, the rash is caused by an allergy to an external substance (cell-mediated immune or type IV reaction); in the second, the cause is wear and tear and/or irritation.

Allergic contact dermatitis

A large number of compounds found in daily life, both in the home and at work, may be responsible for allergic contact dermatitis. Common culprits are:

- metals, e.g. nickel
- topical medicaments (including antibiotics, antihistamines and local anaesthetics), cream and ointment bases and preservatives
- dyes
- plants
- rubber compounds
- in industry, resins, plastics and cement frequently cause problems (Fig. 57.5).

The dermatitis rarely starts after the patient's first exposure to the allergen, and there may be months or years of contact before the reaction occurs.

The first and most important step in the diagnosis of contact allergy is to take a detailed history and note the pattern and distribution of the rash; this will frequently establish the cause. Common patterns include dermatitis under metal fastenings in clothes such as zips and jeans studs (nickel allergy) and under rubber gloves. A rash around the eyes may indicate airborne allergens from plants, nail varnish or strike-anywhere matches (which release phosphorus sesquisulfide vapour), or allergens in local applications of medicaments. Make-up allergy is surprisingly uncommon. If the allergy is severe or uncontrolled, the dermatitis may extend to other areas of the skin and occasionally become generalized.

If confirmation or further investigation is required, patch testing may be useful, unlike skin tests in other types of eczema. A battery of possible allergens is applied to uninvolved skin, usually the back, in small quantities at the appropriate concentration and in the correct vehicle. The skin is examined for an eczematous reaction under the test patches at 48 hours and 96 hours, which indicates delayed hypersensitivity.

Once an allergy has been confirmed, the patient must avoid the allergen, since this type of allergy is lifelong and the dermatitis is likely to persist as long as contact continues.

Primary irritant dermatitis

This is the most common cause of hand eczema and is seen particularly in housewives, nurses, hairdressers, caterers, and those who work with oils and greases in industry. Contact with anything that dehydrates the skin, particularly water, detergents and soaps, and solvents, removes the natural protective oils from the skin, allowing evaporation of water and penetration of irritants. The longer the skin is exposed to such insults, the more likely is the development of dermatitis. Atopics are particularly prone to this problem, especially on the hands.

No allergy is involved in this type of dermatitis and therefore patch testing is not usually indicated unless a co-existing allergy is suspected or needs to be excluded.

Other eczemas

Seborrhoeic eczema

This involves the areas of the body with a high density of sebaceous glands, i.e. the face, scalp and upper trunk, and occurs after puberty, when these glands become active (Fig. 57.6). It is due to an overgrowth of *Pityrosporum ovale,* a yeast that is a normal commensal on the skin. The skin is red, with greasy yellow scales, and the scalp shows severe dandruff.

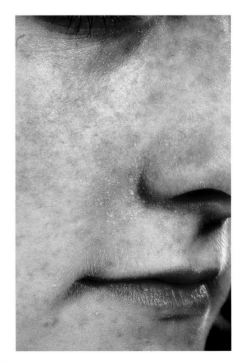

Figure 57.6 Seborrhoeic eczema in a teenager.

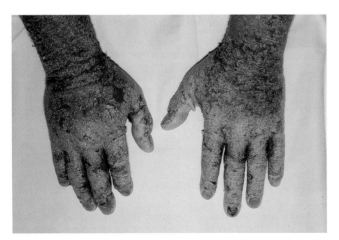

Figure 57.5 Contact dermatitis to cement in a building worker.

An infantile version of the disease may occur in the first months of life, causing 'cradle cap' on the scalp and a shiny red rash in the folds of the skin and in the napkin area. This recovers in a few weeks or months.

Discoid eczema

As the name suggests, this occurs in circular patches. These characteristically occur on the forearms and lower legs, and are intensely itchy. As a result, they are frequently excoriated and become secondarily infected.

Varicose/stasis eczema

This is usually the result of varicose veins, venous stasis and oedema in the lower leg, particularly around the ankle, and may progress to varicose ulceration. The patient with varicose eczema is particularly at risk of developing allergic contact dermatitis to topical medicaments such as antibiotics and vehicles, and to rubber in compression bandages.

Asteatotic eczema

This means 'lacking in oil' and is typically found in the elderly, in whom the skin becomes overdry, perhaps aggravated by the use of soap.

Treatment

The same basic principles of treatment apply regardless of the type of eczema.

Emollients

The mainstay of eczema treatment is the use of liberal quantities of moisturizers as, in all types, the basic problem is the loss or deficiency of the skin's lipid layer. Adequate use of emollients will reduce the requirement for topical steroid, both in quantity and potency. Soap should be avoided if at all possible, and a soap substitute such as an emollient cream should be applied before, during and after bathing or showering. In addition, a bath oil or emulsifying ointment added to the water may be very helpful in hydrating the skin. Despite long-established clinical experience, there have been very few controlled trials to confirm the effectiveness of emollients (Charman 2000).

If the patient is prone to secondary infection of the skin, reinfection via organisms in the emollient tub may be avoided by supplying a preparation in a pump dispenser.

It is very important that sufficient quantities of moisturizer be supplied; the minimum weekly requirement for an infant is 50 g, for a 10 year old 100 g, and for an adult 200 g.

Topical corticosteroids

Eczema is an inflammatory and immunologically mediated condition, so specific treatment must be anti-inflammatory and directed at modifying the immune response, which in many cases means corticosteroids, normally used topically.

Topical steroids, developed over the past 50 years, have revolutionized the treatment of inflammatory dermatoses, particularly the eczemas. Modification of the first compound, hydrocortisone, has produced large numbers of more potent drugs. Unfortunately, with time and increasingly extensive usage of topical fluorinated steroids, it is apparent that the greater the potency of the steroid, the greater its potential for adverse effects (Table 57.1). Epidermal atrophy (thinning), telangiectasia (prominent surface blood vessels), striae (stretch marks) and premature ageing due to collagen loss, rosacea and exacerbation of skin infection are frequently seen. Rarely, pituitary–adrenal axis suppression may occur, and reduced growth rates in children after prolonged use have been reported. As a result of publicity in both the medical and popular press during the 1970s and 1980s, primary care doctors and their patients are now only too well aware of the potential hazards of steroid usage. This can result in some patients receiving inadequate treatment. Others may use topical steroids inappropriately as emollients. The aim of topical steroid therapy is to control the eczema using a potent application if necessary, under close medical supervision, and then to maintain control using a drug of the lowest effective potency.

Choice of preparation

Potency Topical steroids are classified by potency into four groups:

- very potent (group 1) – Dermovate, Halciderm Topical, Nerisone Forte
- potent (group 2) – betametasone valerate 0.1%, Betacap, Bettamousse, Betnovate, Cutivate, Diprosone, Elocon, Locoid, Locoid Crelo, Metosyn, Nerisone, Propaderm, Synalar
- moderately potent (group 3) – Betnovate RD, Eumovate, Haelan, Modrasone, Synalar 1 in 4 dilution, Ultralanum Plain
- mildly potent (group 4) – hydrocortisone 0.1–2.5%, Dioderm, Efcortelan, Mildison.

The clinical potency generally correlates with the frequency and severity of adverse effects after prolonged usage. The newer potent steroids appear to have lower potential for systemic absorption

Table 57.1 Side effects of topical steroids

Local	Systemic
Skin atrophy, striae	Suppression of pituitary–adrenal axis
Telangiectasia	Growth retardation in children
Increased susceptibility to skin infection	Osteoporosis
Contact allergy to steroids	
Rosacea	
Tachyphylaxis	
Rebound of eczema on steroid withdrawal	

and may produce fewer long-term side effects, but this has yet to be fully evaluated in long-term studies. However, they do have the advantage of being effective in once-daily applications, which is convenient for the user. Group 4 steroids are most suitable for use on thin skin, such as the face and flexures, and for maintenance therapy in children. Preparations of increased potency may be needed to control acute exacerbations of the eczema and on areas where the horny layer and epidermis are naturally thicker, for example on the palms of the hands and soles of the feet.

Base Topical steroids are available in ointment, cream and oily cream formulations and as aqueous or alcoholic lotions, gel and mousse for use on the scalp. In general, dry eczemas should be treated with ointments and weeping areas with creams. Where the scalp is inflamed or excoriated an alcoholic lotion may be uncomfortable and the use of a cream or mousse preparation preferred.

Allergies Some constituents of the bases can occasionally cause allergic reactions. The most common culprits are propylene glycol and lanolin in ointments, and parabens, ethylene diamine and chlorocresol in creams. In addition, allergy to the steroid molecules is being increasingly recognized. These factors must be taken into account when choosing a preparation for a particular patient.

Antibiotic/antiseptic additives Chronic low-grade infection is common in eczema and dermatitis, and this may be exacerbated by using a steroid alone. Significant infection is best managed with oral antibiotics. Topical steroid/antibiotic combinations should be avoided as the topical antibiotics can prove to be potent sensitizers, although chlortetracycline is an exception. Chronic infection can be controlled using a topical steroid/clioquinol combination of appropriate potency, which is antiseptic rather than antibiotic.

Quantities

It is important to monitor the topical steroid consumption of the patient, to ensure that there is not overusage and, equally, that treatment is adequate. In many cases only localized areas of the body need treatment but in a widespread eczema, an adult may need up to 170 g per week for a twice-daily application, and an infant 35 g (Table 57.2).

Table 57.2 Minimum quantity (grams) of topical application required for twice-daily treatment for 1 week

Age	Whole body	Trunk	Both arms and legs
6 months	35	15	20
4 years	60	20	35
8 years	90	35	50
12 years	120	45	65
Adult (70 kg)	170	60	90

Other topical immunomodulators

Recently two calcineurin inhibitors have been introduced as topical agents for the treatment of atopic eczema. As calcineurin is a cytoplasmic enzyme involved in the activation of T-lymphocytes, it plays an important role in the initiation of immune inflammation. Therefore inhibition of calcineurin has an anti-inflammatory effect.

The macrolide antibiotics, tacrolimus and pimecrolimus, are of sufficiently low molecular weight to penetrate the stratum corneum of the skin, particularly when its barrier function is impaired in eczema. They do not produce cutaneous atrophy, even with long-term application, so they can be more readily used on face and flexures than topical steroids. Their greatest value appears to be the control and maintenance of eczema in a steady state. Concerns about their use and long-term side effects are mainly related to possible increase in skin infections, skin cancer and lymphoma. Infection rates in trials to date are no higher than expected and the risk of skin cancer remains under review.

Tacrolimus

In comparative trials, tacrolimus has been shown to be comparable in efficacy to potent (group 2) topical steroids such as betametasone valerate (Hanifin et al 2001) and in children superior to hydrocortisone acetate 1% (Reitamo et al 2002). It is available only as an ointment. At the beginning of treatment it may produce a burning sensation in the skin; however, this rarely disturbs the patient greatly and wears off with continued use. Systemic absorption is negligible.

Pimecrolimus

This agent is less potent than tacrolimus but penetrates the stratum corneum more efficiently. It is available as a cream. Pimecrolimus appears to inhibit flares of atopic eczema, and reduces the requirement for topical steroids to control acute episodes (Kapp et al 2002).

Antibiotics

Wherever possible, swabs should be taken from infected skin before starting oral antibiotics. The antibiotic of choice to cover *Staphylococcus aureus* is normally erythromycin or flucloxacillin, which should be given for a minimum of 10 days. Chronic infection may occasionally require long-term treatment.

Herpes simplex virus infection should be treated promptly with aciclovir, orally if the problem is widespread or the patient is ill, to prevent a marked deterioration of atopic eczema.

Drying agents

In vesicular or weeping eczema the blisters and oozing areas are dried using potassium permanganate baths, soaks or wet compresses. Crystals or tablets are added to warm water to produce a purplish-pink colour, and the skin soaked for at least 15 minutes if possible. This appears to have an astringent and antiseptic effect. It will, however, stain the bath and is therefore most suitable for use in hospital, or mixed in a bowl for use on localized areas.

Antihistamines

Pruritus (itching) is often the most distressing feature of eczema, and the patient may benefit from the short-term use of a sedative antihistamine at night. In this situation the newer, non-sedative antihistamines have little value. Topical antihistamines are potent sensitizers and have no place in the management of eczema.

Coal tar preparations

Although less cosmetically acceptable than other topical preparations, tar is an effective antipruritic. It is chiefly used at night in impregnated bandages to occlude the limbs in atopic children, both for symptomatic relief and to prevent scratching. Ichthammol is used in the same way.

Tar creams and ointments are useful in the treatment of discoid eczema, which is often resistant to topical steroids.

There has recently been concern about the safety of tar, based on animal testing and industrial experience, but this has not been borne out in decades of clinical use.

Bandaging

In children with atopic eczema, occlusion with bandages has long been used to prevent scratching and to keep ointments and creams in contact with the skin. Wet wrapping, a technique involving the application of emollients and steroids under a double layer of conforming tubular bandage, keeps the inner layer moist. It can be very effective, and also soothing because of the cooling effect of evaporation. Specialist nurses can train parents to apply these dressings at home.

Once the acute phase has been treated, compression bandaging or graduated support stockings are probably the single most effective method of controlling varicose eczema.

Topical imidazoles

Ketoconazole as a shampoo or cream will reduce the population of *Pityrosporum ovale* on the skin, and thus control seborrhoeic eczema and dandruff. The disease runs a chronic, relapsing course, so regular or intermittent use is usually necessary. Other imidazoles can also be used.

Systemic therapies

Systemic steroids

Oral corticosteroids are used as a short-term measure in the treatment of acute eczemas, to bring the condition rapidly under control. Acute exacerbations of atopic eczema, acute allergic contact dermatitis and erythrodermic eczema, where the skin is red and hot all over the body, may require this type of management.

With the advent of other immunosuppressive agents, the need for long-term treatment of eczema with oral steroids is now very rare.

Ciclosporin

This drug is extremely effective in the treatment of chronic severe eczema and at present is used mainly in adult patients, although its use in children is increasing. The therapeutic range is 2.5–5 mg/kg. The eczema tends to relapse when the drug is stopped, but intermittent courses can be very useful in keeping the condition manageable. It is an immunosuppressant, so patients must be carefully monitored for signs of infection. The main adverse reactions are hypertension and renal impairment but these are reversible if the dose is reduced or the drug stopped. A number of drugs interact with ciclosporin and must be used with caution (Table 57.3). There are concerns about the long-term risks of developing skin cancers on light-exposed areas of

Table 57.3 Interactions with drugs used in the treatment of psoriasis and eczema

	Interacting drug	Outcome
Methotrexate	Aspirin	Increased plasma concentration and toxicity of methotrexate
	NSAIDs	Increased plasma concentration and toxicity of methotrexate
	Probenecid	Increased plasma concentration and toxicity of methotrexate
	Phenytoin	Increased bone marrow toxicity
	Sulfonamides	Increased toxicity
	Trimethoprim	Increased antifolate effect of methotrexate
Azathioprine	Allopurinol	Enhanced effect and toxicity of azathioprine
	Warfarin	Inhibition of anticoagulant effect
	Cimetidine	Enhanced myelosuppression
	Indometacin	Increased risk of leucopenia
Ciclosporin	NSAIDs	Increased risk of nephrotoxicity
	Aminoglycosides	Increased risk of nephrotoxicity
	Co-trimoxazole	Increased risk of nephrotoxicity
	Ciprofloxacin	Increased risk of nephrotoxicity
	Ketoconazole	Increased plasma concentration of ciclosporin
	Itraconazole	Increased plasma concentration of ciclosporin
	Erythromycin	Increased plasma concentration of ciclosporin
	Oral contraceptives	Increased plasma concentration of ciclosporin
	Calcium channel blockers	Increased plasma concentration of ciclosporin
	Phenytoin	Decreased plasma concentration of ciclosporin
	Carbamazepine	Decreased plasma concentration of ciclosporin
	Rifampicin	Decreased plasma concentration of ciclosporin
Acitretin	Methotrexate	Increased plasma concentration of methotrexate

the body. This underlines the importance of using this drug for short-term treatment wherever possible.

Topical preparations of ciclosporin have so far proved disappointing in treating eczema due to poor skin penetration, as a result of its high molecular weight.

Azathioprine

This antimitotic drug is used as a steroid-sparing agent, or alone, in cases of severe, treatment-resistant eczema, at a dose of 50–150 mg per day. It acts more slowly than ciclosporin but is widely used for long-term treatment. It suppresses the bone marrow and the immune system and patients must be monitored with regular blood tests.

Other immune modulators

Interferon-γ has been used in cases of severe refractory eczema but has unpleasant flu-like side effects. Methotrexate has also been used in unresponsive, adult atopic eczema but has never been evaluated in clinical trials.

Evening primrose oil

This has proved disappointing in clinical trials, but may occasionally have a place in the treatment of resistant eczema, especially where extreme dryness is the major problem (Munn 1999).

Phototherapy

Some atopic patients benefit from the use of PUVA (the combination of oral psoralen and ultraviolet A) or UVB, particularly in the dry, chronic stages (Krutmann 2000). Narrow-band UVB therapy is now becoming widely available and may be as effective and safer than PUVA. Potential side effects of all types of phototherapy include burning, premature ageing of the skin and increased risk of skin cancer. Patients attend for two or three treatments per week, usually for several weeks, and courses may be repeated at intervals.

Other therapies

Diets

These are not used routinely in the management of atopic eczema as they are only of value in very few cases. They should only be used under the supervision of a dietitian.

Chinese herbal medicine

Traditional Chinese herbal medicines are prescribed and made up on an individual basis for the patient. A standardized form has been devised by a Chinese practitioner in collaboration with Great Ormond Street Hospital for Sick Children in London. The active principle and constituents are unknown, and the treatment is therefore only available on a named patient basis. It has been shown to be effective in atopic eczema, but possible side effects include liver disturbance, so patients are monitored regularly with blood tests. The treatment has been evaluated but conflicting results have been obtained (Fung et al 1999).

Alternative therapies

These include psychotherapy, hypnotherapy, yoga and reflexology, which may help individual patients, usually atopic adults.

Patient care

It is important to recognize that eczema affects many aspects of a patient's life and has considerable effects on the family. Apart from the appearance and discomfort of the rash, the irritability and loss of sleep, there may be notable limitations on the patient's activities, and assistance in treating and overcoming the problems may be needed from primary care doctors, dermatologists, nurses, pharmacists and teachers. Advice and help through contact with other patients and their families together with information on the latest dressings, treatments, clothing, etc. can be obtained from the local branch of the National Eczema Society or via their website (www.eczema.org). The parents of atopic children need to understand that prescribed treatments are designed to control rather than cure the condition, and that the majority of atopics gradually improve during childhood and need to be treated until their eczema naturally resolves. They should not be afraid to use prescribed topical steroids if they are necessary and used under medical supervision.

Cool cotton clothing is the most suitable for eczema sufferers, and soap powders are probably not a problem if used in a modern washing machines with efficient rinsing programmes. However, leave-in fabric conditioners are best avoided. House dust mite precautions are advisable in many atopics, particularly if they also suffer from asthma or allergic rhinitis. In cases of allergic contact dermatitis, avoidance of the known allergen is the treatment of choice, as continued exposure will result in persistence of the rash, despite medication.

Eczema patients should aim to lead as normal a life as possible, and schools and employers can help to achieve this. Emollients applied regularly at break times, with assistance if necessary, make an enormous difference to the state of the skin. A child's self-image can be enhanced if other children are encouraged to accept the eczema, and not to regard it as infectious.

Career discussions are advisable at an early stage with atopics and their parents to avoid later disappointment. Even if the eczema has apparently settled, exposure to water, detergents, oils, greases and degreasers may result in a recurrence, particularly on the hands, which may ultimately result in loss of a job. For this reason occupations such as nursing, hairdressing, catering and handling machinery are unwise choices for an atopic. Therefore clean, dry jobs should be considered in preference.

A treatment algorithm for eczema is outlined in Figure 57.7.

PSORIASIS

Aetiology

Psoriasis is a chronic condition which may affect the skin and joints. In the skin it is seen as a red scaly rash that affects between 1% and 3% of the population in Europe and North America. There is a genetic predisposition to the disease; over 70% of patients

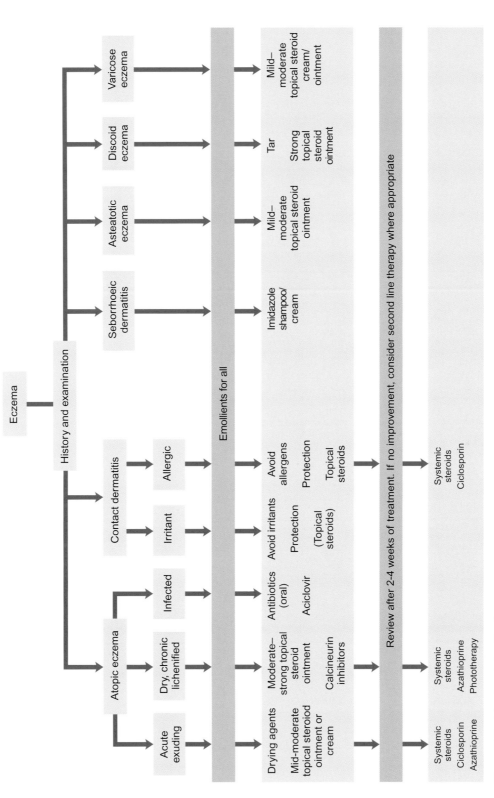

Figure 57.7 A treatment algorithm for eczema.

have a family history. HLA typing shows a preponderance of certain antigens, including DR7 and CW6. In recent years there has been progress in understanding the precise genetic determinants of the disease but it remains a complex field and different types of psoriasis may have different genetic characteristics. Certain non-hereditary factors also appear to contribute by precipitating an attack. These include the following:

Infection

Streptococcal infections, particularly in the upper respiratory tract, may be followed 10–14 days later by an attack of psoriasis. This is particularly common in children and may be the first presentation of the disease, in a typical guttate pattern (see below).

Patients with psoriasis who develop AIDS may have a severe flare of the rash.

Koebner phenomenon

An injury to the skin, for example a cut, burn, scratch or operation scar, may subsequently cause psoriasis to develop at that site, which may later spread to other areas.

Lithium, chloroquine and β-blockers

These drugs, given to treat dipolar affect disorder, rheumatological disorders and cardiovascular disease, respectively, may provoke a flare of psoriasis in susceptible patients.

Stress

An association between stress, either emotional or physical, and psoriasis is frequently claimed, but is difficult to confirm or refute.

Alcohol and smoking

Excess alcohol consumption may aggravate psoriasis, and psoriasis is known to be associated with high rates of alcoholism but it may be difficult to establish cause and effect. There is also a high correlation between smoking and pustular psoriasis of the palms and soles.

Pathogenesis

Many skin changes occur in psoriasis, which may be either the cause or effect of the disease.

Histologically, the epidermis is thickened (acanthosis), the granular layer is absent and epidermal cell nuclei are seen persisting in the horny layer (parakeratosis). In the dermis, the dermal capillaries are dilated, tortuous and closer to the surface of the skin than normal.

Large numbers of inflammatory cells are present in all layers of the skin; granulocytes are predominant and form microabscesses in the epidermis. Langerhans cells and lymphocytes are also increased.

In dynamic terms, the main abnormality is increased epidermal cell turnover, about 10 times the normal rate. The histological

changes have led to a number of hypotheses regarding how hyperproliferation occurs. The presence of lymphocytes and Langerhans cells has suggested an immunological cause, with mediators, cytokines, being released by these cells, recruiting more inflammatory cells to the process and thus increased stimulation of epidermal cell turnover. Some studies, however, suggested that epidermal cells themselves produce the cytokines that promote their own proliferation, and attract lymphocytes. Changes in the structure of the dermal blood vessels also occur, possibly as a result of mediator activity. None of these observations or theories is mutually exclusive, but their relationship to the underlying genetic defect is as yet unknown.

Clinical features

The typical psoriatic lesion is a red, scaly, sharply demarcated plaque, which may be of any size and may affect any part of the body. However, the most common sites are the extensor surfaces of the elbows (Fig. 57.8) and knees, the sacrum and the scalp. Hands and feet are frequently involved. The scale is silvery and easily scraped off, revealing tiny bleeding points.

Psoriasis is not characteristically itchy but may be when very inflamed, rapidly spreading or involving the palms and soles.

The natural history of psoriasis is that it tends to appear for the first time in young adults, although it may start at any time from infancy to old age, and runs a chronic, relapsing course. Treatment is aimed at controlling the current attack, not curing the psoriasis, and will not influence the future disease progress.

A number of different patterns of psoriasis occur, and these are described below.

Guttate psoriasis

This means 'drop-like', describing the multiple small plaques all over the body which occur, particularly in children, after streptococcal sore throats (Fig. 57.9). This type is usually self-limiting after a few weeks.

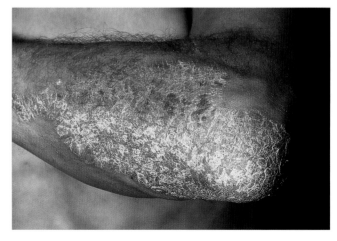

Figure 57.8 Chronic scaly plaque psoriasis on an elbow.

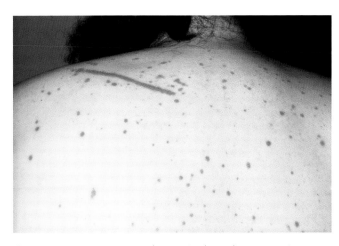

Figure 57.9 Guttate psoriasis showing Koebner phenomenon in scratch mark.

Chronic plaque psoriasis

Medium or large plaques occur on the trunk and limbs, and may be very persistent.

Psoriasis of the scalp

Involvement of the scalp may be as demarcated plaques or may involve the whole scalp, extending into the hairline (Fig. 57.10). The scale is white, thick and chalky, and hair loss may occur when the scalp is thickly scaled. Hair should recover if the scale is cleared and kept under control.

Psoriasis of the nails

The nails are frequently affected in psoriasis and in some cases this may be the only evidence of the disease. The changes include pitting, onycholysis (separation of the nail from its bed) and hyperkeratosis under the nail, which can be uncomfortable and disfiguring in some patients. The changes in psoriatic nails are very resistant to treatment.

Psoriasis of the palms and soles

At these sites there is sharp demarcation of the involved areas, which are inflamed and very scaly and may contain sterile pustules of large pin-head size (Fig. 57.11). These dry up into brown spots, and the affected skin then becomes thickened and fissured. As a result, secondary infection, with accompanying itch and pain, is common.

Flexural psoriasis

When psoriasis occurs in the flexures, such as the axillae, groins, submammary areas and genitalia, the demarcation is still present but the affected areas are glazed rather than scaly, and bright red.

Erythrodermic and generalized pustular psoriasis

These are severe and potentially life-threatening forms of the disease but fortunately they are uncommon. The patient is sick, the whole skin surface is involved and very inflamed, the pustules are sterile and may coalesce to form sheets of pus.

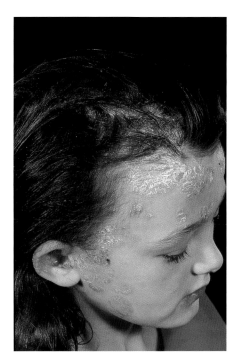

Figure 57.10 Chalky scaling of scalp psoriasis extending on to the face.

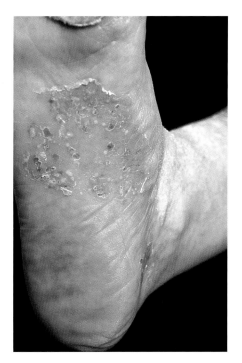

Figure 57.11 Pustular psoriasis of the sole.

Psoriatic arthropathy

The arthritis associated with psoriasis occurs in about 5% of psoriatics. It is of a similar type to rheumatoid arthritis but the rheumatoid factor is negative. Several patterns are recognized.

Distal arthritis

This type involves the terminal interphalangeal joints of the fingers and toes, and is associated with nail changes.

Large joint involvement

Here a single large joint, such as the hip or knee, may be involved, and the arthritis is destructive.

Sacroiliitis/spondylitis

The changes here are similar to ankylosing spondylitis, with the sexes equally affected. There is a strong association with HLA-B27.

Treatment

Many patients with psoriasis need little treatment, as their disease is minimal. Emollients may be all that is necessary to prevent drying and fissuring of the elbows and knees. Other patients may simply prefer not to treat their skin, as the process is laborious, time consuming and frequently messy.

Many of the treatments still used today are historical, and therefore empirical, and have never been subjected to controlled trials. More modern therapies, directed at reducing epidermal cell turnover, have been more critically tested. Different types of psoriasis may respond best to different treatments.

Topical therapy

Emollients

These may be all that is needed in very mild cases. Rest and soothing applications are essential in the management of erythroderma, although the patient may also need systemic therapy.

Topical steroids

These are widely used, and probably overused, in the treatment of psoriasis. They are of most value in acutely inflamed plaques, controlling inflammation and preparing the way for other treatments. They are not as effective on chronic scaly plaques.

Mild, group 4 steroids are helpful on the face and flexures, where dithranol, tar and calcipotriol may be irritant. More potent steroids are frequently used on the hands and feet, possibly in combination with clioquinol if the skin is fissured or with salicylic acid if there is hyperkeratosis. Potent steroid preparations are commonly used on scalp psoriasis, often producing an unsatisfactory effect. This is because lotions and creams do not efficiently penetrate thick scale. Therefore the scalp should first be prepared with a keratolytic such as salicylic acid. Aqueous and alcoholic lotions cause stinging and burning on inflamed scalps, and a cream, ointment or mousse may be preferable. Short-term use of potent topical steroids on large areas of psoriasis, although anti-inflammatory, may result in a rebound flare when the steroid is discontinued. This results in continuation of the steroid and, ultimately, unwanted side effects.

Dithranol

For many years, dithranol has been the main psoriasis treatment in hospital. It has a number of disadvantages that until recently made it impractical to use at home, including staining skin, clothing and bath fittings. It burns the skin, especially the clinically normal skin surrounding psoriatic plaques, and it is usually unsuitable for use on the face, flexures or acutely inflamed psoriasis.

Ingram regimen   This remains the standard psoriasis regimen used in most in patients treated in UK hospitals. Dithranol is applied in Lassar's paste, a stiff vehicle designed to prevent dithranol from spreading onto uninvolved skin, starting at a concentration of 0.1% and, if no burning occurs, increasing the strength every few days, normally up to 2%. The paste is covered with stockinette tubular dressings, left on for 24 hours, then washed off in a bath with a coal tar additive. This is followed by treatment with UVB (short-wave ultraviolet light), before reapplication of dithranol. Daily treatment will clear most psoriasis in 2–3 weeks.

Short-contact regimens   It is now known that sufficient dithranol penetrates the skin in 20–30 minutes to have a similar effect as 24-hour applications. When applied for a short time, higher concentrations can be used which cause less burning and staining. Therefore keeping dithranol off normal skin is not as critical. These factors have enabled some patients to use a cream formulation of dithranol at home, applied for 20–30 minutes per day and then bathed or showered off. The starting concentration is usually 0.5%, increasing every 5 days, if tolerated, to 3%.

Coal tar

This has been used in numerous mixtures over many years, in combination with emollients, salicylic acid and topical steroids, However, it has beome less popular in most UK centres with the advent of cleaner, less smelly treatments. In addition, restrictions on manufacturing in hospital and community pharmacies have greatly reduced the number and variety of preparations available. Attempts to purify coal tar to make it more cosmetically acceptable have resulted in loss of potency. Coal tar compounds are now mostly used on guttate and scalp psoriasis, and localized pustular psoriasis of the palms and soles.

The efficacy of tar in psoriasis is enhanced when used with UVB and the tar may be used as a bath additive before irradiation.

There is a theoretical risk of carcinogenesis from the long-term use of tar preparations. However, this is not supported in clinical practice, despite long-established use in dermatology, although there are few published data on the subject.

Salicylic acid

This is useful to reduce scale, in preparation for other treatments. It can be mixed with dithranol (as in Lassar's paste), coal tar, emollients, steroids and shampoos.

Vitamin D analogues

Calcipotriol is a popular outpatient treatment for psoriasis, available as an ointment, cream and scalp lotion. It is colourless, odourless and does not stain. It is more effective than tar, but may be more irritant. In addition, it is more effective than short-contact dithranol cream, and also causes less staining and burning. It seems to have similar efficacy in psoriasis to 0.1% betametasone ointment; it causes more irritation but no long-term skin atrophy. It should not be used on the face, where it may cause dermatitis. It does not cause hypercalcaemia provided that the weekly dose does not exceed 100 g. Another vitamin D analogue, tacalcitol, is used for the once-daily treatment of chronic plaque psoriasis (Van de Kerkhof et al 1996), as is calcitriol. They are both suitable for use on the face, being less irritant than calcipotriol.

The efficacy of topical calcipotriol is enhanced in a combination preparation with betametasone, but there are concerns about long-term use and the possibility of steroid side effects, such as skin atrophy.

Ultraviolet light (UVB)

Many patients report that they are better in the summer or after a sunny holiday. Artificial UVB (wavelength 290–320 nm) is therefore used therapeutically, usually in combination with tar or vitamin D analogues, and also in conjunction with short-contact dithranol in outpatient dressings units in some hospital dermatology departments.

Narrow-band UVB (wavelength 311–313 nm) is available in many dermatology units, and appears to be more effective than conventional UVB and possibly as effective as PUVA (see below). It is thought that there may be fewer long-term side effects and this is being evaluated.

Topical treatment of psoriasis at special sites

Scalp Mild scalp psoriasis may be controlled simply by regular use of a tar shampoo. More thickly scaled scalps may require overnight application to the hair roots of an ointment or cream containing salicylic acid; one of the most effective is based on coconut compound ointment. On the following day the scales are loosened with a toothcomb and then shampooed out with a coal tar shampoo or suitable detergent. This regimen is messy but more effective than aqueous or alcoholic lotions, and usually more comfortable. It does, however, require considerable time and commitment from the patient and family.

Nails Once fungal infection of the nails has been excluded as the main differential diagnosis, there is little treatment that can be offered. Intralesional steroid injections into the nail bed and phototherapy have both been tried, with disappointing results. If the patient is on systemic therapy for psoriasis there may be some improvement in the nails. However, in most cases any improvement is most likely to be spontaneous.

Systemic therapy

Indications for the use of systemic therapy include severe and widespread psoriasis, failure or intolerance of topical treatment, and rapid relapse of psoriasis after clearance.

PUVA

PUVA was developed to bridge the gap in therapy between traditional messy applications and toxic systemic drugs. It still has a valuable role in the treatment of moderate to severe chronic plaque psoriasis, despite increasing evidence of long-term side effects. Psoralens are drugs that are activated by long-wave ultraviolet light (UVA, wavelength 320–400 nm) to interfere with DNA synthesis, and thus reduce epidermal cell turnover. Two psoralens are available for PUVA treatment in the UK, 8- and 5-methoxypsoralen; neither has a product licence, so patients are treated on a named patient basis. The psoralen is either taken by mouth 2 hours before exposure to UVA, allowing the drug to reach its maximum concentration in the skin, or applied topically, usually in a bath containing the drug, immediately before exposure. The initial exposure time is calculated by previous light testing, and the time increased as tolerated by the patient as the course progresses. The treatment is normally given twice weekly, until clearance or significant improvement is achieved, usually in about 6 weeks. This is accompanied by a tan. Unless the psoriasis is severe and relapsing, maintenance therapy is avoided to minimize long-term side effects. Further courses can be given subsequently, if necessary, and total cumulative dosage of UVA must be carefully monitored (British Photodermatology Group 1994).

Adverse effects PUVA should be avoided in pregnancy. Nausea is the most common side effect and is worst on the day of treatment. Pruritus and drying of the skin are also frequent problems. Ageing of the skin and the development of melanoma and non-melanoma skin cancer are the major long-term risks; this depends on the skin type of the patient (fair, type 1 skins suffer most) and the total cumulative dose of UVA. Those who have had in the past or are currently taking immunosuppressant therapy are also at increased risk.

The eyes are always protected with suitable UVA screening spectacles from the time of taking the tablet until 12 hours after UVA treatment, to avoid the possibility of developing cataracts.

In some units bath PUVA is preferred as this avoids the systemic side effect of nausea and makes the wearing of sunglasses unnecessary.

Cytotoxic drugs

These drugs all have toxic effects on the bone marrow and germ cells, and must be avoided at conception and in pregnancy. Their use should be supervised by a dermatologist.

Methotrexate This folic acid antagonist is the most popular cytotoxic drug in use for severe psoriasis, including acute generalized pustular psoriasis, and is the most effective treatment for psoriatic arthritis. It is given in a once-weekly, low-dose regimen, usually orally but occasionally intramuscularly to avoid side effects, following a test dose of 2.5 mg. The therapeutic dose is normally up to 30 mg weekly (Roenigk et al 1988).

Some patients complain of nausea and other gastrointestinal side effects, together with fatigue and lassitude, for up to 48 hours after the weekly dose. This may be eased with regular metoclopramide, and folic acid 5 mg per day on the non-methotrexate days can also be very helpful.

Acute toxic effects occur due to the effect on the folic acid metabolism of rapidly dividing cells in the bone marrow and gastrointestinal tract, resulting in marrow suppression or gastrointestinal bleeding. They can be reversed by folinic acid rescue (120 mg of folinic acid over 12–24 hours intravenously or intramuscularly in divided doses, followed by 15 mg/kg orally every 6 hours for 48 hours) which opposes the folate antagonist effect of methotrexate. These adverse effects are more likely to occur in the elderly with poor renal function, so a creatinine clearance test should be performed before the start of treatment and the dose reduced if renal function is impaired. The full blood count should be monitored regularly.

Liver toxicity, producing a hepatitic pattern in the liver function tests, may occur and progress to fibrosis and cirrhosis in the long term unless the drug is reduced or stopped. Regular liver function tests are therefore performed, together, in some centres, with procollagen III enzyme levels. A liver biopsy is recommended if there are sustained or significant abnormalities. Patients are strongly advised to abstain from drinking alcohol while they remain on the drug.

Several commonly used drugs interact with methotrexate (see Table 57.3), so a careful drug history is necessary, and the patient and the primary care doctor should be warned of contraindicated medication.

Hydroxycarbamide This drug has similar effects on the bone marrow and germ cells to methotrexate, but not the hepatic toxicity. It needs to be used continuously, as relapse occurs when the drug is stopped. Previous treatment with hydroxycarbamide appears to increase the risks of development of skin cancer in patients receiving PUVA.

Immunosuppressant drugs

Ciclosporin This is an effective treatment for severe psoriasis in doses lower than those used to prevent rejection of transplanted organs; it is used in a range 2.5–5 mg/kg daily. Renal function and blood pressure are monitored regularly and any rise in creatinine or blood pressure reversed by a reduction in dosage, drug treatment of hypertension or cessation of the drug. Relapse may occur when the drug is stopped, but intermittent therapy is preferred to maintenance, as this should reduce the long-term risks of skin cancers, lymphomas and solid tumours. Patients should also be warned to avoid overexposure to the sun, and should not receive concurrent PUVA or UVB therapy.

Systemic corticosteroids These have little place in the treatment of psoriasis, except in the management of life-threatening erythroderma. In fact, systemic steroids, or their withdrawal, may provoke an acute generalized pustular psoriasis.

Acitretin

This second-generation oral retinoid is used in the treatment of severe resistant psoriasis, acute pustular psoriasis and palmoplantar psoriasis. It is available on hospital prescription only, due to its teratogenic effects, and women of childbearing age must use effective contraception during treatment and for 2 years after its cessation. Therefore, wherever possible it is better to find an alternative treatment in these patients. Acitretin enhances the action of PUVA and allows a reduction in UVA dosage while providing a protective effect against malignant change in the skin. This combination therapy is known as Re-PUVA. Acitretin may cause abnormalities in liver function tests and plasma lipids, and these are monitored and adjustments in dosage made or advice about a low-fat diet given. There may be effects on bone maturation, so acitretin is avoided if at all possible in children.

The most common adverse effect seen in all patients is dry skin, especially on the lips, and in some people the mucous membranes of the eye and nose may also be affected. There may be considerable hair loss, but this and all other side effects are dose related and reversible.

Biologic agents

A proportion of patients with moderate or severe psoriasis are either unsuitable for or resistant to the second-line medications described. For these patients, there is now the possibility of treatment with 'biologics', molecules genetically engineered to block specific steps in the pathogenesis of psoriasis, targeting T-cell receptors, antigen-presenting cells, cytokines and adhesion molecules. They are also used in rheumatoid and psoriatic arthritis. Currently, there are two main groups of agents used in psoriasis:

- drugs targeting the cytokine TNF-α, e.g. infliximab, etanercept, adalimumab
- drugs targeting T-cells or antigen-presenting cells, e.g. efalizumab, alefacept.

Etanercept, efalizumab and infliximab have been licensed in the UK for the treatment of moderate-to-severe psoriasis. They are given by injection and require monitoring of blood counts, liver and renal function. Guidelines are available for the selection of patients and use of these drugs (Smith et al 2005).

Photodynamic therapy

This treatment requires the application of a photosensitizing drug, 5-aminolaevulininc acid (ALA), which causes local accumulation of protoporphyrin IX. This compound is then activated by irradiation with visible light, resulting in tissue destruction. Studies have shown this to be effective for localized plaque psoriasis (Boehncke et al 1994); side effects seem to be confined to a burning sensation at the site of treatment. However, it is not widely used and is time consuming. In addition, it is only performed by specialist nurses and is only suitable for isolated plaques of psoriasis.

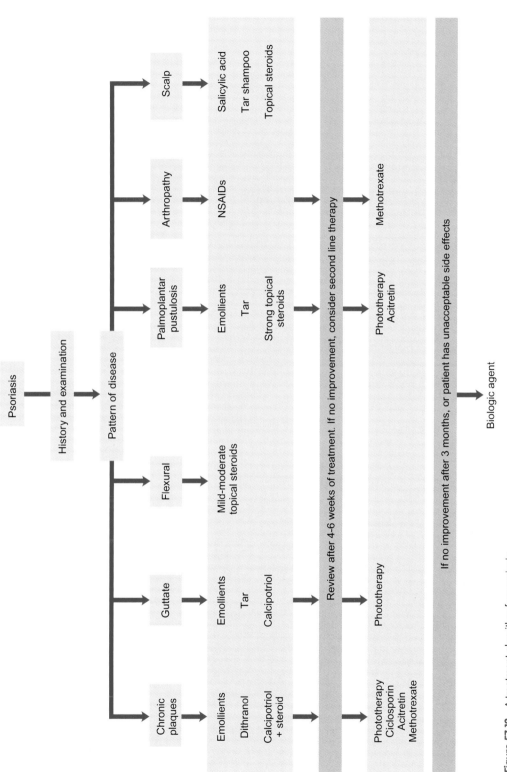

Figure 57.12 A treatment algorithm for psoriasis.

Table 57.4 Common therapeutic problems in eczema and psoriasis

Problem	Result
Topical treatments are frequently messy and sticky	Patients are reluctant to use them
Water-based creams contain preservatives and may cause stinging on inflamed skin	Children will resist their use and become distressed at treatment time
Topical treatment is time consuming for patients and their families/carers	Treatments may be missed
Methods of application and amount to use often not well explained	Treatment is inadequate
Patients or parents may be frightened by publicity about the side effects of topical steroids	Treatment may be inadequate or non-existent
Dithranol stains skin, fabric and hardware a purple-brown colour	Bathrooms may be ruined if short contact therapy is used carelessly
Emollients may not emulsify completely with water	Outflow from bath or shower may become blocked, and washing machines damaged
Topical treatments are hard work and may take many weeks to show results	Patients become discouraged
Systemic therapies all have significant side effects	Patients have to attend clinics regularly for monitoring of tests, blood pressure, etc.

Future therapies

Research for the future will continue to be targeted at immunotherapy for psoriasis. T-cells, antigen-presenting cells, cytokines and adhesion molecules all appear to play important roles in the pathogenesis of psoriasis and future drugs, either topical or systemic, will be designed either to suppress or block their actions.

Patient care

Psoriasis is a chronic disease, which in its mild form is little more than a nuisance. In moderate and severe cases, however, it may become extremely distressing for the patient and socially unacceptable. The patient tends to be very conscious of the appearance of the rash and the fact that it leaves a trail of silvery scales in its wake. This is probably at its worst when the patient undresses, causing a 'snowstorm' of scales, which increases the dusting and vacuuming required at home. When the joints are involved there is pain, often severe, and later deformity of the joints concerned. If the skin of the hands and feet is affected, fissuring and resultant

infection and pain may make work impossible, either because of exacerbation by the friction of manual work or because of the health risks in catering, nursing or personal contact. In some cases the embarrassment is just too great for the sufferer to stay at work.

Psoriatics can be greatly helped by doctors, nurses, pharmacists and other health professionals. An explanation that the disease is inherited and not infectious is often helpful; although there is no cure the disease can be controlled so that the individual can lead a normal life. It may be reassuring to know that if things are out of control an admission to hospital or a course of daily treatment in an outpatient therapy unit is available.

It must be emphasized that a responsibility lies with the patient to apply or take any treatment regularly to ensure maximum benefit, and to attend regularly for follow-up and monitoring in a clinic for systemic treatment. Patients whose psoriasis tends to clear in the summer months should be encouraged to take advantage of any natural sunshine.

Information on the entitlement to benefits to replace clothing ruined by ointments or washing machines worn out by constant use is available. The Psoriasis Association (www.psoriasis-association.org.uk) provides an excellent local service covering this and many other aspects, together with practical advice from fellow sufferers on day-to-day problems.

A treatment algorithm for psoriasis is presented in Figure 57.12.

Common therapeutic problems in the management of eczema and psoriasis are outlined in Table 57.4.

CASE STUDIES

Case 57.1

A 3-year-old child was brought to the hospital dermatology clinic with widespread, dry atopic eczema, from which she had suffered from the age of 6 months. She had always been a poor eater and restless sleeper due to the itch of her eczema. She had also been treated repeatedly for bacterial infection of her skin. Her normal skin treatment was 1% hydrocortisone cream. Her parents had been advised by their health visitor and other health professionals to keep bathing to a minimum, because of the discomfort caused. They were very keen to have tests performed, to identify the cause of the eczema, and to decide on a cure.

Question

What advice could be given to the child's parents?

Answer

Time should be spent explaining to the parents that eczema is a disease whose cause is not known, but it is likely to improve spontaneously through childhood. It will probably leave the child with little more than dry skin by her teens. Skin tests will therefore not contribute to the management in childhood and may cause discomfort which may frighten the child. It should be emphasized that the eczema will be controllable through development of a suitable regimen of regular treatment. The importance of bathing with plenty of emollient on the skin and in the water, which makes it comfortable, in additional to applications of emollient as necessary, should be reinforced. A topical steroid ointment of moderate potency, with an antiseptic added if the eczema is infected, should be used to control the eczema. The potency can subsequently be reduced for maintenance, or changed to a topical calcineurin inhibitor. Systemic antibiotics may also help.

If this regimen does not produce a marked improvement in 2 weeks, a short admission to hospital or daily visits to a treatment unit may help both the child and the parents, as they can be given advice and tuition in methods of topical treatment application and bandaging.

Case 57.2

A 3-year-old child was brought by her mother to her primary care doctor's surgery because of very persistent facial eczema. Aqueous cream and 0.5% hydrocortisone cream had previously been prescribed, but the little girl screamed whenever the aqueous cream was used on her skin. Also her mother was very concerned about the use of topical steroids and their long-term effects. She was thus not using either medication and the child was receiving no effective treatment.

Question

What advice can be given, or alternative treatment prescribed?

Answer

As aqueous cream is mainly composed of water, it is an unstable formulation and liable to bacterial contamination unless preservatives are added. These frequently cause stinging, especially on broken or inflamed skin. The emollient/soap substitute could therefore be changed to one with a higher oil content and consequently lower preservative level. Emulsifying ointment and similar proprietary products would be more comfortable to use.

The problem of active treatment is more difficult to solve, because of the mother's concerns over steroid use. The primary care doctor can explain that of all topical steroids, hydrocortisone is the least potent, and associated with the lowest potential to damage skin. They can also discuss that it may be more damaging to the child's skin and psyche to leave her untreated with hydrocortisone than to use the cream on a short-term basis until the eczema settles. However, topical calcineurin inhibitors are now available, and it could be explained to the mother that these are not steroids and will not cause skin thinning. If the primary care doctor is experienced in their use, then pimecrolimus cream or tacrolimus 0.03% ointment could be prescribed. The mother should be warned that a minority of children may have a temporary burning sensation in the skin when the treatment begins. However, this is rarely severe enough for the treatment to be discontinued. Alternatively, the child could be referred to the local hospital dermatology department for advice and initiation of treatment which, if successful, can then be continued by the primary care doctor.

Case 57.3

A 17-year-old girl was referred to the clinic with a 6-month history of severe hand dermatitis. She had been a trainee hairdresser since leaving school, and the problems with her hands had started within a few months of commencing work. Her hands were now dry, fissured, painful and itchy, but improved when she had more than a week's holiday from work. As a child, she had mild atopic eczema and asthma, which had appeared to improve when she was about 8 years old.

Question

What is the cause of this girl's problems, and how can they be managed?

Answer

This girl is an atopic and should have been advised at an early stage that a career in hairdressing would risk development of dermatitis. She will be prone to both irritant and allergic contact dermatitis, which may be caused by water, shampoos and perming and colouring chemicals. She needs to be patch tested to try to determine the cause, although both types of reaction may be involved.

She should stop work for a while, as this has been shown to improve her condition, and her hands should be treated intensively with emollients and barrier creams. Potent topical steroid ointment may be necessary until the dermatitis is under control, and thereafter emollients alone should continue, to maintain the normal barrier function of the skin.

Most importantly, she should be encouraged to change occupations to a clean, dry job where her hands will be at less risk from ongoing dermatitis. In future she will have to protect her hands from domestic chores with cotton-lined rubber gloves.

Case 57.4

A 32-year-old man with lifelong eczema is working under great pressure as a management executive, and his eczema has been deteriorating steadily over several months. He has used emollients and topical steroids in adequate quantities and has had several courses of oral antibiotics when the eczema appeared to be secondarily infected. None of this has had a sustained effect, and he cannot afford to have time off work to be admitted for hospital treatment. His sleep is disturbed and tiredness is beginning to affect his daily activities.

Question

What are the options for treatment for this man?

Answer

This patient needs effective treatment before the eczema becomes erythrodermic. Systemic medication should bring the problem under control, and three might be considered: first, as a short course, high-dose systemic steroids should have a rapid effect and can be reduced over a week or two. If it is anticipated that a few weeks or months of treatment may be needed, since his stress is ongoing, then ciclosporin would be a better choice as the side effects can be monitored and detected at an early stage with blood pressure readings and blood tests. This treatment can be tailed off when the situation seems to be under control. If long-term systemic management is necessary, azathioprine might be considered. However, it takes much longer than the other two drugs to take effect and it may be at least a month before any obvious relief of symptoms, so treatment might initially be combined with prednisolone. In the long term, however, azathioprine will not cause hypertension, renal impairment, obesity, osteoporosis or skin atrophy, and it can be monitored with simple blood tests.

Case 57.5

A 55-year-old woman presents at the clinic with a history of chronic plaque psoriasis from the age of 16 and she has never been clear of the disease. She has had numerous topical treatments over the years, none of which has been particularly effective. She was markedly intolerant of dithranol. Over the previous 2 years she has gradually developed arthritis in her finger joints, with early signs of deformity. She has tried a number of pain killers and NSAIDs but these have not relieved her pain and stiffness.

Question

What would be the best treatment for this patient's problems?

Answer

Providing that there are no contraindications, methotrexate would be the most suitable single treatment to control this lady's psoriasis of both the skin and joints. She should be advised to stop her NSAIDs and to take paracetamol as a short-term alternative, and also to avoid alcohol. If her blood count and liver function tests are normal 1 week after a 2.5 mg test dose of methotrexate, a weekly dose of 10 mg can be given, initially with further weekly monitoring of the blood tests. The dose can be adjusted every 2–3 weeks until improvement occurs. The skin should show clearance over about 6–12 weeks, but the joints may take longer to respond. Once this has happened, the lowest dose that controls symptoms can be continued as maintenance, with 3-monthly blood tests.

Case 57.6

A 24-year-old man presents at the clinic with a 10-year history of plaque psoriasis affecting his elbows, knees and sacral area, with a few small plaques elsewhere. He is otherwise fit and well, but embarrassed by the appearance of his skin when he regularly plays football. He has tried Betnovate RD ointment (0.025%), which smoothed the plaques a little, and calcipotriol ointment, which removed the scale from the plaques but did not clear them.

Question

What treatment could this patient try next?

Answer

With relatively few plaques to treat, this patient might respond very well to short-contact dithranol creams. In most patients these can be started at a concentration of 0.5%, which can be increased to 1%, 2%, and 3%, every 5–7 days, depending on how well the skin tolerates the treatment. The effect can be enhanced by UVB therapy twice weekly in a dermatology department for up to 8 weeks. The usual staining and burning with dithranol are minimized by short-contact therapy, and any discoloration fades quickly after the treatment is stopped.

The patient should be warned, however, that dithranol may stain fabrics and bathroom suites, especially where the surface has been damaged or roughened. Dark-coloured towels and underwear are advisable while dithranol is being used.

Case 57.7

A 45-year-old man has become increasingly disabled with palmoplantar pustular psoriasis; he has frequent crops of inflamed pustules on the palms and soles, which dry up to form crusts and scaling followed by painful fissuring of the skin. This has made his job as a joiner increasingly difficult and he has had prolonged periods of sick leave; he is afraid that he could be made redundant. He has tried emollients, topical steroid applications and tar and steroid combinations, with only temporary relief.

Question

What are this patient's options for treatment?

Answer

This can be a chronic and very disabling condition for manual workers, and this patient may benefit from systemic therapy.

Oral acitretin works very well in this condition and can be given intermittently or long term if the patient's fasting lipids and liver function tests remain normal. A rise in lipids may be controlled by diet or medication or reversed by stopping the drug. The major side effect of retinoids is dry skin, so regular emollient treatment will have to continue.

If there are contraindications to acitretin, an effective alternative is hand and foot PUVA. A convenient way of using psoralen on the hands and feet is to soak them in psoralen solution for 20 minutes; they are then irradiated with UVA, and this treatment is done twice or three times weekly. This avoids the disadvantages of wearing UVA-screening glasses after oral psoralen on the day of treatment; the main disadvantage is having to attend hospital regularly. Long-term side effects on the relatively thick skin of hands and feet seem to be fewer than on thinner skin elsewhere.

Re-PUVA, combining acitretin with PUVA, can be very effective and reduces the required dose of both therapies.

The major advantage to the patient of both acitretin and PUVA is that he should be able to continue working, using simple emollients only on the skin.

Case 57.8

A 24-year-old woman has had psoriasis since the age of 13, and her skin has never been clear in that time. Her teenage years were ruined by embarrassment and discomfort due to her skin disease, and she had 12 admissions to hospital by the age of 20. She is an intelligent girl, who has been determined to do well in life, but had to revise for her GCSEs in a hospital ward.

By the age of 18, her skin was so difficult to control, despite a wide range of topical treatments and many courses of UVB, that systemic treatment became necessary. Ciclosporin was relatively contraindicated, as she has had so much UVB, and the combination predisposes to the formation of skin cancers. Acitretin is avoided in young women of this age group, due to its teratogenicity and long half-life in the body. She was therefore started on methotrexate, which she tolerated well, and her skin cleared initially. However, the psoriasis gradually became uncontrolled, despite steady increase in the methotrexate dose, and she was once again in a spiral of outpatient treatment attendances and regular admissions to hospital. Her absences from work were also putting her job at risk.

Question

What more can be offered to this young woman?

Answer

As she has had all the topical and systemic treatment appropriate available for her age and condition, she is therefore eligible to be considered for treatment with a biological agent. Pretreatment baseline blood tests and screening for infection were carried out. Funding was obtained from her Primary Care Trust and she was commenced on etanercept, 25 mg by subcutaneous injection twice weekly, which she was taught to self-administer. Within 2 weeks, her psoriasis was clearing and after 12 weeks, she was virtually clear and felt better and more confident than she had for many years. She has now stopped the injections and her progress is being observed; if she relapses, further courses of etanercept can be prescribed.

Case 57.9

A 16-year-old boy has thick plaques of psoriasis on his scalp, producing dense scaling, which is matting his hair. He has tried to use steroid scalp applications, but they appear to have no effect. He is now starting to lose some hair with the scales, and he and his mother are very worried.

Question

What treatment will clear his scalp?

Answer

Aqueous and alcoholic scalp applications will not penetrate thick scale and therefore a keratolytic such as salicylic acid is required. Preparations such as 2% sulfur and salicylic acid in aqueous cream or coconut compound ointment are rubbed into the hair roots and left for a minimum of 2–3 hours, and sometimes overnight. They are then removed with a tar or tar and salicylic acid shampoo, and the process repeated every day until the scalp is clear. There may be some additional hair loss due to hair being firmly adherent to the scale, but this will recover once the scalp is free of scale. Once clear, the scalp can then be treated with a steroid preparation on a daily basis to help to keep it scale free, but the salicylic acid treatment may have to be repeated at intervals.

REFERENCES

Boehncke W H, Sterry W, Kaufmann R 1994 Treatment of psoriasis by topical photodynamic therapy with polychromatic light. Lancet 343: 801
British Photodermatology Group 1994 British Photodermatology Group guidelines for PUVA. British Journal of Dermatology 130: 246-255
Charman C R 2000 Atopic eczema. Clinical Evidence 3: 797-808
Fung A Y, Look P C, Chong L Y et al 1999 A controlled trial of traditional Chinese herbal medicine in Chinese patients with recalcitrant atopic dermatitis. International Journal of Dermatology 38: 387-392
Hanifin J M, Ling M R, Langley R et al 2001 Tacrolimus ointment for the treatment of atopic dermatitis in adult patients I. Efficacy. Journal of the American Academy of Dermatology 44: S28-S38
Kapp A, Papp K, Bingham A et al 2002 Long-term management of atopic dermatitis in infants with topical pimecrolimus, a non-steroid anti-inflammatory drug. Journal of Allergy and Clinical Immunology 110: 277-284
Krutmann J 2000 Phototherapy for atopic dermatitis. British Journal of Dermatology 25: 553-557

Munn S 1999 Use of γ-linolenic acid in atopic dermatitis. CME Bulletin of Dermatology 2: 20-22
Roenigk H H Jr, Auerbach R, Maibach H I et al 1988 Methotrexate in psoriasis: revised guidelines. Journal of the American Academy of Dermatology 19: 145-156
Reitamo S, Van Leent EJ, Ho V et al 2002 Efficacy and safety of tacrolimus ointment compared with that of hydrocortisone acetate in children with atopic dermatitis. Journal of Allergy and Clinical Immunology 109: 539-546
Smith C H, Anstey A, Barker J et al 2005 British Association of Dermatologists guidelines for the use of biological interventions in psoriasis. British Journal of Dermatology 153: 486-497
Van de Kerkhof P C, Werfel T, Haustein U F et al 1996 Tacalcitol ointment in the treatment of psoriasis vulgaris: a multicentre, placebo-controlled, double-blind study on efficacy and safety. British Journal of Dermatology 135: 758-765

FURTHER READING

Berth-Jones J, Maibach H I 2004 Eczema and contact dermatitis. Health Press, Oxford
Breuer K, Werfel T, Kapp A 2005 Safety and efficacy of topical calcineurin inhibitors in the treatment of childhood atopic dermatitis. American Journal of Clinical Dermatology 6: 65-77
Brown S, Reynolds N J 2006 Atopic and non-atopic eczema. British Medical Journal 332: 584-588

Buxton P 2003 ABC of dermatology, 4th edn. BMJ Books, London
Ghaffar S A, Clements S E, Griffiths C E 2005 Modern management of psoriasis. Clinical Medicine 5: 564-568
Judge M 2005 Atopic eczema: a modern epidemic. Clinical Medicine 5: 559-563
Williams H C (ed) 2000 Atopic dermatitis. Cambridge University Press, Cambridge

58 Pressure sores and leg ulcers

R. Anderson

Pressure sores

A pressure sore may be defined as any break in skin integrity that results from sustained pressure on the body, with or without the additional stresses of shear and friction. Other patient-specific factors may contribute to skin damage and affect healing ability. The terms 'bed sore' and 'decubitus ulcer' have been used, but these imply that damage can only occur when lying down, whereas the sitting position can equally produce ulceration. The term 'pressure ulcer' is preferable as without pressure the condition cannot develop and, although often sore to the patient with intact sensation, in those with neurological impairment there is no associated soreness.

Pressure ulcers result in high costs to the individual and the health services, with treatment costs for a Grade 4 ulcer estimated to cost £40 000 (Gethin et al 2005). The overall cost of treating pressure ulcers in the UK NHS has been estimated to be £2.1 billion.

In the UK national guidance has been issued on pressure ulcer risk assessment and prevention (NICE 2003) and the management of pressure ulcers in primary and secondary care (NICE 2005).

Epidemiology

Pressure damage can occur in patients whether they are cared for in hospital or the community, and is a distressing and expensive problem to manage. Studies of prevalence have revealed that 5–32% of patients may suffer from pressure ulcers at any one time depending on the patient population studied. Few community-based prevalence studies have been done but a prevalence of 4–7% has been reported. In the hospice setting a prevalence of 21–37% has been reported. Incidence studies in hospitals have indicated ranges from 2% in 12 months to 66% over 18 months in elderly individuals with hip fractures.

Aetiology

Various factors play a role in the development of pressure ulcers.

Pressure

Excess pressure on the skin results in the ischaemia of underlying tissue by mechanical compression of the vascular supply. The critical factor is when pressure on the skin exceeds the average arteriolar pressure (25 mmHg).

Sustained pressure on tissues is most damaging. Low pressure applied for long periods is worse than high pressure for short periods, and some alternating-pressure beds work on a high-pressure/short-time cycle principle. Portable equipment is available to measure pressure beneath patients so that the most suitable support equipment (mattress, cushion or chair) can be chosen. However, this approach is not in widespread use.

Numerous pieces of equipment are promoted to prevent pressure ulcers, including fluidized beds and specialized cushions. All patients at risk should have ready access to appropriate preventive equipment, whether in hospital or community settings. The need for high-specification foam mattresses with pressure-relieving properties for all vulnerable patients has been stressed in national guidance (NICE 2005). Alternating-pressure or other high-technology systems should also be considered to assist repositioning for certain high-risk individuals, even though evidence for enhanced effect over foam mattresses is not yet available.

Risks to 'sitting' patients are sometimes less well recognized. Those sitting in chairs or wheelchairs should be regularly checked for weight distribution, positional alignment and feet support and provided with additional supporting overlays as appropriate. The following are inappropriate as pressure-relieving aids: sheepskins, whether synthetic or natural, doughnut-style devices such as ring cushions, and water-filled gloves.

Shear

All shearing forces will also involve some pressure, but shear caused by patients sliding down beds or chairs will damage the superficial skin layers with resultant stretching of blood vessels, possible thrombosis and damage to the dermis.

Friction

Friction between skin and sheets or seating may cause ulceration by mechanically rubbing off outer layers of skin. Soft and uncreased linen, towels and dressings should be used. Massage and vigorous application of skin preparations should be avoided.

Moisture

In the presence of moisture, due to urine, sweat or faeces, pressure ulcer formation is more likely as skin becomes macerated and traumatized. The excessive use of barrier creams may overmoisten skin and exacerbate the problem, as may some moisture-retentive dressings.

Combined forces

If shear and friction are applied together, the tissues attached to bony structures move under shear while the epidermal layers may move in the opposite direction due to friction between the skin and supporting surfaces.

The effect of the three combined forces of shear, friction and pressure can result in ulcer formation at lower pressures than would be normally anticipated.

Patient factors and risk assessment

Various concurrent problems constitute risk factors for pressure ulcer development and these are summarized in Table 58.1. Pressure ulcers may occur at any age, including childhood, particularly when patient mobility and activity are reduced. It is therefore important that all patients at risk should have their pressure ulcer risk assessed on admission to hospital, and be regularly reviewed. Similarly, chronically ill patients in the community must be monitored. The need for accurate assessment, grading of pressure ulcers and ongoing monitoring in at-risk patients cannot be overemphasized.

Various risk assessment scales are available but these must be used in conjunction with clinical judgement. It is also essential that the scale in use has been tested for relevance in the population under care. The reliability of the various scales and their respective sensitivities have been investigated (Pancorbo-

Table 58.1 Risk factors for the development of pressure ulcers

Increasing age
Reduced mobility and activity
Poor nutrition, especially if linked with severe anaemia
Diabetes
Obesity
Cardiac failure
Osteomyelitis
Orthopaedic problems
Drug addiction
Malignancy/cytotoxic therapy
Neurological disorders

Hidalgo et al 2006). Aspects taken into consideration within the various scales include: physical condition; mental condition; activity; mobility; incontinence; nutrition; predisposing diseases; age; and concurrent medication.

Common sites of occurrence

Although any area of the body subjected to unrelieved pressure may ulcerate, certain sites are more susceptible to damage. The five classic locations for pressure ulcers are:

- sacrum
- buttocks (ischial tuberosity)
- hips (greater trochanter)
- heel
- lateral malleolus of foot.

The significance of position in relation to pressure ulceration site is shown in Table 58.2.

Pressure ulcers can occur in less common locations that also depend on the position of the patient and include the ear, scalp, elbows and genitalia. In infants and young children pressure injury is more likely on the occipital scalp than the sacrum (Willock et al 2000).

Signs of pressure damage

Various warning signs on the skin should immediately indicate the need for additional precautions. After sustained pressure, the skin initially turns red due in part to histamine release. This redness is termed blanching erythema and if gently pressed, it will whiten (or blanch). If pressure is relieved at this stage, the skin should return to normal. There are, however, hazards of using erythema as a diagnostic tool since variation in the degree of applied pressure can affect the result as well as potentially inflict further damage.

Table 58.2   Relationship between position of patient and area at risk of developing a pressure ulcer

Position of patient	Risk areas
Supine	Scapula Sacrum Heels
Prone	Chest Patellae Anterior surface of tibia
Sidelying	Femoral trochanters Malleoli
Sitting	Ischial tuberosities Sacrum Femoral trochanters (posterior surface)

It is recommended that pressure ulcers should be graded using the European Pressure Ulcer Advisory Panel (EPUAP) classification system (available at www.epuap.org/puclas/theory_classification_epuap.html). Ulcers classified at Grade 2 or above should be reported as a local clinical incident to ensure thorough review of the reasons for development and the necessary steps identified and put in place to prevent reoccurrence.

EPUAP's grading for pressure damage subsequent to initial blanching erythema is as follows.

- *Grade 1: non-blanchable erythema.* Continuous pressure initially leads to non-blanching erythema. In this situation when the affected area is pressed it will remain red, indicating that a pressure ulcer is developing.
- *Grade 2: blistering.* The next clinical sign of progression is blistering.
- *Grade 3: superficial ulcer.* With sustained pressure there will be progression to a superficial ulcer.
- *Grade 4: deep ulcer.* A deep ulcer can quickly develop and may be masked by an area of hard, black necrotic tissue, termed an eschar. An eschar may break down and putrify, with formation of a strong odour, usually due to the presence of anaerobic bacteria

Where skin is thin and bony prominences are superficial, progressive damage and full skin thickness necrosis may be the first identified sign, with underlying bone and muscle exposed to view. To promote healing it will be necessary to remove the necrotic material (debride), either chemically or surgically, resulting in a deeper ulcer, which can distress patient and carer. Large volumes of exudate may be produced, particularly if infection is present.

Within deep cavities there may be sinus formation, i.e. narrow tracks may form, which lead into deeper tissue. In such cavities, careful selection of treatment is required to avoid damage to underlying tissue. In patients who have suffered with chronic pressure ulcers, long-standing sinuses may exist, visible on the surface of the skin as only a narrow, often leaking, opening. This generally indicates an unhealed cavity below in which there is risk of abscess formation and chronic infection.

Investigations

If a sinus exists, it is important to establish the extent of the tracking within the body tissue, and this can only be achieved by radiological investigation (a sinogram). The sinogram may indicate the need for surgical intervention to open up the area, drain and treat it as appropriate.

Chronic wounds, especially if abnormal in appearance, should be biopsied, since malignancy can develop in non-healing wounds. A cauliflower-like appearance, suggestive of squamous cell carcinoma, will bleed very readily. This should not be confused with overgranulation, which can occur spontaneously during healing and may be precipitated by specific dressings, e.g. hydrocolloids. This tissue is also very friable, bleeding readily if traumatized.

Treatment

Urgent treatment of pressure ulcers is essential. Unfortunately there is little evidence from randomized controlled trials to support specific treatment applications. There is, however, considerable evidence to demonstrate the dangers of excessive pressure. Any mechanism which can reduce pressure as well as shear and friction should be considered. Realistic objectives should be established as some pressure ulcers will never heal but may be made more acceptable for patients and carers.

Deep, infected pressure ulcers carry a high risk of morbidity due to septicaemia. Treatment priorities must be based on the degree of pressure damage and the need for surgical or other intervention and have regard to overall prognosis and predisposing factors. Pressure ulcers on heels can impede rehabilitation by severely restricting mobility.

A multidisciplinary approach to treatment will consider all aspects of care and will involve:

- a dietitian, to ensure optimum nutrition for patients with pressure damage, and those at risk
- a doctor, to assess overall prognosis and patient management
- a nurse, to regularly assess the risk of individual patients and their pressure points, establish a turning/moving routine, appropriate dressing changes and the provision of moral support to patients and carers
- a pharmacist, to aid rational product selection and ensure availability and assist with product familiarity
- a physiotherapist, to improve and encourage patient mobility and advise on supplementary healing techniques
- an occupational therapist, to select the most appropriate support surface and aids to minimize additional tissue stresses.

Physiotherapists may treat pressure ulcers with ultraviolet or ultrasound therapy, often in conjunction with topical preparations. Ultrasound may be performed with dressings in situ, while ultraviolet therapy requires removal of the dressing. Caution is needed if enzymatic debriding agents are in use as these are easily inactivated.

Tissue viability nurses (TVNs) are now employed in many areas to co-ordinate a consistent approach to wound care, including pressure ulcer prevention and treatment, and to advise on the care of patients with complex ulcers.

Wound management

A holistic approach is essential in pressure ulcer care. Topical applications are only part of treatment, and often surgical intervention will be required to speed healing. No single product is normally suitable for all stages of ulceration. As the ulcer changes, so should the product. However, a fair trial of a given treatment is essential with accurate documentation to explain reasons for choice. Staff education should emphasize the benefits of co-ordinated wound management strategies.

Clinical infection

Before commencing treatment, any clinical infection should be identified. All wounds will show bacterial growth if swabbed, but this is only significant if present in sufficient numbers to produce clinical infection. When assessing a wound it is necessary to consider whether:

- there is pus formation
- the patient is pyrexial and feeling unwell
- there is surrounding cellulitis, i.e. inflammation of the surrounding skin and tissues with associated heat
- there is likely to be infection involving bone.

If any of the above factors are present, a swab should be taken from the deep part of the wound to determine the appropriate systemic antibiotic to prescribe. If there is no indication that a clinical infection is present, a swab is not necessary.

Treatment selection

The optimal wound care product should

- create a moist environment without maceration
- remove excess exudate from the wound surface
- provide a barrier to micro-organisms
- be sterile
- be non-adherent and easily removed
- be free of particulate contamination
- be non-toxic, non-allergenic and non-sensitizing
- be thermally insulating
- allow gaseous exchange
- be easy to use for health professionals and carers
- have acceptable characteristics, e.g. odour free
- be cost-effective
- be available in a wide range of sizes for hospital and community use.

Products such as lint, gauze and gamgee do not fulfil these requirements due to:

- limited absorbency
- rapid saturation with wound exudate which can strike through to the dressing surface, increasing the risk of infection
- adherence
- potential for pain and bleeding on removal
- tendency to lift newly formed cells from the wound surface.

A protocol for ulcer treatment decision making can be devised, based on the stages of ulceration and characteristics of available products. The position of the pressure ulcer will also influence the decision as there may be a need for a secondary (covering) dressing.

Table 58.3 outlines management options for pressure ulcer categories at different stages of healing.

When determining optimum treatment it is necessary to consider the following questions.

- Is the wound clean?
- Is there excessive exudate?
- Is sloughy tissue present?
- Is the wound clinically infected?
- Is the wound malodorous?

Many traditional cleansing agents such as hypochlorite solutions and hydrogen peroxide are now recognized as having harmful effects.

Wounds should only be cleaned to aid removal of:

- excessive exudate
- pus
- loose necrotic or sloughy tissue.

Ideally a warmed sodium chloride solution (0.9%) should be used. Cold solutions can lower the wound surface temperature below body temperature and impair new cell formation.

Methicillin-resistant *Staphylococcus aureus* (MRSA)

If MRSA is identified in the wound, special precautions are needed in the hospital and care home situation. Although MRSA can occur in wounds which are apparently healing normally, cross-infection to other patients is a risk and some could develop fatal clinical infections. Various options have been tried to both aid healing and reduce the risk of cross-infection. Sterile maggots have been used to eradicate MRSA from individual wounds. Local policies should guide management of such patients.

Odorous wounds

Although pseudomonal infections can cause odour, the most likely cause is anaerobic bacteria. Charcoal dressings will mask and absorb odour if changed before the charcoal layer is saturated. The preferred approach is eradication of the odour-producing anaerobes using metronidazole, given orally 200–400 mg three times a day. If poorly tolerated, a topical metronidazole gel can be used. This route may also be used to avoid the disulfiram-like reaction of metronidazole with alcohol, although the reaction is still theoretically possible even with topical application.

The resolution of the odour, through oral or topical use, is normally dramatic and reassuring for the patient. Prolonged use may result in resistant anaerobes.

Debridement of the ulcer

Surgical debridement is preferred but is not always practical or available for community patients. Previous national guidance (NICE 2001) recommended selection of the most cost-effective product. It is now accepted that there is insufficient evidence to determine this (NICE 2005), with more studies

Table 58.3 Management options for pressure ulcers at different stages

Type of wound	A Epithelializing	B Granulating	C(i) Exuding (light to medium)	C(ii) Exuding (moderate to high)	D Necrotic (dry[a]/moist)	E Sloughy	F Malodorous
Superficial break	Non-adherent dressing	Non-adherent dressing or thin hydrocolloid	Foam film or hydrocolloid or alginate	Foam film, alginate or silicone dressing[b]	Hydrocolloid or hydrogel	Hydrocolloid or hydrogel	Charcoal dressing or metronidazole gel[c]
Partial/full thickness		Hydrocolloid	Foam film or hydrocolloid or alginate	Foam film, alginate or silicone dressing[b]	Hydrocolloid or hydrogel	Hydrocolloid or hydrogel or fibrous hydrocolloid[d]	Charcoal dressing or metronidazole gel[c]
Cavity/sinus (only loose packing recommended for sinuses, with careful removal). A sinogram will identify any tracking		Hydrogel	Alginate ribbon or hydrogel	Alginate ribbon or silicone dressing[b]	Hydrogel or fibrous hydrocolloid[d]	Hydrogel or fibrous hydrocolloid[d]	Charcoal dressing or metronidazole gel[c]

[a] For dry necrotic areas, a fibrous hydrocolloid is inappropriate.
[b] Mepitel, a silicone dressing, can remain in place for up to 14 days with only an outer absorbent dressing being changed as necessary. Education of users and carers is crucial to cost-effective use of this dressing.
[c] Oral metronidazole should be considered before topical gel for eradication of odour-producing anaerobes, but may be poorly tolerated and the alcohol restriction may be inappropriate.
[d] Aquacel, a modified fibrous hydrocolloid, can remain in place for up to 7 days and is suitable for exuding slough/necrotic wounds.
N.B. If clinical infection is present, appropriate systemic antibiotics will be required. Do not confuse with wound colonization. Do not swab the wound unless clinical signs of infection are present.

required on cost-effectiveness, quality of life and objective measures of dressing performance. In the interim practitioners are advised to create the optimum wound-healing environment using modern dressings in preference to basic dressing types.

The biosurgical approach, using sterile maggots of the green bottle fly, is now used in early management by some practitioners. Sharp debridement is a technique practised more widely by nurses in the USA and may increase in the UK with appropriate training. When chemical or biosurgical approaches are used, including enzymatic preparations and povidone-iodine containing preparations, review dates should be set to assess effectiveness and avoid prolonged use. Excessive use of iodine or povidone-iodine containing products should be avoided, particularly in anyone with a history of thyroid disorder. Reconstitution and application of preparations such as Varidase require great care to avoid early inactivation.

Characteristics of pressure ulcer products

Hydrocolloids Hydrocolloids (e.g. Comfeel and Granuflex) are available as self-adhesive sheets, although if used on the sacrum and buttocks they may need to be taped in place, even if the specially shaped sacral dressings are used. All hydrocolloids contain carboxymethylcellulose with some additionally incorporating pectin and gelatin, the latter being responsible for an unpleasant odour noticeable at dressing changes even in the absence of clinical infection.

Hydrocolloid dressings liquefy at the wound surface, hydrating soft sloughy tissue and encouraging wound healing. In wounds with low exudate, hydrocolloids may remain in place for 7 days. If left in place on a black eschar, marked softening of the necrotic tissue will occur. Different degrees of gaseous permeability are claimed for the various products and caution should be observed regarding their use in the presence of anaerobic infection.

Overproduction of granulation tissue may occur beneath hydrocolloids. If this occurs their use should be discontinued. The excess tissue may be reduced by compression bandaging if appropriate or by use of a particular polyurethane foam dressing, Lyofoam. An alternative is the application of 0.25% silver nitrate solution daily for 5–7 days. Thereafter, epithelialization should be encouraged with an alternative category of dressing appropriate to the wound type.

Modified hydrocolloids (e.g. CombiDERM, Aquacel) These are suitable for medium to heavily exudating wounds and may remain in place for up to 7 days but intially may need more frequent changes. CombiDERM's central wound contact pad contains exudate-retaining polyacrylate granules, while Aquacel is composed of hydrocolloid fibres and sodium carboxymethylcellulose, but no gelatin and hence has no odour.

Hydrogels Hydrogels (e.g. Intrasite, Purilon) require a secondary covering dressing, whether the gel or conformable sheet versions are used. Gel formulations are particularly useful for cavity pressure ulcers.

Hydrogels consist of a hydrophilic polymer in an aqueous base and serve to hydrate the wound surface and lift slough and necrotic tissue while encouraging moist wound healing. Initially, the gel is normally changed daily, extending to every 3 days in cleaner wounds. Hydrogel-hydrocolloid (e.g. GranuGel) and hydrogel-alginate (e.g. SeaSorb) formulations can stay in place

for longer. Hydrogels may be used on black eschars after scoring of the eschar to assist penetration but tend to be rather more rapidly effective on wounds covered with softer necrotic or sloughy tissue. They are inappropriate for heavily exuding wounds. If excessive amounts of gel are applied to an ulcer, maceration will occur at the wound edge with whitening of the surrounding skin.

Alginates Alginates (e.g. Kaltostat and Sorbsan) are available in a flat or rope form. Most require a secondary dressing but some newer forms incorporate an adhesive border to aid retention on lightly exuding wounds.

The available dressings consist of either calcium alginate alone or a combination of sodium and calcium alginate and differing proportions of mannuronic and guluronic acid. The difference in composition determines the gelling properties of the dressings at the wound surface. In contact with wound exudate, the dressing is very absorbent and forms a moist gel over the wound surface. This forms better if the dressing can remain in place for 48 hours.

Alginates are therefore only suitable for exuding wounds, not for dry wounds or eschars where no gelling will occur. In a heavily exuding wound, daily changes may be needed initially but these can be reduced as the exudate lessens, and an alternative dressing may then be considered. The haemostatic properties of some of these dressings may be useful in controlling bleeding on granulating pressure ulcers, when daily changes are likely to be needed. Depending on the gelling properties, the dressings are removed from the wound with sterile saline or lifted off with forceps.

Foam films Dressings in this category (e.g. Allevyn and Lyofoam) include self-adhesive options but some must be held in place with tape. Either may be inappropriate on fragile skin. Medium to high absorbency makes them suitable for exuding wounds. Due to the nature of the dressing, lateral absorption of exudate occurs, avoiding the vertical strike-through of traditional dressings. The dressing is initially changed daily. Inspection will reveal if this is inadequate because seepage of exudate will be seen at the edges of the dressing. In wounds producing less exudate, some of the dressings may remain in place for up to 7 days, encouraging healing in a moist environment. Foams generally show low adherence to the wound surface but saline may be needed to assist removal.

Cavity dressings These are available mainly in ribbon form for loose packing into deeper ulcers, with probes provided with some products to assist in depth assessment. Most are conformable alginates or fibrous hydrocolloids.

Allevyn cavity wound dressing is foam based and available in various shapes, whose usefulness depends on size and shape of the ulcer and fit of the dressing.

Film dressings Film dressings (e.g. OpSite and Cutifilm) are self-adhesive and are inappropriate for use on elderly fragile skin, which can easily be damaged by incorrect application and removal. The films are semipermeable, allowing evaporation of some water vapour, but exudate accumulates beneath and may irritate and macerate the surrounding skin. They are widely used to reduce friction over pressure points in at-risk patients when they may be left in place for several days. Careful attention must be paid to the manufacturer's instructions for application and removal of each different film dressing to avoid inflicting skin damage.

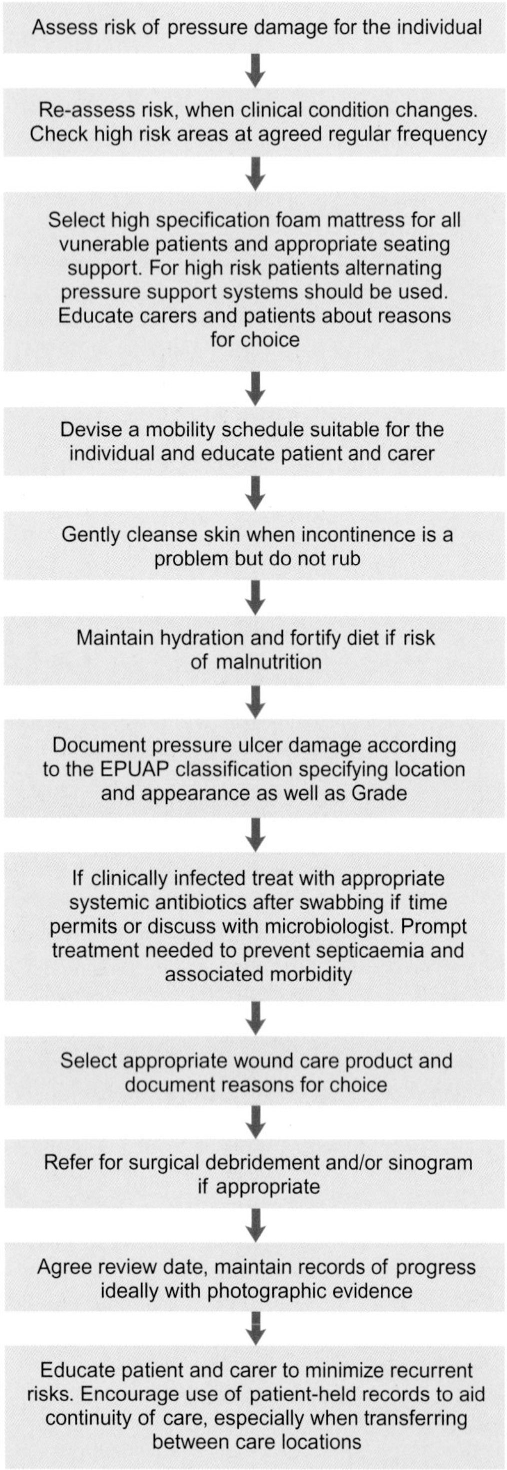

Assess risk of pressure damage for the individual

↓

Re-assess risk, when clinical condition changes.
Check high risk areas at agreed regular frequency

↓

Select high specification foam mattress for all
vunerable patients and appropriate seating
support. For high risk patients alternating
pressure support systems should be used.
Educate carers and patients about reasons
for choice

↓

Devise a mobility schedule suitable for the
individual and educate patient and carer

↓

Gently cleanse skin when incontinence is a
problem but do not rub

↓

Maintain hydration and fortify diet if risk
of malnutrition

↓

Document pressure ulcer damage according
to the EPUAP classification specifying location
and appearance as well as Grade

↓

If clinically infected treat with appropriate
systemic antibiotics after swabbing if time
permits or discuss with microbiologist. Prompt
treatment needed to prevent septicaemia and
associated morbidity

↓

Select appropriate wound care product and
document reasons for choice

↓

Refer for surgical debridement and/or sinogram
if appropriate

↓

Agree review date, maintain records of progress
ideally with photographic evidence

↓

Educate patient and carer to minimize recurrent
risks. Encourage use of patient-held records to aid
continuity of care, especially when transferring
between care locations

Figure 58.1 Key practice points for pressure ulcer prevention and management.

Soft silicone wound contact dressings These products (e.g. Mepitel) can remain in place for up to 7 days and often longer, simply changing the outer dressing which can be of the perforated absorbent type (e.g. Mepore) placed over the silicone gel net of Mepitel. These products are of specific use in blistering skin conditions where non-adhesion is critical but also have a place in exuding pressure sores and in some exuding leg ulcers where compression bandaging may be inappropriate and where infrequent dressing changes are desirable if possible.

Silicone dressings have also developed to include inherent absorbency. If used correctly, the higher unit costs of silicone dressings can prove worthwhile in relation to speed and effectiveness of healing.

Silver dressings Silver is now incorporated into a range of interactive wound care products, including alginates, hydrocolloids, charcoal dressings, films and foams, all with very different release characteristics and changing frequencies to reduce risk of saturation of the silver component. Products vary in silver release and more research is needed to clarify the optimal silver concentration to achieve minimal systemic absorption and to avoid local deposition.

Larval or maggot therapy The sterile larvae of the green bottle fly are accepted as a useful addition to the care of pressure ulcers (Thomas 2002). They can debride successfully in a short time and patient acceptability has been helped by media coverage. Neglected wounds can provide habitats for natural maggots. The sterile versions can be applied in a controlled manner to necrotic and sloughy wounds at an early stage with the aim of progression to healing. In practice, they are often used late in the life of sloughy ulcers providing a major challenge, often with less successful outcomes. Education of health professionals, as well as patients and carers, is crucial to their effective use and comprehensive information on application and removal is available from the LarvE website (www.pobiotic.org). Larvae must be treated well and not overheated or saturated with cleaning solution. Certain hydrogels can adversely affect the larvae. Patients should be warned that the larval therapy may be painful and additional analgesia may be necessary, especially for the initial applications (Steenvoorde et al 2005).

Key steps in the prevention and management of pressure ulcers are summarized in Figure 58.1 and some of the common therapeutic problems encountered in the management of pressure ulcers are presented in Table 58.4.

Table 58.4 Common therapeutic problems in the management of pressure ulcers

Inconsistencies between risk assessment schemes used in different settings

Failure to reassess risk as patient's condition changes

Limited availability of preventive equipment and assessments of suitability

Use of the same wound management product for too long with infrequent reviews

Combined use of interactive wound management products

Limited use of portable documentation

Inappropriate use of interactive products, e.g. on non-healing heavily exuding ulcers needing daily changes

Leg ulcers

A leg ulcer is any break in skin integrity on the lower leg, normally caused by an underlying circulatory disorder or specific medical condition, even if reported as being initiated by trauma. Many leg ulcers are chronic in nature, with some patients having suffered for 30–40 years. Treatment must be directed at the underlying cause rather than simply the break in the skin.

Epidemiology

It has been estimated that 1% of the population have chronic leg ulcers, with 70% of patients developing the leg ulcer before the age of 65 years and 25% before the age of 45 years.

Over the age of 50 years, women are more commonly affected. Approximately 75% of healed ulcers may eventually recur. Most leg ulcer patients are managed in the community at a cost estimated at between £2700 and £5200 per patient per year. The most recent estimation of annual cost to the UK health service is between £300 and £600 million. With the advent of more specialist leg ulcer treatment clinics and clinical specialists, and with accurate diagnosis and assessment, it may be possible to reduce overall costs and healing times.

Aetiology

There are a number of different types of leg ulcer, which can be classified according to the underlying causation:

- venous
- arterial
- arteriovenous
- diabetic
- autoimmune ulcers.

Venous ulcers

Venous ulcers account for >80% of all leg ulcers. They occur as a result of failure of the calf muscle pump, i.e. the calf muscles which squeeze deep venous blood upwards from the legs back to the heart. This pump will not function effectively if there is a backflow of blood from the deep veins to the superficial veins in the leg. Backflow may occur due to fatigue or incompetence of the valves in the deep veins and in the perforating veins which connect the superficial and deep veins (Fig. 58.2A).

Restricted mobility may also predispose to venous ulceration. During walking, the action of the foot striking a solid surface facilitates venous return while the ankle movement involved in normal walking alternately contracts and relaxes the calf muscle.

As backflow of blood occurs into the superficial veins and capillaries, leakage of fluid occurs into the interstitial space and oedema results. Haemosiderin from red cell breakdown is deposited in the tissues, causing a characteristic brown coloration, particularly in the gaiter or lower area of the leg. Fibrinogen leaks from capillaries and is converted to fibrin, forming a fibrin 'cuff' around the capillaries which may also reduce tissue oxygenation. In the affected area the skin becomes friable as oedema progresses and any slight trauma can precipitate ulceration.

The original cause of perforator valve incompetence may be a deep vein thrombosis which could have occurred many years previously. In elderly women this can often be traced back to a pregnancy. Patients with valve incompetencies may have a history of varicose veins and approximately 3% of patients with varicosities go on to suffer leg ulcers. Clinical practice guidelines

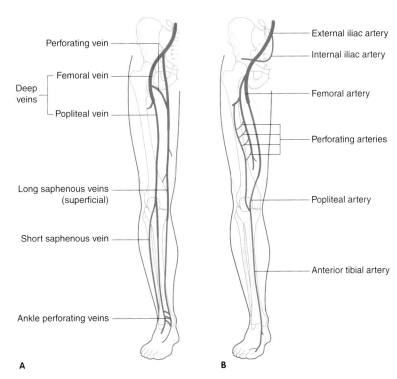

Figure 58.2 **A** Venous circulation: lower limb. **B** Arterial circulation: lower limb.

(SIGN 1998) have reviewed available evidence in this area of care and helped to standardize management of patients with venous ulcers and distinguish this from the approaches needed in treating patients with ulcers of differing aetiology.

Arterial ulcers

The arterial circulation is illustrated in Figure 58.2B. Arterial ulcers arise in a different manner from venous ulcers. Blood fails to reach the superficial tissues as a result of atherosclerosis affecting the medium and large arteries of the lower leg. Oxygen supply to the arterioles is therefore inadequate and breakdown of skin results in a painful ulcer.

An arterial embolism will similarly produce ulceration but in a more rapid and dangerous manner.

Arteriovenous ulcers

Lower leg ulcers may result from a combination of both venous and arterial incompetence and a mixed picture of clinical signs will be seen.

Diabetic leg ulcers

Diabetes is associated with approximately 5% of all leg ulcers. The ulcers are typically ischaemic in nature as a result of diabetic vascular disease which affects the small distal arteries, particularly in the weight-bearing areas such as the feet.

Autoimmune leg ulcers

The most common causative factor in this category is rheumatoid arthritis which is present in 8% of patients with leg ulcers. Although associated immobility will limit calf muscle pump activity, the ulceration primarily occurs through arteritis of the small vessels and consequent ischaemia.

Other leg ulcers

Several other conditions may be associated with leg ulcer formation in patients, including burns, infections, haematological disease, lymphoedema and vasculitis. Malignancy can develop in chronic non-healing ulcers or the ulcer may begin as a malignant manifestation. As with chronic pressure ulcers and other non-healing skin problems, biopsy is recommended for long-standing leg ulcers.

The practitioner should be aware that a small number of ulcers may be self-inflicted, or an existing ulcer may be further damaged by the patient to maintain contact with healthcare staff (the 'social ulcer phenomenon').

Clinical signs

In determining the cause of a leg ulcer, observation of clinical signs is important, together with an accurate history from the patient or carer. The characteristic clinical features of venous and arterial ulcers are shown in Table 58.5. Diabetic ulcers often look similar to arterial ulcers. However, in the diabetic ulcer foot pulses may be present if only the microcirculation is

Table 58.5   Clinical features of venous and arterial ulcers

Venous	Arterial
Occur in gaiter area (generally above medial malleolus)	Occur around malleolus or on the foot, toes or heels
Often large and shallow with flat edges and copious exudate	Punched-out appearance with steep edges often deep with little exudate. Muscle and tendon exposure occurs
Generalized oedema of leg may be present	Local oedema may occur
Dark staining of lower leg due to red blood cell breakdown	Skin staining rare
Sensitive to touch but not normally very painful unless clinically infected or oedematous. Infection common in chronic venous ulcers	Very painful, especially at night or if leg is elevated. Relieved by hanging leg out of bed/ sleeping in a chair. Pain may be severe on exercise due to muscle tissue ischaemia
Foot pulses are present and foot is warm. Surrounding varicose eczema is common	Foot pulses reduced or absent. Foot is cold and shiny with hair loss and degeneration of toe nails. Foot may whiten on elevation and colour when dependent

damaged while if the deeper arterial system is damaged, as in arterial ulcers, these pulses are absent. The patient with a diabetic ulcer does not always complain of pain, due to loss of sensation resulting from diabetes-induced peripheral neuropathy.

Diagnostic investigation

Before treatment is started, the extent of venous and arterial damage should be determined by use of a portable Doppler machine. This permits calculation of the patient's ankle–brachial pressure index (ABPI) by comparing brachial and ankle systolic pressures:

$$\text{ABPI} = \frac{\text{systolic blood pressure in the ankle}}{\text{systolic blood pressure in the arm}}$$

The ABPI index should be greater than 1 in people with undamaged arteries.

If compression bandaging is applied to the leg of patients with an ABPI below 0.8, the arterial circulation will be compromised, tissue necrosis may result and amputation could be required. Light compression may be used in patients with an ABPI of between 0.8 and 0.9 and some specialist centres have used this in patients with lower ABPIs. Erroneous readings can occur in diabetics and compression bandaging should only be used with great caution in such patients.

Pulse oximetry is increasingly being used as an additional diagnostic and assessment tool to determine appropriateness for compression therapy. This measures oxygenation of fingers and toes, remains a non-invasive technique and can increase the accuracy of assessment for some patients when used in conjunction with clinical judgement.

Ulcer treatment

The treatment regimen should be holistic in approach and aim to:

- correct the circulation
- provide pain relief
- protect and treat the surrounding skin
- prevent and treat any infection
- heal the ulcer
- prevent any recurrence.

Correction of circulation

If a patient presents with a venous ulcer and severe oedema, total bed rest is required. The affected limb should be elevated above the height of the hip and preferably the heart. If mild oedema is present elevation of the limb at night, achieved by raising the foot of the bed, may resolve the problem.

Venous return to the heart should be encouraged by improving the calf muscle pump. Exercise should be encouraged to the limit of the patient's ability. If severely restricted, regular walking on the spot can help and immobile patients can be taught ankle exercises which may be practised when lying down or sitting. In combination with exercise, graduated compression bandaging applied from the base of the toes to the knee is essential. Various multilayered compression systems have been used in trials, consisting of a non-adherent dressing immediately over the ulcer area followed by orthopaedic padding to protect the bony prominences of the ankle. Other layers may include:

- crepe bandage to hold padding in place
- class 3a compression bandage
- cohesive outer layer to retain bandages and provide additional compression.

There is no conclusive evidence from randomized controlled trials to confirm that layered systems are more efficient than any other high-compression systems. When interpreting studies it is important to ensure that identical parameters have been compared. Some workers have considered the time to complete healing, i.e. all ulcers healed in all patients, while others have looked at the percentage of individual ulcers healed.

In the absence of strong evidence it has been suggested that cost differences between available methods cannot be overlooked. The layered components or single-layer systems are usually applied weekly but in cases of oedema more frequent changes may be needed as the limb changes shape. Cohesive components cannot be reused but crepe and compression layers can be washed and reapplied. Patient acceptance varies, especially as the layered systems will not fit into a normal shoe. The correct application of such bandaging is crucial to its success. Incorrect bandaging and its inappropriate use can cause limb necrosis, and is therefore worse than no bandage at all.

In a patient with an arterial ulcer it is essential that the extent of arterial damage is diagnosed and compression bandaging is often

avoided. However, specialist assessment may advise reduced layer compression depending on circulatory status.

In severe arterial damage, only light bandaging may be possible to hold dressings in place and afford limited protection. Gentle exercise should be encouraged, limbs should be kept warm, and smoking discouraged. Surgical assessment is important to establish prognosis and the potential for surgical intervention.

There is no clear evidence to support the use of the majority of vasodilators in improving arterial blood flow and hence treating ulceration, although oral pentoxyfylline may prove to be beneficial in certain ulcer types. Tissue engineered skin applied beneath compression has been investigated and demonstrated some benefit.

Pain relief

This is an often neglected area of leg ulcer management. Venous ulcers are not generally considered painful but may become extremely painful when first elevated. In addition, applications of compression and the healing process itself can be painful. Regular analgesia may be needed, with an additional dose prior to the dressing change. Anti-inflammatory drugs may help but can interfere with the healing process. Patients with arterial ulcers sometimes require strong analgesia, such as an opioid, particularly at night, when cramping pains may be severe. Opioids may also be needed for some patients with venous ulcers. A topical anaesthetic cream, e.g. Emla, is advocated by some centres but caution is required as there is a risk of local sensitization.

Protection and treatment of surrounding skin

Minimal medication should be applied to a venous ulcer as the surrounding skin is usually extremely sensitive due, in part, to varicose eczema, and also to chronic application of assorted medicaments. Barrier creams often contain lanolin and hydroxy-benzoate preservatives to which the patient may be allergic and which may exacerbate the underlying problem.

Medicated paste bandages (e.g. Icthopaste, Steripaste) or stockings (e.g. Zipzoc) with a zinc oxide base may be used over the chosen ulcer preparation to treat the surrounding chronic eczema and sensitive skin. These can be placed over the primary ulcer dressing prior to application of layered compression. There is a need to be aware of differences in preservative and lanolin content, both of which can cause sensitization, and gelatin content which can cause bandages to harden and impair movement.

In patients with severe eczema on the tissue surrounding the ulcer, a steroid preparation may be needed but care must be taken to avoid contact with the ulcer. Patch testing to identify the causative agent for the eczema may be necessary. Weeping eczema may respond to potassium permanganate soaks and there has been a resurgence of use of eosin and silver nitrate as additional astringents by some specialists.

If the surrounding skin of venous ulcers is dry with crusting scales of dead skin (hyperkeratosis), application of olive oil may be helpful.

The skin surrounding an arterial ulcer is often shiny and easily traumatized. Rubbing in topical medicaments should be avoided.

58

Infection

Most ulcers will be colonized with micro-organisms and if swabbed, bacteria will be identified. However, only clinical infection is significant. The presence of pus with accompanying odour and the presence of cellulitis in surrounding tissues all indicate the presence of infection. The patient is often unwell and systemic antibiotic therapy is essential. To prevent build-up of exudate and debris in such ulcers, cleansing with water or saline is important. Soaking the leg in warm water is often also soothing for the patient.

Healing the ulcer

Without treatment of the underlying condition, topical applications will be ineffective, or effective in the short term only.

If a venous ulcer is present, a simple primary dressing can be covered with graduated compression bandaging which aims to correct the circulatory problem, as described earlier. In between, a paste bandage could be used if the surrounding skin condition is compromised.

Arterial ulcers may be improved with a primary dressing selected from Table 58.3, depending on the ulcer assessment, held in place if necessary with light, non-elastic bandaging.

However, recurrence and further ulceration are common. Surgical intervention may improve circulation in some cases.

Prevention of recurrence

For all patients with an ulcer, education and support are essential to prevent recurrence of the problem if and when healing occurs. When a venous ulcer heals, protection is essential together with prescription of accurately fitted, below-knee class II or III compression stockings to avoid future breakdown. These can be obtained in standard sizes but made-to-measure are preferable to achieve an accurate fit and particularly for legs of difficult shape. They should be renewed every 3–6 months and air-dried to maintain elasticity. Class III stockings have been shown to reduce recurrence rates more effectively but class II are better tolerated. Use for a minimum of 5 years is advised. Patients should be reviewed regularly to encourage compliance with treatment, regular exercise, good nutrition, weight control and appropriate skin care (Vowden & Vowden 2006). There is as yet no firm trial evidence to confirm the optimal approach but strategies are based on expert opinion and should be individualized to motivate patients.

Arterial ulcers must be protected with a light protective dressing to reduce the risk of external trauma when recently healed. Full compression should be avoided.

Community leg ulcer clinics

There is some evidence that leg ulcer patients are best managed in specialist community leg ulcer clinics. These clinics are staffed by specially trained community nurses, ideally with access to a vascular surgeon for the referral of patients with arterial ulcers and ulcers of mixed aetiology. Excellent ulcer healing rates have been achieved in these clinics. Recurrence rates also appear to be dramatically reduced as patients receive ongoing education

about the care of their leg and are often motivated by their peers. An alternative approach, especially in rural areas, is utilization of community nurse practitioners to provide leg ulcer management on an ongoing basis to motivate and encourage the individual.

Some common therapeutic problems in the treatment of leg ulcers are listed in Table 58.6 whilst Figure 58.3 outlines key practice points in leg ulcer management.

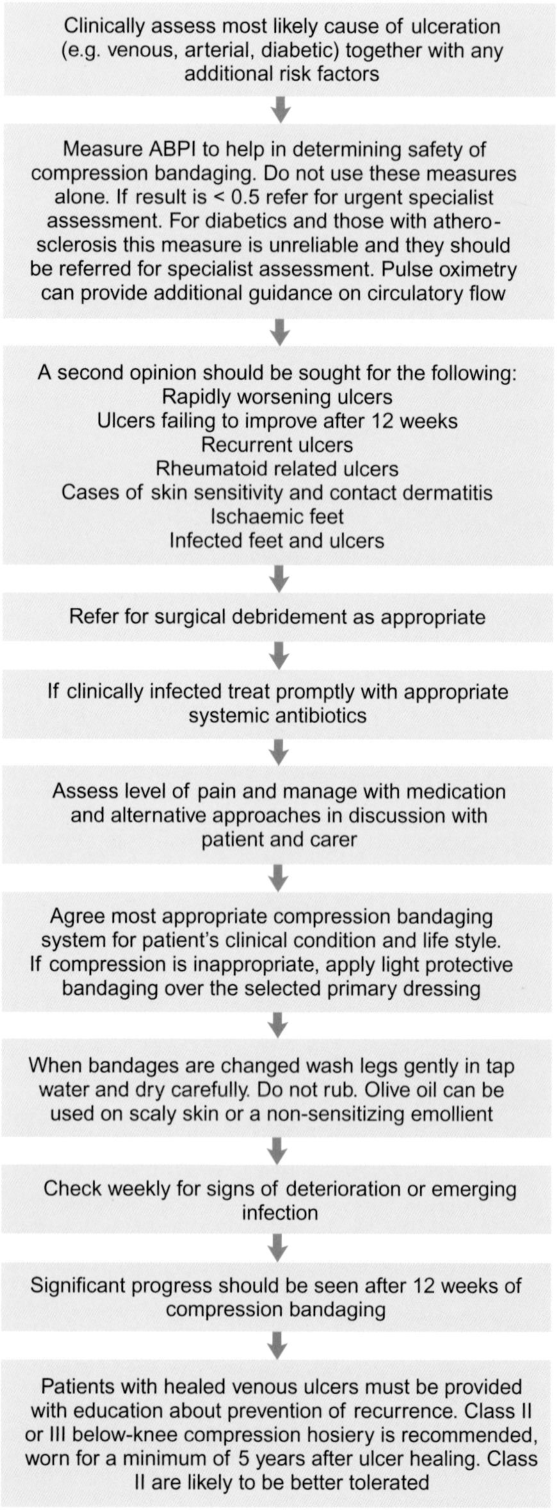

Clinically assess most likely cause of ulceration (e.g. venous, arterial, diabetic) together with any additional risk factors

Measure ABPI to help in determining safety of compression bandaging. Do not use these measures alone. If result is < 0.5 refer for urgent specialist assessment. For diabetics and those with atherosclerosis this measure is unreliable and they should be referred for specialist assessment. Pulse oximetry can provide additional guidance on circulatory flow

A second opinion should be sought for the following:
Rapidly worsening ulcers
Ulcers failing to improve after 12 weeks
Recurrent ulcers
Rheumatoid related ulcers
Cases of skin sensitivity and contact dermatitis
Ischaemic feet
Infected feet and ulcers

Refer for surgical debridement as appropriate

If clinically infected treat promptly with appropriate systemic antibiotics

Assess level of pain and manage with medication and alternative approaches in discussion with patient and carer

Agree most appropriate compression bandaging system for patient's clinical condition and life style. If compression is inappropriate, apply light protective bandaging over the selected primary dressing

When bandages are changed wash legs gently in tap water and dry carefully. Do not rub. Olive oil can be used on scaly skin or a non-sensitizing emollient

Check weekly for signs of deterioration or emerging infection

Significant progress should be seen after 12 weeks of compression bandaging

Patients with healed venous ulcers must be provided with education about prevention of recurrence. Class II or III below-knee compression hosiery is recommended, worn for a minimum of 5 years after ulcer healing. Class II are likely to be better tolerated

Figure 58.3 Key practice points for leg ulcer management.

Table 58.6 Common problems in the management of leg ulcers

Reliance on ABPI measurement without adequate clinical assessment when considering bandaging

Inadequate education and support for patients to reduce risk of ulcer recurrence

Unnecessary use of costly interactive dressings beneath compression therapy

Limited use of accessible, portable documented history

The way forward for pressure and leg ulcer management

Compression therapy is likely to remain the mainstay of venous ulcer therapy but research may aid selection of simpler, more universally acceptable regimens which will achieve and maintain adequate pressure. Suitable approaches for those with arterial damage need to be determined by research.

As growth factors and other tissue engineered products are developed, specific treatments will target different ulcer types, including pressure ulcers. Becaplermin, a recombinant human platelet-derived growth factor, is licensed only for use in diabetic neuropathic foot ulcers and only if used in conjunction with good wound care measures, which includes debridement. Dermal replacements have also been developed, e.g. Dermagraft. However, both approaches are costly, with limited data on long-term safety. Earlier use of larval therapy for debridement is likely for both pressure ulcers and sloughy, necrotic leg ulcers, but use of a pain management protocol is advised (Steenvorde et al 2005). As technology develops, regular review of pain control must remain a cornerstone of wound management.

The integrated multiprofessional team approach is crucial to effective management of patients who are unfortunate enough to experience ulceration of either classification.

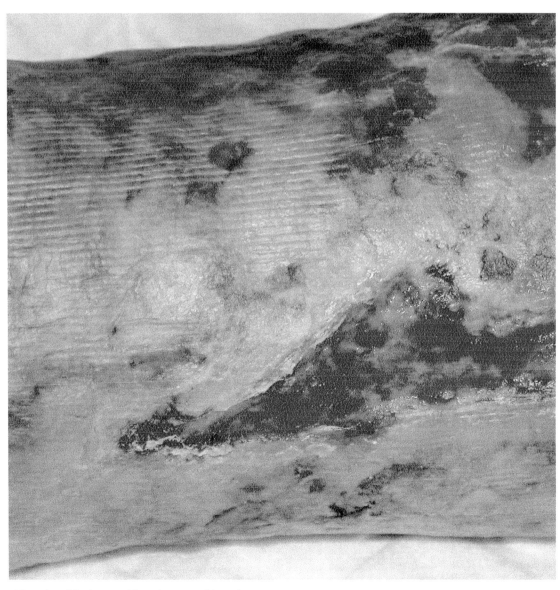

Figure 58.4 Ulceration of the inner and frontal aspects of the gaiter area.

CASE STUDIES

Case 58.1

An 82-year-old patient has ulceration of the inner and frontal aspects of the gaiter area (Fig. 58.4).

Questions

1. What is the most likely cause of the ulceration?
2. What is the cause of the brown discoloration?
3. What action and advice could help?

Answers

1. From the position and appearance, these are likely to be venous ulcers caused by reduced venous return resulting from damage to the valves in the deep veins and the superficial perforator veins. The ulcers are shallow with flat edges and some slough.
2. The brown discoloration is caused by haemosiderin release as red cells break down in the compromised venous system, which is then deposited in tissues.
3. The slough should autodebride with appropriate compression bandaging, after ensuring adequate circulation by ABPI measurement/ pulse oximetry and clinical assessment of pedal pulses and appearances of the feet and legs.

    An interactive wound product could be utilized beneath compression, particularly if exudate is a problem. A foam film or fibrous hydrocolloid would be suitable if exudate is medium to high. In the absence of exudate, a hydrocolloid could be suitable. Care with application and taping is important in view of likely skin sensitivity.

    Protection from further damage is important as this area is easily retraumatized as the ulcers heal. Motivation to wear compression stockings to prevent risk of recurrence after healing should be discussed.

Case 58.2

A 54-year-old paraplegic has a sacral pressure ulcer extending down to the left buttock (Fig. 58.5).

Questions

1. What should be the key concern in planning care for this patient?
2. What are the key concerns in selecting a product(s) to manage this ulcer?

Answers

1. Relief of pressure to prevent further tissue damage and a review of how this has developed to such a degree. This should be documented as a clinical incident and key carers interviewed to try and track the ulcer's development and identify potential intervention points to assist future care. A history of the care of the ulcer will help determine the original size.

    An assessment of the surrounding redness is crucial. Is erythema developing due to continuing tissue trauma? Is this an indication of the original size of the ulcer or of the cavern beneath and developing cellulitic tissue?
2. An assessment of the concerns of the patient in relation to the wound should be a priority.

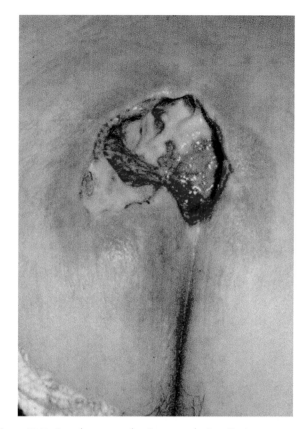

Figure 58.5 Sacral pressure ulcer in a paraplegic patient.

The wound is likely to produce copious exudate as it is of an excavating type. This will probably cause major distress and use of an absorbent product with an ability to conform to the cavity is a priority. A fibrous hydrocolloid cavity dressing, such as Aquacel, could be useful but this has to be held in place preferably by a dressing which extends beyond the sensitive area. The superficial sloughing at the edge of the wound must also be managed, either with the same product, if that area is sufficiently moist, or with a template of hydrocolloid unless clinically infected.

Case 58.3

A 62-year-old lady has an ulcer with mixed appearance on her malleolar area (Fig. 58.6).

Questions

1. What is the likely ulcer type and why?
2. Why is the edge white in appearance?
3. What are the options for assessment and treatment?

Answers

1. This is likely to be arterial in origin due to the position, the punched-out appearance and absence of haemosiderin staining. It should be noted that the colouring immediately around the ulcer has probably been caused by multiple applications of different products.
2. The white appearance around the ulcer is caused by maceration of the tissue by moisture-retentive products such as hydrogels when applied

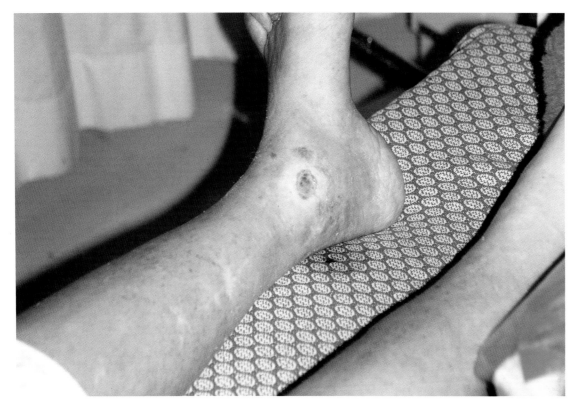

Figure 58.6 Malleolar ulcer with mixed appearance.

in excessive amounts. This impedes the healing process but arterial ulcers are anyway often slow to heal, if they heal at all.

3. Depending on the pedal pulses, it may be possible to apply light compression to aid healing. However, if clinical judgement linked with ABPI and pulse oximetry suggest that circulation is compromised, this will make use of any compression dangerous and a topical desloughing agent should be selected as an alternative to the hydrogel which has been applied in excessive amounts. A hydrocolloid could remain in place for 7 days to help with autodebriding but arterial ulcers often become cyclical in their production of slough. Larval therapy could be concentrated on this small area, within a hydrocolloid barrier. However, larvae can be particularly painful on arterial ulcers and adequate analgesia should be prescribed.

4. The ulcer must be protected from possible trauma.

Case 58.4

A 60-year-old lady has a pressure ulcer on her left buttock which has been treated and shows healthy areas as well as areas for concern (Fig. 58.7).

Question

What remains a problem with the wound appearance and what action should be taken?

Answer

The ulcer has been much larger and considerable healing has been achieved. A persistent area of pale slough may impede the healing process but there appears to be granulation tissue forming in the cavity. Closer inspection and possible biopsy would be advised to exclude any likelihood of squamous cell carcinoma which can develop in a chronic wound which is slow to heal and which is also friable and granular in appearance. Sharp debridement could be more efficient in removing slough than hydrogel application, which can also macerate the surrounding skin. The upper pale edge of the wound may be caused by over-spill of the hydrogel onto the surrounding skin.

A review of support surfaces should be urgently sought as the lower area of reddening could be a precursor to further skin damage or could be due to exudate leaking from the ulcer.

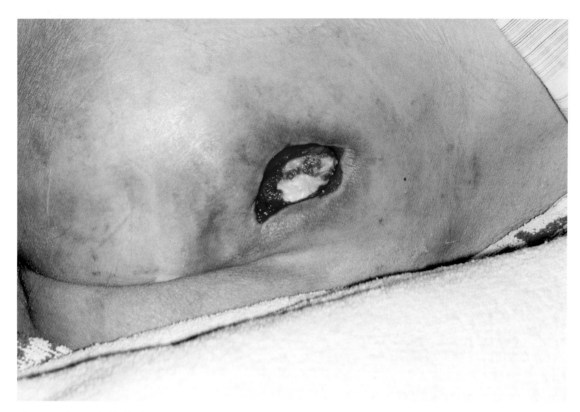

Figure 58.7 Pressure ulcer on left buttock.

REFERENCES

Gethin G, Jordan-O'Brien J, Moore Z 2005 Estimating costs of pressure area management based on a survey of ulcer care in one Irish hospital. Journal of Wound Care 14: 162-165

National Institute for Clinical Excellence 2001 Guidance on the use of debriding agents and specialist wound care clinics for difficult to heal wounds. National Institute for Clinical Excellence, London. Available online at: www.nice.org.uk/pdf/

National Institute for Clinical Excellence 2003 Pressure ulcer risk assessment and prevention. Clinical Guideline 7. National Institute for Clinical Excellence, London. Available online at: www.nice.org.uk/pdf/CG7

National Institute for Clinical Excellence 2005 The management of pressure ulcers in primary and secondary care. Clinical Guideline 29. National Institute for Clinical Excellence, London. Available online at: www.nice.org.uk/pdf/CG029fullguideline.pdf

Pancorbo-Hidalgo P L, Garcia-Fernandez F P, Lopez-Medina I M et al 2006 Risk assessment scales for pressure ulcer prevention: a systematic review. Journal of Advanced Nursing 54: 94-110

Scottish Intercollegiate Guideline Network 1998 The care of patients with chronic leg ulcers Guideline 26. Scottish Intercollegiate Guideline Network, Edinburgh. Available online at: www.sign.ac.uk/guidelines

Steenvorde P, Budding T, Oskam J 2005 Determining pain levels in patients treated with maggot debridement therapy. Journal of Wound Care 14: 485-488

Thomas S 2002 Use of maggots in the care of wounds. Hospital Pharmacist 2002: 267-271. Available online at: www.pharmj.com/pdf/hp/200210/hp

Vowden K R, Vowden P 2006 Preventing venous ulcer recurrence: a review. International Wound Journal 3: 11-21

Willock J, Hughes J, Tickle S et al 2000 Pressure sores in children – the acute hospital perspective. Journal of Tissue Viability 10: 59-62

FURTHER READING

Abbade L P, Lastoria S 2005 Venous ulcer: epidemiology, physiopathology, diagnosis and treatment. International Journal of Dermatology 44: 449-456

Bouza C, Munoz A, Amate J M 2005 Efficacy of modern dressings in the treatment of leg ulcers: a systematic review. Wound Repair and Regeneration 13: 218-229

Grey J E, Harding K G, Enoch S 2006 Venous and arterial leg ulcers. British Medical Journal 11: 347-350

Lyder C H 2003 Pressure ulcer prevention and management. Journal of the American Medical Association 289: 223-226

Morgan D A 2004 Formulary of wound management products, 9th edn. Euromed Communications, Haslemere

Nelson E A, Cullum N, Jones J 2006 Venous leg ulcers. Clinical Evidence 13: 2607-2626

Reichenberg J, Davis M 2005 Venous ulcers. Seminars in Cutaneous Medicine and Surgery 24: 216-226

Royal College of Nursing 2001 The management of patients with venous leg ulcers: report of the National Audit Pilot Project. Royal College of Nursing, London

APPENDICES

Medical abbreviations

AAA	abdominal aortic aneurysm		aortic pressure
	acute anxiety attack		apical pulse
AAAAA	aphasia, agnosia, apraxia, agraphia and alexia		appendectomy
Ab	antibody		artificial pneumothorax
abd.	abdomen (abdominal)	APB	atrial premature beat
	abduction	APC	activated protein C
ABE	acute bacterial endocarditis		atrial premature contraction
ABG	arterial blood gases	APP	amyloid precursor protein
ABMT	autologous bone marrow transplant	APSAC	anisoylated plasminogen streptokinase activated complex
ABVD	adriamycin (doxorubicin), bleomycin, vinblastine, dacarbazine	APTT	activated partial thromboplastin time
ACAT	acylcholesterol acyltransferase	AR	aortic regurgitation
ACBS	aortocoronary bypass surgery		apical/radial (pulse)
ACE	angiotensin-converting enzyme	ARB	angiotensin receptor blocker
acid phos.	acid phosphatase	ARDS	adult respiratory distress syndrome
ACR	albumin:creatinine ratio	ARF	acute renal failure
ACT	activated clotting time	AS	aortic stenosis
AD	Alzheimer's disease		arteriosclerosis
ADC	AIDS dementia complex	A–S attack	Adams–Stokes attack
ADH	antidiuretic hormone	5-ASA	5-aminosalicylic acid
ADL	activities of daily living	ASB	asymptomatic bacteriuria
ADP	adenosine diphosphate	ASCA	anti Saccharomycs cerevisiae antibodies
ADR	adverse drug reaction	ASD	atrial septal defect
ADU	acute duodenal ulcer	ASLO titre	antistreptolysin-O titre
A&E	accident and emergency	AST	aspartate transaminase
AED	antiepileptic drug	ATG	antithymocyte globulin
AF	atrial fibrillation	ATN	acute tubular necrosis
AFB	acid-fast bacillus	AUC	area under the curve
AFP	α-fetoprotein	AUR	acute urinary retention
AGL	acute granulocytic leukaemia	AV	aortic valve
AGN	acute glomerulonephritis		atrioventricular
AHA	autoimmune haemolytic anaemia	A-V	arteriovenous
AHD	autoimmune haemolytic disease	AVR	aortic valve replacement
AIDS	acquired immune deficiency syndrome		augmented V lead, right arm (ECG)
AK	above knee	AVS	arteriovenous shunt
ALA	aminolaevulinic acid	A & W	alive and well
ALD	alcoholic liver disease	AXR	abdominal x-ray
ALF	acute liver failure		
ALG	antilymphocyte globulin	BACUP	British Association of Cancer United Patients
ALL	acute lymphocytic leukaemia	BBB	bundle branch block
ALT	alanine transaminase	BBBB	bilateral bundle branch block (ECG)
	argon laser trabeculopasty	B Bx.	breast biopsy
AMA	against medical advice	BCAA	branched-chain amino acid
AMI	acute myocardial infarction	BCG	bacille Calmette–Guérin
AML	acute myeloid leukaemia	BDA	British Diabetic Association
AMP	adenosine monophosphate	BE	base excess
ANA	antinuclear antibody	BEACOPP	bleomycin, etoposide, adriamycin (doxorubicin), cyclophosphomide, Oncovin (vincristine), procarbazine, prednisolone
ANC	absolute neutrophil count		
ANF	antinuclear factor	BEAM	carmustine, etoposide, cytarabine, melphalan
ANP	atrial natriuretic peptide	BG	blood glucose
anti-HbAb	anti-hepatitis B antibody	BIA	bioelectrical impedence analysis
A & O	alert and oriented	BJ protein	Bence-Jones protein
A & P	anterior and posterior	BKA	below knee amputation
	auscultation and percussion	BM	bowel movement
AOB	alcohol on breath	BMI	body mass index
AP	alkaline phosphatase	BMT	bone marrow transplant
	angina pectoris	BNO	bowels not open
	antepartum	BOR	bowels open regularly
	anterior pituitary	BP	bypass
	anteroposterior		blood pressure

BPA	British Paediatric Association
BPD	bronchopulmonary dysplasia
BPH	benign prostatic hyperplasia
BS	blood sugar
	bowel sounds
	breath sounds
BSA	body surface area
BW	body water
	body weight
Bx.	biopsy
C	complement
$C_1, C_2, \ldots$	cervical vertebrae 1, 2, ...
CA	cancer
	carcinoma
	cardiac arrest
	coronary artery
Ca	carcinoma
CABG	coronary artery bypass graft
CAD	coronary artery disease
CAH	chronic active hepatitis
CAP	community-acquired pneumonia
CAPD	continuous ambulatory peritoneal dialysis
CAT	computed axial tomography
CAVH	continuous arteriovenous haemofiltration
CBA	cost–benefit analysis
CBT	cognitive behaviour therapy
CC	chief complaint
	current complaint
CCF	congestive cardiac failure
CCU	coronary care unit
CEA	cost-effectiveness analysis
CF	cardiac failure
	complement fixation
	cystic fibrosis
CFT	complement fixation test
CGL	chronic granulocytic leukaemia
CGN	chronic glomerulonephritis
CHB	complete heart block
CHD	coronary heart disease
CHF	congestive heart failure
CHM	Commision on Human Medicines
CHO	carbohydrate
CHOP	cyclophosphamide, hydroxydaunorubicin (doxorubicin), Oncovin (vincristine), prednisolone
CHOP-R	cyclophosphamide, hydroxydaunorubicin (doxorubicin), Oncovin (vincristine), prednisolone, rituximab
CI	cardiac index
	cerebral infarction
CINV	chemotherapy-induced nausea and vomiting
CIVA	centralized intravenous additive
CK	creatine kinase (same as CPK)
CKD	chronic kidney disease
CL	clubbing
Cl_{Cr}	creatinine clearance
CLD	chronic liver disease
	chronic lung disease
CLL	chronic lymphocytic leukaemia
CMA	cost minimization analysis
CML	chronic myelocytic leukaemia
CMV	cytomegalovirus
CNS	central nervous system
CO	cardiac output
c/o	complains of
CoA	co-enzyme A
COAD	chronic obstructive airways disease
COD	cause of death
COG	closed angle glaucoma
COLD	chronic obstructive lung disease
COP	capillary osmotic pressure
COPD	chronic obstructive pulmonary disease
COX	cyclo-oxygenase
C & P	cystoscopy and pyelogram
CP	cor pulmonale
	creatine phosphate

CPA	cardiopulmonary arrest
	cerebellar pontine angle
CPAP	continuous positive airway pressure
CPD	continuous peritoneal dialysis
CPK	creatine phosphokinase
CPN	chronic pyelonephritis
CPPV	continuous positive pressure ventilation
CPR	cardiopulmonary resuscitation
CPZ	chlorpromazine
CR	cardiorespiratory
	clot retraction
	colon resection
	complete remission
	conditional reflex
	crown–rump
CRD	chronic renal disease
CRF	chronic renal failure
	corticotrophin-releasing factor
CRP	C-reactive protein
C & S	culture and sensitivity
CSF	cerebrospinal fluid
CSH	chronic subdural haematoma
CSM	carotid sinus massage
	cerebrospinal meningitis
CSP	carotid sinus pressure
CSR	Cheyne-Stokes respiration
	correct sedimentation rate
CSS	carotid sinus stimulation
	central sterile supply
CSU	catheter specimen of urine
CT	circulation time
	clotting time
	computed tomography
	Coombs' test
	coronary thrombosis
cTnI	cardiac troponin I
cTnT	cardiac troponin T
CTZ	chemoreceptor trigger zone
CUA	cost–utility analysis
CUG	cystourethrogram
CV	cardiovascular
	central venous
	cerebrovascular
	contingent valuation
CVA	cerebrovascular accident (stroke)
	costovertebral angle
CVD	cardiovascular disease
CVP	central venous pressure
CVVH	continuous venovenous haemofiltration
Cx	cervical, cervix
CXR	chest x-ray
d	dead
	deceased
DAFNE	(insulin) dose adjustment for normal eating
DBP	diastolic blood pressure
D/C	discontinue
D & C	dilation and curettage
DDx.	differential diagnosis
DEXA	dual energy x-ray absorptiometry
DH	drug history
DIC	disseminated intravascular coagulation
DIP	drug-induced parkinsonism
DIT	di-iodotyrosine
DKA	diabetic ketoacidosis
DLBCL	diffuse large B cell lymphoma
DLE	discoid lupus erythematosus
	disseminated lupus erythematosus
DM	diabetes mellitus
	diastolic murmur
DMARDS	disease-modifying antirheumatic drugs
DNA	did not attend (outpatients)
DOA	dead on arrival
DOB	date of birth
DOD	date of death

DOE	dyspnoea on exertion		FUO	fever of unknown origin
DOTS	Directly Observed Treatment Short course TB programme		FVC	forced vital capacity
DRE	digital rectal examination		Fx.	fracture
DROP	dyslipidaemia, insulin resistance, obesity and high blood pressure		GA	general anaesthesia
				general appearance
D/S	dextrose and saline		GABA	γ-aminobutyric acid
DTI	direct thrombus imaging		$GABA_A$	γ-aminobutyric acid A
DSM	*Diagnostic and Statistical Manual of Mental Disorders*		GAD	glutamic acid decarboxylase
			Gamma-GT	γ-glutamyl transferase
DTP	diphtheria, tetanus, pertussis (vaccine)		GB	gallbladder
DTs	delirium tremens			Guillain–Barré (syndrome)
DU	diagnosis undetermined		GBM	glomerular basement membrane
	duodenal ulcer		G-CSF	granulocyte-colony stimulating factor
DUB	dysfunctional uterine bleeding		GDM	gastrointestinal diabetes mellitus
DUE	drug use evaluation		GF	glomerular filtration
D5W	dextrose 5%			gluten-free
D & V	diarrhoea and vomiting		GFR	glomerular filtration rate
DVT	deep vein thrombosis		GGT	γ-glutamyl transpeptidase (transferase)
Dx.	diagnosis		GIK	glucose, insulin and potassium
DXT	deep x-ray therapy		GI	gastrointestinal
			GLA	γ-linolenic acid
EBV	Epstein–Barr virus		GM seizure	grand mal seizure
ECBV	effective circulating blood volume		GN	glomerulonephritis
ECF	extracellular fluid		GNDC	Gram-negative diplococci
ECFV	extracellular fluid volume		GnRH	gonadotrophin-releasing hormone
ECG	electrocardiogram		GORD	gastro-oesophageal reflux disease
ECHO	echocardiogram		grav.	gravid (pregnant)
	echoencephalogram		GRE	glycopeptide-resistant enterococci
ECMO	extracorporeal membrane oxygenation		GS	general surgery
ECT	electroconvulsive therapy			genital system
EDD	expected date of delivery		GTN	glyceryl trinitrate
EDV	end-diastolic volume		GTT	glucose tolerance test
EEG	electroencephalogram		G6PD	glucose-6-phosphate dehydrogenase
EENT	eyes, ears, nose and throat		GU	gastric ulcer
EGFR	epidermal growth factor receptor			genitourinary
E/I	expiration–inspiration ratio			gonococcal urethritis
ELBW	extremely low birth weight		GUS	genitourinary system
ELISA	enzyme-linked immunosorbent assay		GVHD	graft-versus-host disease
EM	ejection murmur			
EMG	electromyogram		HAA	hepatitis-associated antigen
EN	erythema nodosum		HAP	hospital-acquired pneumonia
ENT	ears, nose and throat		HAS	human albumin solution
ER	(o)estrogen receptor		HAV	hepatitis A virus
EP	ectopic pregnancy		HB	heart block
ERCP	endoscopic retrograde cholangiopancreatography		Hb (Hgb)	haemoglobin
ESHAP	etoposide, methylprednisolone, cytarabine, cisplatin		HbA_1	glycated haemoglobin
			HBA_{1c}	glycated haemoglobin
ESM	ejection systolic murmur		HBA_2	haemoglobin found in β-thalassaemia carriers
ESN	educationally subnormal		HBAg	hepatitis B antigen
ESP	end-systolic pressure		HbS	sickle haemoglobin in sickle cell disease
ESR	erythrocyte sedimentation rate		HBsAG	hepatitis B surface antigen
ESRF	end-stage renal failure		HBD	hydroxybutyrate dehydrogenase
ET	endotracheal tube		HBDH	hydroxybutyrate dehydrogenase
ETT	exercise tolerance test		HBGM	home blood glucose monitoring
			Hct. (hct.)	haematocrit
FAS	fetal alcohol syndrome		HCV	hepatitis C virus
FB	finger breadths		HDL	high-density lipoproteins
FBS	fasting blood sugar		HDL-C	high-density lipoprotein
FCE	finished consultant episode		HDT	high-dose therapy
FeNa	fractional excretion of sodium		HER1	human epidermal growth factor receptor type 1
FEV	forced expiratory volume		HER2	human epidermal growth factor receptor type 2
FEV_1	forced expiratory volume in 1 second		HF	heart failure
FFA	free fatty acids		HHV	human herpes virus
FFP	fresh frozen plasma		5-HIAA	5-hydroxyindolacetic acid
FH	familial hypercholesterolaemia		Hib	*Haemophilus influenzae* type b
	family history		HIE	hypoxic-ischaemic encephalopathy
FHH	familial hypocalciuric hypercalcaemia		HIT	heparin induced thrombocytopaenia
FMD	fludarabine, mitoxantrone, dexamethasone		HIV	human immunodeficiency virus
FOB	faecal occult blood		H & L	heart and lungs
FP	frozen plasma		HLA	human lymphocyte antibody
FRC	functional reserve capacity		HMD	hyaline membrane disease
	functional residual capacity		HMMA	4-hydroxy-3-methoxymandelic acid
FSH	follicle-stimulating hormone		hMPV	human metapneumovirus
FT_4	free thyroxine		h/o	history of
FTI	free thyroxine index			

HO	house officer
HONK	hyperosmolar non-ketotic hyperglycaemia
HPEN	home parenteral and enteral nutrition
HPI	history of present illness
HPN	home parenteral nutrition
HPV	human papilloma virus
HR	heart rate
HRS	hepatorenal syndrome
HRT	hormone replacement therapy
HS	half strength
	Hartmann's solution
	heart sounds
HSA	human serum albumin
HSV	herpes simplex virus
5-HT	5-hydroxytryptamine (serotonin)
HT, HTN	hypertension
HUS	haemolytic uraemic syndrome
HVA	homovanillic acid
HVD	hypertensive vascular disease
Hx.	history
IADHS	inappropriate antidiuretic hormone syndrome
IBC	iron binding capacity
IBD	inflammatory bowel disease
IBS	irritable bowel syndrome
IC	intercostal
	intracerebral
	intracranial
ICA	islet cell antibody
ICE	ifosfamide, carboplatin, etoposide
ICD	*International Classification of Diseases*
ICF	intracellular fluid
ICH	intracerebral haemorrhage
ICM	intracostal margin
ICS	intercostal space
ICU	intensive care unit
ID	intradermal
IDDM	insulin-dependent diabetes mellitus
IDL	intermediate-density lipoprotein
IDL-C	intermediate-density lipoproteins
IDP	intradialytic parenteral nutrition
IEP	immunoelectrophoresis
IFRT	involved field radiotherapy
Ig	immunoglobulin
IGT	impaired glucose tolerance
IHC	immunohistochemistry
IHD	ischaemic heart disease
IHR	intrinsic heart rate
IMI	inferior myocardial infarction
IMP	impression
Inf. MI	inferior myocardial infarction
INR	international normalized ratio
IOP	intraocular pressure
IPF	idiopathic pulmonary fibrosis
IPI	International Prognostic Index
IPP	intermittent positive-pressure inflation with oxygen
IPPB	intermittent positive-pressure breathing
IPPV	intermittent positive-pressure ventilation
IRDS	idiopathic respiratory distress syndrome
ISA	intrinsic sympathomimetic activity
ISDN	isosorbide dinitrate
ISI	International Sensitivity Index
ISMN	isosorbide mononitrate
IT	intrathecal(ly)
ITT	insulin tolerance test
IUCD	intrauterine contraceptive device
IUD	intrauterine death
	intrauterine device
i.v.	intravenous
IVD	intervertebral disc
IVH	intraventricular haemorrhage
IVP	intravenous push
	intravenous pyelography
IVSD	interventricular septal defect
IVU	intravenous urography

J	jaundice
JVD	jugular venous distension
JVP	jugular venous pressure
KA	ketoacidosis
KCCT	kaolin-cephalin clotting time
KLS	kidney, liver, spleen
KS	Kaposi's sarcoma
KUB	kidneys, ureters, bladder
L	left
	lower
	lumbar
L_1, L_2, …	lumbar vertebrae 1, 2, …
L & A	light and accommodation
LA	left arm
	left atrium
	local anaesthesia
LABA	long acting β-adrenoceptor agonist
LAD	left anterior descending
LADA	latent autoimmune diabetes in adults
LBBB	left bundle branch block
LBM	lean body mass
LBW	low birth weight
LCAT	lecithin-cholesterol acyltransferase
LCT	long-chain triglyceride
LD, LDH	lactate dehydrogenase
LDL	low-density lipoprotein
LDL-C	low-density lipoprotein
LFT	liver function test
LH	luteinizing hormone
LHRH	luteinizing hormone-releasing hormone
LIF	left iliac fossa
LK	left kidney
LKS	liver, kidney, spleen
LKKS	liver, kidneys, spleen
LL	left leg
	left lower
	lower lobe
LLL	left lower lobe
	left lower lid
LLQ	left lower quadrant
LMN	lower motor neurone
LMP	last menstrual period
LMWH	low molecular weight heparin
LN	lymph node
LNG-IUS	levonorgestrel intrauterine system
LNMP	last normal menstrual period
LOM	limitation of movement
LP	lumbar puncture
Lp(a)	lipoprotein a
LPA	left pulmonary artery
LS	left side
	liver and spleen
	lumbosacral
	lymphosarcoma
LSD	lysergic acid diethylamide
LSK	liver, spleen, kidneys
LSM	late systolic murmur
LT	leukotriene
LTC	long-term care
LTOT	long-term oxygen therapy
L & U	lower and upper
LUL	left upper lobe
LUQ	left upper quadrant
LV	left ventricle
LVDP	left ventricular diastolic pressure
LVE	left ventricular enlargement
LVEDP	left ventricular end-diastolic pressure
LVEDV	left ventricular end-diastolic volume
LVET	left ventricular ejection time
LVF	left ventricular failure
LVH	left ventricular hypertrophy
LVP	left ventricular pressure
L & W	living and well

M	male
	married
	metre
	mother
	molar
	murmur
MABP	mean arterial blood pressure
MAC	*Mycobacterium avium* complex
MAI	*Mycobacterium avium-intracellulare*
MALT	mucosal-associated lymphoid tissue
MAMC	mid-arm muscle circumference
MARS	molecular adsorbent recycling system
MAO-A	monoamine oxidase A
MAO-B	monoamine oxidase B
MAOI	monoamine oxidase inhibitor
MAP	mean arterial pressure
MBC	minimum bactericidal concentration
MBP	mean blood pressure
MCH	mean corpuscular cell haemoglobin
MCHC	mean corpuscular cell haemoglobin concentration
MCP	metacarpophalangeal (joint)
MCT	medium-chain triglycerides
MCV	mean corpuscular cell volume
MD	mitral disease
	muscular dystrophy
MDI	metered-dose inhaler
MDM	mid-diastolic murmur
MDMA	methylene dioxymethamphetamine, ecstasy
MDRD	modification of diet in renal disease formula for GFR estimation
MDRST	multidrug-resistant *S. enterica* serovar typhi
MDRTB	multidrug-resistant tuberculosis
MEN	multiple endocrine neoplasia
met.	metastatic (metastasis)
MGN	membranous glomerulonephritis
MH	medical history
	menstrual history
MHPG	methoxyhydroxyphenylglycerol
MHRA	Medicines and Healthcare products Regulatory Agency
MI	myocardial infarction
	mitral incompetence
MIC	minimum inhibitory concentration
MID	multi-infarct dementia
MIRU	mycobacterial interspersed repetitive unit typing
MIT	monoiodotyrosine
ML	middle lobe
	midline
MMR	measles, mumps, rubella
MODY	maturity-onset diabetes of the young
MOPP	mustine, Oncovin (vincristine), procarbazine, prednisolone
MOTT	mycobacteria other than tuberculosis
M:P	milk-to-plasma ratio
MPJ	metacarpophalangeal joint
MR	mitral regurgitation
MRA	magnetic resonance angiography
MRD	minimal residual disease
MRDM	malnutrition-related diabetes mellitus
MRI	magnetic resonance imaging
MRSA	meticillin-resistant *Staphylococcus aureus*
MS	mitral stenosis
	multiple sclerosis
	musculoskeletal
MSSA	meticillin-sensitive *Staphylococcus aureus*
MSL	midsternal line
MSU	midstream urine specimen
MTI	minimum time interval
MTP	metatarsophalangeal
MUD	matched unrelated donor
MV	minute volume
	mitral valve
MVP	mitral valve prolapse
MVPP	mustine, vinblastine, procarbazine, prednisolone
MVR	mitral valve replacement

N	normal
NAD	no appreciable disease
	normal axis deviation
	nothing abnormal detected
NAG	narrow angle glaucoma
NAI	neuraminidase inhibitor
NAPQI	*N*-acetyl-*p*-benzoquinoneimine
NARI	noradrenergic reuptake inhibitor
NARTI	nucleoside analogue reverse transcriptase inhibitor
NaSSA	noradrenergic and specifc serotonergic antidepressant
NBM	nil by mouth
NEC	necrotizing enterocolitis
NG	nasogastric
NHL	non-Hodgkin's lymphoma
NIDDM	non-insulin-dependent diabetes mellitus
NKHA	non-ketotic hyperosmolar acidosis
NLPHL	nodular lymphocyte-predominant Hodgkin's lymphoma
NMR	nuclear magnetic resonance
NMS	neuroleptic malignant syndrome
NNRTI	non-nucleoside reverse transcriptase inhibitor
NOF	neck of femur
NS	nephrotic syndrome
	nervous system
	normal saline
	no specimen
NSAID	non-steroidal anti-inflammatory drug
NSFTD	normal spontaneous full-term delivery
NSR	normal sinus rhythm
NSU	non-specific urethritis
NT	nasotracheal (tube)
N & T	nose and throat
NTS	nucleus tractus solitarius
N & V	nausea and vomiting
NVD	nausea, vomiting, diarrhoea
O	oedema
O & A	observation and assessment
O/A	on admission
OA	osteoarthritis
OAD	obstructive airway disease
OAG	open angle glaucoma
OB	occult blood
OD	overdose
O & E	observation and examination
O/E	on examination
OGTT	oral glucose tolerance test
OH	occupational history
OHT	ocular hypertension
OI	opportunistic infection
OKGA	ornithine salt of α-ketoglutaric acid
OLT	orthoptic liver transplantation
OPA	outpatient appointment
OPD	outpatient department
OT	occupational therapy
PA	pernicious anaemia
	pulmonary artery
P & A	percussion and auscultation
PaCO$_2$	arterial carbon dioxide tension
PACG	primary angle-closure glaucoma
PAF	platelet-activating factor
PAH	pulmonary artery hypertension
PaO$_2$	arterial oxygen tension
pANCA	perinuclear antineutrophil cytoplasmic antibodies
PAPS	primary antiphospholipid syndrome
PAS	*P*-aminosalicylic acid
	pulmonary artery stenosis
PAT	paroxysmal atrial tachycardia
PAWP	pulmonary artery wedge pressure
PB	premature beats
PBC	primary biliary cirrhosis
PBI	protein-bound iodine
PBSCT	peripheral blood stem cell transplantion
PCA	patient-controlled analgesia
PCAS	patient-controlled analgesia system

PCO_2	partial pressure of carbon dioxide
PCR	polymerase chain reaction
PCS	portocaval shunt
PCV	packed cell volume
PD	peritoneal dialysis
PDA	patent ductus arteriosus
PE	physical examination
	pleural effusion
	pulmonary embolism
PEARLA	pupils equal and react to light and accommodation
PEF	peak expiratory flow
PEFR	peak expiratory flow rate
PEG	percutaneous endoscopic gastrostomy
PEJ	percutaneous endoscopic jejunostomy
PEM	prescription event monitoring
PERLA	pupils equal, react to light and accommodation
PERRLA	pupils equal, round, react to light and accommodation
PET	position emission tomography
PF	peak flow
PFR	peak flow rate
PFT	pulmonary function test
PG	prostaglandin
PH	past history
	patient history
	personal history
	prostatic hypertrophy
	pulmonary hypertension
PI	present illness
	protease inhibitor
PICC	peripherally inserted central catheter
PID	pelvic inflammatory disease
PIP	proximal interphalangeal joint
PIVD	protruded intervertebral disc
PJB	premature junctional beat
PJC	premature junctional contraction
PJP	*Pneumocystis jiroveci* pneumonia
PKU	phenylketonuria
PL	product licence
PMDD	premenstrual dysphoirc disorder
PMH	past medical history
PMI	past medical illness
PMN	polymorphonucleocyte
PMS	premenstrual syndrome
	postmenopausal syndrome
PMT	premenstrual tension
PMV	prolapsed mitral valve
PN	percussion note
	peripheral nerve
	peripheral neuropathy
PND	paroxysmal nocturnal dyspnoea
	postnasal drip
PO_2	partial pressure of oxygen
POAG	primary open-angle glaucoma
POMR	problem-oriented medical record
PONV	postoperative nausea and vomiting
PPAR-γ	proliferative-activated receptor-γ
PPD	purified protein derivative
PPH	postpartum haemorrhage
PPI	proton pump inhibitor
PPNG	penicillinase-producing *Neisseria gonorrhoeae*
PPV	positive-pressure ventilation
PROM	premature rupture of membranes
PR	per rectum
	progestogen receptor
PRCA	pure red cell aplasia
PS	pulmonary stenosis
	pyloric stenosis
PSA	prostate-specific antigen
PSG	presystolic gallop
PSGN	poststreptococcal glomerulonephritis
PSVT	paroxysmal supraventricular tachycardia
PT	parathyroid
	paroxysmal tachycardia
	physical therapy
	physical training

	posterior tibial (pulse)
	prothrombin time
PTC	percutaneous cholangiogram
PTH	parathyroid hormone
PTT	partial thromboplastin time
PTTK	partial thromboplastin time kaolin
PTU	propylthiouracil
PU	pass urine
	per urethra
	peptic ulcer
PUD	peptic ulcer disease
	pulmonary disease
PUO	pyrexia (fever) of unknown origin
PUVA	psoralen and ultraviolet A radiation
PV	vaginal examination (per vagina)
P & V	pyloroplasty and vagotomy
PVB	premature ventricular beat
PVC	premature ventricular contraction
PVD	peripheral vascular disease
PVP	pulmonary venous pressure
PVT	paroxysmal ventricular tachycardia
Px.	past history
	prognosis
QALY	quality-adjusted life-year
R	respiration
RA	renal artery
	rheumatoid arthritis
	right arm
	right atrial (atrium)
RAST	radio-allergosorbent test
RBBB	right bundle branch block
RBC	red blood cell
	red blood (cell) count
RBS	random blood sugar
R-CVP	rituximab, cyclophosphamide, vincristine, prednisolone
RDS	respiratory distress syndrome
REMS	rapid eye movement sleep
Re-PUVA	PUVA treatment with retinoids
RF	renal failure
	rheumatic fever
	rheumatoid factor
RFT	respiratory function tests
RHF	right heart failure
Rh factor	rhesus factor
rhuEPO	recombinant human erythropoietin
rhuGM-CSF	recombinant human granulocyte-macrophage colony-stimulating factor
RHL	right hepatic lobe
RIF	right iliac fossa
RIMA	reversible inhibitor of monoamine oxidase type A
RK	right kidney
RL	right leg
	right lung
RLC	residual lung capacity
RLD	related living donor
RLL	right lower lobe (lung)
RLQ	right lower quadrant (abdomen)
RP	radial pulse
RPI	resting pressure index
RQ	respiratory quotient
RR	respiratory rate
RR & E	round, regular and equal (pupils)
RS	respiratory system
RSF	rheumatoid serum factor
RSV	respiratory syncytial virus
RTA	road traffic accident
rt-PA	recombinant plasminogen activator
RUL	right upper lobe
RUQ	right upper quadrant
RV	residual volume
	right ventricle
RVH	right ventricular hypertrophy

SA	sinoatrial (node)
	Stokes–Adams (attacks)
	surface area
SAH	subarachnoid haemorrhage
SARS	severe acute respiratory syndrome
SARS CoV	severe acute respiratory syndrome-associated
	coronovirus
SB	seen by
	shortness of breath
SBE	subacute bacterial endocarditis
	shortness of breath on exertion
SBO	small bowel obstruction
SBP	spontaneous bacterial peritonitis
sCT	spiral computed tomography
SCU	*see* SCUF
SCUF	slow continuous ultrafiltration
SDD	selective decontamination of the digestive tract
SEM	systolic ejection murmur
SGOT	serum glutamate-oxaloacetate transaminase
SGPT	serum glutamate-pyruvate transaminase
SH	social history
SIADH	syndrome of inappropriate antidiuretic hormone
SIDS	sudden infant death syndrome
SLE	systemic lupus erythematosus
SNRI	serotonin-noradrenaline reuptake inhibitor
SOA	swelling of ankle(s)
SOAP	subjective, objective, assessment, plan
SOB	short of breath
SOBOE	short of breath on exertion
SP	systolic pressure
SPA	suprapubic aspiration
SPC	Summary of Product Characteristics
SR	sinus rhythm
	sustained release
SSI	surgical site infection
SSRI	selective serotonin reuptake inhibitor
ST	sinus tachycardia
stat.	immediately (Latin: statim)
STD	sexually transmitted disease
	sodium tetradecyl sulfate
STS	serological tests for syphilis
SV	stroke volume
SVI	stroke volume index
SVT	supraventricular tachycardia
SWS	slow-wave sleep
Sx.	symptoms
T	temperature
T_3	tri-iodothyronine
T_4	thyroxine
TAGvHD	transfusion-assisted graft-versus-host disease
TB	tuberculosis
TBA	to be administered
	to be arranged
TBG	thyroid-binding globulin
TBI	total body irradiation
TBW	total body weight
T & C	type and cross-match
TC	total capacity
	total cholesterol
	tricarboxylic acid cycle
TCA	tricyclic antidepressant
TDM	therapeutic drug monitoring
TEN	toxic epidermal necrolysis (Lyell's syndrome)
TENS	transcutaneous electrical nerve stimulation
TF	tissue factor
TFTs	thyroid function tests
TGs	triglycerides
TH	thyroid hormone (thyroxine)
THA	tetrahydroaminoacridine
THC	tetrahydrocannabinol
TIA	transient ischaemic attack
TIBC	total iron-binding capacity
TIMP	tissue inhibitor of metalloproteinases

TIPSS	transjugular intrahepatic portosystemic shunting
TLC	total lung capacity
	tender loving care
TLS	tumour lysis syndrome
TNF	tumour necrosis factor
TNF-α	tumour necrosis factor-α
t-PA	tissue plasminogen factor
TPMT	thiopurine methyl transferase
TPN	total parenteral nutrition
TP & P	time, place and person
TPR	temperature, pulse, respiration
TRABs	thyroid receptor antibodies
TRH	thyrotrophin-releasing hormone
TSF	triceps skinfold thickness
TSH	thyroid-stimulating hormone
TTA	transtracheal aspiration
TTO	to take out (to take home)
TUIP	transurethral incision of the prostate
TUR	transurethral resection
TURB	transurethral resection of the bladder
TURP	transurethral resection of the prostate
TV	tidal volume
TVN	tissue viability nurse
Tx.	transfusion
	treatment
T & X	type and cross-match
UBIC	unsaturated iron-binding capacity
UC	ulcerative colitis
U & E	urea and electrolytes
UFH	unfractionated heparin
URTI	upper respiratory tract infection
US	ultrasound
UTI	urinary tract infection
UVA	ultraviolet A
UVB	ultraviolet B
VC	vital capacity
	vulvovaginal candidiasis
VD	venereal disease
VDRL	Venereal Disease Research Laboratory
	(test for syphilis)
VEGF	vascular endothelial growth factor
VF	ventricular fibrillation
VHD	valvular heart disease
VLBW	very low birth weight
VLDL	very low-density lipoprotein
VMA	vanillyl mandelic acid
VNTR	variable number of tandem repeats typing
VP	venous pressure
VPC	ventricular premature contraction
V/Q	ventilation-perfusion ratio
VS	vital signs
VT	ventricular tachycardia
VTE	venous thromboembolism
VTEC	verotoxin-producing *E. coli*
VUR	vesicoureteric reflux
WBC	white blood cell
	white blood count
WCC	white cell count
WHO	World Health Organization
WPW	Wolff–Parkinson–White (syndrome)
WR	Wassermann reaction
WTA	willingness to accept
WTP	willingness to pay
ZE	Zollinger–Ellison (syndrome)
ZIG	zoster immune globulin
ZPP	zinc protoporphyrin

Useful website when searching for the definition of abbreviations:
www.medilexicon.com/extsearch.php?searchtype=acronym&
username=pharmale

Glossary

acanthosis nigricans: diffuse velvety acanthosis with grey, brown or black pigmentation, chiefly in axilla and other body folds, occurring in an adult form, often associated with an internal carcinoma and in a benign, nevoid form, more or less generalized.

achlohydria: absence of hydrochloric acid from maximally stimulated gastric secretion.

acropachy: clubbing of the fingers and toes with distal periosteal bone changes and swelling of the overlying soft tissues.

addisonian crisis: the symptoms that accompany an acute onset or worsening of Addison's disease, including fatigue, nausea and vomiting, loss of weight, hypotension, fever and collapse.

adenomyosis: penetration of an endometrial tissue into the myometrium.

agenesis: absence of an organ.

amphipathic: molecules containing groups with characteristically different properties, e.g. both hydrophilic and hydrophobic properties.

amphoteric: having opposite characters, i.e. capable of acting as an acid and a base.

anoxaemia: reduction of blood oxygen content below physiological levels.

anthropometry: the science which deals with the measurement of the size, weight and proportions of the human body.

aphakia: no lens.

aplasia cutis: localized failure of development of skin.

apnoea: cessation of breathing.

arachnoiditis: inflammation of the arachnoidea, a delicate membrane interposed between the dura mater and the pia mater.

ataxia telangectasia: hereditary disorder with severe progressive cerebellar ataxia, associated with oculocutaneous telangectasia, sinopulmonary disease with frequent respiratory infections and abnormal eye movements.

atelectasis: incomplete expansion of a lung.

atretic: without an opening; characterized by atresia.

azoospermia: absence of spermatozoa in the semen, or failure of formation of spermatozoa.

bacteriuria: the presence of bacteria in the urine.

Barrett's oesophagus: a precancerous condition in which normal cells lining the oesophagus are replaced with abnormal cells that may develop into an adenocarcinoma.

bronchiectasis: characterized by dilation of the small bronchi and bronchioles, associated with the presence of chronic pulmonary sepsis. It presents as a chronic cough, often with the production of large amounts of purulent, foul-smelling sputum, and may eventually lead to repeated episodes of pneumonia and respiratory failure.

bronchoalveolar lavage: a procedure performed during bronchoscopy in which the bronchial tree is literally washed (lavaged) with a small volume of sterile saline. The saline is then collected and sent for microbiological or cytological examination.

bronchoscopy: the procedure in which a flexible fibreoptic endoscope is inserted into the bronchial tree to allow direct visualization of the bronchi and, if required, the collection of specimens for microbiology or histology.

Budd–Chiari syndrome: symptomatic obstruction or occlusion of the hepatic veins, usually of unknown origin but probably caused by neoplasms, strictures, liver disease, trauma, systemic infections or haematological disorders.

cachectic: a profound and marked state of general ill health and malnutrition.

cardiogenic emboli: emboli originating from the heart; caused by abnormal function of the heart.

carpal tunnel syndrome: a complex of symptoms resulting from compression of the median nerve in the carpal tunnel, with pain and burning or tingling paraesthesias in the fingers and hand, sometimes extending to the elbow.

cataract: an opacity of the crystalline lens of the eye.

cavitation: formation of cavities. For example, in the lungs when the liquefied centre of a tuberculous lesion drains (usually into a bronchus).

Charcot's arthropathy: a destructive arthropathy (disease of any joint) with impaired pain perception or position sense.

cholelithiasis: the presence or formation of gallstones.

chondrocyte: a mature cartilage cell embedded in a lacuna (a small pit or hollow cavity) within the cartilage matrix.

Christmas disease: haemophilia B.

Churg–Strauss syndrome: allergic granulomatosis.

Chvostek's sign: spasm of the facial muscles elicited by tapping the facial nerve in the region of the parotid gland, seen in tetany.

coarctation of the aorta: a localized malformation characterized by deformity of the aortic media, causing narrowing, usually severe, of the lumen of the vessel.

cognitive: pertaining to cognition; that operation of the mind by which we become aware of objects of thought or perception; it includes all aspects of perceiving, thinking and remembering.

corneal arcus: crescentic deposition of lipids in the cornea.

cor pulmonale: persistent lung damage eventually leads to increased blood pressure in the pulmonary arteries (pulmonary hypertension), which in turn leads to stress on the right ventricle, right ventricular hypertrophy and heart failure. This process is known as cor pulmonale.

cryptogenic: obscure, doubtful or unascertainable origin.

cytotoxin: a toxin or antibody that has a specific toxic action upon cells of special organs.

denudation: removal of the epithelial covering from any surface.

diarthrodial joint: a joint characterized by mobility in a rotary direction.

dimorphic: occurring in two distinct forms.

disseminated intravascular coagulation (DIC): in this condition vigorous activation of the clotting cascade causes widespread intravascular deposition of fibrin and consumption of clotting factors and platelets. There are numerous potential triggers for this process, including severe sepsis, burns, massive transfusion and placental abruption.

diverticulosis: the presence of circumscribed pouches or sacs of variable size called diverticula that occur normally or are created by herniation of the lining mucous membrane through a defect in the muscular coat of a tubular organ such as the gastrointestinal tract.

Dubin–Johnson syndrome: familial chronic form of non-haemolytic jaundice due to a defect in the excretion of conjugated bilirubin and other organic anions.

Dupuytren's contracture: shortening, thickening and fibrosis of the palmar fascia, producing a flexion deformity of a finger. The term also applies to a flexion deformity of a toe.

dyschezia: difficult or painful evacuation of faeces from the rectum.

dyskinesia: impairment of the power of voluntary movement, resulting in fragmentary or incomplete movements.

dyspareunia: difficult or painful intercourse.

dyspnoea: difficult or laboured breathing.

dystonia: disordered tonicity of muscle.

dysuria: painful or difficult urination.

eclampsia: convulsions and coma occurring in a pregnant or puerperal woman, associated with hypertension, oedema and/or proteinuria.

electrodiathermy: heating of the body tissues due to their resistance to the passage of an electric current

elliptocytosis: a hereditary disorder in which the majority of erythrocytes are elliptical in shape, and characterized by varying degrees of increased red cell destruction and anaemia.

emphysema: a state in which the alveoli of the lung become dilated, possibly with destruction of the alveolar walls, leading to large empty air spaces which are useless for gas exchange. It is often seen accompanying chronic bronchitis but may be due to inherited disorders such as α_1-antitrypsin deficiency.

encephalopathy: any degenerative disease of the brain.

endophthalmitis: inflammation involving the ocular cavities and their adjacent structures.

enterostomy: the formation of a permanent opening into the intestine through the abdominal wall.

enterotoxin: a toxin arising in the intestine.

episcleritis: inflammation of the loose connective tissue forming the external surface of the sclera.

Epstein–Barr virus: a herpes virus originally isolated from Burkitt lymphomas and believed to be the aetiological agent in infectious mononucleosis or closely related to it.

euthymic: normal state of thymus

faecal: occult blood in the stools. Called 'occult' because it is partly digested and therefore no longer red in colour. Usually detected by means of a chemical test.

Fanconi's anaemia: a rare hereditary disorder, transmitted in a recessive manner and having a poor prognosis, characterized by pancytopenia, hypoplasia of the bone marrow, and patchy brown discoloration of the skin due to the deposition of melanin, and associated with multiple congenital anomalies of the musculoskeletal and genitourinary systems.

fastidious organism: organism which will only grow with specialist culture media or under certain physiological conditions.

feculent: having dregs or a sediment.

fistula: an abnormal passage or communication, usually between two internal organs or from an internal organ to the surface of the body.

foreign body giant cells: giant cells resembling Langhan's giant cells, having clusters of nuclei scattered in an irregular pattern throughout the cytoplasm, characteristic of granulomatous inflammation due to invasion of the tissue by a foreign body.

gastroschisis: congenital fissure of the abdominal wall not involving the site of insertion of the umbilical cord, and usually accompanied by protrusion of the small and part of the large intestine.

glomerulonephritis: nephritis characterized by inflammation of the capillary loops in the glomeruli of the kidney.

glossitis: inflammation of the tongue.

gonioscopy: estimate of the width of the eye chamber angle, measured using a slit-lamp.

granuloma: a tumour-like mass or nodule of granulation tissue, with actively growing fibroblasts and capillary buds; it is due to a chronic inflammatory process associated with infectious disease or with invasion by a foreign body.

Guillain–Barré syndrome: acute febrile polyneuritis.

haematuria: blood in the urine.

haem(at)opoiesis: the formation and development of blood cells.

Harris Benedict equation: equation first developed in 1919 to predict basal energy expenditure.

haustral: pertaining to the haustra of the colon, denoting sacculations in the wall of the colon produced by adaptation of its length.

Heberden's nodes: gelatinous cysts or bony outgrowths on the dorsal aspects of the distal interphalangeal joints.

Heinz bodies: inclusion bodies in red blood cells resulting from oxidative injury to and precipitation of haemoglobin, seen in the presence of certain abnormal haemoglobins and erythrocytes with enzyme deficiencies.

Henoch–Schönlein purpura: an acute or chronic vasculitis primarily affecting skin, joints and the gastrointestinal and renal systems.

hepatorenal syndrome: development of renal failure secondary to liver disease.

Hirschsprung's disease: congenital megacolon.

Horner's syndrome: sinking in of the eyeball, ptosis of the upper eyelid, slight elevation of the lower lid, constriction of the pupil, narrowing of the palpebral fissure, anhidrosis and flushing of the affected side of the face; caused by paralysis of the cervical sympathetic nerves.

Horton's syndrome: migrainous neuralgia; also called paroxysmal nocturnal cephalalgia.

Huntington's chorea: a rare hereditary disease characterized by chronic progressive chorea and mental deterioration terminating in dementia. The age of onset is variable but usually occurs in the fourth decade of life.

hyaline membrane: a layer of eosinophilic hyaline material lining the alveoli, alveolar ducts and bronchioles, found at autopsy in infants who have died of respiratory distress syndrome of the newborn.

hypersplenism: a condition characterized by exaggeration of the inhibitory or destructive functions of the spleen, resulting in deficiency of the peripheral blood elements, singly or in combination, hypercellularity of the bone marrow, and usually splenomegaly.

hypophonic: reduced volume of speech.

hypovolaemia: abnormally reduced volume of circulating fluid in the body/plasma.

ileus: obstruction or lack of smooth muscle tone in the intestines.

immunoblastic: pertaining to or involving the stem cells (immunoblasts) of lymphoid tissue.

index case: the first detected case in a particular series that prompts investigation into other patients.

interstitial nephritis: inflammation of the renal interstitial tissue resulting from arterial, arteriolar, glomerular or tubular disease which destroys individual nephrons.

intussusception: the prolapse of one part of the intestine into the lumen of an immediately adjoining part.

Jod–Basedow syndrome: thyrotoxicosis produced in a patient with goitre, when given a bolus of iodine.

Kayser–Fleischer ring: a grey-green to red-gold pigmented ring at the outer margin of the cornea, seen in progressive lenticular degeneration and pseudosclerosis.

koilonychia: dystrophy of the fingernails, in which they are thin and concave, with edges raised.

Kussmaul's respiration: air hunger.

kwashiorkor: insufficient protein provision.

labyrinthitis: inflammation of the labyrinth; otitis interna.

laminectomy: excision of the posterior arch of a vertebra.

laparoscopy: examination of the interior of the abdomen by means of a laparoscope.

Lesch–Nyhan syndrome: rare disorder of purine metabolism due to deficiency of the enzyme hypoxanthine-guanine phosphoribosyl-transferase and characterized by physical and mental retardation, self-mutilation of fingers and lips by biting, choreoathetosis, spastic cerebral palsy and impaired renal function.

leucocytosis: total white cell count in excess of 11×10^9/L.

lichenoid: resembling the skin lesions designated as 'lichen' – the name applied to many different kinds of papular skin diseases in which the lesions are typically small, firm papules that are usually set very close together.

lipaemia retinalis: retinal deposition of lipid.

lipohypertrophy: thickening of subcutaneous tissues at injection sites because of recurrent injection in the same area.

livedo reticularis: a peripheral vascular condition characterized by a reddish blue netlike mottling of the skin and extremities.

Lyme disease: a multisystem tick-borne disorder caused by the spirochaete *Borrelia burgdorferi*. Clinical manifestation includes an erythematous macule followed by systemic disorders such as arthralgias, myalgias and headache followed by neurological manifestations, cardiac involvement and a migratory polyarthritis.

lymphadenopathy: disease of the lymph nodes.

lymphoblastic: pertaining to a lymphoblast.

maculopapular: an eruption consisting of both macules (areas distinguishable by colour from their surroundings, e.g. spots) and papules (small circumscribed, superficial, solid elevations of the skin).

malleolus medialis: the rounded protruberance on the medial surface of the ankle joint.

malrotation: abnormal or pathological rotation.

marasmus: insufficient energy provision.

melaena: the passage of dark stools stained with blood pigments or with altered blood.

menorrhagia: excessive and prolonged uterine bleeding occurring at the regular intervals of menstruation.

microalbuminuria: small amounts of albumin present in the urine.

miliary: literally, resembling small round millet seeds. Miliary tuberculosis is so called because the chest radiograph usually shows miliary speckling.

morbilliform: resembling the eruption of measles.

mucositis: inflammation of a mucous membrane.

mycosis fungoides: a rare, chronic, malignant, lymphoreticular neoplasm of the skin and, in the late stages, the lymph nodes and viscera, marked by the development of firm, reddish, painful tumours that ulcerate.

myelofibrosis: replacement of the bone marrow by fibrous tissue occurring in association with a myeloproliferative disorder or secondary to another disorder.

myoglobulinuria: presence of myoglobin in the urine.

myomas: fibroids, common benign tumours of the myometrium.

myometrium: the muscular layers of the uterus that contract spontaneously throughout the menstrual cycle.

myopathy: unexplained muscle soreness or weakness.

myositis: inflammation of a voluntary muscle.

necrobiosis lipoidica: a dermatosis usually occurring in diabetics characterized by necrobiosis (swelling and distortion of collagen bundles in the dermis) of the elastic and connective tissue of the skin, with degenerated collagen occurring in irregular patches, especially in the upper dermis.

nephrolithiasis: formation of uric acid calculi in the kidneys.

nocturia: waking at night to pass urine.

nystagmus: involuntary rapid movement of the eyeball, which may be horizontal, vertical, rotatory or mixed.

obligate intracellular pathogen: an organism that cannot be cultured using artificial media since it requires living cells for growth.

oliguria: diminished urine output.

onycholysis: separation of the nail from its bed.

oophorectomy: removal of an ovary or ovaries.

ophthalmopathy: any disease of the eye.

opsonization: the rendering of bacteria and other cells subject to phagocytosis.

orosomucoid: α_1-acid glycoprotein, a glycoprotein occurring in blood plasma.

orthopnoea: difficult breathing except in an upright position.

orthoptic: correcting obliquity of one or more visual axis.

Osler's nodes: small, raised, swollen tender areas, about the size of a pea and often bluish in colour but sometimes pink or red, occurring most commonly in the pads of the fingers or toes, in the palm or the soles of the feet.

osteomalacia: reduced mineralization.

osteophyte: a bony or osseous outgrowth.

pallidotomy: a stereotaxic surgical technique for producing lesions in the globus pallidus or extirpation of it by other means.

palmar striae: yellow raised streaks across the palms of the hands.

pancytopenia: deficiency of all cell elements of the blood.

panmyelopathy: a pathological condition of all the elements of the bone marrow.

paroxysmal nocturnal dyspnoea: difficult or laboured breathing at night that recurs in paroxysms.

pericarditis: inflammation of the fibrous sac (pericardium) that surrounds the heart and the roots of the great vessels.

petechial: characterized by pinpoint, non-raised, round, purplish red spots caused by intradermal or submucous haemorrhage.

phaeochromocytoma: a tumour of chromaffin tissue of the adrenal medulla or sympathetic paraganglia. The cardinal symptom that represents the increased secretion of adrenaline and noradrenaline is hypertension, which may be persistent or intermittent.

phagocytosis: the engulfing of micro-organisms, cells and foreign particles by phagocytes.

phlebitis: inflammation of a vein.

pica: a craving for unnatural articles of food.

pneumaturia: passage of urine charged with air.

polycythaemia rubra vera: a myeloproliferative disorder in which the abnormal bone marrow overproduces red blood cells (white cells and platelets may also be raised).

polymorphic: occurring in several or many forms.

polyp: a protruding growth from a mucous membrane.

pompholyx: a skin eruption on the sides of the fingers, toes, palms or soles, consisting of discrete round intraepidermal vesicles 1 or 2 mm in diameter, accompanied by intense itching and occurring in repeated self-limited attacks lasting 1 or 2 weeks.

porphyria: any of a group of disturbances of porphyrin metabolism, characterized by marked increase in formation and excretion of porphyrins or their precursors.

pretibial myxoedema: localized myxoedema associated with preceding hyperthyroidism and exopthalmus, occurring typically on the anterior (pretibial) surface of the legs where mucin deposits as plaques and papules.

priapism: persistent, abnormal erection of the penis, usually without sexual desire, and accompanied by pain and discomfort.

Prinzmetal's angina: a variant of angina pectoris in which the attacks occur during rest.

proptosis: a forward displacement or bulging, especially of the eye.

pseudophakia: false lens.

pyruvate kinase deficiency: a deficiency in the glycolytic (metabolic) pathway of red blood cells that results in haemolysis.

Raeder's syndrome: a syndrome consisting of the Horner syndrome but without loss of sweating on the affected side of the face.

Reed–Sternberg cells: giant histiocytic cells, typically multinucleate, most often binucleate; the nuclei are enclosed in abundant amphophilic cytoplasm and contain prominent nucleoli.

retinopathy: any non-inflammatory disease of the retina.

retroperitoneal fibrosis: deposition of fibrous tissue in the retroperitoneal space, producing vague abdominal discomfort, and often causing blockage of the ureters with resultant hydronephrosis and impaired renal function.

retrosternal: situated or occurring behind the sternum.

Reye's syndrome: an acute and often fatal childhood syndrome of encephalopathy and fatty degeneration of the liver, marked by rapid development of brain swelling and hepatomegaly and by disturbed consciousness and seizures.

rhabdomyolysis: dissolution of muscle associated with excretion of myoglobin in the urine.

Roth's spots: round or oval white spots sometimes seen in the retina early in the course of subacute bacterial endocarditis.

Rotor's syndrome: chronic familial non-haemolytic jaundice differing from Dubin–Johnson syndrome in the lack of liver pigmentation.

sarcoidosis: a chronic, progressive, generalized granulomatous reticulosis of unknown aetiology, involving almost any organ or tissue.

Schofield equation: an equation to predict basal metabolic rate; may be used to estimate the total calorie intake required to maintain current body weight.

sclerotherapy: the injection of sclerosing solutions in the treatment of haemorrhoids or varicose veins.

scotoma: an area of depressed vision within the visual field, surrounded by an area of less depressed or of normal vision.

Sézary syndrome: generalized exfoliative erythroderma produced by cutaneous infiltration of reticular lymphocytes and associated with intense pruritus, alopecia, oedema, hyperkeratosis, pigment and nail changes.

Shy–Drager syndrome: orthostatic hypotension, urinary and rectal incontinence, anhidrosis, atrophy of the iris, external ophthalmoplegia, rigidity, tremor, loss of associated movements, impotence, atonic bladder, generalized weakness, fasciculations, and neuropathic muscle wasting.

sickle cell anaemia: a hereditary haemolytic anaemia occurring almost exclusively in black people, characterized by arthralgia, acute attacks of abdominal pain, ulcerations of the lower extremities and with sickle-shaped erythrocytes in the blood.

Sjögren's syndrome: a symptom complex of unknown aetiology, usually occurring in middle-aged or older women, in which keratoconjunctivitis is associated with pharyngitis sicca, enlargement of the parotid glands, chronic polyarthritis and xerostomia.

sloughing material: soft, gel-like material often found in ulcer bases. Composed of tissue exudate and cellular debris.

spherocytosis: the presence of spherocytes (thick, almost spherical, red blood cells) characterized by abnormal fragility of erythrocytes, jaundice and splenomegaly.

splinter haemorrhages: linear haemorrhages beneath the nail.

steatosis: fatty degeneration.

stenosis: narrowing or stricture of a duct or canal.

Stevens–Johnson syndrome: a severe form of erythema multiforme in which the lesions may involve the oral and anogenital mucous membranes in association with constitutional symptoms, including malaise, prostration, headache, fever, arthralgia and conjunctivitis.

subchondral: beneath a cartilage.

subluxation: an incomplete or partial dislocation.

supranuclear palsy: pseudobulbar paralysis.

sympathetic ileus: failure of gastrointestinal motility secondary to acute non-gastrointestinal illness, e.g. hyaline membrane disease or septicaemia.

tamponade: surgical use of the tampon; also pathological compression of a part, as compression of the heart by pericardial fluid.

telangiectasia: prominent surface blood vessels.

tendon xanthomas: yellow papules or nodules or lipids deposited in tendons.

tenesmus: straining, especially ineffectual and painful straining at stool or in urination.

tenosynovitis: inflammation of a tendon sheath.

thalassaemia: a heterogeneous group of hereditary haemolytic anaemias that have in common a decreased rate of synthesis of one or more haemoglobin polypeptide chains and are classified according to the chain involved (α, β, γ). The homozygous form (thalassaemia major) is incompatible with life. The heterozygous form (thalassaemia minor) may be asymptomatic or marked by mild anaemia.

thrombocytopenia: decrease in the number of blood platelets.

thrombocytosis: increased number of platelets in blood.

thrombophilia: a tendency to the occurrence of thrombosis.

thromboplastin: phospholipids-protein extract of tissue that promotes the activation of factor X by factor VIII.

tonometry: measurement of intraocular pressure.

tophi: deposits of monosodium urate crystals, typically in subcutaneous and periarticular areas.

trephine: biopsy examination of an intact core of tissue (e.g. liver, bone marrow) obtained through a wide-bore needle.

tropical sprue: a malabsorption syndrome occurring in the tropics and subtropics. Protein malnutrition is usually precipitated by the malabsorption, and anaemia due to folic acid deficiency is particularly common.

Trousseau's sign: spasmodic contractions of muscles provoked by pressure upon the nerves which go to them; seen in tetany.

tuberoeruptive xanthomas: groups of flat or yellowish raised nodules on the skin over joints, especially the elbows and knees.

tuberous sclerosis: congenital familial disease characterized by tumours on the surfaces of the lateral ventricles and sclerotic patches on the surface of the brain and marked clinically by progressive mental deterioration and epileptic convulsions.

tubular cast: a cast formed from gelled protein precipitated in the renal tubules and moulded to the tubular lumen; pieces of these casts break off and are washed out with the urine.

uraemic frost: crystalline area deposited on the skin.

urethral: pertaining to the urethra, the membranous canal conveying urine from the bladder to the exterior of the body.

variant angina: *see* Prinzmetal's angina.

volvulus: intestinal obstruction due to a knotting and twisting of the bowel.

von Willebrand's disease: a lack of or a defective plasma protein (von Willebrand factor) necessary for the adhesion of platelets to vascular elements when a blood vessel is damaged.

Wernicke–Korsakoff syndrome: the co-existence of Wernicke's disease (acute onset of mental confusion, nystagmus, ophthalmoplegia and gait ataxia, due to thiamine deficiency) with Korsakoff's syndrome (a gross disturbance in recent memory, sometimes compensated for by confabulation).

West's syndrome: a form of myoclonus epilepsy with onset in infancy or early childhood and characterized by seizures involving the muscles of the neck, trunk and limbs, with nodding of the head and flexion and abduction of the arms. Mental retardation is common.

Wilson's disease: characterized by progressive accumulation of copper within body tissues, particularly erythrocytes, kidney, liver and brain, and associated with liver and lenticular degeneration.

xanthelasma: yellow plaques or nodules of lipids deposited on eyelids.

xenotransplantation: transplantation of tissue from another species.

xerosis: dry skin.

Index

H

N

Q